PRIMER ON TRANSPLANTATION

SECOND EDITION

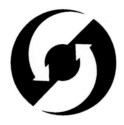

EDITORS

Douglas J. Norman, MD
Professor of Medicine
Division of Nephrology
Director, Transplantation Medicine Program
Medical Director, Laboratory of Immunogenics and Transplantation
Oregon Health Sciences University
Portland, Oregon

Laurence A. Turka, MD
C. Mahlon Kline Professor of Medicine
Chief, Renal-Electrolyte and Hypertension Division
University of Pennsylvania
Philadelphia, Pennysylvania

Managing Editor: Gina Brewer

Printed in the United States of America

ISBN: 0-9660150-1-0

American Society of Transplantation
National Office
17000 Commerce Parkway, Suite C
Mt. Laurel, NJ 08054-2255
Telephone: 856-439-9986
Fax: 856-439-9982
Email: ast@ahint.com
AST Home Page: http://www.a-s-t.org

Last digit is print number: 10 9 8 7 6 5 4 3 2 1

DEDICATION

The second edition of the Primer on Transplantation is dedicated to our wonderful patients who challenge us daily and who, because of their growing numbers, have promoted the emergence of a group of specialists in transplantation, the continuing education of whom is the purpose of this book.

TABLE OF CONTENTS

I. IMMUNOBIOLOGY AND TRANSPLANTATION RESEARCH
Alan M. Krensky, MD

II. PHARMACOLOGY AND IMMUNOSUPPRESSION
Philip F. Halloran, MD

III. ORGAN PROCUREMENT/ECONOMICS
William E. Harmon, MD

IV: MEDICAL COMPLICATIONS OF TRANSPLANTATION
Connie L. Davis, MD

V.   HEART TRANSPLANTATION
Jon A. Kobashigawa, MD

VII. LIVER AND INTESTINAL TRANSPLANTATION
Michael R. Lucey, MD

VIII. LUNG TRANSPLANTATION
Adaani E. Frost, MD

TABLE INDEX

XV

FIGURE INDEX

ACKNOWLEDGEMENTS

The editors would like to acknowledge the hard work of members of the Portland editorial office without whom this second edition of the Primer would not have been possible. Gina Brewer and Denise Askelson were superb in their roles as Managing Editors. Gina Brewer in particular was instrumental in seeing this project through to its completion. Kathleen Kautz did an outstanding job formatting tables and re-drawing a number of figures. The high quality of the Primer is in a very large part due to her dedication and skills in this area. Thanks also goes to Tami McCoy, Alyssa Manwill and Julie McClelland for their invaluable help. The editors would also like to thank Paula Wetzsteon, Supervisor of the Immunogenetics Laboratory, for providing assistance on this project.

SECTION EDITORS

Alan M. Krensky, MD
Shelagh Galligan Professor
Chief, Division of Immunology & Transplantation Biology
Department of Pediatrics
Stanford University School of Medicine
Stanford, California

Philip F. Halloran, MD, PhD
Professor of Medicine and Immunology
Division of Nephrology and Immunology
University of Alberta, Edmonton
Alberta, Canada

William E. Harmon, MD
Associate Professor of Pediatrics, Harvard Medical School
Director, Pediatric Nephrology
Children's Hospital Boston
Boston, Massachusetts

Connie L. Davis, MD
Associate Professor of Medicine
Medical Director of Transplantation
University of Washington
Seattle, Washington

Jon A. Kobashigawa, MD
Clinical Professor of Medicine, Division of Cardiology
University of California
Los Angeles School of Medicine
Medical Director, UCLA Heart Transplant Program
UCLA Medical Center
Los Angeles, California

Bertram L. Kasiske, MD
Professor of Medicine, Division of Nephrology
Department of Medicine
University of Minnesota
Hennepin County Medical Center
Minneapolis, Minnesota

Michael R. Lucey, MD, FRCPI
Professor of Medicine
Associate Chief, Division of Gastroenterology
Director of Hepatology
Medical Director, Liver Transplant Program
University of Pennsylvania
Philadelpha, Pennsylvania

Adaani E. Frost, MD
Associate Professor, Pulmonary Critical Care
Department of Medicine
Baylor College of Medicine
Houston, Texas

AUTHORS

Kareem Abu-Elmagd, MD, PhD, FACS
Professor of Surgery
Director, Intestinal Rehabilitation and Transplantation Center
University of Pittsburgh
Thomas E. Starzl Transplantation Institute
Pittsburgh, Pennsylvania

David Adams, MD, FRCP
Professor of Hepatology, Liver Unit
Queen Elizabeth Hospital
Birmingham, United Kingdom

Linda J. Addonizio, MD
Associate Professor of Pediatrics
Medical Director, Pediatric Cardiac Transplant Program
Columbia University College of Physicians and Surgeons
Babies' and Children's Hospital
New York, New York

Craig J. Baker, MD
Senior Research Fellow
Department of Cardiothoracic Surgery
University of Southern California and Children's Hospital
Los Angeles
Los Angeles, California

Mark L. Barr, MD
Associate Professor of Cardiothoracic Surgery
Department of Cardiothoracic Surgery
University of Southern California and Children's Hospital
Los Angeles
Los Angeles, California

John M. Barry, MD
Professor of Surgery and Chairman
Divisions of Urology and Abdominal Organ Transplantation
Oregon Health Sciences University
Portland, Oregon

William M. Bennett, MD
Medical Director, Solid Organ and Cellular Transplantation
Legacy Good Samaritan Hospital
Portland, Oregon

Sangeeta M. Bhorade, MD
Pulmonary & Critical Care Medicine Program, and Lung
Transplantation Program
Loyola University Medical Center
Maywood, Illinois

Jeffrey A. Bluestone, PhD
A.W. and Mary Margaret Claussen Distinguished Professor
Director, UCSF Diabetes Center
University of California at San Francisco
San Francisco, California

Daniel C. Brennan, MD, FACP
Associate Professor of Medicine
Director, Transplant Nephrology
Washington University School of Medicine
Barnes-Jewish Hospital
St. Louis, Missouri

Kimberly Ann Brown, MD
Liver Transplantation, Henry Ford Hospital
Detroit, Michigan

Ronald W. Busuttil, MD, PhD
Professor and Chief, Division of Liver and Pancreas
Transplantation
Dumont Chair in Transplantation Surgery
Director, The Dumont-UCLA Transplant Center
Los Angeles, California

Darcy Carr, MD
Acting Instructor, Department of Obstetrics and Gynecology
University of Washington Medical Center
Seattle, Washington

Charles B. Carpenter, MD
Professor of Medicine, Harvard Medical School
Brigham and Women's Hospital, Immunogenetics
Boston, Massachusetts

Thomas M. Coffman, MD
Professor of Medicine
Chief, Division of Nephrology
Duke University Medical Center
Durham, North Carolina

David J. Cohen, MD
Associate Professor of Clinical Medicine
Medical Director, Renal Transplantation
Columbia University College of Physicians and Surgeons
Columbia-Presbyterian Medical Center
New York, New York

Angelo M. de Mattos, MD
Assistant Professor of Medicine
Division of Nephrology, Hypertension and Clinical
Pharmacology
Transplantation Medicine Program
Oregon Health Sciences University
Portland, Oregon

Gabriel M. Danovitch, MD
Professor of Clinical Medicine
Medical Director, Adult Kidney and Pancreas Transplantation
University of California, Division of Nephrology
Los Angeles, California

R. Duane Davis, Jr., MD
Director, Cardiothoracic Transplantation
Associate Professor of Surgery
Duke University Medical Center
Durham, North Carolina

Francis L. Delmonico, MD
Professor of Surgery
Harvard Medical School
Medical Director, New England Organ Bank
Director, Renal Transplantation
Massachusetts General Hospital
Newton, Massachusetts

A.J. Demetris, MD
Professor of Pathology
Director, Transplant Pathology
University of Pittsburgh Medical Center
Pittsburgh, Pennsylvania

Steven R. Duncan, MD
Assistant Professor, Department of Immunology
The Scripps Research Institute
Attending Physician, Chest and Critical Care Medicine
Scrips Green Hospital
La Jolla, California

Thomas R. Easterling, MD
Associate Professor, Department of Obstetrics and Gynecology
University of Washington Medical Center
Seattle, Washington

Howard J. Eisen, MD
Professor of Medicine and Physiology
Medical Director, Advanced Heart Failure and Transplant Center
Temple University School of Medicine
Philadelphia, Pennsylvania

Jean Emond, MD
Professor of Surgery
Columbia College of Physicians and Surgeons
Surgical Director: Center for Liver Disease and Transplantation
The New York Presbyterian Hospital
New York, New York

Robert B. Ettenger, MD
Professor, Department of Pediatrics
Head, Division of Pediatric Nephrology
UCLA Center for Health Sciences
Los Angeles, California

Gregory T. Everson, MD
Professor of Medicine
Director, Section of Hepatology
Medical Director of Liver Transplantation
University of Colorado School of Medicine
Denver, Colorado

Harold I. Feldman, MD, MSCE
Associate Professor of Medicine and Epidemiology
Renal, Electrolyte and Hypertension Division
Center for Clinical Epidemiology and Biostatistics
Department of Biostatistics and Epidemiology
University of Pennsylvania School of Medicine
Philadelphia, Pennsylvania

Fatima A.F. Figueiredo, MD, PhD
Fulbright Scholar, Division of Gastroenterology and Hepatology
Mayo Clinic
Rochester, Minnesota

M. Roy First, MD
Professor of Medicine, Division of Nephrology and
Hypertension
Department of Internal Medicine
University of Cincinnati College of Medicine
Cincinnati, Ohio

Daniel P. Fishbein, MD
Division of Cardiology
Heart Failure / Cardiac Transplantation Service
University of Washington Medical Center
Seattle, Washington

Michael C. Fishbein, MD
Professor of Pathology and Medicine
Department of Pathology and Laboratory Medicine
UCLA Medical School
Los Angeles, California

Jay A. Fishman, MD
Associate Professor of Medicine
Clinical Director, Transplant Infectious Disease
Massachusetts General Hospital
Harvard Medical School
Boston, Massachusetts

Ira J. Fox, MD
Associate Professor of Surgery
University of Nebraska Medical Center
Omaha, Nebraska

Adaani E. Frost, MD
Associate Professor, Pulmonary Critical Care
Department of Medicine
Baylor College of Medicine
Houston, Texas

John J. Fung, MD, PhD, FACS
Professor of Surgery
Chief, Division of Transplantation Surgery
University of Pittsburgh
Thomas E. Starzl Transplantation Institute
Pittsburgh, Pennsylvania

James S. Gammie, MD
Assistant Professor
Surgical Director, Cardiac Transplantation/Mechanical
Circulatory Support
University of Massachusetts Medical Center
Division of Cardiothoracic Surgery
Worcester, Massachusetts

Edward R. Garrity, Jr., MD
Professor of Medicine
Pulmonary & Critical Care
Medical Director, Lung Transplantation
Loyola University Medical Center
Maywood, Illinois

Robert S. Gaston, MD
Professor of Medicine, Division of Nephrology
Professor of Surgery, Division of Transplantation
University of Alabama at Birmingham
Birmingham, Alabama

Anderson S. Gaweco, MD, PhD
Assistant Professor of Medicine and Pathology
Loyola University Medical Center
Loyola University Chicago
Maywood, Illinois

Rafik M. Ghobrial, MD, PhD
Assistant Professor of Surgery
Division of Liver and Pancreas Transplantation
Dumont-UCLA Transplant Center
University of California Los Angeles
Los Angeles, California

Thomas A. Gonwa, MD, FACP
Associate Director, Transplant Services
Professor of Transplant Medicine
Baylor University Medical Center
Clinical Associate Professor of Medicine
University of Texas, Southwestern Medical School
Dallas, Texas

Sita Gourishankar, MD
Nephrology Fellow
Division of Nephrology and Immunology
University of Alberta, Edmonton
Alberta, Canada

Philip F. Halloran, MD, PhD
Professor of Medicine and Immunology
Division of Nephrology and Immunology
University of Alberta, Edmonton
Alberta, Canada

Wayne W. Hancock, MD, PhD
Associate Professor of Pathology, Harvard Medical School
Millenium Pharmaceuticals, Inc., Cambridge, MA;
Department of Pathology
Beth Israel Deaconess Medical Center and Harvard Medical
School
Boston, Massachusetts

William E. Harmon, MD
Associate Professor of Pediatrics, Harvard Medical School
Director, Pediatric Nephrology
Children's Hospital Boston
Boston, Massachusetts

J. Harold Helderman, MD
Professor of Medicine and Microbiology and Immunology
Medical Director, Vanderbilt Transplant Center
Vanderbilt University Medical Center
Division of Nephrology
Nashville, Tennessee

Marshall I. Hertz, MD
Professor of Medicine
Pulmonary/Critical Care Medicine Division
University of Minnesota
Minneapolis, Minnesota

Bernhard J. Hering, MD
Assistant Professor of Surgery and Medicine
University of Minnesota
Minneapolis, Minnesota

Jeffrey D. Hosenpud, MD
Head, Transplant Cardiology
St. Luke's Cardiac Transplant Program
Milwaukee, Wisconsin

Sharon A. Hunt, MD
Professor, Cardiovascular Medicine
Cardiac Transplant Program
Stanford University Medical Center
Stanford, California

Aliya N. Husain, MD
Associate Professor of Pathology
Director, Surgical Pathology
Loyola University Medical Center
Loyola University Chicago
Maywood, Illinois

Donald E. Hricik, MD
Professor of Medicine
Chief, Division of Nephrology
Case Western Reserve University
Medical Director of Transplantation Services
University Hospital of Cleveland
Cleveland, Ohio

Bertram L. Kasiske, MD
Professor of Medicine, Division of Nephrology
Department of Medicine
University of Minnesota
Hennepin County Medical Center
Minneapolis, Minnesota

Abdallah G. Kfoury, MD
Assistant Professor of Medicine, Division of Cardiology
Salt Lake City Veterans Affairs Medical Center
Salt Lake City, Utah

Melissa B. King, MD
Assistant Professor of Medicine
Division of Allergy, Pulmonary and Critical Care
University of Minnesota
Minneapolis, Minnesota

James K. Kirklin, MD
Professor of Surgery
University of Alabama at Birmingham
Birmingham, Alabama

Jochen Klupp, MD
Research Professor
Director, Transplantation Immunology
Department of Cardiothoracic Surgery
Stanford University School of Medicine
Stanford, California

Jon A. Kobashigawa, MD
Clinical Professor of Medicine, Division of Cardiology
University of California
Los Angeles School of Medicine
Medical Director, UCLA Heart Transplant Program
UCLA Medical Center
Los Angeles, California

Robert L. Kormos, MD
Associate Professor of Surgery
Director, Artificial Heart Program and Adult Heart
Transplantation
University of Pittsburgh Medical Center
Division of Cardiothoracic Surgery
Pittsburgh, Pennsylvania

Alan M. Krensky, MD
Shelagh Galligan Professor
Chief, Division of Immunology & Transplantation Biology
Department of Pediatrics
Stanford University School of Medicine
Stanford, California

John R. Lake, MD
Professor of Medicine and Surgery
Director, Division of Garstroenterology, Hepatology and
Nutrition
Director, Liver Transplantation Program
University of Minnesota
Minneapolis, Minnesota

Kathleen D. Lake, PharmD, FCCP, BCPS
Director of Clinical Transplant Research and Therapeutics
The Michigan Transplant Center and the
University of Michigan Health Systems
Senior Associate Research Scientist
Departments of Medicine and Surgery
University of Michigan Medical School
Clinical Professor, University of Michigan College of Pharmacy
Division of Nephrology, University of Michigan Medical School
Ann Arbor, Michigan

Hillel Laks, MD
Chairman, Division of Cardiothoracic Surgery
UCLA Medical Center
Los Angeles, California

Christine L. Lau, MD
Senior Assistant Resident in General & Thoracic Surgery
Duke University Medical Center
Durham, North Carolina

Randall G. Lee, MD
Medical Director, Pathology Services
Providence St. Vincent Medical Center
Portland, Oregon

Mary B. Leonard, MD, MSCE
Assistant Professor of Pediatrics and Epidemiology
Division of Pediatric Nephrology
The Children's Hospital of Philadelphia
Center for Clinical Epidemiology and Biostatistics
Department of Biostatistics and Epidemiology
University of Pennsylvania School of Medicine
Philadelphia, Pennsysvania

Xian Chang Li, MD, PhD
Assistant Professor of Medicine
Harvard Medical School
Beth Israel Deaconess Medical Center
Boston, Massachusetts

Susan E. Light, MD
Vice President, Product Development
Quark Biotech, Inc.
Menlo Park, California

Michael R. Lucey, MD, FRCPI
Professor of Medicine
Associate Chief, Division of Gastroenterology
Director of Hepatology
Medical Director, Liver Transplant Program
University of Pennsylvania
Philadelpha, Pennsylvania

Timothy McCashland, MD
Associate Professor of Medicine, Liver Transplant Program
University of Nebraska Medical Center
Omaha, Nebraska

Sue V. McDiarmid, MD
Associate Professor of Pediatrics and Surgery
Director, Pediatric Liver Transplantation
Departments of Pediatrics and Surgery
University of California
Los Angeles Medical Center
Los Angeles, California

Peter N. Madras, MD
Associate Professor of Surgery
Harvard Medical School
Co-Director, Transplant Services
Rhode Island Hospital
Providence, Rhode Island

George B. Mallory, Jr., MD
Associate Professor of Clinical Pediatrics
Washington University School of Medicine
St. Louis Children's Hospital
St. Louis, Missouri
Consultant Physician
Cardiopulmonary Transplantation Programme
Great Ormond Street Hospital for Children NHS Trust
London, United Kingdom

Daniel Marelli, MD
Assistant Clinical Professor, Division of Cardiothoracic Surgery
UCLA Medical Center
Los Angeles, California

Paul Martin, MD
Associate Professor of Medicine
Director, Hepatology
Division of Digestive Diseases and Dumont-UCLA Transplant
Program
University of California at Los Angeles
Los Angeles, California

Howard Todd Massey, MD
Fellow in Cardiothoracic Transplantation
Duke University Medical Center
Durham, North Carolina

Arthur J. Matas, MD
Professor of Surgery, Department of Surgery
University of Minnesota Medical School
Minneapolis, Minnesota

Janet R. Maurer, MD
Head, Section of Lung Transplantation
Department of Pulmonary and Critical Care Medicine
Associate Medical Director, Transplant Center
Cleveland Clinic Foundation
Cleveland, Ohio

K.V. Narayanan Menon, MD, MRCP
Fellow, Division of Gastroenterology and Hepatology
Mayo Clinic
Rochester, Minnesota

Robert E. Michler, MD
Professor and Chief,
Cardiothoracic Surgery and Thoracic Transplantation
Director, Heart Hospital
Ohio State University Medical Center
Columbus, Ohio

Leslie W. Miller, MD
Professor of Medicine
Director, Cardiovascular Division
Department of Medicine
University of Minnesota
Minneapolis, Minnesota

Dilip Moonka, MD
Liver Transplantation, Henry Ford Hospital
Detroit, Michigan

Anthony P. Monaco, MD
Director, Transplant Center
Beth Israel-Deaconess Medical Center
Peter Medawar Professor of Transplant Surgery
Harvard Medical School
Boston, Massachusetts

Randall E. Morris, MD
Professor; Director of Transplantation Immunology,
Cardiothoracic Surgery
Department of Cardiothoracic Surgery
Stanford University School of Medicine
Stanford, California

Paul E. Morrissey, MD
Assistant Professor of Surgery, Brown University
Co-Director, Transplant Services
Rhode Island Hospital
Providence, Rhode Island

Barbara T. Murphy, MD, FRCPI
Assistant Professor of Clinical Medicine
Director of Transplant Nephrology
Renal Division
Mount Sinai School of Medicine
New York, New York

James Neuberger DM, FRCP
Consultant Physician and Professor of Medicine
Liver Unit
Queen Elizabeth Hospital
Birmingham, United Kingdom

John F. Neylan, MD
Vice President, Clinical Research and Development
Transplantation/Immunology
Wyeth-Aherst Research
Radnor, Pennsylvania

Douglas J. Norman, MD
Professor of Medicine
Director, Transplantation Medicine Program
Director, Laboratory of Immunogenetics and Transplantation
Oregon Health Sciences University
Portland, Oregon

Frederick Nunes, MD
Assistant Professor of Medicine, Division of Gastroenterology
University of Pennsylvania
Philadelpha, Pennsylvania

Jonah Odim, MD, PhD
Clinical Instructor, Division of Cardiothoracic Surgery
UCLA Medical Center
Los Angeles, California

Kim M. Olthoff, MD
Assistant Professor of Medicine
University of Pennsylvania Liver Transplantation Program
Philadelphia, Pennsylvania

Ali J. Olyaei, PharmD, BCPS
Assistant Professor of Medicine
Division of Nephrology, Hypertension and Clinical
Pharmacology
Oregon Health Sciences University
Portland, Oregon

Susan M. Ott, MD
Associate Professor, Department of Medicine
University of Washington
Seattle, Washington

Scott M. Palmer, MD
Associate in Medicine
Division of Pulmonary and Critical Medicine
Duke University Medical Center
Durham, North Carolina

Jayan Parameshwar, MBBS, MD, M.phil, FRCP
Transplant Cardiologist, Transplant Unit
Papworth Hospital
Cambridge, United Kingdom

G.A. Patterson, MD
Joseph C. Bancroft Professor of Surgery
Division of Cardiothoracic Surgery
Washington University School of Medicine
St. Louis, Missouri

V. Ram Peddi, MD
Associate Professor of Medicine
Division of Nephrology and Hypertension
Department of Internal Medicine
University of Cincinnati College of Medicine
Cincinnati, Ohio

Israel Penn, MD
University of Cincinnati Medical Center
Department of Surgery
Cincinnati Veterans Affairs Medical Center
Cincinnati, Ohio

John D. Pirsch, MD
Professor of Medicine and Surgery
Director of Medical Transplantation Service
University of Wisconsin Medical School
Madison, Wisconsin

Lorraine C. Racusen, MD
The Johns Hopkins University School of Medicine
Department of Pathology
Baltimore, Maryland

David D. Ralph, MD
Associate Professor of Medicine
Pulmonary and Critical Care Medicine
University of Washington Medical Center
Seattle, Washington

Dale G. Renlund, MD
Professor of Medicine
University of Utah Health Sciences Center
Division of Cardiology
Salt Lake City Veterans Affairs Medical Center
Salt Lake City, Utah

Jorge Reyes, MD, FACS
Professor of Surgery
University of Pittsburgh
Thomas E. Starzl Transplantation Institute
Pittsburgh, Pennsylvania

Camillo Ricordi, MD
Professor of Surgery and Medicine
University of Miami
Miama, Florida

Hugo R. Rosen, MD
Associate Professor of Medicine, Molecular Microbiology, and
Immunology
Division of Gastroenterology/Hepatology
Medical Director, Liver Transplantation Program
Oregon Health Sciences University
Portland Veterans Affairs Medical Center
Portland, Oregon

Jayanta Roy-Chowdhury, MD, MRCP
Professor of Medicine and Molecular Genetics
Albert Einstein College of Medicine
Bronx, New York

Robert H. Rubin, MD, FACP, FCCP
Gordon and Marjorie Osborne Professor of Health Sciences
and Technology
Professor of Medicine, Harvard Medical School
Chief of Surgical and Transplant Infectious Disease
Massachusetts General Hospital
Director, Center for Experimental Pharmacology and
Therapeutics
Harvard-M.I.T. Division of Health Sciences and Technology
Cambridge, Massachusetts

Mark A. Russell, MD
Instructor in Medicine, Department of Dermatology
Vanderbilt University Medical Center
Nashville, Tennessee

Steven Sanislo, MD
Assistant Professor, Department of Opthalmology
Stanford University School of Medicine
Stanford, California

Saad Shaikh, MD
Resident Physician, Department of Opthalmology
Stanford University School of Medicine
Stanford, California

Abraham Shaked, MD, PhD
Professor of Surgery
Chief, Liver Transplant Program
Hospital of the University of Pennsylvania
Philadelphia, Pennsylvania

Eric W. Schneeberger, MD
Fellow, Cardiothoracic Surgery
Ohio State University Medical Center
Columbus, Ohio

Felicia A. Schenkel, RN, BS, CCTC
Senior Cardiothoracic Transplant Coordinator
Department of Cardiothoracic Surgery
University of Southern California School of Medicine
Los Angeles, California

Larry L. Schulman, MD
Associate Professor of Clinical Medicine
Director, Lung Transplant Service
Columbia University, College of Physicians & Surgeons
New York, New York

Fuad S. Shihab, MD
Associate Professor of Medicine
Division of Nephrology and Hypertension
Medical Director, Kidney Transplantation Program
University of Utah Medical Center
Salt Lake City, Utah

Kim Solez, MD
Professor of Pathology, University of Alberta
Director of NKF cyberNephrology
President of Transpath, Edmonton
Alberta, Canada

Michael F. Sorrell, MD
Robert L. Grissom Professor of Medicine
Liver Transplant Program
University of Nebraska Medical Center
Omaha, Nebraska

Randall C. Starling, MD, MPH
Director, Heart Transplant Medical Services
The Cleveland Clinic Foundation
Cleveland, Ohio

Vaughn A. Starnes, MD
Hastings Professor and Chairman
Department of Cardiothoracic Surgery
University of Southern California and Children's Hospital
Los Angeles
Los Angeles, California

Thomas Stasko, MD
Assistant Professor of Medicine, Department of Dermatology
Vanderbilt University Medical Center
Nashville, Tennessee

Theodore I. Steinman, MD
Professor of Medicine, Harvard Medical School
Director, Dialysis Unit
Beth Israel Deaconess Medical Center
Boston, Massachusetts

Lynne Warner Stevenson, MD
Director, Cardiomyopathy and Heart Failure Program
Cardiovascular Division
Brigham and Women's Hospital
Harvard Medical School
Boston, Massachusetts

Robert J. Stratta, MD
Professor of Surgery, Division of Transplantation Surgery
University of Tennessee at Memphis
Memphis, Tennessee

Terry B. Strom, MD
Professor of Medicine, Harvard Medical School
Director of Immunology, Beth Israel Deaconess Medical Center
Boston, Massachusetts

David Sutherland, MD, PhD
Professor of Surgery, University of Minnesota
Minneapolis, Minnesota

Lynda Anne Szczech, MD, MSCE
Assistant Professor of Medicine
Duke Institute of Renal Outcomes Research
Division of Nephrology
Duke University Medical Center
Durham, North Carolina

Victor F. Tapson, MD, FCCP
Associate Professor of Medicine
Division of Pulmonary and Critical Medicine
Medical Director, Duke University Lung Transplant Program
Duke University Medical Center
Durham, North Carolina

David O. Taylor, MD
Associate Professor of Medicine
University of Utah Health Sciences Center
Division of Cardiology
Salt Lake City Veterans Affairs Medical Center
Salt Lake City, Utah

Amir H. Tejani, MD
Professor of Pediatrics and Surgery
New York Medical College
Valhalla, New York

Elbert P. Trulock, MD
Professor of Medicine
Division of Pulmonary and Critical Care Medicine
Washington University School of Medicine
St. Louis, Missouri

Laurence A. Turka, MD
C. Mahlon Kline Professor of Medicine
Chief, Renal-Electrolyte and Hypertension Division
University of Pennsylvania
Philadelphia, Pennsylvania

Wickii T. Vigneswaran, MD
Professor of Surgery
Chief, Thoracic Surgery
Surgical Director, Lung Transplantation Program
Loyola University Medical Center
Maywood, Illinois

Flavio Vincenti, MD
Professor of Clinical Medicine, Kidney Transplant Service
University of California
San Francisco, California

Matthew R. Weir, MD
Professor and Director
Division of Nephrology and Clinical Research Unit
Department of Medicine
University of Maryland School of Medicine
Baltimore, Maryland

Russell H. Wiesner, MD
Professor of Medicine
Medical Director, Liver Transplantation
Mayo Clinic
Rochester, Minnesota

Alan Wilkinson, MD, FRCP
Professor of Medicine
Director, Kidney and Pancreas Transplantation
UCLA School of Medicine
Los Angeles, California

Mohamad H. Yamani, MD
Associate Staff, Department of Cardiology
The Cleveland Clinic Foundation
Cleveland, Ohio

Hasan Yersiz, MD
Assistant Professor of Surgery
Division of Liver and Pancreas Transplantation
The Dumont-UCLA Transplant Center
Los Angeles, California

Carlton J. Young, MD
Assistant Professor of Surgery, Division of Transplantation
University of Alabama at Birmingham
Division of Nephrology
Birmingham, Alabama

James B. Young, MD
Medical Director, Kaufman Center for Heart Failure
Department of Cardiology
The Cleveland Clinic Foundation
Cleveland, Ohio

FOREWORD

We are pleased to be able to offer the second edition of the AST Primer on Transplantation to the transplantation community. The second edition is longer than the first, not because we were not as disciplined this time but because there is an increased base of knowledge about transplantation in the year 2001. Again, with the second edition we have included similar information about kidney, heart, liver and lung transplantation to allow students and practitioners to "see how the other guys do it." However, because there is so much that is common among transplant recipients of the different organs, we have added a new section entitled "Medical Complications of Transplantation." This section covers areas such as heart disease in non-heart transplant patients and liver disease in non-liver transplant patients, as examples. This section has valuable information on topics such as bone, eye and skin diseases and reproduction in transplant patients. The other generic sections of the book include updated information on the immunologic basis of transplantation, tissue typing, pharmacology and immunosuppressive drugs. There is also a new chapter on understanding, interpreting and conducting research in transplantation. In summary, we hope that the second edition of the AST Primer on Transplantation is found to be an important reference for a variety of individuals, students, fellows, faculty and other practitioners who have an interest in this most exciting field – the transplantation of life saving organs into those unfortunate patients who develop end-stage organ disease.

The Editors

Section I

IMMUNOBIOLOGY AND TRANSPLANTATION RESEARCH

1   HISTORICAL OVERVIEW
Laurence A. Turka, MD

IMMUNOLOGY

The earliest recorded attempts at organ or tissue transplantation date back thousands of years. However, modern scientific studies in the field of transplantation trace their beginnings to studies by Emerich Ullmann who, in 1902, performed a successful renal autotransplant in a dog. Shortly thereafter, Alexis Carrel showed that renal autografts in dogs can survive indefinitely, but that renal allografts rapidly cease to function. This seminal work, for which he was awarded a Nobel prize in 1912, led to the concept of histocompatibility; that is, the fact that, even within a species, there are polymorphic genetic systems that encode tissue antigens, and that these alloantigens serve as targets for an immune response that leads to rejection. Carrel saw that the technological capabilities of renal transplantation were now fairly well-developed. Displaying remarkable insight, he believed that, "the power of the organism to eliminate foreign tissue was due to organs such as the spleen or bone marrow," and suggested that, "[all] our efforts must now be directed toward the biological methods which will prevent the reaction of the organism against foreign tissue and allow the adapting of homoplastic grafts to their hosts."

Progress in what we now recognize as the immune response to alloantigens was limited for many years. However, interest in this field was spurred by several events. First, experiments in the 1940s by Sir Peter Medawar demonstrated immunological memory in a skin transplant model. Second, Owen, Medawar and Billingham discovered the phenomenon of neonatal tolerance, demonstrating that it was possible to prevent immune responses to alloantigens. Third, work by Dausset and others defined what the alloantigens were, namely the major histocompatibility complex (MHC), which in humans is called HLA.

More recently, we have seen an explosion of information about how the immune system works. Further studies on the MHC have led to the concept of tissue typing and histocompatibility. Studies in the early 1960s defined the function of lymphocytes and identified separate roles for T cells (cellular immunity) and B cells (humoral immunity). The T cell receptor and immunoglobulins were discovered, and the role of HLA proteins in presenting antigens to T cells were elucidated. X-ray

crystallographic studies have defined the structure of each of these proteins, making possible the fine dissection of structure and function relationships on a three-dimensional level. The revolution in molecular biology ushered in transgenic and knockout mice, and these have helped uncover the normal mechanisms of tolerance induction. These techniques also provide hope that the barriers to xenotransplantation may be surmounted.

In summary, remarkable progress has been made over the last century. It is clear that there are two separate barriers to overcome for successful transplantation: technical problems associated with surgery itself, and immunologic problems as a consequence of the host response to donor antigens. The former issues are reviewed individually by organ in later sections of this textbook. This section concerns itself with defining the immunologic problems. The next section traces efforts to overcome them.

PHARMACOLOGY

Between 1959 and 1962, a series of transplants were performed, primarily in Paris and Boston, in which the recipients received total body irradiation for immunosuppression. There were only isolated successes, and these occurred with sibling grafts. Nonetheless, these rare patients provided encouragement that, if better means of immunosuppression were found, success rates would improve.

In 1959, Dameshek and Schwartz reported studies in which they used 6-mercaptopurine (6-MP) in place of irradiation to precondition patients for bone marrow transplantation. Picking up on this work, Roy Calne showed that 6-MP could be used in place of irradiation for renal transplants in dogs. In 1962, the Paris group reported successful survival of a living-nonrelated renal transplant in which the recipient was treated with 6-MP and intermittent corticosteroids. Concurrently, Calne found that a derivative of 6-MP, azathioprine (Imuran®), was just as effective and less toxic and, in 1962, this drug came into widespread use. By 1963, maintenance azathioprine and corticosteroids became the standard regimen for renal transplantation. By 1966, the introduction of crossmatching by Terasaki and others led to a marked reduction in the occurrence of hyperacute rejection.

Progress was slow but steady for the next decade. Then, in 1978, Calne reported the use of a remarkable new drug, cyclosporine. Within several years, virtually all patients were receiving cyclosporine plus corticosteroids for immunosuppression, in many instances combined with azathioprine. In the early 1980s, muromonab-CD3 (Orthoclone OKT®3) was introduced into clinical practice. This was the first monoclonal antibody licensed for clinical use. It has dramatically improved the treatment of acute rejection episodes.

C. Mahlon Kline Professor of Medicine; Chief, Renal-Electrolyte and Hypertension Division, University of Pennsylvania, Philadelphia, PA

Since then, other new agents have been approved, and still more are in development. This section details the pharmacology and mechanisms of action of these agents, as well as provides an overview of general pharmacologic principles and special considerations of drug treatment that apply in the transplant setting.

2 NORMAL IMMUNE RESPONSES
Laurence A. Turka, MD

Over centuries of evolution, the immune system developed a highly specialized and tightly regulated series of responses, the main function of which is traditionally described as discriminating between self and nonself. Based on the concept that immune responses can be primarily provoked by tissue destruction, it also has been proposed that the immune system senses tissue damage or danger, a distinction that to a large extent may be semantic. In any event, the immune system is responsible for graft rejection. Immunodeficient animals, with either congenital or acquired immunodeficiency, are unable to reject either allogeneic or xenogeneic transplants. Although many cells participate in the immune response to transplanted organs and tissues, T cells have a primary role in graft rejection. Animals that lack T cells, but have otherwise intact and functional immune compartments still cannot reject transplants. This chapter is designed to provide a brief overview of the physiology of normal immune responses, and to serve as a foundation for understanding the pathophysiology of graft rejection. It reviews immune system development; the mechanisms that initiate an immune response; and finally, the mechanisms that regulate, and ultimately terminate a response. Because of their primary role in allograft rejection, T cells are the main focus of this chapter.

CELLS AND DEVELOPMENTAL ASPECTS OF THE IMMUNE SYSTEM

T cells, B cells, natural killer (NK) cells, macrophages, and dendritic cells, all of which are bone marrow-derived, are the primary cellular elements of the immune system (Figure 2-1).

T cells, B cells, and NK cells are thought to arise from a common precursor stem cell. These cells show many similarities in antigen recognition and intracellular signaling, but have distinct immune functions. T cells account for what is termed *cellular immunity*. This includes delayed-type hypersensitivity reactions, cell-mediated lympholysis, and most forms of transplantation reactions such as allograft rejection and graft-vs-host disease, which can be seen as a combination of the first two responses. The hallmark of cellular responses is that lymphocytes act either directly on the target cell, in which case cell-to-cell contact is required

C. Mahlon Kline Professor of Medicine; Chief, Renal-Electrolyte and Hypertension Division, University of Pennsylvania, Philadelphia, PA

(as in cell-mediated lympholysis), or locally through elaborated cytokines, in which case the target cell or antigen must be nearby (as in delayed-type hypersensitivity). B cells form the humoral arm of the immune system. Antibodies produced by B cells circulate throughout the body and are present in secreted fluids and mucosal surfaces. These antibodies can act independently of lymphocytes by fixing complement or targeting cells for phagocytosis, a process termed *opsonization.* Antibody-binding to cells can also serve as a stimulus for cell-mediated lympholysis (eg, antibody-dependent cellular cytotoxicity). NK cells appeared early in the evolution of the vertebrate immune system, and form part of the cellular immune response. Rather than recognizing and reacting to nonself antigens, as do T cells, they appear to lyse cells that fail to express self-antigens. This relatively primitive form of immunity is ineffective against certain types of pathogens such as viruses, but probably contributes to transplantation responses and tumor surveillance.

Macrophages and dendritic cells are nonlymphoid cells of hematopoietic origin that play a crucial role in initiating immune responses by presenting foreign antigens to T cells, a function that can be performed by B cells. In addition to these specialized antigen-presenting cells (APCs), under certain circumstances, non-hematopoietic cells, such as endothelial cells and renal epithelial cells, may also present antigens.

T Cells

T cells are so-named because, in most instances, their development depends on the thymus, an organ that is embryologically derived from pharyngeal pouches. In the absence of a thymus, such as in the nude mice strain, T cells are either absent or extremely rare, and animals are grossly immunodeficient. Once mature T cells are formed, however, they no longer need a thymus, as evidenced by the ability of T cells adoptively transferred to syngeneic nude mice to colonize the animals and function normally. Similarly, incidental thymectomy during corrective cardiac surgery in children does not lead to immunodeficiency. By adulthood, the thymus involutes, producing few, if any, new T cells. While it was once thought that all T cells developed in the thymus, there is increasing evidence for extrathymic development of at least some T cells, although the degree to which these cells are required for normal immune function is not clear.

One of the hallmarks identifying T cells is the T cell receptor for antigen (TCR) itself. The receptor is a heterodimer formed using two of four possible molecules: the α, β, γ, or δ chain. To form the heterodimer, α pairs with β, and γ pairs with δ. Most T cells formed in the thymus use the $\alpha\beta$ heterodimer, and these constitute the majority of cells found in the blood and in peripheral

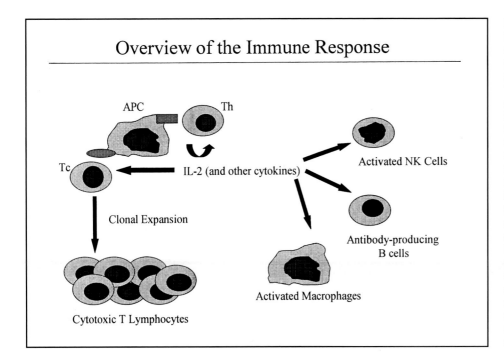

Overview of the Immune Response

APC

Th

Tc

IL-2 (and other cytokines)

Activated NK Cells

Antibody-producing B cells

Clonal Expansion

Activated Macrophages

Cytotoxic T Lymphocytes

Figure 2-1. Overview of the immune response. MHC class II-restricted CD4+ T helper cells (Th) initiate immune responses by secreting cytokines such as IL-2. These cytokines are used in an autocrine fashion by the Th cells themselves, and in a paracrine fashion by the other major subset of T cells, MHC class I-restricted CD8+ cytotoxic T cells (Tc). The latter require activation by antigen in order to respond to cytokines. Since antigen-presenting cells (APCs) bear class I and class II antigens on their surface, they are able to simultaneously stimulate Th and Tc in a three-cell complex. This is an efficient way to sustain a response since cytokines act in local microenvironments. Other immune effector cells present locally such as NK cells, B cells, and macrophages will be activated as well.

lymphoid organs such as lymph nodes and spleen. TCR γδ cells are particularly prominent in the skin and in mucosal surfaces such as the tongue, the vagina, and the intestinal epithelium.

The genes encoding the TCR chains are members of the immunoglobulin supergene family. This is a large family of genes, many of which are found on B, T, and NK cells. While all members of this family share certain features of structural similarity, the TCR genes are most closely related to their B cell homologs, the immunoglobulin (Ig) genes. While soluble immunoglobulin is familiar to us as antibodies, surface immunoglobulin forms the B cell antigen receptor; thus, the similarity between the TCR and Ig genes is not surprising.

The universe of antigens is enormous and, therefore, a diverse repertoire of TCRs and Igs is needed to mount an appropriate response. In theory, this could be accomplished by having a large number of intact TCR and Ig genes contained within the genome, with each T or B cell then selectively activating and transcribing a different one. However, given the numbers of lymphocytes that are generated in humans, well over 10^{10}, this would require more space than exists in the genome. The solution that has evolved uses a limited number of genetic elements to create a relatively limitless repertoire, in large part through a process of genetic rearrangement known as V(D)J recombination. Thus, both TCR and Ig genes are formed through the rearrangement of genetic loci from their germline configuration. The process of rearrangement is cell and lineage-specific, such that TCR loci only rearrange in T cells, and Ig loci rearrange only in B cells.

T cells, through their antigen receptors, recognize foreign proteins in the form of short peptide fragments

(9 to 15 amino acids) presented in the antigen-binding groove of major histocompatibility complex (MHC) molecules (Figure 2-2). Peptide binding to MHC is absolutely required, as unbound peptides will not activate T cells. Two other important features are that the MHC loci are highly polymorphic and the immune response is self-MHC restricted. The latter means that, in general, T cells are only activated by peptides bound to self-MHC molecules, and not to foreign MHC molecules.

Since TCR gene rearrangement is essentially random, a process has evolved whereby T cells that have undergone appropriate TCR rearrangements are selected for further maturation, and T cells of inappropriate specificities are eliminated. This process, known as thymic selection, has two components. In the first, *positive selection*, developing thymocytes receive appropriate signals for maturation only if their TCRs bind MHC. Since only self-MHC molecules are available, it follows that only self-MHC-restricted T cells will mature. In the second component, *negative selection*, T cells with too high an affinity for self-MHC are eliminated. These T cells are believed to be potentially autoreactive, and are destroyed before they mature. Thus, the forces that act on developing T cells in the thymus create a repertoire with intermediate affinity for self-MHC molecules. As a result, these cells are not able to become activated by self-MHC alone, or complexed to a self-peptide, but contain cells with high affinity for self-MHC plus foreign peptide.

While T cells are self-MHC-restricted, a very high proportion of T cells will respond to foreign MHC molecules. In fact, roughly $1/10^5$ to $1/10^6$ T cells will respond to any given nominal antigen (eg, a peptide derived from tetanus toxin or influenza hemagglutinin). The frequency

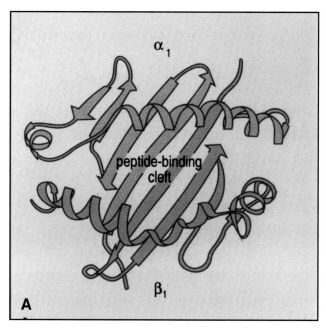

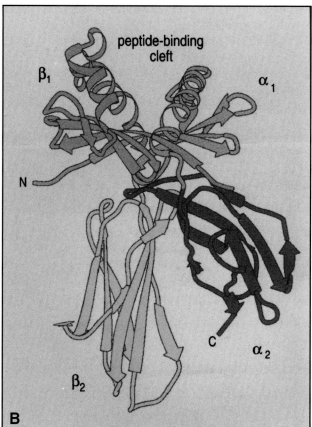

Figure 2-2. Structure of an MHC molecule. The crystal structure of an MHC class I molecule, as solved by x-ray crystallography, reveals a peptide-binding cleft with sides formed by two γ-helices and a floor consisting of a β-pleated sheet. Panel A shows an overhead view of the peptide-binding groove (cleft) and Panel B shows a view from the side of the entire molecule. Reprinted with permission from Janeway CA and Travers P, eds. In: Immunobiology, 3rd ed. Garland Publishing Inc.; New York, NY:1997.

of cells that respond to foreign MHC molecules (alloantigens) is 100 to 1,000-fold higher (up to 1/100 T cells). It is believed this occurs as a consequence of several events. First, as noted above, T cells have intrinsic affinity for self-MHC molecules. Second, the allelic variation among MHC molecules from individual to individual is quite small. This means that different alleles at any given MHC genetic locus can be up to 98% identical, varying at only three to four amino acids. As a result, foreign MHC can "look" remarkably like self-MHC. Third, MHC molecules are each able to bind diverse peptides, meaning that APCs display to T cells a large "choice" of peptide plus MHC molecules. Structurally, these complexes can resemble self-MHC plus peptide. Thus, taking the example of a T cell specific for a tetanus toxoid peptide bound to a self-MHC molecule, there is a significant likelihood (1/100 to 1/1,000) that this T cell will "crossreact" with at least one different peptide presented by a foreign MHC molecule.

While alloantigens can be thought of as a special (and extreme) case of nominal antigens, there is another distinct group of antigens that is capable of activating T cells: *superantigens*. Superantigens, so-named because they activate an extraordinarily high proportion (up to one-third) of T cells, themselves, belong to two categories. The first is made-up of secreted or cell-wall proteins derived from bacteria, such as staphylococcal enterotoxins or toxic shock syndrome toxins. The second category consists of retroviral proteins that are either endogenous to the host genome, or acquired shortly after birth during nursing. Both bacterial and viral superantigens activate T cells almost exclusively through interaction with the TCR β chain, and do not require the α chain for binding. As a result, they lack the fine specificity of "regular" peptide antigens, and instead activate a very large proportion of T cells. Once activated, these T cells secrete inflammatory cytokines. In the case of circulating superantigens, the large number of responding T cells secreting diverse cytokines causes the severe systemic illness known as toxic shock syndrome.

B Cells

In birds, B cells develop in a discrete organ known as the bursa of Fabricius. Mammals do not have a bursa however, and there is no single discrete organ of B cell development that functions as a homolog to the thymus for T cells. Instead, B cells develop at multiple sites including the liver, bone marrow, and spleen.

Although their immunological functions are quite distinct, there are an extraordinary number of parallels between T cells and B cells including development, receptor structure, tolerogenic mechanisms, and signaling. One of the most important similarities is apparent from the nomenclature of the gene family to which the TCR belongs (ie, the immunoglobulin supergene family).

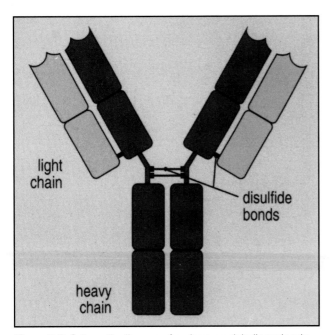

Figure 2-3. Schematic diagram of an immunoglobulin molecule. The immunoglobulin molecule consists of two light chains and two heavy chains. Disulfide bonds link each light chain to a heavy chain and the heavy chains to each other. The distal ends of each light chain-heavy chain pair form an antigen binding site. The proximal ends of the heavy chain bind to Fc receptors on phagocytic cells. Reprinted with permission from Janeway CA and Travers P, eds. In: Immunobiology, 3rd ed. Garland Publishing, Inc.; New York, NY:1997.

Ig genes, expressed exclusively in B cells, are the prototype for a large number of immunologically important genes, including the TCR. Secreted Ig gene products are antibodies, the basis for humoral immunity (Figure 2-3). Membrane-bound Ig gene products are B cell receptors for antigen (BCR), the B cell "equivalent" of the TCR.

The processes of B cell development, selection, and elimination or inactivation of autoreactive cells are very similar to those for T cells, in that B cells with high-affinity for self-antigens can be deleted or inactivated during maturation. These events are not be elaborated upon further in this text. There are, however, two important processes that are unique to B cells: isotype switching and affinity maturation.

ISOTYPE SWITCHING. There are five primary classes (isotypes) of immunoglobulin: IgM, IgD, IgG, IgE, and IgA, as determined by the constant region the heavy chain uses, the μ, δ, γ, ϵ, or α segments, respectively (Table 2-1). Mature *naive* B cells express both IgM and IgD on their surface, the only instance in which B cells express more than one Ig isotype. Both IgM and IgD function as BCRs for antigen. After activation, the B cell undergoes a process of isotype switching to either IgG, which has several subclasses (IgG1, IgG2a, IgG2b, and IgG3), IgE, or IgA as part of further differentiation and expansion.

SOMATIC MUTATION AND AFFINITY MATURATION. Following immunization with an antigen, B cells are able to undergo somatic point mutations in their Ig genes. The purpose of somatic mutation is to refine the Ig repertoire further. The mutation process itself is essentially random, therefore some mutated Ig genes will have unchanged antigen affinity, some will have higher antigen affinity, while others will have lower antigen affinity. Since B cell expansion, maturation and survival are dependent upon continued antigen stimulation, those B cells whose somatic mutations have led to high-affinity Ig genes will have a selective survival advantage. The result is affinity maturation during the immune response.

NK Cells

NK cells are capable of lysing a variety of viral-infected and tumor cells in vitro. They are variably classified as lymphocytes and are clearly distinct from either T or B cells, but their precise lineage is not known. It is hypoth-

Table 2-1. General Properties of Immunoglobulins

Property	Immunoglobulin Isotype				
	IgM	IgG	IgA	IgE	IgD
Usual form	pentamer or hexamer	monomer	monomer or dimer	monomer	monomer
Valence	10, 12	2	2, 4	2	2
Half-life (days)	10	21	6	2	3
Complement activation Classical pathway Alternate pathway	yes no	yes no	no yes	no no	no no
Binds to phagocytes	yes	no	no	no	no
Binds to mast cells through Fc receptors	no	no	no	yes	no

esized that they represent the remnant of a primitive form of immunity, one that arose prior to the development of the TCR. One of the most interesting aspects of NK-mediated cytotoxicity is that, unlike cytotoxic T cells, which are activated to kill upon specific recognition of antigen, NK cells seem constitutively able to kill many cell types, but are inactivated if the target expresses self-MHC class I molecules. Thus, this is a form of self-nonself recognition.

Specialized Antigen-Presenting Cells

For reasons detailed later in this chapter, immune responses are initiated most effectively, perhaps even exclusively, when antigen is presented to T cells by specialized, or "professional," APCs. Monocytes or macrophages, dendritic cells, and activated, but not resting B cells are all professional APCs and have certain shared characteristics including hematopoietic origin, expression of class II MHC molecules, and ability to provide costimulatory signals (see below) to T cells. Professional APCs are also highly efficient at capturing antigen for subsequent presentation to T cells. Macrophages and dendritic cells do this through phagocytosis. B cells capture foreign antigen through their surface immunoglobulin molecules that serve as their antigen receptors. Once antigen binds to surface Ig, the Ig-antigen complex is internalized. All three cell types are able to degrade internalized antigens by proteolysis and process them into peptide fragments which are capable of being recognized by T cells. The efficiency of these three types of professional APCs differs, with dendritic cells being the most potent and activated B cells the least. Some of the factors responsible for differential antigen-presenting capacity include the density of MHC molecules and costimulatory molecules on the APC.

Anatomically, these cells are well-situated to capture and subsequently present antigens. Both dendritic cells and macrophages are widely distributed throughout body organs and tissues. In particular, dendritic cells are thought to be sentinel cells of the immune system, and in some instances have acquired distinct names when located within distinct tissues. For example, dendritic cells in the epidermal layer of the skin are known as Langerhans' cells. It is thought that these cells are responsible for initiating many immune responses. In the case of transplantation, depletion of dendritic cells from tissue or organ grafts such as thyroid cells, pancreatic islet cells, or kidneys, can greatly prolong graft survival in animals, and in some instances lead to antigen-specific tolerance.

Nonhematopoietic Cells with Immune Function

A variety of cells, whose primary functions are nonimmunologic, may be active participants in immune responses as well. Recently, a great deal of attention has been focused on endothelial cells. In studies using human endothelial cells isolated from umbilical cords, as well as with porcine endothelial cells, it appears that these cells are capable of supporting immune responses in many of the same ways as professional APCs. This includes the expression of MHC class II molecules and costimulatory molecules, and the secretion of proinflammatory cytokines. In the case of transplantation, this feature of endothelial cells contributes to the high relative immunogenicity of vascularized organ allografts compared with tissue grafts. It also promotes the endothelium as a target for rejection.

INITIATING THE RESPONSE TO FOREIGN ANTIGEN

To respond to a foreign antigen, the immune system, especially T cells, must first "see" the antigen. As noted above, T cells, through their TCRs, recognize foreign peptides in the antigen-binding groove of MHC molecules. It is an historical curiosity of interest to transplantation immunologists that these genes, which are critically important for immune responses in general, were discovered because the ability of inbred strains of mice to reject organ and tissue transplants segregated primarily with this genetic locus, hence its role in histocompatibility. In humans, the MHC class I genes expressed on the cell surface consist of HLA-A, HLA-B, and HLA-C loci, and cell surface class II genes are the HLA-DR, HLA-DP, and HLA-DQ loci.

Alleles at all these loci are codominantly expressed, and the loci are highly polymorphic. This means that two randomly chosen individuals will always have multiple HLA disparities. The ability of T cells to react to foreign HLA molecules is the major stimulus for transplant rejection. The biology of the MHC is reviewed further in Chapter 3.

Antigen Presentation

MHC genes are subdivided into two classes, I and II, based on genetic and structural homology. Although there are some well-noted exceptions, in general, these two classes have distinct functions in immune homeostasis, with class I molecules presenting endogenous antigens, and class II molecules presenting exogenous antigens. Distinct systems have evolved for targeting endogenous vs exogenous antigens to the appropriate subcellular compartments, and for loading them onto class I or class II molecules, respectively. The teleological reasons for this compartmentalization have been debated. In any event, class II molecules are important for initiating immune responses to foreign proteins. As such, it is appropriate that they are found primarily on APCs. Class I molecules are found on all cells, and primarily present endogenous (ie, cytosolic) antigens. They are important for immune surveillance against cells that have been infected or altered in some way that leads to the production of novel or foreign proteins (eg, by a virus or by malignant transformation).

Mature T cells are subdivided based on reciprocal expression of either the CD4 or CD8 glycoproteins. CD4+ T cells have MHC class II-restricted TCRs, and CD8+ T cells are MHC class I-restricted in their antigen recognition. This means that recognition of exogenous antigens processed by APCs is almost entirely dependent on CD4+ cells. One can think then of MHC class II molecules and CD4+ T cells as being of primary importance in the response to extracellular antigens including parasites, many bacteria, and intact virus particles. The response of CD4+ cells may be to produce cytokines that support the expansion and differentiation of B cells into antibody-producing plasma cells (humoral immunity), or to produce proinflammatory cytokines that activate macrophages and CD8+ cytotoxic T lymphocytes (cellular immunity). In the former case, antibodies can serve to neutralize and/or opsonize extracellular pathogens. In the latter case, cytotoxic T lymphocyte (CTL) function also will require recognition of intracellular antigens presented on MHC class I molecules.

Anatomic Sites of Antigen Encounter and Sensitization

In considering immune responses, it is often useful to separate the response into two phases: the initiation phase and the effector phase. Most antigens are encountered first in nonimmune tissues. Thus, although the bulk of lymphocytes are in the spleen and lymph nodes, it is unusual for a foreign antigen to make its first entrance into the body at those sites. More typically, initial sites of encounter are the skin, respiratory tract, or gastrointestinal tract. Upon first exposure of the skin to an antigen, resident APCs of dendritic lineage, which in the skin are called Langerhans' cells, take up and process the protein into antigenic peptides for display on MHC class II molecules. The dendritic cells also undergo maturation, and in doing so, upregulate and/or newly express a variety of activation markers and cell surface proteins important to support the activation of T cells. Most importantly, dendritic cells leave the skin and migrate to regional lymph nodes where they can present the antigen to T cells. The importance of this phenomenon is illustrated by the fact that depletion of dendritic cells from the skin markedly blunts, sometimes completely, the response to applied antigens. It is in the peripheral lymphoid tissue that CD4+ (helper) T cells first respond to antigen by elaborating a variety of cytokines, thus, completing the initiation phase of the immune response. Following this, activated effector cells, both T and B lymphocytes, as well as macrophages and NK cells, migrate out of the lymph nodes to the site of antigen where they actually effect their response. Thus, one can think of immune responses being initiated within the lymphoid tissue, but being effected at a distal site. An exception to this is the response to alloantigens, where to a limited extent the presence of large numbers of donor-type APCs can lead to the recruitment and activation of T cells within the graft itself.

T Cell Activation

As recently as 15 years ago, very little was known about T cell surface receptors, and even less was known about the signaling pathways that coupled activation of the surface receptors to intracellular responses. Today, the picture is much clearer.

TCR ENGAGEMENT: SIGNAL 1. The T cell receptor for antigen (TCR) is a heterodimer of two closely related members of the immunoglobulin gene superfamily. Signal transduction through the TCR relies on an associated group of proteins known as CD3. Together, they form the TCR/CD3 complex. Once the TCR binds antigen, a cascade of pathways is activated. Many of the most proximal signals are transduced through cytosolic protein tyrosine kinases. However, studies over the last decade have established that these signals initiated through the TCR are not sufficient to enable cells to traverse the cell cycle, proliferate, and produce cytokines. A second costimulatory signal is needed.

COSTIMULATION: SIGNAL 2. Studies of T cell activation requirements over the past ten years have demonstrated that TCR stimulation by itself not only fails to lead to proliferation, but in the absence of a costimulatory signal, actually induces anergy in the T cell (Figure 2-4), a state in which the cell is nonresponsive, even to appropriate stimuli (ie, signals 1 plus 2). In vitro studies suggest that anergy can persist for up to several weeks. Additional studies have shown that costimulatory signals not only prevent anergy induction, but also up-regulate cell survival genes of the bcl-2 family, most notably bcl-xL. Furthermore, TCR engagement without costimulation can lead not only to anergy induction, but also to increased and accelerated T cell apoptosis. At present, it is unclear to what extent T cell anergy vs T cell apoptosis is responsible for the marked blunting of T cell immune responses observed in vivo when costimulatory signals are absent. However, it is likely that both mechanisms contribute to this phenomenon, perhaps with anergy preceding apoptosis.

A large number of molecules has been demonstrated to some degree to mediate costimulation, when this is "liberally" defined as synergism with TCR stimulation for proliferation. Most prominent in this list would be the T cell surface molecules LFA-1 (CD11a/CD18) and CD2.

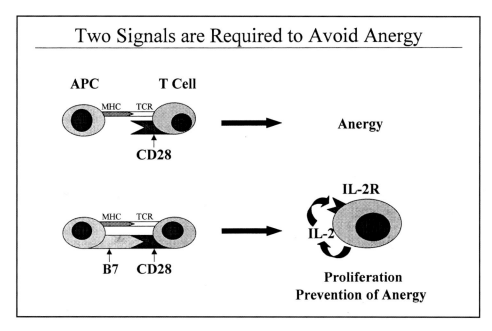

Two Signals are Required to Avoid Anergy

Figure 2-4. T cell stimulatory requirements. Stimulation through the T cell receptor alone induces anergy in T cells (top). A second (costimulatory) signal, such as that delivered through the CD28-to-B7 interaction, is required for induction of cytokine gene expression, proliferation, and prevention of anergy (bottom). In some instances, anergy may precede, or be superceded by, apoptosis (not shown).

However, neither of these pathways have been shown to prevent anergy induction in T cells. At present, the best characterized pathway that clearly prevents anergy induction is that which is mediated by the CD28 surface receptor (Figure 2-4). Activation of the CD28 pathway provides costimulation for proliferation and cytokine production, as well as prevents anergy induction. CD28 has at least two natural ligands that have been cloned, B71 (CD80) and B7-2 (CD86). Both are expressed almost exclusively on activated APCs (Figures 2-4 and 2-5). Their presence on APCs is crucial for full T cell activation. Their absence on non-APCs may be an important mechanism to maintain peripheral tolerance, because potentially autoreactive T cells with TCRs directed against self-antigens would be anergized by contact with those antigens on non-APCs, rather than activated by them (Figure 2-5).

As noted above, in the absence of costimulation, TCR ligation fails to induce a sustained T cell response, indicating that, in addition to preventing anergy induction and promoting cell survival, CD28 costimulation can be important in the primary T cell response to antigen. There are several mechanisms by which this occurs, including induction of cytokine gene expression, stabilization of cytokine gene transcripts, and increasing the "sensitivity" of the T cell to low concentrations of antigen by promoting clustering of T cell receptor activation complexes on the cell surface.

In addition to CD28, activated T cells express a homologous molecule called CTLA-4. Studies in CD28-knock-out mice demonstrate that, unlike CD28, CTLA-4 does not deliver a stimulatory signal to the cell interior, but instead transduces a negative one, which may be important in terminating immune responses.

Consistent with this, in some experimental systems, blockade of signals through CTLA-4 can prevent the induction of tolerance.

There is at least one other pathway in addition to CD28 that appears to be important for costimulation in vivo. This pathway, the subject of intense ongoing investigation, is mediated through the CD40 molecule on APCs that binds to CD40-ligand (CD40L, recently named CD154) on activated T cells. Stimulation of CD40 on APCs induces expression of B7 molecules (the ligands for CD28). However, numerous studies indicate that this is not the only mechanism by which the CD40-to-CD154 pathway supports immune responses. For example, CD40 engagement activates APCs to secrete proinflammatory cytokines such as IL-12 and up-regulate adhesion molecules. CD40 activation of B cells promotes B cell survival, proliferation, and antibody production. There is little evidence, however, that CD154 itself transduces a direct costimulatory signal to the T cell. Therefore, most investigators believe that the effects of the CD154-to-CD40 pathway on T cells are mediated indirectly by activation of APCs. Recent studies indicate that a molecule related to CD154, called 4-1BB, may transduce a costimulatory signal to T cells, explaining, perhaps, why mice deficient in CD28 can still mount some protective immune responses.

T Cell Effector Function

As referenced above, in most instances the number of T cells that react to a given antigen is quite small. Furthermore, previously unstimulated T cells, so-called *naive* T cells, are inefficient at making cytokines and killing target cells. Therefore, observable immune responses generally require clonal expansion and differentiation of responding T cells (Figure 2-6). These

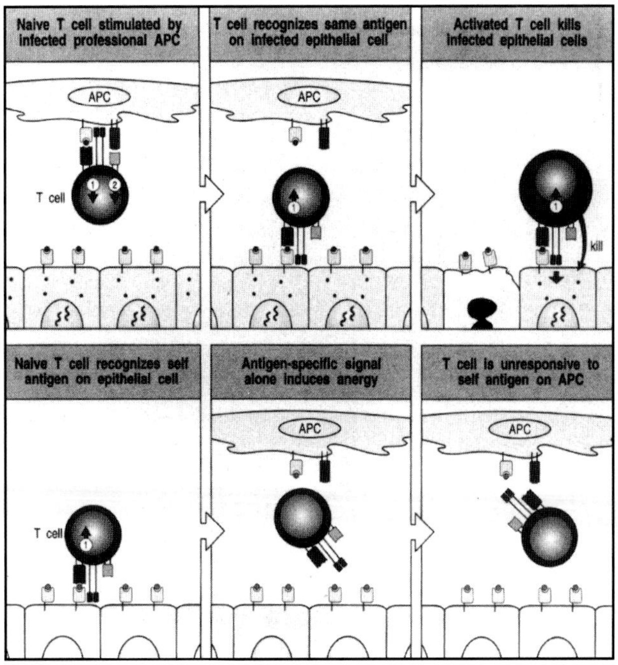

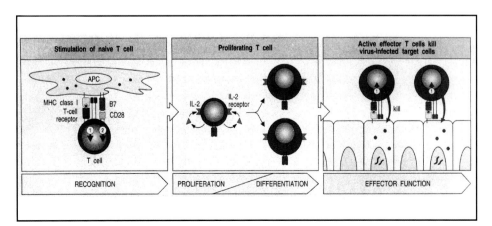

Figure 2-5. The requirement for two signals to activate T cells is important in preventing autoimmunity. In the example shown here, one of viral infection, a T cell becomes activated by stimulation with a viral peptide presented by an APC (eg, a macrophage or a dendritic cell), and at the same time receives a co-stimulatory signal (top left panel, indicated by the numbers 1 and 2). This T cell then proliferates and differentiates into effector cells, which are capable of recognizing viral antigens on virally-infected cells. The mature effector cell does not need costimulation, and is therefore capable of responding to viral antigens expressed by non-APCs, such as epithelial cells (top middle and top right panels). In contrast, if a T cell first encounters an antigen on an epithelial cell, engagement of the TCR without a costimulatory signal, which only APCs can provide, will induce anergy or apoptosis in the T cell. If the T cell survives, it will be unable to respond to that antigen even if subsequently presented by an APC (bottom panels). It is thought that the requirement of T cells for costimulation, plus the inability of non-APCs to provide costimulation, is important for immune homeostasis by preventing potentially autoreactive T cells, which escaped thymic selection from causing autoimmune disease. Reprinted with permission from Janeway CA and Travers P., eds. In: Immunobiology, 4th ed. Garland Publishing, Inc.; New York, NY:1999.

processes are largely driven by cytokines. Furthermore, some of the cytokines that support T cell proliferation and differentiation also are important in the immune effector functions of T cells. The list of cytokines is large and growing. Table 2-2 outlines selected cytokines, their source, and their effects. What follows is a consideration of three important effects of cytokines, listed by the target cell rather than the cytokine itself.

CTL DIFFERENTIATION AND FUNCTION. With a few minor exceptions, virtually all CTLs are MHC-class I-restricted CD8+ cells. Unlike CD4+ T cells that make large amounts of cytokines, CD8+ T cells make far less and, therefore, are often dependent on cytokines produced locally by CD4+ cells. IL-2 seems to be their most important growth factor, and provision of exogenous recombinant IL-2 to isolated CD8+ T cells can make up for much of the deficit seen by removal of the CD4+ population.

Activated CTLs possess two mechanisms to kill their targets, both of which require cell-to-cell contact (Figure 2-7). The first mechanism is through perforin and granzymes, proteins found in most CTLs and NK cells. Perforin, like complement components, has the capacity to induce transmembrane pores in the target cell, leading to target cell lysis. Although it was originally thought that membrane lysis by perforin was the sole mediator of CTL killing, it is now known that a second mechanism of CTL killing, the Fas pathway, exists. Fas (CD95) is a member of the tumor necrosis factor (TNF) receptor family, and is the surface mediator of a pathway that, when activated, induces the cell to undergo programmed cell death through apoptosis. Many cells express Fas, and activated CTLs express Fas ligand. Both mechanisms of killing are available to CTLs in vivo.

B CELL HELP. The B cell response to most well-studied protein antigens requires T cell help. The stimulatory requirements for B cells and the ways in which B and T cells interact are reviewed below.

Figure 2-6. Clonal expansion precedes differentiation to effector function. Following activation of naive T cells by antigen plus costimulation (through CD28), T cells proliferate then differentiate in response to cytokines such as IL-2. This expanded population of activated T cells is then able to carry out effector functions, such as cytotoxicity. Reprinted with permission from Janeway CA and Travers P., eds. In: Immunobiology, 4th ed. Garland Publishing, Inc.; New York, NY:1999.

Table 2-2. Selected Cytokines and Their Effects

Cytokine*	Cell of Origin	Action(s)
IL-1α and IL-β	Macrophages, epithelial cells	Proinflammatory†
IL-2	T cells	T and B cell growth and survival factor
IL-3	T cells	Hematopoiesis
IL-4	T cells, mast cells, basophil	B cell activation, T cell growth factor, induces Th2 responses
IL-5	T cells, mast cells	Eosinophil growth factor
IL-6	T cells, macrophages	Proinflammatory
IL-7	Stromal cells in thymus and marrow	Growth or maintenance factor for immature T and B cells
IL-8‡	Macrophages	Leukocyte chemotaxis
IL-10	T cells, macrophages	Suppresses macrophage functions, supports Th2 responses
IL-12	APCs	NK cell growth or activation factor, induces Th1 responses
IL-15	non-T cells	same as IL-2
IFN-γ	T cells, NK cells	Activates macrophages, increases MHC expression, induces IL-12 production
TNF	T cells, macrophages, NK cells	Proinflammatory
TGF-β	Macrophages, T cells	Antiinflammatory

*IL indicates interleukin; IFN-interferon; TNF, tumor necrosis factor; and TGF, transforming growth factor.
†Pro-inflammatory and anti-inflammatory actions include effects on vasodilatation, leukocyte recruitment, antigen presentation, etc.
‡IL-8 is a part of the chemokine family, other members of which including MIP-1α, MIP-1β, MCP-1, and RANTES also are strong chemo attractants for leukocytes.

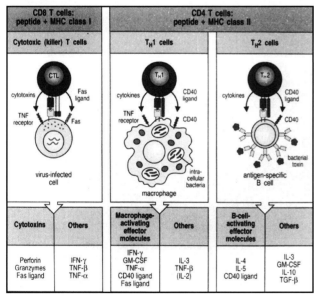

Figure 2-7. Mechanisms of T cell effector function. CD8 T cells are predominantly cytotoxic T cells that kill their targets directly following cell-to-cell contact. This effect is mediated through perforin, granzymes and/or Fas ligand. CD4 T cells of the Th1 (T helper 1) subtype are specialized for activation of macrophages, an effect they exert through the production of IFN-γ and other cytokines. They also have cytotoxic capacity, which is mediated through Fas ligand. Unlike CD8 cytotoxic T cells, they do not release perforin or granzymes. CD4 T cells of the Th2 subtype provide help for B cell antibody production. This is done through secretion of B cell growth factors such as IL-4, and through cell-to-cell interactions involving CD40 and CD40 ligand. Reprinted with permission from Janeway CA and Travers P, eds. In: Immunobiology, 3rd ed. Garland Publishing, Inc.; New York, NY:1997.

MACROPHAGE ACTIVATION. The activated macrophage is one of the most important mediators of many types of immune responses, especially delayed-type hypersensitivity (DTH) and related cellular immune reactions. Resting macrophages must be activated in order to exert their full inflammatory and cytopathic effects. IFN-γ, produced by T cells, is particularly important in this process (Figure 2-7). It enhances phagocytosis; stimulates macrophages secretion of the proinflammatory agents TNF and IL-1; stimulates production and secretion of tissue proteases and reactive oxygen products, such as superoxide and nitric oxide, which are important mechanisms for the cytopathic effect of macrophages; and upregulates MHC expression on macrophages.

B Cell Activation

T-INDEPENDENT ANTIGENS. In general, B cell responses to antigen require T cell help. However, some types of antigen (ie, those containing repetitive epitopes) are highly efficient at crosslinking membrane Ig, the B cell receptor for antigen. These antigens, most commonly bacterial capsular polysaccharides, deliver such potent signals to the B cell that, unlike most protein antigens, T cells are not required for the B cell response. Therefore, these antigens are called T-independent antigens.

COGNATE INTERACTIONS AND COSTIMULA-TORY SIGNALS. Most B cell antigens are probably not able to crosslink Ig extensively and, therefore, are unable by themselves to activate B cells. They depend on a process known as T cell-to-B cell cognate help. In this instance, the antigen binds to the B cell surface Ig, is internalized, and presented to CD4+ T cells on B cell MHC class II molecules. The T cell-to-B cell contact initiated in this way also allows the B cell surface receptor CD40 to bind to its ligand on the T cell (known as CD40-ligand). Signals through CD40 act in concert with T cell-derived cytokines to activate the B cell (Figure 2-7).

ANTIBODY SECRETION. Following appropriate activation and signaling, previously naive B cells secrete IgM and proceed through one of two pathways: development into memory cells, or differentiation into antibody-secreting plasma cells. The latter is frequently accompanied by somatic mutation and isotype switching to IgA, IgG, or IgE, although some plasma cells do not class-switch and secrete IgM. This process occurs over a period of two to three weeks, and the initial antibody response in a naive animal is IgM, with subsequent maturation to IgG and IgA. Some of the distinctions between Ig isotypes are outlined in Table 2-1. Antibodies can function in several different ways, varying by isotype. These mechanisms include fixation of complement, opsonization for phagocytosis by FcR+ cells, opsonization for lysis by cells capable of antibody-dependent cellular cytotoxicity, and induction of eosinophil degranulation.

REGULATING THE RESPONSE TO FOREIGN ANTIGEN
Migration and Adhesion of Immune Cells

As sophisticated as the mechanisms of immunologic recognition may be, they will be of little avail unless lymphocytes and other immune effector cells have access to the inflammatory site. It is exceedingly rare for foreign antigens to be located primarily and initially in peripheral lymphoid tissue. Almost always, they are introduced into the body elsewhere (eg, skin, mucosal surfaces). While there are normally few lymphocytes resident in most parenchymal organs and tissues, during an immune response the number of cells that become localized to the site of inflammation increases substantially. It is through the expression and regulation of adhesion molecules that this process takes place.

The molecules that regulate adhesion fall into three primary families: selectins, integrins, and immunoglobulin superfamily proteins.

SELECTINS AND "ROLLING" OR "TETHERING". When an inflammatory process occurs, leukocytes need

to get to the inflammatory site (Figure 2-8). They are, however, unable to access that site directly, as it is hidden behind endothelium. Although normally leukocytes are rushing through the bloodstream, local vasodilation in response to inflammation increases the volume of blood flow and, at the same time, decreases the flow rate. As cells flow more slowly, they have a greater chance of reacting with the endothelium and adhering to it. Nonetheless, leukocytes adhere poorly to resting endothelial cells. However, in response to inflammatory stimuli such as the macrophage products TNF and IL-1, both lymphocytes and endothelial cells up-regulate selectins on their cell surface. The ligands for the selectins are sugars (eg, sialylated or sulfated Lewis blood group antigens X and A). These sugars can be found on any one of a number of proteins expressed by lymphocytes and endothelia, and thus, each cell type bears both selectins and selectin-ligands. Selectins mediate transient adhesion of the lymphocyte to the

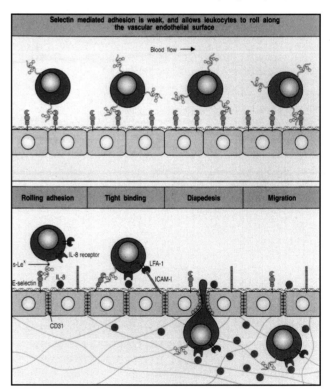

Figure 2-8. A model for cell adhesion and migration. Inflammatory mediators such as TNF induce the expression of selectins on endothelial cells. The relatively weak interaction of selectins with their ligands such as sialyl Lewis X (s-Le^X) is sufficient for transient adhesion of the leukocyte. This adhesion, however, is broken by shear forces of blood flow, reestablished distally, broken again, etc., so that the leukocyte rolls along the endothelium. Triggering of the cell through chemokines such as IL-8 induces high affinity in the integrin LFA-1 for its ligand ICAM-1. This is a strong adhesive interaction, which withstands shear forces of the bloodstream. Subsequently, the leukocyte migrates through the endothelium. Reprinted with permission from Janeway CA and Travers P, eds. In: Immunobiology, 3rd ed. Garland Publishing, Inc.; New York, NY:1997.

endothelium so that the cell appears to roll along the surface of the blood vessel, a phenomenon also termed "tethering."

CHEMOKINES AND TRIGGERING. Lymphocytes slowed down by selectin interactions come into more prolonged contact with the endothelium. As a result, lymphocytes are stimulated by chemokines, a group of small proinflammatory molecules produced by endothelia, fibroblasts, platelets, and monocytes. Once secreted, chemokines such as IL-8 associate with cell-surface proteoglycans on endothelial cells such as CD44 through their heparin-binding domains. This retains the chemokines locally, enabling them to activate lymphocytes and neutrophils as they roll by. When the chemokines bind to their receptors on leukocytes, they trigger the adhesive function of integrins.

ADHESION. The integrin family of molecules are $\alpha\beta$ heterodimers formed by noncovalent association. The ligands for one of the first known and best characterized integrins, LFA-1, are the immunoglobulin superfamily gene members ICAM-1, -2, and -3. LFA-1 is expressed on most leukocytes. ICAM-1 is weakly expressed on resting endothelium, but induced by activation with IL-1 and TNF. Thus, they form a potent adhesion pair to enable leukocytes to adhere to endothelia at the sites of inflammation. An important property of integrins such as LFA-1 is that their baseline state is one of low-affinity for their ligands. This prevents unnecessary adhesion of leukocytes to normal endothelium. Activation of the LFA-1-bearing cell, such as by chemokines, triggers the transition of LFA-1 to a high-affinity state for ICAM-1, leading to tight adhesion of the leukocyte to the endothelial cell.

TRANSMIGRATION. This is the final step required to get the leukocyte to the site of inflammation, and occurs rapidly after adhesion. Both the transient nature of integrin triggering, as well as shedding of cell surface selectin molecules assist in detaching the leukocyte from the vessel wall. The events that take place during actual locomotion or transmigration remain poorly understood.

Th1 and Th2 Responses

During the 1980s, increasing numbers of cytokines secreted by T cells and macrophages were identified. In studies examining cytokine production by T cell clones, Mosmann and colleagues made the surprising discovery that many murine CD4+ T cell clones could be subdivided into two categories based on the cytokines they produced. The so-called Th1 (for T helper-type 1) clones produced IL-2 and IFN-γ, while Th2 clones produced IL-4, IL-5, and IL-10 (Figures 2-7 and 2-9). As the effects

of these cytokines became known, it was apparent that the subdivision of production correlated with a categorization of function, namely, that the cytokines produced by Th1 clones provided help for cellular immune responses while Th2-derived cytokines provided help for humoral responses. Thus, the Th1-derived cytokines are growth and maturation or activation factors for cytotoxic T lymphocytes and NK cells (especially IL-2), and macrophages (particularly IFN-γ). In contrast, Th2 cytokines perform similar functions for B cells. Interestingly, Th1 cytokines not only promote cellular responses, but they tend to inhibit humoral responses, and the opposite is true of Th2 cytokines. Therefore, they seem to be mutually antagonistic pathways, although as expected, there are exceptions. The original findings arose out of the murine system using T cell clones, but most researchers report similar findings in humans using both T cell clones and "normal" (uncloned) T cells as well.

Emergence of Memory Cells

Although there is only a patchy understanding of how immunologic memory is generated or maintained, this phenomenon is used frequently because it forms the basis for vaccination. The principle of immunologic memory is that the immune response to a previously seen antigen is both faster and more effective than the response to a new antigen. There are probably several reasons for this. First, lymphocytes can be subdivided based on their cell surface phenotype into naive and memory cells. Naive cells are those that have never encountered their target antigens and, therefore, have never been stimulated. Memory cells are those that have been stimulated, survived, and matured into a memory phenotype. The signals that instruct a lymphocyte to become a memory cell are not known. As might be expected, newborn mammals have predominantly naive cells, with the proportion of memory cells increasing with age. One of the reasons that a recall response to antigen is more robust than an initial response is that memory cells seem to be more easily activated than naive cells and, in addition, make more cytokines than activated naive cells. A second basis for immunologic memory is precursor frequency. Sensitive assays using tetrameric complexes of MHC plus peptide have shown an increase in the frequency of antigen-reactive cells following exposure to an antigen. A third mechanism for immunologic memory is used only by the B cell compartment, namely, affinity maturation. As detailed above, exposure to antigen leads to refinement of the antibody repertoire with selection of high-affinity antibody-producing B cells. Thus, antibody production in a memory response is significantly more effective than in a primary response.

A corollary of memory cell development is memory cell survival. The best understood mechanism by which

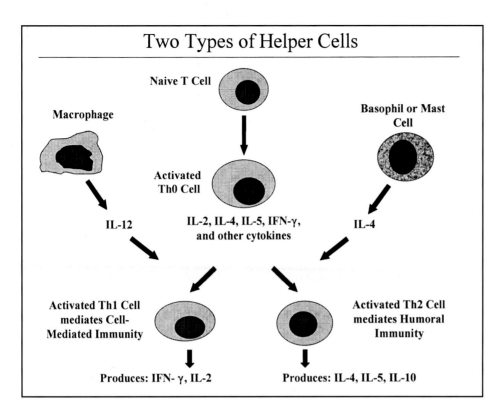

Two Types of Helper Cells

Naive T Cell

Macrophage

Basophil or Mast Cell

Activated Th0 Cell

IL-12

IL-2, IL-4, IL-5, IFN-γ, and other cytokines

IL-4

Activated Th1 Cell mediates Cell-Mediated Immunity

Activated Th2 Cell mediates Humoral Immunity

Produces: IFN-γ, IL-2

Produces: IL-4, IL-5, IL-10

Figure 2-9. Two types of T-helper cells. When a previously unactivated ("naive") T cell is stimulated, it secretes low levels of virtually all T cell-derived cytokines. This is frequently referred to as a Th0 cell. Further differentiation is largely under the control of exogenous cytokines. IL-12, produced by activated antigen-presenting cells, strongly directs T cells toward the Th1 phenotype. These cells produce IFN-γ and IL-2 and direct cell-mediated immunity. IL-4, believed to be initially produced by basophils and/or mast cells, directs T cells toward the Th2 phenotype. Th2 cells, responsible for providing B cell help for humoral immunity, secrete IL-4, IL-5, and IL-10.

this occurs is through expression of the antiapoptotic genes Bcl-2 and Bcl-xL, which are induced primarily by IL-2 and CD28 stimulation, respectively, following T cell activation. Expression of these genes inhibits cell death from apoptosis, an event to which cycling T and B cells are susceptible. Signals for cell survival are also delivered tonically though periodic interactions of T cells with self-MHC molecules plus self-peptide. While the signal generated by this interaction is not sufficient to support a T cell immune response, through unknown means it promotes T cell survival.

Terminating the Immune Response

For the organism to survive, it is as important to terminate the immune response, when appropriate, as it was to initiate it. Since antigen stimulation triggers lymphoid proliferation, in the absence of cell death, repeated encounter with pathogens would lead to massive continued expansion of the lymphoid pool, turning us into giant lymph nodes. Nonetheless, until recently, the mechanisms by which immune responses are terminated have been sorely neglected. However, interest in this area has been rekindled recently. As it is now understood, lymphocytes are constantly dying during the course of an immune response, only to be replaced by new ones (Figure 2-10). When antigen is gone, normally no new ones are generated and the response is ended. Failure to eliminate cells normally means the response may continue even in the absence of antigen, and this can have serious adverse consequences.

The fact that withdrawal of antigen ends a response means that the immune response is not inherently self-sustaining, but requires continued "initiation" through encounters with antigen. The first step, therefore, to ending an immune response is to destroy the source of antigen. Depending on the nature of the pathogen, this might be through engulfment and digestion of bacteria by macrophages and neutrophils, lysis of virally-infected cells by CTLs, or antibody-mediated destruction of target organisms. In any event, when the inciting antigen is gone, there will be no more initiating stimulus to induce growth factor production, cell proliferation, and cell activation.

However, what about the expanded and activated effector cell population that already exists? At first glance it might seem that these cells are irrelevant, since in the absence of antigen they will do little harm. In fact, this is not the case. A significant amount of immune-mediated tissue injury is promiscuous (ie, antigen nonspecific). There are several reasons for this. First, some mediators of injury, such as macrophages, do not have antigen receptors and act relatively indiscriminately to destroy local tissues. Second, high cytokine levels can activate some T and NK cells even in the absence of antigen stimulation. Therefore, in a mixed population of lymphocytes at an inflammatory site, high levels of cytokines produced by cells responding to an antigen can trigger activation in some cells that are not antigen-specific. If some of these cells are actually self-reactive, an autoimmune response will ensue. Third, antibodies can cause disease by being

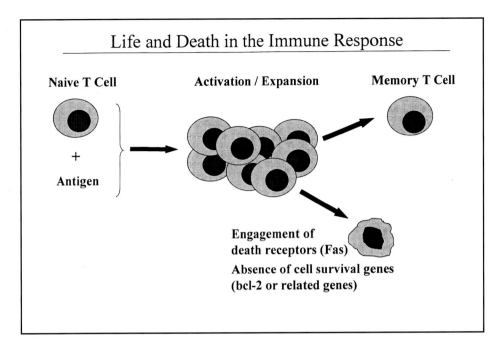

Figure 2-10. Life and death in the immune response. Following challenge with antigen, a small number of antigen-specific T cells undergo clonal activation and expansion, becoming a large population of effector cells (both helper and cytotoxic T cells). After a period of time, the majority of these cells undergo programmed cell death through a variety of mechanisms, leaving behind a small number of antigen-specific memory cells. Under conditions of antigen persistence, this scenario is continually repeated and a dynamic equilibrium is reached. When the antigen is no longer present, the stimulus for expansion is removed, and the T cell population returns to roughly its baseline level. Similar processes and considerations apply to B cell stimulation and B cell memory.

nonspecifically trapped in certain susceptible target tissues, such as synovia and glomeruli, leading to immune complex-mediated arthritis and glomerulonephritis.

It should be evident then, that elimination or inactivation of immune response cells, once they are no longer needed, is both desirable and necessary. This is accomplished largely through induction of programmed cell death in the responding cells. Activated T cells express two genes important for this process: Fas and Fas ligand. Engagement of Fas by its ligand triggers a death signal leading to apoptosis of the cell. Since T cells express both genes, elimination of T cells can be through "fratricide" or "suicide." The importance of these genes for immune homeostasis is highlighted by two interesting mouse mutations: *lpr* (lymphoproliferation) and *gld* (generalized lymphadenopathy), in which mice homozygous for the mutant gene exhibit profound lymphadenopathy with accumulation of abnormal T cells. Both *lpr* and *gld* mice develop autoimmune disease reminiscent of lupus, with autoimmune arthritis and immune complex-mediated glomerulonephritis that lead to eventual death by uremia. *lpr* mice are deficient in Fas, and *gld* mice have defective Fas ligand. Thus, each of these two genes is required for the "normal" death of T cells as immune responses are terminated. Clearly, not all responding cells die. A minority of T and B cells survive as memory cells. Increasing data suggests that sensitivity to Fas-mediated apoptosis may be negatively regulated by cell survival genes such as bcl-2 and bcl-xL, and thus, these genes may be important in the development of immunological memory.

RECOMMENDED READING

Steinman RM. The dendritic cell system and its role in immunogenicity. Annu Rev Immunol. 1991;9:271-296.

Pober JS, Cotran RS. Immunologic interactions of T lymphocytes with vascular endothelium. Adv Immunol. 1991;50:261-302.

Weiss A, Littman DR. Signal transduction by lymphocyte antigen receptors. Cell. 1994;76(2):263-274.

Janeway CH, Bottomly K. Signals and signs for lymphocyte responses. Cell. 1994;76(2):275-285.

June CH, Bluestone JA, Nadler LM, Thompson CB. The B7 and CD28 receptor families. Immunol Today. 1994;15(7):321-31.

Pleiman CM, D'Ambrosio D, Cambier JC. The B-cell antigen receptor complex: structure and signal transduction. Immunol Today. 1994;15(9):393-399.

Sprent J. T and B memory cells. Cell. 1994;76(2):315-322.

Imhof BA, Dunon D. Leukocyte migration and adhesion. Adv Immunol. 1995;58:345-416.

Thompson CB. Apoptosis in the pathogenesis and treatment of disease. Science. 1995;267(5203):1456-1462.

Nagata S, Goldstein P. The Fas death factor. Science. 1995;267(5203):1449-1456.

3 IMMUNE RESPONSE TO ALLOGRAFTS

Alan M. Krensky, MD

When an organ (or tissue) from one individual is transplanted into a second, genetically nonidentical individual of the same species, a series of cellular and molecular events are initiated, which if left unchecked, result in rejection of the graft. This "allogeneic" response involves a variety of overlapping mechanisms that evolved to discriminate self from nonself, and is directed at foreign antigens present in the graft. The most important of these foreign antigens are the human leukocyte antigens (HLA) encoded within the major histocompatibility complex (MHC) on chromosome 6. In normal immune responses, T lymphocytes recognize foreign antigens when presented as peptide fragments in association with self-HLA molecules (Chapter 2). In organ transplants, the precise molecular nature of the alloantigen is less certain. Most likely, nonself HLA is recognized in a variety of forms. Despite this fundamental difference, the cascade of events in transplant rejection appears to be essentially the same as the one that occurs against any foreign invader. These processes lead to recognition and destruction of the invader, followed by healing of the remaining viable tissue.

NATURE OF THE ALLOANTIGEN

The dominant form of alloantigen is the nonself HLA molecule complexed with a variety of different peptides in its antigen binding groove. The frequency of precursor cells for an alloresponse is very strong: 100 to 1,000 times as strong as the response to standard nonself antigens, such as viral peptides presented in the context of self-HLA. In addition to, and perhaps because of, an unusually high frequency of precursor cells, the alloresponse, unlike the response to most other antigens, is not dependent on "priming" (ie, previous exposure) for an initial immune response. Rather, the primary response to foreign HLA molecules is rapid and strong. Any strategies to prevent allorecognition must take into account these cardinal observations.

Several theories have been proposed to explain the strength of the alloresponse. These include the natural high affinity of T cell receptors for HLA molecules; the high density of alloantigens on the surface of cells; the large numbers of potential peptide-HLA combinations

Shelagh Galligan Professor; Chief, Division of Immunology & Transplantation Biology, Department of Pediatrics, Stanford University School of Medicine, Stanford, CA.

recognized as nonself; and the potential for molecular mimicry (crossreactivity).

MECHANISM OF ALLORECOGNITION

Two major models of alloantigen recognition have been proposed (Figure 3-1). In direct allorecognition, donor T lymphocytes recognize foreign HLA molecules directly, without processing via antigen-presenting cells. Recognition is probably due to the inherent natural affinity of T cell receptors for HLA molecules. This process is best understood in the context of positive and negative selection. As described in Chapter 2, T lymphocytes are educated to distinguish self from nonself in the thymus. T lymphocytes with too high an affinity for self-HLA are deleted (negative selection), while those with proper affinity for self-HLA are selected for maturation and exported to the peripheral immune system (positive selection). This process insures adequate affinity between self-HLA and the T cell receptor repertoire in order to allow a competent immune response to a variety of foreign proteins. It does not, however, account for the "unnatural" encounter with nonself HLA that takes place in transplantation. Since developing T cells with high affinity for nonself HLA would not have been eliminated during ontogeny, high-affinity T cell receptors for nonself HLA should persist in the periphery. It is these cells that are thought to predominate in the alloimmune response.

Bevan and Matzinger proposed that alloreactivity is due to the large number of antigenic complexes that can be formed by the combination of self and nonself cellular antigens recognized in the context of nonself HLA. Although the role of antigenic peptide in the HLA groove was not appreciated when this theory was first proposed, it is now clear that the variety of peptides that can associate with the groove of any single HLA type (allele) may help to account for the complexity of the alloresponse.

An unresolved issue in this regard is the importance of particular peptides in the nonself HLA groove in allorecognition. As described in Chapter 2, most, if not all HLA molecules expressed on the cell surface contain peptides in their grooves. Although it is clear that alloantigens are recognized as nonself HLA with peptide present, the precise role of the individual peptide is uncertain. Several different possibilities exist and there are data to support all of them (Table 3-1). Allogeneic T cells may recognize a particular peptide, a family of peptides, or any peptide may suffice. It is also possible that peptides may not be required at all (empty HLA).

It is clear that T cell recognition is affected by conformational changes that occur some distance from the peptide-binding groove, as has been shown in studies employing site-directed mutagenesis of HLA molecules. In addition, T cell recognition is affected by single amino

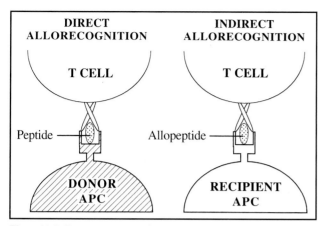

Figure 3-1. Two mechanisms for allorecognition. Direct allorecognition involves recognition of foreign HLA with a variety of potential peptides present in the antigen-presentation groove. In contrast, indirect allorecognition involves recognition of specific foreign HLA sequences as peptides in the context of self-HLA.

acids in the bound peptide. Such changes can either up-regulate or down-regulate the immune response. An active immune response can be changed to no immune response (passive indifference) or to the induction of tolerance (active antigen-specific nonresponsiveness).

Molecular mimicry is another theory proposed to account for the strength of the allogeneic immune response. This model suggests that a particular HLA molecule-peptide complex resembles another, different HLA molecule-peptide complex (HLA 1 + X = HLA 2 + Y), or that a given nonself HLA may mimic self-HLA plus peptide (HLA 1 = HLA 2 + X). Despite several examples of such mimicry, its relative importance in the overall immune response to foreign or nonself HLA is unproven.

A second form of allorecognition also exists. In indirect allorecognition, fragments of foreign HLA molecules are recognized as antigenic peptides bound in the groove of self-HLA molecules (Figure 3-1). This is the same mechanism of presentation involved in the recog-

Table 3-1.
Molecular Nature of the Alloantigen Recognized by T Lymphocytes

Various peptides suffice
HLA molecule with peptide present but peptide is irrelevant to response
Specific peptide is necessary but may be expressed with several HLA types
Peptide is specific for the HLA type (faithfully HLA-dependent)
HLA molecule with no peptid present (empty)

nition of "natural" antigens (Chapter 2). Although numerous observations have shown that indirect allorecognition occurs and that it is relevant to transplant rejection, it is not yet clear how indirect allorecognition could account for the strength of the alloimmune response, the high precursor frequency, or the lack of need for priming. Therefore, although indirect allorecognition likely contributes to the alloimmune response, it is almost certain that direct allorecognition predominates.

CELLULAR EVENTS

The initiating event in any antigen-specific immune response is antigen presentation (Chapter 2). In order for T lymphocytes to recognize foreign proteins, such antigens must normally be degraded into peptide fragments and presented in association with HLA molecules. As indicated above, it is possible that this important step is not required for transplant rejection. Nevertheless, even in transplant rejection, the involvement of antigen-presenting cells is necessary. Antigen-presenting cells

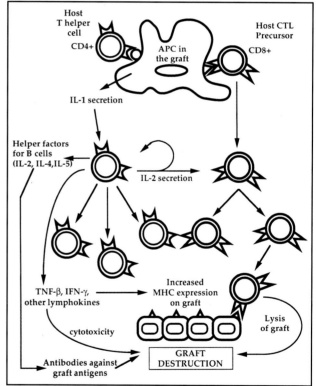

Figure 3-2. Cellular and molecular events involved in transplant rejection. Recipient CD4+ helper T lymphocytes recognize HLA class II molecules on the surface of the graft and secrete lymphokines (helper factors). CD8+ precursor cytotoxic T lymphocytes (CTL) recognize HLA class I molecules, and in conjunction with stimulation by helper factors, become cytotoxic. B cells, activated by donor HLA molecules and lymphokines, differentiate into antibody secreting plasma cells producing antibodies against donor antigens. Reprinted with permission from Krensky AM, Clayberger C. Prospects for induction of tolerance in renal transplantation. Pediatr Nephrol. 1994;8(6):772-779. Copyright© 1994, Springer-Verlag.

express HLA class II molecules: HLA-DR, DP, and DQ. Such molecules either present peptide antigen to, or are directly recognized by CD4+ helper T lymphocytes (Figure 3-2). Whether or not specific peptide fragments are required, it is clear that HLA class II molecules are important for induction of the alloimmune response. A proviso is that rejection can occur without class II differences. When this type of rejection occurs clinically, however, it is generally weak. In instances where it occurs experimentally, it is usually due to the contrived nature of experimental models used (ie, "knockout" or congenic mice).

Donor cells express HLA molecules on their surface. HLA class II antigens are recognized by CD4+ helper T lymphocytes while HLA class I antigens are recognized by CD8+ cytotoxic T lymphocytes. Since organ transplants are vascularized organs, recipient effector cells must traverse the vascular endothelium in order to reach the graft. For this to occur, they must first recognize the vascular endothelium as foreign. Since resting vascular endothelium does not express HLA class II molecules unless it is somehow damaged or activated, it may not be the stimulus that initiates the antigraft response.

Passenger leukocytes are donor hematopoietic cells that are passively transferred in the organ. These cells can then exit the transplanted organ and enter into recipient-draining lymph nodes. There, these donor cells (direct allorecognition) and/or their isolated antigens (indirect allorecognition) are recognized by the recipient immune cells. Circulating CD4+ cells recognize the foreign antigen in the lymph node and are activated to proliferate and differentiate. These helper T cells release cytokines (Table 3-2), initiating an immune response. Antigen-specific T cells increase in number and enter the peripheral blood stream. Locally, in the lymph node, cytotoxic T lymphocytes (CTL) specific for donor HLA class I, also become sensitized, increase in number, and enter the periphery. Since the graft vessels express HLA class I antigens, such CTL may directly recognize the graft as foreign and damage it. These cells may cause release of gamma interferon, a cytokine that induces expression of HLA class II molecules. Together, recognition of nonself HLA class II by CD4+ cells and nonself HLA class I by CD8+ CTL initiate the antigen-specific immune response.

Until recently, relatively little was understood about entry of blood borne monocytes and activated T cells into the site of a graft. Typically, cell-mediated rejection is characterized by a cellular infiltrate containing a variety of cell types, including both antigen-specific and non-

Table 3-2. Selected Cytokines Involved in Transplant Rejection

Cytokine	Biologic Action(s)
IL-1αβ (interleukin)	enhances B and T cell activation, induces fever, induces acute phase reactants, induces fibroblast proliferation
IL-2	induces T cell, B cell, and NK cell growth and differentiation
IL-4	T and B cell growth factor
IL-5	eosinophil growth and differentiation, B cell proliferation
IL-6	B cell differentiation
IL-8	neutrophil chemotaxis
IL-9	T cell stimulation
IL-10	inhibition of antigen presentation and γ-interferon production
IL-12	potentiates γ-interferon production
IL-13	inhibits IL-1, TNF, IL-6 and IL-8 production, enhances γ-interferon production
TNF-αβ (tumor necrosis factor)	stimulates fibroblasts, macrophages, neutrophils
IFN-γ (interferon)	activates macrophages, induces HLA class I and II
TGF-β (transforming growth factor)	inhibits proliferation of B and T cells, inhibits macrophage activation, stimulates fibroblast growth factor
RANTES (regulated upon activation, normal T expressed, and secreted)	monocyte, T lymphocyte chemoattractant and activator
MIP-1αβ (macrophage inflammatory proteins)	monocyte, T lymphocyte chemoattractant and activator

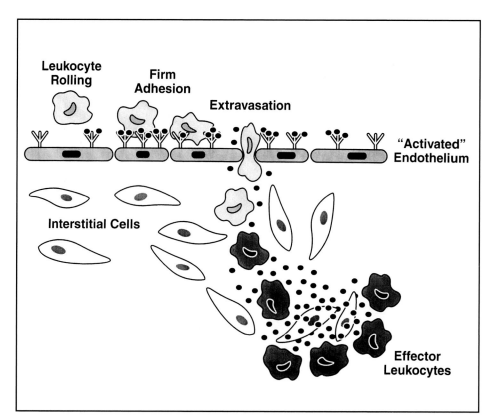

Figure 3-3. Monocytes and T lymphocytes move from the blood to the graft. Monocytes and T lymphocytes roll along activated endothelium by adhering to selectins. Cytokines and inducible adhesion molecules induce firm adhesion and entry into the site of inflammation. For example, RANTES, a chemoattractant cytokine shown here, is made by fibroblasts and epithelial cells in response to IL-1 and TNF produced by tissue macrophages. RANTES binds to glycosaminoglycans along the endothelium and leads to firm adhesion via *haptotaxis* for monocytes and T cells. Monocytes and T lymphocytes extravasate from the bloodstream into the graft via chemotaxis. Once inside the graft, T lymphocytes are activated and produce additional RANTES, enhancing the inflammatory response.

specific T cells. Resident macrophages, once activated, release interleukin-1 and tumor necrosis factor (Table 3-2). These cytokines induce the expression of RANTES (regulated upon activation, normal T expressed, and secreted) in tubular epithelial cells and fibroblasts. RANTES is a member of a large family of chemoattractant cytokines (chemokines), which are fundamentally important in attraction of cells into an inflammatory infiltrate and their subsequent activation. IL-8 is another member of this family, involved in granulocyte attraction and activation.

A three-step model has been proposed to explain entry of the cellular infiltrate into the graft (Figure 3-3). Selectins are constitutive and inducible lectin-like molecules on the vascular endothelium that lead monocytes and leukocytes to roll along the vessel wall. Chemokines, like RANTES, are released from the inflamed tissue and bind to the vessel wall. If such soluble factors were merely released into the bloodstream, they would quickly be washed downstream. Instead, they are firmly bound to glycosaminoglycans on the vascular endothelium. Via a process termed *haptotaxis*, leukocytes are attracted along the solid matrix of the vessel wall. Chemokines also induce the expression of cell surface molecules leading to firm adhesion to the vessel wall. The up-regulation of adhesion molecules, of the integrin and immunoglobulin supergene families, on the leukocytes and the vascular endothelium contribute to antigen recognition and

diapedesis through the vessel wall (Table 3-3). The same chemokines responsible for haptotaxis along the vessel wall are involved in chemotaxis of the cells through the tissue to the site of injury. Molecules such as RANTES induce the release of metalloproteinase by the leukocytes, allowing them to digest extracellular matrix in order to move through the tissues. Once confronted with foreign antigen in the graft, previously activated T cells are capable of releasing proinflammatory cytokines

Table 3-3.
Selected Adhesion Molecules Involved in the Leukocyte-Endothelial Interaction

Receptor-Ligand Pair*		Biologic Action(s)
Molecule	Ligand(s)	
LFA-1	ICAM-1,2,3	Leukocyte adherence, migration and activation
VLA-4	VCAM-1	Leukocyte adherence, migration and activation
E-selectin	s-Le^X	Leukocyte rolling
P-selectin	s-Le^X	Leukocyte rolling
L-selectin	PNAd	Leukocyte rolling

*LFA indicates lymphocyte-function-associated; ICAM, intercellular adhesion molecule; VLA, very late antigen; VCAM, vascular cell adhesion molecule; s-Le^X, sialyl Lewis X; and PNAd, peripheral node addressin.

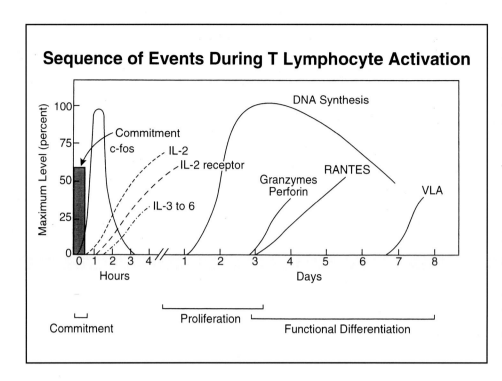

(helper T cells) or directly killing the foreign cells (cytotoxic T cells). Naive T cells attracted nonspecifically by the chemokine trail will become activated if they express T cell receptors which recognize the foreign antigens.

Differentiation of naive T cells takes approximately three to five days (Figure 3-4). If the T cell receptor engages an HLA-peptide complex for which it has sufficient affinity, a series of intracellular biochemical events at the T cell surface are initiated. Various kinases are activated, calcium is released from both intracellular stores and the extracellular space, and a phosphatidyl inositol pathway is activated. These signals work through a kinase or phosphatase network to induce the binding of regulatory proteins to the enhancer regions of specific genes in the T cell nucleus, triggering the transcription of genes involved in proliferation and differentiation.

Within hours of activation, helper T cells release factors involved in T cell (IL-2, IL-4, IL-5) and B cell (IL-4, IL-6, IL-8) growth and differentiation (Table 3-2).

EFFECTOR MECHANISMS
Cytotoxic T Lymphocytes

When precursors for cytolytic T lymphocytes (CTL) recognize HLA class I antigens in the presence of T cell growth factors, they differentiate into fully competent CTL (Figure 3-2). CTL lyse targets via two separate pathways (Figure 3-5). One mechanism involves secretory granules that contain complement-like molecules (perforin), serine esterases (granzymes), and a new lytic molecule related to amebapores (granulysin). The second system is an apoptotic process involving the interaction of cell surface molecules, Fas and Fas ligand. The secre-

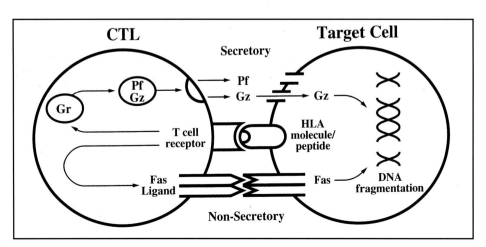

tory pathway depends upon calcium-dependent degranulation of specific cytolytic granules contained within the antigen-specific CTL. Perforin and granzymes released into the local environment between the CTL and the target cell lyse the target but spare the effector cell. Granzymes may enter the target cell through polyperforin pores and direct osmotic lysis, as well as DNA fragmentation. In contrast, the nonsecretory pathway (ie, involving Fas and Fas ligand) occurs in the absence of calcium and does not involve perforin or granzymes. Fas is a transmembrane 48kD glycoprotein, which shares homology with TNFα and is capable of transmitting an apoptotic signal via activation of the caspase cascade. Crosslinking of Fas by antibody or binding to its natural ligand (Fas ligand) induces cell death, characterized in its latest stages by cell fragmentation.

B Lymphocytes

Another major effector cell type is the B lymphocyte. B cells express immunoglobulin molecules on their surface; these molecules function both as antigen-specific receptors and as effector molecules. Precursor B cells are triggered by specific antigen and the B cell growth and differentiation factors discussed above. They mature into plasma cells, which release large amounts of soluble antibody specific for the triggering antigen. Antibodies can directly damage the graft via complement binding or by involving so-called *K* cells to induce antibody-dependent, cell-mediated cytotoxicity (ADCC). Such humoral (antibody) responses can occur rapidly, within seconds, and account for hyperacute rejection. This apparent paradox, the immediate appearance of humoral immunity, is due to the fact that antibodies capable of recognizing graft antigens can be present prior to transplantation. Such preformed antibodies commonly recognize HLA or blood group antigens, or other polymorphic antigens encountered during earlier blood transfusions. In addition, there is the potential for crossreactivity, whereby antibodies directed at one antigen may also bind another.

Granulocytes and Natural Killer Cells

Much less is understood about the involvement of other immune effector cells in transplant rejection, but both granulocytes and natural killer (NK) cells are present in cellular infiltrates and may contribute to graft rejection. Recent advances in understanding the role of chemokines in attracting granulocytes into the site of inflammation (similar to schema in Figure 3-3), and the role of HLA as a negative modulator of NK cell-mediated cytolysis (Figure 3-6) provide new insights into the potential involvement of these so-called *antigen nonspecific* effector cells.

TRANSPLANT REJECTION
Hyperacute Rejection

If preexisting antibodies to blood groups, HLA, or other polymorphic antigens expressed on the graft are present in the recipient, they can immediately bind to the graft and activate complement or cytolytic K cells. Platelets and fibrin are deposited, granulocytes and monocytes infiltrate, and fibrinoid necrosis of the vessel wall ensues (Figure 3-7A). Hyperacute rejection has largely been eliminated by routine crossmatch prescreening.

Acute and Subacute Rejection

Cellular infiltrates characterize both acute and subacute rejection. As described above, HLA differences trigger the recruitment of monocytes and T lymphocytes which result in rapid graft damage and destruction (Figures 3-7B, 3-7C, and 3-7D). Eosinophils, granulocytes, macrophages, and NK cells may variably also be present.

Chronic Rejection

In chronic rejection, graft damage, by the immune events detailed in this chapter, occurs very slowly, unlike the more rapid acute rejection. Extracellular matrix is destroyed by inflammatory proteases and debris is phagocytosed by macrophages and granulocytes. Fibroblasts undergo morphologic changes and produce scar formation by elaborating collagen, fibronectin, and proteoglycans, which are organized into new extracellu-

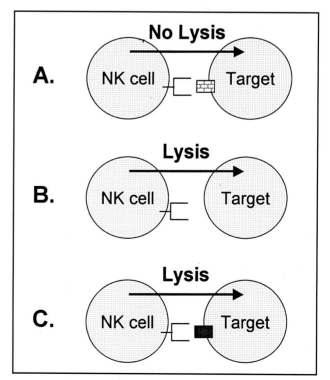

Figure 3-6. NK cells recognize HLA molecules. NK cells do not lyse cells expressing self-HLA (a), but can lyse cells expressing no HLA (b), or nonself HLA (c).

lar matrix. These highly regulated events probably evolved to maintain the structural integrity of damaged organs, but in this circumstance result instead in progressive graft dysfunction and eventual loss. Cytokines produced by macrophages and lymphocytes, including platelet-derived growth factor (PDGF) and basic fibroblast growth factor (bFGF), induce smooth muscle proliferation, and narrowing blood vessels (Figures 3-7E and 3-7F). Thus, the response to injury, as well as the injury itself, contribute to the loss of graft function. This chronic form of rejection is resistant to current therapies and may even be induced by some of the drugs currently in use. As grafts survive longer due to progress with immunotherapy and improved care, chronic rejection has become an increasingly important problem (Table 3-4). At present, chronic rejection is the major barrier to indefinite graft survival in renal transplantation and the only therapy is re-transplantation.

SUMMARY AND CONCLUSIONS

The immune response to allografts is directed at foreign HLA molecules and is only a variation on the normal immune response designed to discriminate self from nonself. As progress in understanding the basic cellular and molecular mechanisms involved in transplant acceptance and rejection is made, there is new hope for the development of better immunosuppressive regi-mens, and, eventually, attainment of specific tolerance. Only when we can reproducibly induce and maintain organ-specific tolerance will there truly be a cure for end-stage disease.

RECOMMENDED READING

Auchincloss H Jr., Sachs DH. Xenogeneic Transplantation. Annu Rev Immunol. 1998;16:433-470.

Busch R, Mellins ED. Developing and shedding inhibitions: how MHC class II molecules reach maturity. Curr Opin Immunol. 1996:8(1):51-58.

Clements JL, Koretzky GA. Recent developments in lymphocyte activation: linking kinases to downstream signaling events. J Clin Invest. 1999;103(7):925-929.

Crabtree GR. Generic signals and specific outcomes: signaling through Ca2+, calcineurin, and NF-AT. Cell. 1999;96(5):611-614.

Davis MM, Boniface JJ, Reich Z, et al. Ligand recognition by alpha beta T cell receptors. Annu Rev Immunol. 1998;16:523-544.

Krammer PH. CD95 (APO-1/Fas)-mediated apoptosis: live and let die. Adv Immunol. 1999;71:163-210.

Krensky AM, Weiss A, Crabtree G, Davis MM, Parham P. Mechanisms of disease: T-lymphocyte-antigen interactions in transplant rejection. N Engl J Med. 1990;322(8): 510-517.

Krensky AM, Clayberger C. The nature of allorecognition. Curr Opin Nephrol Hypertens. 1993;2(6):898-903.

Krensky AM, Clayberger C. Structure of HLA molecules and immunosuppressive effects of HLA derived peptides. Intl Rev Immunol. 1996;13(3):173-185.

Lanier LL. NK cell receptors. Annu Rev Immunol. 1998;16:359-393.

Table 3-4.
Incidence of Chronic Rejection in Selected Organs

Organ	Incidence*
Kidney	15%
Liver	5%
Heart (coronary artery atherosclerosis)	40%
Lung (obliterative bronchiolitis)	50%

*Incidence data are from Stanford University Medical Center.

Table 3-5. Cells of the Immune System

T Cell	Subdivided into helper cells that initiate immune responses through the production of cytokines, and cytotoxic cells that lyse target cells expressing foreign proteins.
B Cell	Differentiates into plasma cells that produce antibodies. Also serves to present antigen to helper T cells.
NK Cell	A primitive immune effector that kills target cells that fail to express self-proteins.
Macrophage	Mediates nonspecific inflammation and tissue destruction when activated by T cell-derived cytokines. Also presents antigen to helper T cells.
Dendritic Cell	Specialized-type antigen-presenting cell that is particularly potent at capturing and presenting antigens.

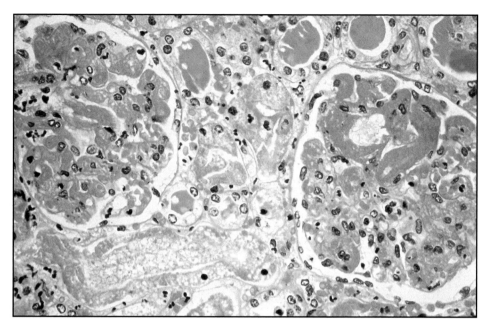

Figure 3-7A. Pathology of renal transplant rejection. Hyperacute rejection with glomerular thrombosis, glomerular and peritubular capillary infiltration, and tubular coagulation necrosis. In: Jamison RL, Wilkinson R eds. Nephrology. New York, NY: Chapman & Hall; 1997.

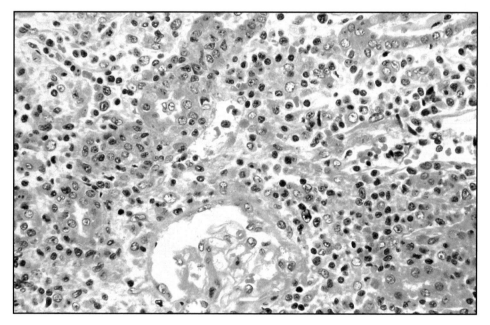

Figure 3-7B. Pathology of renal transplant rejection. Acute cellular interstitial rejection with pleomorphic inflammatory infiltrate and prominent tubulitis. In: Jamison RL, Wilkinson R eds. Nephrology. New York, NY: Chapman & Hall; 1997.

Pamer E, Cresswell P. Mechanisms of MHC class I – restricted antigen processing. Annu Rev Immunol. 1998;16:323-358.

Pober JS, Cotran RS. Immunologic interactions of T lymphocytes with vascular endothelium. Adv Immunol. 1991;50:261-302.

Sayegh MH, Turka LA. The role of T-cell costimulatory activation pathways in transplant rejection. N Engl J Med. 1998;338(25):1813-1821.

Springer TA. Traffic signals for lymphocyte recirculation and leukocyte emigration: the multistep paradigm. Cell. 1994;76(2):301-314.

Stockinger B. T lymphocyte tolerance: from thymic deletion to peripheral control mechanisms. Adv Immunol. 1999;71:229-265.

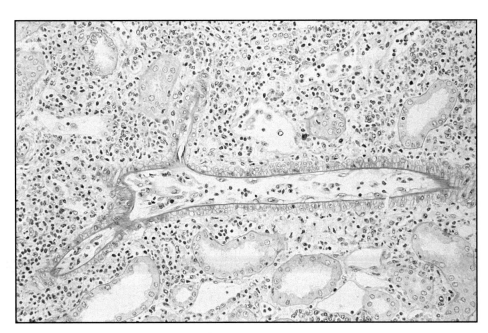

Figure 3-7C. Pathology of renal transplant rejection. Acute cellular rejection with interstitial and vascular infiltration. In: Jamison RL, Wilkinson R eds. Nephrology. New York, NY: Chapman & Hall; 1997.

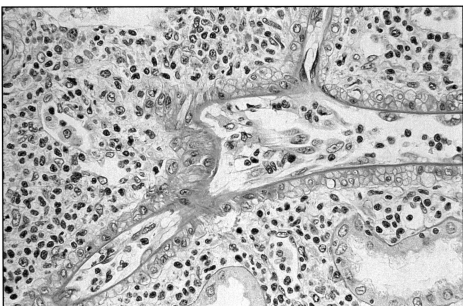

Figure 3-7D. Pathology of renal transplant rejection. Higher power of Figure 3-7C shows subendothelial infiltration by mononuclear cells and endothelial cell injury. In: Jamison RL, Wilkinson R eds. Nephrology. New York, NY: Chapman & Hall; 1997.

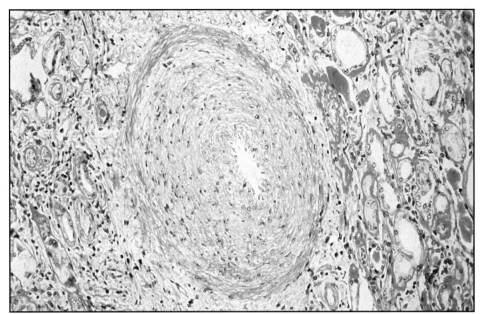

Figure 3-7E. Pathology of renal transplant rejection. Chronic vascular rejection and tubulo-interstitial rejection with marked proliferative endarteritis ("onion-skinning"), severe tubular atrophy and interstitial fibrosis. In: Jamison RL, Wilkinson R eds. Nephrology. New York, NY: Chapman & Hall; 1997.

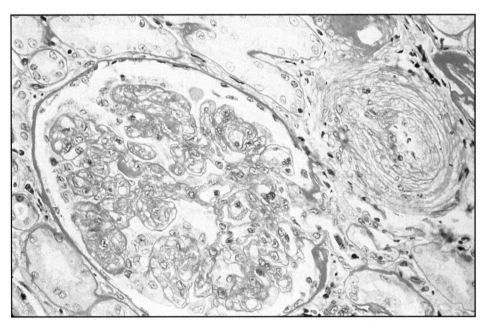

Figure 3-7F. Pathology of renal transplant rejection. Chronic transplant glomerulopathy and transplant rejection with proliferative arteriolitis and capillaritis. In: Jamison RL, Wilkinson R eds. Nephrology. New York, NY: Chapman & Hall; 1997.

4 INFLAMMATORY RESPONSE TO ALLOGRAFTS

Thomas M. Coffman, MD

An intense inflammatory response within the transplant is a defining feature of acute allograft rejection. This response is triggered by the specific interactions between T cells with donor alloantigens that have been described in previous chapters. These specific molecular interactions provoke a vigorous and complex inflammatory response. While this response consists of an array of cellular elements, its nature and intensity are regulated by the actions of soluble inflammatory mediators. These mediators play a critical role in the pathogenesis of both acute and chronic allograft rejection.

Inflammatory mediators in rejection act in several distinct capacities. First, they promote the recruitment and accumulation of inflammatory cells into the graft. Second, components of the inflammatory response may act directly on T cells to modulate their functions. Finally, the inflammatory response is an important effector pathway that causes graft dysfunction and injury directly. These effector mechanisms may be especially important in vascularized organ grafts. This chapter reviews the inflammatory response to allografts, and three systems that play key roles in rejection: chemokines, lipid mediators derived from arachidonic acid, and complement.

ACUTE REJECTION IS AN INFLAMMATORY RESPONSE

Acute rejection is an intense inflammatory response that is focused within the confines of the engrafted organ. Acute rejection may be accompanied by the classic signs of inflammation including rubor (due to vascular congestion), edema, fever, pain, and loss of function. However, immunosuppressive therapies may modify the appearance of some or all of these signs. The inflammatory response that occurs in acute rejection is most analogous to classical delayed-type hypersensitivity (DTH) reactions. DTH models serve as a reasonable starting point for understanding the organization and regulation of graft inflammation.

The trigger for DTH responses is the interaction of T cells, usually of the CD4+ phenotype, with antigen. The character of the DTH response was originally defined by observing the kinetics of inflammation following injection of antigen into the skin. Unlike allergic

responses that occur within minutes, or immune complex reactions that become apparent within hours, DTH reactions peak in two to three days following antigen injection. These reactions are characterized by edema and altered vascular permeability, along with prominent infiltration by a combination of antigen-specific and nonspecific T cells, B cells, and macrophages. DTH reactions are organized by the actions of a number of soluble mediators including the proinflammatory cytokines IL-1, γ-interferon, and TNF-α.

Inflammatory mechanisms in transplant rejection are complex and the relative importance of the individual pathways that organize and regulate alloimmune responses have not been rigorously defined. Nonetheless, there is clear evidence that DTH mechanisms contribute to the pathogenesis of rejection and graft injury. The result of these reactions is the accumulation of a mixed population of inflammatory cells within the graft. Because of the nonspecific nature of these recruitment processes, only a small minority of the infiltrating T cells is antigen-specific. However, the localization and activation of a combination of potent, nonspecific effector systems within the graft contributes to the development of allograft injury.

EARLY RECRUITMENT OF INFLAMMATORY CELLS INTO THE TRANSPLANT

In experimental models using untreated, nonsensitized recipients, T cells are not detected within heart or kidney allografts until two to three days after transplant. As depicted in Figure 4-1, inflammatory cells enter the graft through a series of interactions with the endothelial cells of the donor organ. These interactions may be facilitated by ischemic injury associated with the transplant procedure. For example, renal ischemia causes a dramatic increase in γ-interferon production that enhances expression of adhesion molecules and MHC antigens in the kidney. Clinical observations that ischemic injury and delayed graft function are associated with a higher incidence of severe acute rejection episodes suggest that this nonspecific tissue injury can substantially enhance the intensity of alloimmune responses.

Leukocyte trafficking from the circulation into a site of inflammation such as a rejecting allograft is accomplished through a series of molecular interactions between leukocytes and endothelial cells (Figure 4-1). In the first step of this process, inflammatory cells contact and roll on the endothelium. This loose and transient adhesion of the leukocyte with the endothelium is primarily mediated by the selectin family of adhesion molecules: L-selectin, E-selectin, and P-selectin. L-selectin is expressed by most classes of circulating leukocytes with the exception of a subset of memory T cells. P-selectin is

Professor of Medicine; Chief, Division of Nephrology, Duke University Medical Center, Durham, NC

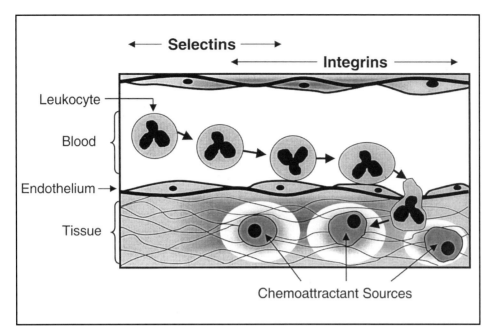

Selectins

Integrins

Leukocyte

Blood

Endothelium

Tissue

Chemoattractant Sources

Figure 4-1. Interactions between leukocytes and endothelial cells regulate the accumulation of inflammatory cells in the rejecting allograft. These events involve a series of activation and adhesion processes including the initial rolling and then transient adhesion of the leukocyte to endothelium mediated by the selectin family of adhesion molecules. A firm adhesion of leukocytes to endothelial cells is promoted through binding of integrins expressed on inflammatory cells to their ligands expressed on endothelium. Soluble chemoattractant molecules promote the activation of integrin molecules, and are also involved in facilitating extravasation of cells across junctional spaces in the endothelium and guiding these cells to their final destinations.

expressed by platelets and both P-selectin and E-selectin are expressed on endothelial cells. Expression of these selectins on endothelium is rapidly up-regulated after exposure to inflammatory mediators such as TNF-α, LPS, and IL-1. In this way, activation of the endothelium by products of inflammation promotes leukocyte adhesion.

Integrins such as lymphocyte function antigen-1 (LFA-1, αLβ2), and very late activation antigen-1 (VLA-4, α4β1) that are expressed on inflammatory cells bind to their respective endothelial counter-receptors, the intercellular adhesion molecules (ICAMs): vascular cell adhesion molecule-1 (VCAM-1), and mucosal addressin cell adhesion molecule-1 (MAdCAM-1). This firm adhesion is facilitated by increases in the number of ICAM-1 and VCAM-1 molecules induced by IL-1, TNF-α, and lipid mediators such as leukotrienes. The integrins must also be activated through conformational changes that are conferred by interactions of leukocytes with E-selectin, or through the direct action of chemokine molecules. The binding of leukocyte integrins with their endothelial ligands establishes firm contact between the two cells, but this interaction is not permanent. Many of these inflammatory cells will eventually traverse the junctional spaces in the endothelium guided to their final destinations in the graft interstitium by gradients of chemoattractants, such as chemokines and leukotriene B4.

CHEMOKINES

In addition to selectins and integrins, several classes of soluble factors have been implicated in the initial steps of homing, adhesion, and extravasation of lymphocytes in sites of inflammation. Among these factors, molecules belonging to a large family called chemokines may play a

critical role. The name *chemokine* is derived from the properties of these proteins to function both as chemoattractants, to attract leukocytes, and as cytokines, to directly activate leukocytes. Chemokines are relatively small proteins with basic, heparin-binding structures. More than 40 chemokines and 14 chemokine receptors have been identified to date.

The chemokines are structurally homogeneous proteins with 20% to 70% homology at the amino acid level. These small proteins, averaging 8 to 10 kd in size, have four conserved cysteines that form two essential disulfide bonds. Subfamilies of chemokines can be defined according to the positions of the N-terminal cysteines (Table 4-1). In CXC chemokines (or α-chemokines), there is one amino acid separating the N-terminal cysteines. The CXC chemokines can be further divided into those that contain a glu-leu-arg amino acid sequence near the N-terminus, and those that do not. CXC chemokines containing this sequence are chemotactic for neutrophils, whereas those lacking this sequence are chemotactic for lymphocytes. Chemokines within these subfamilies tend to have overlapping functions. Interleukin-8 is the prototypic CXC chemokine, and is a strong chemoattractant for neutrophils, but not monocytes.

In CC chemokines (also called β-chemokines), there is no intervening amino acid between the N-terminal cysteines. In general, β-chemokines do not act on neutrophils, but are chemoattractive for monocytes, eosinophils, basophils, and lymphocytes with variable degrees of selectivity. Based on structural homologies, β-chemokines can be further subdivided into two groups: the monocyte chemoattractant protein (MCP)-eotaxin family, and all other CC chemokines.

Table 4-1. The Chemokine Families

CXC Chemokines (α-chemokines)	CC Chemokines	C Chemokine (β-chemokines)	CX$_3$C Chemokines

Containing glu-leu-arg:
  IL-8
  GCP-2
  GRO-α, -β, -γ
  ENA-78
  NAP-2
  LIX
 	
Not containing glu-leu-arg:
  MIG
  IP-10
  I-TAC
  SDF-1
	MCP-eotaxin Family:
	  MCP-1, -2, -3, -4, and -5
	  Eotaxin
	Others:
	  MIP-1α, -1β, -3α, -3β
	  RANTES
	  TARC
	  I309
	  HCC-1
		Lymphotactin	Fractalkine (human)
			Neurotactin (mouse)

While the CXC and CC chemokines comprise the largest subgroups of known chemokines, other structurally distinctive chemokine subfamilies have been described. The C-chemokine lymphotactin possesses only two cysteines while the CX$_3$-C chemokine, fractalkine, has three intervening amino acids between the N-terminal cysteines. In the fractalkine molecule, the chemokine domain sits on a mucin-like stalk. This structure seems to facilitate the ability of fractalkine to also function as an adhesion molecule.

The actions of chemokines upon leukocytes are mediated by G protein-coupled chemokine receptors (Table 4-2). Most chemokine receptors are coupled to the G$_{\alpha I}$ family of G proteins, and thus are inhibited by pertussis toxin. Many chemokine receptors bind more than one chemokine and several chemokines bind more than one receptor (Table 4-2). This provides a molecular basis for the redundancy and versatility that characterize the chemokine system. However, CXC-chemokine receptors (CXCRs) only bind CXC-chemokines, and CC-chemokine receptors (CCRs) only bind CC-chemokines. This suggests that the secondary structure conferred by the N-terminal cysteines plays a key role in determining the specificity of ligand-receptor interactions. Cellular responses to chemokines are determined by expression of chemokine receptors on the target cell populations, and chemokine receptor expression by T cells is further regulated by cytokines such as IL-2. In addition, certain chemokine receptors (CXCR4, CCR5, CX$_3$CR1) serve as coreceptors for HIV entry into cells.

During inflammation, expression of chemokines and their receptors are induced or modulated, and with the appropriate stimulus virtually any cell can produce chemokines. Thus, in transplant rejection, it is likely that both recipient and donor tissues elaborate chemokines.

Chemokines have a number of cellular effects that are potentially relevant to promoting inflammation in rejecting allografts. These include the up-regulation and activation of integrins on leukocytes that were reviewed above, potent chemoattractant properties, and an ability to directly activate leukocyte effector functions. Examples of leukocyte effector functions that are induced by chemokines include the stimulation of respiratory burst and degranulation in neutrophils by CXC chemokines, and the induction of cytokine release from macrophages and monocytes by CC chemokines such as MCP-1, MIP-1α, and MIP-1β.

While the "classical" chemoattractants such as N-formyl peptides, leukotriene B4, and platelet activating

---

Table 4-2.
Chemokine Receptors and Their Ligands

Receptor	Ligands
CXCR1	IL-8, GCP-2
CXCR2	IL-8, GRO-α/β/γ, NAP-2, ENA78, GCP-2
CXCR3	IP-10, MIG
CXCR4	SDF-1
CXCR5	SCA-1/BLC
CCR1	RANTES, MIP-1α, MCP-3, -4
CCR2	MCP-1, -2, -3, -4, -5
CCR3	Eotaxin, RANTES, MCP-2, -3, -4
CCR4	TARC, RANTES, MIP-1α, MCP -1
CCR5	RANTES, MIP-1α, MIP -1β
CCR6	LARC/MIP-3β
CCR7	ELC/MIP-3β
CCR8	I-309
CX$_3$CR1	Fractalkine/neurotactin

factor act on multiple leukocyte subsets, chemokines exhibit chemotactic specificity for restricted cell populations. Their ability to stimulate adhesion, and then to attract specific subsets of leukocytes provides a potential mechanism for regulating the selective accumulation of cells in sites of inflammation. The chemoattractive properties of chemokines are probably enhanced through their ability to bind to glycosaminoglycan molecules. For example, chemokines that are bound and immobilized by heparan sulfate molecules on endothelial cell surfaces may be more efficiently presented to rolling leukocytes. Moreover, such a system avoids dilution by blood flow and would maintain chemokine molecules in the immediate vicinity of the inflammatory response. Substrate-bound gradients of chemokines may also be more effective in directing cellular migration toward the site of inflammation.

Chemokines in Allograft Rejection

While there are a number of theoretical reasons to suggest that chemokines may participate in inflammation associated with rejection, evidence to support such a role is primarily indirect and consists of demonstrations of enhanced chemokine production in rejecting allografts. In human allograft tissue, enhanced expression of chemokines such as RANTES, ENA-78, MIP-1α, MIP-β, IL-8, and MCP-1 has been detected. For example, Pattison and associates demonstrated expression of RANTES mRNA and protein in a series of kidney allografts during acute rejection episodes. Expression of RANTES in these rejecting grafts was localized to infiltrating mononuclear cells and renal tubular epithelial cells, while RANTES protein was also detected on endothelial surfaces. The principal chemokines that are expressed in acute rejection are those that interact with the CCR1 and CCR5 receptors (ie, MIP-1α, MIP-β, and RANTES). Since these receptors are primarily expressed by T cells and monocytes that are also the major cellular components of acute rejection, this association may have functional significance.

Based on these demonstrations of enhanced production of chemokines in rejecting grafts, a role for chemokines in regulating intragraft inflammation has been proposed. Chemokines that act on T lymphocytes may influence the recruitment of immunocompetent cells into the rejecting graft while other chemokines may regulate accumulation of macrophages and monocytes in the graft, and thus influence the development of both acute and chronic rejection. Because of their multiple and relatively selective effects to promote immune responses and inflammation, chemokines are attractive targets for therapeutic interventions to prevent graft injury associated with rejection. However, such approaches are potentially limited by the large number of chemokines and their overlapping functions. The efficacy and feasibility of such therapies are being explored.

LIPID MEDIATORS DERIVED FROM ARACHIDONIC ACID

A number of biologically active mediators are produced from the metabolism of arachidonic acid, a 20 carbon polyunsaturated fatty acid that is a normal constituent of plasma membrane phospholipids. Metabolites of arachidonic acid, called eicosanoids, are synthesized through the coordinated actions of several specific enzyme pathways. Two of these pathways are illustrated in Figure 4-2: the cyclooxygenase pathway that produces prostaglandins (PG) and thromboxane (TX) A_2, and the 5-lipoxygenase pathway that produces leukotrienes. While other enzymatic cascades for arachidonic acid metabolism have been identified, this review focuses on the cyclooxygenase and 5-lipoxygenase pathways since their functions in inflammation are well-characterized, and both have been shown to contribute to the pathogenesis of graft rejection.

As illustrated in Figure 4-2, arachidonic acid is released from membrane phospholipids through the actions of phospholipases such as phospholipase A2 (PLA_2). The activities of phospholipases are regulated by hormones and cytokines. For example, IL-1 and TNF-α stimulate PLA_2 activity, while corticosteroids inhibit its actions. The release of free arachidonic acid from esterified precursor lipids is the rate-limiting step in eicosanoid synthesis.

Eicosanoids are rapidly metabolized in vivo to inactive end products. Therefore, they must act as autocrine or paracrine mediators exerting their most concentrated effects in the tissues where they are produced. In allograft rejection, enhanced production of arachidonic acid metabolites coincides with the appearance of inflammatory cells in the graft, and the absolute levels of eicosanoid production generally parallel the intensity of the rejection response. Because mature T cells do not synthesize eicosanoids, they must be produced by other infiltrating cell populations such as macrophages and platelets. In addition, cells from the graft may contribute to lipid mediator synthesis. For example, endothelial cells are an important source of prostacyclin (PGI_2) while renal tubular cells and glomerular mesangial cells are capable of producing large amounts of PGE_2. The cellular actions of eicosanoids are mediated by specific cell surface receptors that belong to the G protein-coupled receptor family.

Cyclooxygenase Metabolites in Rejection

In the cyclooxygenase (COX) pathway, COX enzymes convert arachidonic acid to the endoperoxides PGE_2 and PGH_2. These endoperoxide intermediates are then further metabolized to form prostaglandins and thromboxane through the actions of specific synthase enzymes. COX exists in two isoforms, COX-1 and COX-2. COX-1 is constitutively expressed in most cells, whereas the

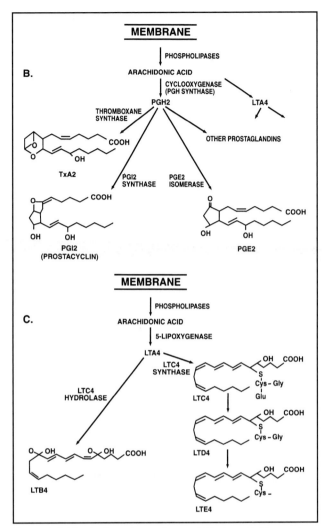

Figure 4-2. Metabolic pathways for arachidonic acid. The cyclooxygenase or PGH synthase pathway produces both prostaglandins and thromboxane A_2 from arachidonic acid substrate. This pathway is inhibited by nonsteroidal antiinflammatory drugs. The 5-lipoxygenase pathway produces two classes of leukotrienes with distinct biological effects: the peptidoleukotrienes (LTC_4, LTD_4, and LTE_4), which have a number of vascular and endothelial effects, and LTB_4, a potent chemoattractant that promotes adhesion of leukocytes to endothelial cells.

expression of COX-2 is more restricted and tends to be up-regulated in inflammatory states. Both COX isoforms are inhibited by standard nonsteroidal antiinflammatory drugs (NSAIDs), and a new class of specific COX-2 inhibitors has been recently released for clinical use. While distinct roles for COX-1 and COX-2 in rejection have not been identified, COX metabolites have a number of biological actions that modulate inflammation in the rejecting organ transplant. For example, TxA_2 is a potent vasoconstrictor that stimulates platelet aggregation. Within the allograft, TxA_2 causes reduced blood flow and promotes vascular occlusion. TxA_2 may also facilitate certain immune responses such as allospecific cytotoxicity. In contrast, PGE_2 and PGI_2 have actions

that tend to oppose those of TxA_2. These prostaglandins inhibit platelet aggregation and are potent vasodilators. In T cells and macrophages, PGE_2 generally suppresses proliferation and effector functions. Thus, in inflammatory responses including rejection, the final effect of eicosanoids will depend on the relative amounts of the individual prostaglandins or thromboxanes that are produced within the local micro environment.

Among the cyclooxygenase metabolites, a pathogenetic role for TxA_2 in rejection has been most clearly established. A role for TxA_2 in rejection was first suggested by the clinical studies of Foegh and associates that demonstrated enhanced urinary excretion of thromboxane metabolites in renal allograft recipients during episodes of acute rejection. Subsequent studies in several animal models demonstrated enhanced production of prostaglandins and thromboxane by rejecting allografts. Furthermore, agents that reduce the production of thromboxane or block the TxA_2 receptor improve function and prolong survival of various types of allografts including kidney, heart, and skin. Since thromboxane antagonists have little effect on the number of inflammatory cells within the graft, the major effect of thromboxane in vascularized grafts is probably due to local effects on blood flow and vascular integrity. In addition, thromboxane may directly modulate the intensity of certain T cell responses.

Enhanced production of prostaglandins such as PGE_2 and prostacyclin is also observed in rejecting allografts. As indicated above, these compounds have a number of biological functions that would tend to suppress T cell functions and be cytoprotective for cells within the graft. The relevance of these effects in rejection has been suggested by studies showing that generalized inhibition of cyclooxygenase has detrimental effects on graft function. However, specific roles for individual prostaglandins in rejection have been difficult to establish because of a lack of specific pharmacological antagonists. This may be facilitated by the recent generation of a series of mouse lines with targeted disruption of individual prostaglandin receptor genes.

5-Lipoxygenase Products in Rejection

Leukotrienes are the final products of the 5-lipoxygenase (5-LO) pathway of arachidonic acid metabolism (Figure 4-2). In this pathway, 5-LO converts arachidonic acid to leukotriene A_4, which can be metabolized through two enzymatic pathways to produce compounds with distinct biological effects: LTB_4, and the peptidoleukotrienes (LTC_4, LTD_4, and LTE_4). LTB_4 is a potent chemoattractant promoting adhesion of leukocytes to endothelial cells and facilitating the production of cytokines such as IL-1, IL-2, and γ-IFN. The peptidoleukotrienes, which were previously known as the slow-reacting substance of anaphylaxis, are potent vasoconstrictors that can alter vascular permeability and promote expression of integrins on endothelial cells.

Because expression of 5-LO is restricted to cells of myeloid lineage, production of leukotrienes within a rejecting graft requires the presence of macrophages, neutrophils or eosinophils. The observation that enhanced production of leukotrienes in rejection correlates with the appearance of inflammatory cell infiltrates within the graft is consistent with this notion. In experimental models of kidney and heart transplantation, pharmacological leukotriene antagonists improve allograft function and survival suggesting that enhanced production of leukotrienes contributes to graft destruction. Moreover, a comparison of the effects of 5-LO inhibition with blockade of peptidoleukotriene receptors in kidney allografts indicates that LTB_4 and the peptidoleukotrienes contribute to different components of the rejection response; peptidoleukotrienes directly promote vascular and endothelial injury, while LTB_4 enhances MHC class II antigen expression and facilitates inflammatory cell infiltration. During acute rejection, actions of LTB_4 and the peptidoleukotrienes both contribute to allograft injury and dysfunction.

In summary, a role for arachidonic acid metabolites in the pathogenesis of rejection has been established based on experiments showing enhanced production of eicosanoids by rejecting grafts and beneficial effects of specific eicosanoid antagonists in several models of rejection. Some of these mediators have proinflammatory effects and constitute an effector limb that contributes to graft injury and dysfunction, while others may modulate and inhibit graft inflammation. Therapies that favorably alter the balance of eicosanoid production in the graft may provide useful additions to current immunosuppressive strategies.

COMPLEMENT

The complement cascade is a recognition and effector system of humoral immunity. Its effector functions include the capacity to cause lysis and destruction of target cells, along with the ability to induce and promote inflammation. The proinflammatory actions of complement include chemotactic effects, alterations of vascular permeability, and direct activation of mast cells and neutrophils. As shown in Figure 4-3, there are two pathways for activating the complement system: the classical and alternative pathways. The classical pathway is activated when antibodies bind antigens, and this is the pathway most clearly involved in graft rejection. Through the alternative pathway, complement can be activated in the absence of antibody.

The C3 protein plays a central role in both the classical and alternative pathways for complement activation (Figure 4-3). Once C3b is generated, it promotes opsonization or leads to cell lysis by activating terminal complement components that form the membrane attack complex (MAC), the lytic effector mechanism. The first step in generation of the MAC is cleavage of C5 by C5 convertases to form C5a and C5b. C5b is incorporated into the MAC, while C5a is released and acts as a potent anaphylatoxin and chemotactic factor. C4a and C3a have similar, although less potent, proinflammatory activities. The actions of C3a, C4a, and C5a are mediated by specific cell surface receptors. Receptors for C3a and C4a are found on mast cells, basophils, lymphocytes, and smooth muscle cells. In addition to mast cells and basophils, the C5a receptor is also expressed on neutrophils, endothelial cells, and monocytes or macrophages.

Because of the potent destructive and proinflammatory properties of complement, tight regulation of the complement cascade is necessary. Regulation is accomplished through the actions of two types of complement regulatory proteins. The first are circulating plasma proteins, such as C1 inhibitor, C4-binding protein, and factor H, which inhibit complement in the plasma phase. The second are proteins such as decay accelerating factor (DAF), membrane cofactor protein (MCP), and CD59, which are membrane bound, and thus, exert protective effects on the cells that express them. They function to directly protect the host tissues against injury that might be caused by complement activation. These membrane-

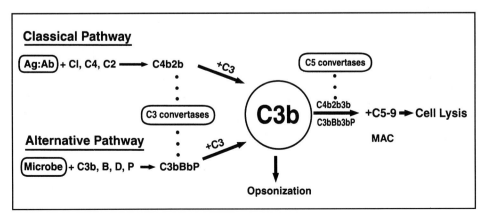

Figure 4-3. The classical and alternative pathways for complement activation. The classical pathway is activated when antibodies bind antigens, while through the alternative pathway, complement can be activated in the absence of antibody. C3b plays a central role in both the classical and alternative pathways. Reprinted with permission from Liszewski MK, Atkinson JP. The complement system. In: Paul WE, ed. Fundamental Immunology, 3rd ed. New York, NY; Raven Press 1993.

associated proteins function in a species-specific manner, a fact that has special relevance to hyperacute xenograft rejection as discussed below.

Complement in Allograft Rejection

In clinical transplantation, a role for the complement system is most clearly seen in hyperacute allograft rejection. In hyperacute rejection, circulating preformed antibodies against donor HLA antigens bind to the transplanted organ resulting in widespread complement activation. This activation of complement causes diffuse vascular injury, thrombosis, and destruction of the grafts within a matter of minutes to hours. Happily, routine pretransplant crossmatching has virtually eliminated this devastating problem.

In acute allograft rejection, contributions of antibody and complement are more subtle and have been more difficult to demonstrate. Nonetheless, several clinical studies have described patients with episodes of acute rejection that are characterized by predominate vascular involvement with endothelial swelling, medial edema or fibrinoid necrosis, and granulocyte infiltration. Complement can often be demonstrated in these vascular lesions, and such rejections are often associated with circulating antibodies against donor MHC class I antigens. These rejection episodes are typically resistant to standard anti-lymphocyte therapies and often result in early graft loss.

Beyond these clinical observations, there is some experimental evidence to suggest that antibody and complement may contribute to graft injury and inflammation in rejection. For example, acute rejection can be initiated by passive transfer of alloantibodies in several rat strains, and rats with a genetic C6 deficiency have been found to reject cardiac allografts more slowly than controls. Studies by Russell and associates have also suggested a role for complement in chronic rejection. These investigators found that repeated transfer of immune serum to immunodeficient mice causes chronic vascular lesions in cardiac allografts. These lesions contain antibody and complement along with a prominent macrophage infiltrate, suggesting that alloantibodies plus complement are sufficient to produce the vascular lesions that characterize chronic rejection.

Complement in Xenograft Rejection

Based on the acute shortage of human donor organs, there has been an emerging interest in the potential use of nonprimates, such as the pig, as a source of organs for transplantation. However, a major hurdle preventing the clinical application of xenotransplantation is hyperacute xenograft rejection. Similar to hyperacute allograft rejection, hyperacute rejection of a xenograft begins immediately after blood flow to the graft is established and it is characterized by interstitial hemorrhage and diffuse thrombosis. Once initiated, the process invariably destroys the graft within minutes to hours. In pig-to-primate xenografts, hyperacute rejection is initiated through the binding of natural antibodies, present in the serum of humans and other primates, to Galα1-3Gal sugar moieties on endothelial cell surfaces. Binding of these xenoreactive antibodies to this antigen activates complement through the classical pathway. The pathogenic relevance of complement activation in this disorder has been demonstrated by the efficacy of maneuvers that prevent or limit complement activation to ameliorate hyperacute rejection.

As mentioned above, the activity of complement regulatory proteins such as DAF are highly species-specific. Thus, porcine DAF that is naturally expressed on porcine endothelial cells is a poor inhibitor of human complement proteins. Because of these incompatibilities, it was suggested that some aspects of hyperacute xenograft rejection may be attributed to a failure of the complement regulatory proteins expressed on the xenograft to control the recipient's complement cascade. Based on this concept, several transgenic animal models have been developed, which express human complement regulatory proteins with the expectation that organs from such animals would resist injury by heterologous complement. In fact, when organs from transgenic pigs expressing human DAF and CD59 are transplanted into primate hosts, there is striking protection from hyperacute xenograft rejection. The prolonged survival of these transgenic pig organs further underscores the importance of the complement system in hyperacute xenograft rejection and raises hopes for future clinical applications of xenotransplantation.

RECOMMENDED READING

Baggiolini M. Chemokines and leukocyte traffic. Nature. 1998;392(6676):565-568.

Baldwin WM 3rd, Pruitt SK, Brauer RB, Daha MR, Sanfilippo F. Complement in organ transplantation. Contributions to inflammation, injury, and rejection. Transplantation. 1995;59(6):797-808.

Butcher EC, Picker LJ. Lymphocyte homing and homeostasis. Science. 1996;272(5258):60-66.

Foegh ML, Winchester JF, Zmudka M, et al. Urine i-TXB2 in renal allograft rejection. Lancet. 1981;2(8244):431-434.

Gladue RP, Coffman TM. Potential roles for chemokines in transplant rejection. In: Herbert CA, ed. Chemokines in Disease: Biology and Clinical Research. 1st ed. Totowa, NJ: Humana Press; 1998:159-168.

Halloran PF, Broski AP, Batiuk TD, Madrenas J. The molecular immunology of acute rejection: an overview. Transpl Immunol. 1993;1(1):3-27.

Luster AD. Chemokines: chemotactic cytokines that mediate inflammation. New Engl J Med. 1998;338(7):436-445.

Moore FD, Jr. Therapeutic regulation of the complement system in acute injury states. Adv Immunol. 1994;56:267-299.

Pattison J, Nelson P, Huie P, et al. RANTES chemokine expression in cell-mediated transplant rejection of the kidney. Lancet. 1994;343(8891):209-211.

Parker W, Saadi S, Lin SS, Holzknecht ZE, Bustos M, Platt JL. Transplantation of disordant xenografts: a challenge revisited. Immunol Today. 1996;17(8):373-378.

Robinson LA, Steeber DA, Tedder TF. The selectins in inflammation. In: Gallin JI, Snyderman R, eds. Inflammation: Basic Principles and Clinical Correlates. 3rd ed. Philadelphia, PA: Lippincott Williams & Wilkins; 1999:571-583.

Russell PS, Chase CM, Winn HJ, Colvin RB Coronary atherosclerosis in transplanted mouse hearts. II. Importance of humoral immunity. J Immunol. 1994;152(10):5135-5141.

Springer TA. Traffic signals for lymphocyte recirculation and leukocyte emigration: the multistep paradigm. Cell. 1994;76(2):301-314.

Spurney R, Coffman T. The role of eicosanoids in transplant rejection. In: Ruffolo RR, Hollinger MA, eds. Inflammation: Mediators and Pathways. New York, NY: CRC Press; 1995:129-145.

5   MECHANISMS OF TOLERANCE

Xian Chang Li, MD, PhD
Terry B. Strom, MD

Organ transplantation offers a tremendous opportunity for rehabilitation among patients with end-stage organ disease. In the past two decades, remarkable progress has been made in delineating the molecular basis of T cell activation, and powerful immunosuppressive agents have been developed to combat allograft rejection. Hence, organ transplant recipients enjoy more frequent engraftment and a better quality of life. However, immunosuppressive drug regimens do not universally prevent transplantation rejection, and certainly do not uniformly create a state of allograft tolerance. New immunosuppressive protocols have drastically curbed the incidence of overt acute allograft rejection and early graft failure. Unfortunately, long-term graft survival has not improved appreciably since the early 1970s. Current immunosuppressive protocols have made no impact on the incidence of subclinical acute rejection or the tempo of chronic rejection. Furthermore, the immunosuppressive drugs used in the clinic to repress allograft rejection are broadly immunosuppressive, and often have life-threatening toxic effects such as increased incidence of opportunistic infections, malignancy, and metabolic disorders. Thus, the acquisition of allograft tolerance, a state of permanent engraftment in the absence of global immunosuppression, remains the "holy grail" and a practical need in clinical transplantation.

THE DEFINITION OF TOLERANCE

Immunologic tolerance is traditionally defined as a state of antigen-specific unresponsiveness in the absence of immune system ablation. Transplantation tolerance is often defined as donor-specific unresponsiveness that persists despite cessation of immunosuppressive therapy. Thus, tolerance is manifested as acceptance of subsequent donor allografts in a host that retains the ability to reject third party allografts.

Transplantation tolerance is rarely due, in all measures, to passive unresponsiveness to an allograft by the host. Tolerance is an actively acquired and highly regulat-

Xian Chang Li, MD, PhD, Assistant Professor of Medicine, Harvard Medical School, Beth Israel Deaconess Medical Center, Boston, MA

Terry B. Strom, MD, Professor of Medicine, Harvard Medical School; Director of Immunology, Beth Israel Deaconess Medical Center, Boston, MA

ed process. Although the precise nature underlying allograft tolerance is still not firmly established, it is now clear that allograft tolerance is a multifaceted process involving multiple cellular components evolving over time, which enables the induction and maintenance of a tolerant state.

On the basis of the cellular components involved, tolerance is often classified as B cell tolerance or T cell tolerance. As T cell tolerance is most pertinent to transplantation, the focus of this chapter is on T cell tolerance. In the circumstance in which intrathymic deletion of developing antigen-specific T cells is involved, tolerance is classified as central tolerance. In contrast, tolerance created in fully mature hosts in the absence of massive intrathymic deletion is classified as peripheral tolerance.

CENTRAL TOLERANCE

Central tolerance refers to a tolerant state established primarily in the thymus through clonal deletion of developing antigen-reactive T cells. Central tolerance is the principal mechanism that enables eradication of autoreactive T cells and self-tolerance. Creation of central tolerance requires extensive deletion of immature developing T cells in the thymus that are potentially auto-aggressive; a process called *negative selection*. T cells that have low-affinity T cell receptors (TCR) to self-MHC, but are tolerant to self-antigens, are allowed to mature (*positive selection*). The fine details of thymic selection are extremely complex and beyond the scope of this review; however, the outcome of the positive and negative intrathymic selection processes is the establishment of a T cell repertoire that is self-MHC-restricted and self-tolerant.

T cell precursors arising from bone marrow stem cells migrate to the cortex of the thymus where they proliferate into thymocytes. At this stage, thymocytes are firmly committed to the T cell lineage, but they do not express the mature T cell phenotype. Expression of a clonotypic TCR is mandatory for full thymocyte maturation, and intrathymic selection process can proceed, as selection for life or death of developing thymocytes is dictated by the TCR specificity and affinity. The vast majority of thymocytes (>90%) die of "neglect" in the thymic cortex due to nonproductive gene rearrangements of their TCRs. Only thymocytes that express a functional TCR can survive and proceed to the next stage of development during which they express both CD4 and CD8 accessory molecules. CD4+CD8+ thymocytes (intrathymic double positive thymocytes) then acquire the capacity to interact with antigen-presenting cells (APC) that express self-MHC molecules bearing self-antigenic peptides. This MHC-peptide complex is recognized by the TCR, and signals transduced through the TCR constitute a key element in selection of developing thymocytes. Double positive thymocytes are hypersensitive to strong TCR signaling. In contrast to mature T cells in the periphery, where stimulation through the TCR leads to robust T cell activation, strong TCR stimulation of double-positive thymocytes causes rapid apoptotic cell death. Thus, potentially autoreactive double positive thymocytes that express a TCR with high affinity to a self-MHC-peptide complex are eliminated via programmed cell death or apoptosis (ie, negative selection). Only those double positive thymocytes (1% to 2%) that express a TCR with low or moderate affinity to a self-MHC-peptide complex are rescued from programmed cell death (ie, positive selection), and are allowed to undergo further differentiation and maturation (Figure 5-1).

Both intrathymic bone marrow-derived APCs (eg, dendritic cells and macrophages) and thymic epithelial cells are critical for the intrathymic selection process. Some have proposed that bone marrow-derived APCs are the principal cell type mediating negative selection, whereas thymic epithelial cells are vital to the positive selection. This distinction, however, is somewhat controversial. Nevertheless, positively selected double positive thymocytes then differentiate into CD4 or CD8 single-positive T cells. Subsequently, CD4 and CD8 single-positive T cells migrate to the medulla of the thymus from which they migrate to the lymphoid tissues in the periphery as mature T cells.

MHC class I and MHC class II molecules expressed on thymic APCs impart distinct effects on the maturation of CD4+ and CD8+ T cells. Maturation of CD4+ T cells requires the expression of MHC class II molecules on thymic APCs, whereas maturation of CD8+ T cells requires the expression of MHC class I molecules. The stringent requirement of MHC class I and MHC class II

molecules for the development of CD4 and CD8 single-positive T cells is elegantly demonstrated by the creation of MHC class I or MHC class II knockout mice. Mice deficient for MHC class I or class II molecules exhibit impaired intrathymic development of CD8+ and CD4+ T cells, respectively.

The precise biochemical signals that govern the positive and negative selection of double positive thymocytes remain enigmatic. Double-positive thymocytes manifest remarkable down-regulation of CD4 and CD8, and up-regulation of CD5, CD69 and IL-2 receptor just prior to apoptotic cell death. Under in vitro conditions, strong TCR stimulation of double-positive thymocytes initiates a cascade of events including activation of protein tyrosine kinases; hydrolysis of phosphatidylinositol; sustained elevation of intracellular Ca^{2+}; activation of protein kinase C; and induction of various transcriptional factors. It is clear that apoptosis of thymocytes requires transcriptional activation and new protein synthesis. Although expression of several intracellular apoptotic and anti-apoptotic mediators such as bcl-2, bcl-xL, p53, nur77, and caspases are directly relevant to T cell apoptosis, the downstream events involved in activating and regulating these anti-apoptotic and pro-apoptotic molecules are still poorly understood.

The processes of thymic selection have been exploited in experimental models. Tolerance to allografts across full MHC barriers can be achieved in adult rodents by creation of hematopoietic chimerism where deletion of donor-specific alloreactive T cells in the thymus, occurring as a consequence of interaction with donor-derived APCs, is a principal mechanism of toler-

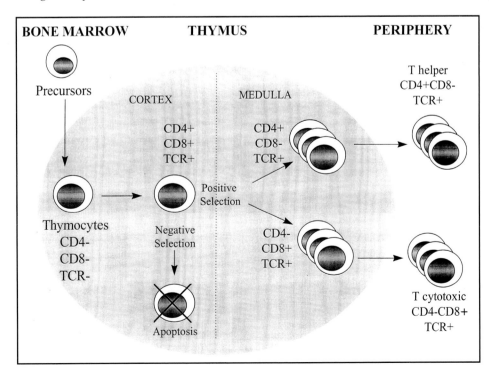

BONE MARROW   **THYMUS**   **PERIPHERY**

Precursors

CORTEX   MEDULLA

CD4+   CD4+
CD8+   CD8-
TCR+   TCR+

Positive
Selection

Thymocytes
CD4-
CD8-
TCR-

Negative
Selection

CD4-
CD8+
TCR+

Apoptosis

T helper
CD4+CD8-
TCR+

T cytotoxic
CD4-CD8+
TCR+

Figure 5-1. Thymic selection of developing T cells. Thymocytes without functional TCRs are "neglected"; those with high-affinity TCRs for self-MHC or peptide complex are deleted via apoptosis; and those with low-affinity TCRs are selected for maturation.

ance induction (ie, central allograft tolerance). Protocols aimed at establishment of permanent chimerism and induction of central allograft tolerance often entail aggressive ablation of recipient's immune system such as total body irradiation, massive depletion of peripheral T cells, and subsequent reconstitution of recipient animals with donor or mixed donor and recipient bone marrow cells. T cell precursors and APCs arising from the donor bone marrow cells repopulate the thymus of recipient animals. As donor T cells develop in the thymus, T cell clones reactive to the donor alloantigens are deleted upon interaction with donor bone marrow-derived APCs. Thus, a T cell repertoire that is tolerant to the donor alloantigens is created. Chimeric hosts can accept any tissues from the donor without any immunosuppression. Interestingly, this strategy can be successfully adopted to create stable xenograft tolerance by reconstitution of recipients with xenogeneic bone marrow cells. Thus, this form of allograft tolerance is remarkably robust and can even withstand the most stringent test of tolerance.

More recently, the same principle has been used to create central allograft tolerance by intrathymic injection of allogeneic cells or allogeneic peptides. Requirements that produce allograft tolerance by intrathymic injection of allogeneic cells often involve extensive depletion of mature T cells in the periphery. Although the precise mechanisms involved in the creation of tolerance via intrathymic injection of antigens are still poorly understood, depletion of mature peripheral T cells may create "space" for T cells to undergo development in the thymus and to repopulate the periphery of the host. As T cells develop in the alloantigen-loaded thymus, T cell clones that are reactive to the donor alloantigens may be selectively deleted, and a T cell repertoire that is tolerant to the alloantigens may be created.

Several critical questions remain to be answered regarding central tolerance. Despite massive deletion of maturing T cells in the thymus to purge potential autoreactive T cell clones, intrathymic deletion is by no means complete. Often, there are some autoreactive T cells in the periphery. Similarly, peripheral T cells from tolerized animals created by immune ablation and bone marrow reconstitution strategy can exhibit anti-donor CTL activity in vitro. Thus, a requirement for peripheral mechanisms to control the cytodestructive potential of T cell clones that have escaped the negative selection in the thymus is evident.

PERIPHERAL TOLERANCE

Peripheral tolerance refers to a tolerant state that is primarily established in the absence of intrathymic selection. Creation of peripheral tolerance often involves qualitative modification in the activation program of fully mature antigen-reactive peripheral T cells. The mechanisms involved in the induction and maintenance of peripheral tolerance have defied attempts at simple categorization. Despite the recent advance in the understanding of the molecular and biochemical aspects of T cell activation, detailed knowledge about the precise nature of peripheral allograft tolerance is still lacking. Indeed, it is believed that peripheral tolerance may not be a uniform process. Several forms of peripheral tolerance may exist.

It is also believed that peripheral tolerance is induced and maintained by a series of distinct but interrelated mechanisms. Depending on the experimental systems used and the tolerizing therapies employed, different mechanisms may come into play at different times with evolution of tolerance, although one particular mechanism may predominate over another in a given model system. Table 5-1 summarizes various mechanisms that have been implicated as contributing to or governing peripheral tolerance.

Clonal Deletion

Many believed that, unlike central tolerance, peripheral tolerance did not entail T cell deletion. Although exposure of mature T cells to antigen generally evokes a rapid and often vigorous immune response, it is now clear that, eventually, most of the effector T cells generated in the immune response are subsequently eliminated via activation-induced cell death (AICD). In a variety of situations, apoptotic cell death of mature T cells following

Table 5-1. Possible Mechanisms of Tolerance

1. Although deletion is primarily confined to developing thymocytes, mature peripheral T cells can also undergo apoptosis following robust immune activation leading to deletion of antigen-specific T cells.
2. Antigen-specific T cells can be functionally inactivated in the absence of T cell deletion, a process called clonal anergy. As with other forms of nondeletional T cell tolerance, anergy can be reversed by providing exogenous T cell growth factors.
3. Tolerance can occur as a result of vigorous immune activation under certain milieu leading to immune deviation.
4. Peripheral tolerance can be established by active suppression of antigen-reactive T cells by other T suppressor or T regulatory cells.

robust and ongoing immune activation can lead to, or at least contribute to, a state of antigen-specific tolerance. For example, in vivo administration of staphylococcal enterotoxin B (SEB), a bacterial superantigen (sAg), into recipient mice provokes vigorous proliferation and clonal expansion of TCR Vβ8-expressing T cells, followed by extensive deletion (>60%) of the activated Vβ8-expressing T cells. The remaining Vβ8-expressing T cells are functionally tolerant and do not respond to antigen, to re-challenge with SEB, or to TCR crosslinking by specific mAbs. Similarly, injection of high-dose lymphocytic choriomeningitis virus (LCMV) into recipient mice provokes a rapid and robust T cell proliferative response, which is followed by deletion of LCMV-activated T cells. The recipient mice become tolerant to the virus as manifested by the persistence of LCMV in the hosts. In ovalbumin (OVA)-specific TCR transgenic mice, injection of OVA subcutaneously, in complete Freunds adjuvant, primes OVA-specific T cells to develop into memory-like T cells without noticeable T cell deletion. In contrast, profound AICD is induced when the OVA peptide is introduced into the TCR transgenic mice intravenously without adjuvant, and the mice usually become tolerant to OVA upon subsequent challenge.

T cell tolerance via apoptotic cell death can be part of a stepwise, multi-staged process. This is elegantly demonstrated in MHC class I molecule K^b transgenic mice crossed with K^b specific TCR transgenic mice. These double transgenic mice express very low levels of K^b antigen in the liver, and T cells specific to the K^b antigen are functionally tolerant in vivo. These mice can permanently accept K^b positive skin allografts. T cells that are tolerant to the K^b antigen exhibit profound TCR downregulation without detectable T cell deletion; however, these tolerant T cells can still mount a vigorous proliferative response to the K^b antigen in vitro. Induction of a high level of K^b expression in the liver of these transgenic mice results in exhaustive antigen-specific T cell deletion and complete functional tolerance (ie, both in vitro and in vivo). Thus, T cells that are rendered antigen-unresponsive following initial antigen encounter remain susceptible to deletional signals upon subsequent exposure to higher doses of antigen or stronger antigenic stimulation.

Although not definitively proven, it is believed that T cell AICD is necessary, albeit not sufficient, to create peripheral allograft tolerance in the absence of lymphoablative treatment. There is compelling evidence that apoptosis of activated alloreactive T cells in certain microenvironments may contribute to the induction, maintenance, and regulation of peripheral allograft tolerance. Certain tissues and organs such as cornea, testis, placenta, and to some extent, the liver, enjoy a state of immune privilege (ie, they are not rejected by MHC-mismatched recipients). The expression of Fas ligand, which triggers apoptotic cell death of invading host lymphocytes, confers the privileged status in these situations. For example, Fas ligand expressing testis was not rejected when transplanted under the renal capsule into fully MHC-mismatched recipient mice. In striking contrast, testis from Fas ligand deficient *gld* mice was vigorously rejected. A similar finding was reported in a mouse model of corneal transplants where apoptosis of infiltrating host lymphocytes was the principal mechanism of prolonged allograft survival. Transplantation of syngeneic myoblasts genetically engineered to express Fas ligand, together with pancreatic islet allografts, protected the islet allograft from rejection. Protection of islet allografts has also been observed by cotransplantation of Fas ligand-expressing Sertoli cells. Furthermore, in a donor bone marrow-induced, skin tolerant model, expression of functional Fas ligand on the bone marrow cells is required for a apoptotic process leading to the deletion of alloreactive T cells and the establishment of skin allograft tolerance. Compelling evidence concerning the requirement for AICD in transplantation tolerance has emerged from the study of IL-2 knockout mice and bcl-xL transgenic mice as allograft recipients. These mice have profound, albeit distinct, defects in T cell apoptotic events that affect antigen-activated T cells. Induction of allograft tolerance in these mice has proven to be extremely difficult through use of noncytolytic tolerizing therapies.

Clonal Anergy

Clonal anergy refers to a state of nondeletional, and often a reversible form of T cell unresponsiveness. Anergy is readily induced in vitro by TCR engagement in the absence of CD28 imparted costimulation, or stimulation of T cells with altered TCR ligands (partial TCR agonists). Anergy induced in this manner is characterized by a profound inhibition in the ability of anergic T cells to produce IL-2 upon secondary challenge with antigen in the presence of optimal costimulation. Thus, cells that normally produce and use IL-2 in vitro for proliferation, including Th1, Th0, and CD8 clones, are unable to enter the cell cycle and become incompetent for proliferation. However, at least some anergic T cell clones can enter the cell cycle and proliferate in response to exogenous IL-2. Such anergy can be reversed by provision of exogenous IL-2 in the culture system, although reversal of the anergic state is not immediate, and multiple rounds of cell divisions are required to gain fully functional recovery.

Antigen-specific T cell anergy can be induced in normal CD4+ T cells in vivo. Persistence of anergic T cells has been demonstrated in mice after in vivo administration of tolerizing doses of bacterial sAgs, Mls-1a, and peptide antigens that do not cause deletion of antigen-reactive T cells. In many cases, CD4+ T cells anergized in vivo are resistant to stimulation with exogenous IL-2, which is in striking contrast to the behavior of T cell clones anergized in vitro. This difference may reflect the constitutive expression of high-affinity IL-2 receptor on T cell clones, but not on normal T cells. In CD4+ T cells anergized in vivo, the proliferative response to other cytokines including IL-12 dependent events is also blocked. CD4+ T cells anergized in vivo, and Th1 clones anergized in vitro also exhibit a profound defect in the expression of CD40 ligand. CD40 ligand is expressed on activated CD4+ T cells and can deliver critical costimulatory signals for T cell activation. The impaired CD40 ligand expression by anergic T cells may aid to the development of antigen-specific tolerance in vivo.

At the biochemical level, certain forms of T cell anergy are associated with a defect in TCR-mediated signaling events. In Th1 clones anergized in vitro, and CD4+ T cells anergized in vivo, decreased TCR ζ chain and ZAP-70 phosphorylation, as well as an abnormal ζ chain-to-ZAP-70 association have been clearly demonstrated. The defect in tyrosine phosphorylation of key signaling proteins in anergic T cells is correlated with stable changes in the expression of tyrosine kinases *lck* and *fyn*. The decreased enzymatic activity of *lck* coupled with a constitutively active form of *fyn* may result in a defect in downstream signaling events in T cell activation pathways. In anergic Th1 cell clones, a transcriptional block in IL-2 gene expression is evident, and this defect is localized to the AP-1 binding sites in the IL-2 enhancer. Perhaps changes in activation of early tyrosine kinases may alter the phosphorylation status of *fos* and *jun* components of the AP-1 complex by preventing MAP kinases ERK-1 and ERK-2 activation.

In certain model systems, T cell anergy has been implicated as an essential component of allograft tolerance; however, the reversible nature, at least in some forms of T cell anergy, suggests that anergy is unlikely to be a robust mechanism for maintenance of peripheral allograft tolerance.

Immune Deviation

Antigen-activated CD4+ T helper cells can differentiate into at least two distinct phenotypes. Th1 cells produce IL-2, IFN-γ, and TNF-β, and are often manifested during T cell-dependent cytopathic immunity including allograft rejection. In contrast, Th2 cells secrete IL-4, IL-5, IL-6 and IL-10, and are the classical T helper cells for the provision of B cell help in antibody production. Differentiation into Th1 phenotype requires IL-12 that is produced primarily by activated macrophages and dendritic cells, while Th2 differentiation is primarily IL-4-dependent. In addition to distinct cytokine profiles and effector functions, Th1 and Th2 cells also express distinct sets of chemokines and homing receptors. Th1 cells express CXCR3, whereas Th2 cells selectively express CCR3 and CCR4 chemokine receptors. Thus, they respond to a distinct array of chemokines. Moreover, Th1 cells express functional ligands for P and E selectins that allow their selective accumulation in Th1-dominated inflammatory sites such as sensitized skin and arthritic joints. Th2 cells do not express ligands for P and E, and accumulate in Th2-dominated allergic inflammatory sites.

As the Th1 and Th2 paradigm holds that the fate of an immune response is determined as a consequence of whether the Th1 or Th2 is in control of the other, it has been proposed that a Th1 to Th2 immune deviation may be beneficial in certain Th1-mediated pathologic processes. Indeed, a Th1 to Th2 deviation is highly beneficial in several models of T cell-dependent autoimmunity.

Allograft rejection in unmodified recipients is consistently, albeit not universally, associated with a Th1 pattern of immune activation. Moreover, allograft recipients treated with certain tolerizing immunosuppressive regimens often manifest a Th2-type response during the treatment period. Nonetheless, IL-2 or IFN-γ deficient hosts reject allografts despite strong expression of IL-4, and IL-4-deficient allograft hosts can be permanently engrafted under the cover of select immunosuppressive protocols. Furthermore, attempts to induce permanent engraftment or to create a state of tolerance to MHC-mismatched allografts through administration of long-acting Th2 cytokines (ie, IL-4Ig and IL-10Ig fusion proteins) or immune deviation via application of IL-12 antagonists have failed. Interestingly, certain tolerizing regimens failed to produce allograft tolerance in IL-4 knockout hosts. Furthermore, neutralizing IL-4 during the induction phase of cardiac allograft tolerance completely abolished the capacity of T cells to adoptively transfer allograft tolerance to naive secondary recipients. It is believed that the differing impact of Th1 to Th2 immune deviation on the outcome of alloimmunity and autoimmunity can be explained by the fact that alloimmune and autoimmune responses differ in at least two interrelated ways. First, the host response to MHC-mismatched allografts includes responses to directly presented foreign (donor) MHC antigens (ie, direct antigen presentation), while autoimmunity is characterized by indirect presentation of autoantigens upon self-MHC molecules. Second, rejection of MHC incompatible allografts activates more T cell clones than typical autoimmune responses. These factors may explain the paradoxical ability of Th1 to Th2 immune deviation to curtail T cell-dependent autoimmunity, a process that is conducted by a small number of T cell clones, while failing to blunt the polyclonal T cell-dependent response to MHC-mismatched allografts. Indeed, a Th1 to Th2 immune deviation produces islet allograft tolerance only when the donor and recipient are mismatched for the minor histocompatibility barriers, or when rejection is dependent on indirect presentation of donor alloantigens, suggesting an unequivocal role of Th2 cells in regulation of allograft tolerance under certain highly restricted conditions. Recent experiments in MHC-mismatched models indicate that Th1 to Th2 immune deviation is helpful, but not sufficient, for creation of a tolerant state.

Active Immunosuppression

It has been long known that in allograft models of peripheral tolerance, donor-specific allograft prolongation or tolerance can be achieved in passive transfer systems, ie, T suppressor cells exist. In tolerant models, T cells that elaborate immune suppressive mediators often present at the site of antigen stimulation. More recently, the phenomena of *infectious allograft tolerance* and *linked immunosuppression* are well documented in many transplantation models.

Mice tolerized against skin allografts mismatched for multiple minor histocompatibility antigens can be readily induced by nondepleting anti-CD4 plus anti-CD8 mAbs. The tolerant state can be transferred to a cohort of naive recipients bearing the original skin allografts in the absence of the initial tolerizing therapy. This suppression operates in the primary tolerant hosts if fresh alloreactive T cells are introduced into the tolerant recipients, or if cells are transferred from tolerant mice to naive recipients. This type of infectious tolerance is critically dependent on CD4+ T cells. Tolerant T cells can recruit other antigen-specific T cells into the pool of regulatory T cells. The potency of the immune system to generate such powerful regulatory T cells has been demonstrated in the fully MHC-mismatched cardiac allograft model. Tolerance created by the anti-CD4 plus anti-CD8 mAbs against cardiac allografts can be passed on to naive unmanipulated recipients for more than ten generations. Clearly, this type of tolerance is a self-perpetuating process. Interestingly, such regulatory CD4+ T cells can also confer tolerance to a third party MHC-mismatched cardiac allograft as long as the graft is from a F1-hybrid mouse that is crossed with the tolerant strain, a phenomenon called *linked immunosuppression.* Clearly, infectious allograft tolerance is remarkably potent, it becomes self-sustaining, and can be passed on by a population of CD4+ T cells that act to suppress the generation of any CD4+ and CD8+ effector cells either to the same antigen, or to different antigens presented in the context of donor APCs to which the host is tolerant. Consequently, naive CD4+ T cells also become tolerant upon recognition of alloantigens and gain the ability to suppress further generations of T cells.

Despite these intriguing observations, the precise identity of such regulatory T cells, the specificity of the antigens recognized by such cells, and the precise mechanism by which tolerance occurs remain elusive. Attempts to clone these suppressor T cells have generally failed, and no specific cell surface markers are known to distinguish such regulatory cells from other cell types. However, there is ample evidence to suggest that infectious allograft tolerance is driven by some forms of cytokine-mediated immune deviation. For example, skin allograft tolerance across multiple minor histocompatibility barriers can be created by nondepleting anti-CD4 and anti-CD8 mAbs, which is a tolerizing protocol that reliably creates infectious tolerance. This model of tolerance can be partially impaired by neutralizing IL-4, suggesting that an IL-4-driven process, possibly a Th2-dominant immune activation, is critical in this model. Moreover, the ability of CD4+ T cells from tolerized hosts to passively transfer allograft tolerance was severely compromised by blocking IL-4 during the induction of allograft tolerance in the primary recipients, although blocking IL-4 had no impact on the survival of cardiac allografts in the primary hosts.

Perhaps a Th2-dominant response is only an epiphenomenon, as neonatal tolerance and oral tolerance that inevitably manifest strong Th2 response can be induced in mice deficient for IL-4 or IL-10. In certain models, tolerance is achieved in both Th1 and Th2 subsets simultaneously, leaving a population of T cells that produce only transforming growth factor β (TGF-β), and this subset of TGF-β-producing T cells was recently named Th3. Interestingly, high levels of TGF-β are produced in the anterior chamber of the eye upon direct antigen challenge, an effect which is often associated with antigen-specific tolerance. Such TGF-β-producing CD4+ T cells (Th3) have also been found in oral tolerant models. The power of TGF-β as a critical regulatory cytokine is highlighted by the finding that mice with targeted gene mutation of TGF-β 1 exhibit widespread multifocal inflammatory disease.

Recently, CD4+ T cell clones have been generated that produce a novel pattern of cytokines distinct to either Th1, Th2 or Th3. These CD4+ T cell clones produce TGF-β and various amounts of IL-10, but not IL-4, and therefore are termed *T regulatory cells* (Tr). Tr cells or Th3 cells can effectively prevent autoimmunity in certain autoimmune disease models. The cytokine requirements for generating regulatory cells in vivo, and the precise nature by which they function to suppress ongoing immunity is still poorly understood.

A UNIFYING CONCEPT

Although a clear road map leading to the acquisition of true transplantation tolerance is still lacking, establishment of classical allograft tolerance is a process that is active, stepwise and highly regulated. Multiple stages often result in achieving stable peripheral allograft tolerance, and different mechanisms evolve at different stages over time that enable the creation of stable allograft

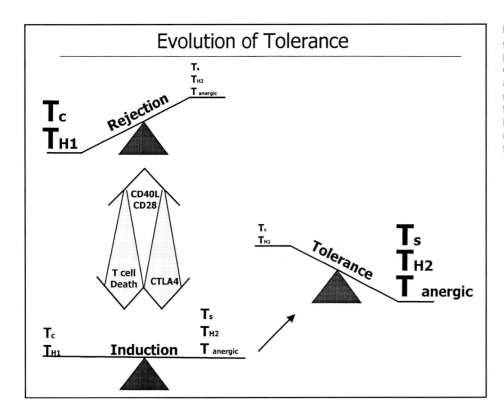

Figure 5-2. Evolution of allograft tolerance. A deletional process to reduce the mass of cytopathic alloreactive clones and preservation of CTLA-4 negative signals is critical in the tolerance induction phase. Development of an immunoregulatory process is essential for tolerance maintenance

tolerance. In allograft hosts that achieve donor-specific tolerance, the process culminating in the acquisition of tolerance can be divided into three time-related and mechanism-related stages: (1) tolerance induction, (2) ignorance, and (3) tolerance maintenance (Figure 5-2).

Tolerance Induction

This is the period in which the hosts are treated with immunosuppressive drugs. Prolonged engraftment can be readily induced by a variety of protocols including: (1) administration of mAbs targeting cell surface molecules such as CD4, CD8, CD25, LFA-1 or the TCR; (2) blockade of the costimulation pathways of T cell activation; (3) institution of pharmacological drug including steroids, rapamycin, cyclosporine; and (4) donor-specific transfusion. Although immunosuppressive reagents, alone or in combination, can drastically prolong allograft survival, the impact of different regimens on the acquisition of true allograft tolerance can be strikingly different. It is hypothesized that the unusually large clone size of alloreactive T cells requires rapid T cell death to reduce the mass of alloreactive T cells in order to achieve tolerance. Reduction of some cytopathic Th1 clones to levels such that the alloimmune response can be contained by regulatory means is a likely prerequisite for tolerance induction. Thus, a deletional process in the inductive phase may be instrumental to the subsequent acquisition of true allograft tolerance. Therapies that enable T cell death either by administration of cytolytic reagents or by promoting AICD may constitute a critical compo-

nent in the inductive therapy. Also, preservation of CTLA-4-imparted negative signals in T cell activation is also essential during the inductive therapy. The inductive therapy should also foster the development of immune regulatory cells over time, or qualitative changes in T cell reactivity (eg, Th2 immune deviation). As generation of regulatory T cells during immune activation is an active process, therapies that completely suppress the immune activation may preclude the development of stable allograft tolerance, although graft survival can be prolonged through continuous immune suppression.

Ignorance

Following the cessation of successful inductive therapy, the initial allograft rejection is transiently suppressed and the host response enters the ignorance phase. This phase of tolerance induction is often metastable and fragile as the cytopathic anti-donor response is contained, however, a robust tolerant state has not yet been firmly established. Rejection can be unleashed via re-challenging the recipients with large doses of exogenous T cell growth factors such as IL-2, or re-challenging the hosts with a second donor-specific allograft or donor-derived APC. For example, in an islet model of allograft tolerance, systemic administration of IL-2 in the early stage of tolerance induction completely abolished the tolerant status achieved via costimulation blockade; however, IL-2 had no impact on islet allograft tolerance when the tolerant state was well established. The reversibility in the ignorance phase suggests that

T cell anergy may be actively involved. Hence, strategies that stabilize the anergic state, or prevent bystander immune activation or activation by tissue-derived T cell growth factors (IL-7 and IL-15), are clearly important for ensuring development of the robust form of regulatory process that maintains the tolerant state.

Tolerance Maintenance

True allograft tolerance is achieved at this stage as a challenge with donor tissues can no longer elicit graft rejection, although third party tissues are readily rejected. Maintenance of stable allograft tolerance often requires an active immunoregulatory process. In certain models, allograft tolerance can be adoptively transferred at this stage to naive secondary recipients by T cells harvested from tolerized hosts. Hence, a potent immunoregulatory process is achieved in the maintenance phase of peripheral allograft tolerance. Persistence of alloantigens in transplant recipients is an absolute prerequisite for maintenance of peripheral allograft tolerance. Following removal of the primary allografts from the tolerized hosts, the tolerance status to the original donor allografts is often lost, and the recipients regain the capability of rejecting the donor strain allografts. Similarly, creation of stable mixed hematopoietic chimerism results in permanent donor-specific allograft tolerance and the tolerant status is often lost when the donor bone marrow-derived cells are depleted from the recipient mice. Thus, regulatory T cells that maintain the tolerance state require continuous presence of alloantigens.

CLINICAL IMPLICATIONS

Peripheral allograft tolerance can be readily and reproducibly induced in various rodent experimental models using inbred donor and recipient strains. Unfortunately, an understanding of the underlying mechanisms is far from complete, and our current immunosuppressive protocols to implement such an approach, clinically, are far from perfect. While the transplant community celebrates the success of intermediate term engraftment in the clinic, achieved with prolonged immunosuppression, it should also be remembered that our current immunosuppressive protocols do not create true allograft tolerance. It is critically important to analyze therapeutic protocols in the context of the multistep nature of tolerance induction. There is evidence to suggest that some of the current immunosuppressive regimens causing global immunosuppression actually hinder the acquisition of allograft tolerance. Hence, as more and more reagents are added to the immunosuppressive list, careful analysis of their therapeutic compatibility will undoubtedly aid in the design of better immunosuppressive protocols to promote the creation of true allograft tolerance.

RECOMMENDED READINGS

Ikuta K, Uchida N, Friedman J, Weissman IL. Lymphocyte development from stem cells. Annu Rev Immunol. 1992;10:759-783.

Sykes M. Chimerism and central tolerance. Curr Opin Immunol. 1996;8(5):694-703.

Posselt AM, Barker CF, Tomaszewski JE, Markmann JF, Choti MA, Jaji A. Induction of donor-specific unresponsiveness by intrathymic islet transplantation. Science. 1990;249(4974):1293-1295.

Arnold B, Schonrich G, Hammerling GJ. Multiple levels of peripheral tolerance. Immunol Today. 1993;14(1):12-14.

Bellgrau D, Gold D, Selawry H, Moore J, Franzusoff A, Duke RC. A role for CD95 ligand in preventing graft rejection. Nature. 1995;377(6550):630-632.

George JF, Sweeney SD, Kirklin JK, Simpson EM, Goldstein DR, Thomas JM. An essential role for Fas ligand in transplantation tolerance induced by donor bone marrow. Nat Med. 1998;4(3):333-335.

Jenkins MK. The role of cell division in the induction of clonal anergy. Immunol Today. 1992;13(2):69-73.

Perez VL, Van Parijs L, Biuckians A, Zheng XX, Strom TB, Abbas AK. Induction of peripheral T cell tolerance in vivo requires CTLA-4 engagement. Immunity. 1997;6(4):411-417.

Salojin KV, Zhang J, Madrenas J, Delovitch TL. T-cell anergy and altered T-cell receptor signaling: effects on autoimmune disease. Immunol Today. 1998;19(10):468-473.

Quill H. Anergy as a mechanism of peripheral T cell tolerance. J Immunol. 1996;156(4):1325-1327.

Mosmann TR, Coffman RL. Th1 and Th2 cells: different patterns of lymphokine secretion lead to different functional properties. Annu Rev Immunol. 1989;7:145-173.

Constant SL, Bottomly K. Induction of Th1 and Th2 CD4+ T cell responses: the alternative approaches. Annu Rev Immunol. 1997;15:297-322.

Strom TB, Roy-Chaudhury P, Manfro R, et al. The Th1/Th2 paradigm and the allograft response. Curr Opin Immunol. 1996;8(5):688-693.

Bushell A, Niimi M, Morris PJ, Wood KJ. Evidence for immune regulation in the induction of transplantation tolerance: a conditional but limited role for IL-4. J Immunol. 1999;162(3):1359-1366.

Li XC, Zand MS, Li Y, Zheng XX, Strom TB. On histocompatibility barriers, Th1 to Th2 immune deviation, and the nature of the allograft responses. J Immunol. 1998;161(5):2241-2247.

Cobbold S, Waldmann H. Infectious tolerance. Curr Opin Immunol. 1998;10(5):518-524.

Weiner HL, Friedman A, Miller A, et al. Oral tolerance: immunologic mechanisms and treatment of animal and human organ-specific autoimmune diseases by oral administration of autoantigens. Annu Rev Immunol. 1994;12:809-837.

Letterio JJ, Roberts AB. Regulation of immune responses by TGF-beta. Annu Rev Immunol. 1998;16:137-161.

Tran HM, Nickerson PW, Restifo AC, et al. Distinct mechanisms for the induction and maintenance of allograft tolerance with CTLA4-Fc treatment. J Immunol. 1997;159(5):2232-2239.

Larsen CP, Elwood ET, Alexander DZ, et al. Long-term acceptance of skin and cardiac allografts after blocking CD40 and CD28 pathways. Nature. 1996;381(6581):434-438.

6   BASIC IMMUNOGENETICS
Charles B. Carpenter, MD

MAJOR HISTOCOMPATIBILITY COMPLEX
Background

Immunogenetics is the study of genes that have polymorphic variants of particular relevance to the immune system. Some of these are antigenic and provide forbidding barriers to blood transfusion and tissue transplantation. The presence of a single system of linked genes that provokes the vigorous rejection of skin grafts between members of different inbred mouse strains was discovered by Snell over 50 years ago. It was named H-2, as it was the second in a series of genes that provoked graft rejection. Only H-2 differences led to rejection times of six to eight days in normal recipients, in comparison to weeks with H-1, H-3, H-4, etc. differences. Analogous genes are present in all mammals, birds, and bony fishes. The term *major histocompatibility complex* (MHC) is the general term for the H-2-like system, called *HLA* in humans. The MHC is a closely-linked group of genes that encode molecules of crucial importance to the generation of antigen-specific T cell and IgG responses to antigens from the microbial world. In the 1960s, Benacerraf showed that the ability to make an immune response to polypeptide antigens was genetically controlled, and the locus was proven to be H-2 by McDevitt. In the 1970s, Zinkernagel and Doherty demonstrated that T cells recognize peptide antigens on the surface of antigen-presenting cells (APCs) only if both cells share the same H-2. They correctly inferred that each T cell must recognize both the antigen and self-MHC. On a parallel track, starting with Dausset's demonstration of transfusion-induced antibodies to white blood cells in the 1950s, human studies revealed the presence of a completely analogous system, later to be called HLA. The strength of alloimmunity to MHC antigens is due to the high density of MHC molecules on tissue cells, and to the T cell preoccupation with binding to self-MHC, the only physiological way that T cell antigen receptors can function. As noted in Chapter 4, some T cell clones bind to the polymorphic surface of intact allo-MHC molecules directly, while other clones "see" polymorphic peptide fragments presented by self-MHC (*indirect pathway*). This chapter focuses on the nature of HLA polymorphisms and their role in clinical transplantation.

Professor of Medicine, Harvard Medical School, Brigham and Women's Hospital, Immunogenetics, Boston, MA

Structure of MHC Molecules

The process of antigen presentation to T cells by so-called *professional* APCs, such as monocytes, macrophages, B lymphocytes, and dendritic cells, uses two structurally different classes of MHC molecules. Class I molecules are present on most cells of the body, although not on human red blood cells, while class II molecules are restricted to the APCs. Endothelium and epithelium, when activated, may also express class II. The polymorphic antigenic sites on these molecules are a small proportion of the total protein sequence.

Human MHC class I molecules of importance in transplantation are HLA-A, HLA-B, and HLA-C, each encoded by a separate genetic locus (Figure 6-1). These molecules are identical in general structure and consist of two polypeptide chains, the larger of which traverses the cell membrane (Figure 6-2). This heavy chain (44 kilodaltons [kda]) is divided into three extracellular domains designated as $\alpha1$, $\alpha2$, and $\alpha3$. The other chain is not membrane-inserted and associates noncovalently to support the heavy chain in a stable configuration for peptide-binding and T cell recognition. This smaller protein (11.5 kda) is β_2-microglobulin, encoded on chromosome 15. The surface formed by the $\alpha1$ and $\alpha2$ domains faces away from the cell surface and is the location of the peptide-binding site and the allelic polymorphisms. A large number (>20) of additional class I loci are mapped between HLA-B and HLA-A, and in the region to the right of HLA-A. These play no defined role as MHC alloantigens.

Each class II antigen consists of two membrane-inserted glycosylated polypeptides designated α (34 kda) and β (28 kda). The extracellular portion of the α chain is divided into two domains designated $\alpha1$ and $\alpha2$. The extracellular portion of the β chain is also divided into two domains: $\beta1$ and $\beta2$. In contrast with class I, the peptide-binding and polymorphic external surface of class II is composed of the distal domains of each chain, $\alpha1$ and $\beta1$. The two polypeptide chains interact noncovalently to form a structure very similar to that of class I (Figure 6-2). There are three sets of class II molecules having varying degrees of importance to alloimmunity: HLA-DP, HLA-DQ, and HLA-DR (Figure 6-1).

When the crystal structure of MHC molecules became available in 1987, a clearer understanding of MHC structure-function relationships was made possible. MHC class I and class II molecules each have a 2 to 3nm x 1nm x 1nm groove on the external face of the molecule, which is bounded by α-helices along the sides and with β-sheets forming the base (Figure 6-3). Quite remarkably, the carbon backbones of class I and II molecules are virtually superimposable; therefore, it is the amino acid side chains that provide the different configurations for peptide binding. Indeed, the regions of hypervariability that induce alloimmunization are located primarily along the sides and base of the groove, indicating that they determine various shapes, charges, and hydrophobicity regions for the selection of peptides for presentation to T cells.

Functional Aspects

As noted in Chapter 2, CD8 and CD4 accessory molecules on T cells bind specifically to MHC class I and II, respectively. Therefore, one can assume that for direct recognition, class I antigen mismatches will expand CD8 effector cells, principally cytotoxic T cells, and that class II mismatches yield expanded clones of CD4 helper cells. Class II-expressing APCs degrade molecules that have been endocytosed or pinocytosed from the extracellular space or, in the case of B cells, are bound to surface immunoglobulins before internalization. The class II system is therefore involved with defense against extracellular infectious agents, and also soluble alloantigens in a transplant situation. Hence, peptide fragments of MHC class I molecules originating in the same or surrounding cells can also end up in the groove of class II molecules for recognition by CD4 T cells.

Genetics and Polymorphisms

GENE ORGANIZATION. MHC genes are related to immunoglobulins, T cell receptors, and adhesion molecules, all of which are members of the immunoglobulin

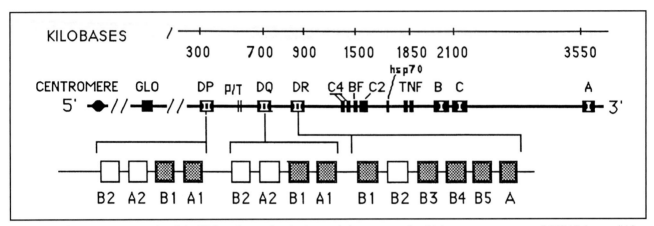

Figure 6-1. Diagram, not to scale, of the HLA region on the short arm of chromosome 6, which encompasses over 3,000 kilobases (kb) of nucleotides. Toward the right end are the class I genes, HLA-A, -B, and -C, while class II genes are toward the left end of the region. In between are genes for some of the complement components, heat shock protein hsp70, and tumor necrosis factors α and β. There are multiple class II genes for each of the components of the heterodimers for HLA-DR, -DQ, and -DP molecules. A and B refer to the genes for the respective α and β chains. Pseudogenes, not expressed, are shown as open boxes. Each HLA-DR molecule is encoded by a monomorphic A chain in association with one of four B chains, of which B1 encodes the HLA-DR1 to -DR18 molecules. HLA-DQ and HLA-DP molecules consist of polymorphic A and B chains, although in each case the B chains are more polymorphic. Other loci in the region do not have sequence similarity to HLA, but are of interest: P/T, in the class II region, represents two sets of proteosome LMP genes, which proteolyze proteins in a controlled manner to make peptides of eight to ten amino acids, while the TAP genes encode chaperone molecules, which transport these peptides for loading on MHC class I molecules. This diagram omits a large number of genes, including many class I-like and others of unknown function. Reprinted by permission of Blackwell Science, Inc. from Carpenter CB. Histocompatibility systems. In: Ginns LC, Cosimi AB, Morris PJ, Eds. Transplantation. Boston, MA; Blackwell Science: 1999.

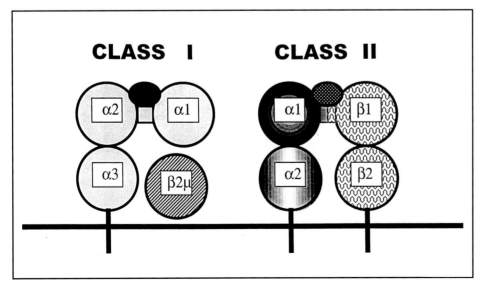

Figure 6-2. The domains of MHC class I and II molecules are schematized to show that class I consists of a 3 domain heavy chain (α1, α2, α3) inserted into the cell membrane, and noncovalently associated with a light chain, β2-microglobulin. The view is horizontal to the cell membrane showing the side aspect of the molecule. The binding groove for peptide (dark symbol) is composed of portions of the the α1 and α2 domains. Class II molecules consist of two chains, α and β, both of which are inserted into the cell membrane. The external domains form a peptide-binding groove very similar to that of class I, one-half of the external surface being formed by each of the chains.

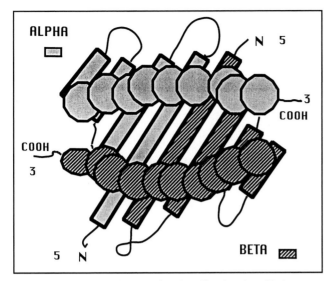

Figure 6-3. A ribbon diagram of a class II molecule, with the two chains shown in different shading. This top view, showing the molecule facing away from the cell surface, exposes the peptide-binding groove. The α-helices form the sides, and the β-sheets form the floor of a 2 to 3nm x 1nm x 1nm groove that binds peptides. The polymorphic amino acids shown in Figure 6-5 are located along the edges and floor of the groove where their different side chains determine the binding characteristics of a given allele.

supergene family. HLA class I and II genes are in separate clusters on the short arm of the sixth chromosome. The loci appear to have arisen by gene duplication in the very distant evolutionary past (Figure 6-1). Class I genes (A, B, and C) encode a single heavy chain, while there are two genes for each of the class II molecules DP, DQ, and DR, consisting of α and β chains. A feature of HLA-DR, shared with analogous genes in other mammals, is that polymorphism occurs only on the β chain, while the other class II loci provide polymorphisms on both α and β chains. The α chains of either HLA-DP or HLA-DQ do not associate with the β chains of the other locus, but the inherited maternal and paternal α and β gene products of each locus do form heterodimers that do not exist in either parent. This phenomenon may play a role in some autoimmune diseases, but is not yet clearly shown to matter in transplantation, possibly because HLA-DP and HLA-DQ antigens are relatively weak antigens in comparison to HLA-DR. The chromosomal space between the HLA class I and II loci is fairly large and contains a large number of other genes, some of which are relevant to the immune response, such as: some of the complement components (C2, C4, and BF); TNFα and β; heat shock protein hsp70; and genes for molecules involved in

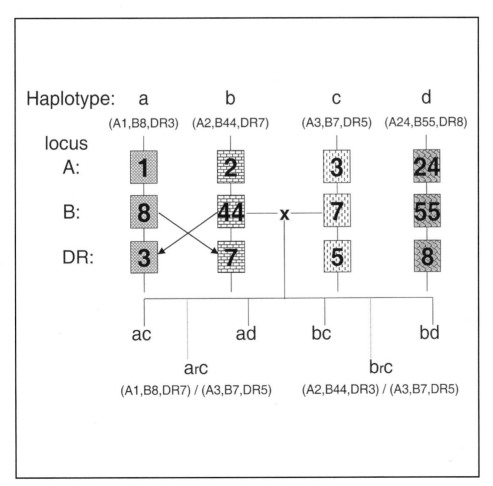

Figure 6-4. Segregation of HLA haplotypes in an illustrative family. Only the HLA-A, -B, and -DR loci are shown, labelled for the allele present. The haplotypes are assigned as *a* and *b* for one parent, *c* and *d* for the other. The expected combinations found in the children are shown as *ac, ad, bc, bd*. For any given child, the chance of having an HLA-identical sibling is 25% (eg, *ac* and *ac*); of having a totally mismatched sibling is 25% (eg, *ac* and *bd*); and of having a one HLA haplotype-matched sibling is 50%. Also, either parent to any child is always a one HLA haplotype match. When a recombination, or crossover, has occurred during germline meiosis, illustrated here between B and DR, a recombinant (r) haplotype can be inherited. In this illustration, the two possible haplotypes from a single recombination are shown at the bottom as a_{rc} and b_{rc}. When alleles are shared by chance for a locus, it may not be possible to detect such an event. An example would be if DR3 were present on *a* and *b*. High-resolution molecular typing is usually able to distinguish minor differences in the two DR3 genes.

antigen processing. The practice of assigning the designation class III to the complement genes is being dropped, because structural and functional homologies to MHC are lacking.

INHERITANCE. HLA antigens are inherited in simple Mendelian-dominant fashion, and since they are linked, they pass as a block from generation to generation. Each child will have a set of half maternal and half paternal antigens. Each of these sets of linked genes is called a *haplotype.* There are four possible haplotype combinations among children with the same mother and father, with the chances of HLA identity between any two siblings being 25%, total nonidentity being 25%, and one haplotype identity being 50% (Figure 6-4). Genetic recombination occurs at various sites in the HLA region; for example, a rate of 0.7% between class I and II, and 0.6% between HLA-A and -C in each generation. In general, assignment of HLA identity in a family does not require precise typing of every antigen because of the usual inheritance of whole haplotypes; however, antigens that are closely related can be mistyped when serological techniques are employed. The mixed lymphocyte culture test in which recipient T cells confront and proliferate to donor class II-bearing cells is very sensitive in detecting the lack of proliferation when the cells are from HLA-identical siblings, and has been used for many years as a confirmatory bioassay. It is used infrequently now because HLA class II molecular typing can provide the same information.

Because of the relatively low rate of gene recombination, an HLA haplotype may remain linked together for many generations. If an ethnic group's population has expanded, many individuals will have inherited haplotypes from a single or limited number of ancestors. Eventually, over many generations one expects that alleles will, by accumulation of recombination events, be associated on haplotypes in a random manner, at which point the genes are said to be in equilibrium. Before that

happens, one may discern a phenomenon called *linkage disequilibrium* or Δ, expressed as the excess of a combination such as HLA-B8 with HLA-DR3, which is the most prevalent combination Δ in northern Europeans. There are not a large number of such Δs, however, and none have been shown in African populations.

Polymorphisms

The original definition of the large number of HLA antigens in populations was based on serology using antisera obtained from multiparous women. Anti-HLA antibodies develop as a normal phenomenon in pregnancy, but only a small fraction (1% or less) of these sera are suitable for HLA typing. Molecular DNA-based techniques have been in development and are now being brought on-line in the clinical laboratory. The number of alleles found by molecular typing is much greater than with serology (Table 6-1). When the amino acid sequences of some of the MHC alleles were obtainable in the 1980s, it became apparent that there were relatively small regions of variability along the length of a typical MHC domain of 90 amino acids, that an *antigen* could be the result of differences in more than one of these sites, and that some of the motifs may be shared with other alleles (Figure 6-5).

Nomenclature

HLA is the "logo" for the human MHC, comparable to H-2 for the mouse and RT1 for the rat. The adoption of HLA was a compromise between competing terminologies, and approved by the World Health Organization as the designation to be used for this genetic system. The letters do not stand for particular words, such as "human leukocyte antigen," a confusing term to those who work with a large number of non-MHC human leukocyte antigens that have the CD designations. Alleles are now fully named according to nucleotide sequencing. Class I is relatively simple; for example, HLA-A*0201 is A2, first variant, A*0202 for second variant, etc. The logo HLA may be omitted when the context is clear. Class II is genetically more complicated, especially DR, which has several β chain genes, and only one of these (B1) encodes the classical DR1 to 18 antigens, which have been shown to be important for kidney transplantation; for example, DRB1*0101 is the first variant of DR1, and DRB1*0102 is its second. DR2 has been divided (split) into 2 versions, DR15 and DR16, and each of these has two variants yielding DRB1*1501, DRB1*1502, DRB1*1601, DRB1*1602 (Figure 6-5). Other entirely separate DR molecules are expressed as well in different haplotypes. DRB3, DRB4, and DRB5 encode the DR52, DR53, and DR51 molecules, respectively (Figure 6-1). HLA-DP and -DQ molecules are allelic for both α and β chains. Both DQA and DQB designations must, therefore, be made, and the notation for these, for

Table 6-1.
Numbers of Defined HLA Alleles

Locus	Serology	DNA Sequenced
A	28	83
B	60	185
C	10	42
DRB1	21	184
DRB3,4,5	3	32
DQA	0	18
DQB	9	31
DPA	0	10
DPB	6	78

example, is DQA*0301 and DQB*0201. The number of molecularly-defined alleles is shown in Table 6-1, and far exceed the number of serological equivalents.

HLA Antigen Matching in Renal Transplantation

In the early 1970s it was shown that living-related donor transplantation of kidneys was influenced in a major way by the degree of HLA haplotype matching, thereby proving that HLA was the MHC in humans. The best results were obtained with HLA-identical sibling donors, having 90% 1-year graft survivals, and half-lives of 20 to 25 years thereafter. Haplo-identical combinations were less successful, with 70% 1-year survivals and a 12-year half-life, while unrelated cadaveric cases attained only a 50% 1-year survival and a half-life of seven to eight years. At that time the methodology for HLA typing was very limited, but a negative MLR was excellent evidence of HLA identity, and analysis of one haplotype identity was based upon parent-to-child combinations. Since then, there has been steady improvement in the one-year graft survival figures in all categories, to the point now that it takes a large number of cases to discern a difference at one year after transplantation among these three levels of compatibility; however, the half-lives for the three categories have remained close to historical values (Table 6-2). Definition of the HLA system has been evolving also; for example, in the 1970s there was no knowledge of HLA-DR, and large scale application of mandatory

matching criteria did not begin until the early 1980s in Europe, and in 1987 in the US. Analysis of tens of thousands of cadaveric kidney transplants in the past decade shows that the half-life of cadaveric kidney survival after the first year varies in a statistically significant way with the number of incompatibilities for the six antigens of only the HLA-A, -B, and -DR loci (Table 6-2), without consideration of HLA-C, HLA-DQ, and HLA-DP. The great experiment initiated by the United Network for Organ Sharing (UNOS) was to see if matching for these three loci among unrelated donors and recipients would equal the results obtained with HLA-identical family donors. Unrelated cadaveric donors completely matched for HLA-A, -B, and -DR (six antigens) with recipients having their first transplant were shown in the first prospective series in 1992 of 1,000 cases distributed through the UNOS system to have 20-year half-lives and projected 10-year survivals of 65%, vs 7.7 years and 34% for cases with five to six mismatches (Table 6-2). Since this result was close to that obtained with HLA-identical siblings, it became the top priority for organ sharing nationally. In registry data with large numbers of patients, a graded beneficial matching effect for lesser degrees of match is present, but is less impressive than results with the full six-antigen match. Frequently, in serological typing only, one antigen is identified for one of the loci, and is termed a "blank." When this is present in the donor, it may be assumed not to be a mismatch. Since the UNOS criteria

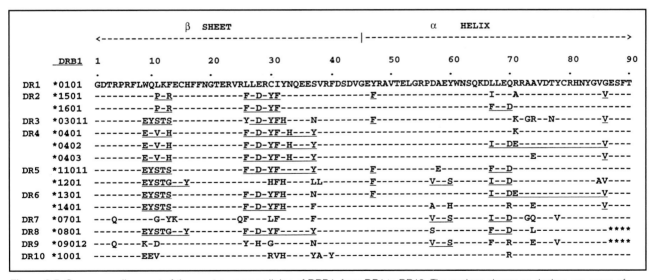

Figure 6-5. Sequence alignment of the most common alleles of DRB1, from DR1 to DR10. The regions shown as dashes are areas of identity with the reference sequence (DRB*0101) at the top. The 90 amino acids comprising the β1 domain of DRB1 is shown in single-letter code from 5' to 3', left to right. The first half represents the β-sheet, and the second half the α-helical portion. The main hypervariable regions are in the vicinity of residues 10, 30, 47, 56 to 60, and 67 to 86. Amino acids that are shared with at least one other allele are underlined to show that some polymorphic segments are utilized in several alleles; for example, EYSTS in *03011, *11011, *1301, *1401, and EYSTG in *1201 and *0801. The first three alleles of DR4 are shown to illustrate how these closely related variants are identical in the β-sheet, but have a few single amino acid differences in the α-helix. The distal domains of class I HLA-A, -B, -C, and class II HLA-DQ and -DP show similar regions of variability, although each locus has a unique sequence signature in its constant regions. The locus-specific constant regions provide a means for selective PCR amplification of DRB1 DNA, for example. Subsequent analysis with specific probes or restriction enzymes can then characterize the polymorphisms.

Table 6-2. Effect of HLA Mismatching on Kidney Graft Survival*

Donors	Mismatches*	Half-Life (Years)	10-Year Graft Survival (%)
Living-Related Donors (HLA-identical)	0	24.0	74
Cadaveric Donors 1992 (6 antigen-match)	0	20.3	65
1996 (0 antigen-mismatch)	0	14.0	57
Living-Related Donors (1 HLA haplotype)	3	12.0	54
Living-Unrelated Donor (spouse)	4	12.0	54
Cadaveric Donors	1 to 6	9.0	40
	1 to 2	10.4	45
	3 to 4	8.4	38
	5 to 6	7.7	34

*Total number of antigens considered were 6 (2 As, 2 Bs, and 2 DRs)

were changed in 1996 to permit the no-mismatch cases to be mandated for sharing, the results have declined somewhat, but are still superior to the average cadaveric result for half-life of graft survival (Table 6-2). It is now established that application of molecular techniques for typing can greatly improve accuracy, and allow selection of only those cases that are truly compatible. With regard to more detailed extended typing of individual variants obtainable by molecular typing, such is not needed for organ transplantation, although it is important for unrelated bone marrow transplantation, and for clinical research into defining mismatches that may be predicted to be of low immunogenicity.

Factors other than tissue mismatching of cadaveric transplants can reduce the overall rate of success. This point is illustrated by the results with living unrelated donor transplants, which have short ischemic times and come from carefully evaluated donors. These kidneys provide results comparable to one haplotype-matched family donors, when they might be expected to be in the less successful range of three to four antigen-mismatched cadaveric donors (Table 6-2).

An important fact of clinical immunogenetics is that mismatches for each of the three HLA loci do not have equal influence on outcomes. UNOS data show that mismatches for HLA-A do not exert a deleterious effect until after the first year of engraftment, and an analysis from Eurotransplant shows further that DR incompatibility is important during the first six months, B incompatibility effects last up until two years, and A incompatibility first shows its effects after three years.

In order to provide improved chances for the 80% of patients who cannot be HLA matched, various schemes to include more patients, particularly ethnic groups who do not match well with the northern European population, have been proposed. The first scheme was based upon the CREG (crossreactive groups) phenomenon seen with antisera that contain antibodies that identify "public" antigens that are common to groupings of the "private" antigens shown in Table 6-3. These patterns are not easily explained by amino acid sequences, but the existence of human antibodies that define them suggests that they do mark antigens that play a role in rejection. If CREG groups were to be used for matching, their lower frequency would make it easier to declare a match.

OTHER HISTOCOMPATIBILITY SYSTEMS

Minor Histocompatibility Antigens (minor H)

As single incompatibilities in the mouse, minor H are characterized by skin graft rejection times of 60 to 100 days, while H-2 incompatibility evokes rejection in six to eight days. Multiple minor incompatibilities can be additive, and can equal the strength of H-2, especially when the recipient has been previously immunized to the donor. Another general feature of minor H systems is the lack of an antibody response to them, in contrast to the strong cellular cytotoxic T cell response that develops. Minor H are restricted by MHC class I antigens, meaning that the attacking and target cells must share an MHC class I antigen. The only human minor H specificity that can be easily identified is in cases where the cytotoxicity of female effector cells occurs only on male target cells that bear a shared class I antigen. This minor H is antigen encoded by the male Y chromosome. Minor H systems, as defined in inbred mice, are peptides, and priming requires help from CD4+ cells in order to develop the CD8+ response. Some progress is being made in defining several human minor H systems.

A possible future role in organ transplantation would be to assess patients having repeat transplants for the likelihood of sensitization to minor H, based upon genotyping for minor H incompatibilities, and consideration of donor and recipient class I HLA alleles as restricting elements.

Monocyte-Endothelial Antigens

Not all non-MHC antigens are minor H. There are tissue-restricted antigenic systems that may generate antibody responses of potential harm to the graft. HLA-identical sibling recipients can generate antibodies that

Table 6-3. Serologically-Defined HLA Antigens

Broad Antigen	Splits*	Crossreactive Groups (CREGs)†						
A1		A1C1	A1C2	A1C3				
A3		A1C1	A1C2	A1C3				
A11		A1C1	A1C2	A1C3				
A2					A2C1	A2C2	A2C3	
A9	A23,24	A1C1				A2C2		
A10	A25,26	A1C1		A1C3	A2C1			A28C
A19	A29,30,31,32,33,74	A1C1		A1C3				A28C
A28								A28C
A29	A68,69				A2C1	A2C2		A28C
A36		A1C1						
B5	B51,52	B5C						
B7			B7C					
B8				B8C				
B12	B44,45				B12C			
B13			B7C					
B14	B64,65			B8C				
B15	B62,63,75,76,77	B5C						
B16	B38,39			B8C		B22C		
B17	B57,58	B5C						
B18		B5C		B8C				
B21	B49,50	B5C			B12C			
B22	B54,55,56		B7C			B22C		
B27			B7C					
B35		B5C						
B37								
B40	B60,61		B7C		B12C			
B41					B12C			
B42			B7C			B22C		
B47			B7C					
B48			B7C					
B59				B8C				
B70	B71,72	B5C						
DR1								
DR2	DR15,16							
DR3	DR17,18							
DR4								
DR5	DR11,DDR12							
DR6	DDR13,DR14							
DR7								
DR8								
DR9								
DR10								
DQ1	DQ5,6							
DQ2								
DQ3	DQ7,8,9							

*Distinct antigens closely related to the original "parent" broader grouping.
†CREGs are complex serological patterns, unrelated to splits, for which there is evidence of shared immunogenicity.

bind to donor endothelium, and also to monocytes, and in some cases skin. A high graft failure rate may occur if transplants are done in the face of such a positive cross-match. The difficulty has been in defining this system at a molecular and genetic level, and it is further compounded by a lack of useful typing antisera, and the extreme difficulty in applying crossmatch techniques in tissue typing laboratories, since it appears that only some cases have antibodies that crossreact with monocytes.

ABH Blood Groups

In the clinical setting, the donor and recipient major red blood cell groups are considered first, and appropriate matching for these is taken for granted. However, no review of immunogenetics would be complete without a few words about these polysaccharide antigens that are expressed on the endothelium. Attempts to cross the barrier against natural anti-A and anti-B blood group antibodies has a high risk of hyperacute rejection. Group "O" means lacking A or B, but the basic polysaccharide structure called "H" is still present. The matching rules apply as in blood banking; however, the group O "universal" donor is a special situation. Organ procurement organizations have had to restrict such donors to O recipients to avoid putting the list of waiting O recipients at a disadvantage. The genes controlling ABH expression are not linked to HLA. In working up family members as kidney donors, one must be prepared for the disappointment of finding HLA-identical pairs who have a forbidden ABH incompatibility.

In lifesaving emergent transplant situations with heart, lung, or liver recipients, plasmapheresis to reduce the anti-A and anti-B titer has been employed with some success. A state of adaptation in which a rising titer no longer harms the graft can occur if the graft is sustained for several days. A similar phenomenon of adaptation has been reported in some experimental xenograft studies with discordant antibodies.

RECOMMENDED READING

Brown JH, Jardetzky TS, Gorga JC, et al. Three-dimensional structure of the human class II histocompatibility antigen HLA-DR1. Nature. 1993;364(6432):33-39.

Carpenter CB. Histocompatibility systems. In: Ginns LC, Cosimi AB, Morris PJ, eds. Transplantation. Boston, MA: Blackwell Science Inc. 1999:60-78.

Takemoto S, Terasaki PI, Cecka JM, Cho YW, Gjertson DW. Survival of nationally shared HLA-matched kidney transplants from cadaveric donors. N Engl J Med. 1992;327(12):834-839.

Zantvoort FA, D'Amaro J, Persijn GG, et al. The impact of HLA-A matching on long-term survival of renal allografts. Transplantation. 1996;61(5):841-844.

Takemoto SK, Terasaki PI. Evaluation of the transplant recipient and donor: molecular approach to tissue typing, flow cytometry and alternative approaches to distributing organs. Curr Opin Nephrol Hypertens. 1997;6(3):299-303.

Mytilineos J, Scherer S, Opelz G. Comparison of RFLP-DR beta and serological HLA-DR typing in 1500 individuals. Transplantation. 1990;50(5):870-873.

Mytilineos J, Lempert M, Middleton D, et al. HLA class I DNA typing of 215 "HLA-A, -B, -DR zero mismatched" kidney transplants. Tissue Antigens. 1997;50(4):355-355.

Carpenter CB. HLA class I DNA typing in organ transplantation. Tissue Antigens. 1997;50(4):322-325.

Doxiadis II, Smits JM, Schreuder GM, et al. Association between specific HLA combinations and probability of kidney allograft loss: the taboo concept. Lancet. 1996;348(9031):850-853.

Pfeffer PF, Thorsby E. HLA-restricted cytotoxicity against male-specific (H-Y) antigen after acute rejection of an HLA-identical sibling kidney: clonal distribution of the cytotoxic cells. Transplantation. 1982;33(1):52-56.

Simpson E, Roopenian D. Minor histocompatibility antigens. Curr Opin Immunol. 1997;9:655-661.

7 CLINICAL IMMUNOGENETICS
Douglas J. Norman, MD

Clinical immunogenetics encompasses activities conducted in the tissue typing laboratory. These are: (1) tissue typing, which determines the ABO and HLA types of donors and recipients; (2) detection of anti-HLA antibodies in the sera of prospective transplant recipients; and (3) performing assays, known collectively as the crossmatch, which detect the presence of antibodies that specifically bind to the cells of a prospective donor. ABO compatibility is essential for the survival of transplanted organs. Minimizing HLA antigen mismatches improves the survival of kidney, pancreas and heart allografts. A negative crossmatch, indicating the absence of donor-directed antibodies, is key to the immediate survival and quality of function of kidney, pancreas and heart allografts. Interestingly, neither antigen matching nor the presence of anti-donor antibodies appear to have any important effect on the outcome of liver transplantation.

TISSUE TYPING
ABO Blood Group Typing

ABO blood group antigens are present on most tissues, in differing amounts, and serve as targets of naturally occurring IgM and IgG antibodies. Hyperacute rejection occurs in patients with a high titer of anti-A or anti-B antibodies who are given an incompatible organ. The standard of practice in organ transplantation is to avoid incompatible donor-recipient combinations. United Network for Organ Sharing (UNOS) regulations have gone further by requiring ABO identity, which prevents blood group O organs from being used for group A recipients. Group A recipients' waiting times for transplant are already the shortest.

A_2 INTO O, AND A_2 AND A_2B INTO B BLOOD TYPES. Blood group A has several subtypes, and one of these, A_2, is present in significantly lower amounts than A_1 on red cells and other tissues. Consequently, organs from blood group A_2 donors can be used successfully in group O and B recipients. A caveat for using A_2 kidneys is that the IgG anti-A antibody titer (conventionally, this has been the anti-A_1 titer) should be less than 1:8. Moreover, if the IgM titer is greater than 1:8, it may be useful to perform plasmapheresis immediately before,

Professor of Medicine; Director, Transplantation Medicine Program; Director, Laboratory of Immunogenetics and Transplantation, Oregon Health Sciences University, Portland, OR

and twice on successive days after transplantation. If renal dysfunction occurs after transplantation and the anti-A antibody titer has increased by two or more dilutions, plasmapheresis can be used again.

Typing for Major Histocompatibility Complex (MHC) Antigens

MHC GENE EXPRESSION. The MHC contains genes whose products are important targets of the alloimmune response. These are known as HLA. Class I HLA gene products are A, B and C. Class II HLA gene products are DP, DQ and DR. As detailed in Chapter 6, HLA genes are highly polymorphic. Through a process of recombination and gene transfer, multiple different nucleotide sequences for each gene have evolved. Since each gene has multiple different alleles, there are millions of possible combinations of HLA types. HLA-A, -B and -DR are generally typed for the purpose of sharing cadaveric kidneys. While HLA-C, -DP and -DQ are immunogenic, and are also targets of the alloimmune response, it is impractical to attempt to match for all of the antigens among unrelated individuals. Even with a mandatory national kidney sharing program, only approximately 15% of the cadaveric transplants performed in the US are mismatched for zero A, B and DR molecules. In families in which one sibling desires to be a donor for another, matching for the A, B and DR alleles on one chromosome usually results in matching for the other MHC genes as well, so there is little need to directly type for the others.

To use matching of HLA for organ allocation, techniques to accurately type HLA are needed. The terms *high-resolution* and *low-resolution* are used to indicate the precision with which HLA typing is achieved. High-resolution typing can identify single amino acid differences among HLA molecules that appear to be identical using low-resolution techniques. For bone marrow transplantation, using unrelated donors, the precision of typing is very important. Therefore, high-resolution techniques are used. Low-resolution techniques are sufficient for solid organ transplantation. When using low-resolution techniques, it is still rare to find perfect matches among the 35,000 patients on the kidney transplant waiting list for the small number of cadaver organ donors that become available each year. Among siblings and other relatives who wish to donate a kidney to a family member, low-resolution techniques are also sufficient to identify two, one or zero haplotype-matched donors.

METHODS USED FOR HLA TYPING
Typing the HLA Gene Products. The classical, low-resolution methods for HLA typing are serological techniques that employ antibodies capable of detecting the HLA molecules expressed on the surfaces of cells. The

HLA phenotype of an individual is determined by the HLA molecules that are displayed on the cell surface. Monospecific anti-HLA antibodies, produced in some people as a result of a natural immune response to transfusions, pregnancy and tissue transplantation, are used for phenotyping. The assays used for serological typing rely on the ability of these antibodies to bind to and kill, via complement activation, lymphocytes that express the specific HLA molecule. The technique for complement-dependent cytotoxicity assays will be detailed later in this chapter. Serological techniques are approximately 98% accurate in identifying class I molecules correctly, but only about 85% accurate in typing class II molecules. Sharing of kidneys via the UNOS point system relies heavily on HLA matching, so a more accurate method for typing class II is needed. This need is met by typing HLA genes directly.

Typing HLA Genes. Three techniques are used for typing HLA genes. All use polymerase chain reaction (PCR) technology to amplify the HLA genes, making ample material available for typing. The first technique is called the SSP or sequence specific primer technique. Primers specific for the different alleles of an HLA gene of interest (eg, HLA-DQ 1, 2, 3, etc.) are added, in multiple separate tubes, to the DNA of the person being typed. A control primer for a universally present gene is also added to each tube. The DNA is amplified using a PCR technique. Only if the specific allele is present in the individual's DNA, will two products from one tube be amplified. The contents of the tubes are put in separate lanes on a gel, and an electric current is applied to separate the DNA fragments according to their size. If both primers successfully anneal to and amplify their target nucleotide sequences, two bands of DNA are seen in the lane used for the contents of that tube. Most of the tubes yield lanes with only the single band representing the control gene. SSP can be used for both high-resolution and low-resolution typing and is the most commonly used technique for solid organ transplantation. The primers used determine the resolution of the typing. Low-resolution typing uses primers that will amplify all the subtypes of an HLA allele (eg, DRB1*0401 through 0424 to identify DRB1*04, also known as DR4). For high-resolution typing, primers specific for each subtype are used, requiring many more primers and tubes.

The second technique is called the SSOP or sequence specific oligonucleotide probe technique. *Probes,* or nucleotide sequences specific for the different alleles of an HLA gene are separately placed on a membrane. Using PCR and the appropriate broad primer, multiple copies of the entire HLA gene of interest (eg, HLA-DR) are obtained from the person being typed. The amplified DNA is labeled with any substance that allows for its detection and flooded onto the membrane con-

taining the specific, separately located probes. After an appropriate time to allow the annealing of DNA to a probe, the nonannealed DNA is washed off the membrane. The location of the labeled DNA on the membrane determines the specific HLA type of the patient. SSOP is commonly used for high-resolution typing.

The third technique uses a DNA sequencer that determines the actual nucleotide sequence of the HLA gene of interest. This high-resolution technique relies on expensive equipment, is very useful for unrelated bone marrow transplantation, but is unnecessary for solid organ transplantation.

IMPORTANCE OF HLA MATCHING. Matching for HLA is highly useful in kidney transplantation. Approximately 30% of kidney transplants are now performed using living donors. When the option is available, the living donor with the best HLA match to the recipient is chosen. HLA-identical, or two haplotype-matched, sibling donors are clearly superior to all other donors for achieving long-term graft survival. The half-life of these grafts (25 to 30 years) is twice as long as the next best match. Among living donors, including unrelated donors, graft survival is worse with each mismatch for the six HLA-A, -B and -DR molecules. Mismatches for HLA also affect graft survival from cadaveric donors. There is a mandatory requirement to share cadaver kidneys for a recipient who has no mismatches for HLA-A, -B and -DR. Morever, the point system established by UNOS for allocating cadaver kidneys locally and regionally is heavily based on the number of mismatched HLA antigens. Matching for HLA also has a significant impact on the survival of heart allografts. Heart allocation is not based on HLA, because ABO and size matching, as well as patient illness status have priority for allocation. Accounting for these leaves only a small number of potential local recipients for whom adding HLA matching criteria would be futile. In addition, hearts cannot be shipped long distances because of a limited allowable ischemia time. HLA matching also has relevance in pancreas transplantation, but it appears to have none in liver transplantation.

Some people are homozygous for an HLA allele. That is, the gene is the same on both chromosomes. It is a convention in solid organ transplantation to refer to a *mismatch* rather than to a *match* when comparing donor and recipient HLA types. The immune response to an allograft is only directed one way, from the recipient to the donor. Therefore, only the HLA antigens that the recipient sees as different, or mismatched from his own are important. An example is illustrated in Figure 7-1, which demonstrates the value of referring to a mismatch rather than to a match. Alex and Sage are a four antigen-match (A2, B7, B8, DR3) as are Alex and Abbie (A1, A2, B8, DR3). If Alex is the recipient, however, Sage, who is a

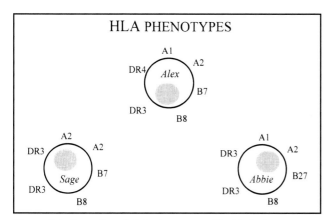

Figure 7-1. Examples of HLA phenotypes. The HLA phenotype is the expression of the HLA gene products or HLA molecules on the surface of cells such as lymphocytes. This figure illustrates the use of "match" and "mismatch" terminology when referring to organ donors and recipients. The preferred term is "mismatch" especially when either the donor or recipient are homozygous for an HLA allele. Homozygosity refers to the expression of the same allele at a specific gene locus on both chromosomes. For example, in this figure Sage is homozygous for HLA-A2 and HLA-DR3, and Abbie is homozygous for HLA-DR3. Assume that Alex is a prospective recipient, and Sage and Abbie are possible donors. Both Sage and Abbie are matched with Alex for 4 HLA antigens (Sage: A2, B7, B8, DR3; Abbie: A1, A2, B8, DR3). However, when Alex looks at Abbie he sees one mismatched antigen (B27). When he looks at Sage he sees no mismatched antigens. Sage is the preferred donor. If Sage was the prospective recipient, Alex and Abbie are both two antigen-mismatches (Alex: A1, DR4; Abbie: A1, B27). Early kidney graft failure is more common when mismatches for HLA class II molecules are present than when mismatches for class I molecules are present. Abbie is the preferred donor for Sage.

zero antigen-mismatch, is the better choice as a donor. Abbie is a one antigen-mismatch (B27). The donor with the fewer mismatches is always the better choice. The antigens that are mismatched also matter. If Sage was the recipient, Abbie would be the best donor even though both Alex and Abbie are two antigen-mismatches for Sage. DR mismatches are more important to avoid than A or B mismatches. The UNOS point system for kidney allocation assigns points according to the number of mismatched HLA antigens.

DETECTING THE PRESENCE OF ANTI-HLA ANTIBODIES

Anti-HLA antibodies are made following exposure to blood transfusions, pregnancy or tissue transplants. These antibodies are potentially dangerous in transplantation because they can react with HLA molecules on the endothelia of a transplanted organ's blood vessels, including glomerular capillaries, causing inflammatory endotheliitis, fibrin deposition, clotting and irreversible ischemic damage to the organ. It is useful to know whether a patient has anti-HLA antibodies before he or she is placed on the waiting list.

The presence of anti-HLA antibodies determines the patient's risk status. A patient with a high level of broadly reactive anti-HLA antibodies, referred to as a sensitized patient, requires the use of a sensitive assay at the time of transplant to ensure the absence of antibodies directed against a prospective donor. The presence of antibodies, even if specific anti-donor antibodies are not present, predicts earlier, more frequent and more severe rejection episodes. Thus, stronger immunosuppression (ie, antilymphocyte antibodies for induction, mycophenolate mofetil for maintenance) and closer surveillance for rejection are warranted.

The level of antibodies predicts how long a patient may need to wait for a transplant. Sensitized patients wait a very long time because antibodies that will react with most donors are present. For such a patient, a donor who is mismatched for few, if any, HLA antigens must be found. The absence of any antibodies predicts a much earlier transplant. In the US, there is a nationally mandated kidney allocation scheme. In this scheme, additional points are assigned to a patient with antibodies that react with 80% or more of a standard lymphocyte panel because, for them, it is normally difficult to find a donor. If an antibody is ever found in a patient's serum that reacts with a specific HLA antigen, donors with that HLA antigen are avoided. Even if that antibody is not present in a patient's current serum, it is assumed that memory cells exist and that the specific antibody will be made again, after the patient encounters that HLA antigen on the transplanted organ.

The work done in the tissue typing laboratory can be simplified by knowing a patient's level of antibodies prior to listing the patient. The final crossmatch performed using a donor's cells and a potential recipient's sera consists of two, three and sometimes four different assays. It is impractical to perform all of these assays each time a sensitized patient is considered for transplant. Instead, the sera of sensitized patients are placed on screening trays. The least sensitive assay is used to determine which patients, if any, have a negative result with a donor. All of the assays are then performed using the sera of these and some of the nonsensitized patients. Only a few nonsensitized patients at the top of the list, based on points assigned for level of antigen-mismatch and time waiting, need to be crossmatched with a donor. Nonsensitized patients are unlikely to test positive in the crossmatch assays. Since only two kidneys are available per donor, it is impractical to perform a crossmatch on more than five or six nonsensitized patients. Finally, it is important to identify sera with anti-HLA antibodies for use in the pretransplant crossmatch. A periodic performance of assays to detect antibodies will identify which sera should be used in the crossmatch. Currently, it is required that an assay must be performed to detect anti-HLA antibodies a minimum of every three months on all patients waiting for a cadaveric kidney transplant.

Techniques Used to Detect the Presence of Anti-HLA Antibodies

CONVENTIONAL METHODS. Anti-HLA antibodies are conventionally called panel reactive antibodies, or PRA. Historically, the earliest method for detecting antibodies used a panel of lymphocytes selected from 40 to 60 individuals who were chosen to represent the widest variety of HLA antigens possible. The breadth of antibodies present in a patient's serum is determined by counting the number, or percent, of individuals in the panel whose cells are killed. A PRA of 50% indicates that a patient has antibodies in his or her serum that react with the cells from 50% of the individuals selected for the panel. Today, there are a variety of assays used to detect anti-HLA antibodies. These assays determine whether anti-HLA antibodies are present, the breadth of antibodies present, and/or the specificity of antibodies present.

The classical assays for detecting antibodies rely on their ability to kill target cells by activating complement. These are called cytotoxicity assays. The necessary components for these assays are live target cells, serum from a patient, a source of complement, and a vital dye to detect cell death. Target cells can be either peripheral blood lymphocytes, of which 80% to 90% are T cells, or an enriched population of B cells (eg, chronic lymphocytic leukemia [CLL] cells). The specifics of the three common cytotoxicity assays used, the NIH standard, the antiglobulin-enhanced, and the B cell-enriched, are reviewed in more detail below. The cytotoxicity assays can determine the breadth of antibodies, known as the percent PRA, and also the specificity of antibodies present. One disadvantage of this type of assay is that it generally cannot determine for certain if broadly reactive antibodies are directed to HLA or to some other molecules that reside on lymphocytes. The importance of making this distinction is that some molecules on lymphocytes might not be on organ cells. Another disadvantage is that it cannot easily differentiate between IgG and IgM antibodies. IgM antibodies are generally considered benign and are often auto-antibodies induced by drugs and not directed to HLA molecules. Dithiothreitol (DTT), which destroys IgM, is often used to differentiate between IgG and IgM, however, it can dilute and cause a weak IgG antibody to disappear.

NEWER METHODS. Newer methods for detecting anti-HLA antibodies use soluble HLA molecules that are bound to plastic trays, beads or strips. The soluble HLA molecules are obtained from the intact cells of HLA typed individuals. The advantage of assays that use HLA molecules is that the antibodies detected in a patient's serum are known to be directed to HLA and not to molecules that have no importance in transplantation. The assays used to detect antibodies are either enzyme-linked immunoabsorption (ELISA) or flow cytometry assays. Both assays can determine with reasonable accuracy whether anti-HLA antibodies are present, can measure their breadth or the percent PRA, can differentiate between IgG and IgM antibodies, and can determine if the antibodies are directed to HLA class I molecules, class II molecules, or both. Only the ELISA assays can determine the specificity of anti-HLA antibodies. Individuals whose cells are selected for harvesting HLA molecules represent a spectrum of HLA types.

The flow cytometry assay uses beads with adherent HLA molecules. An aliquot of beads contains either class I or class II HLA molecules from a large number of typed individuals who also represent a spectrum of HLA types. After incubation with a patient's serum and xeno anti-human antibodies labeled with a fluorochrome, the beads are passed through a flow cytometer. The percent PRA equivalence is determined by the intensity of light emitted from the fluorochromes on the cells. Increasing numbers of antibodies directed to different HLA molecules will cause increased light emission.

THE PRETRANSPLANT CROSSMATCH

The most important activity in the tissue typing laboratory is performing the crossmatch, which detects donor-directed antibodies in the sera of a potential transplant recipient. The crossmatch is primarily aimed at preventing hyperacute rejection, an immediate and devastating immunological event. A secondary purpose of the crossmatch, using more sensitive techniques, is detecting antibodies that can gradually destroy a graft during the first year after transplant, or that can predict the occurrence of early or advanced rejection episodes. The crossmatch in cadaver donor transplantation is performed immediately before a transplant for the purpose of selecting, from among a number of potential recipients, those who have no anti-donor antibodies. The crossmatch for living donor transplantation is performed to select, from among a number of volunteer donors, one or more whose cells do not react with the potential recipient's serum.

A current serum sample and selected sera from the past are always tested in the crossmatch. Past sera are selected if anti-HLA antibodies were found on routine screening. Generally, the one or two samples with the highest PRA are selected. These sera can be tested using four different crossmatch assays. A review of each of these follows below.

The NIH Standard Crossmatch Technique

The NIH standard crossmatch has been used, with some minor variations, since the late 1960s. This is the least sensitive but most specific of the assays. A positive result using this technique suggests the presence of anti-HLA class I antibodies, is highly predictive of hyperacute rejections, and is an absolute contraindication to transplantation of kidney, pancreas and heart allografts. A negative result cannot predict long-term success, however, since the standard assay fails to detect small amounts of anti-class I or anti-HLA class II antibodies (Figure 7-2). The presence of complement-activating anti-donor antibodies creates pores in donor cell membranes causing them to expand with extracellular water and vital dye. Live cells remain small and exclude the vital dye. Table 7-1 shows the original data demonstrating the specificity of this assay. Eighty percent of kidney grafts failed immediately in patients with a positive test result. However, the 15% immediate graft loss seen even when the test was negative demonstrates its

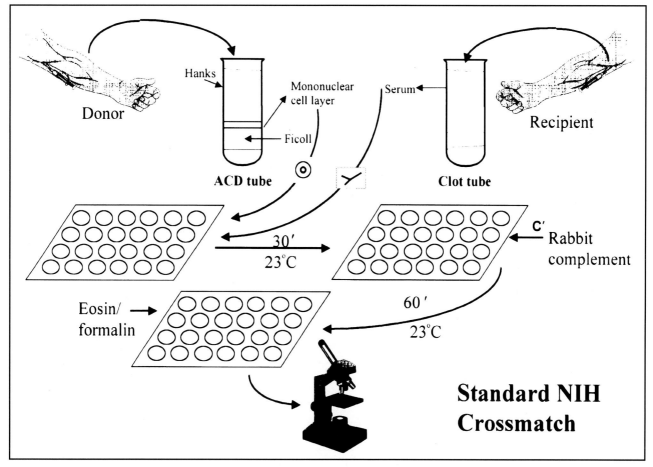

Figure 7-2. The NIH Standard Crossmatch Technique. This is a cytotoxicity assay that has three main components: donor cells, recipient serum and complement. Donor cells are obtained from an anticoagulated (ACD indicates acid citrate dextrose) sample of blood separated into a mononuclear cell layer, and a plasma and red cell layer using Ficoll-Hypaque and centrifugation. The mononuclear cell layer is aspirated, washed and suspended in a standard solution. The cells are placed in microtiter plates. Recipient serum is obtained from a clot tube and added, in different dilutions, to the cells in the plates. Cells and serum are incubated for 30 minutes at room temperature. Rabbit serum is then added as a source of complement and the trays are incubated for an additional hour at room temperature. Formalin is then added to stop the reaction, and a vital dye such as eosin is added to help differentiate between live and dead cells. The trays are placed on an inverted phase microscope and evaluated by a technologist for the presence of live or dead cells. Each well, which contains a different serum or a different dilution of that serum, or a positive or negative control, is read separately and scored for percent-cytotoxicity.

For the antiglobulin-enhanced crossmatch, the cells are washed three times after the first 30 minute incubation, and then the anti-human antibodies and rabbit serum are added together and incubated with the cells for one hour at room temperature. Formalin and eosin dye are then added and the trays are evaluated in the same way.

For the B cell-enriched crossmatch, B cells are isolated using metallic beads, with attached anti-class II antibodies, and a magnet. The B cells are washed and labeled with carboxyfluorescein diacetate (CFDA) and added to microtiter plates with recipient serum. The cells and serum are incubated at 37 degrees for 60 minutes. Rabbit serum is added and the trays are incubated for an additional two hours at room temperature. Ethidium bromide is then added, the trays are incubated for an additional five minutes and then washed three times before being viewed using a fluorescence microscope. Live cells are small, contain CFDA, and exclude ethidium bromide. Dead cells are larger, the ethidium bromide has entered the cells, and the CFDA has leaked out.

lack of sensitivity. Only four percent of grafts failed in patients who did not have any detectable anti-HLA antibodies in sera screened in the weeks before transplant.

The Anti-Human Globulin-Enhanced Crossmatch Technique

Since the standard crossmatch technique lacks sensitivity, additional assays are used. One of these is the anti-human globulin (AHG)-enhanced technique. The key to making this assay more sensitive is the addition of an anti-human immunoglobulin antibody. The purpose of this assay is to enhance the ability of antibodies to lyse target cells. Anti-donor antibodies may not be able to lyse donor cells using the NIH standard assay because they are inefficient, or present in insufficient amounts to activate complement. Goat (or other xeno antibody) anti-human immunoglobulin-heavy and -light chain antibodies will bind to any human antibodies that are bound to donor cells, and will provide the necessary crosslinking to activate complement. Table 7-2 shows

data indicating that this is a more sensitive technique than the NIH standard assay. Among both primary and regrafted cadaveric donor kidney recipients in whom a standard crossmatch was negative, the one-year graft survival rate was significantly better when the AHG assay was also negative. Generally, the antibodies that cause the AHG assay to be positive when the standard assay is negative are not present in amounts large enough to cause hyperacute rejection. However, their presence influences graft survival and, therefore, transplantation should be avoided when the AHG crossmatch is positive.

The B Cell-Enriched Crossmatch Technique

Another assay that adds additional sensitivity to the crossmatch is the B cell-enriched crossmatch. B cells express both HLA class I and II molecules. As indicated above, and also in Chapter 6, class I molecules are present on the endothelial and interstitial cells of a transplanted organ and are the primary targets of the alloimmune

---

Table 7-1. Role of the NIH Standard Crossmatch in Kidney Transplant Outcomes

Graft Survival	Recipients with Anti-HLA Antibodies			Recipients without Anti-HLA Antibodies
	Positive Crossmatch	No Crossmatch	Negative Crossmatch	
Immediate Failure	24 (80%)	6 (26%)	4 (15%)	4 (2.4%)
Failure < 3 months	0	6	4	32
Failure > 3 months	1	3	7	22
Survival < 3 months	2	2	1	6
Survival > 3 months	3 (10%)	6 (26%)	11 (41%)	104 (62%)
Total Patients	30	23	27	168
	80			

Patel R, Terasaki PI. Significance of the positive crossmatch test in kidney transplantation. N Engl J Med. 1969;280(14):735-739.

Table 7-2. Role of Anti-Human Globulin Enhanced Crossmatch on One-Year Kidney Transplant Outcomes. All patients had negative NIH standard crossmatches.

Cadaveric Kidney Donor Recipients	Negative NIH Standard Crossmatch			P-Value
	All Patients	Anti-human Globulin Crossmatch		
		Negative	Positive	
	2-Year Graft Survival			
First Transplants	81% (N=166)	82% (N=151)	67% (N=15)	<0.01
Re-transplants	64% (N=70)	77% (N=48)	36% (N=22)	<0.01

Kerman RH, Kimball PM, Van Buren CT, et al. AHG and DTE/AHG procedure identification of crossmatch-appropriate donor-recipient pairings that result in improved graft survival. Transplantation. 1991;51(2):316-320.

response. Class II molecules have a limited tissue distribution but are present in small amounts on venous endothelium, and can be expressed on injured endothelial and interstitial cells. Antibodies to HLA class II can influence graft survival. However, they are not efficiently detected using the standard or AHG techniques because resting T cells do not express class II molecules and the target cells used in those assays are mostly T cells. Eighty to ninety percent of peripheral blood lymphocytes are T cells. The use of a technique that uses an enriched population of donor B cells as targets allows for the detection of anti-donor class II antibodies. Table 7-3 shows that the use of an assay using B cells as targets can improve graft survival. Among the entire group of cadaveric and living donor recipients with a negative standard crossmatch, the group with a negative, compared with positive, B cell crossmatch had significantly better two-year graft survival. Despite these data and others like it, not all transplant programs use a B cell crossmatch. This is because, in general, anti-donor class II antibodies have a delayed effect on graft survival. However, there have been case reports of anti-HLA class II antibodies causing hyperacute rejection. An approach to transplantation that favors the most conservative use of organs would include a B cell crossmatch. An approach that emphasizes patient access to transplantation might have only a limited use of the B cell crossmatch. Ultimately, if grafts fail early, patient access to transplantation will become even more limited. This is because patients with failed grafts are usually relisted to an already growing waiting list.

The Flow Cytometry Crossmatch Technique

The above assays, which add more sensitivity to the crossmatch, subtract specificity. The diminished specificity is evident when observing the outcomes of grafts in patients who were found to have a positive result in either the AHG or B cell-enriched crossmatches (see tables). Certainly, not all of the grafts failed, even at one

and two years. In contrast, 80% of grafts failed immediately in the group with a positive NIH standard crossmatch. The explanation for the diminished specificity of these assays is that, in some cases, they detect antibodies that might not be directed to HLA and therefore will not react with the allograft, or they detect antibodies that are present in small enough amounts that they can be overcome by the use of strong immunosuppression.

The final assay to be reviewed is the most sensitive and least specific of all the techniques. This assay is able to detect even the smallest amount of recipient antibodies that can bind to a donor's cells. Goat (or other xeno antibody) anti-human immunoglobulin antibodies, labeled with a fluorochrome, are added to a tube in which donor cells and recipient serum have incubated together. The xeno antibodies will bind to recipient antibodies that are bound to donor cells. The fluorochrome present on the xeno antibody will become activated by the laser beam and emit photons when the cells are passed through a flow cytometer. The intensity of the light emitted from a sample of donor cells is directly related to the amount of anti-donor antibodies present in a recipient's serum. Even when the standard AHG and B cell-enriched crossmatches are negative, the flow crossmatch can still detect additional antibodies directed to donor cells. Figure 7-3 shows results of retrospective flow crossmatches in 171 patients with negative crossmatches using standard, AHG and B cell-enriched techniques. A number of these patients had significant anti-donor antibodies, as is evident by the intensity of light emitted by the cells in the assay.

Because of its lack of specificity, the flow crossmatch is not routinely used prospectively to determine the suitability of a donor for a recipient. However, there are two situations in which a pretransplant flow crossmatch (FXM) can be useful. The first is for patients who are being transplanted for a second time and whose first graft failed within three months of transplant. Graft survival is significantly better with the second transplant if, in addition to the standard and AHG and B cell-enriched

Table 7-3. Role of B Cell-Enriched Crossmatch on Two-Year Kidney Transplant Outcomes. All patients had negative standard crossmatches.

B Cell Crossmatch Result	Recipients with Anti-HLA Antibodies						All	
	Cadaver		Nonidentical Relative		Identical Relative			
	N	Survival	N	Survival	N	Survival	N	Survival
Positive	33	60%	13	57%	7	71%	56	68%
Negative	37	88%	61	82%	37	100%	137	88%
P-Value	0.015		0.144		0.001		0.001	

Morrow CE, Sutherland DE, Fryd DS, et al. Renal allograft survival in patients with positive B cell crossmatch to their donor. Ann Surg. 1984;199(1):75-78.

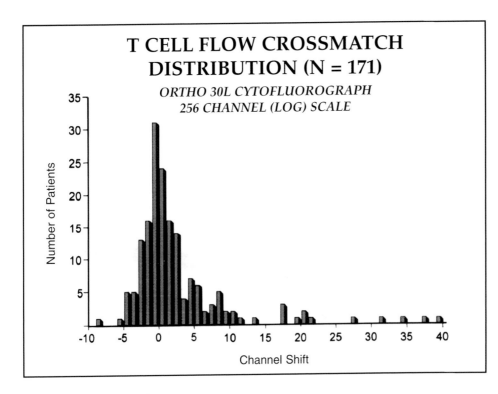

T CELL FLOW CROSSMATCH DISTRIBUTION (N = 171)

ORTHO 30L CYTOFLUOROGRAPH
256 CHANNEL (LOG) SCALE

Figure 7-3. T Cell Flow Crossmatch Distribution. One hundred seventy-one patients who had negative NIH standard, AHG-enhanced and B cell-enriched crossmatches had retrospective flow crossmatches performed following cadaveric kidney transplantation. The results are shown in this figure. The "channel shift" refers to the increase in fluorescence (photons) emitted from donor cells incubated with recipient serum compared to a control serum. A channel shift of greater than zero suggests that there are antibodies in a recipient's serum that are bound to donor cells. A channel shift of greater than ten confirms that there are such antibodies. Sixteen (9%) of these patients were confirmed to have anti-donor antibodies in their sera at the time of transplantation. A few had a high titer of these antibodies, which caused no reaction in the cytotoxicity assays.

crossmatches, the FXM is negative. The second situation is when the cadaver donor cells available to use in the cytotoxic crossmatches are already dead. This makes it impossible to use any complement-dependent cytotoxicity assays for the crossmatch. However, the FXM does not require live cells and can be performed, when necessary, instead of the cytotoxicity assays.

LOGISTICS OF TISSUE TYPING FOR SPECIFIC ORGANS
Kidney
For kidney transplantation, the rules of the various regulating agencies (eg, UNOS, American Society of Histocompatibility [ASHI], Healthcare Financing Administration [HCFA]) dictate which tests to use and how often they need to be performed. A PRA should be determined every three months on all patients on the cadaveric kidney waiting list. A current serum must be used in any crossmatches performed with potential donor cells. Unless a patient has been transfused or seriously ill, any serum obtained in the previous 30 days is generally satisfactory for the current serum. Most programs require that a fresh serum sample must be sent to the laboratory monthly. A pretransplant crossmatch is required in all cases before a donor kidney can be assigned to a particular recipient. A pretransplant crossmatch must include the standard and a more sensitive crossmatch such as the AHG crossmatch. If a patient had been sensitized in the past but currently has few, if any, anti-HLA antibodies, it may be reasonable to disregard the previous sera in the crossmatch. The current serum

must be negative in the crossmatch, including the B cell-enriched crossmatch. Moreover, previously transplanted patients should have a negative flow crossmatch with the current serum. For patients who are being considered for a second or subsequent transplant, the HLA class II antigens of the previous donors should be avoided. This is not true for class I antigens. Also, since the survival of second grafts is worse than for first grafts, antigen match criteria should be stricter.

Heart
For heart transplantation, a prospective crossmatch is necessary if anti-HLA antibodies have been identified in the prospective recipient's serum. In practice, only about 10% of patients will require a prospective crossmatch. Most of the immunogenetics laboratory work is done during the work-up of the patient before he or she is placed on the waiting list. An AHG technique is used for detecting anti-HLA antibodies. In addition, any patient who has been transfused with blood, as well as recipients of ventricular assist devices, should have a prospective crossmatch until six to eight weeks after the event. If no anti-HLA antibodies have developed, it is no longer necessary to do a prospective crossmatch. All women who have tested negative for cytotoxic anti-HLA antibodies on the standard panel tests should have a PRA determined using the flow cytometry and beads method or ELISA technique. If any antibodies are detected using either of these methods, fresh sera should be tested monthly for cytotoxic antibodies while they are on the waiting list.

Pancreas

Criteria for crossmatching prospective pancreas transplant recipients are similar to those for kidney transplants because most of the time a kidney and pancreas are transplanted together.

Liver

Neither tissue matching nor crossmatching are required for liver transplantation.

CONCLUSION

Successful outcomes in transplantation are dependent upon the clinical immunogenetics evaluation and pretransplant testing. This chapter has covered the three key activities conducted in the tissue typing laboratory: tissue typing, detecting the presence of anti-HLA antibodies, and the pretransplant crossmatch. The transplant physician and surgeon need to understand the basic concepts of clinical immunogenetics so they can appreciate the importance of the work conducted in the clinical laboratory. The best transplant programs are those with a highly cooperative relationship between the clinical immunogenetics laboratory and the clinical transplant service.

RECOMMENDED READING

Krensky AM. The HLA system, antigen processing and presentation. Kidney Intl. 1997;58:S2-S7.

Cecka JM. The role of HLA in renal transplantation. Hum Immunol. 1997;56(1-2):6-16.

Dyer PA, Claas FH. A future for HLA matching in clinical transplantation. Eur J Immunogenet. 1997;24(1):17-28.

Takemoto SK, Terasaki PI. Evaluation of the transplant recipient and donor: molecular approach to tissue typing, flow cytometry and alternative approaches to distributing organs. Curr Opin Nephrol Hypertens. 1997;6(3):299-303.

Carpenter CB. HLA class I DNA typing in organ transplantation. Tissue Antigens. 1997;50(4):332-335.

Feucht HE, Oplez G. The humoral immune response towards HLA class II determinants in renal transplantation. Kidney Int. 1996;50(5):1464-1475.

Cook DJ, El Fettouh HIA, Gjertson DW, et al. Flow cytometry crossmatching (FCXM) in the UNOS kidney transplant registry. Clinical Transplants 1998; UCLA Tissue Typing Laboratory. Los Angeles, CA. 413-419.

8   XENOTRANSPLANTATION

Wayne W. Hancock, MD, PhD

Xenotransplantation (ie, transplantation between species) is far from being a standard clinical procedure, with the very limited exceptions of use of acellular porcine heart valves or pig skin for temporary skin coverage following massive burns. However, knowledge of xenotransplantation is relevant to transplant professionals for at least one major reason, the lack of an adequate organ supply.

As reported by the United Network for Organ Sharing (UNOS) in the 1998 Annual Report for the US Scientific Registry for Transplant Recipients and the Organ Procurement and Transplantation Network, 4,327 patients died in 1997 while waiting for an organ transplant. Despite continuing advances in medicine and technology, the demand for organs dramatically outweighs the supply of organ donors. From 1989 to 1998, the number of patients on the waiting list increased at a rate of 14% per year, while the total number of transplants increased by only 6% per year. At these rates, in 2005, the waiting list will be approximately 166 thousand patients long, the bulk of which will be prospective renal transplant recipients.

There are additional reasons for development of clinical xenotransplantation. First, the donor can be engineered such that a xenograft may fulfill more than can be accomplished by an allograft. For example, a diabetic with renal failure might be given a renal xenograft into which insulin-producing cells were genetically engineered. Second, some conditions leading to organ failure can recur in an allograft but not in a xenograft. Thus, a liver xenograft is considered resistant to recurrence of Hepatitis B or other hepatatrophic human viruses. Third, the xenograft can be obtained under optimal conditions, be of an ideal size, and have minimal or no preservation injury.

This chapter reviews the main limitations to xenotransplantation, beginning with hyperacute rejection, which can destroy a vascularized xenograft within minutes in one of the most violent immunologic responses known. Since hyperacute rejection can be overcome, the principles, pathophysiology and remaining barriers to vascularized xenografts are described, followed by a brief consideration of biocompatibility and infectious risks.

Associate Professor of Pathology, Harvard Medical School; Millennium Pharmaceuticals, Inc., Cambridge, MA; Department of Pathology, Beth Israel Deaconess Medical Center and Harvard Medical School, Boston, MA

HISTORY OF XENOTRANSPLANTATION

Scientific reports of xenotransplantation, or heterotransplantation as it was known until the 1970s, were first published over 90 years ago. Princeteau, in 1905, placed slices of rabbit kidney in the nephrotomy of a child with renal failure and noted an immediate increase in urine output and cessation of vomiting, though the patient died of pulmonary complications on day 16. In 1906, Jaboulay tried xenografting with vascular anastomosis of a pig kidney, and in a second case, a goat kidney, into the antecubital space, but neither graft functioned, apparently due to vascular thrombosis. In 1910, Unger grafted the kidneys of a nonhuman primate into a man with renal failure, but the patient died at 32 hours with venous thromboses. Neuhof, in 1923, transplanted the kidney of a lamb into a patient dying of mercury poisoning; the patient died nine days later, apparently of nonrenal causes. Scientific interest declined in the 1920s, as it became clear that transplants were subject to a powerful immune response.

In the 1950s, as immunosuppressive drugs were developed and allografting between twins was shown to overcome renal failure and provide a good quality of life, interest in transplantation was renewed. However, problems with organ procurement and limited knowledge of organ preservation severely curtailed development of allograft programs. Thus, groups led by Reemtsma, Starzl and others began programs of experimental xenotransplantation using chimpanzees, or baboons, who gave far less satisfactory results as donors. A series of patients who were maintained on dialysis were offered the choice of supportive therapy: an allograft (living-related or cadaveric) if and when available, or a xenograft. The longest xenograft survival (still unsurpassed) was in a patient who, in 1963, received a chimpanzee renal graft and died, with normal renal function, of an unexplained intercurrent illness after nine months. Soberingly, at post-mortem, histologic evidence of chronic rejection was noted.

Based on such experience, a consensus was reached between the groups active in the field that, compared to baboons or Rhesus monkeys, the chimpanzee was the best choice as a nonhuman primate donor. However, even in the 1960s, only minuscule numbers of chimpanzees were available for this purpose, and this situation became worse in later years as the chimpanzee was listed as an endangered species. By 1965, chronic dialysis and cadaveric transplantation became available, and in the absence of effective means to control xenograft rejection, all groups discontinued their clinical xenograft studies.

CHOICE OF A DONOR SPECIES AND RISK OF ZOONOSES

Given the restrictions on use of chimpanzees, other species have received attention as potential sources of organs for human xenotransplantation. Baboons are approximately 30 times as plentiful as chimpanzees, but major barriers exist to the use of any subhuman primates. None of these species do well in captivity; all have long gestation times and few offspring; and their use is expensive, leads to widespread objections on ethical and social grounds, and may be associated with risks of infections. The US Food and Drug Administration's Biological Response Modifiers Advisory Committee (BRMAC), in hearings completed in July 1995, evaluated the public health significance of clinical trials using xenogeneic tissues. Summaries and recommendations from these hearings were published in the Federal Register, and guidelines and legislation to regulate application of xenotransplantation remain under review. With the background of the HIV epidemic and recent Ebola virus outbreaks, the BRMAC expressed concern over the potential for inadvertent transmission of infectious agents that would pose a threat to the recipient, health care workers, their contacts, and potentially, the general community. BRMAC considered that primate donors pose the greatest risk for transmission of latent or intracellular organisms, including retroviruses.

Seeking an alternative, most investigators have settled on use of pigs as xenograft donors. Over 90 million pigs are raised and slaughtered in the US each year. In contrast to nonhuman primates, pigs breed well in captivity, have large litters, and their use raises few objections in the broad community. BRMAC considered that use of pig tissues for xenotransplantation was less likely to introduce new pathogens to humans, given the already close and prolonged contact with these species. The FDA regulatory guidelines for xenotransplantation are expected to: (1) promote development of animal sources of donor organs, which are free of zoonotic disease; (2) place responsibility for ensuring the quality of donor tissues on the supplier; (3) urge transplant teams to independently monitor the microbial status of donor tissues; and (4) provide long-term follow-up of patients and their contacts for development of diseases of public health significance.

CONCORDANT VS DISCORDANT SPECIES COMBINATIONS

Use of pigs as xenograft donors is problematic since pig xenografts elicit hyperacute rejection if transplanted into primate recipients. Calne suggested the use of the terms *concordant* and *discordant* to describe the relationship of various species with regard to xenografting, with the emphasis on the outcome following revascularization. Concordant combinations, including nonhuman primate-to-man, typically take several days to reject, whereas discordant combinations, such as pig-to-nonhuman primate, are subject to a violent response and fulminant hyperacute rejection within minutes to very few hours of transplantation.

IMMUNOBIOLOGY OF DISCORDANT XENOGRAFT REJECTION

With the exception of a pig liver that was transplanted into a patient with end-stage liver failure, who survived less than 24 hours, all relevant data has so far arisen from pig-to-nonhuman primate transplantation, plus from ex

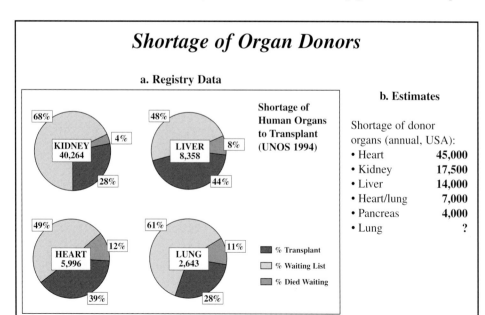

Figure 8-1. The impetus for the development of xenotransplantation as a clinical option is the shortage of allograft organ donors for transplantation. UNOS data (left) give the numbers of patients on waiting lists for organ transplants in the US, and show the breakdown as to those receiving a transplant vs those still awaiting, or dying while awaiting, a transplant. These are conservative estimates of the numbers of patients who would benefit from a transplant, since only those accepted into transplant programs are shown. Estimates by Roger Evans (Mayo Clinic) of the unmet need for organ allografts (right) indicate considerably greater numbers of transplants could be performed if organ supply was not the limiting factor.

vivo perfusion or cell culture studies. Humans have pre-formed, or so-called *xenoreactive natural antibodies* (XNA) directed against nonprimate species. These XNA, which include IgM, IgG and probably IgA classes appear to arise in early neonatal life following colonization of the large bowel by coliform bacteria. The majority of XNA recognize carbohydrate moieties associated with the bacterial cell wall and are polyreactive, binding many similar but nonidentical residues.

Demonstration of the presence of such XNA among humans, apes and Old World monkeys (catarrhines), but not other species, including New World monkeys (platyrrhines), provided the key to understanding the outcome of discordant xenografts involving humans or baboon recipients. The majority, but not all, of human XNA are directed against a terminal carbohydrate of linear B-type, Galα1,3-Galβ1GlcNAc-R, where a galactosyl residue is linked to another galactosyl residue (α-gal), which in turn is linked to anN-acetyl-glucosaminyl residue. This process is controlled by a glucosidase, galactosyl transferase. Since galactosyl transferase is not found in humans, the carbohydrate epitope expressed on coliform bacteria is perceived as foreign,

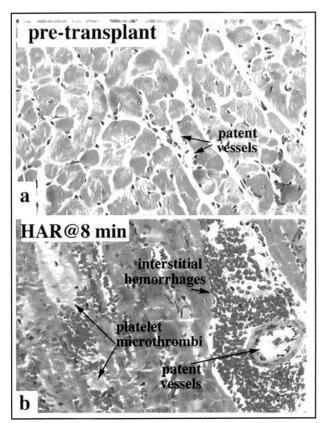

Figure 8-2. In contrast to (a) the pretransplant biopsy, which shows normal morphology, (b) hyperacute rejection at eight minutes posttransplant of a pig-to-baboon cardiac xenograft demonstrates interstitial hemorrhages and platelet microthrombi (arrows); in both groups, large vessels remain patent (Paraffin sections, H&E).

and antibodies (so-called *natural antibodies*) are produced against it. As this same carbohydrate residue is found on pig cells, humans have naturally occurring anti-pig antibodies (ie, XNA). Similar crossreactivities account for the presence of antibodies against ABO blood group antigens without prior sensitization to those antigens. This is in contrast to the situation with HLA where only patients with prior exposure to blood transfusions, pregnancy or transplants have anti-HLA antibodies.

Several groups are attempting to "knockout" expression of the α1,3 galactosyl transferase gene in pig cells as a strategy to markedly diminish their immunogenicity following xenotransplantation. The use of antisense technology has shown that this step can largely abrogate the cytotoxicity of human serum to pig cells in vitro, and if development of a suitable pig stem cell line is achieved, targeting of this gene by homologous recombination is planned. However, initial studies indicate that targeted deletion of the gene in mice did not significantly affect the survival of mouse xenografts transplanted into nonhuman primate recipients; apparently, such mice showed a terminal N-acetyl-fructosamine epitope, which is also recognized by human XNA, indicating that, as with much of xenotransplantation, many unforeseen obstacles are present.

An alternate approach is the genetic modification of α-gal expression. By upregulating expression of H-transferase, an enzyme which competes for similar substrates as galactosyl-transferase, in transgenic pigs, the expression of α-gal-containing molecules may be reduced; however, the efficacy of this procedure has yet to be tested rigorously in vivo. Given that decreasing the immunogenicity of pig tissues for primate recipients by manipulation of the donor animal is of uncertain value, various groups have gone on to consider "downstream" events and potential sites for therapeutic intervention. The pathobiology of discordant xenograft rejection is considered next, plus strategies to interrupt various points of the primate immune response.

PATHOBIOLOGY OF HYPERACUTE REJECTION

Following revascularization of a pig xenograft in a non-human primate recipient such as the baboon, the classical features of hyperacute rejection are engorgement and discoloration of the organ, and by light microscopy, interstitial hemorrhages with platelet microthrombi (Figure 8-2). Immunohistologic analysis shows dense deposition of various immunoglobulins and multiple complement components throughout the vascular bed consistent with the presence of host XNA directed against carbohydrate moieties on endothelial and other cells, and activation of complement via the classical pathway (Figure 8-3). Although early studies emphasized the predominance of IgM deposition, recent studies have established that deposition of IgG and IgA also occur. This is more than a trivial point, since the presence of IgA antibodies provides a mechanism for activation of the alternate pathway of complement (Figure 8-4). Indeed, several alternate pathway components, including properdin and Factor B, can be shown to co-localize with intragraft IgA during development of hyperacute rejection. In rodent models such as the well-studied guinea pig-to-rat combination, alternate pathway activation, regardless of XNA deposition, is the key mechanism of hyperacute rejection. Regulation of the complement system, which is central to an understanding of modern genetic approaches to control of hyperacute rejection, is shown in Figure 8-5 and Table 8-1, and is considered in the following sections.

Platelets

Hyperacute rejection involves the activation and degranulation of platelets through multiple mechanisms, including: (1) local generation of complement fragments (C5b-C9); (2) C3a- and C5a-induced mast cell degranulation, histamine and serotonin release, with local generation of platelet-activating factor (PAF); (3) FcR signaling upon exposure to deposited XNA; and (4) ischemic injury and endothelial cell retraction with platelet GP1b interaction with subendothelial matrix-bound vWF. Thus, even in the absence of complement activation, there are multiple signals to stimulate platelets. An additional factor may include the very rapid loss of endothelial ecto-ADPase, which normally main-

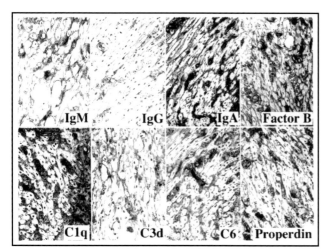

Figure 8-3. Hyperacute rejection of a pig-to-baboon cardiac xenograft is associated with dense endothelial deposition of IgM, IgG and IgA classes of XNA, leading to activation of both classical (C1q) and alternate (factor B, properdin) complement pathways. Both pathways activate C3 and lead to generation of the terminal pathway, as demonstrated here by endothelial localization of C6 (Cryostat sections, immunoperoxidase).

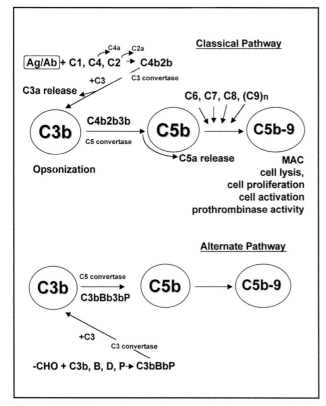

Figure 8-4. Dual routes for complement activation as a result of antigen binding by IgM or IgG (classical pathway, upper panel), or carbohydrate (-CHO) or IgA activation of the alternate pathway (lower panel). Each pathway has a respective C3 and C5 convertase. Events common to each pathway, from generation of C3b onward, are shown only in the upper panel.

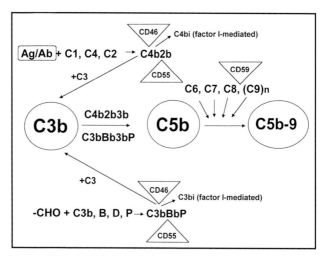

Figure 8-5. Principal sites of action of key regulators of complement activation (CD46, CD55, CD59), whose properties are detailed in Table 8-1, are shown in triangles. These molecules are of particular interest because of their relative species specificity and use in development of transgenic pigs in which their high level of expression results in abrogation of hyperacute rejection despite the depostion of immunoglobulins and early complement components.

Table 8-1. Human Regulators of Complement Activation (RCA Molecules)*

RCA	Size	Membrane	Distribution	Actions
CD35 (CR1)	190-280 kD	Transmembrane	Blood cells except platelet	Decay – accelerating and cofactor activity
CD46 (MCP)	55-70 kD	Transmembrane	All cells except RBC	Cofactor for factor I-mediated cleavage of C3b, C4b
CD55 (DAF)	70 kD	GPI-linked	All cells	Inhibits C3 and C5 convertases, and enhances their dissociation
CD59	18-20 kD	GPI-linked	All cells	Inhibits insertion of C8 and C9 into membrane-attack complex

* The RCA listed (whose sites of action are shown in Figure 8-5) are those being tested or currently used in experimental models and are likely to reach clinical usage; additional RCA that are not discussed include CD21 (CR2), C4bp and factor H.

tains a nonthrombogenic state at the endothelial surface (Figure 8-6). Loss of ecto-ADPase expression occurs as a result of ischemia and reperfusion injury, complement activation and other factors, and contributes to the development of hyperacute rejection. Although platelet microthrombi formation and their physical disruption of blood perfusion through the microvasculature may not be great enough to cause rapid graft dysfunction, platelet aggregation and activation lead to fibrin deposition, a hallmark and key effector mechanism of hyperacute rejection. In addition, as detailed in the next section, if hyperacute rejection is avoided, subsequent development of delayed xenograft rejection can be linked to platelet activation in the early posttransplant period.

Coagulation

Rapid assembly of coagulation factors on the platelet surface occurs through several related events. Receptors for factor V are up-regulated upon platelet activation, and platelet membrane phospholipids are exposed as a result of microparticle formation, facilitating the binding and assembly of a prothrombinase complex. Platelets also

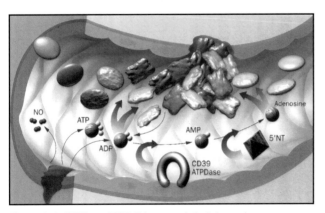

Figure 8-6. ATPDase (CD39) is an endothelial membrane-enzyme, which by degrading ATP and ADP limits local platelet aggregation. Rapid loss of ATPDase during inflammatory events contributes to platelet aggregation and thrombosis.

degranulate, resulting in high local concentrations of fibrinogen and other coagulation factors present in α-granules. Lastly, the trigger to platelet aggregation provided by thrombin or collagen results in release of ADP and serotonin. The combined effects of local platelet aggregation and activation are activation of coagulation and dense fibrin deposition, causing graft ischemia and rapid, progressive loss of organ function. A key role for coagulation, as powerful as that of complement, can be demonstrated in ex vivo perfusion systems.

Type I Endothelial Activation

Knowledge of endothelial responses during hyperacute rejection is very limited, whereas considerably more is known of the effects of XNA, complement and thrombin on cultured endothelial cells. Endothelial responses during HAR do not involve gene activation or protein synthesis, and are, therefore, examples of what is termed type I endothelial activation.

Summary of Hyperacute Rejection

As depicted in Figure 8-7, immediately upon revascularization of a discordant xenograft, complement activation begins on the surface of endothelial cells. The anaphylatoxins C3a and C5a are generated, and act locally on basophils and mast cells to release histamine and cause degranulation of platelets, including serotonin. Within seconds, histamine and serotonin bind to receptors on endothelial cells, stimulate surface expression of PAF and P-selectin, and cell contraction. PAF causes a dramatic increase in vascular permeability and endothelial cells contraction, resulting in sludging of platelets and RBC within the microcirculation. Endothelial cell retraction exposes underlying vWF, basement membranes and collagen to plasma components, including platelets and the contact activator, Hageman factor. Together, these events result in stasis, platelet aggregation, coagulation, fibrin deposition, and interstitial hemorrhages, which rapidly reduce compliance, such that a vascularized xenograft typically fails within minutes of engraftment. However, in some cases, grafts survive for a few hours such that neutrophil accumulation occurs in response to intragraft generation of chemotactic factor such as C3a and C5a.

OVERCOMING HYPERACUTE REJECTION

Given the complex involvement of antibody, complement, coagulation and other inflammatory pathways in mediation of xenograft rejection, identification of the key events that are of therapeutic significance is clearly essential. For the pig-to-nonhuman primate xenograft combination, complement is by far the most effective therapeutic target, but the blocking of complement is itself not sufficient to achieve significant long-term survival (more than a few days). XNA depletion, through various combinations of splenectomy, plasmapheresis, absorption with soluble trisaccharides, organ perfusion, and additional anti-B cell-directed immunosuppression has shown the important role of antibody, inde-

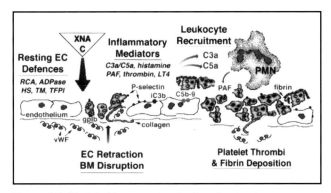

Figure 8-7. Model of hyperacute rejection showing key components. On the left are two "resting" endothelial cells (EC) serving to maintain a barrier between the intravascular space and organ parenchyma. EC normally express several proteins with antithrombotic actions, including thrombomodulin (TM), antithrombin III, tissue factor pathway inhibitor (TFPI), and the ectoenzyme ATPDase, which efficiently degrades platelet-derived ADP, thus inhibiting amplification pathways, which result in platelet plug formation. Heparan sulphate on the EC also binds superoxide dismutase, which degrades reactive oxygen species. Recipient XNA and complement activate porcine EC, leading to their retraction and development of interstitial hemorrhages. In addition, exposure of subendothelial molecules such as von Willebrand factor (vWF) allows adhesion and spreading of platelets through the interaction of platelet receptor GP1b with vWF. The activation of platelets, with increased expression of P selectin (also on EC) and GPIIbIIIa, is accompanied by release of inflammatory mediators, including platelet activating factor (PAF), thrombin and the leukotrienes (eg, LTB4). The loss of ADPase activity with EC activation permits ADP to accumulate, which promotes platelet aggregation, leading to platelet thrombi. Fibrin is deposited consequent to loss of molecules from the surface of the activated EC that normally maintain anticoagulation, and the interaction of fibrin(ogen) with the GPIIbIIIa receptor on the activated platelets.

pendent of complement, in development of hyperacute rejection in the pig-to-nonhuman primate combination (Figure 8-8). However, regardless of the protocol, antibody targeting has been incomplete, difficult to maintain, and has at very best, prolonged xenograft survival only modestly in a handful of isolated cases (ie, from several hours to 14 to 15 days). Similarly, the effects of targeting the coagulation system alone, or inflammatory mediators such as PAF, although often resulting in statistically significant effects compared to controls (eg, up to a few hours prolongation of graft survival), are not biologically meaningful.

Targeting the complement pathway using cobra venom factor or one of several alternate agents, such as soluble complement receptor type I (sCR1), FUT-175 or K76COOH, is about equally effective as, but more reproducible than, targeting of XNA, typically providing several days of survival; however, there are important limitations. For example, the toxicity associated with use of agents such as cobra venom factor renders them unsuitable for clinical usage. In addition, these agents are extremely expensive and prone to eliciting neutralizing antibodies. Hence, with the realization that the arcane world of complement includes multiple regulators of complement activation (RCA) (Table 8-1, Figure 8-4), and that such RCA are, to a large extent, species-specific, genetic approaches to manipulation of the organ donor have received great attention. The main human RCA are CD46 (membrane cofactor protein) and CD55, which regulate expression of C3 convertase, and CD59 (homologous restriction factor) which blocks insertion of C9 into the developing membrane attack complex of complement. The principle of this approach has been demonstrated in vitro, wherein transfected

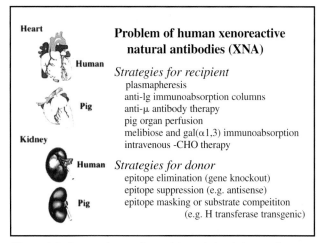

Heart

Human

Pig

Kidney

Human

Pig

Problem of human xenoreactive natural antibodies (XNA)

Strategies for recipient
   plasmapheresis
   anti-Ig immunoabsorption columns
   anti-μ antibody therapy
   pig organ perfusion
   melibiose and gal(α1,3) immunoabsorption
   intravenous -CHO therapy

Strategies for donor
   epitope elimination (gene knockout)
   epitope suppression (e.g. antisense)
   epitope masking or substrate compeititon
      (e.g. H transferase transgenic)

Figure 8-8. Approaches to the problem of circulating preformed XNA in patients about to receive a pig xenograft; unfortunately, none result in more than short-term XNA depletion or prolongation of survival and, in the case of strategies for the recipient, are frequently associated with rebound to higher than normal XNA levels.

pig cells show dramatically increased resistance to complement-mediated lysis in the presence of human serum, but the key point has been to develop transgenic pigs expressing human RCA and to test this approach in vivo.

In late 1992, Astrid, the world's first transgenic pig, was born. Astrid was heterozygous for human CD55 and became the founder pig of a large herd at Cambridge University. In initial studies, organs (heart or kidney) from pigs homozygous for human RCA such as CD55, when transplanted into unmodified baboon recipients, survived about 130 hours, in contrast to normal controls that reject within minutes to a few hours. Hence, expression of human RCA on pig endothelial cells can abrogate hyperacute rejection following xenotransplantation. Although initial pigs transgenic for CD55 had unpredictable and often low tissue expression, the application of new vectors now allows adequate expression of this transgene in the endothelium of pigs. In particular, the use of mini-genes whose expression is driven by the human ICAM-2 promoter has proven very successful. The extent to which use of immunosuppressive agents such as cyclophosphamide can usefully extend xenograft survival, when pig donors transgenic for one or other human RCA are employed, is somewhat controversial. There are only very limited data available from such addition of immunosuppression, and successful prolongation appears to have been achieved only at the expense of high toxicity in the recipient.

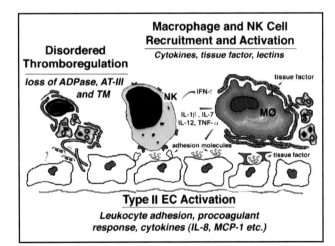

Figure 8-9. Delayed xenograft rejection (DXR) and thrombosis of the vasculature are multicellular processes. Thrombosis takes place based both on events that are a part of type I activation, and on the expression of tissue factor (TF) by infiltrating macrophages and graft endothelial cells. Platelet aggregates form based on the mechanisms illustrated in Figure 8-7. Multiple chemokines produced by activated EC recruit (and activate) leukocytes. Activated monocytes and NK cells likely contribute to inflammation through their elaboration of toxic products, cytokines and direct, cell-mediated events, amplifying organ injury; the graft is rejected based on the inflammatory and thrombotic consequences of these events.

IMMUNOPATHOLOGY OF DELAYED XENOGRAFT REJECTION (DXR)

If hyperacute rejection is avoided by depleting XNA or complement, xenografts are rejected in days instead of minutes to hours, by a process referred to as delayed xenograft rejection (DXR) (Figure 8-9). DXR may appear a rather uninformative term, when compared to terms such as hyperacute, acute or chronic rejection, which have clear morphologic features and, at least in the case of the first two conditions, a considerable body of knowledge regarding the contribution of humoral and cellular immune responses to their development. By contrast, large vessels in DXR are typically uninvolved so that it cannot be described as a classic vascular rejection and, since T cells are not essential to the process, it cannot be described as classical cellular rejection. Hence, DXR merely indicates the typical timing of rejection in recipients which are, in effect, de-complemented, whether through use of cobra venom factor or analogous agent, or through use of donors expressing RCA, but otherwise unmodified. It is important to remember that hyperacute rejection and DXR represent parts of a continuum. Some of the components of hyperacute rejection, such as platelet activation or immunoglobulin deposition, do not typically result in hyperacute rejection if complement activation is avoided, and yet these responses, as well as activation of coagulation and endothelial cell responses, may contribute to development of DXR.

DXR occurs in large and small animal models of discordant xenograft rejection, and is characterized by progressive infiltration over several days of mononuclear cells, primarily monocytes and NK cells; development of focal infarcts and interstitial hemorrhages; widespread activation of coagulation within the microvasculature; and cessation of graft function (Figure 8-10). Such a picture is not simply a delayed form of vascular rejection. Vascular rejection involves inflammation of large- and medium-sized arteries, often with fibrinoid necrosis, thrombosis and neutrophil infiltration of the vessel wall, which are absent in DXR. Moreover, the same events are seen in XNA-depleted recipients, necessitating consideration of other components of the host response.

Leukocytes

During development of DXR, over 75% of intragraft leukocytes are mononuclear phagocytes, with additional contributions from NK cells (10% to 20%) and only very small numbers (approximately 5%) of T cells until at least several days posttransplant. The presence of T cells or XNA is not essential for DXR in complement-depleted rats, but it has been difficult to determine the actual roles of macrophages and NK cells. Moreover, the progressive infiltration by T cells may contribute to

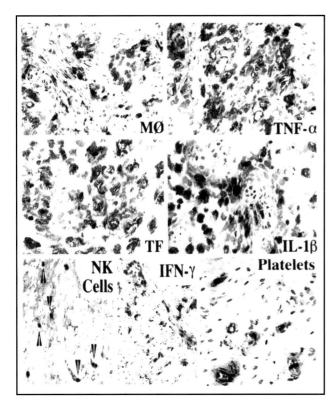

Figure 8-10. Immunopathology of DXR in a pig cardiac xenograft at day five posttransplant in decomplemented primate recipient, showing dense macrophage infiltration plus lesser numbers of NK cells, along with examples of their respective cytokine products, such as TNF-α, IL-1β, and IFN-γ. Macrophages, and endothelial cells, show induction of the procoagulant, tissue factor (TF), and the microvasculature is associated with widespread platelet microthrombi. DXR can be accompanied by significant numbers of T cells, but at least experimentally can readily occur in T cell-deficient recipients (Cryostat sections, immunoperoxidase).

xenograft rejection in at least some models. Infiltrating macrophages produce large amounts of TNF-α and IL-1β during DXR, as well as IL-7, IL-12, iNOS and various chemokines. Some monokines, such as IL-1β and IL-6 are likely to act only on host cells (eg, contributing to systemic fever and acute phase response). Others, like TNF-α, appear to act across species, and the upregulation of adhesion molecules is consistent with such effects. TNF-α also has direct, toxic effects on myocardial cells. IL-7 and IL-12 are relevant to NK cell recruitment and activation, with IL-12 playing a key role in induction of IFN-γ production, and xenografts display extraordinarily dense IFN-γ expression during development of DXR. However, the extent to which IFN-γ acts across species is controversial and appears to depend upon the species combinations involved. Nevertheless, since IFN-γ is the most potent activator of macrophages known, regardless of direct effects across species barriers, the action of IFN-γ on host macrophages is likely to be dramatic.

Endothelial Responses During DXR

Analysis of serial samples from small and large animal models has demonstrated considerable evidence of endothelial cell activation during discordant xenograft rejection. Endothelial responses, which are so-called Type II in nature since they involve gene induction and protein synthesis, include the following: (1) shift to a procoagulant state, with downregulation of surface thrombomodulin and induction of tissue factor, consistent with dense local fibrin deposition; (2) induction of leukocyte adhesion molecules, including, progressively, E-selectin, ICAM-1 and VCAM-1; and (3) production of chemokines such as MCP-1, as well as other cytokines. The significance of endothelial activation in DXR is controversial. On one hand, these are "downstream" events, which are present in essentially any inflammatory response, albeit to a more florid extent than usual. On the other hand, the ability to genetically engineer the donor animal suggests the potential for modulating endothelial responses by genetic approaches.

Summary of DXR

Once hyperacute rejection is overcome, xenografts show progressive mononuclear and endothelial cell activation, cytokine expression, platelet and fibrin deposition, and rejection within a few days. Logically, DXR may be caused by infiltrating mononuclear cells and/or the consequences of endothelial cell activation. NK cells could be present secondary to direct recognition of xenogeneic endothelial cells, and either NK cells or macrophages could be present through FcR binding of IgG bound to endothelial cells, lectin interactions or chemokine production. Once present and activated, mononuclear cell products, including cytokines and tissue factor, contribute to coagulation, damage surrounding endothelial cells, and depress myocardial contractility. The factors that result in activation of endothelium in DXR are not well-defined. However, following stimulation, activated endothelial cells contribute to inflammation and thrombosis (Figure 8-9).

OVERCOMING DXR

Current reports involving xenografts from pigs transgenic for human RCA to nonhuman primate recipients show that DXR can be overcome, and xenograft survival prolonged in a few cases to greater than 60 days, when recipients also are treated with high-dose cyclophosphamide and steroids. Such therapy induced leukopenia and thrombocytopenia, and recipients typically suffered from diarrhea and weight loss associated with gastrointestinal toxicity and infections (eg, mixed CMV and candidial oesphagitis, duodenitis) as a consequence of the immunosuppression. Biopsies of xenografts showed normal histology, including a lack of any leukocyte infiltrate, platelet thrombi or interstitial hemorrhages, and normal organ function.

Hence, initial results with transgenic pigs expressing human RCA show that hyperacute rejection can be readily overcome. Although these results are the first major triumph of gene therapy in the field of organ transplantation, but that additional, nonclinically acceptable immunosuppression is required to overcome development of DXR and, presumably T cell-mediated xenograft rejection. The challenge is to develop a protocol for the use of such pigs that will allow long-term survival without compromising the host. Further genetic manipulation of the donor appears a likely area for progress, with the eventual strategy of crossing pigs expressing human RCA with those expressing other genes, or with those in which certain genes have been silenced. Likely candidates are listed in Table 8-2. These include over-expression of an H-transferase to decrease gal(α1,3)gal expression; regulated expression of an inhibitor of endothelial cell activation, for example, through over-expression of an inhibitor of NFκB; and eventually, possible development of "self-pigs" bearing

human MHC genes of the recipient, potentially in conjunction with knockout of swine MHC class I antigens and tolerance-inducing protocols. Progress on some form of galactosyl transferase knockout in pigs is also likely within the next few years.

CHALLENGES FOR THE FUTURE

Faced with the almost evangelical fervor of proponents of xenotransplantation advocating immediate clinical trials of organs from the currently available transgenic pigs, plus awareness of the crisis in organ donation rates vs numbers of patients, it is important to ponder for a second the things we do not yet know. None of the trials of very small numbers of pig-to-primate xenografts have yet addressed biocompatibility issues. Data on the basic physiology of pig organ function following xenografts are not known, nor are the more subtle factors such as hormone (eg, erythropoietin) production, ability to grow in the host, hemodynamic factors, and, as occurred in early studies using chimpanzee donors, the potential for rapid development of chronic rejection. An additional major concern that must be overcome prior to clinical consideration of xenotransplantation is the

Table 8-2. Genetic Manipulations of the Pig Organ Donor to Promote Xenotransplantation

Target	Concept	Comment	When?
Transgenic expression of human RCA	Expression of human CD46, CD55 or CD59 on pig cells will locally regulate assembly of complement cascade.	Prevents HAR, but without additional massive immunosuppression, xenografts reject in 4 to 5 days; alternate vectors to increase endothelial expression (eg, ICAM-2) are under evaluation.	Testing underway
Transgenic H-transferase	α1,2 Fucosyltransferase over expression may compete with endogenous α1,3 galactosyl transferase.	May usefully be combined with pigs transgenic for RCA.	Testing underway
Transgenic expression of inhibitors of endothelial activation	Regulated endothelial expression of IκB, a natural inhibitor of NFκB, or a dominant negative mutant of an NFκB subunit.	Strategy to inhibit NFκB, a key transcription factor essential for inducible gene expression in endothelial cells; regulation of inhibitor achieved in vivo through use of tetracycline-sensitive promoter.	2 to 3 years
Yeast artificial chromosome (YAC) transfer of human genes	Large portions (~150-300 kb) of human chromosome carrying desired transgene.	May be used to achieve position-independent expression of multiple human genes; in long-term could be used to introduce human MHC genes into donor pig, creating "self-pig".	2 to 3 years
α1,3 Galactosyl transferase deletion	Block expression of pig Galα1,2 Gal residues recognized by human XNA.	Requires isolation of a pig stem cell line; other sugars may still bind XNA.	2 to 3 years
Swine MHC (SLA) deletion	Block pig expression of pig MHC genes to facilitate tolerance induction.	Requires isolation of a pig stem cell line; pig β2-microglobulin cloned so targeting of swine class I feasible; class II genes have very restricted expression and may be less important.	2 to 3 years

capacity to transmit infectious agents. Since the grafts, and any pathogens, are placed deep within immuno-suppressed individuals, Fishman has suggested use of the term *xenosis* rather than simply zoonosis. Many possible agents could induce xenoses in a patient, such that donor pigs will likely be subject to intense microbiologic scrutiny prior to use. However, of particular concern is the possibility of transmission of pig endogenous retro-viruses (PERV). The extent to which PERV transmission to human cells can occur is currently a major area of investigation. In the coming years, far more attention will likely be paid to such issues, as well as to the estab-lishment of pathogen-free colonies, before clinical trials will be considered worthwhile.

RECOMMENDED READING

Bach FH, Robson SC, Winkler H, et al. Barriers to xeno-transplantation. Nat Med. 1995;1(9):869-873.

Cooper DK, Koren E, Oriol R. Oligosaccharides and discordant xenotransplantation. Immunol Rev. 1994;141:31-58.

Cozzi E, White DJ. The generation of transgenic pigs as potential organ donors for humans. Nat Med. 1995;1(9):964-966.

Hancock WW. The past, present and future of renal xenotransplantation. Kidney Int.1997;51(3):932-944.

Platt JL, Logan JS. Use of transgenic animals in xeno-transplantation. Transplant Rev. 1996;10:69-77.

Rooney IA, Atkinson JP. Using membrane-bound complement regulatory proteins to inhibit rejection. Xenotransplantation. 1993;1:29-35.

Starzl TE, Valdivia LA, Murase N, et al. The biological basis of and strategies for clinical xenotransplantation. Immunol Rev. 1994;141:213-244.

Sykes M, Lee LA, Sachs DH. Xenograft tolerance. Immunol Rev. 1994;141:245-276.

Section II

PHARMACOLOGY AND IMMUNOSUPPRESSION

9 HISTORICAL OVERVIEW OF PHARMACOLOGY AND IMMUNOSUPPRESSION

Philip F. Halloran, MD, PhD
Sita Gourishankar, MD

THE CONCEPT OF IMMUNOSUPPRESSION

Awareness of inflammation as a mechanism of disease long predated the understanding of the elements of the specific immune response. The development of adreno-corticotropic hormone (ACTH) and corticosteroids led to the demonstration, in 1950, that inflammatory diseases could be improved by adrenal steroids, as shown in rheumatoid arthritis, nephrotic syndrome, and allergic conditions. Thus, it was natural to apply glucocorticoids to prevent or reverse the severe inflammation of experimental graft rejection. Some human kidney transplants performed in the 1950s received little or no immunosuppression, with predictably tragic consequences. Knowledge of immunosuppression lagged behind surgical skill, so the first kidney transplants were performed using identical twin donors, which were not at risk for rejection. By the late 1950s, the first attempts to use whole body irradiation to prolong transplant survival were reported.

INTRODUCTION OF AZATHIOPRINE, ANTILYMPHOCYTE GLOBULIN, AND PHYSICAL MEASURES

Immunosuppressive options that would allow for successful cadaveric transplantation emerged at the end of the 1950s. Elion and Hitchings developed 6-mercapto-purine (6-MP) and azathioprine (AZA), for which they received a 1988 Nobel prize. Schwartz and Dameschek demonstrated that 6-MP could alter the immune response to an allograft. It is interesting to note that these pioneers thought that the state of immunosuppression they were inducing was immunologic tolerance, a claim made for almost every immunosuppressive drug introduced since. By the early 1960s, the practice of

Philip F. Halloran, MD, PhD, Professor of Medicine and Immunology, Division of Nephrology and Immunology, University of Alberta, Edmonton, Alberta, Canada

Sita Gourishankar, MD, Nephrology Fellow, Division of Nephrology and Immunology, University of Alberta, Edmonton, Alberta, Canada

using glucocorticoids in conjunction with AZA had been initiated, with high-dose steroid used to reverse rejection, permitting only limited success in cadaver transplantation. The first application of antilymphocyte globulin (ALG) was in the 1960s. Efforts at immune cell depletion included thoracic duct drainage, irradiation, thymectomy and splenectomy.

By the late 1970s, those centers that had access to effective antilymphocyte antibodies, such as Minnesota antilymphocyte globulin, were reporting improved survival rates. However, the overall survival of cadaver kidneys was still less than 50% at one year, and many patients experienced severe steroid side effects. Graft survival for other organs remained poor, and only kidney transplants were performed in significant numbers.

THE CYCLOSPORINE ERA

The discovery of cyclosporine (CsA), its first clinical use in 1978, and its growing application in the early 1980s changed transplantation as few other developments have. Results in this era were also improved with widespread access to effective polyclonal antilymphocyte antibodies and, later, muromonab-CD3, which reduced reliance on high-dose steroids. Many improvements in medical, surgical, anesthetic, and intensive care management also improved clinical results. Significant interest and investment in transplantation permitted large-scale trials. The growth in the transplantation of hearts, livers, pancreases and lungs created the transplantation programs of the present day. Studies of the mechanism of action of CsA led rapidly to the realization that CsA blocks the transcriptional activation of IL-2 and other cytokines in T cells. This was a significant contribution to the basic science of T cell activation.

MUROMONAB-CD3 MONOCLONALS

The development of mouse monoclonal antibodies was based on the work of Milstein and Kohler (Nobel prize, 1984). Anti-CD3 was shown to be effective in reversing and controlling acute rejection, but soon it was being deployed as an induction therapy to prevent rejection.

TACROLIMUS, MYCOPHENOLATE MOFETIL, RAPAMYCIN, AND ANTI-CD25

Tacrolimus differed from other drugs in that much of its early development occurred in liver transplants, rather than in kidneys. It was surprising that tacrolimus acted by the same mechanism as CsA, and that each required binding to abundant intracellular binding protein to create a complex that inhibited the enzyme calcineurin. These observations triggered much basic research. Studies of the calcineurin pathway led to the discovery of a new class of transcription factors, the nuclear factor of activated T cells (NF-AT). By the late 1980s, tacrolimus was introduced for use in organ transplants.

Mycophenolate mofetil was an agent derived from the older drug mycophenolic acid, which was specifically selected for development as an inhibitor of de novo purine synthesis in lymphocytes. It was found to be highly effective in combination with CsA at preventing acute rejection in humans. Rapamycin (or sirolimus) had been discovered in the 1970s as an antifungal, but the potential of its immunosuppressive properties for commercial development was not recognized until the late 1980s. By the 1990s rapamycin was in development as a clinical immunosuppressive in combination with CsA, and large-scale trials had demonstrated its potential and led to its approval for use in kidney transplantation.

THE PRESENT AND THE FUTURE

As the millennium begins, new humanized or chimeric protein products are becoming available. Anti-CD25s have been released for prevention of renal transplant rejection. Novel agents, such as anti-CD40 ligand, CTLA4Ig, and humanized anti-CD3, hold promise, but must prove their superiority to the present drugs. Anti-CD40 ligand was in Phase 1 and 2 studies, but has been withdrawn at present. A fully humanized anti-CD3 is in Phase 2 trials as a replacement for murine monoclonal muromonab-CD3. CTLA4Ig has shown efficacy in psoriasis and is slated to go into Phase 1 in renal transplanta-tion. The potential of agents to block chemokine receptors is being explored experimentally. Gene therapy and antisense oligonucleotides are producing interesting experimental results. New classes of agents such as FTY720, peptides and antisense oligonucleotides will be evaluated to determine their potential, which remains unknown in humans.

The new priority is reduction in toxicity with equivalent efficacy. The establishment of safer and more effective protocols using the recently introduced agents is needed. Concern regarding infections, cancer, cardiovascular risks, and specific toxicities of the agents dominates the clinical agenda. Those laboratories developing new agents are faced with the task of finding a niche in transplantation that will generate sufficient return on investment to cover the costs of development of new drugs.

Immunosuppression would be aided by better laboratory measurement of the immunologic state, immunologic injury, and stability. The current use of organ function as a surrogate for immunologic information is analogous to using end-organ damage in hypertension instead of measuring blood pressure. Ideally, measurements of the immune mechanisms of disease, and the effects of the agents on those mechanisms, must be developed.

The field of immunosuppression is driven by the mandate of making transplantation more effective. These technologies should find an increased application in other areas of medicine (ie, lupus, glomerulonephritis, arthritis, and vasculitis) where immunologic injury remains poorly controlled, and where therapies are often still based on the drugs of the 1950s.

Finally, studies in human populations now emphasize the importance of nonimmune factors in graft outcome (eg, age, blood pressure, lipid abnormalities, brain death-related injury). New interventions to ameliorate the effects of these influences would be welcome.

RECOMMENDED READING

Allison AC, Eugui EM. Immunosuppressive and long-acting anti-inflammatory activity of mycophenolic acid and derivative, RS-61443. Br J Rheumatol. 1991;20(S2):57-61.

Amlot PL, Rawlings E, Fernando ON, et al. Prolonged action of a chimeric interleukin-2 receptor (CD25) monoclonal antibody used in cadaveric renal transplantation. Transplantation. 1995;60(7):748-756.

Borel JF, Feurer C, Gubler HU, Stahelin H. Biological effects of cyclosporin A: a new antilymphocytic agent. Agents Actions. 1976;6(4):468-475.

Calne RY, White DJG, Thiru S, et al. Cyclosporin A in patients receiving renal allografts from cadaver donors. Lancet. 1978; 2(8104-8105):1323-1327.

Table 9-1. A Time Line of Immunosuppression

Year	Immunosuppressive Milestones
1950	Benefits of glucocorticoid therapy on immune-mediated diseases
1959	6-mercaptopurine and azathioprine
1968	Polyclonal antilymphocyte globulin
1975	Murine monoclonal antibody production
1976	First report of immunosuppressive properties of cyclosporine
1976	First report of immunosuppressive properties of rapamycin
1978	First clinical use of cyclosporine
1981	Introduction of murine monoclonal anti-CD3 to reverse rejection
1987	Description of tacrolimus
1989	First clinical results with tacrolimus
1991	First report of clinical use of mycophenolate mofetil
1998	First report of clinical use of rapamycin

Cosimi AB, Colvin RB, Burton RC, et al. Use of monoclonal antibodies to T cell subsets for immunologic monitoring and treatment in recipients of renal allografts. N Engl J Med. 1981;305(6):308-314.

Elion GB, Hitchings GH. Metabolic basis for the actions of analogs of purines and pyrimidines [review]. Adv Chemother. 1965;2:91-177.

Groth CG, Backman L, Morales JM, et al. Sirolimus (rapamycin)-based therapy in human renal transplantation: similar efficacy and different toxicity compared with cyclosporine. Sirolimus European Renal Transplant Study Group. Transplantation. 1999;67(7):1036-1042.

Hakimi J, Mould D, Waldmann TA, Queen C, Anasetti C, Light S. Development of Zenapax: a humanized anti-Tac antibody. In: Harris WJ, Adair JK, eds. Antibody Therapeutics. Boca Raton, Fla.; CRC Press, Inc.; 1997: 277-300.

Hench PS. The reversibility of certain rheumatic and non-rheumatic conditions by the use of cortisone or of the pituitary adrenocorticotropic hormone. Ann Intern Med. 1952;36:1-38.

Hume DM, Merrill JP, Miller BF, Thorn GW. Experiences with renal homotransplantation in the human: report of nine cases. J Clin Invest. 1955;34:327-382.

Kahan BD, Podbielski J, Napoli KL, Katz SM, Meier-Kriesche HU, Van Buren CT. Immunosuppressive effects and safety of a sirolimus/cyclosporine combination regimen for renal transplantation. Transplantation. 1998;66(8):1040-1046.

Kino T, Hatanaka H, Miyata S, et al. FK-506, a novel immunosuppressant isolated from a *streptomyces*. II. Immunosuppressive effect of FK-506 in vitro. J Antibiot. 1987;40(9):1256-1265.

Kirk AD, Harlan DM, Armstrong NN, et al. CTLA4-Ig and anti-CD40 ligand prevent renal allograft rejection in primates. Proc Natl Acad Sci USA. 1997;94(16):8789-8794.

Kohler G, Milstein C. Continuous cultures of fused cells secreting antibody of predefined specificity. Nature. 1975;256(5517):495-497.

Linsley PS, Wallace PM, Johnson J. Immunosuppression in vivo by a soluble form of the CTLA-4 T cell activation molecule. Science. 1992;257(5071):792-795.

Marunaka Y, Niisato N, Shintani Y. Protein phosphatase 2B-dependent pathway of insulin action on single Cl-channel conductance in renal epithelium. J Membr Biol. 1998;161(3):235-245.

Medawar PB, Sparrow EM. The effects of adrenocortical hormone, adrenocorticotrophic hormone, and pregnancy on skin transplantation immunity in mice. J Endocrinol. 1954;11:78-82.

Murgia MG, Jordan S, Kahan BD. The side effect profile of sirolimus: a phase I study in quiescent cyclosporine-prednisone-treated renal transplant patients. Kidney Int. 1996;49(1):209-216.

Schwartz R, Dameshek W. Drug-induced immunological tolerance. Nature. 1959;183:1682-1683.

Schwartz R, Dameshek W, Donovan J. The effects of 6-mercaptopurine on homograft reactions. J Clin Invest. 1960;39:952-958.

Sehgal SN, Baker H, Vézina C. Rapamycin (AY-22,989), a new antifungal antibiotic. II. Fermentation, isolation and characterization. J Antibiot. 1975;28(10):727-732.

Sollinger HW, Eugui EM, Allison AS. RS-61443: mechanism of action, experimental and early clinical results. Clin Transplant. 1991;5:523-526.

Starzl TE, Todo S, Fung J, Demetris AJ, Venkataramanan R, Jain A. FK 506 for liver, kidney, and pancreas transplantation. Lancet. 1989;2:1000-1004.

Starzl TE, Marchioro TL, Porter KA, Iwasaki Y, Cerilli GJ. The use of heterologous antilymphoid agents in canine renal and liver homotransplantation and in human renal homotransplantation. Surg Gyne Obs. 1967;124(2):301-308.

Vézina C, Kudelski A, Sehgal SN. Rapamycin (AY-22,989), a new antifungal antibiotic. I. Taxonomy of the producing streptomycete and isolation of the active principle. J Antibiot. 1975;28(10):721-726.

10 BASIC PRINCIPLES OF PHARMACOLOGY

Kathleen D. Lake, PharmD, FCCP, BCPS

Understanding the basic precepts of pharmacology is very important, as health care practitioners are faced with making decisions regarding the use of highly effective but potentially toxic agents in their patients. The recent advances in therapeutics have extended the lives of many patients who would not be alive today without the administration of complicated medication regimens. However, it is not unusual to find patients with chronic conditions receiving eight to ten different medications, some of which are used to treat the adverse effects of their life-sustaining medications (ie, antihypertensive and lipid-lowering agents to treat the hypertension and hyperlipidemia associated with cyclosporine therapy). It is also becoming increasingly evident that these complicated medication regimens can contribute to the overall cost of health care if they are not managed correctly. Other factors, such as patient compliance and quality of life derived from the drug therapy regimens, can influence therapeutic outcomes. The complexity of today's pharmacotherapy regimens mandates a thorough understanding of pharmacology and its domains to promote the optimal use of medications.

Pharmacology can be defined as understanding how drugs act within the body to produce their therapeutic effects. The interactions between the drug and the body can be classified by the concepts of *pharmacokinetics* (simply stated, what the body does to the drug) and *pharmacodynamics* (what the drug does to the body). Toxicology is the portion of pharmacology that focuses on the undesirable effects of a given agent. Therapeutic drug monitoring incorporates the pharmacokinetic data obtained from patients with the application of pharmacodynamic concepts, and this has improved the ability of clinicians to maximize efficacy while minimizing the toxicity of various pharmacologic agents. *Pharmacoeconomics* is a relatively new discipline that has evolved because of increasing health care costs. This entity attempts to analyze the overall cost of drug therapy (ie, not just the cost

Director of Clinical Transplant Research and Therapeutics, The Michigan Transplant Center and the University of Michigan Health Systems; Senior Associate Research Scientist, Departments of Medicine and Surgery, University of Michigan Medical School; Clinical Professor, University of Michigan College of Pharmacy, Division of Nephrology, University of Michigan Medical School, Ann Arbor, MI

of the drug) relative to the actual benefit derived from the therapy, and can be described by various techniques including cost-benefit, cost-effectiveness, and cost-minimization analyses. A number of other techniques, including quality-adjusted-life-years analysis method, attempt to put a dollar value on the years of life that are extended or the associated improvement in quality of life.

PHARMACOKINETICS

The study of pharmacokinetics is an attempt to mathematically describe the behavior of a drug in the body and is characterized by its absorption, distribution, metabolism and elimination. It is important to remember that the response to a drug is related to the concentration at a target organ receptor site. The receptor concentration can seldom be measured, whereas it is much easier to measure the concentration in the blood. There is usually a much better relationship between drug concentration in plasma and the intensity of the pharmacologic effect than there is between a given dose and these effects. It is this relationship that supports the use of pharmacokinetic monitoring for those drugs with narrow therapeutic indices.

Absorption

In practical terms, it would be ideal to administer a drug directly to its intended site of action, however, other than topical administration of ointments to skin and intracardiac administration of some agents, most drugs are administered into one body compartment and must distribute to their sites of action. But before a drug can move to its site of action, it must be absorbed, unless it is administered intravenously, to reach the systemic circulation. Absorption can be described by two concepts, *rate* and *extent.*

RATE OF ABSORPTION. The rate of absorption is determined by the site of administration and the drug formulation, and is usually only important in emergency settings or single-dose administration of agents (eg, hypnotics) where therapeutic concentrations need to be achieved immediately. In these settings, drugs must be administered intravenously to ensure immediate onset of pharmacologic effect. Drugs administered by other routes (eg, intramuscularly, subcutaneously, orally, rectally) typically have delayed absorption as they must cross biologic membranes to reach the systemic circulation. For instance, agents administered orally must pass through the gastrointestinal tract wall into the systemic circulation before exerting a pharmacologic effect; this may take one to two hours or longer to achieve peak concentrations. Other than in emergency situations, alterations in the rate of absorption (ie, decreased gastrointestinal motility) are usually less of a concern than factors altering the extent of absorption.

EXTENT OF ABSORPTION. The extent of absorption is influenced by a number of factors. In simple terms, absorption of an oral drug is defined as the fraction of a dose that is dissolved and subsequently absorbed from the intestine. However, a number of other factors determine how much actually reaches the systemic circulation before the drug ultimately elicits its pharmacologic effect. Some drugs, such as acyclovir, are too lipophilic to be absorbed readily. Other drugs such as vancomycin and the aminoglycosides are too water soluble to be absorbed. A number of drugs are actually metabolized in the gastrointestinal tract by the cytochrome P450 iso-enzymes before absorption can occur, and this is usually referred to as presystemic metabolism. In addition, a counter transport protein, p-glycoprotein, located in the gastrointestinal tract, can decrease the amount of drug available for absorption, and this action may explain some of the poorer bioavailability reported previously with the Sandimmune® formulation of cyclosporine. A number of compounds with poor absorption character-istics are administered as inactive pro-drugs, which require conversion to biologically active metabolites before they can elicit their pharmacologic effects. Two such immunosuppressive agents administered as pro-drugs include azathioprine, which following absorption is rapidly converted by plasma esterases to 6-mercapto-purine, and mycophenolate mofetil, which is rapidly de-esterified to mycophenolic acid. In addition, a num-ber of gastrointestinal diseases, including diarrhea and radiation of the abdomen, may reduce absorption of orally administered drugs. Drug absorption is frequently reduced in the elderly because of age-related decreases in intestinal motility and the number of mucosal cells.

FIRST PASS METABOLISM. Once the oral drug is absorbed and reaches the hepatic venous portal system, it is delivered to the liver in high concentrations before tissue distribution occurs. Metabolism in the liver can further decrease the amount of drug available for distrib-ution to the systemic circulation. Some drugs are also excreted into the bile and may undergo enterohepatic recirculation, allowing the parent compound to be absorbed again. This effect can be observed as a second peak when concentrations are measured over the entire dosing interval. To avoid the first pass effect, drugs can be administered by other routes such as sublingually or by inhalation.

Bioavailability

It is important to make a distinction between the terms *absorption* and *bioavailability.* Bioavailability refers to the fraction of the dose that actually reaches the systemic

circulation following administration by any route. Following oral administration, this reflects the amount remaining after losses from incomplete absorption and from presystemic metabolism that occurs either in the gut and/or first pass metabolism in the liver. Some oral drugs have good absorption but low bioavailability. Bioavailability is the more important parameter for pre-dicting pharmacotherapeutic effects as it is the measure of total systemic exposure.

Distribution

After a drug is absorbed or injected into the systemic cir-culation, it may be distributed into other body fluids and tissues.

The rate and extent of drug distribution in the body varies according to a number of factors including blood flow, the solubility of the agent (hydrophilicity vs lipophilicity) in various body tissues, and its degree of protein binding within the plasma.

Plasma protein binding is defined as the percentage of drug present in plasma that is bound reversibly to plasma proteins such as albumin, lipoproteins and alpha-1-acid-glycoprotein. The importance of protein binding relates to the fact that only the unbound or free circulating fraction of a drug is able to cross cellular membranes and elicit pharmacologic responses (Figure 10-1). The concentration of unbound drug in blood is probably more important pharmacologically than the total (bound plus unbound) concentration. An equilibrium exists between protein-bound drug and unbound drug, and it is the unbound drug that provides the driving force for distribution of the agent to body tis-sues and reflects the concentration of drug at its site of action. Once the drug leaves the bloodstream and dis-tributes to the tissue, it may become tissue-bound, remain unbound or be inactivated or eliminated by the tissue.

Mycophenolate mofetil (Cellcept®), valproic acid (Depakene®), salicylates, and warfarin sodium (Coumadin®, Panwarfin®) are examples of drugs that bind to albumin. Acidic drugs typically bind to albumin, whereas many basic drugs bind to alpha-1-acid-glycoprotein, such as lidocaine (Xylocaine®), quinidine, propranolol (Inderal®), phenothiazines, tricyclic antide-pressants, narcotic analgesics, and many cancer chemo-therapeutic agents. Alpha-1-acid-glycoprotein is an acute-phase reactant that is released in high concentra-tions during times of stress or inflammation. Increased concentrations have been reported following surgery, burns and myocardial infarction, and in patients with chronic pain, cancer or antiinflammatory disorders. These acute changes may affect the amount of free drug available to exert both desired therapeutic actions and toxic effects. Some of the other differences in side effect profiles may be explained by different binding character-

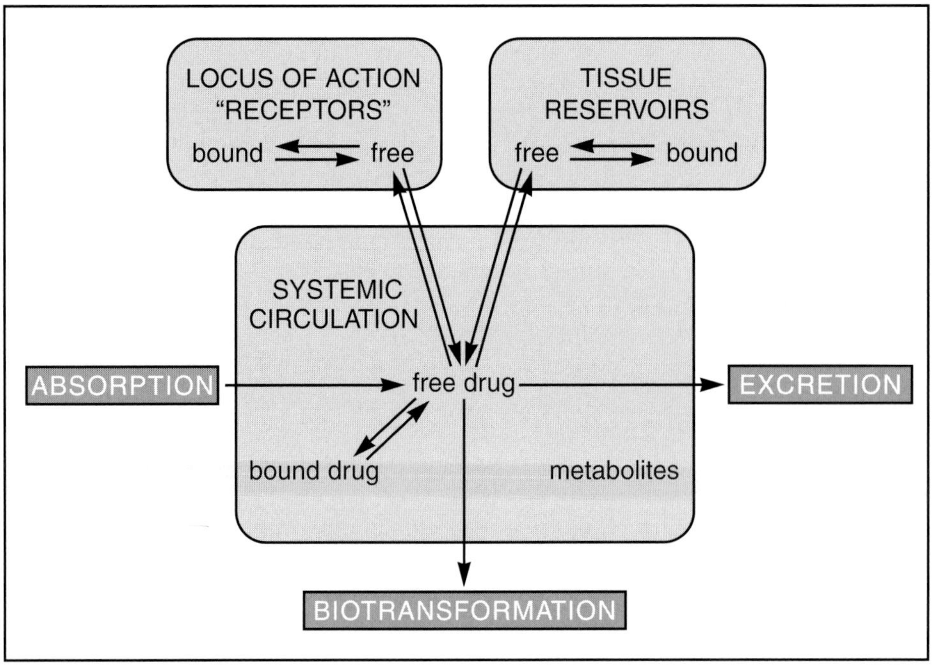

Figure 10-1. Schematic representation of the interrelationship of the absorption, distribution, binding, biotransformation, and excretion of a drug and its concentration at its locus of action. Reproduced with permission from Benet L. Pharmacokinetics: the dynamics of drug absorption, distribution, and elimination. In: Hardman, Goodman, Gilman, eds. The Pharmacologic Basis of Therapeutics, 9th Ed. New York, NY: The McGraw-Hill Companies; 1992.

istics of the immunosuppressive drugs. Tacrolimus (Prograf®) binds to alpha-1-acid-glycoprotein, and this may explain its lower propensity to cause hyperlipidemia compared to cyclosporine, which binds to lipoproteins.

Metabolism or Elimination

Metabolism is typically thought of as a means to facilitate elimination of lipid soluble drugs from the body; however, a number of compounds with poor absorption characteristics are administered as inactive pro-drugs, which require conversion to biologically active metabolites before they can elicit their pharmacologic effects. Two such immunosuppressive agents administered as pro-drugs include azathioprine, which is rapidly converted by plasma esterases to 6-mercaptopurine, and mycophenolate mofetil, which is rapidly de-esterified to mycophenolic acid.

The primary role of metabolism is to terminate the pharmacologic activity of the low molecular weight, lipid soluble compounds, and to convert them into more water soluble substances allowing for excretion in the urine or feces. The reactions of drug metabolism can be divided into two phases: phase I, which involves oxidation, reduction or hydrolysis; and phase II, which involves conjugation or synthetic reactions with endogenous donor molecules such as glucuronic acid, sulfate, glutathione, amino acids, and acetate. Phase I reactions are more important in reducing or terminating the biological effect, altering the drug in such a way that it is no longer able to interact with its specific target site. Products of phase I metabolism frequently serve as substrates for phase II reactions and allow the metabolites to be finally eliminated in the urine or feces.

Of the phase I reactions, those catalyzed by cytochrome P450-dependent mixed-function oxidase system predominate. There are multiple forms of cytochrome P450, subject to influence by a wide variety of genetic, environmental, physiological and pathological factors. The most important of these effects include induction, in which there is increased synthesis or decreased breakdown of P450, which occurs with compounds such as anticonvulsants (eg, phenytoin), hydrocarbons in cigarette smoke, alcohol, and tuberculostatic agents (eg, rifampin). Induction results in increased elimination of the drug and a decrease in its efficacy (eg, patients receiving concomitant cyclosporine (CsA) and rifampin may require a tripling of their CsA dosage to maintain therapeutic levels). Smoking can induce cytochrome P450 enzyme activity such that smokers often require larger doses of some drugs (eg, theophylline) compared with nonsmokers. Following discontinuation of an enzyme inducer, reversal of the inductive effects may take weeks to months, whereas inhibitory effects are usually dependent on the drug being physically detectable. Ethanol in acute high doses often inhibits the metabolism of other drugs; however, when taken chronically, produces hepatic enzyme induction, and finally following chronic use, can cause hepatic dysfunction impairing the metabolism of other drugs. Ethanol interactions with diazepam and warfarin are complex and can alter both metabolism and pharmacologic activity.

Inhibition of CYP450 is also important, reducing the elimination of one or both compounds and potentially aggravating the toxicity of a given agent. Some drugs act as highly competitive, specific inhibitors of a single form of P450 (eg, ketoconazole's affect on cyclosporine's metabolism by CYP4503A), whereas others depend on several enzymes and others act as relatively nonspecific inhibitors of P450 (eg, cimetidine). Specific drug interactions with immunosuppressants are addressed in more detail in a later chapter.

Even though the liver is thought of as the predominate site for drug metabolism, it is important to remember that other tissues and organs are also responsible for the biotransformation of drugs. The small intestine has a high concentration of CYP450 isoenzymes and is an important site for presystemic metabolism of commonly used immunosuppressant agents such as cyclosporine and tacrolimus. Other organs with significant metabolic activity include the kidneys, skin and lung. The kidney can excrete drugs by glomerular filtration or by such active processes as proximal tubular secretion. Drugs can also be eliminated in the bile produced by the liver or air expired by the lungs.

Pharmacokinetic Concepts

The three most important parameters are *clearance*, a measure of the body's ability to eliminate a drug; *volume of distribution*, a measure of the apparent space in the body available to contain the drug; and *bioavailability*, the fraction of drug absorbed into the systemic circulation.

CLEARANCE. Clearance is a pharmacokinetic parameter that describes the capability of a patient to eliminate a drug. This parameter relates the rate of elimination of a drug relative to its serum concentration. The concept of total body clearance takes into consideration all possible routes of elimination (renal, hepatic, and other organs) and is useful when designing drug regimens. Clearance can vary depending on organ dysfunction, age, gender and genetic makeup.

Most drugs follow linear pharmacokinetics, which means that serum concentrations change proportionally with changes in dosing (ie, doubling the dose results in a doubling of the serum concentration), and that the rate of elimination is also linear. This simple technique cannot be applied to several commonly used drugs, including phenytoin and ethanol, since their elimination processes are saturable (nonlinear) and can lead to rapidly increasing drug concentrations after small increases in dose.

Half-Life ($T_{1/2}$) . The term that usually describes the elimination rate of the drug in the body is the *half-life*, which is the time it takes for the plasma or blood concentration to decline by 50% (eg, it takes the same amount of time for a serum concentration to decline from 400 ng/mL to 200 ng/mL as it does to decline from 200 ng/mL to 100 ng/mL).

Half-life is a useful pharmacokinetic concept in that it determines the time required to achieve steady-state, and can also be used to determine the amount of desired serum concentration fluctuation in a given dosing interval. Typically, it takes three to five half-lives to reach steady-state concentrations for a given dosing regimen; application of this concept becomes important when determining whether a patient's drug concentration is being measured at steady-state for a given dosage (Figure 10-2). Similarly, following discontinuation of a medication, it takes five to seven half-lives for the drug to be completely eliminated from the system. For medications with short half-lives (eg, two to three hours), the drug is usually eliminated within 24 hours of discontinuation, whereas some of the newer serotonin re-uptake inhibitor (SSRI) antidepressants (eg, the half-life of fluoxetine's active metabolite norfluoxetin is more than six

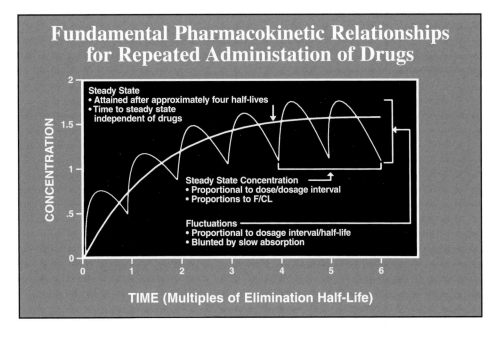

Figure 10-2. Fundamental pharmacokinetic relationships for repeated administration of drugs. Reproduced with permission from Benet L. Pharmacokinetics: the dynamics of drug absorption, distribution, and elimination. In: Hardman, Goodman, Gilman, eds. The Pharmacologic Basis of Therapeutics, 9th Ed. New York, NY: The McGraw-Hill Companies; 1992.

days) may have detectable concentrations and exert pharmacologic effects for up to a month or more following discontinuation (eg, when switching from fluoxetine [Prozac®] to an monoamine oxidase inhibitor, it is recommended that the patient wait five weeks before starting the new medication).

When selecting dosing intervals, half-life can be used to determine whether large or small variations are desired between the peak and trough concentrations. Drugs with narrow therapeutic indices may need to be dosed more frequently to avoid toxicity from high peak concentrations and lack of efficacy associated with too low trough concentrations (eg, a drug dosed at an interval equal to its half-life would have a 50% difference between its peak and trough concentration, whereas one dosed less frequently would be expected to have more variation in interval concentrations). For some drugs, it is better to maintain a steady-state concentration and minimize the fluctuation in serum concentrations, similar to an intravenous continuous infusion; in this setting, it is preferable to administer drugs in a sustained-release formulation.

VOLUME OF DISTRIBUTION

The apparent volume of distribution (Vd) is a proportionality constant that relates the amount of the drug in the body to the plasma concentration and rarely corresponds to an actual physiologic compartment. Drugs that are lipophilic have large Vds (eg, CsA, 4.3 l/kg; digoxin 6.7 l/kg; tricyclic antidepressants 15 to 30 l/kg) whereas hydrophilic compounds have small Vds (tobramycin, 0.2 l/kg). A patient's own Vd is rarely known, unless a pharmacokinetic profile is performed with multiple drug concentrations measured around a dosing interval, but average values can be used to calculate a loading dose for a patient to achieve a given serum concentration. Based on the ability of drugs to distribute into the various tissues, sometimes it is necessary to make dosage adjustments that are patient-specific (eg, for obese patients, it may be necessary to calculate a lean body weight for dosing purposes if a drug does not distribute into fat).

Disease states that alter albumin (eg, liver disease, nephrotic syndrome, malnutrition, burns, cancer) or other endogenous protein concentrations may complicate the use of therapeutic drug monitoring, as the measured total serum concentration (bound plus unbound) of a drug may be low while the free fraction remains therapeutic. Changes in the percentage of a drug bound to plasma proteins rarely have clinical consequences as a new equilibrium is usually achieved unless drug input is increased or clearance of the unbound drug is impaired. Problems arise, however, when practitioners attempt to restore total drug levels to those achieved with normal albumin concentrations (eg, the therapeutic range for

phenytoin (Dilantin®) is 10 μg/mL to 20 μg/mL with a normal free fraction of 10% (eg, 1 μg/mL to 2 μg/mL). However in patients with low albumin concentrations, a so-called *subtherapeutic* level of 5 μg/mL to 10 μg/mL may correspond to a therapeutic free fraction of 1 μg/mL to 2 μg/mL). Toxicity associated with an elevated free fraction occurs when one attempts to restore the patient's drug level to that identified as the normal therapeutic range. As most drug assays do not distinguish free from bound drug concentrations, it is important to remember that free fraction monitoring is useful for drugs such as phenytoin and valproic acid for patients with low albumin levels. This is especially important for drugs that exhibit nonlinear pharmacokinetics (eg, phenytoin), because a small increase in dose may result in a disproportionate increase in measured drug concentration. It has recently been suggested that free fraction monitoring for mycophenolate mofetil, which is 97% protein-bound, may be a more useful indicator of its therapeutic effect on IMPDH inhibition.

In addition to diseases that can affect binding of drugs to plasma proteins, if a patient is given two highly protein-bound drugs, they may compete for the same binding sites and displace one or both of the agents from those sites. This does not usually create a problem, unless one of the agents has a narrow therapeutic index; transient change in unbound concentration occurring immediately after the dose of the displacing drug could be of concern.

BIOAVAILABILITY. The bioavailability of different formulations or products is an important concept to understand when switching formulations of medications. Intravenous medications are usually considered to be 100% bioavailable, unless a salt formulation is administered (eg, aminophylline = 80% theophylline), whereas various oral formulations of a drug will exhibit different degrees of bioavailability. If a drug has good oral bioavailability (>90% bioavailable), dosage adjustments are not necessary when converting between oral and intravenous (IV) formulations. Conversely, when the magnitude of difference between bioavailability of formulations is great, such as in the case of intravenous and oral cyclosporine, major dosage adjustments are necessary to avoid toxicity or loss of efficacy (eg, when converting from oral CsA to IV, the IV dosage should be reduced to approximately 25% of the oral dosage). Even with oral products, bioavailability can vary somewhat among different dosage forms of the same drug (eg, liquid, tablet and capsule formulations of a given medication).

Bioequivalence . The determination of bioequivalence of two or more products is based on comparing the bioavailability of those products under identical conditions. This term has become relevant in the transplant community now that generic agents are available for a number of immunosuppressants (eg, CsA, azathioprine and prednisone). For a generic drug to be FDA approved (ie, receive an AB rating), it must meet standards for bioequivalence and come within a specified rate and extent of absorption of the original formulation used in clinical trials. Ironically, if a generic drug or even a different formulation of a brand-name drug (eg, Neoral® as compared to Sandimmune® CsA) demonstrates better bioavailability than the original product, it cannot be deemed bioequivalent. A number of misconceptions exist surrounding generic substitution and this is one area where passion and promotion rather than actual data play an important role regarding the substitution of FDA-approved generic equivalents for brand-name medicines. Since passage of the Waxman-Hatch amendments in 1962, few, if any, documented cases of nonequivalence between generically approved drugs and their brand-name equivalent have been reported. In fact, of the first 224 generic drugs approved, the observed mean difference in bioavailability between generic and innovator product was only 3.5%.

PHARMACODYNAMICS

Pharmacodynamics is the study of the relationship between concentration of a drug, the biochemical and physiologic effects of the drug and the biologic response obtained in a patient. For some diseases, a therapeutic response is easy to detect and it is not necessary to perform drug concentration monitoring. In patients with hypertension, blood pressure reduction is simple to monitor. In other disease states, therapeutic endpoints are much more difficult to observe, and the signs of medication inefficacy and toxicity may be difficult to recognize clinically. In some situations, the lack of efficacy may be detected only by the occurrence of undesirable "breakthrough events" such as in patients who have epilepsy, where there is a high intrinsic variability of seizure activity and where the likelihood of a seizure in a given patient is unpredictable. Another example is the prevention of acute allograft rejection, where the level of immune reactivity is hard to detect until a florid reaction is underway and significant damage to the graft has occurred. Chronic rejection is even more problematic since the changes are so subtle and the histologic effects irreversible.

Combining pharmacokinetic monitoring with the assessment of patient outcomes is based on the fact that a relationship between drug concentration and effect was identified in clinical pharmacology studies. Attempts are then made to apply this knowledge to patient care (Figure 10-3). This method can be limited by the fact that drug concentrations in the blood or plasma may not accurately reflect the concentrations achieved at the actual site of drug action. For those drugs exhibiting high degrees of protein binding, the issue of whether the free fraction or the total concentration should be monitored is also a topic of debate. Another confounding factor is that the analytical assays (eg, immunoassays) may measure both parent and crossreactive metabolites, and the metabolite may not contribute to overall efficacy. Finally, the major problem that exists with pharmacodynamic monitoring is that there is not one method to assess the cumulative effect of combination therapy. It certainly would be far easier to make clinical correlations between pharmacodynamic effect and drug concentrations if patients received only one drug that affected their immune systems. The lack of correlation with drug concentration monitoring and outcome variables for some agents is most likely influenced by the background immunosuppression provided by the other agents in the immunosuppressive cocktail. And even if pharmacodynamic monitoring techniques are identified for specific drugs, identification of a technique that measures the cumulative pharmacodynamic effect of combination therapy is highly desirable.

Pharmacodynamic monitoring is not performed routinely in the clinical setting, as it is very difficult to determine the concentration of a drug at a specific receptor site. Examples of pharmacodynamic monitoring that have been studied for immunosuppressive drugs include: measuring calcineurin activity for CsA; inosine monophosphate dehydrogenase activity for mycophenolic acid; thiopurine methyltransferase activity for azathioprine's metabolite; 6-mercaptopurine, and the activity of a P70 S6 kinase in lymphocytes for rapamycin.

TOXICOLOGY

Toxicology is the aspect of pharmacology that deals with adverse effects of drugs. Toxicity associated with specific serum concentrations can usually be managed by making appropriate dosage reductions. In other situations, toxicity may overlap with concentrations needed for effectiveness, and then the risks vs benefits of dosage adjustments must be considered. In this situation, it may be preferable to add a second agent in an attempt to optimize efficacy while minimizing toxicity. This is, in fact, the basis for combination therapy with multiple immunosuppressive agents used by most solid organ transplant programs.

Toxicity can vary on a spectrum that ranges from minor side effects to life-threatening consequences. Most adverse effects fall somewhere in the middle and can complicate therapy and increase the overall cost of managing the patient if the side effects necessitate the addition of more medications. As more medications are added to the regimen, the risk for additional or additive toxicities and drug interactions also increases. Impair-

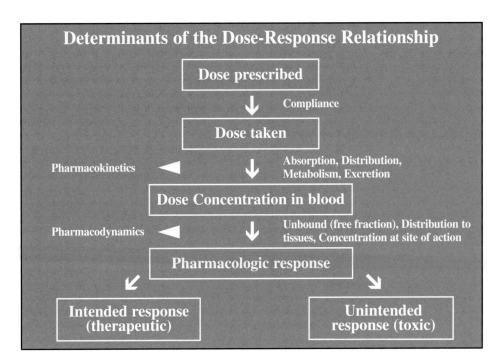

Figure 10-3. Determinants of the dose-response relationship.

ment of quality of life and the added cost burden for additional drug therapy or treatments need to be considered when selecting primary regimens for patients. Recent data suggest that for some chronic conditions, health care expenditures are greater for the drug-related toxicities than the direct cost of the original therapy. Patients should be queried about which adverse effects they are able or willing to tolerate, as noncompliance can become a factor if the side effects are either disfiguring (eg, hirsutism, alopecia, severe acne) or impair day-to-day functioning (eg, impotence, orthostatic hypotension, drowsiness). If alternative agents are available, it is far better to design a regimen that facilitates compliance rather than one that only offers efficacy.

PRINCIPLES OF THERAPEUTICS

Each year, a number of new medications are approved by the FDA and practitioners are faced with the dilemma of how to incorporate these agents into existing therapeutic regimens. Marketing efforts by the pharmaceutical industry to both health care providers and now directly to consumers are increasing the pressure to use new agents rather than existing products. However, it is important for the practitioner to determine what is best for his or her patients based on scientific evidence rather than marketing strategies. Evidence-based medicine has become the buzzword of current times as practitioners are faced with decisions regarding the use of older and usually less expensive agents vs new, more costly drugs. Large, randomized, prospective controlled clinical trials designed to evaluate the safety and efficacy of a new medication or intervention serve as the foundation for these studies. Practitioners are still challenged by the fact

that not all randomized prospective clinical trials provide useful answers to today's clinical questions, especially if irrelevant control groups are used that do not reflect contemporary practice or long-term follow-up is not performed. The latter is becoming an issue in transplantation, for as more agents become available, it is unlikely that a large number of patients will continue on a specific regimen for five to ten years. However, it is important to put these trials into perspective and realize that a difference exists between the reported efficacy of a new medication for a given population as compared to effectiveness of the medication in an individual patient.

Efficacy is the percentage of patients that can be expected to respond partially or totally, and/or tolerate a complete course of therapy under ideal conditions. Most clinical trials designed to study the safety and efficacy of a new agent are performed under ideal conditions (ie, rigorous exclusion criteria prohibit high-risk patients such as those with multiple disease states and complicated drug therapy regimens). In contrast, *effectiveness* is the percentage of patients who can be expected to respond partially or totally, and/or tolerate a complete course of therapy in the usual clinical practice setting. This partially explains why some adverse effects of recently approved medications are not detected until these agents are used in large numbers of patients who have multiple conditions and require complex drug regimens.

Because of the limitations of the existing scientific data and the complexity of current drug therapy regimens, a number of tools (eg, algorithms, treatment guidelines and decision analysis models) have been developed to assist the practitioner in making sound medical decisions. These tools are typically based on consensus conferences and analyses using evidence-based medicine, however, they too are limited by the timeliness with which they can be created.

THERAPEUTIC DRUG MONITORING

Ideally, drugs used for the transplant patient would be efficacious, safe and simple to use. However, even though the currently available agents are quite effective at preventing acute rejection in transplant patients, they all possess dose-limiting side effects, some of which occur well within the given therapeutic range. In addition, intrapatient and interpatient pharmacokinetic variability necessitates monitoring to ensure that adequate concentrations are present to maintain efficacy. Therapeutic drug monitoring facilitates the quantification of each patient's pharmacologic response. This process is based on the generation of evidence that a relationship exists between a given concentration and the drug producing a desired effect and not producing unwanted effects. When both are accomplished, the desired pharmacotherapeutic benefits will usually be realized.

The old adage, "treat the patient and not the drug level," should be at the forefront of practitioner's minds as a number of factors must be considered when interpreting the results of a drug level measurement (Figure 10-4).

Therapeutic Range

This concept is defined as the range of concentrations within which the pharmacologic response is produced and adverse effects are avoided in most patients. For practical purposes, the therapeutic range is useful as an initial goal of therapy and as a parameter for monitoring

drug therapy when the pharmacologic effects are not easy to identify. In general, as serum concentrations rise, more patients exhibit the desired pharmacologic effect, but they also may experience an increased incidence of adverse effects. The relationship between concentration and incidence of toxicity varies for different toxic effects. It is important to remember, however, that the therapeutic range is based on population data. A particular patient may achieve the desired effect at a low concentration, or may require a concentration higher than the population's therapeutic range to achieve the desired effect. When the relationship between drug concentration and effect in an individual patient is known, that information is more useful than knowledge of therapeutic range for the population. A particular patient may experience adverse effects at a concentration well below the therapeutic range. In addition, it is important to remember that there may be a low incidence of idiosyncratic or hypersensitivity reactions that are independent of drug concentration.

For most drugs in clinical use, the desired effect is obtained in a large percentage of patients at concentrations that cause few serious toxic effects. However, there are also a limited number of medications that are considered to have a narrow therapeutic range (or window or interval). Within the US Code of Federal Regulations (21CFR320.33), a definition exists for narrow therapeutic "ratio" drugs such that: (1) there is less than a twofold difference in median lethal dose (LD 50) and median effective dose (ED50) values; or (2) there is less than a twofold difference in the minimum toxic concentrations and minimum effective concentrations in the blood; and (3) safe and effective use of the drug products requires

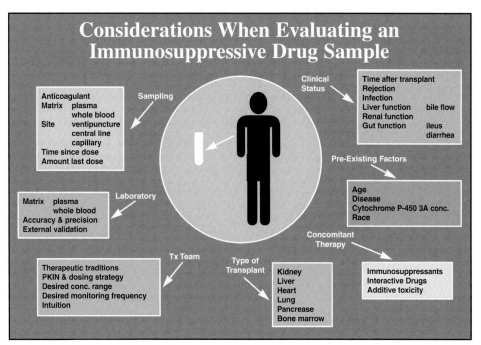

Figure 10-4. Considerations when evaluating an immunosuppressive drug sample. Adapted and reprinted with permission from Lindholm A, Sawe J. Pharmacokinetics and therapeutic drug monitoring of immunosuppressants. Ther Drug Monit. 1995;17(6):570-573.

careful dosage titration and patient monitoring. Not all medications that have so-called *therapeutic* ranges necessarily meet the strict definitions as listed in (1) and (2) above, but therapeutic monitoring is still useful in individualizing drug therapy regimens.

Sampling Techniques for Therapeutic Drug Monitoring

TROUGH CONCENTRATION MONITORING. Measurement of trough concentrations, which are usually reached just before administration of the next dose, offers several advantages: it provides a reliable and reproducible assessment of the lowest effective concentration during a given dosing interval, it is easy to perform (ie, can be done daily and as an outpatient), and it is the standard acceptable method for monitoring most drugs. Limitations of trough level monitoring are that: (1) it is only a rough estimation of what is occurring during the rest of the dosing interval; (2) not all drugs exhibit a good correlation between trough concentration and pharmacodynamic effect; and (3) if the result is inconsistent with what is expected or if the sample is missed, there are no additional data points available, and the patient will need a repeat study.

AREA UNDER THE CURVE MONITORING AND ABBREVIATED AREA UNDER THE CURVE. Traditional area under the curve (AUC) monitoring involves sampling over the entire dosing interval (eg, eight to 12 samples drawn over 12 hours). The advantages of AUC monitoring are that a concentration-time profile is available for analysis, pharmacokinetics parameters (eg, volume of distribution, clearance, half-life) can be calculated, and even if one sample is omitted, an adequate number of specimens is available. The disadvantages include the fact that AUC monitoring requires patients to spend prolonged periods of time at the hospital, is not practical to perform on a daily basis or as an outpatient, and is costly.

An abbreviated AUC involves less frequent sampling (eg, two to four specimens) over a dosing interval. This technique offers several advantages in that it is more convenient, less costly and can possibly be performed on an outpatient basis. Limitations of this method are that a very strong correlation must exist between the preselected time points and pharmacodynamic effect, and if samples are not drawn correctly, the data are almost impossible to interpret and extrapolations to concentration-effect time curves are weakened.

PEAK CONCENTRATION MONITORING. When a drug is given orally, one must allow time for absorption to occur, and even though it is assumed that most drugs achieve their peak concentrations within one to two

hours, it is still difficult to know when a peak concentration should be drawn. A serum concentration measured too soon after an oral dose may not accurately reflect the concentration after complete drug absorption. Again, in most cases, measurement of trough concentrations is recommended to avoid this problem with long-term oral therapy. After an intravenous drug dose is administered, the drug remains in high concentration in the blood for a short time until it can equilibrate into the tissues. In most cases, the high serum concentrations measured before tissue penetration has occurred are not related to clinical effect. The relationship between drug serum concentrations and pharmacologic effect (ie, pharmacodynamics) is known only when the serum concentration is in equilibrium with the tissue concentration.

TOXICITY. If toxicity is suspected, the serum concentration of a drug should be measured at that moment. Prior to the development of sustained release theophylline preparations, some patients exhibited signs of toxicity (eg, tremors, palpitations) associated with high peak concentrations, yet exhibited signs and symptoms of inadequate therapy associated with subtherapeutic trough concentrations at the end of the dosing interval. A high serum concentration with symptoms of possible toxicity helps to validate the suspicion of a drug effect. In this situation, measurements should be made without regard to whether the patient is at steady-state or the time of dose administration.

Assays

For TDM to be useful on a clinical basis, analytical techniques must exist that have adequate sensitivity and specificity for detection of a compound. In addition, the preferred media (whole blood or plasma) for sampling must be identified. Due to temperature-dependent effects on equilibrium between plasma and whole blood, the latter has been selected as the preferred media for immunosuppressants such as CsA and tacrolimus. The various analytical techniques offer advantages and disadvantages: HPLC is considered the "gold standard" for measurement of parent compound and metabolites, however, it is a more complicated procedure and can be time prohibitive if many samples need to be performed at the same time. Immunoassays (EMIT, RIA) offer the advantage of relatively quick performance, but a disadvantage is that immunoassays are not as sensitive and crossreactivity may occur between the parent compound and its metabolites.

Drug concentrations are studied for most immunosuppressants during clinical development, however, a good correlation between efficacy and drug concentration is not always identified. Some of the early clinical studies have been limited by analytical techniques that lack sensitivity and specificity rather than a poor correlation with efficacy. The current assay for measuring tacrolimus concentrations provides a much better correlation between trough concentrations and pharmacodynamic effect.

Indications for Therapeutic Drug Monitoring

EFFICACY. Patients can often be treated more effectively with fewer drugs if the dosage regimen of each is optimized. Since the application of therapeutic drug monitoring, epilepsy is well-controlled by a single drug in many more patients than before. Also, the fewer drugs used, the less probability of serious adverse drug reactions or interactions. Compliance also tends to be better when fewer drugs are prescribed and dosage is less frequent. Therapeutic drug monitoring can be useful in making correlations with patient outcomes and identifying patient-specific *therapeutic ranges*. Practitioners are often challenged by situations in which the patient has therapeutic levels yet exhibits signs of toxicity or inefficacy. In these cases, it becomes prudent to individualize therapy according to the patient response and not rely solely on a drug concentration.

Measuring serum drug concentrations can also be used to identify the optimal dose for some drugs with wider therapeutic indices and avoid excessive dosing of patients to achieve the same desired therapeutic effect. This would reduce the patient's exposure to potential toxicity and reduce the overall cost. A good example is vancomycin that, when originally marketed, was dosed in a standard regimen (eg, 1.0 gm every 12 hours or 500 mg every six hours) until blood level monitoring demonstrated that the majority of adults achieve effective concentrations when doses are administered less frequently. These patients did not necessarily exhibit overt toxicity with the standard regimen, but appropriate therapy was administered at a lower cost.

COMPLIANCE. Serum concentration monitoring can also be useful for the practitioner to assess patient compliance with a drug regimen. However, it is important to remember that poor compliance is not the only cause of subtherapeutic drug concentrations; for example, rapid elimination or poor absorption, drug interactions or increased dosage requirements, as is the case with adolescent growth, could also be responsible. Some noncompliant patients may actually have supratherapeutic concentrations as they attempt to give themselves a loading dose on the day prior to checking their drug levels.

DRUG INTERACTIONS. Therapeutic drug monitoring is mandatory when two drugs known to interact (eg, CsA and ketoconazole) are administered simultaneously. Drug concentration monitoring can also be useful to identify the presence of unknown or suspected drug concentrations when two or more drugs with the potential to interact are administered.

SUMMARY

The application of the understanding of pharmacology, pharmacokinetics and pharmacodynamics is very important when dealing with transplant patients. Due to the complexity of the medication regimens for transplant patients and the consequences of suboptimal drug therapy, practitioners should take advantage of the available tools to optimize drug therapy regimens.

RECOMMENDED READING

Winter ME, ed. Basic Clinical Pharmacokinetics, 3rd ed. Spokane, WA; Applied Therapeutics, Inc.: 1994.

Evans WE, Schentag JJ, Jusko WJ, eds. Applied Pharmacokinetics: Principles of Therapeutic Drug Monitoring, 3rd ed. Spokane, WA; Applied Therapeutics, Inc.: 1992.

Johnson L, Bootman JL. Drug-related morbidity and mortality: a cost-of-illness model. Arch Intern Med. 1995;155(18):1949-1956.

Lown KS, Mayo RR, Leichtman AB, et al. Role of intestinal P-glycoprotein (mdr1) in interpatient variation in the oral bioavailability of cyclosporine. Clin Pharmacol Ther. 1997;62(3):248-260.

Aronoff GR, ed. Drug Prescribing in Renal Failure: Dosing Guidelines for Adults. American College of Physicians; Philadelphia, Pa: 1999.

Benet LZ, Goyan JE. Bioequivalence and narrow therapeutic index drugs. Pharmacotherapy. 1995;15(4):433-440.

Murphy JE. Generic substitution and optimal patient care [editorial]. Arch Intern Med. 1999;159(5):429-433.

Yatscoff RW, Aspeslet LJ, Gallant HL. Pharmacodynamic monitoring of immunosuppressive drugs. Clin Chem. 1998;44(2):428-432.

Shaw LM, Nicholls A, Hale M, et al. Therapeutic monitoring of mycophenolic acid. A consensus panel report. Clin Biochem. 1998;31(5):317-322 .

Meier-Kriesche HU, Kaplan B, Brannan P, Kahan BD, Portman RJ. A limited sampling strategy for the estimation of eight-hour Neoral® areas under the curve in renal transplantation. Ther Drug Monit. 1998;20(4):401-407.

Primmett DR, Levine M, Kovarik JM, Mueller EA, Keown PA. Cyclosporine monitoring in patients with renal transplants: two- or three-point methods that estimate area under the curve are superior to trough levels in predicting drug exposure. Ther Drug Monit. 1998;20(3):276-283.

Oellerich M, Armstrong VW, Kahan B, et al. Lake Louise Consensus Conference on cyclosporin monitoring in organ transplantation: report of the consensus panel. Ther Drug Monit. 1995;17(6):642-654.

Braun F, Schutz E, Christians U, et al. Pitfalls in monitoring tacrolimus (FK 506). Ther Drug Monit. 1997;19(6):628-631.

Alak AM. Measurement of tacrolimus (FK506) and its metabolites: a review of assay development and application in therapeutic drug monitoring and pharmacokinetic studies. Ther Drug Monit. 1997;19(3):338-351.

Jusko WJ, Thomson AW, Fung J, et al. Consensus document: therapeutic monitoring of tacrolimus (FK-506). Ther Drug Monit. 1995;17(6):606-614.

Shaw LM, Sollinger HW, Halloran P, et al. Mycophenolate mofetil: a report of the consensus panel. Ther Drug Monit. 1995;17(6):690-699.

Yatscoff RW, Boeckx R, Holt DW, et al. Consensus guidelines for therapeutic drug monitoring of rapamycin: report of the consensus panel. Ther Drug Monit. 1995;17(6):676-680.

Shaw LM, Annesley TM, Kaplan B, Brayman KL. Analytic requirements for immunosuppressive drugs in clinical trials. Ther Drug Monit. 1995;17(6):577-583.

Schumacher GE, Barr JT. Economic and outcome issues for therapeutic drug monitoring in medicine. Ther Drug Monit. 1998;20(5):539-542.

11 PRINCIPLES AND OVERVIEW OF IMMUNOSUPPRESSION

Philip F. Halloran, MD, PhD
Sita Gourishankar, MD

INTRODUCTION: IMMUNOSUPPRESSION VS TOLERANCE

Clinical immunosuppression is the control of undesirable immune responses while avoiding, if possible, the complications of immunodeficiency – infection and malignancy. The effect can be achieved by ablation (ie, damaging immune tissue and killing lymphocytes); by altering lymphocyte location and traffic; or by altering lymphocyte function. These interventions may be physical or pharmacologic, and may or may not be reversible. In practice, immunosuppression is usually achieved by using immunosuppressive drugs (ISDs) that reversibly suspend lymphocyte functions.

Ideally, transplants between unrelated persons *(allografts)* or species *(xenografts)* would be accepted as self by the host. The host immune system would be induced to be specifically unresponsive to the antigens of the graft *(immunological tolerance)*. Tolerance is antigen-specific unresponsiveness, induced by previous exposure to the antigen. Tolerance avoids the need to suppress host defense with the attendant risks of infection and cancer, and to use drugs that produce collateral damage to host organs and tissues. True tolerance should be stable and durable over many years.

Although many experimental protocols have been proposed, tolerance can only be achieved by a successful transplantation of allogeneic bone marrow bearing the antigens of the donor. This establishes significant (ie, 1% or more) numbers of donor stem cells in the host. This state can be termed *chimerism,* recalling the chimera in Greek mythology, wherein tissues of multiple organisms lived in one individual. In practice, achieving a successful bone marrow transplant across HLA differences is not possible as a routine clinical procedure. Chimerism should be distinguished from *microchimerism,* which is the persistence of small (ie, one per 10,000) numbers of

Philip F. Halloran, MD, PhD, Professor of Medicine and Immunology, Division of Nephrology and Immunology, University of Alberta, Edmonton, Alberta, Canada

Sita Gourishankar, MD, Nephrology Fellow, Division of Nephrology and Immunology, University of Alberta, Edmonton, Alberta, Canada

donor marrow cells in the host. Spontaneous microchimerism occurs frequently after transplants, pregnancies, and transfusions. However, microchimerism does not establish tolerance, although it may somewhat reduce the responsiveness of the host immune system. Thus, no current procedure can establish robust and durable tolerance with acceptable morbidity. We are left with immunosuppression.

In reality, organ transplantation with ISDs is successful because, in the first few months, the organ evokes an adaptation of the host immune response to the antigens of the graft – a state of partial unresponsiveness to antigen. Thus, heavy immunosuppression is required early, but the doses are reduced after several months. To remain stable, this state of partial adaptation requires persistence of the graft and continued immunosuppression. Occasionally, people with organ transplants can completely discontinue ISDs for long periods of time with no rejection, probably reflecting a state of specific and nonspecific unresponsiveness. The ability to discontinue ISDs without rejection is sometimes used to define tolerance in an operational sense, but the withdrawal of ISDs in humans creates an inherently unstable state. Most persons who discontinue their ISDs eventually reject and ultimately lose their grafts. In the current state of the art, complete withdrawal of ISDs can only be regarded as suitable when one is prepared to accept the loss of the organ.

THE IMMUNE RESPONSE

The basic principles of the host recognition and response to foreign antigens are discussed in Section I, Chapter 2, and are summarized here as a backdrop for discussing the mechanism of action of ISDs. The principal elements to consider are outlined in Table 11-1.

The competence of the immune system is based on the organization of lymphoid tissues and the functional state of the antigen-presenting system and of the antigen-specific lymphocytes. Antigens can induce a response, can induce unresponsiveness, or can be ignored. The usual rules for response are that freely-circulating antigens evoke unresponsiveness, locally-expressed antigens in normal tissue are ignored, and locally-expressed antigens in stressed, injured, or inflamed sites evoke immune responses.

There is much more to transplant survival than immunity (Figure 11-1, Table 11-1). The organ transplant is, by definition, an area of stress. The organ itself is like a used car, carrying its stresses from the original owner. Then it experiences many types of acute injury in the transplant process, especially in the brain dead donor. This combination of chronic injury (ie, age) and acute injury (ie, brain death) can be considered as "input" (Figure 11-1). Injury decreases graft survival: in most organs, measures of nonspecific injury are associated with reduced survival of the transplant. One example is the reduced survival of kidney transplants from brain dead individuals compared with those from living donors. This could reflect the direct effects of injury, or the tendency of injury to evoke the immune response. Injury evokes a complex program of inflammation called the *injury response.* The injury response increases the expression of many genes in the graft, including chemokines, cytokines, growth factors, MHC molecules, and adhesion molecules, followed by a mononuclear cell infiltrate. The injury response is not an immune response, but can mimic rejection. Moreover, the injury response may increase the antigen-presenting mechanisms of the host, and thus may facilitate rejection. Independent of input and immune-inflammatory stress, the transplant experiences chronic stresses in the recipient, such as hypertension, obesity, drug toxicity, and hyperlipidemia.

The immune response is initiated when donor antigens on antigen-presenting cells (APCs) (typically monocytes, macrophages and dendritic cells) from the host or the donor trigger the host T cells (typically CD4 T cells) (Figures 11-2, 11-3). Donor antigen triggering of host T cell receptors (TCRs) is called *signal 1.* TCRs signal through a transduction apparatus known as the *CD3 complex.* Presentation of donor antigen by host APCs is termed *indirect,* and by donor APCs is called *direct.* The APCs also provide costimulation (*signal 2*) which increases the strength and duration of signal 1. The majority of signal 2 is due to B7-1/B7-2 on the APC binding to CD28 on the T cells. T cell activation can increase signal 2; activated T cells express CD40 ligand (CD40L) which can activate the APC by engaging CD40 on the APC. There are many other effects of CD40L, such as helping B cells to switch to IgG production.

Activation of signal 1 and 2 leads to signals through the calcium-calcineurin pathway and the MAP kinase

---

Table 11-1. Determinants and Events in Graft Recognition

Injury
    Chronic: age, hypertension
    Acute: brain death, ICU, removal, preservation, implantation, reperfusion

Immune recognition
    TCR triggering
    Costimulation
    Activation via the CN and MAP kinase pathways lead to activated cytokine expression
    Trigger cytokine receptors (ie, IL-2R)
    TOR pathway
    Signaling pathways to cell cycle
    De novo synthesis of purines and pyrimidines
    Clonal expansion
    Development of effector pathways

Resolution, adaptation, and memory

The fate of the graft: determinants of long-term function and survival
    Workload (eg, recipient size, race, sex)
    Blood pressure
    Lipid abnormalities
    Drug toxicity (ie, nephrotoxicity)
    Infectious agents

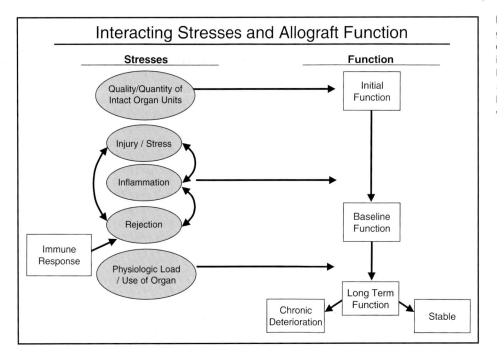

Figure 11-1. The fate of an allograft reflects initial quality of the organ *(input),* the immune and inflammatory stresses, and the long-term workload and stress *(load)* on the graft. The early baseline function correlates well with long-term survival.

pathway. Calcineurin activates the nuclear factor of activated T cells (NF-AT) family of transcription factors. Calcineurin dephosphorylates serines in the NF-ATs, which causes NF-ATs to move into the nucleus and bind specific DNA binding sites in promoters of cytokine genes. This is one of the key mechanisms activating cytokine transcription. The MAP kinase pathways activate transcription factors, such Jun and Fos, which form the AP-1 complex. The activation of many transcription factors initiate the transcription of cytokine genes, including growth factors such as IL-2 and proinflammatory factors such as IFN-γ. Depending on the types and degrees of signaling, full activation of the T cell may occur, or T cells may undergo partial activation, apoptosis, or anergy.

IL-2 signals through its specific receptor, one component (the α chain) of which is CD25. IL-2 and other T cell growth factors engage receptors that deliver the signal which activates the cell cycle *(signal 3)*. One of the critical pathways for signal 3 requires the enzyme TOR (target of rapamycin) (Figures 11-2, 11-3). TOR controls the translation of mRNAs for proteins, which regulate the cycle. Cell cycling in lymphocytes requires the de novo synthesis of purines, controlled by the enzyme inosine monophosphate dehydrogenase (IMPDH), which controls GMP synthesis. GMP levels are critical because GMP deficiency and AMP excess shuts down the de novo pathway of biosynthesis of purines, which are selectively required for the proliferation of T and B lymphocytes.

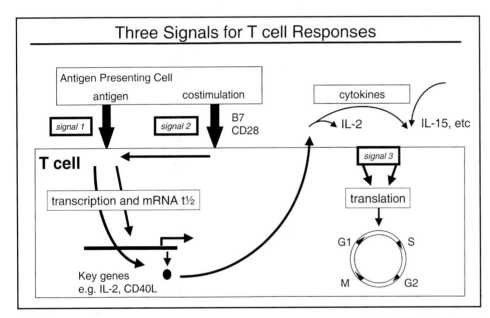

Figure 11-2. Three signals for the T cell response. The antigen-presenting cell presents antigen (MHC plus peptide) and co-stimulation (ie, B7 molecules). Antigen (signal 1) and costimulation (signal 2) together produce intense and prolonged activation of the T cell, resulting in the activation of the transcription of cytokine genes and a prolongation of the half-life of cytokine mRNAs. Certain cytokines such as IL-2 activate signal transduction pathways leading to the cell cycle. One of the critical events on the cell cycle is the activation of translation of certain pre-existing mRNAs.

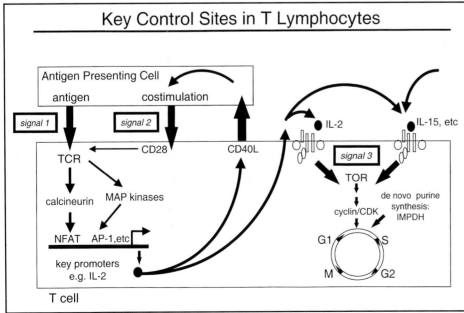

Figure 11-3. Some of the principal mediators in T cell activation. Shown are the TCR (T cell receptor), CD28, calcineurin, MAP kinases, NF-AT, AP-1, leading to production of cytokines. The steps in the cytokine pathways include activation of cytokine receptors, with associated tyrosine kinases, activation of TOR (target of rapamycin), and activation of cyclin/cyclin-dependent kinase control mechanisms leading to progression from G1 to S phase. As lymphocytes enter the S phase, they require de novo synthesis of purines, by a pathway in which IMPDH is the limiting step.

As the immune response builds, CD4 and CD8 T cells home to the graft by virtue of expression of chemokines, adhesion molecules, and foreign MHC antigens by the endothelium of the graft. Mononuclear cells enter the interstitium by crossing the endothelium of the microcirculation. Typical acute rejection requires tissue invasion by mononuclear cells, including T cells (many of which are activated), monocytes and macrophages, B cells and plasma cells, and varying numbers of other cell types. The antigen-specific lymphocytes recruit and activate nonspecific cells such as macrophages. In some cases, unusual pictures emerge such as neutrophil infiltration, particularly when antibody and complement are operating.

Many genes involved in inflammation are regulated by the nuclear factor – κB (NF-κB) family of transcription factors. These are proteins that reside in the cytosol in resting cells, bound to inhibitors called IκB. When inflammation is activated (ie, by cytokines such as TNF-α) IκB is degraded, releasing NF-κB, which moves into the nucleus, engages specific sequences in DNA, and activates transcription of many genes.

The immune response leads to three effector mechanisms: cytotoxic T lymphocytes (CTL), delayed type hypersensitivity (DTH), and alloantibody. CD8 T cells recognize donor class I HLA products to become CTL. CD4 T cells recognize donor-derived MHC peptides in the groove of recipient class II molecules, and develop the ability to recruit and activate nonspecific inflammatory cells whose products then cause the DTH process. CD4 T cells also help B cells to produce IgG, by binding via CD40L to CD40 on the B cell, thereby directing the immunoglobulin class switch from IgM to IgG production by the B cell. Preformed antibody can destroy the graft rapidly, a process termed *hyperacute rejection*. Alloantibody appearing posttransplant can mediate acute rejection, particularly in the first days of the transplant.

The diagnostic feature of acute rejection in a biopsy is invasion of the endothelium of the vessels *(endothelialitis)* and invasion of the parenchymal structures, associated with injury to the cells in these locations. For example, kidney rejection takes the form of tubulitis, and liver rejection displays bile ductulitis, as mononuclear cells invade the respective epithelia. Whether the parenchymal injury is mediated by CTL or by DTH is not clear; the mechanisms of rejection are T cell-dependent, but the molecular mechanism of the pathologic lesions remains undefined. (Note: Sometimes tubulitis and inflammation are found in renal biopsies with no clinical evidence of rejection. This may be the response to injury, and should not be considered "subclinical rejection".)

The T cell response is programmed to self-terminate, and will tend to do so if the graft is not rejected. The mechanisms involve antigen-driven apoptosis; expression of CTLA4 to terminate cytokine production; and other mechanisms leading to anergy. (Note: apoptosis may also follow antigen withdrawal but that is a different mechanism.) It is here that immunosuppression and tolerance converge. The clinician uses tools to prevent rejection, while trying to permit (or ideally promote) adaptations that attenuate the clonal response, which leads to acute rejection. Thus, most acute rejection occurs in the first three months, and immunosuppression can be reduced after the first few months.

The degree of adaptation to the graft varies among individuals, and is usually neither complete nor durable. Responsiveness usually persists, necessitating long-term immunosuppression. Moreover, responsiveness may be reactivated by intercurrent events, such as infections. Late deterioration of the graft may reflect either immune or nonimmune mechanisms. One of the powerful influences on long-term graft function and survival is the age of the donor, which may determine the ability of the tissue to withstand the stress of brain death and the transplantation process.

GENERAL FEATURES OF IMMUNOSUPPRESSION

Immunosuppression can be achieved by ablation of lymphocytes or lymphoid tissue, sequestration of lymphocytes, or altered function of lymphocytes. Ablation of lymphoid tissue can severely impair the immune response. In the past, whole body irradiation, lymphoid tissue irradiation, surgical ablation of lymphoid tissue (eg, thymectomy, splenectomy) and destruction of lymphocytes by thoracic duct drainage have been employed. Some current immunosuppressives and some experimental agents work by destruction of lymphocytes, followed by recovery. In general, the process of depletion of lymphocytes, followed by recovery in the presence of antigen, favors unresponsiveness to antigens encountered during recovery. Depletion strategies work, but the available methods tend to have excessive morbidity. The degree to which a depleted system truly recovers to normal function is questionable, especially in older persons. Sequestration and altered traffic of lymphocytes may be a component of the action of many immunosuppressives, including some in development. However, the mainstay of immunosuppression is the use of ISDs that interfere with lymphocyte functions.

The principal characteristics of ISDs are their potency, selectivity, reliability of delivery, durability, and reversibility. One could also consider patient acceptance, compliance, and cost. Potency of an immunosuppressive requires inhibition of a process that is required by the immune response, either in development or during the immune response. Other cells have similar requirements as the immune response (eg, DNA synthesis, cell respiration). Selectivity reflects the degree to which the targeted process is required by the immune response, but not by other tissues. Ideally, the mechanism targeted is needed solely by the immune system, or is more important to immune cells than to other cells. (Note: selectivity could also be achieved by targeting a drug uniquely to lymphocytes and thus avoiding effects on other cells.)

As guides to the potency and selectivity of a biochemical process for the immune system, one can look at spontaneous mutations that affect the process in humans, or at spontaneous or targeted mutations in mice (ie, knockout mice). The identification of the mechanism of action of known immunosuppressive drugs also leads to an understanding of targets for new immunosuppressives.

Reliability describes consistent drug delivery. Durability means the potential for reuse or continued use in the same host. Reversibility reflects the extent to which the immune system recovers from the intervention. If the intervention structurally alters lymphoid tissue, recovery may take months. Moreover, it must not be assumed that all injury to the immune system is reversible. Deficits may persist indefinitely after treatment is stopped, especially in older people, and alter severe depletion. This is a consideration with some new experimental treatments that alter immune tissue, or that severely deplete T cells.

IDENTIFYING ESSENTIAL STEPS: MUTATIONS, KNOCKOUTS, AND MECHANISMS OF ESTABLISHED ISDS

One can control the immune response by interventions at rate-limiting steps. To identify the critical points, one can learn from the study of human immunodeficiencies,

spontaneous or induced mutations in animals (ie, knockout mice), and the action of immunosuppressive drugs. Many immunodeficiencies can now be explained on the basis of mutations in genes affecting pathways essential for immune responses. The immunodeficiencies are often difficult to interpret because of impaired immune system development as well as function. The list of genetic mutations known to produce severe immunodeficiency is growing, due to studies of human primary immunodeficiencies and the ability to create knockout mice. Some processes previously considered vital, such as IL-2 expression, have been shown in knockout mice to be partially redundant. Again, this is useful information when developing immunosuppressives that affect IL-2.

The study of the mechanism of action of empirically developed ISDs has often led to the identification of key steps in the immune response (Figure 11-4). The role of calcineurin and TOR in T cells was identified by studying the action of ISDs. The problem of studying drug effects is that a drug can have more than one action.

THE CLASSES OF ISDS

A classification of ISDs is presented in Table 11-2 and the current status is listed in Table 11-3.

Small Molecule ISDs

Small molecule drugs typically act on intracellular targets. The first small molecule drugs were the glucocorticosteroids (GC), followed by the antimetabolites, such as azathioprine, made by modifying a purine. Subsequently, the discovery of other small molecule ISDs has been similar to the discovery of antibiotics: screening compounds produced by microorganisms. The ISDs

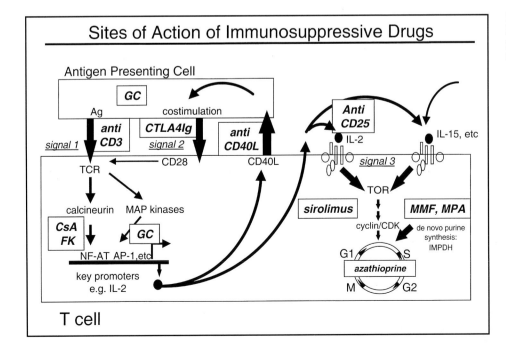

Figure 11-4. A map of the postulated site of action of some of the principal immunosuppressives. GC indicates glucocorticoid.

identified in this way have been those that act on highly conserved enzyme systems such as calcineurin, TOR, and IMPDH. That explains why these agents act on the same targets in lymphocytes as in microorganisms. Cyclosporine (CsA), tacrolimus (FK), rapamycin, and mycophenolate mofetil (MMF) are examples of the usefulness of this strategy.

There is great potential in structure-based drug design. However, no small molecule drug to date has been created by structure-based drug design (ie, using structural information about the target molecule). Many inhibitors of key enzymes can be created in this way, but they often inhibit something unexpected.

Protein ISDs

The protein-based drugs are targeted against extracellular or membrane molecules of the immune system, and have a very high potential for selectivity and potency. Protein immunosuppressives have been used in renal transplantation since the introduction of antilymphocyte globulin (ALG) or antithymocyte globulin (ATG). ALG and ATG are prepared by injecting human lymphoid cells into animals (ie, horses, goats, or rabbits), which then make antibodies against the human immune proteins. The resulting globulin preparations are purified by absorption to reduce toxic activities (eg, antiplatelet antibody). Polyclonal antibodies against human lymphocytes remain effective with repeated use, perhaps because they contain such a diverse array of immunoglobulins, in such relatively large quantities, that the host cannot neutralize them. In rare cases, allergies to the foreign proteins can develop.

Mouse monoclonal antibodies are produced by inducing mice to produce antibodies, then fusing their spleen cells with myelomas to create hybridomas. Then, the hybridoma producing the desired specificity is selected. The development of mouse monoclonals per-

---

Table 11-2. A Classification of Immunosuppressive Therapies

Physical therapies

Irradiation, total lymphoid irradiation, UV irradiation
Thoracic duct drainage
Thymectomy, splenectomy
Other depleting therapies

Pharmaceutical therapies

Small molecule drugs
Glucocorticosteroids

Immunophilin binding drugs
calcineurin inhibitors: cyclosporine, tacrolimus
TOR inhibitors: rapamycin, RAD

Inhibitors of de novo nucleotide synthesis
Purine synthesis: IMPDH inhibitors
Mycophenolic acid
Mycophenolate mofetil
Mizorbine (only in Japan)
Pyrimidine synthesis: DHODH inhibitors
Brequinar
Leflunomide
Azathioprine, antimetabolites
Cyclophosphamide
Deoxyspergualin

FTY720
Protein drugs
Antibodies against immune proteins
polyclonal ALG
murine monoclonals
humanized murine monoclonals
Fusion proteins using natural properties
solubilized ligands: eg, P selectin ligand, CTLA4Ig
solubilized receptors: IFN-γ Receptor
Immunotoxins
IL-2 -targeted toxins
Anti-CD3 targeted toxins
IVIg
Peptides
Oligonucleotides
Gene therapy

Table 11-3. Immunosuppressive Drugs Currently in Clinical Use or Trials in Transplantation

Polyclonal ALG/ATG
Murine monoclonal anti-CD3; Humanized anti-CD3
Glucocorticosteroids
Cyclosporine, tacrolimus
Humanized or chimeric monoclonal anti-CD25
(Anti-CD40 ligand: on hold)
Rapamycin (sirolimus), RAD
MMF, mycophenolic acid
Azathioprine
Leflunomide
(FTY720: phase I in normals)

Others at or near human phase I:
ICAM-1 Antisense oligonucleotide
Humanized Anti-LFA-1
Soluble P selectin ligand (PSGL)

Agents which have been in human trials
Murine anti-ICAM-1
Murine anti-LFA-1
Brequinar
Deoxyspergualin

mitted the introduction of anti-CD3. However, human hosts make antibodies against mouse monoclonals, which can severely limit the continued or future use of the drug (ie, the durability). Recently, the technology was developed to engineer the mouse monoclonals to be "nearly human". The human IgG framework (constant regions) are substituted for the mouse framework, but the mouse antigen-binding regions are retained. This can be achieved by retaining the entire mouse V region, creating a "chimeric" monoclonal. Alternatively, one can leave only the mouse complementarity determining regions, creating a "humanized" monoclonal. Humanized or chimeric monoclonal antibodies do not seem to be limited by host antibody responses.

Fusion proteins such as CTLA4Ig represent a new class of agents. Fusion proteins use the natural ligand for a molecule to define specificity, but add the Fc portion of human IgG to confer stability and effector functions. CTLA4Ig retains the specificity of CTLA4, but with the stability and effector functions of the Fc portions of human IgG. Engineering existing natural ligands, such as CTLA4, overcomes the problem of the very short half-lives of most injected natural proteins. Soluble P selectin ligand (PSGL) has also been engineered in the form of a fusion protein to block P selectin.

The number of monoclonal antibodies and fusion proteins that can be generated is almost unlimited. The key is to select the right target and the correct protein for development, and hope that it will perform favorably in clinical trials.

PROTEINS VS SMALL MOLECULES

Proteins and small molecule drugs each have their advantages and disadvantages. Proteins have very high specificity and potentially few side effects but cannot cross membranes and are limited to interactions with surface molecules. They must be administered parenterally, but they may have very long half-lives.

Small molecule drugs (*xenobiotics*) cross membranes freely and usually inhibit enzymes. To date, only a limited number of targets have been found for such molecules. The targets tend to be highly conserved proteins. Designer molecules targeting the other potential target enzymes and transporters in cells are possible, but to date have been limited by unforeseen side effects.

OTHER POSSIBLE DRUGS

Peptides, antisense oligonucleotides, and gene therapy all have possible applications in immunosuppression. Peptides (ie, 10mers) may be either random or derived from naturally-occurring proteins, such as the HLA molecule. Unfortunately, the fact that a peptide sequence occurs in a particular protein does not predict whether or how it will act in cells. Peptides have not yet

been shown to have dose-dependent reliable immunosuppressive effects, but remain an active area of research.

Oligonucleotides may be derived from the antisense sequence of a specific gene such as adhesion molecule ICAM-1. Such agents could potentially alter expression of the targeted gene in a variety of ways (eg, by causing mRNA degradation, by interfering with promoter function). They may also have completely unexpected effects, unrelated to the gene from which their sequence was derived. The utility of antisense oligonucleotides remains promising, but unproven.

Gene therapy could have many applications in immunosuppression, by conferring transient local production of an immune response modifier in a targeted tissue (eg, CTLA4Ig). To date, this approach has been limited by the available vectors for introducing the gene.

IMMUNOSUPPRESSION VS IMMUNODEFICIENCY

The complications of immunodeficiency (eg, cancer, infection) can be avoided in immunosuppression by limiting either the duration or the intensity. Limiting the duration is important when one uses intense immunosuppression such as anti-CD3. Thus, the number of days on such agents should be carefully monitored. Limiting the dose and number of maintenance agents ensures the safety of maintenance agents such as CsA.

EFFECTS OF IMMUNOSUPPRESSIVE DRUGS

ISDs have three types of effects: therapeutic effects (ie, immunosuppression); *immunodeficiency toxicities* (ie, increased infection and malignancies); and *nonimmune toxicities* (eg, nephrotoxicity, hyperlipidemia, diabetes).

One goal in immunosuppression is to avoid immunodeficiency effects. Immunodeficiency causes certain characteristic infections (eg, *pneumocystis* pneumonia, CMV) and malignancies such as B cell lymphomas that reflect the uncontrolled action of infectious agents such as Herpes group viruses. Immunodeficient complications are related more to the overall intensity of immunosuppression, and to the duration of maximal depleting immunosuppression (ie, with anti-CD3). Specific prevention greatly reduces the frequency of these complications (ie, prevention of *pneumocystis* by trimethoprim-sulfamethoxazole). However, it is also important to limit the amount of immunosuppression to what is justifiable for that patient.

Nonimmune toxicity is usually agent-specific and is due to undesirable effects of the drug in other organs. The mechanism mediating nonimmune toxicity is often the same as that which mediates immunosuppressive effects (eg, calcineurin, TOR, IMPDH). Examples include:

endothelial damage (HUS) and nephrotoxicity of calcineurin inhibitors; marrow toxicity of mycophenolate; and hyperlipidemia of rapamycin. In many cases the molecular basis of the toxicity is unknown, but has been inseparable from the therapeutic effect.

QUANTITATIVE VIEW OF IMMUNOSUPPRESSION: SATURATION VS PARTIAL INHIBITION

Suppression of the T cell response can be near complete or partial. Near total suppression can be obtained by saturating an essential target, as occurs with anti-CD3. The longer this is sustained, the greater is the incidence of opportunistic infection and lymphoproliferative disease. The number of days of therapy with anti-CD3 or polyclonal ALG should be strictly limited.

Partial inhibition of immune activation can be achieved by partial inhibition of an essential mechanism (eg, calcineurin) or by complete inhibition of a semi-redundant mechanism (eg, CD25).

THE ACTION OF SPECIFIC ISDS (TABLE 11-2)
Glucocorticosteroids

Glucocorticosteroids (GC) have been used as immunosuppressive agents since the beginnings of transplantation, for their immunosuppressive and antiinflammatory properties. GC are used for induction, maintenance, and for treatment of acute rejections. Their exact mechanisms of action are not understood, but include suppression of macrophage function, reduction of cytokine production and adhesion molecule expression, induction of lymphocyte apoptosis, inhibition of leukocyte transmigration through blood vessels, and altered leukocyte traffic.

The principal molecular effects of GC are mediated through the GC receptor (GR). GC influence the rate of transcription of specific genes encoding for important proteins in the immune and inflammatory responses. The GR is a member of a superfamily of nuclear receptors which serve as ligand-regulated transcription factors. GRs are present in the cytoplasm of all cells. In the absence of GC, the GRs in the cytoplasm are in an inactive form, in a large complex of proteins that contain heat shock proteins, hsp90, hsp70 and hsp56. GC bind to GR, dissociating hsp from the receptor and forming an active GC-GR complex. This complex migrates to the nucleus and dimerizes. The dimer binds to the GC response element (GRE) in the promoters of the target genes, where interaction between the corticosteroid receptor complex, the CRE, and other transcription factors or coactivators leads to either induction or suppression of gene transcription (ie, cytokines).

GC can also affect gene transcription by DNA binding, or by interacting directly with other transcriptional factors even without DNA binding. The most important transcription factors regulated by GC are activator protein-1 (AP-1) and NF-κB. These transcription factors play an important role in the induction of numerous immunoregulatory genes. NF-κB is regulated in part by the ability of GC-GR to induce expression of IκB (Chapter 14e).

GC are both antiinflammatory and immunosuppressive. Some effects are mediated through the release of a regulatory protein, lipocortin, which is an inhibitor of phospholipase A2. Lipocortin inhibits the production of inflammatory mediators such as leukotrienes and prostaglandins via phospholipase A2.

The side effects of GC therapy contribute significantly to the morbidity of transplantation. They include posterior subcapsular cataracts, avascular necrosis of the femoral heads, acne, Cushingoid features, increased risk of infections, osteoporosis and growth retardation in children. Other frequently encountered side effects include diabetes mellitus, hypertension, poor wound healing, and skin thinning. Curiously, there is little evidence that steroids predispose to malignancy.

ANTI-CD3 MONOCLONALS

Mouse monoclonal anti-CD3 has been in use for nearly two decades, but humanized anti-CD3 is now in clinical trials. Anti-CD3 binds to ε component of the CD3 complex associated with TCR. Anti-CD3 triggers, and then disrupts or blocks, the TCR-CD3 complex. The immunosuppression seems to be due to a combination of T cell lysis, T cell sequestration, and disrupted function due to the loss of the TCR-CD3 complex.

The first effect of anti-CD3 is to trigger the TCR-CD3 complex, releasing TNF-α, IFN-γ, and other mediators. TCR-CD3 triggering produces the first dose effect, or cytokine release syndrome: fever, chills, muscle aches, "flu-like" symptoms, gastrointestinal symptoms, plus occasional acute pulmonary edema, acute renal failure, and encephalopathy. Anti-CD3 is used for reversal of acute rejection and also for induction by IV for seven to 14 days. The murine monoclonal anti-CD3 is highly effective in reducing CD3 counts and creates potent T cell suppression: for several days there is virtually no T cell function. However, it evokes anti-mouse antibody production by the host, which neutralizes the antibody. The characteristics of a humanized monoclonal anti-CD3 are under investigation in phase 1-2 trials.

THE CALCINEURIN INHIBITORS

Calcineurin inhibitors cyclosporine (CsA) and tacrolimus (here abbreviated FK, recalling its original code name FK506) are usually given by mouth and rapidly distribute to many cell types. They cross cell membranes freely and bind to abundant and ubiquitous binding proteins termed cyclophilins (CP) and FK-binding proteins (FKBP), respectively. Each drug thus creates a specific complex: CsA:CP and FK:FKBP. The complex is the actual drug. The complex targets the calcium-regulated phosphatase calcineurin (Figure 11-5). The complex binds to calcineurin and prevents it from engaging its substrates, such as NF-ATs. The CsA:CP or FK:FKBP prevents the dephosphorylation of NF-ATs and thus prevents cytokine transcription (Figure 11-5). While this is believed to be the principal mechanism of action of both CsA and FK, other effects of calcineurin may also contribute to the immunosuppressive action.

The toxicities of CsA and FK are both similar and different. Both drugs are nephrotoxic, neurotoxic, and diabetogenic. The nephrotoxicity is probably related to a role for calcineurin in renal vasomotion, such that CN inhibitors produce vasoconstriction. The exact mechanism is not known. The short-term manifestation is vasoconstriction and the long-term effect is interstitial fibrosis, tubular atrophy, and a characteristic pattern of nodular hyalinization of the afferent arteriole. CsA also causes hirsutism, gum hyperplasia, hypertension and hyperlipidemia. FK is more likely to cause neurotoxicity and diabetes, and tends to cause hair loss. Hypertrophic cardiomyopathy has been reported in children on FK therapy. How these mechanisms relate to calcineurin inhibition is not known.

CTLA4Ig

CTLA4Ig binds to B7-1 and B7-2 on APCs and prevents these molecules from triggering CD28. This acts to suppress immune responses. Trials in psoriasis suggest that CTLA4Ig is a safe and moderately effective immunosuppressive in humans. In addition, antigen (signal 1) in the absence of signal 2 may be prone to cause anergy rather than response, and theoretically should lead to a state of partial tolerance. This is observed in some animal models. However, it is not yet clear that this is a general outcome:

tolerance was not seen in experimental immunizations in humans in a psoriasis trial. For the moment CTLA4Ig is a promising ISD with interesting potential benefits, which must be proven in human transplant trials.

ANTI-CD40L

Humanized monoclonal against CD40L produced promising results in organ transplants in mice and in monkeys. CD40L deficiency in humans and mice produces immunodeficiency with hyper IgM, due to inability of B cells to "class switch" from IgM to IgG. Anti-CD40L in mice and monkeys produced very long-term survival of allografts. Initial trials in humans have been held, due to concern about thrombosis and more rejection than had been anticipated. The thrombosis may be related to CD40L expression on activated platelets. It is not yet known whether anti-CD40L is an effective immunosuppressive in humans.

THE ANTI-CD25S

One humanized monoclonal, anti-CD25 (daclizumab), and one chimeric monoclonal, anti-CD25 (basiliximab), are in clinical use. They bind to CD25 (IL-2Rα) in the high-affinity IL-2R complex which is expressed on activated T cells. They may have several effects: blockade or even disruption of the IL-2R on activated T cells, reducing T cell proliferation; and depletion of some activated T cells. The anti-CD25s are similar in their effect, and have a long t1/2-like human IgG (21 days) once CD25 is saturated. This achieves mild immunosuppression, and is useful in prophylaxis against rejection, using interval dosing to saturate the CD25 for four to 16 weeks.

THE TOR INHIBITORS

Sirolimus (rapamycin), a relative of FK, is a macrolide product of a soil organism found in Easter Island (Rapa Nui) and is related to the "mycin" antibiotics. RAD is a

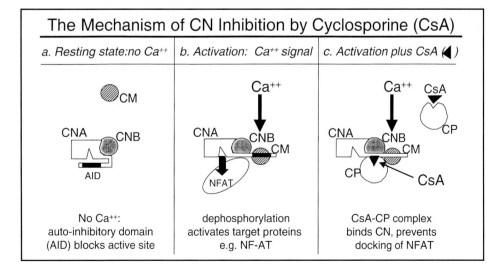

Figure 11-5. The mechanism of CN inhibition by CsA showing the resting state, the state of activation of the T cell, and the effect of CsA. In the resting state, CN is inactive due to blockade of the active site by the autoinhibitory domain. When the T cell is activated, the high intracytosolic calcium causes calmodulin to bind, removing the autoinhibitory domain and permitting CN to engage and act on its substrates, such as NF-AT. When CsA engages cyclophilin (CP) it forms a complex that binds to CN and hinders access of the substrate to the active site. The action of tacrolimus is similar, as a complex with FKBP.

similar molecule to rapmycin, differing in only small details. Rapamycin binds to and inhibits FKBP, but does not inhibit calcineurin. The rapamycin:FKBP complex inhibits cell activation and division driven by some (but not all) cytokine receptors. Unlike CsA or FK, rapamycin blocks IL-2-mediated signal transduction and cell proliferation and blocks lymphocyte responses to IL-4, IL-7, IL-15, and other cytokines and growth factors. It prevents the activation of the kinase enzyme TOR (also known as FRAP and RAFT among other names) (Figure 11-6). TOR is critical in transducing a signal from cytokine receptors to the mechanisms controlling cell division. TOR autophosphorylates and activates itself. TOR activation leads to the translation of many mRNAs, which are required for cycling. TOR activation activates ribosomal enzyme p70S6 kinase, and inhibits 4E-BP1, an inhibitor of the elongation of polypeptide chains. Both of these actions promote protein synthesis, and thus, rapamycin inhibits synthesis of these proteins. Rapamycin has an interaction with CsA that may increase the therapeutic and toxic effects of CsA.

THE IMPDH INHIBITORS

MMF ($C_{23}H_{31}NO_7$) (MW 433.51), a semi-synthetic 2-(4-morpholino)ethyl ester of mycophenolic acid, was developed to simulate a metabolic error in de novo purine synthesis in lymphocytes. In the 1970s it was established that severe combined immunodeficiency without neurologic damage occurred when humans lacked adenosine deaminase (ADA), but HGPRT deficiency had brain dysfunction with no immune deficit. Thus, lymphocytes used de novo purine synthesis, whereas other tissues, such as the brain, used the salvage pathway. MPA was identified as a potential drug to

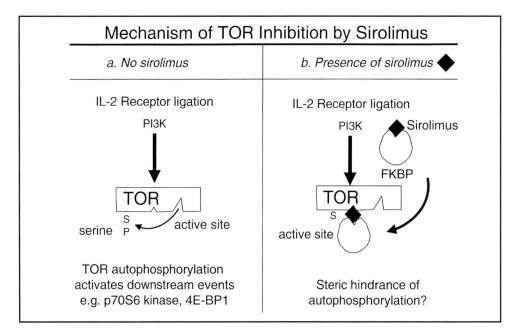

Figure 11-6. Mechanisms of TOR-inhibition by sirolimus. In the absence of sirolimus, the IL-2 receptor ligation leads to autophosphorylation of TOR. In the presence of sirolimus and FKBP, the function of TOR is inhibited. This may also interfere with the interaction of TOR with other proteins. PI3K indicates phosphatidyl inositol 3-OH kinase, which is activated by the IL-2 receptor.

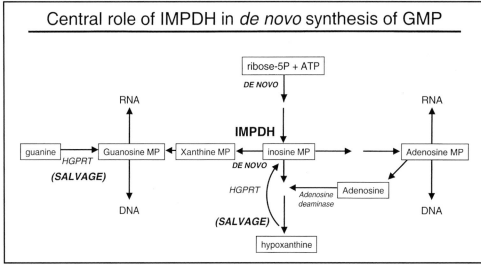

Figure 11-7. The key role of IMPDH in balancing the G. to A nucleotides synthesized by the de novo pathway. Salvage is adequate for other cell types, but not for proliferating lymphocytes, which must have de novo synthesis.

replace azathioprine on the basis of increased potency and selectivity. MMF is a morpholinoethyl (mofetil) ester derivative of MPA. The mofetil moiety increases the bioavailability of MPA in man. MMF is rapidly and completely adsorbed and is hydrolysed by esterases to yield the active drug, MPA.

MPA inhibits inosine monophosphate dehydrogenase (IMPDH), the rate-limiting enzyme in the de novo synthesis of guanosine monophosphate (GMP) (Figure 11-7). MPA blocks proliferative responses of T and B lymphocytes, inhibiting antibody formation and the generation of cytotoxic T cells and the delayed type hypersensitivity response. MPA effects are selective for lymphocytes because most other cell types use the salvage pathway to recycle existing purines. Salvage is not adequate for lymphocytes, however.

MPA inhibits IMPDH noncompetitively, but reversibly. MPA is not a nucleoside analogue. MPA is metabolized to the glucuronide (MPAG), the principal metabolite, by glucuronosyl transferase, which is inactive and is excreted mainly by the kidney.

AZATHIOPRINE

Azathioprine is a derivative of 6 mecaptopurine (6MP) and releases 6MP in vivo. 6MP is metabolized to TIMP. TIMP is incorporated as a purine into DNA, interfering with DNA replication, but it may also interfere with purine synthesis. The effects of azathioprine are less selective than those of MMF, and include leukopenia, anemia, thrombocytopenia, and megaloblastoid changes. It is currently used with CsA or FK, plus steroids.

Azathioprine acts mainly as an antiproliferative agent, with a number of potential effects on the synthesis of DNA. TIMP can potentially interfere with the synthesis of guanylic and adenylic acids from inosinic acid by inhibiting the enzymes adenylosuccinate synthetase, adenylosuccinate lyase and inosine monophosphate dehydrogenase. TIMP itself is converted to thioguanylic acid, a precursor for thiodeoxyguanosine triphosphate, which is incorporated into the developing strands of DNA and interferes with DNA synthesis. TIMP interferes with the synthesis of co-enzymes such as nicotinamide mononucleotide-adenyl transferase. Finally, the thiopurine ribonucleotides can potentially act as feedback inhibitors of the initial steps in the de novo purine synthesis pathway by inhibiting the enzyme glutamine phosphoribosyl pyrophosphate amidinotransferase. However, it is likely that the main action of azathioprine is on DNA synthesis, not on purine synthesis. Azathioprine suppresses the proliferation of activated B and T lymphocytes, and reduces the number of circulating monocytes by arresting the cell cycle of promyelocytes in the bone marrow.

OTHER AGENTS

Leflunomide is an immunosuppressive drug that is believed to act by inhibition of de novo pyrimidine synthesis by inhibiting the rate-limiting enzyme DHODH. The action is thus parallel, in some respects, to MPA. It is released for rheumatoid arthritis and may go into trials in organ transplantation. Brequinar is also believed to be an inhibitor of DHODH.

FTY720 is an interesting new agent that causes massive depletion of lymphocytes from the peripheral blood of animals within two hours of administration. It may cause sequestration of the lymphocytes to the mucosa-associated lymphoid tissues, such as the gut. It is not yet clear whether it produces apoptosis. It is in phase I testing in humans.

IVIg is useful in treating alloantibody-mediated rejection since it can suppress alloantibody production in some cases. The mechanism of action is presumably through Fc receptors. In fact the exact mechanism of IVIg effects remains unclear, but the increased catabolism of IgG is the most likely explanation.

Peptides derived from immune proteins have been used to block immune responses. No peptide to date has shown consistent dose-dependent benefit in animal or human experiments, but some have shown promising preliminary results.

Antisense oligonucleotides have potential as drugs: the theory is that they bind to specific mRNA and cause it to be degraded. One agent showing promising preclinical results is an antisense oligonucleotide against ICAM-1.

HOW MUCH IMMUNOSUPPRESSION IS ENOUGH?

There are distinct levels of immunosuppression. The initial period after transplantation requires intense immunosuppression. The immune response is very active, and the injured graft is very immunogenic. This is called the induction period. Some clinicians favor heavy immunosuppression with protein ISDs (eg, anti-CD3, polyclonal ATG) in the induction period. High doses of small molecule ISDs (ie, combinations of calcineurin inhibitors, MMF or rapamycin or azathioprine, and GC) are also effective in the induction period. A new option in induction is anti-CD25, which has mild immunosuppressive effects, but great safety.

The reversal of acute rejection – especially severe rejection – also requires very intense immunosuppression. High doses of GC are effective, but severe rejection may require intense immunosuppression with anti-CD3 or polyclonal ALG or ATG. Such therapies can virtually abolish T cell responsiveness for a short period.

After three to six months, an adaptation occurs between the immunosuppressed host and the graft, greatly reducing the probability of rejection. Long-term immunosuppression (maintenance) must be incomplete, to preserve vital host defense functions that control opportunistic infection and malignancy. Thus, maintenance immunosuppression involves significant, but partial, inhibition of immune function. Partial inhibition is currently achieved two ways. The first is by using small molecule drugs that only partially inhibit immune function, such as CsA. Partial effects can also be produced by saturating a partially redundant molecule such as the IL-2 receptor α chain with anti-CD25, but the application of this to long-term maintenance therapy has not been established. Maintenance immunosuppression currently involves small molecule drugs such as CsA or FK, in combination with MMF, rapamycin, or azathioprine, and/or steroids. When using subsaturation, as with the calcineurin inhibitors, one must be concerned about monitoring the drug levels. However, when saturation is achieved (ie, anti-CD25 monoclonals) one need not monitor levels, only the time until the drug levels will decline on the basis of the dose and the half-life.

RECOMMENDED READING

Abrams JR, Lebwohl MG, Guzzo CA, et al. CTLA4Ig-mediated blockade of T-cell costimulation in patients with psoriasis vulgaris. J Clin Invest. 1999;103(9):1243-1252.

Auphan N, Didonato JA, Rosette C, Helmberg A, Karin M. Immunosuppression by glucocorticoids: inhibition of NF-kappa B activity through induction of I kappa B synthesis. Science. 1995;270(5234):286-290.

Beretta L, Gingras AC, Svitkin YV, Hall MN, Sonenberg N. Rapamycin blocks the phosphorylation of 4E-BP1 and inhibits cap-dependent initiation of translation. EMBO J. 1996;15(3):658-664.

Blazar BR, Taylor PA, Panoskaltsis-Mortari A, et al. Blockade of CD40 ligand-CD40 interaction impairs CD4+ T cell-mediated alloreactivity by inhibiting mature donor T cell expansion and function after bone marrow transplantation. J Immunol. 1997;158(1):29-39.

Bowman JS 3d, Angstadt JD, Waymack JP, Jaffers GJ. A comparison of triple-therapy with double-therapy immunosuppression in cadaveric renal transplantation. Transplantation. 1992;53(3):556-559.

Chung J, Kuo CJ, Crabtree GR, Blenis J. Rapamycin-FKBP specifically blocks growth-dependent activation of and signaling by the 70 kappa D S6 protein kinases. Cell. 1992;69(7):1227-1236.

Elion GB. The pharmacology of azathioprine. Ann NY Acad Sci. 1993;685:400-407.

Eugui EM, Allison AC. Immunosuppressive activity of mycophenolate mofetil. Ann NY Acad Sci. 1993;685:309-329.

Kahan BD, Gibbons S, Tijpal N, Stepkowski SM, Chou TC. Synergistic interactions of cyclosporine and rapamycin to inhibit immune performances of normal human peripheral blood lymphocytes in vitro. Transplantation. 1991;51(1):232-239.

Karin M. New twists in gene regulation by glucocorticoid receptor: is DNA binding dispensable? Cell. 1998;93(4):487-490.

Kirk AD, Harlan DM, Armstrong NN, et al. CTLA4-Ig and anti-CD40 ligand prevent renal allograft rejection in primates. Proc Natl Acad Sci USA. 1997;94(16):8789-8794.

Kuo CJ, Chung J, Fiorentino DF, Flanagan WM, Blenis J, Crabtree GR. Rapamycin selectively inhibits interleukin-2 activation of p70 S6 kinase. Nature. 1992;358(6381):70-73.

Larsen CP, Elwood ET, Alexander DZ, et al. Long-term acceptance of skin and cardiac allografts after blocking CD40 and CD28 pathways. Nature. 1996;381(6581):434-438.

Linsley PS. Distinct roles for CD28 and cytotoxic T lymphocyte-associated molecule-4 receptors during T cell activation? J Exp Med. 1995;182(2):289-292.

Linsley PS, Wallace PM, Johnson J, et al. Immunosuppression in vivo by a soluble form of the CTLA-4 T cell activation molecule. Science. 1992;257(5071):792-795.

Lorenz MC, Heitman J. TOR mutations confer rapamycin resistance by preventing interaction with FKBP12-rapamycin. J Biol Chem. 1995;270(46):27531-27537.

Scheinman RI, Cogswell PC, Lofquist AK, Baldwin AS, Jr. Role of transcriptional activation of I kappa B alpha in mediation of immunosuppression by glucocorticoids. Science. 1995;270(5234):283-286.

Schreiber SL, Crabtree GR. The mechanism of action of cyclosporin A and FK506. Immunol Today. 1992;13(4):136-142.

Timmerman LA, Clipstone NA, Ho SN, Northrop JP, Crabtree GR. Rapid shuttling of NF-AT in discrimination of Ca2+ signals and immunosuppression. Nature. 1996;383(6603):837-840.

Ullman KS, Northrop JP, Admon A, Crabtree GR. Jun family members are controlled by a calcium-regulated, cyclosporin A-sensitive signaling pathway in activated T lymphocytes. Genes Dev. 1993;7(2):188-196.

12 COMMONLY USED DRUGS AND DRUG INTERACTIONS

Ali J. Olyaei, PharmD, BCPS
Angelo M. de Mattos, MD
William M. Bennett, MD

During the last two decades, the introduction of new drugs and advances in the understanding of immuno-pharmacology and the immunobiology of allograft rejection have led to major achievements in the field of transplantation. These have included a decrease in the incidence of rejection, adverse immunosuppressive drug reactions and severe infection episodes. Consequently, long-term outcomes of transplantation have improved.

Since many transplant patients are prescribed multiple medications to sustain the transplant and to treat concurrent conditions, it is imperative for caregivers to be aware of potential drug interactions and to monitor these appropriately. This chapter will provide information on drug interactions involving those drugs commonly used in transplant recipients to help clinicians avoid harmful drug interactions. Transplant recipients are a heterogenous group whose individual responses to drugs may vary. The tables in this chapter will provide guidelines for dosing of these drugs. Drugs are listed according to their pharmacologic or therapeutic classification. Generic names appear alphabetically in columns and recommended dosages for oral agents are listed in brackets. Appropriate starting and maximum doses are included, as well as guidelines for drug administration in patients with impaired renal function. Finally, each table has a comment section containing precautions and warnings.

DRUG INTERACTIONS

Drugs having wide therapeutic indicies usually interact without any clinically significant interactions, but this is not true for drugs with narrow therapeutic indicies, such as some immunosuppressive drugs. Drug interactions are generally categorized as pharmacokinetic, pharma-

codynamic, or a combination of both. Pharmacokinetic drug interactions include changes in absorption, distribution, metabolism and renal excretion. Pharmacodynamic drug interactions may lead to additive or synergistic toxicities. When an adverse drug interaction is detected, an alternative therapy should be considered or the dose or schedule of one of the drugs should be adjusted and drug levels or toxicities should be monitored closely. Tables 12-1 and 12-2 summarize common and clinically important drug-drug interactions and their management.

Pharmacokinetic drug-drug interactions are common in transplant recipients. A drug may bind to or otherwise decrease the gastrointestinal absorption of an immunosuppressive drug. Only drugs that alter the extent, but not the rate, of immunosuppressive drug absorption are clinically important. For example, food decreases the rate of absorption of mycophenolate mofetil without any significant effect on its area under-the-curve (AUC) drug levels. A decrease in rate of absorption is clinically insignificant and mycophenolate can be taken with or without food. In contrast, food significantly reduces both the rate and extent of tacrolimus absorption. Thus, tacrolimus should be taken on an empty stomach. Gastrointestinal prokinetic agents, cisapride and metoclopramide, increase gastrointestinal motility and, consequently, can increase bioavailability and serum concentration of cyclosporine and tacrolimus. Cholestyramine and antacids may interfere with absorption of mycophenolate and tacrolimus, leading to a decrease in blood concentration. These drug-drug interactions can be avoided by taking immunosuppressive agents two to three hours before cholestyramine or antacids.

Cyclosporine and tacrolimus are metabolized by the IIIA-4 subfamily of cytochrome P450 (CYP-450). There are high concentrations of CYP IIIA-4 enzymes in the endoplasmic reticulum of hepatocytes and enterocytes. CYP IIIA-4 isoenzymes account for 30% of the cytochrome enzymes in the liver and 70% of the cytochrome enzymes in the gastrointestinal tract. They are responsible for 30% to 40% of the metabolism of all drugs in humans. All patients have different basal concentrations of CYP IIIA-4 isoenzymes in their livers and gastrointestinal tracts. Differences in CYP IIIA-4 iso-enzyme activity have been observed between the very young and old and also between men and women. Unfortunately, there is no specific test to measure or identify patients with high or low concentration of CYP IIIA-4 isoenzymes. CYP IIIA-4 isoenzymes are responsible for the metabolism of several important classes of drugs that are commonly used in transplant recipients. Examples of these classes include azole antifungal drugs, calcium channel blockers, antihistamines, anticonvulsants, certain antimicrobials and corticosteroids.

Ali J. Olyaei, PharmD, BCPS, Assistant Professor of Medicine, Division of Nephrology, Hypertension and Clinical Pharmacology, Oregon Health Sciences University, Portland, OR

Angelo M. de Mattos, MD, Assistant Professor of Medicine, Hypertension and Clinical Pharmacology, Transplantation Medicine Program, Oregon Health Sciences University, Portland, OR

William M. Bennett, MD, Medical Director, Solid Organ and Cellular Transplantation, Legacy Good Samaritan Hospital, Portland, OR

Table 12-1. Cyclosporine and Tacrolimus Drug Interactions

Drug	Mechanism	Effects	Severity	Comments
Acetazolamide	Decrease clearance	Increase CsA/FK level	3	May cause acidosis
Acyclovir	Crystallization in renal tubules	Nephrotoxicity	4	Avoid dehydration Infuse over one hour
Amikacin	Synergistic nephrotoxicity	Nephrotoxicity	3	Monitor aminoglycoside level very close Target Amikacin level peak 30 to 40 and trough less than ten
Amiloride	Decrease K+ secretion	Hyperkalemia	3	Avoid in transplant recipients
Amiodarone	Decrease clearance	Nephrotoxicity	3	Very slow onset and offset
Amlodipine	Decrease clearance	Increase CsA/FK level	4	10% to 15% increase in CsA/FK level
Amphotericin B	Synergistic nephrotoxicity	Nephrotoxicity	3	Require hydration and electrolyte monitoring
Atorvastatin	CsA decreases clearance of statins	Myopathy, rhabdomyolysis	3	Monitor CPK carefully
Carbamazepine	Increase clearance	Decrease CsA/FK level	3	Slow onset (may take up to seven days)
Carvedilol	Decrease clearance	Increase CsA/FK level	3	May cause toxicity
Cerivastatin	CsA decreases clearance of statins	Myopathy, rhabdomyolysis	3	Require close CPK monitoring
Chloroquine	Decrease clearance	Increase CsA/FK level	3	
Cholestyramine	Increase clearance	Decrease CsA/FK level	4	Separate doses by three hours
Cimetidine	Inhibit creatinine secretion	Increase serum creatinine	4	Use other H_2 antagonist agents (ranitidine, famotidine and nizatidine)
Ciprofloxacin	Decrease CsA effects on IL-2	Pharmacodynamic antagonism	4	May increase risk of rejection
Clarithromycin	Decrease clearance	Increase CsA/FK level	2	Azithromycin is the preferred agent
Colchicine		Increase neurotoxicity	3	Gastrointestinal dysfunction and neuromyopathy
Co-trimoxazole	Inhibit creatinine secretion	Increase serum creatinine	4	Preferred agent for PCP
Digoxin	CsA may decreases clearance of digoxin	Increase digoxin level	3	Monitor digoxin level closely
Diltiazem	Decrease clearance	Increase CsA/FK level	3	Monitor CsA/FK level closely
Enalapril	Renal dysfunction in RAS	Increase serum creatinine	3	May cause anemia Use for treatment of posttransplant erythrocytosis
Erythromycin	Decrease clearance	Increase CsA/FK level	2	Azithromycin is the preferred agent
Fluconazole	Decrease clearance	Increase CsA/FK level	3	Increase LFTs Monitor levels carefully
Fluvoxamine	Decrease clearance	Increase CsA/FK level	2	Monitor levels carefully
Fosinopril	Renal dysfunction in RAS	Nephrotoxicity	3	May cause elevation of Scr
Fosphenytoin	Increase clearance	Decrease CsA/FK level	3	Monitor levels carefully
Ganciclovir	Synergistic nephrotoxicity	Nephrotoxicity	3	Avoid dehydration
Gentamicin	Synergistic nephrotoxicity	Nephrotoxicity	3	Monitor blood concentrations very closely
Griseofulvin	Unknown	Decrease CsA/FK level	3	Decreased CsA effectiveness
Itraconazole	Decrease clearance	Increase CsA/FK level	3	Monitor levels carefully Decrease dosage 50% to 85%
Ketoconazole	Decrease clearance	Increase CsA/FK level	3	Monitor levels carefully Decrease dosage 25% to 75%
Lovastatin	CsA decreases clearance of statins	Myopathy, rhabdomyolysis	3	Require close CPK monitoring
Methyl-prednisolone	Decrease clearance	Increase CsA/FK level	3	Only high doses
Methyltestosterone	Decreased cyclosporine metabolism	Increase CsA/FK level	3	May cause toxicity
Metoclopramide	Decrease gastric emptying time	Increase CsA/FK level	3	Increase peak and AUC by 25% to 50%
Metronidazole	Decrease clearance	Increase CsA/FK level	4	Monitor CsA/FK levels
Nafcillin	Increase CsA/FK clearance	Decrease CsA/FK level	3	Monitor CsA/FK levels
Nefazodone	Decrease CsA/FK clearance	Increase CsA/FK level	3	Monitor CsA/FK levels
Nicardipine	Decrease CsA/FK clearance	Increase CsA/FK level	3	Monitor CsA/FK levels
NSAIDs	Synergistic nephrotoxicity	Nephrotoxicity	3	CsA/FK induced vasoconstriction is influenced by prostaglandins inhibition

(Continued on next page)

Table 12-1. Cyclosporine and Tacrolimus Drug Interactions *(continued)*

Drug	Mechanism	Effects	Severity	Comments
Octreotide	Decrease intestinal absorption of CsA/FK	Decrease CsA/FK level	3	Monitor CsA/FK levels
Phenobarbital	Increase CsA/FK clearance	Decrease CsA/FK level	3	Slow onset slow off-set
Phenytoin	Increase CsA/FK clearance	Decrease CsA/FK level	3	Monitor CsA/FK levels
Pravastatin	CsA decreases clearance of statins	Myopathy, rhabdomyolysis	3	Monitor CPK carefully
Rifabutin	Increase CsA/FK clearance	Decrease CsA/FK level	3	Monitor CsA/FK levels rifabutin is a less potent hepatic enzyme inducer than rifampin
Rifampin	Increase CsA/FK clearance	Decrease CsA/FK level	2	Monitor CsA/FK levels
Sildenafil	Increase FK level	Decrease CsA/FK level	4	
Simvastatin	CsA decreases clearance of statins	Myopathy, rhabdomyolysis	4	Monitor CPK carefully
Spironolactone	Decrease K+ secretion	Hyperkalemia	3	Avoid
Terbinafine	Decrease CsA/FK clearance	Increase CsA/FK level	3	Monitor CsA/FK levels
Ticlopidine	Increase CsA/FK clearance	Decrease CsA/FK level	3	Monitor CsA/FK levels
Tretinoin	Inhibit tretinoin metabolism	Increase tretinoin toxicity	3	
Triamterene	Decrease K+ secretion	Hyperkalemia	3	Avoid
Valacyclovir	Hemolytic uremic syndrome	Renal Dysfunction	3	Acyclovir or famciclovir are preferred agents for treatment of HSV and VZV

1) Avoid combination
2) Usually avoid (use only no other alternative agents available)
3) Monitor closely
4) No action needed (the risk of ADR is small)

Table 12-2. Azathioprine and Mycophenolate Drug-Drug Interactions

Drug	Mechanism	Effects	Severity	Comments
ACE-inhibitors	Synergistic myelosuppression	Anemia, neutropenia	3	Increase bone marrow toxicity
Acyclovir	Increase AUC of MMF	Not significant	4	
Allopurinol	Inhibit xanthine oxidase	Severe neutropenia	2	Decrease azathioprine dose by 75%, monitor blood count closely
Antacids	Decrease absorption of MMF	Decrease efficacy	3	
Cholestyramine	Decrease absorption of MMF		3	Increase bone marrow toxicity
Ganciclovir	Synergistic myelosuppression	Anemia, neutropenia	3	
TMP/SMX	Synergistic myelosuppression	Anemia, neutropenia	3	

1) Avoid combination
2) Usually avoid (use only no other alternative agents available)
3) Monitor closely
4) No action needed (the risk of ADR is small)

Both induction and inhibition of CYP IIIA-4 isoenzymes may complicate drug therapy in transplant recipients. The times to onset and offset of CYP IIIA-4 interactions are related to the half-life of each drug and the half-life of enzyme production. However, for individual patients, it is very difficult to predict the onset and offset of the interaction. Phenytoin and rifampin are examples of drugs that induce CYP IIIA-4 enzymes. Phenytoin has a half-life of approximately 18 hours and requires four to five days to induce CYP IIIA-4 isoenzymes effectively. Rifampin has a shorter half-life and can induce CYP IIIA-4 isoenzymes within two days. Both drugs can decrease cyclosporine or tacrolimus blood concentra-

tions to substantially subtherapeutic levels. Ketoconazole, erythromycin and nifedipine are examples of drugs that inhibit CYP IIIA-4.

A drug can inhibit CYP IIIA-4 by competitive inhibition for the binding site or by permanent inhibition of the CYP IIIA-4 isoenzymes. The affinity and intensity of binding are different for each drug. Ketoconazole and erythromycin are two very potent inhibitors and nifedipine is a very weak inhibitor of CYP IIIA-4. Clinically significant drug interactions can cause nephrotoxicity, hypertension, neurotoxicity and allograft rejection.

There are a large number of potential pharmacodynamic or additive toxicities with immunosuppressive drugs. The concomitant use of cyclosporine or tacrolimus with acyclovir, aminoglycosides, amphotericin B, ganciclovir, nonsteroidal antiinflammatory drugs and vancomycin can result in increased nephrotoxicity. Cimetidine and trimethoprim may increase serum creatinine without any structural or functional effect on kidney function. These agents interfere with the secretion of creatinine. Cyclosporine may also interact with HMG-CoA reductase inhibitors and increase the blood concentration of HMG-CoA reductase inhibitors by fourfold to 20-fold. This is a serious drug-drug interaction that can cause rhabdomyolysis, acute renal failure and allograft loss. Calcium channel blockers and phenytoin cause gingival hyperplasia, which is usually not severe and is tolerated by most patients. The risk of gingival hyperplasia increases substantially when these agents are given with cyclosporine. Changing from cyclosporine to tacrolimus will alleviate gingival hyperplasia. Excessive hair growth can result from the concurrent use of minoxidil and cyclosporine. Again, changing from cyclosporine to tacrolimus will benefit most patients. Cyclosporine and tacrolimus can cause mild to moderate hyperkalemia. The additional use of ACE-inhibitors and potassium-sparing diuretics can result in severe or life-threatening hyperkalemia. These agents should be employed with caution in transplant recipients.

Use of myelosuppressive agents such as ganciclovir and sulfamethoxazole-trimethoprim (SMX-TMP) may increase the incidence for myelosuppression associated with the use of mycophenolate and azathioprine. Allopurinol, a structural isomer of hypoxanthine, inhibits xanthine oxidase, the enzyme that catalyzes 6-mercaptopurine, an active moiety of azathioprine. Since severe myelosuppression can occur when these agents are used concomitantly, the azathioprine dose should be reduced 60% to 75% whenever allopurinol is used and a complete blood count should be monitored.

ANTI-INFECTIVE AGENTS
Antibacterials
A multitude of antibacterial agents are used for the prophylaxis and treatment of the common infections seen in transplant patients. SMX-TMP or TMP alone have been used for the prophylaxis (low-dose) and treatment (high-dose) of *P. carinii* pneumonia. SMX-TMP competitively inhibits renal tubular secretion and therefore can raise serum creatinine and potassium. SMX-TMP can also cause myelosuppression and interstitial nephritis. Monitoring of complete blood counts and renal function is indicated with its prolonged use. Pentamidine is used as an alternative agent in patients with a history of sulfa allergy. When given intravenously, pentamidine, like other nephrotoxic agents, may potentiate the nephrotoxicity of cyclosporine and tacrolimus. In addition, pentamidine may cause hypotension and hypoglycemia. Ciprofloxacin has been implicated in an increased incidence of renal transplant rejection via mechanisms still not fully understood.

Erythromycin and clarithromycin are known inhibitors of cytochrome CYP IIIA-4. Their use requires appropriate cyclosporine and tacrolimus dose adjustment and close blood level monitoring. Aminoglycoside antibiotics are nephrotoxic, especially when used in combination with calcineurin inhibitors, diuretics, amphotericin B, or vancomycin. As discussed above, rifampin, an inducer of CYP IIIA-4, results in a dramatic decrease in cyclosporine and tacrolimus blood levels. Isoniazid, nafcillin and rifabutin also decrease the levels of calcineurin inhibitors by the same mechanism, but to a lesser degree.

Dose adjustments of most drugs are required when renal or hepatic dysfunction are present and drugs that depend on those organs for metabolism or elimination are being used (see Table 12-3).

Antiviral Drugs
Prophylaxis of reactivation and treatment of symptomatic herpes virus infections is accomplished with the use of acyclovir, famciclovir or valacyclovir. Acyclovir has been shown to increase the AUC of MMF. The clinical relevance of such an effect is questionable. High-dose acyclovir, as used in the treatment of varicella-zoster infection, can induce renal dysfunction by crystallization of the drug inside the renal tubules. Hemolytic anemia has been described with the use of valacyclovir in renal transplant recipients.

Ganciclovir, which is used for either prophylaxis or treatment of CMV, can induce myelosuppression, when azathioprine and MMF are being used. Nephrotoxicity from ganciclovir has been described in transplant patients. The absolute oral bioavailability of ganciclovir is approximately 5%. Taking oral ganciclovir with food enhances its oral bioavailability. Foscarnet should only be used in patients with documented ganciclovir-resistant strains of CMV. During foscarnet treatment, serum creatinine and electrolytes should be monitored carefully. Amantadine and rimantadine, used in the treatment of influenza virus infections, do not appear to interact with immunosuppressive drugs. Dosage adjustment for most antiviral agents is indicated in the presence of renal dysfunction (see Table 12-3).

Antifungal Therapy
Despite the introduction of several new classes of antifungal agents, amphotericin B has remained the "gold standard" for the treatment of invasive mycoses. The major dose-limiting, specific organ toxicity of amphotericin B is nephrotoxicity. Nephrotoxicity from amphotericin B is caused by a decrease in renal blood flow and

Table 12-3. Common Antimicrobial Agents Used in Solid Organ Transplant Recipients

Drugs	Normal Dose	% Of Renal Excretion	Dosage Adjustment in Renal Failure			Comments
			GFR >50	GFR 10-50	GFR <10	
Antimicrobial Agents						
Aminoglycoside						Nephrotoxic, ototoxic, may prolong the neuromuscular blockade effect of muscle relaxants
Gentamicin	2 mg/kg q8hrs	95%	60% to 90% q12hrs	30% to 70% q24hrs	20% to 30% q24hrs	Peak 6 to 8, Trough <2
Tobramycin	2 mg/kg q8hrs	95%	60% to 90% q12hrs	30% to 70% q24hrs	20% to 30% q24hrs	Peak 6 to 8, Trough <2
Netilmicin	2 mg/kg q8hrs	95%	60% to 90% q12hrs	30% to 70% q24hrs	20% to 30% q24hrs	Peak 6 to 8, Trough <2
Amikacin	7.5mg/kg q12hrs	95%	60 to 90% q12hrs	30% to 70% q24hrs	20% to 30% q24hrs	Peak 6 to 8, Trough <2
Cephalosporin						Coagulation abnormalities, transitory elevation of BUN, rash and serum sickness-like syndrome
Oral Cephalosporin						
Cefaclor (Rx 250, 500, liquid Sus)	250 to 500 mg tid	70%	100%	100%	50%	Ibid
Cefadroxil (Rx 250, 500, liquid Sus)	500 to 1 gm bid	80%	100%	100%	50%	Ibid
Cefixime (Rx 200, 400, liquid Sus)	200 tp 400 mg q12h	85%	100%	100%	50%	Ibid
Cefpodoxime (Rx 100, 250, liquid Sus)	200 mg q12 hrs	30%	100%	100%	100%	Ibid
Ceftibuten (Rx 400)	400 mg 24 hrs	70%	100%	100%	50%	Ibid
Cefuroxime (Rx 250, 500, liquid Sus)	250 to 500 mg tid	90%	100%	100%	100%	Ibid
Cephalexin (Rx 250, 500, liquid Sus)	250 to 500 mg tid	95%	100%	100%	100%	Ibid
Cephradine (Rx 250, 500, liquid Sus)	250 to 500 mg tid	100%	100%	100%	50%	Ibid
IV Cephalosporin						
Cefamandole	1 to 2 gm IV q6-8hrs	100%	q6hrs	q8hrs	q12hrs	Ibid
Cefazolin	1 to 2 gms IV q8hrs	80%	q8hrs	q12hrs	q12 to 24hrs	Ibid
Cefepime	1 to 2 gms IV q8hrs	85%	q8 to 12hrs	q12hrs	q24hrs	Ibid
Cefmetazole	1 to 2 gms IV q8hrs	85%	q8hrs	q12hrs	q24hrs	Ibid
Cefoperazone	1 to 2 gms IV q12hrs	20%	No renal adjustment is required.			Ibid
Cefotaxime	1 to 2 gm IV q6-8hrs	60%	q8hrs	q12hrs	q12 to 24hrs	Ibid
Cefotetan	1 to 2 gm IV q12hrs	75%	q12hrs	q12 to 24hrs	q24hrs	Ibid
Cefoxitin	1 to 2 gm IV q6hrs	80%	q6hrs	q8 to 12hrs	q12hrs	Ibid
Ceftazidime	1 to 2 gms IV q8hrs	70%	q8hrs	q12hrs	q24hrs	Ibid
Ceftriaxone	1 to 2 gms IV q24hrs	50%	No renal adjustment is required.			Ibid
Cefuroxime	705-1.5gms IV q8hrs	90%	q8hrs	q8 to 12hrs	q12 to 24hrs	Ibid
Penicillin						Bleeding abnormalities hypersensitivity
Oral Penicillin						
Amoxicillin (Rx 125, 250, 500, liquid Sus)	500 mg po tid	60%	100%	100%	50% to 75%	Ibid
Ampicillin (Rx 125, 250, 500, liquid Sus)	500 mg po q6hrs	60%	100%	100%	50% to 75%	Ibid
Dicloxacillin (Rx 125, 250, 500, liquid Sus)	250 to 500 mg po q6hrs	50%	100%	100%	50% to 75%	Ibid
Penicillin V (Rx 125, 250, 500, liquid Sus)	250 to 500 mg po q6hrs	70%	100%	100%	50% to 75%	Ibid
IV Penicillin						
Ampicillin	1 to 2 gms IV q6hrs	60%	q6hrs	q8hrs	q12hrs	Ibid
Nafcillin	1 to 2 gms IV q4hrs	35%	No renal adjustment is required.			Ibid
Penicillin G	2 to 3 million Units IV q4hrs	70%	q4-6hrs	q6hrs	q8hrs	Ibid
Piperacillin	3 to 4 gms IV q4 to 6hrs		No renal adjustment is required.			Ibid
Ticarcillin/clavulanate	3.1 gm IV q4 to 6hrs					Ibid

Continued on next page

Table 12-3. Common Antimicrobial Agents Used in Solid Organ Transplant Recipients *Continued*

Drugs	Normal Dose	% Of Renal Excretion	Dosage Adjustment in Renal Failure			Comments
			GFR >50	GFR 10-50	GFR <10	
IV Penicillin (continued)						
Piperacillin/tazobactam	3.375 gm IV q6 to 8hrs					Ibid
Quinolones						Photosensitivity, food, dairy products, tube feeding and A1(OH)3 may decrease the absorption of quinolones
Ciprofloxacin (Rx: 250, 500, 750, Sol)	200 to 400 mg IV q24hrs	60%	q12hrs	q12-24hrs	q24hrs	Ibid
Levofloxacin (Rx: 250, 500)	500 mg po qd	70%	q12hrs	250 q12hrs	250 q12hrs	Ibid
Norfloxacin (Rx: 400)	400 mg po q12hrs	30%	q12hrs	q12 to 24hrs	q24hrs	Ibid
Ofloxacin (Rx: 200, 300, 400)	200 to 400 mg po q12hrs	70%	q12hrs	q12 to 24hrs	q24hrs	Ibid
Miscellaneous Agents						
Azithromycin (Rx: 250, Sus)	250 to 500 mg po qd	6%	No renal adjustment is required.			No drug interaction with CsA/FK
Clarithromycin (Rx: 250, 500, Sus)	500 mg po bid	20%	No renal adjustment is required.			Pseudomembranous colitis
Clindamycin (Rx: 75, 150, 300, Sus)	150 to 450 mg po tid	10%	No renal adjustment is required.			Increase CsA/FK level: avoid in transplant patients
Erythromycin (Rx: 250, 500, Sus)	250 to 500 mg po qid	15%	No renal adjustment is required.			Increase CsA/FK level: avoid in transplant patients
Imipenem/cilastatin	250 to 500 mg IV q6hrs	50%	500 mg q8hrs	250 to 500 q8-12hrs	250 mg q12hrs	Seizure
Meropenem	1gms IV q8hrs	65%	1 gms q8hrs	0.5 to 1gms q12hrs	0.5 to 1 gms q24hrs	
Metronidazole (Rx: 250, 500)	500 mg IV q6hrs	20%	No renal adjustment is required.			Peripheral neuropathy, increase LFTs, disulfiram reaction with alcoholic beverages
Pentamidine (Rx: 300)	4 mg/kg per day	5%	q24hrs	q24hrs	q48hrs	Inhalation may cause bronchospasm, IV administration may cause hypotension, hypoglycemia and nephrotoxicity
Rifampin (Rx: 150, 300)	300 to 600 mg po qd	20%	No renal adjustment is required.			Decrease CsA/FK level
Trimethoprim / Sulfamethoxazole (Rx: SS or DS)	one po bid	70%	q12hrs	q12hrs	q24hrs	Increase serum creatinine
Vancomycin	1 gm IV q12hrs	90%	q12hrs	q24 to 36hrs	q48 to 72hrs	Nephrotoxic, ototoxic, may prolong the neuromuscular blockade effect of muscle relaxants. Peak 30, trough 5 to 10
Vancomycin (Rx: 125, 250 mg)	125-250 mg po qid	0%	100%	100%	100%	Oral vancomycin is indicated only for the treatment of *C. difficile*
Antifungal Agents						
Amphotericin B	0.5 mg to 1.5 mg/kg per day	<1%	No renal adjustment is required.			Nephrotoxic, infusion related reactions, give 250 cc NS before each dose
Amphotec®	4 to 6 mg/kg per day	<1%	No renal adjustment is required.			
Abelcet®	5 mg/kg per day	<1%	No renal adjustment is required.			
AmBisome®	3 to 5 mg/kg per day	<1%	No renal adjustment is required.			
Azoles and other antifungals						Increase CsA/FK level
Fluconazole (Rx: 50, 100, 150, 200, Sus)	200 to 400 mg IV qd/bid	70%	100%	100%	50%	
Itraconazole (Rx: 100, liquid)	200 mg q12hrs	35%	100%	100%	50%	Poor oral absorption
Ketoconazole (Rx: 200)	200 to 400 mg po qd	15%	100%	100%	100%	Hepatotoxic
Miconazole	1,200 to 3,600 mg/day	1%	100%	100%	100%	

Continued on next page

Table 12-3. Common Antimicrobial Agents Used in Solid Organ Transplant Recipients
Continued

Drugs	Normal Dose	% Of Renal Excretion	Dosage Adjustment in Renal Failure GFR >50	GFR 10-50	GFR <10	Comments
Antiviral Agents						
Acyclovir (Rx: 200, 400, 800, Sus)	200 to 800 mg po 5x/day	50%	100%	100%	50%	Poor absorption
Amantadine (Rx: 100, 200, oral Sus)	100 to 200 mg q12hrs	90%	100%	50%	25%	
Famciclovir (Rx: 125, 250, 500)	250 to 500 mg po bid to tid	60%	q8hrs	q12hrs	q24hrs	VZV: 500 mg po tid HSV: 250 po bid
Foscarnet	40 to 80 mg IV q8hrs	85%				Nephrotoxic, neurotoxic, hypocalcemia, hypophosphatemia, hypomagnesemia and hypokalemia
Ganciclovir IV	5 mg/kg q12hrs	95%	q12hrs	q24hrs	2, 5 mg/kg qd	Granulocytopenia and thrombocytopenia
Ganciclovir PO (Rx: 250, 500)	1,000 mg PO tid	95%	1000 mg tid	1000 mg bid	1000 mg qd	Oral ganciclovir should be used ONLY for prevention of CMV infection. Always use IV ganciclovir for the treatment of CMV infection
Lamivudine (Rx: 100, 150)	150 mg po bid	80%	q12hrs	q24hrs	50 mg q24hrs	For hepatitis B
Ribavirin (Rx: 200)	500 to 600 mg q12hrs	30%	100%	100%	50%	Hemolytic uremic syndrome.
Valacyclovir (Rx: 500, 1000)	500 to 1,000 mg q8hrs	50%	100%	50%	25%	Thrombotic thrombocytopenic purpura/hemolytic uremic syndrome. Avoid in transplant recipients

tubular dysfunction. Amphotericin-induced nephrotoxicity can be potentiated by sodium depletion and the use of other nephrotoxic agents. Since most transplant patients receive several nephrotoxic agents such as cyclosporine/tacrolimus, ganciclovir, trimethoprim, pentamidine and aminoglycosides, renal insufficiency may be observed in up to 80% of these patients. In addition, amphotericin B may cause electrolyte disorders that require close monitoring of serum magnesium and potassium. Several different new lipid-based amphotericin B preparations are now available. These formulations have shown a lower rate of nephrotoxicity when compared to the standard formulation of amphotericin B. In general, the antifungal activity of lipid-based amphotericin B formulations is similar to that of conventional therapy. The incidence of nephrotoxicity and administration-associated adverse drug reactions (eg, fever, chills) are significantly lower with lipid-based amphotericin B. Among all lipid-based amphotericin B formulations, liposomal amphotericin is the least nephrotoxic and fewer patients require dose reduction or discontinuation due to adverse drug reactions. Liposomal amphotericin B may be more efficacious than the standard formulation of amphotericin B for the treatment of CNS fungal infections.

Azole antifungal agents (ie, ketoconazole, fluconazole and itraconazole) have been used extensively in transplant patients. Ketoconazole and itraconazole are not recommended for the treatment of systemic fungal infections in seriously ill patients and are only available as oral formulations (an intravenous formulation of itraconazole is under investigation). Normal gastric acidity is required for absorption of these agents. H_2 antagonists and proton pump inhibitors (eg, omeprazole, lansoprazole) can reduce adequate absorption of ketoconazole and itraconazole.

Fluconazole is pharmacokinetically and therapeutically superior to ketoconazole in many respects and should be used for the treatment of invasive candida infections. Although itraconazole is an effective agent against histoplasmosis, blastomycosis, aspergillosis and cryptococcosis, amphotericin B is generally used for severe life-threatening infections with these species. Itraconazole is commonly used as a "wrap up" therapy in transplant patients after four to six weeks of amphotericin B. Azole antifungal agents are potent inhibitors of cytochrome P450 hepatic metabolism. Plasma concentration of cyclosporine/tacrolimus should be monitored closely to avoid potential toxicities. Cardiac dysrhythmias may occur in patients taking these agents with cisapride or some of the non-sedative antihistamines. The concomitant use of azole antifungal agents and cisapride or terfenadine is not recommended because cardiac dysrhythmias may occur.

ANTIHYPERTENSIVE AGENTS

Hypertension is a common complication affecting an estimated 60% to 75% of these patients. Calcium channel blockers, angiotensin-converting enzyme (ACE)-inhibitors, Beta blockers and diuretics are the most commonly used antihypertensive agents for the treatment of hypertension following transplantation (Table 12-4).

Calcium Channel Antagonists

Calcium channel blockers (CCBs) inhibit entrance of calcium into the smooth-muscle of arterioles and cause vasodilation. The major renal hemodynamic effects of CCBs are decreased mean arterial pressure and renal vascular resistance (RVR), and increased renal blood flow and glomerular filtration rate (GFR). Calcium channel blockers are considered the drugs of choice for the

Table 12-4. Antihypertensive Agents

| Drugs | Normal Doses | | % Of Renal Excretion | Dosage Adjustment in Renal Failure | | | Comments |
	Starting Dose	Maximum Dose		GFR >50	GFR 10-50	GFR <10	
ACE-Inhibitors							Hyperkalemia, acute renal failure, angioedema, rash, cough, anemia and liver toxicity
Benazepril (Rx: 5, 10, 20, 40)	10 mg qd	80 mg qd	20%	100%	75%	25% to 50%	
Captopril (Rx: 12.5, 25, 50, 100)	6.25 to 25 mg po tid	100 mg tid	35%	100%	75%	50%	
Cilazapril	1.25 mg po qd		80%	100%	50%	25%	
Enalapril (Rx: 2.5, 5, 10)	5 mg qd	20 mg bid	45%	100%	75%	50%	
Fosinopril (Rx: 10, 20, 40)	10 mg po qd	40 mg bid	20%	100%	100%	75%	
Lisinopril (Rx: 2.5, 10, 20, 40)	2.5 mg qd	20 mg bid	80%	100%	50% to 75%	25% to 50%	
Ramipril (Rx: 1.25, 2.5, 5, 10)	2.5 mg qd	10 bid	15%	100%	50% to 75%	25% to 50%	
Trandolapril (Rx: 1, 2, 4)	1 to 2 mg qd	4 mg qd					
Angiotensin II Receptors Antagonists							Hyperkalemia, angioedema (less common than ACE-inhibitors
Losartan (Rx: 25, 50)	50 mg qd	100 mg qd	100%	100%	100%	100%	
Valsartan (Rx: 80, 160)	80 mg qd	160 mg bid					
Candesartan (Rx: 4,8, 16, 32)	16 mg qd	32 mg qd					
Irbesartan (Rx: 75, 150, 300)	150 mg qd	300 mg qd					
Beta Blockers							Decrease HDL, mask symptoms of hypoglycemia, bronchospasm, fatigue, insomnia, depression and sexual dysfunction
Atenolol (Rx: 25, 50, 100)	25 mg qd	100 mg qd	90%	100%	75%	50%	
Carvedilol (Rx: 3.125, 6.25, 12.5, 25)	3.125 mg po tid	25 mg tid	2%	100%	100%	100%	
Esmolol (IV only)	50 mcg/kg per min	300 mcg/kg per min	10%	100%	100%	100%	
Labetalol (Rx: 100, 200, 300)	50 mg po bid	400 mg bid	5%	100%	100%	100%	
Nadolol (Rx: 20, 40, 80, 120, 160)	80 mg qd	160 mg bid	90%	100%	50%	25%	
Propranolol 40 to 160 mg tid (Rx: 10, 20, 40, 60, 80, 90)	320 mg/day	<5%	100%	100%	100%		
Sotalol (Rx: 80, 120, 160, 240)	80 bid	160 mg bid					
Calcium Channel Blockers							Dihydropyridine: headache, ankle edema, gingival hyperplasia and flushing Non-dihydropyridine: bradycardia, constipation, gingival hyperplasia and AV block
Amlodipine (Rx: 2.5, 5, 10)	2.5 po qd	10 mg qd	10%	100%	100%	100%	
Diltiazem (Rx: 30, 60, 90, 120)	30 mg tid	90 mg tid	10%	100%	100%	100%	
Felodipine (Rx: 2.5, 5, 10)	5 mg po bid	20 mg qd	1%	100%	100%	100%	
Isradipine (Rx: 5, 10)	5 mg po bid	10 mg bid	<5%	100%	100%	100%	

Continued on next page

Table 12-4. Antihypertensive Agents *Continued*

Drugs	Normal Doses		% Of Renal Excretion	Dosage Adjustment in Renal Failure			Comments
	Starting Dose	Maximum Dose		GFR >50	GFR 10-50	GFR <10	
Nicardipine (Rx: 20, 30)	20 mg po tid	30 mg po tid	<1%	100%	100%	100%	
Nifedipine XL (Rx: 30, 60, 90)	30 qd	90 mg bid	10%	100%	100%	100%	Avoid short-acting nifedipine formulation
Nimodipine (Rx: 30)			10%	100%	100%	100%	
Nisoldipine (Rx: 10, 20, 30, 40)	20 mg qd	30 mg bid	10%	100%	100%	100%	
Verapamil (Rx: 40, 80, 120)	40 mg tid	240 mg/day	10%	100%	100%	100%	
Diuretics							Hypokalemia/hyperkalemia (potassium sparing agents), hyperuricemia, hyperglycemia, hypomagnesemia, increase serum cholesterol.
Acetazolamide (Rx: 125, 250, 500)	125 mg po tid	500 mg po tid		100%	100%	Avoid	Ibid
Amiloride (Rx: 5)	5 mg po qd	10 mg po qd	50%	100%	100%	Avoid	Ibid
Bumetanide (Rx: 0.5, 1, 2)	1 to 2 mg po qd	2 to 4 mg po qd	35%	100%	100%	100%	Ibid
Ethacrynic Acid (Rx: 25, 50)	50 mg po qd	100 mg po bid	20%	100%	100%	100%	Ibid
Furosemide (Rx: 20, 40, 80, Sol)	40 to 80 mg po qd	120 mg po tid	70%	100%	100%	100%	Ibid
Metolazone (Rx: 2.5, 5, 10)	2.5 mg po qd	10 mg po bid	70%	100%	100%	100%	Ibid
Spironolactone (Rx: 25, 50, 100)	100 mg po qd	300 mg po qd	25%	100%	100%	Avoid	Ibid
Torsemide (Rx: 5, 10, 20)	5 mg po bid	20 mg qd	25%	100%	100%	100%	Ibid
Miscellaneous Agents							
Clonidine (Rx: 0.1, 0.2, 0.3, TTS1, TTS-2, TTS-3)	0.1 po bid/tid	1.2 mg/day	45%	100%	100%	100%	Sexual dysfunction, dizziness, postal hypotension
Digoxin (Rx: 0.125, 0.25, Sol)	0.125 mg qod/qd	0.25 mg po qd	25%	100%	100%	100%	
Hydralazine (Rx: 10, 25, 50, 100)	10 mg po qid	100 mg po qid	25%	100%	100%	100%	Lupus-like reaction
Minoxidil (Rx: 2.5, 10)	2.5 mg po bid	10 mg po bid	20%	100%	100%	100%	Pericardial effusion, fluid retention, hypertrichosis and tachycardia
Nitroprusside	1 mcg/kg per min	10 mcg/kg per min	<10%	100%	100%	100%	Cyanide toxicity
Amrinone	5 mcg/kg per min	10 mcg/kg per min	25%	100%	100%	100%	
Dobutamine	2.5 mcg/kg per min	15 mcg/kg per min	10%	100%	100%	100%	
Milrinone	0.375 mcg/kg per min	0.75 mcg/kg per min		100%	100%	100%	

treatment of posttransplant hypertension for many reasons. It has been postulated that calcium channel blockers may protect against cyclosporine-induced nephrotoxicity, perfusion injury, and delayed graft function, and improve long-term graft survival. The use of calcium channel blockers following renal transplantation has been associated with a lower serum creatinine and greater urine output. In addition, calcium channel blockers may improve graft survival by inhibiting T cell activation and all other incidents of rejection. All calcium channel blockers are vasodilators and, therefore, have the potential to cause dizziness, flushing, and headache. A combination of dihydropyridine derivatives (ie, nifedipine, amlodipine, isradipine, nicardipine, nimodipine, felodipine) and steroids may cause or aggravate edema. Fast-acting calcium channel blockers produce a rapid reduction in blood pressure, which stimulates baroreceptors and may activate the sympathetic nervous system. Retrospective studies in nontransplant patients with advanced heart disease suggest that some fast-acting calcium channel blockers (dihydropyridines) are associated with increased mortality. The same has not been shown with agents with a slow onset of action. Verapamil and diltiazem depress cardiac function and should be used with caution in transplant recipients who have left ventricular and AV nodal dysfunction. Amlodipine, verapamil, diltiazem and nicardipine may increase cyclosporine and tacrolimus levels, and dosages should be monitored closely.

ACE-inhibitors

ACE-inhibitors are effective agents for the treatment of hypertension. The primary renal hemodynamic effect of ACE-inhibitors is vasodilation of the efferent arteriole, which is mediated through suppression of the renin-angiotensin-aldosterone system. Since cyclosporine causes vasoconstriction of the afferent arteriole, its use with an ACE-inhibitor can significantly compromise the renal blood flow and GFR of the renal allograft. ACE-inhibitors, together with cyclosporine, may cause hyperkalemia. ACE-inhibitors are most beneficial when hypertension is caused by the native kidneys. In patients experiencing posttransplant erythrocytosis, they can lower the hematocrit as well as treat hypertension. ACE-inhibitors have been shown to be effective in controlling hypertension associated with chronic allograft rejection. Experimental data suggest that ACE-inhibitors and angiotensin II receptor antagonists (losartan) can reduce cyclosporine-induced chronic nephropathy.

Diuretics

In uncomplicated nontransplant patients, diuretics and beta-adrenergic antagonists (beta blockers) are preferred drugs for the treatment of hypertension. No comparative studies using diuretics have been conducted in transplant patients. Undesirable metabolic side effects of diuretics include glucose intolerance, hyperlipidemia and electrolyte imbalances. Gynecomastia, ototoxicity and sexual dysfunction may also occur. A diuretic is an excellent choice in a transplant patient with excess fluid and sodium concentration. Sodium loading, food-with-drug interactions and drug interactions (eg, nonsteroidal antiinflammatory drugs) may lessen the effectiveness of diuretic therapy. Loop diuretics can cause hypocalcemia and thiazide diuretics can induce hypercalcemia. Loop diuretics can exacerbate hyperparathyroidism and post-transplant bone disease associated with prednisone. Cyclosporine, tacrolimus, ACE-inhibitors, SMX-TMP and beta blockers are also associated with hyperkalemia. Hyperuricemia and hypomagnesemia are frequent complications of both cyclosporine and tacrolimus therapy. The extended use of both diuretics and calcineurin inhibitors may require close electrolyte monitoring to avoid gout and cardiac mortality associated with low levels of magnesium. Ethacrynic acid is the only diuretic that can be used safely in patients with a history of a sulfa allergy. Diuretics should be considered the preferred agents for treatment of posttransplant hypertension in patients with evidence of sodium and extracelluar fluid overload.

Beta Blockers

Beta blockers have no clinically relevant effects on GFR or renal vascular resistance in nontransplant patients. Beta blockers inhibit the release of renin and angiotensin system products. Cyclosporine may increase sympathetic activity resulting in tachycardia and hypertension and beta blockers are known to antagonize the action of catecholamines at beta adrenergic receptors. Beta blocker drugs may cause hyperglycemia or mask the symptoms of hypoglycemia, complicating the treatment of hypertension in diabetic renal transplant recipients. They may also exacerbate hyperlipidemia disorders by increasing cholesterol levels in renal and heart transplant recipients. Beta-adrenergic blocking drugs reduce morbidity and mortality following an acute myocardial infarction (MI) or in patients with coronary artery disease. These benefits in transplant patients with a history of MI or coronary artery disease outweigh the risk of adverse drug reactions or potential synergistic toxicity with immunosuppressive drugs. Therefore, these agents should be considered the drugs of choice in patients with posttransplant hypertension and a history of coronary artery disease. If beta-adrenergic blocking drugs need to be discontinued, these agents should be tapered slowly over a two week period to avoid rebound hypertension.

ANTIHYPERLIPIDEMIC AGENTS

Approximately 60% to 70% of solid organ transplant recipients develop hyperlipidemia following transplantation. Hyperlipidemia and atherosclerosis are established risk factors for premature cardiovascular events or death in transplant recipients with a functioning allograft. Several clinical studies in transplant recipients have demonstrated a positive correlation between a reduction in LDL or an increase in HDL and a decrease in morbidity and mortality associated with hyperlipidemia. Transplant recipients, like nontransplant patients, have the same or even higher risk of coronary artery events. A rise in cholesterol levels begins as early as the first three months following transplantation. Cyclosporine, steroids, allograft failure, cytomegalovirus (CMV) infection and/or immunological responses may contribute to posttransplant hyperlipidemia/atherosclerosis. The incidence of hyperlipidemia is lower among recipients of tacrolimus when compared to cyclosporine. Serum cholesterol can be lowered by a combination of decreasing dietary intake of cholesterol and use of lipid lowering agents or conversion from cyclosporine to tacrolimus.

Fibric acid derivatives (eg, gemfibrozil, fenofibrate) are effective agents in reducing total triglyceride levels (Table 12-5). The major side effects of these agents include an increased risk of myositis when used in combination with HMG-CoA reductase inhibitors and immunosuppressive drugs. Bile acid sequestrants (cholestyramine, colestipol) and niacin are effective agents in reducing total cholesterol and LDL cholesterol. These agents lower cholesterol by interrupting the enterohepatic circulation of bile acids. However, potential drug-drug interactions with immunosuppressive agents and gastrointestinal side effects limit their routine use in transplant recipients. Bile acid sequestrants reduce the absorption of immunosuppressive agents by binding the drugs in the gastrointestinal tract. Side effects that limit the use of niacin in transplant patients include flushing, itching, hepatotoxicity, hyperglycemia, peptic ulcer disease, and hyperuricemia. The frequency of these side effects may be increased when used with immunosuppressive drugs. For example, hepatotoxicity may be increased when niacin is used with cyclosporine. Hyperglycemia may be increased when niacin is used with tacrolimus; peptic ulcer disease may be increased with the use of steroids; and hyperuricemia may be increased with the use of either cyclosporine or tacrolimus.

HMG-CoA reductase inhibitors are generally considered the initial drugs of choice when drug therapy is indicated for the management of hyperlipidemia in transplant recipients. HMG-CoA reductase inhibitors reduce total cholesterol by inhibiting the rate limiting enzyme in cholesterol synthesis, up-regulating LDL receptors and thus increasing LDL uptake from the circulation. In addition, these agents may have some immunosuppressive effects. Pravastatin has been shown to improve allograft survival and decrease acute rejection in heart transplant recipients. Adverse drug reactions in transplant patients include elevation of liver function tests and myositis. The concurrent use of HMG-CoA reductase inhibitors and cyclosporine has resulted in rhabdomyolysis and acute renal failure. To reduce the incidence and severity of any adverse effects, HMG-CoA reductase inhibitors should be given in reduced doses. Patients should be advised of the signs and symptoms of myopathy and asked to report promptly any unexplained muscle pain, tenderness or muscle weakness. Creatine phosphokinase (CPK) concentrations should be monitored.

ANTICOAGULATION

Since allograft thrombosis is a significant complication of organ transplantation, anticoagulation is indicated in certain patients. Low doses of standard unfractionated heparin and low molecular weight heparin (eg, deltaprin, enoxaprin) are indicated during the course of muromonab-CD3 for induction. Warfarin therapy for four to six weeks is the most recommended protocol following kidney transplantation in recipients at high risk for graft thrombosis because of the presence of antiphospholipid antibodies or other hypercoagulable states. In most cases, low-dose heparin therapy does not affect the usual coagulation cascade. However, an individual transplant recipient's sensitivity to low-dose heparin therapy varies greatly and there is no simple laboratory test available to predict which patients are at high risk of complications. The major adverse drug reactions of heparin therapy are bleeding and thrombocytopenia. Patients should be assessed for bleeding tendencies when heparin is prescribed as a thromboprophylactic protocol. Ticlopidine and clopidogrel are antiplatelet agents that inhibit collagen-induced platelet aggregation. Ticlodpine may cause severe life-threatening hematological abnormalities. The use of this agent is highly discouraged in transplant recipients. Aspirin or clopidogrel should be considered for reducing the risk of fatal or nonfatal thrombotic stroke in transplant patients (Table 12-6).

Table 12-5. Antihyperlipidemic Agents

| Drugs | Normal Doses | | % Of Renal Excretion | Dosage Adjustment in Renal Failure | | | Comments |
	Starting Dose	Maximum Dose		GFR >50	GFR 10-50	GFR <10	
Atorvastatin (Rx: 10, 20, 40)	10 mg/day	80 mg/day	<2%	100%	100%	100%	Liver dysfunction, myalgia and rhabdomyolysis with CsA/FK
Cholestyramine (Rx: 4 gm)	4 gm bid	24 gm/day	None	100%	100%	100%	Schedule CsA/FK 3 hrs after the dose, N/V and constipation
Colestipol (Rx: 5 gm)	5 gmbid	30 gm/day	None	100%	100%	100%	Schedule CsA/FK 3 hrs after the dose, N/V and constipation
Fluvastatin (Rx: 20, 40)	20 mg daily	80 mg/day	<1%	100%	100%	100%	Liver dysfunction, myalgia and rhabdomyolysis with CsA/FK
Gemfibrozil (Rx: 300, 600)	600 bid	600 bid	None	100%	100%	100%	Hyperglycemia, rhabdomyolysis, elevation of LFTs
Lovastatin (Rx: 10, 20, 40)	5 mg daily	20 mg/day	None	100%	100%	100%	Liver dysfunction, myalgia and rhabdomyolysis with CsA/FK
Pravastatin (Rx: 10, 20)	10 to 40 mg daily	80 mg/day	<10%	100%	100%	100%	Liver dysfunction, myalgia and rhabdomyolysis with CsA/FK
Simvastatin (Rx: 5, 10, 20, 40, 80)	5 to 20 mg daily	20 mg/day	13%	100%	100%	100%	Liver dysfunction, myalgia and rhabdomyolysis with CsA/FK

ANTI-ULCER MEDICATIONS

Peptic ulcer disease, gastrointestinal bleeding, acid reflux disorders, pancreatitis, diarrhea, nausea and vomiting are commonly reported in transplant recipients. These complications may be aggravated by the use of glucocorticoids, azathioprine, tacrolimus and mycophenolate. Glucocorticoids increase acid secretion and may worsen pre-existing peptic ulcer diseases or acid reflux disorders following transplantation. Ranitidine, famotidine, lansoprazole and omeprazole are generally safe and effective in the treatment of peptic ulcer disease and acid reflux disorders (Table 12-7). Cimetidine should be avoided because of several drug-drug interactions with other agents such as cyclosporine, ciprofloxacin, theophylline and warfarin. Aluminum-based antacids may reduce the absorption of mycophenolate and tacrolimus.

Table 12-6. Antiplatelets/Anticoagulation Agents

| Drugs | Normal Doses | | % Of Renal Excretion | Dosage Adjustment in Renal Failure | | | Comments |
	Starting Dose	Maximum Dose		GFR >50	GFR 10-50	GFR <10	
Aspirin (81, 325, 500, 650, 975)	81 mg/day	325 mg/day					GI irritation and bleeding tendency
Clopidogrel (Rx: 75)	75 mg/day	75 mg/day	50%	100%	100%	100%	
Dalteparin (Rx: 2500, 5000)	2,500 units Sq /day	5,000 units Sq /day	Unknown	100%	100%	100%	
Enoxaparin (Rx: 30, 40, 60, 70, 80, 100)	20 mg/day	30 mg bid	8%	100%	100%	50%	1 mg/kg q12hrs for treatment of DVT. Check anti-factor Xa activity four hours after second dose in patients with renal dysfunction. There are some evidence of drug accumulation in renal failure.
Ticlopidine (Rx: 250)	250 mg bid	250 mg bid	2%	100%	100%	100%	Decrease CsA level and may cause severe neutropenia & thrombocytopenia
Warfarin (Rx: 1, 2, 2.5, 3, 4, 5, 6, 7.5, 10)	5 mg/day	Adjust per INR	<1%	100%	100%	100%	Monitor INR very closely. Start at 5 mg/day. 1 mg Vit. K IV over 30 minutes or 2.5 to 5 mg po can be used to normalize INR.

Table 12-7. Gastrointestinal Agents

| Drugs | Normal Doses | | % Of Renal Excretion | Dosage Adjustment in Renal Failure | | | Comments |
	Starting Dose	Maximum Dose		GFR >50	GFR 10-50	GFR <10	
Anti-ulcer Agents							
Cimetidine (Rx: 100, 200, 300, 400, 800, Sol)	300 mg po tid	800 mg po bid	60%	100%	75%	25%	Multiple drug-drug interactions; beta blockers, sulfonylurea, theophylline, warfarin, etc
Famotidine (Rx: 20, 40, Sol)	20 mg po bid	40 mg po bid	70%	100%	75%	25%	Headache, fatigue, thrombocytopenia, alopecia
Lansoprazole (Rx: 15, 30)	15 mg po qd	30 mg bid	None	100%	100%	100%	Headache, diarrhea
Nizatidine (Rx: 75, 150, 300)	150 mg po bid	300 mg po bid	20%	100%	75%	25%	Headache, fatigue, thrombocytopenia, alopecia
Omeprazole (Rx: 10, 20, 40)	20 mg po qd	40 mg po bid	None	100%	100%	100%	Headache, diarrhea
Ranitidine (Rx: 75, 150, 300, Sol)	150 mg po bid	300 mg po bid	80%	100%	75%	25%	Headache, fatigue, thrombocytopenia, alopecia
Other Agents							
Metoclopramide (Rx: 5, 10, Sol)	10 mg po tid	30 mg po qid	15%	100%	100%	50-75%	Increase CsA and tacrolimus blood concentration neurotoxic
Misoprostol (Rx: 100, 200)	100 mcg po bid	200 mcg po qid		100%	100%	100%	Diarrhea, N/VAbortifacient agent
Sucralfate (Rx: 1, Sol)	1 gm po qid	1 gm po qid	None	100%	100%	100%	Constipation, decrease absorption of MMF

HYPOGLYCEMIC AGENTS

Diabetes may occur early after or several years following transplantation. Approximately 10% of all nondiabetic patients may develop insulin-dependent diabetes and require daily insulin therapy following transplantation. If insulin is required, a ratio of long-acting (NPH or Lente) to short-acting (Regular) of 2:1 is preferred. Two-thirds of the total dose should be given in the morning, and 1/3 of the total dose at dinner and bedtime. Short-acting agents should be given at dinner time and long-acting at bedtime.

Approximately 50% of transplant patients respond to oral hypoglycemic agents. Table 12-8 shows the most commonly used oral hypoglycemic agents in transplant recipients. Sulfonylureas reduce hepatic glucose production, improve basal insulin secretion and increase the sensitivity of insulin receptors. The main limitation of sulfonylureas is hypoglycemia. This is best avoided by educating and encouraging patients not to skip meals after taking sulfonylureas. In addition, sulfonylureas should be started at the lowest possible dose and increased incrementally every seven days.

Metformin inhibits hepatic gluconeogenesis and increases glucose uptake by muscle. Although very rare, the most serious complication of metformin is lactic acidosis. Renal impairment (Scr >1.4 mg/dL), liver dysfunction and cardiovascular decompensation may precipitate lactic acidosis. In general, the use of metformin in transplant recipients is strongly discouraged. Alpha-glucosidase inhibitors (eg, acarbose) delay carbohydrate absorption and blunt postprandial hyperglycemia. The major side effects of acarbose are abdominal fullness, increased intestinal flatulence and diarrhea. Acarbose should be started at a dose of 25 mg orally three times a day with the first mouthful of food. Finally, thiazolidinediones (eg, troglitazone) improve insulin-responsiveness of muscle cells and decrease insulin resistance. Transplant recipients may experience a clinically relevant decrease in cyclosporine/tacrolimus concentrations after the initiation of troglitazone therapy. Although troglitazone is not metabolized by the cytochrome P450 IIIA-4

isoenzyme family, it is an inducer of these enzymes, which are responsible for the metabolism of cyclosporine. Fulminant hepatic failure and increased serum aminotransferase concentrations have been associated with the use of troglitazone. Liver function tests should be monitored closely.

MISCELLANEOUS AGENTS

Antihistamines and decongestants are valuable interventions that may reduce the severity of symptoms of the common cold. Nonsedative antihistamine agents such as terfenadine and astemizole rarely have caused life-threatening arrhythmias due to their accumulation in cardiac tissue. Fexofenadine and loratadine are devoid of fatal cardiotoxicity and should be considered for transplant patients.

High-dose aspirin and nonsteroidal antiinflammatory agents (NSAIDs) should be avoided in transplant recipients. These agents may significantly worsen bleeding time, preexisting hypertension, gastritis and impaired renal function. The concurrent use of NSAIDs and cyclosporine/tacrolimus may result in increased serum creatinine, nephrotoxicity and cyclosporine blood concentration. The renal impairment in transplant patients is frequently reversible following discontinuation of the NSAIDs. NSAIDs may decrease renal blood flow and prostaglandin production and cause sodium and water retention. These effects are of greatest clinical importance in patients with impaired renal function. In addition, NSAIDs may attenuate the effect of certain antihypertensive agents including diuretics, beta blockers and clonidine. The most common side effects of NSAIDs involve the gastrointestinal tract and include gastritis and dyspepsia. Acetaminophen is an effective agent for the treatment of mild to moderate pain. Short-term treatment with acetaminophen has no adverse effects on renal function, hepatic function or cyclosporine tacrolimus pharmacokinetic properties. Most clinical data suggests that acetaminophen provides analgesic effects comparable to aspirin and other NSAIDs.

Table 12-8. Hypoglycemic Agents

Drugs	Normal Doses		% Of Renal Excretion	Dosage Adjustment in Renal Failure			Comments
	Starting Dose	Maximum Dose		GFR >50	GFR 10-50	GFR <10	
Acarbose (Rx: 25, 50, 100)	25 mg tid	100 mg tid	35%	100%	50%	Avoid	Abdominal pain, N/V and Flatulence
Glipizide (Rx: 5, 10)	5 mg qd	20 mg bid	5%	100%	50%	50%	
Glyburide (Rx: 1.25, 2.5, 5)	2.5 mg qd	10 mg bid	50%	100%	50%	Avoid	
Metformin (Rx: 500, 850)	500 mg bid	2,550 mg/day (bid or tid)	95%	100%	Avoid	Avoid	Lactic acidosis
Repaglinide (Rx: 0.5, 1, 2)	0.5 to 1 mg	4 mg tid					
Troglitazone (Rx: 200, 300, 400)	200 mg qd	600 mg qd	3%	100%	100%	100%	Decrease CsA level, Hepatotoxic.

Hyperuricemia and gout have been reported in 85% of renal transplant recipients receiving cyclosporine tacrolimus therapy, as compared with 30% of transplant patients receiving azathioprine and steroids. Cyclosporine and tacrolimus interfere with the tubular excretion of uric acid. Risk factors for hyperuricemia include impaired renal function and concomitant use of diuretics. Allopurinol is the drug of choice in patients with overproduction of uric acid and a history of uric acid stones or renal impairment. Azathioprine is metabolized in the blood to 6-mercaptopurine, which is metabolized by xanthine oxidase in the liver to inactive 6-thiouric acid. Therefore, the inhibition of xanthine oxidase by allopurinol may result in azathioprine toxicities (eg, leukopenia, anemia, nausea, vomiting). A dosage reduction of 60% to 75% of the normal dose of azathioprine is recommended in the presence of concomitant allopurinol therapy.

CONCLUSION

New medications and immunosuppressive drugs are continually being introduced to the market. As the number of different agents increases, drug-drug interactions become more common. Many of these interactions cause a slight increase or decrease in drug concentrations, which are clinically insignificant. However, several drug-drug interactions can result in an undesirable clinical toxicity and, rarely, life-threatening outcome. Proper assessment of clinically important drug interactions is critical when new medications are prescribed to transplant recipients. A benefit-vs-risk analysis should be employed during the drug selection process. Understanding drug interactions in transplant patients may prevent unwanted toxicities, allograft rejection, and may even save a patient's life.

RECOMMENDED READING

Campana C, Regazzi MB, Buggia I, Molinaro M. Clinically significant drug interactions with cyclosporin. Clin Pharmacokinet. 1996;30(2):141-179.

Mignat C. Clinically significant drug interactions with new immunosuppressive agents. Drug Saf. 1997;16(4):267-278.

Jones TE, Morris RG. Diltiazem does not always increase blood cyclosporin concentration. Br J Clin Pharmacol. 1996;42(5):642-644.

Kennedy DT, Hayney MS, Lake KD. Azathioprine and allopurinol: the price of an avoidable drug interaction. Ann Pharmacother. 1996;30(9):951-954.

Seifeldin R. Drug interactions in transplantation. Clin Ther. 1995;17(6):1043-1061.

Lake KD, Canafax DM. Important interactions of drugs with immunosuppressive agents used in transplant recipients. J Antimicrob Chemother. 1995;36(Suppl B):11-22.

Olyaei AJ, de Mattos AM, Norman DJ, Bennett WM. Interaction between tacrolimus and nefazodone in a stable renal transplant recipient. Pharmacotherapy. 1998;18(6):1356-1359.

Rossi SJ, Schroeder TJ, Hariharan S, First MR. Prevention and management of the adverse effects associated with immunosuppressive therapy. Drug Saf. 1993;9(2):104-131.

Trotter JF. Drugs that interact with immunosuppressive agents. Semin Gastrointest Dis. 1998;9(3):147-153.

Matsuda H, Iwasaki K, Shiraga T, Tozuka K, Hata T, Guengerich FP. Interactions of FK506 (tacrolimus) with clinically important drugs. Res Commun Mol Pathol Pharmacol. 1996;91(1):57-64.

Morris-Stiff G, Jurewicz A, Balaji V, et al. Conversion from cyclosporin to tacrolimus in a patient with prolonged acute tubular necrosis. Transpl Int. 1997;10(5):398-400.

Seifeldin RA, Marcos-Alvarez A, Gordon FD, Lewis WD, Jenkins RL. Nifedipine interaction with tacrolimus in liver transplant recipients. Ann Pharmacother. 1997;31(5):571-575.

Fishman JA, Rubin RH. Infection in organ-transplant recipients. N Engl J Med. 1998;338(24):1741-1751.

Elliott WJ. Traditional drug therapy of hypertension in transplant recipients. J Hum Hypertens. 1998;12(12):845-849.

Curtis JJ. Treatment of hypertension in renal allograft patients: does drug selection make a difference? Kidney Int Suppl. 1997;63:S75-S77.

Jenkins GH, Singer DR. Hypertension in thoracic transplant recipients. J Hum Hypertens. 1998;12(12):813-823.

Zeier M, Mandelbaum A, Ritz E. Hypertension in the transplanted patient. Contrib Nephrol. 1998;124:146-157.

Schwartz L, Augustine J, Raymer J, Canzanello V, Taler S, Textor S. Nurse management of posttransplant hypertension in liver transplant patients. J Transplant Coord. 1996;6(3):139-144.

Singer DR, Jenkins GH. Hypertension in transplant recipients. J Hum Hypertens. 1996;10(6):395-402.

Dairou F. Lipid disorders and cardiovascular risks in nephrology. Nephrol Dial Transplant. 1998;13(Suppl 4):30-33.

Jindal RM. Post-transplant hyperlipidaemia. Postgrad Med J. 1997;73(866):785-793.

Olyaei AJ, de Mattos AM, Bennett WM. Switching between cyclosporin formulations. What are the risks? Drug Saf. 1997;16(6):366-373.

Ballantyne CM, el Masri B, Morrisett JD, Torre-Amione G. Pathophysiology and treatment of lipid perturbation after cardiac transplantation. Curr Opin Cardiol. 1997;12(2):153-160.

Arnadottir M, Berg AL. Treatment of hyperlipidemia in renal transplant recipients.. Transplantation. 1997;63(3): 339-345.

Kobashigawa JA, Kasiske BL. Hyperlipidemia in solid organ transplantation. Transplantation. 1997;63(3): 331-338.

de Mattos AM, Olyaei AJ, Bennett WM. Pharmacology of immunosuppressive medications used in renal diseases and transplantation. Am J Kidney Dis. 1996;28(5): 631-667.

Alkhunaizi AM, Olyaei AJ, Barry JM, et al. Efficacy and safety of low molecular weight heparin in renal transplantation. Transplantation. 1998;66(4):533-534.

Langnas AN. Budd-Chiari syndrome: decisions, decisions. Liver Transpl Surg. 1997;3(4):443-445.

du Buf-Vereijken PW, Hilbrands LB, Wetzels JF. Partial renal vein thrombosis in a kidney transplant: management by streptokinase and heparin. Nephrol Dial Transplant. 1998;13(2):499-502.

Salat C, Holler E, Gohring P, et al. Protein C, protein S and antithrombin III levels in the course of bone marrow and subsequent liver transplantation due to veno-occlusive disease. Eur J Med Res. 1996;1(12):571-574.

Troppmann C, Gruessner AC, Benedetti E, et al. Vascular graft thrombosis after pancreatic transplantation: univariate and multivariate operative and nonoperative risk factor analysis. J Am Coll Surg. 1996;182(4):285-316.

Kuypers DR, Vanrenterghem Y. Prophylaxis of cytomegalovirus infection in renal transplantation Nephrol Dial Transplant. 1998;13(12):3012-3016.

Schmaldienst S, Horl WH. Bacterial infections after renal transplantation. Contrib Nephrol. 1998;124:18-33.

Fevery J. Liver transplantation: problems and perspectives. Hepatogastroenterology. 1998;45(22):1039-1044.

Loertscher R. Management issues in renal transplantation. Transplant Proc. 1998;30(5)1723-1725.

Beyga ZT, Kahan BD. Surgical complications of kidney transplantation. J Nephrol. 1998;11(3):137-145.

Grossman RA. Care of the renal transplant recipient: a field guide for the generalist. Dis Mon.1998;44(6): 269-282.

Patenaude YG, Dubois J, Sinsky AB, et al. Liver transplantation: review of the literature. Part 3: Medical complications. Can Assoc Radiol J. 1997;48(5-6):333-339.

Jindal RM, Sidner RA, Milgrom ML. Post-transplant diabetes mellitus. The role of immunosuppression. Drug Saf. 1997;16(4):242-257.

Reich D, Rothstein K, Manzarbeitia C, Munoz S. Common medical diseases after liver transplantation. Semin Gastrointest Dis. 1998;9(3):110-125.

Rao VK. Posttransplant medical complications. Surg Clin North Am. 1998;78(1):113-132.

13 DESIGN AND INTERPRETATION OF CLINICAL TRIALS IN TRANSPLANTATION

Mary B. Leonard, MD, MSCE
Lynda Anne Szczech, MD, MSCE
Harold I. Feldman, MD, MSCE

Evaluation of the safety, tolerability and beneficial effects of immunosuppressive therapies is an important focus of research in transplantation. Investigators rely on the performance of clinical trials to provide valid estimates of the therapeutic effect. After delineating the general principles of clinical research, this chapter describes the methods of designing, conducting and analyzing clinical trials in transplantation. Finally, meta-analysis of clinical trials is reviewed. Although not intended to exhaustively cover all methodological considerations relevant to the conduct of clinical trials, the concepts covered are intended to enhance the readers' skills in the critical appraisal of published research.

GENERAL PRINCIPLES OF CLINICAL RESEARCH
Efficacy vs Effectiveness

The evaluation of the effects of drugs may examine efficacy or effectiveness. Studies of efficacy evaluate the effects of drugs under ideal experimental conditions that optimize compliance and provide close clinical monitoring. Studies of effectiveness evaluate the effects of drugs when administered in the context of usual clinical care outside of a research setting. For example, an immunosuppressive drug given under experimental conditions might prove efficacious in preventing allograft rejection in study subjects. However, in clinical care, compared to

Mary B. Leonard, MD, MCSE, Assistant Professor of Pediatrics and Epidemiology, Division of Pediatric Nephrology, The Children's Hospital of Philadelphia, Center for Clinical Epidemiology and Biostatistics, Department of Biostatistics and Epidemiology, University of Pennsylvania School of Medicine, Philadelphia, PA

Lynda Anne Szczech, MD, MCSE, Assistant Professor of Medicine, Duke Institute of Renal Outcomes Research, Division of Nephrology, Duke University Medical Center, Durham, NC

Harold I. Feldman, MD, MCSE, Associate Professor of Medicine and Epidemiology, Renal, Electrolyte and Hypertension Division, Center for Clinical Epidemiology and Biostatistics, Department of Biostatistics and Epidemiology, University of Pennsylvania School of Medicine, Philadelphia, PA

a controlled research setting, monitoring for drug toxicity and practices geared toward optimizing drug adherence are often less intensive. If patients outside of the research setting have less success adhering to the prescribed dosing regimen, a drug's effectiveness will be less than its demonstrated efficacy. Drug efficacy is best studied in a randomized clinical trial. Studies of efficacy draw on the theoretical framework underlying virtually all scientific experimentation. The design of these studies is guided by the goal of isolating the effects of drugs by controlling for variations in other factors across comparison groups. For example, the ideal experiment would create the circumstance wherein study groups differed only with respect to their immunosuppressive regimen.

The current drug approval process in the US includes preclinical animal testing followed by three phases of clinical testing. Phase 1 and 2 trials are generally conducted on a small number of healthy subjects and patients who have the disease, respectively. These trials provide information on pharmacokinetics and relatively common adverse reactions. Phase 3 testing is performed on a larger number of patients in order to evaluate a drug's efficacy and to gather more information on safety. Under the 1962 Kefauver-Harris Amendment to the Food, Drug and Cosmetic Act of 1939, proof of a drug's efficacy and safety is required prior to marketing for its intended use. This legislation specifically requires that randomized, well-controlled clinical trials be conducted prior to drug approval. Effectiveness is best studied when the drug is prescribed after marketing. These post-marketing surveillance, or phase 4, studies, frequently focus on both effectiveness and toxicity of drugs in the clinical setting.

Basic Study Designs

Analytical studies explicitly compare a drug treatment to a control drug or no drug at all. Analytical studies can be divided into two paradigms (Table 13-1): those using an experimental research model (clinical trials) and those studying treatment strategies existing in the clinical community (observational research).

In clinical trials, the treatment assignment of each subject is determined by the study design. Patient care is altered as a direct consequence of the research, and subsequent clinical outcomes are examined in relation to these interventions. When subjects are randomly allocated to treatment, clinical trials have the unique ability to reduce bias in the interpretation of the relative efficacy of treatments by balancing the study's treatment groups with respect to characteristics that are measurable and, importantly, those that are not.

Patient outcomes are observed in relation to clinical practice in observational research. Comparison groups frequently differ by characteristics in addition to drug treatment, thereby creating opportunities for bias in the

Table 13-1. Research Paradigms

Clinical Trials
Patient care is delivered according to the research protocol
Clinical outcomes are examined in relation to specific experimental interventions
Example: nonrandomized clinical trials, randomized controlled trials
Observational Research
Patient care is delivered according to prevailing clinical practice
Experimental interventions are not implemented
Clinical outcomes are examined in relation to variations in clinical practice
Example: cohort studies, case-control studies

assessment of drug efficacy. The two most common observational study designs are cohort and case-control studies. In a cohort study, investigators sample a population (cohort) and determine the exposures (different immunosuppressive protocols) of each individual at the beginning of follow-up. Subsequent clinical outcomes are then compared across subgroups of the cohort that have been treated in different ways. Case-control studies compare patients who have experienced a particular disease outcome (eg, early allograft failure) to controls who have not experienced that disease outcome, with respect to the frequency of antecedent exposures (eg, immunosuppressive treatments).

Error in the Evaluation of Research Findings

Both random and systematic errors may compromise studies of treatment and clinical outcomes. Minimizing random error increases precision, while minimizing systemic error increases validity. Error can also be characterized according to the direction of the incorrect inference that is created. A type I error, or false-positive, occurs when a study concludes there is an association between treatment and outcome when, in fact, one does not exist. A type II error, or false-negative, occurs when a study concludes that there is no association but, in fact, one does exist. For example, Figure 13-1 demonstrates the possible findings in a study comparing drug A and drug B in the prevention of allograft loss. The principles of study design derive from the goal of reducing systematic and random error, and improving the likelihood of achieving a true positive or true negative result.

RANDOM ERROR. Statistical testing permits calculation of the probability that random error accounts for the results observed in any individual study. Both *P*-values and confidence intervals (CIs) are measures of random variation that may contribute to the observed differences between the randomized study groups. The *P*-value represents the probability of observing a difference in outcomes across study groups (eg, greater allograft survival among patients receiving a new experimental drug, compared to standard therapy) due to chance, when in truth, the experimental and standard therapies do not lead to different rates of allograft survival. Statistical analysis also permits representation of the precision of a study's findings: the CI about the study's observed findings (eg, the relative risk [RR]) indicates the plausible range of findings within which the truth lies. Increasing the size of the study population reduces the magnitude of random error, improves the precision of the findings, and reduces the width of the CI.

The randomized clinical trial should have an adequate sample size to detect the potentially small, but clinically significant differences between the treatment groups. Unduly small trials are limited in their ability to detect statistically significant differences between treatments, and may be misinterpreted as demonstrating that the treatments do not differ, which could be a false-negative conclusion. The statistical power of a trial is the probability that it will detect a difference between treatment groups, if one truly exists. A larger sample size, a greater number of clinical outcomes observed in the study group, and similar-sized comparison treatment groups all increase the power (and decrease the risk of type II error) of a study to detect an effect (eg, RR) of any size. In studies of survival (allograft or patient), increasing the duration of follow-up is a common strategy to increase the power of the study.

SYSTEMATIC ERROR. Systematic error, or bias, may occur as a result of differences across study groups with respect to the way participants are selected for a study, or the manner in which information is obtained, reported,

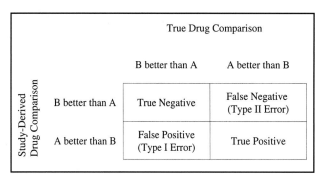

Figure 13-1. Error in Inferences: classification of study results comparing drugs A and B, according to the true relative effects of drug A and B.

or interpreted. Such consistent differences can falsely create (false-positive) or mask (false-negative) an appearance of effectiveness of treatment. Systematic error can be reduced through proper study design and data analysis. Study design elements that reduce systematic error include restricted inclusion criteria, matched comparison groups, standardized protocols for acquiring data on exposures and outcomes, and random allocation to treatment. When systematic error can be reduced through data analysis, it is referred to as *controlling for confounding*. Analytical techniques that control for confounding (eg, stratified analysis and multivariable regression) adjust the comparisons between treatment groups for imbalance in prognostic (confounding) factors that have been measured, such as age. In designing a study, one should consider and measure potential confounding factors to adjust for their effects during data analysis. Confounding factors that are unknown or difficult to measure cannot be adjusted for, and may be important sources of systematic error, especially in observational research.

Observational studies of drug efficacy present the special methodological problem of confounding by indication, in which clinical characteristics that lead to the implementation of specific therapies are also important prognostic factors. Thus, it may become difficult or impossible to separate the effects of specific treatments from the effects of the clinical characteristics that dictated the use of those treatments. Confounding by indi-

cation is not a problem in randomized clinical trials, where administration of treatments is dictated by the study protocol and not by patient characteristics.

OVERVIEW OF ERROR IN A CLINICAL TRIAL.

Figure 13-2 summarizes the potential sources of error in the enrollment of subjects into a randomized clinical trial. The target population in a drug trial is the patient group that may benefit from the new drug and to which the investigators expect the results of the particular trial to be generalized. The desired study population, whether literally sampled or not, is viewed as a figurative sample of the larger target population. The patients who are randomized to treatment ideally represent an unbiased sample of the target population. However, random and systematic error, as indicated in the figure, can threaten the representativeness of study subjects who are randomly allocated to each treatment. For example, if a particular desired study population consists of all patients in a given transplant center, these individuals may not represent the target transplant population of all transplant recipients. Systematic differences in patient characteristics across centers, such as those that arise from distinct referral patterns and regional differences in socioeconomics, can threaten the generalization of a trial's findings. Specific evaluation of the representation of the target population by the study population may be useful in assessing a trial's generalization. A second source of systematic error arises when members of the desired

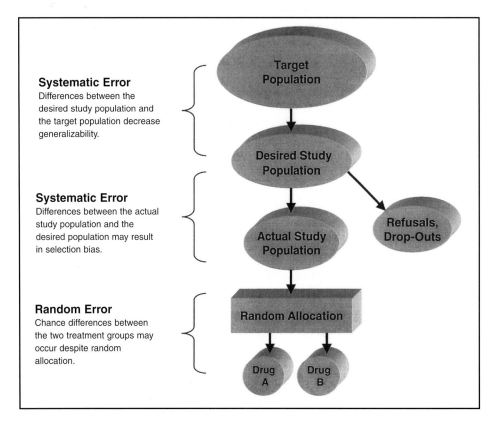

Figure 13-2. Sources of random and systematic error in a randomized clinical trial.

Systematic Error
Differences between the desired study population and the target population decrease generalizability.

Systematic Error
Differences between the actual study population and the desired population may result in selection bias.

Random Error
Chance differences between the two treatment groups may occur despite random allocation.

Target Population

Desired Study Population

Actual Study Population

Refusals, Drop-Outs

Random Allocation

Drug A

Drug B

study population decline participation, or drop out prior to randomization. These individuals may differ in their response to treatment, and their necessary exclusion further threatens the generalization of a trial's findings.

Random error may occur when subjects are randomly assigned to study groups. By chance, it is possible that the groups will not be balanced with respect to health status or other important prognostic characteristics, especially when a trial is small. Such random imbalances may alter the observed relationship between treatment and outcome. Statistical tests specifically evaluate the probability that observed differences across treatment groups arose from such random imbalances.

ISSUES IN THE DESIGN AND CONDUCT OF CLINICAL TRIALS
Types of Clinical Trials: Comparative Trials and Equivalence Trials
As the field of transplantation immunopharmacology advances, new agents are introduced with the hope for greater efficacy in the prevention of allograft loss. One example has been the addition of mycophenolate mofetil (MMF) to cyclosporine-based immunosuppression for renal transplantation. Most clinical trials in transplantation are *comparative* trials designed to demonstrate greater efficacy of a new regimen as compared to standard therapy. However, if the new treatment is expected to match the efficacy of the standard treatment, but has advantages in safety, convenience, or cost, then, the objective of a trial is to show equivalent efficacy – a so-called *equivalence* trial.

A familiar example of an equivalence trial in transplantation is the comparison of the safety, tolerability, and efficacy of microemulsion cyclosporine to traditional cyclosporine. Another example is the evaluation of generic substitutes for immunosuppressive drugs. Generic substitution is a key issue in transplantation because transplant drugs are expensive and the consequences of poorly-controlled immunosuppression are serious.

Unique methodological problems may hinder or compromise equivalence trials. First, in an equivalence trial, conventional statistical tests of significance may have little relevance; failure to detect a difference does not necessarily imply equivalence, especially if the CIs are wide. When comparing a new drug to a standard drug, it is necessary to show that the new drug is sufficiently similar to the standard to be clinically indistinguishable. The approach used by the FDA to assess the equivalence of generic drugs to brand-name drugs examines the 90% CI around the difference between the mean effects of the generic and brand-name drug (eg, for pharmacokinetic measures). For equivalence to be presumed, the upper and lower boundaries of the CI must not exceed (±) 20% of the brand-name drug's mean value. Second, poor compliance, or other blurring of the differences between the treatment groups will increase the likelihood of falsely asserting equivalence. Therefore, equivalence trials generally need to be larger than their comparative counterparts and the standard of conduct needs to be especially high.

Clinical Trial Study Designs: Parallel, Crossover, and Factorial Design
The most common study design in transplantation is the parallel, or noncrossover design (Table 13-2). In this design, study participants are assigned to receive only

---

Table 13-2. Key Attributes of Clinical Trial Study Designs

Parallel

Study subjects are allocated either to an intervention group or a control group and are followed prospectively to assess study outcomes

Crossover

Each study subject receives both the intervention and control treatment consecutively, serving as his or her own control

Ideally, the order in which the treatments are administered is randomized

Inferences are based on the assumption that the effects of the first treatment do not carry over into the period of the second treatment

Inappropriate for studies of mortality or disease resolution

Factorial

Multiple hypotheses are tested in a single trial

Allows examination of combinations of therapies

Must consider impact of interactions

one of the study treatments. Study participants are allocated to either the control group or intervention group. Each patient is then followed prospectively to assess the study outcomes for a predetermined period of follow-up. This is the simplest trial design, but requires larger sample sizes than some alternative designs. Randomized immunosuppression trials addressing patient and allograft survival have generally used this design.

Crossover studies use each study participant as their own control. By evaluating the same subject at different times in the presence and absence of the therapy under study, the variability among subjects can be avoided. Therefore, the differences in outcome between the intervention and treatment can be detected with a smaller sample size. The order of administration of study therapies should be selected at random for each patient. Sufficient time must be allowed between administration of the treatment and comparison therapies to allow the effects to dissipate and to avoid carryover effects. This study design is very efficient for studying the efficacy of therapies intended to reduce the frequency or severity of chronic, recurrent problems, such as hypertension or hyperlipidemia. However, crossover studies are not appropriate for evaluating the long-term efficacy of therapeutic measures whose impact may remain for a lengthy interval following discontinuation. This design is not suitable for most immunosuppressive trials focused on the clinical outcomes of patient or allograft survival because an individual's long-term allograft function may be highly dependent on the initial antirejection therapy. Randomized crossover studies, however, have been used successfully to compare immunosuppressive drug pharmacokinetics and tolerability, in addition to evaluating antihypertensive and cholesterol-lowering agents among transplant recipients.

Factorial designs provide a mechanism to test multiple hypotheses simultaneously in a single trial with a relatively small increase in cost, effort, and number of subjects. A clinical trial to test two hypotheses may use a 2 X 2 factorial design, in which subjects are first randomized to a set of treatments to address the first hypothesis, and then are subsequently randomized to a second set of treatments to address the second hypothesis. The North American Pediatric Renal Transplant Cooperative Study (NAPRTCS) Cooperative Clinical Trials in Pediatric Transplantation (CCTPT) is currently using this approach to: (1) determine the efficacy of induction therapy with a monoclonal T cell antibody (muromonab-CD3)) compared to intravenous cyclosporine among kidney and transplant recipients, and (2) compare maintenance oral cyclosporine metabolism when administered as either the traditional or microemulsion formulation. At entry into the study, patients were randomly assigned to receive either muromonab-CD3 or intravenous cyclosporine induction. Patients were then further randomized to receive one of the two forms of cyclosporine. Thus, the children are allocated to one of four treatment regimens (Figure 13-3): intravenous cyclosporine induction and maintenance microemulsion cyclosporine (I); intravenous cyclosporine induction and maintenance traditional cyclosporine (II); muromonab-CD3 induction and maintenance microemulsion cyclosporine (III); or muromonab-CD3 induction and maintenance traditional cyclosporine (IV).

When considering a factorial design, the possibility of an interaction between treatment regimens must be considered. For example, the relative effect of microemulsion cyclosporine vs traditional cyclosporine may differ among patients receiving intravenous cyclosporine (groups I and II) compared to those receiving muromonab-CD3 induction (groups III and IV), mandating that each group be examined separately. Although identification of interactions may be informative when they occur, the necessity of performing these subgroup analyses limits the functional sample size and, therefore, the power of the analysis.

Formulation of the Research Question

THE INTERVENTION. Every clinical trial requires operational definitions of the experimental treatment, comparative treatment, and clinical outcomes. The active assignment of study participants to either the experimental or comparison treatment invokes ethical and feasibility concerns. Ethics dictate that the experimental and comparison treatments be consistent with the health care needs of the participants. Therefore, there should be sufficient evidence from prior animal studies and observational research supporting the experimental treatment's therapeutic potential; specifically, that the benefits plausibly outweigh the risks. However, there must also be sufficient doubt about the treatment's efficacy to justify withholding it from a portion of study participants. The choice of the comparison treatment will

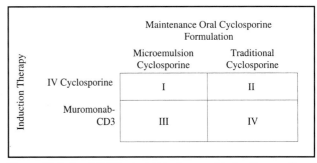

Figure 13-3. The 2 X 2 Factorial Design used in the Cooperative Clinical Trials in Pediatric Transplantation. To compare the efficacy of induction therapy with muromonab-CD3 to intravenous cyclosporine, compare groups I and II to III and IV. To compare maintenance oral cyclosporine metabolism when administered as either the traditional or microemulsion formulation, compare groups I and III to II and IV.

be dictated by current medical practice. In drug trials for transplantation, the intervention may be a new immunosuppressive drug, or different regimens of combination therapy. Finally, feasibility dictates that the intervention must be acceptable to the physicians and patients.

Clinical trials in renal transplantation have become more complex as new agents and combination therapies have become available. For example, the trials in the early 1980s compared cyclosporine to azathioprine and steroids. More recent trials compared different doses and combinations of tacrolimus, cyclosporine, MMF, azathioprine, steroids and antithymocyte globulin. The progressive complexity of the comparative regimens illustrates the evolution of standard therapy in clinical practice. The optimal manner for using many of these medications has not yet been determined.

STUDY OUTCOMES. The primary study outcome measure should be specified when the trial is planned, before the start of data collection. The primary outcome should be clinically important and easy to diagnose or observe without measurement error. In transplantation, allograft and patient survival are the most relevant outcomes and the earliest trials focused on these endpoints. However, one of the primary factors limiting the power of a clinical trial is the number of endpoints observed during the study interval. When clinical trials of cyclosporine were initiated in the late 1970s, efficacy was easier to demonstrate because at the end of one year, 40% of renal allografts had failed and mortality rates were also high. One-year kidney survival now exceeds 85% in most centers and patient survival is often greater than 95%, greatly limiting the statistical power of trials studying these outcomes. The present-day practical dilemma this creates in designing clinical trials comes from the improved clinical outcomes in the standard therapy groups. For example, the six month cumulative allograft loss in the groups receiving standard immunosuppression in the MMF intervention trial was only 8%.

As the traditional endpoints of patient and allograft survival have dramatically improved, it has become progressively more difficult to prove the superiority of a new regimen. Consequently, more recent trials have adopted an intermediate endpoint, such as biopsy-proven acute rejection that occurs more frequently than allograft loss. The utility of rejection as an alternative endpoint was based on evidence that early acute rejection episodes in most solid organ transplantation are associated with late chronic rejection and allograft loss over the long term.

The use of intermediate endpoints in clinical trials of transplantation has been controversial. The clinical outcomes of patient death or allograft loss are discrete and clear-cut. For example, allograft loss in kidney transplantation can be defined as nephrectomy, re-transplantation, or permanent return to dialysis for six or more consecutive weeks. However, the outcome termed *biopsy-proven acute rejection* is graded and significantly more prone to measurement error. In some patients, a core biopsy cannot be obtained or does not fulfill the Banff rejection criteria, despite treatment for acute rejection based on clinical signs and symptoms alone. Raising more questions about intermediate endpoints, an MMF trial that showed a statistically significant decrease in biopsy-proven acute rejection in the first six months subsequently demonstrated a trend toward more rejection in the MMF groups between six and 12 months. This potentially indicates a lesser long-term beneficial effect of MMF than implied by the six month data.

Control of Systematic Error
SELECTION OF A STUDY POPULATION. As shown in Figure 13-2, the desired study population is a representative sample of the target population. The eligibility and exclusion criteria used to define the target population are established to ensure a sufficient frequency of outcome events, and to reduce the variability of the study population by restricting the types of patients who are enrolled. The target population may be restricted by clinical site, age, sex, or other characteristics that may modify the occurrence of clinical outcomes in the study. These strategies that increase the precision of study results can diminish generalization of a study's findings to a broader target population.

The enrolled study subjects are dictated by the investigator's recruitment strategies and the willingness of patients to participate, and therefore, may differ from the target population in a systematic way. Selection bias occurs when the observed effect of the treatment is different in those who entered into the study than in those who would have been eligible but did not participate. Those who participate in a clinical trial are likely to differ from those who refuse to participate in ways that may also affect the development of the clinical outcome under study. Therefore, the baseline characteristics of subjects who were eligible, but refused to participate should be compared to those of the patients that enrolled. This may identify differences between participants and nonparticipants in a particular clinical trial. Methods of recruitment may also introduce bias if the identification of individual subjects for inclusion in the study is related to factors that affect the clinical outcome under study. For example, studies relying on patient referrals may be affected by individual physician's perceptions and belief in the study, and by differences in patient management. Many types of selection bias cannot be controlled for in the analysis; therefore, prevention of bias by appropriate subject selection is critical.

BLINDING. The aim of any trial is to collect data that are free of systematic error. Whenever possible, clinical trials in transplantation should employ blinding (or masking) with respect to the treatment assignment until data collection is complete. Blinding protects against bias in treatment, data gathering, reporting of symptoms, and subject compliance. Ideally, the patients and any individuals gathering information throughout the study interval should be blinded to the treatment assignment. The term *single-blinded* is used to characterize a trial in which only the subjects are unaware of the treatment assignment. A *double-blind* trial is one in which neither the patient nor the physician responsible for treatment are aware of the treatment assignments.

Blinding patients to treatment assignment helps to assure comparable compliance across treatment groups and to avoid biased perceptions of symptoms used to assess the safety and tolerability of a medication. Blinding of the treating physician and research staff prevents knowledge of the treatment assignment from systematically leading to the differential administration or withholding of study medications or other aspects of medical care, such as the performance of diagnostic procedures. Knowledge of treatment assignment may also bias the collection of study data such as physical examination findings, queries about symptoms, administration of questionnaires, abstraction of medical records, and interpretation of diagnostic test results. Blinding is particularly important when the outcomes are subjective, such as the occurrence of acute rejection in a transplant allograft. Whenever possible, unblinded, single-blinded, and double-blinded studies should be designed so that the data collection and interpretation is performed by individuals who are unaware of the treatment status.

OPTIMIZING COMPLIANCE. Even blinded studies may be compromised by noncompliance with the study procedures by the investigators, research staff, and subjects. The effect of noncompliance is to make the study groups more alike, which has the result of decreasing the ability of the trial to detect differences in treatment benefits and adverse events. Monitoring compliance is important since the interpretation of the study results will be affected by knowledge of the degree of noncompliance. Compliance may be improved by the use of a preliminary run-in phase in which patients who demonstrate poor compliance are made ineligible for randomization.

ALLOCATION OF STUDY INTERVENTIONS. Random allocation to study interventions assures that individual subjects have the same chance of receiving each of the possible interventions and that the probability of one subject receiving an intervention is independent of the probability of another subject receiving the same intervention. This strategy maximizes the probability that the groups receiving the different interventions are comparable. Randomization does not lead to identical distributions of characteristics (eg, age, gender); however, as the study size increases, the study groups become more comparable.

Randomization may be simple, stratified, or blocked. Simple randomization results in random treatment allocation without taking into account any patient characteristics that may affect clinical outcomes. Simple randomization is analogous to a coin-flip and is routinely accomplished using a table of random numbers or computer generated randomization list. Alternatively, investigators may stratify trial participants into groups based on the presence or absence of potentially important prognostic variables assessed prior to randomization. Simple randomization is then conducted within each stratum. For example, trials for the prevention of acute rejection may exclude patients with a history of previous transplantation, or may stratify patients according to first or second renal transplant. Stratified randomization improves the statistical power of the study to detect a treatment effect because the variability in the outcome is decreased within each stratum, particularly in studies with fewer than 50 subjects per treatment group. Generally, it is not practical to stratify on more than two or three variables.

ISSUES IN ANALYSIS AND INTERPRETATION

The goal of the analysis of clinical trials is to compare the rates of the outcome of interest in the treatment and control groups. The analysis must include an estimation of the role of chance, bias, and confounding in any observed differences between treatment groups. The use of randomization tends to distribute evenly both known and unknown confounders between the treatment groups. However, chance may result in treatment groups that are not alike with respect to these confounders, especially when the sample size is small. Therefore, the initial step in the analysis of a clinical trial is to compare the subject characteristics across treatment groups with respect to the baseline characteristics, including potentially important risk factors for the outcome of interest. Multivariable analyses may be necessary to adjust for chance baseline differences in prognostic variables.

Modes of Analysis: *Intention-to-Treat* and *As-Treated*

Although it may seem intuitively appealing to exclude from analysis subjects who either were noncompliant, provided poor-quality data, or discontinued a study medication prematurely, such exclusions undermine the principles of randomization. This may create imbalance in prognostic factors across study groups. Patients who fail to comply or drop out are rarely representative of the entire study population. Importantly, they often have a systematically different response to therapy and their exclusion serves to bias the estimate of the treatment effect. Once subjects are excluded, there are no adequate tools of data analysis that permit control for imbalance in the unknown confounders. Given these concerns, the most valid analytical approach for the principal analysis is to use the intention-to-treat dictum: "once randomized, always analyzed."

Subgroup analyses (eg, as-treated analyses) may be useful adjuncts to the primary intention-to-treat analysis. However, only baseline characteristics should be used to define subgroups for analysis rather than information gathered after the study began. Ideally, subgroup analyses should be specified during the design of the study to avoid the problem of multiple analytical comparisons. That is, multiple analyses may generate false-positive associations, simply due to chance. While subgroup analyses may assist in the development of hypotheses for future investigations, they must be interpreted with caution.

The ultimate goal of all clinical trials in transplantation is to provide definitive answers regarding the risks and benefits of therapy. Randomized, double-blind clinical trials have been widely used to study drug efficacy in transplantation. Those trials that are sufficiently large, randomized, and carefully designed, implemented, analyzed and interpreted provide the strongest evidence on which to make judgments about the impact of therapy. Nonetheless, individual randomized clinical trials may not provide definitive information regarding the efficacy of treatment. In particular, when this plausibly occurred because individual trials were small and had low statistical power, meta-analysis of multiple trials may provide important supplemental information about drug efficacy.

META-ANALYSIS IN TRANSPLANTATION
Definition and Overview of Meta-Analysis
Meta-analysis is a structured, quantitative review of previously completed studies that allows the examination of a larger sample size of patients, thereby increasing statistical power to estimate a treatment effect. Meta-analysis can be viewed as an observational study using completed trials as the individual subjects. It is more objective than the traditional, qualitative literature review as it mathematically combines individual study results taking into account study sample size, as well as more subjective issues of quality, bias, and strength of study design. This methodology is especially useful when studies disagree with regard to magnitude or direction of effect,

when sample sizes are individually too small to detect a modest but clinically important effect, or when performing a large trial is too costly.

Meta-analyses most commonly use data abstracted from the published reports of individual studies but may also be performed using patient-level data from each original trial. As a research tool, meta-analysis of patient-level data offers several advantages over meta-analysis of published literature. Meta-analysis of patient-level survival data can take into consideration censored or incomplete follow-up even if the published reports do not, thereby permitting estimates of true survival rates. Additionally, the use of patient-level data can provide information on additional variables that are important predictors of outcome. Each trial can be assessed for balance of these factors across treatment arms, and analyses can be adjusted for confounding factors not typically possible with meta-analyses using published data. Finally, use of patient-level data may permit subgroup analyses that are often not possible using original published reports.

Despite these benefits, the validity of conclusions from meta-analyses may be limited by flaws in individual studies' designs, publication bias, and heterogeneity among studies. Variation in individual study quality can affect the summary measure of a meta-analysis, most often biasing results against finding a difference in treatment. Publication bias may also affect the results of a meta-analysis, typically creating a bias toward demonstrating a treatment effect. The extent to which studies disagree in terms of magnitude or direction of effects is termed *heterogeneity*. When the extent of heterogeneity is larger than can be attributed to random chance, the theoretical basis for combining study results in a meta-analysis may be undermined.

Methods of Meta-Analysis
While an exhaustive discussion of the methods of meta-analysis is beyond the scope of this chapter, and can be obtained from a number of published references, several points deserve emphasis. A goal of meta-analysis is to summarize a treatment effect in an objective and critical manner. However, bias may be introduced during the process of selecting studies for inclusion, data abstraction, or data analysis. To limit bias introduced by selective inclusion of studies, criteria for eligibility should be defined prior to performing a literature search. A thorough search for both published and unpublished studies should be performed, although the inclusion of unpublished studies into a meta-analysis has been debated. Data abstraction from each included study should focus on information regarding patient outcome and study quality. Scales designed to assess study quality often include information on methods of randomization, withdrawals from the analysis, blinding, and assurance

of baseline comparability of prognostic factors across study groups. Studies of insufficient quality may be excluded from some analyses. To minimize subjective interpretation of data from individual studies, data abstraction should be replicated by at least one additional reader.

Once data are reliably abstracted from individual studies, the treatment effects are combined as a weighted average to produce a single summary measure. These summary measures typically include the odds ratio, which estimates the relative risk of a clinical outcome such as mortality at specified time points. One of the most common techniques of combining individual study results is the Mantel-Haenszel test, in which studies contribute to the summary measure inversely proportional to the variance associated with their individual results. Because larger studies generally have a smaller variance, they are weighted more heavily. Depending on the assumptions made about the sources of variation between summary measures for individual studies, either fixed-effects or random-effects statistical models can be used. While fixed-effects models assume that study designs are essentially comparable and that their results differ due to sampling alone, the random-effects models assume some of the variation in the results across studies is due to differences in study protocols or study populations. Random-effects models are typically preferred and provide larger CIs in the presence of inter-study variability.

The variability or heterogeneity among the individual studies' results may occur due to chance or may be caused by systematic differences in study design (eg, differences in eligibility criteria for participants, definitions of disease, or variations in treatment). Heterogeneity of study results should be examined prior to pooling data and calculating the summary measure (eg, using a chi-square or F test). To explore for stability of results, sensitivity analyses are often performed by selecting subsets of trials based on study design, study quality, or study protocol, and repeating the principal analyses. Sensitivity analyses can be used to explore clinical controversies about how certain factors (eg, particular characteristics of a population, different levels of exposure, or exposure measurement methods) impact the response to treatment. The stability of these associations across sensitivity analyses can strengthen conclusions of a meta-analysis or provide insight into important variations in treatment effect.

An Example:
Meta-Analysis in Renal Transplantation

Meta-analyses have rarely combined clinical trials in renal transplantation, but are potentially useful to address questions that may require a large number of subjects or extended follow-up. Examples of published meta-analyses include studies investigating the withdrawal of cyclosporine or corticosteroids from maintenance immunosuppression and studies of induction therapy with antilymphocyte antibodies. Prior to each of these meta-analyses, clinical trials studying the effect of these regimens on patient and allograft survival had been inconclusive. These meta-analyses will be reviewed in more detail to exemplify some of the salient features of a meta-analysis.

Following renal transplantation, the withdrawal of steroids as maintenance immunosuppression may result in improvements in hypertension, hyperlipidemia, and glucose intolerance. The withdrawal of cyclosporine has added potential benefit because of its possible role in chronic renal allograft nephropathy. The meta-analyses examining the withdrawal of cyclosporine and prednisone used published studies as the unit of observation.

Kasiske et al (1993) combined ten randomized, controlled trials and seven nonrandomized trials with a total of 1,534 patients to examine rate of rejection and allograft failure following withdrawal of cyclosporine. Although the group of patients from whom cyclosporine was withdrawn experienced an increased rate of rejection as compared to patients treated without interruption in cyclosporine administration, no statistically significant differences in allograft survival were detected (weighted difference in allografts lost per patient-year was -0.009 [95% CI, -0.022 to 0.004; $P=0.19$]). This meta-analysis was based on studies resulting from thorough attempts to identify studies satisfying predetermined inclusion criteria. Although the authors did not search for unpublished data, their search for published studies used the National Library of Medicine's MEDLINE database and the bibliographies of trials found for inclusion. This meta-analysis also highlights the use of sensitivity analyses, both to explore the impact of variations in individual study protocols, and to examine distinct clinical subgroups on the detection of an effect of cyclosporine withdrawal. By selecting subsets of studies according to the use of random allocation of patients to experimental groups, the type of patients excluded (eg, living-related transplant recipients, patients with history of prior transplant), and the specific protocol for cyclosporine withdrawal, these investigators were able to demonstrate greater credibility of their findings. None of these analyses detected a significant impact of withdrawal of cyclosporine, thereby strengthening the conclusions from their principal analysis.

Hricik et al (1993) combined seven randomized, controlled trials with a total of 1,273 patients to examine the effect of steroid withdrawal on patient and allograft survival among renal transplant recipients. This meta-analysis combined three studies testing steroid withdrawal and four studies of steroid avoidance. The pooled odds ratio suggested no significant effect of steroid-free immunosuppression on either patient or allograft survival over a variable period of follow-up. This meta-analysis highlights the importance of testing for heterogeneity in the interpretation of the summary measure. While heterogeneity was not demonstrated among studies assessing patient survival, evidence of heterogeneity did exist with respect to allograft survival, particularly in the group of studies testing steroid avoidance. This heterogeneity may be related to the variable periods of follow-up (ie, six months to five years) across studies, and limits the inferences possible from this analysis regarding the absence of an effect of steroid avoidance on allograft survival.

Szczech et al performed two meta-analyses addressing the effect of antilymphocyte antibody therapy as induction immunosuppression on cadaveric renal allograft survival. The first used data from published reports, and the second used patient-level data. These meta-analyses highlight the potential value of the additional information gained through the use of patient-level data. The meta-analysis of published data combined seven randomized, controlled trials of adult cadaveric renal transplantation assessing the effect of antilymphocyte antibodies in the immediate posttransplant period as compared to control conventional therapy of cyclosporine, azathioprine, and prednisone on two year renal allograft survival. The meta-analysis summary odds ratio was 0.66 (CI: 0.45, 0.96; $P=0.03$) indicating a beneficial effect of induction therapy on allograft survival, a finding suggested but unproven by any individual randomized, controlled trial. Because data for this meta-analysis were obtained from the published reports, a differential benefit across clinical subgroups could not be explored.

Using patient-level data from these published trials, Szczech et al performed a second meta-analysis to examine the impact of induction therapy on allograft survival among clinical subgroups at high risk for allograft failure, and to extend the analysis based on data from published reports from two to five years of follow-up. Demographic, clinical, and survival data were obtained for each patient from five of the seven trials used in the prior meta-analysis. Multivariable Cox proportional hazards regression was used to estimate the pooled adjusted rate ratio for allograft failure comparing antibody induction therapy to conventional therapy. The rate ratio was 0.62 (CI: 0.43, 0.90, $P=0.012$) over two years and 0.82 (CI: 0.62, 1.09, $P=0.17$) over five years, confirming the beneficial effect of induction therapy on allograft survival. Two new findings emerged from this individual-level analysis. First, among patients at high risk for allograft loss, sensitized patients (PRA >20%) derived particular benefit from induction therapy at two years (rate ratio =0.12, CI 0.03, 0.44, $P=0.001$). Second, the effect of induction therapy was most pronounced during the first two years following transplantation, and was attenuated thereafter.

Meta-analysis is a rigorous method to combine the results of previously conducted studies to increase statistical power in the estimation of a treatment effect using either data from published reports or supplemental patient-level data. It offers many advantages over the more qualitative, traditional literature review by more objectively accounting for individual study size, as well as the quality and strength of study designs. The conclusions derived from meta-analyses may be limited by publication bias, flaws in individual study designs, and heterogeneity among studies. A thorough search for published and unpublished studies, sensitivity analyses, and analyses of heterogeneity all assist in the assessment and minimization of these limitations. As rates of allograft failure and acute rejection fall, individual randomized, controlled trials may have increasing difficulty in detecting differences in treatment effect. The ability of meta-analysis to both estimate a treatment effect when individual study sample sizes are too small to do so, and to reconcile differences across studies make it a very useful tool to derive maximal benefit from rigorously performed clinical trials.

RECOMMENDED READING

Anonymous. A randomized clinical trial of cyclosporine in cadaveric renal transplantation. Analysis at three years. The Canadian Multicentre Transplant Study Group. N Engl J Med. 1986;314(19):1219-1225.

Dickersin K, Berlin JA. Meta-analysis: state-of-the-science. Epidemiol Rev. 1992;14:154-176.

Greenland S. Randomization, statistics and causal inference. Epidemiology. 1990;1(6):421-429.

Guyatt GH, Sackett DL, Cook DJ. Users' guides to the medical literature. II. How to use an article about therapy or prevention. A. Are the results of the study valid? JAMA. 1993;270(21):2598-2601.

Guyatt GH, Sackett DL, Cook DJ. Users' guides to the medical literature. II. How to use an article about therapy or prevention. B. What were the results and will they help me in caring for my patients? JAMA. 1994;271(1):59-63.

Halloran P, Mathew T, Tomlanovich S, Groth C, Hooftman L, Barker C. Mycophenolate mofetil in renal allograft recipients: a pooled efficacy analysis of three randomized, double-blind, clinical studies in prevention of rejection. The International Mycophenolate Mofetil Renal Transplant Study Groups. Transplantation. 1997;63(1):39-47.

Hennekens CH, Buring JE. In: Epidemiology in Medicine. Boston, MA: Little, Brown; 1987.

Hricik DE, O'Toole MA, Schulak JA, Herson J. Steroid-free immunosuppression in cyclosporine-treated renal transplant recipients: a meta-analysis. J Am Soc Nephrol. 1993;4(6):1300-1305.

Jones B, Jarvis P, Lewis JA, Ebbutt AF. Trials to assess equivalence: the importance of rigorous methods. BMJ. 1996;313(7048):36-39.

Kasiske BL, Heim-Duthoy K, Ma JZ. Elective cyclosporine withdrawal after renal transplantation: a meta-analysis. JAMA. 1993;269(3):395-400.

Mantel N, Hansel W. Statistical aspects of the analysis of data from retrospective studies of diseases. J Natl Cancer Inst. 1959;22:719-748.

Meinert CL. Clinical Trials: Design, Conduct and Analysis. New York, NY: Oxford University Press; 1986.

Petitti D. Meta-analysis, Decision Analysis, and Cost-effectiveness: Methods for Quantitative Synthesis in Medicine. New York, NY: Oxford University Press; 1994.

Sabatini S, Ferguson RM, Helderman JH, Hull AR, Kirkpatrick BS, Barr WH. Drug substitution in transplantation: a National Kidney Foundation white paper. Am J Kidney Dis. 1999;33(2):389-397.

Sackett DL. Bias in analytic research. J Chronic Dis. 1979;32(1-2):51-63.

Stewart LA, Parmar MK. Meta-analysis of the literature or of individual patient data: is there a difference? Lancet. 1993;341(8842):418-422.

Strom BL. Generic drug substitution revisited. N Engl J Med. 1987;316(23):1456-1462.

Szczech LA, Berlin JA, Aradhye S, Grossman RA, Feldman HI. Effect of anti-lymphocyte induction therapy on renal allograft survival: a meta-analysis. J Am Soc Nephrol. 1997;8(11):1771-1777.

Szczech LA, Berlin JA, Feldman HI. The effect of anti-lymphocyte induction therapy on renal allograft survival: a meta-analysis of individual patient-level data. Ann Intern Med. 1998;128(10):817-826.

14a ACTION, EFFICACY AND TOXICITIES: CYCLOSPORINE

J. Harold Helderman, MD

Cyclosporine (CsA) is a natural, highly aliphatic, cyclic undecapeptide with each of the amino groups bound to a methyl group and to an ethylene bond. Its unique structure explains the pharmacologic peculiarities of the drug including absorptive properties, delivery systems, and dosing. Its wide-spread clinical use in the beginning of the 1980s revolutionized transplant practice by significantly improving early graft survival. For kidney transplantation, 1-year graft survival doubled from around 50% to almost 90% in most transplant centers in the world. Longer-term graft survival, although recently improving, has not been impacted to the same degree by this medication. Not only were early kidney transplant graft outcomes markedly improved, CsA permitted the routine application of transplantation for organ failure to cardiac, hepatic, and pulmonary disease. For nearly two decades it has been the mainstay of immunosuppression, although other agents with similar immunosuppressive mechanisms of action, such as tacrolimus, may be substituted either as primary agent or for intractable problems. Research and discovery in recent years of potent immunosuppressive agents that inhibit other immune pathways may lead to the development of immunosuppressive strategies that avoid agents that function similarly to CsA, however, such approaches remain experimental at this time.

MECHANISM OF ACTION

CsA enters cells in general, and lymphocytes in particular, through diffusion and, at high blood concentrations, through active transport through the LDL-cholesterol receptor. In the cell, CsA is bound to unique carrier proteins called *cyclophilins,* a 17 KD representative of a group of enzymes now called *immunophilins,* which are also important for protein folding (ie, cis-trans peptidyl-prolyl isomerases). The CsA-cyclophilin complex binds to calcium-activated calcineurin, a serine-threonine phosphatase important in the lymphocyte activation cascade (Figure 14a-1). When activated by calcium released in response to alloantigen recognition events, calcineurin catalyzes the dephosphorylation of cytosolic substances, one of which – the nuclear factor of the acti-

vated T cell transcription factor (NFAT) – can enter the nucleus when dephosphorylated and engage several of the NFAT-specific DNA binding sites in the promotor regions of several important T cell growth factors and cytokines such as interleukin-2 (IL-2), interferon-γ (IFN-γ), TNF-α, and costimulatory molecules such as CD40 ligand. The binding of the CsA-cyclophilin complex to calcineurin inhibits its phosphatase activity, prevents the dephosphorylation of NFAT and therefore, the capacity of the NFAT to engage the appropriate promotor sequences in the gene. This, in turn, inhibits the expression of lymphocyte activation-generated cytokines important for the completion of the activation program including downstream signals for DNA synthesis, cell division, protooncogene synthesis, and elaboration of additional growth factors. Thus, lymphocytes responding to alloantigen are frozen at an early stage of the cell cycle permitting antigen-activated cells to potentially return to their quiescent state. In this way, there is inhibition of early antigen recognition events, reduced clonal expansion, and inhibition of the syntheses of a multiplicity of cytokines important for rejection. However, other growth factors and cytokines elaborated by cells other than T cells, that may also engage receptors on the lymphocyte providing signals for cell cycle progression, are not inhibited by CsA. In the setting of IL-7 or IL-15 excess, for example, the lymphocyte activation cascade can be completed even in the presence of CsA, perhaps explaining breakthrough rejection episodes in patients so-treated. The activation of other proinflammatory genes, the most important of which is transform-

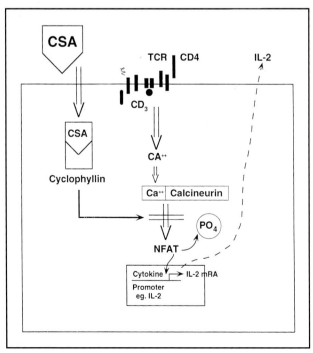

Figure 14a-1. Pathways of immunosuppression flowing from the use of cyclosporine.

Professor of Medicine and Microbiology and Immunology; Medical Director Vanderbilt Transplant Center, Vanderbilt University Medical Center, Division of Nephrology, Nashville, TN

ing growth factor β (TGF-β), is parallel to the inhibition of certain cytokine and growth factor syntheses. TGFβ itself is a potent immunosuppressant and may contribute to the immunosuppressive effects of CsA, however, it has several other actions such as enhancement of matrix formation, increased interstitial fibrosis, and vasoconstriction leading to hypertension, that may explain several of the important toxicities and side effects of this drug (Figure 14a-2).

PHARMACOKINETICS

The chemical structure of CsA predicts its aqueous insolubility that has made its use clinically complicated. Preparations of the drug are delivered in some form of oil base with absorption dependent on adequate gastric emptying, the provision of bile salts, and the formation

of micelles in the gut. The initial formulation of the reagent either as liquid or gel caps (Sandimmune®) has highly erratic absorption characteristics, is importantly affected by the timing and nature of food, requires bile flow, and is poorly absorbed in certain categories of patients, such as children, African-Americans, and diabetics, leading to high intrapatient and interpatient variability. A microemulsion formulation (Neoral®) avoids, generally, interactions with food, does not require bile flow for absorption, has markedly improved absorption characteristics in the poorest absorbers of Sandimmune®, and has, importantly, reduced intrapatient and interpatient drug exposure variability. Recently, generic alternatives to the innovator molecule have begun to penetrate the marketplace. Several generic alternatives with properties similar to Neoral® have been FDA approved as nearly bioequivalent in stable renal transplant recipients. These two generic alternatives have superseded the original generic liquid, SangCya®, which has been withdrawn by the FDA as not bioequivalent in all circumstances. One can predict an array of new generic alternatives finding their way into the clinic with this and other immunosuppressive drugs.

Immunosuppressive efficacy and many of the toxicities and side effects seem best described by total drug exposure as measured by the AUC paradigm (Figure 14a-3). In clinical practice, most transplant programs prescribe CsA in a twice-daily dose, and most of the pharmacokinetic analyses have used a 12-hour AUC measurement to examine efficacy and toxicity. Important variables of this paradigm include the C_{max}, the time to peak (T_{max}), and the C_{min} or 12-hour trough value. In the clinic, most have used the 12-hour trough value to monitor the dosing of the CsA. For the Sandimmune® formu-

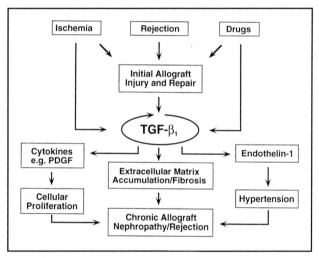

Figure 14a-2. The important role of transforming growth factor on renal injury as adapted from Suthanthiran.

Figure 14a-3. The pharmacokinetic profile of cyclosporin A on a 12-hour dosing schedule. Grevel J, Kahan BD. Ther Drug Monit. 1991;13(2):89-95

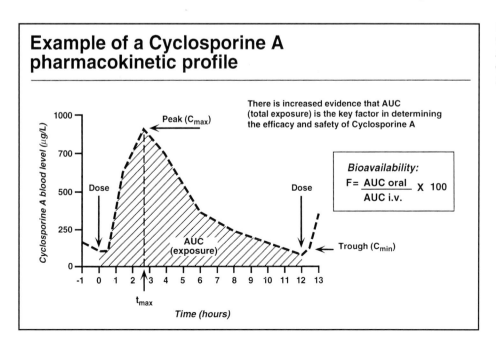

lation, the relationship between the 12-hour trough and the drug exposure by AUC is poor (ie, correlation coefficient or R value of 0.4). For both Neoral® and generic cyclosporine modified, this correlation is better (R=0.8) permitting the trough to be used for dosing the average patient with some degree of confidence. Construction of complete AUC analyses is time-consuming for patients, and expensive, so recent studies have been searching for surrogate measures that predict the AUC with confidence as a means to substitute for the 12-hour trough value as the driver in dosing decisions.

Target 12-hour trough ranges vary with respect to time after engraftment. Most transplant programs have adopted measurements of parent CsA using a monoclonal antibody, which has limited crossreactions with metabolites in a measuring system such as polarizing fluorescence of whole blood specimens. More precise and more difficult to perform, high pressure liquid chromatography methods are relegated to research issues and to special circumstances. With the monoclonal techniques, most clinicians aim for C_{min} ranges in the perioperative period of between 250 ng/mL and 300 ng/mL for kidney transplant recipients, and higher values for life-sustaining organs. Target ranges diminish with time after engraftment. For kidney transplant recipients, values between 125 ng/mL and 150 ng/mL are common one year or more after surgery.

CsA can either be used as part of induction immunosuppression or delayed and used primarily as maintenance immunosuppression. When used for induction, initial doses of cyclosporine modified range between 8 mg/kg per day and 12 mg/kg per day, and are coupled with other agents such as prednisone, mycophenolate mofeteil, or azathioprine. Because of the nephrotoxic propensity of the drug, detailed later in this section, some prefer to avoid the initial use of CsA until glomerular filtration rate (GFR) is well-established and urine flow is evident. For these clinicians, some form of T cell-specific antibody is used initially with the delayed introduction of CsA. Hybrid protocols also exist, in which the decision about initiation of CsA dosing is made on the basis of urine flow in the first or second day posttransplant.

DRUG-TO-DRUG INTERACTIONS

Metabolism of CsA is accomplished primarily by the hepatic P-450 mixed function oxidase enzymes found in microsomes. More recently, similar enzymes have been found in the mucosa of the proximal small bowel and account for interesting interactions of food that alter the enzymatic activity at this site on CsA blood levels. CsA metabolites are considerably less toxic and immunosuppressive than the parent compound. Both parent drug and metabolites are excreted by the liver hepatocyte into the bowel as one route of elimination with renal excre-

tion being a second important step. Hepatic dysfunction may alter drug levels in two ways. Severe hepatocyte dysfunction may not permit P450-induced metabolite formation leading to inordinately high parent compound concentrations in blood for any given dose of CsA, while biliary excretory dysfunction may lead to increased metabolite concentrations in blood that, if measured by crossreacting antibody techniques, may give a spurious picture of exposure to the immunosuppressant parent compound. Importantly, other concomitantly administered drugs that alter the P450 enzymatic activity may lead to derangements in CsA blood levels. Those drugs that enhance enzymatic activity culminate in decreased blood levels, increased dosing requirements, or considerations for decreasing dosing intervals (Table 14a-1). Those drugs that diminish enzymatic activity lead to

Table 14a-1. Cyclosporine Drug Interactions

Ca²⁺ Channel Blockers	
Increases Level	No Effect on Level
Diltiazem Verapamil Nicardipine	Nifedipine Isradipine Amylodipine
Antibiotics	
Increases Level	Decreases Level
Erythromycin Ticarcillin Doxycycline Fluconazole Ketoconazole Tetracycline	Nafcillin Intravenous trimethoprim- sulfamethoxazole (Bactrim) Isoniazid Rifampin
Anticonvulsants	
	Decreases Level
	Phenytoin Phenobarbital Carbamazepine Primidone
Other Drugs	
Increases Level	Decreases Level
Sex hormones Colchicine Metoclopramide Alcohol FK506 Tamoxifen Cimetidine	Omeprazole Sulfinpyrazone

Adapted From McKay, Milford and Sayegh. Clinical Aspects of Renal Transplantation. The Kidney, Vol II, 5th Ed.

increased blood levels, which can culminate in nephrotoxicity on the one hand, or the capacity to lower doses of drug on the other. The list of drugs that interfere with metabolism of CsA and can destabilize blood levels in the chronic maintenance phase of immunosuppression continues to grow. It is important, in the use of this agent, to understand drug-to-drug interactions before any concomitant medication is taken or prescribed.

TOXICITY AND SIDE EFFECTS

A number of important side effects and toxicities have been ascribed to CsA in particular, and to calcineurin inhibitor immunosuppressants in general (Table 14a-1). Several of these side effects are unique to CsA, such as hypertrichosis and gingival hyperplasia, which are markedly enhanced when any of the calcium entry blocker antihypertensive drugs are used in patients receiving CsA. CsA also alters tubular transport properties leading to sodium and water retention, decreased potassium excretion culminating in mild to moderate-mild hyperkalemia, and increased uric acid levels. In the absence of substantial blood concentration elevations or drug exposure as determined by AUC measurements, these electrolyte abnormalities are not usually clinically significant. More important are the neurologic, endocrinologic, hepatic, and renal toxicities. Although less of a problem than with the use of the calcineurin inhibitor tacrolimus, neurologic toxicities are well-described and include fine motor tremor, headache, frank seizures, and even a demyelinating neuropathic syndrome, which is unusual or rare. Hepatic toxicities also track with elevated blood levels and most often are heralded by mild elevation of the liver transaminase enzymes.

The hypertension associated with CsA use is clinically more relevant. As many as 85% of renal transplant recipients will be treated for hypertension in the CsA treatment era. Patients whose dialysis experience did not include hypertension can become hypertensive; patients who were hypertensive during end-stage renal disease can have worse hypertension. The hypertension associated with CsA is multifactorial, and the most important mechanisms are probably related to: (1) increased intracellular calcium concentrations sensitizing resistance vessels; (2) sodium and water retention; and (3) increased sensitivity to adrenergic stimulation. Acute increases in blood pressure can be related to inhibition of the generation of nitric oxide metabolites, elaboration of the vasoconstrictive hormone endothelin, and to acute release of renin leading to angiotensin II generation. Chronically, the renin-angiotensin-aldosterone cascade is actually suppressed; endothelin levels are not explanatory of hypertension; no further inhibition of nitric oxide generation can be measured, and measurable prostaglandin synthesis inhibition seems not to be causally related to persistent hypertension.

The most important toxicity of the calcineurin inhibitor agents and, therefore, for CsA, is nephrotoxicity. Although pathogenetically linked, several distinct clinical syndromes are unique enough to be identified, recognized and explicated. The most common clinical syndrome of CsA nephrotoxicity is acute dose-related, dose-responsive diminution in renal clearance mediated, in general, by intrarenal vasoconstriction, which includes the microvasculature of the kidney and both afferent and efferent arterioles (Figure 14a-4). Histopathologically, findings are generally nonspecific,

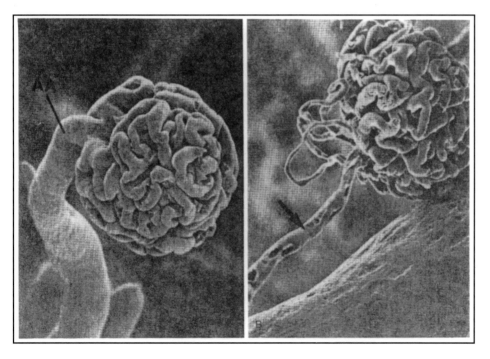

Figure 14a-4. Cast impression of glomerular filtering unit before (left) and after (right) administration of intravenous cyclosporine demonstrating the intense vasoconstrictive properties of the agent. Bennett WM, Elzinga LW, Porter GA. Tubulointerstitial Disease and Toxic Nephropathy. In: Brenner B, Rector F, eds. The Kidney. 4th Ed. Philadelphia, Pa: W.B. Saunders Co.; 1991:1430-1496.

but can include obliterative arteriolopathy with patchy cell necrosis and a peculiar form of isometric vacuolization of the proximal tubule. Occasionally, microcalcification of tubular cells may also be seen. Vasoconstriction may be significant enough to lead to persistent renal failure and can even be the cause of graft loss. In the setting of initial oliguria, CsA may be the cause of delayed graft function after surgical engraftment or even of primary graft nonfunction. A second, relatively distinct clinical syndrome is the result of endothelial injury related to CsA use with microangiopathic hemolytic anemia characterized by thrombocytopenia, an elevated lactic dehydrogenase (LDH), and a progressive fall in hemoglobin associated with peripheral smear evidence for red cell destruction. In this setting, fibrin deposition within arterioles and capillaries, including those of the glomerulus itself, can lead to graft loss. This complication, when it afflicts the glomerulus, may respond in the early phase to dose reduction or discontinuance, and is not invariably recurrent when either CsA is used later in the course, or when the patient is switched to a different calcineurin inhibitor agent. Acute allograft renal artery thrombosis has been thought to be linked to CsA use. This dire complication is reported to occur in 0.5% to 2% of transplant procedures and, anecdotally, has appeared to be increased in the CsA era. Although causality has not been proven, the propensity for these agents to cause endothelial injury permits entertainment of the possibility that transplant artery thrombosis can be one of the rarer forms of CsA nephrotoxicity. The syndrome of chronic renal dysfunction is another distinct clinical nosologic entity characterized morphologically by sclerosis of arterioles and small arteries, and in some by tubulointerstitial fibrosis that occurs in a relatively unique pattern with areas of tubular dropout and fibrosis juxtaposed to relatively normal areas (striped fibrosis). The pathogenesis of this lesion may reflect the impact of prolonged intrarenal ischemia consequent to vasoconstriction of the most vulnerable areas of the graft. Equally interesting is the role of certain profibrogenic cytokines such as transforming growth factor (TGF), the synthesis of which is promoted and enhanced by CsA usage. Recently, TGF has been linked to vasoconstriction, enhancement of angiotensin II, hypertension, and matrix formation with fibrosis explaining many of the side effects of this agent (Figure 14a-2).

RECOMMENDED READING

Kahan BD. Cyclosporine. N Engl J Med. 1989;321(25): 1725-1738.

Kon V, Sugiura M, Inagami T, Harvie BR, Ichikawa I, Hoover RL. Role of endothelin in cyclosporine-induced glomerular dysfunction. Kidney Int. 1990;37(6):1487-1491.

Li B, Sehajpal PK, Khanna A, et al. Differential regulation of transforming growth factor beta and interleukin 2 genes in human T cells: demonstration by usage of novel competitor DNA constructs in the quantitative polymerase chain reaction. J Exp Med. 1991;174(5):1259-1262.

Rao A. NFATp, a cyclosporin-sensitive transcription factor implicated in cytokine gene induction. [Review]. J Leukoc Biol. 1995;57(4):536-542.

Ho S, Clipstone N, Timmermann L, et al. The mechanism of action of cyclosporin A and FK506. [Review] Clin Immunol Immunopathol. 1996;80(3 Pt 2):S40-45.

Bennett WM, Elzinga LW, Porter GA. Tubulointerstitial Disease and Toxic Nephropathy. In: Brenner B, Rector F, eds. The Kidney. 4th Ed. Philadelphia, Pa: W.B. Saunders Co.; 1991: 1430-1496.

Curtis JJ. Hypertension following kidney transplantation. [Review] Am J Kidney Dis. 1994;23(3):471-475.

Halloran PF, Madrenas J. The mechanism of action of cyclosporine: a perspective for the 90's. [Review] Clin Biochem. 1991;24(1):3-7.

Mihatsch MJ, Ryffel B, Gudat F. The differential diagnosis between rejection and cyclosporine toxicity. [Review] Kidney Int Suppl. 1995;52:S63-S69.

14b ACTION, EFFICACY AND TOXICITIES: TACROLIMUS

Leslie W. Miller, MD

Tacrolimus (FK506) is a metabolite of the fungus Streptomycins Tsukubaensis. It is a macrolide lactone that is structurally related to rapamycin. Tacrolimus is lipophilic and has variable absorption after oral administration and poor oral bioavailability. This absorption is not dependent on bile secretion. It is highly bound to plasma proteins and albumin, and mainly metabolized in the liver by the cytochrome P450, CyP384 isoenzyme into at least 15 metabolites. The vast majority of the excretion pathway is biliary tract. Tacrolimus seems to have a preferential pattern of tissue absorption with a relative hierarchy after intravenous administration of lungs →spleen →heart →kidney →pancreas →liver, that is equal to plasma. Lung concentrations may be as high as eight times those of plasma.

The mechanism of action of tacrolimus is virtually identical to that of cyclosporine. Once absorbed across the cell membrane, tacrolimus complexes with a different immunophilin referred to as *FK binding protein (FKBP) 12*. This FKBP-tacrolimus complex then directly inhibits calcineurin and prevents dephosphorylation of the transcription factor NFAT, thus directly inhibiting transcription of critical growth-promoting cytokines. Tacrolimus has been purported to be ten to 100 times more potent than cyclosporine based on in vitro drug concentrations. However, when doses are used that provide equivalent amounts of calcineurin inhibition, tacrolimus seems to have nearly identical potency to cyclosporine. There is a suggestion of increased binding affinity to calcineurin of the tacrolimus-FKBP complex over cyclosporine-cyclophilin.

There have been a large number of studies performed at single centers either describing the results with tacrolimus or comparing its effects to cyclosporine-based immunosuppression, usually to Sandimmune®, rather than the current Neoral® formulation of cyclosporine. This review will focus primarily on the results of large randomized prospective trials in each of the solid organs transplanted and discuss the benefits and complications reported with tacrolimus-based immunosuppression.

Professor of Medicine; Director, Cardiovascular Division, Department of Medicine, University of Minnesota, Minneapolis, MN

LIVER TRANSPLANTATION

Tacrolimus first received FDA approval for use in liver transplantation. There have been two large open-label multicenter randomized trials in liver transplantation, one in the US and one in Europe, that compared the outcome of cyclosporine-based vs tacrolimus-based immunosuppression. It is important to note that in both the US and European comparative trials, the cyclosporine group received triple-drug therapy (ie, prednisone plus azathioprine). In some cases, they also received antilymphocyte antibody therapy. The patients in the tacrolimus arm, however, received only tacrolimus and prednisone, without induction therapy or use of azathioprine.

The US trial examined 478 adults and 51 children, who were randomized 1:1 to tacrolimus or cyclosporine. The actuarial patient survival rates at one year were identical (88% in each group), and graft survival rates were also nearly identical at 82% in the tacrolimus group and 79% in the cyclosporine group. By five years there was still no difference in cumulative patient or graft survival, but the patient half-life survival was significantly longer in the tacrolimus group (25.1 + 5.1 years vs 15.2 ± 2.5, $P=0.049$). Tacrolimus had a significant impact of rejection. Its use was associated with a significant reduction in the incidence of acute rejection (14% vs 32.1%, ($P<0.002$) corticosteroid resistant rejection ($P<0.01$), and refractory rejection (3% vs 15%, $P<0.001$). Both treatments were associated with a low incidence of late acute rejection. There was also a high incidence of adverse events in both adults and children in both treatment arms, but a larger percentage of tacrolimus-treated patients were withdrawn from the study, due primarily to nephrotoxicity and neurotoxicity, both at one year (14% vs 15%, $P= 0.001$) and five years (21% vs 13%). The cumulative dose of corticosteroids for both prophylaxis and rejection was significantly less with tacrolimus than with cyclosporine (90 vs 131 mg/kg per day, $P<0.001$). The 5-year follow-up demonstrated a low incidence of malignancy and serious infection in both groups. A similar number underwent re-transplantation.

The European trial was almost identical in design and number, with a total of 529 patients enrolled, 264 of whom received tacrolimus, and 265 who were treated with cyclosporine. The main difference between the US and European trials was that the US trial excluded patients with significant preoperative risk factors, while they were included in the European trial, including patients with fulminant hepatic failure whose results were similar to the less ill patients.

The European trial also demonstrated virtually identical survival between the two study groups. However, in contrast to the US trial, there was a smaller difference in the incidence of acute rejection (19.4% vs

31.3% in the tacrolimus vs cyclosporine groups respectively, $P=0.04$). Similarly, the incidence of refractory acute rejection was significantly lower in the tacrolimus-treated patients ($P=0.05$), but a smaller difference than the US trial. The incidence of chronic rejection, defined by histologic analysis of liver biopsies, was not examined in the US trial, but was significantly lower in the tacrolimus-treated patients (1.5% vs 5.3%, $P=0.032$) in the European trial. Much like the US trial, lower doses of intravenous, but not oral, corticosteroids were required during maintenance therapy with tacrolimus at one year, and both oral and intravenous doses were lower with tacrolimus at three years ($P<0.05$). The cumulative prednisone dosage was significantly lower at the three year mark in the tacrolimus-treated patients with the difference being approximately 25 mg/kg more steroid in the cyclosporine group ($P=0.003$). At three years, steroid therapy had been successfully withdrawn in 80% of the tacrolimus-treated patients vs 68% of the cyclosporine recipients ($P=0.025$). Overall, there were more re-transplantations required in the cyclosporine-treated patients than in those receiving tacrolimus in the European trial (30 vs 22).

The neurological sequelae associated with use of tacrolimus are well known, and were quite problematic particularly in the first year posttransplant. However, the 3-year follow-up in the US and European multicenter trials showed that there was an increase in the neurological side effects in the cyclosporine-treated patients over 50, compared to those over 50 that received tacrolimus. In particular, convulsions were noted in 4.1% of the cyclosporine patients vs 1.8% in the tacrolimus group. In contrast, headaches were more frequent in the tacrolimus group, 7.5% vs 3.2%.

The combined US and European multicenter trials also demonstrated the reduction in the incidence of hypertension and hyperlipidemia. This overall decrease in "cardiovascular risks" was evident at one year, with mean total cholesterol of 188 in the tacrolimus group compared to 288 in the cyclosporine-treated patients.

One of the leading indications for liver transplantation today is hepatitis C. It has a very high incidence of recurrence and is one of the leading indications for re-transplantation. The US trial did not demonstrate a difference in the outcome of patients who were transplanted for hepatitis C at three years. However, at five years, survival rates were significantly higher in patients with hepatitis C that received tacrolimus.

The largest single center experience with tacrolimus in liver transplantation involved over 1,391 patients, and the use of three different dosing regimens of tacrolimus over a four year period. This cohort was compared to a historical group of 1,212 patients treated with cyclosporine. Patient and graft survival was higher with

tacrolimus compared to cyclosporine with either Euro-Collins or University of Wisconsin preservation solution ($P<0.0005$).

The experience with tacrolimus in pediatric patients has similarly been largely in single center experiences. The one US multicenter trial involved 51 children under 12, 30 of whom received tacrolimus and 21 who received cyclosporine. This study showed similar graft and patient survival rates (80% vs 81% and 70% vs 71%) at one year in the tacrolimus-treated and cyclosporine-treated patients, respectively. Much like the adult US and European trials, the percentage of tacrolimus-treated children free of rejection at one year was more than twice that seen in the cyclosporine group (48% vs 21%) and freedom from use of muromonab-CD3 was higher with tacrolimus (79% vs 68%). The percent of acute rejection was 52% in the tacrolimus-treated patients vs 79% in the cyclosporine-treated patients at one year. Although a large difference, it did not reach statistical significance. The incidence of need for re-transplantation was also similar between the two groups. The cumulative dose of steroids was lower in the tacrolimus group at all time points in the first year, but not statistically significant. The incidence of side effects was similar in both groups, although major neurologic symptoms (coma [1], encephalopathy [2], and convulsions [4]) only occurred in patients receiving tacrolimus. Minor neurologic symptoms were similar in both groups. Serum cholesterol was higher at one year in the cyclosporine group (203 vs 107).

Tacrolimus has also been shown to be an effective agent as rescue therapy for refractory rejection. The US Multicenter Tacrolimus Rescue Trial showed that grafts that developed chronic rejection could be salvaged and had improved function when converted from cyclosporine to tacrolimus. The study involved 386 patients, 300 adults and 86 pediatric patients, and required both clinical and biopsy confirmation for the diagnosis. Patients were treated with tacrolimus plus steroids. There were 234 patients with acute rejection and 124 with chronic rejection. Overall, the patient and graft survival was 64.7% and 79.8% at 1-year. The 1-year incidence of recurrence of rejection was 53.7%. Adverse events occurred in 76.2% of patients, the most common of which were neurotoxicity, nephrotoxicity, and gastrointestinal toxicity. This was particularly true if the conversion was attempted with a bilirubin less than 6, where graft salvage was as high as 80% vs when the bilirubin was greater than 6 which was associated with an only 46% salvage rate.

RENAL TRANSPLANTATION

As with the other solid organs, there have been numerous single center studies examining the effects of tacrolimus in first and second kidney graft recipients, but there have been two prospective randomized multi-center, open-label trials comparing tacrolimus and cyclosporine in renal transplantation. The trials were conducted almost simultaneously and both trials were designed to show equivalency, not superiority. The protocols for these trials included predetermined targets or recommendations for both dose and blood levels of tacrolimus to be followed throughout the study.

The European multicenter trial involved 448 patients randomized in a 2:1 distribution to tacrolimus (N=303) or cyclosporine (N=145). The patient (82.5% vs 86.2%) and graft (93% vs 96.5%) survival was not statistically different between the tacrolimus and cyclosporine groups. However, the incidence of histologically confirmed acute rejection was significantly lower (25.9% vs 45.79%, P<0.001) in the tacrolimus group with an absolute difference of 19.8%. Complications and adverse events were common in both groups and largely reversible. The incidence of elevated creatinine, tremor, diarrhea, hyperglycemia, diabetes, and angina pectoris were higher in the tacrolimus group, whereas acne, gingival hyperplasia, hirsutism, and arrhythmia were more common with cyclosporine. The incidence of new onset diabetes requiring insulin was 8.3% vs 2.2% at one month, but fell to 5.5% and 2.2% at one year.

The US trial randomized 412 patients (205 in the tacrolimus arm and 207 in the cyclosporine arm). The endpoint of this study was patient and graft survival. Unlike all other studies in solid organ transplant, all patients in the US renal study received induction therapy with either ATG or muromonab-CD3 in addition to steroids, azathioprine and either cyclosporine or tacrolimus. One other important advantage of the US renal trial was that it included 27% African-Americans, and 11% Hispanics. All episodes of suspected rejection were evaluated by biopsy, and an independent review panel of pathologists read all biopsies. Ninety-five percent of all suspected rejection episodes defined by specific criteria had histological verification. As with all other major trials of tacrolimus in solid organ transplant recipients, there was no difference in patient (95.6% vs 96.6% in the tacrolimus vs cyclosporine patient survival, respectively) or graft survival (91.2% vs 87.9%, P=0.098) at one or three years. Infection was the number one cause of death in both the tacrolimus and cyclosporine groups.

Tacrolimus was however, associated with a significant reduction in the incidence of acute cellular rejection (30.7% vs 46.6%, P=0.001), and in the requirement for antibody therapy for refractory or severe rejection; (10.7% vs 25.1%, P<0.001). The incidence of Grade 3 or 4 severity by Banff criteria was 0 in the tacrolimus group vs 29.2% in the cyclosporine group, which parallels the incidence of antibody use. Importantly, the difference in rejection was evidenced within three to six months of

transplant. The significant reduction in the incidence of rejection associated with tacrolimus was evident also in African-Americans, (23.2% in the tacrolimus vs 47.9% in the cyclosporine arm; P=0.05). More patients in this study crossed over to tacrolimus from cyclosporine (15.5%) than crossed over to cyclosporine from tacrolimus (77.8%). Twenty-one of the 27 refractory rejection episodes resolved after crossover to tacrolimus, while only one of two refractory rejection episodes resolved after crossover to cyclosporine.

Other side effects that were noted to be significantly greater in the tacrolimus patients include the neurological complications of tremor and paraesthesias, alopecia, and pruritus.

Diabetes has been one of the major side effects of tacrolimus therapy. The US renal trial demonstrated a highly significant (P<0.001) increase in the percentage of patients requiring insulin therapy (19.9% vs 4%) at one year following transplantation. It is of note that 50% of the patients were able to come off insulin by two years posttransplant. Race had an adverse impact on the development of diabetes, with African-American and Hispanic patients noted to be at 3.3 times greater risk for development of diabetes than Caucasian patients in both treatment groups. The development of diabetes was correlated with the dose of tacrolimus and corticosteroids. The starting dose of tacrolimus was 0.3 mg/kg per day, but reduced to 0.18 mg/kg per day at one year. In light of the significant increase in diabetes in the tacrolimus group, a new trial was conducted comparing lower dose tacrolimus from the time of transplantation and either azathioprine or mycophenolate mofetil. The incidence of diabetes in this cohort was only 10.6% at six months with nearly equivalent levels of rejection as in the original US Multicenter Trial.

There are several important cardiovascular benefits with the use of tacrolimus therapy compared to cyclosporine, including reduction in serum cholesterol. The percentage of patients requiring lipid reduction therapy was significantly lower in the tacrolimus group (7.8% vs 14.5%, P=0.031) in the US renal trial. While hypertension has been a demonstrated advantage of tacrolimus in many major multicenter trials, the incidence of hypertension, which was defined pre-study, was nearly identical, 49.8% in the tacrolimus group and 52.2% in the cyclosporine group.

Tacrolimus has been shown to be a potent agent for rescue therapy for patients with refractory rejection on cyclosporine-based immunosuppression. A sub-study of the US Multicenter Trial of Tacrolimus examined the use of tacrolimus in refractory acute renal allograft rejection in 73 patients. Enrollment occurred a mean of 75 days after transplantation. All rejections were biopsied and refractory to corticosteroid therapy. Eighty-one percent had previously received at least one course of antilymphocyte antibody as rejection therapy. The 12-month actuarial patient and graft survival rates were 93% and 75%. Results showed improvement in biopsy grade in 78% of patients, stabilization or no change in 11%, and progressive deterioration in 11%. Risk of progressive deterioration despite conversion to tacrolimus was directly related to the level of serum creatinine at the time of conversion. There were 14 episodes of recurrent rejection following conversion to tacrolimus in ten patients at a median time of 101 days after conversion. None of the recurrent rejection episodes required anti-lymphocyte antibody therapy. Only 15% of the patients had a documented infection, and there was only one case of posttransplant lymphoproliferative disorder diagnosed. Interestingly, treatment outcome did not correlate with tacrolimus blood levels. Tacrolimus was discontinued in 18% of the patients for either progressive, unrelenting, or recurrent rejection, and in an additional 8% due to adverse events, most of which were neurological or gastrointestinal.

There is one study that suggests that tacrolimus may be more cost-effective than cyclosporine. Data from hospital, drug, and professional costs (adjusted to 1996 dollars) from centers participating in the US renal multicenter trial, demonstrated a cost savings of approximately $17,368 per patient over one year for patients on tacrolimus rather than cyclosporine. The source of the cost saving was multifactorial, including factors such as lower incidence of rejection, reduced length of hospital stay, less muromonab-CD3 requirement and lower cost acquisition for tacrolimus and an eventual decrease in professional fees.

There have been no prospective randomized, multicenter trials comparing tacrolimus to cyclosporine in pediatric patients. A recent review of the series at Pittsburgh showed one and four year actuarial patient (99% and 94%) and graft survival rates (98% and 84%) were excellent.

HEART

There have been two multicenter randomized open-label trials comparing tacrolimus-based to cyclosporine-based therapy in heart transplant recipients. The US trial enrolled a total of 85 patients, 39 in the tacrolimus arm and 46 in the cyclosporine arm. The study population included 87% males, 90% of whom were Caucasian, and 55% who had an ischemic etiology. While these demographics are not significantly different from that of the International Heart Transplant Registry, the study provides little insight into results of tacrolimus therapy in other sub-populations. The trial design included use of protocol target levels for both tacrolimus and cyclosporine at all time points during the study. Fifteen percent of the patients were defined as high-risk for

renal insufficiency and were given muromonab-CD3 for the first three days following transplant, and then oral tacrolimus or cyclosporine were initiated. The study used Sandimmune® preparation rather than the current Neoral® preparation of cyclosporine. The results showed no significant difference in survival, incidence of rejection, treatment of steroid-resistant rejection, infection, or renal function at one year of follow-up.

The study did show a significantly lower incidence of hypertension in the tacrolimus group (71% vs 48%, $P=0.05$) with predefined criteria for defining hypertension and initiating therapy. There was also a highly significant reduction in lipids in the tacrolimus group at three, six, and 12 months of follow-up, and a significantly lower requirement for lipid-lowering therapy. There was no difference in the incidence of diabetes between the two groups (19% tacrolimus vs 22% cyclosporine). Eight of the 39 tacrolimus patients dropped out of the study for adverse events, including renal insufficiency, infection, and headaches, while none of the cyclosporine patients were withdrawn from the study.

The European trial involved 82 patients at five centers and was virtually identical to the US trial with the exception of a 2:1 randomization, such that 54 patients received tacrolimus and only 28 patients received cyclosporine. The study population was 88% male and 100% Caucasian with an almost equal frequency of ischemic etiology. The results of this study were also virtually identical to the US trial with no difference demonstrated in survival, incidence of rejection, percent freedom from rejection, steroid resistant rejection, infection, or renal function. Complications included a higher incidence of requirement for ultrafiltration or dialysis and the duration of need for this support in the tacrolimus group, but this did not reach statistical significance. The steroid dose obtained at one year was virtually identical between the two groups.

The European study also confirmed the lower incidence of hypertension in the tacrolimus-treated patients (60% in tacrolimus vs 88% of cyclosporine, $P=0.025$). Although there was a trend toward lower serum lipids in tacrolimus-treated patients, the difference in the requirements for lipid reduction therapy was not significant ($P=0.103$). The incidence of diabetes was also not significantly different at one year of follow-up, although the incidence was lower than that seen in the US trial (7% tacrolimus vs 4.3% in cyclosporine.)

The only other large study comparing cyclosporine vs tacrolimus was a retrospective review performed at the University of Pittsburgh in 243 patients, 125 of whom received tacrolimus and 121 historical controls that received cyclosporine either with ($N=71$) or without ($N=50$) the use of induction therapy. None of the tacrolimus patients received induction therapy.

There was no significant difference in survival in this study. There was however, a significant reduction in the incidence of rejection, freedom from rejection, and steroid resistant rejection in the tacrolimus group compared to either of the cyclosporine arms. The one major adverse effect seen in the tacrolimus group was the incidence of renal insufficiency. The average creatine at one year in the tacrolimus group was 2.1 vs 1.4 in the cyclosporine-treated patients. Eighteen patients in the cyclosporine arm crossed over to receive tacrolimus rescue therapy.

The largest reported series of tacrolimus in pediatric heart transplant recipients was a report describing the series of 49 patients, 38 of whom received tacrolimus as primary therapy and 11 of whom were converted from cyclosporine to tacrolimus for refractory rejection. The authors describe a significant incidence of renal insufficiency, anemia, eosinophilia, and gastrointestinal problems with tacrolimus, but also noted a decrease in hypertension compared to historical controls with cyclosporine-based therapy.

PANCREAS AND KIDNEY/PANCREAS TRANSPLANTATION

There have been no prospective randomized comparisons of cyclosporine-based and tacrolimus-based immunosuppression in pancreas or kidney/pancreas transplantation. The most definitive study to date examining the role of tacrolimus in pancreas transplant recipients was the multicenter trial from the Tacrolimus Pancreas Transplant Study Group, which enrolled 250 patients, both with (77%) and without (23%) simultaneous kidney transplant, all of whom received tacrolimus from the time of transplant. At 18 months of follow-up, the incidence of graft loss and rejection were both low. Patient survival was 95% at 18 months and graft survival was 85% in the 215 patients who did not undergo simultaneous bone marrow transplant. Matched pair analysis from this study showed a higher patient (97% vs 83%) and pancreas graft survival rate (88% vs 71%) for tacrolimus over cyclosporine in patients receiving simultaneous kidney/pancreas transplant (88% vs 73%, $P=0.002$), but not isolated pancreas or pancreas after kidney procedures. Eighty-nine additional patients in this study were converted to tacrolimus from cyclosporine as rescue therapy. Patient and graft survival rates in this group at one year were 96% and 89%.

Tacrolimus has been associated with very good success as rescue therapy with overall 18 month patient and pancreas graft survival rates of 92% and 80% in patients with refractory rejection, with simultaneous kidney/pancreas recipients having the highest graft survival rate. This study also demonstrated a successful conversion from cyclosporine to tacrolimus for patients with signifi-

cant nephrotoxicity. Intravenous tacrolimus has also been used as primary therapy for rejection. The combination of tacrolimus plus mycophenolate mofetil as rescue for rejection or drug toxicity is associated with an even higher rate of patient and graft survival of 97% and 96% at one year follow-up. One important finding in this study was that the incidence of diabetes was <1%. This low incidence was also reported in another study, which suggests that any potential islet toxicity is short-lived and not clinically significant in pancreas transplantation.

LUNG TRANSPLANTATION

To date there have been no prospective, multicenter trials reported comparing tacrolimus and cyclosporine in lung transplant recipients. The largest series is from the University of Pittsburgh involving 133 recipients of single ($N=79$) or bilateral ($N=54$) lung transplantation who were randomized to cyclosporine ($N=67$) or tacrolimus ($N=66$). The one and two year survival rates were not significantly different, although there was a trend toward increased survival in the tacrolimus group. Similarly, there was a trend toward fewer rejection episodes per 100 patient days ($P=0.07$) in the tacrolimus group (0.85 vs 1.09). There was, however, a significant reduction in the incidence of obliterative bronchiolitis with tacrolimus (21.7% vs 38%, $P=0.025$), and an overall greater freedom of development of obliterative bronchiolitis over time, ($P=0.03$). In this study, significantly more cyclosporine-treated patients required crossover to tacrolimus than the reverse, due primarily to refractory rejection (six of the nine patients converted to tacrolimus). The overall incidence of infection in this study was very similar, although there was a significantly higher incidence of bacterial infection in the cyclosporine treated patients ($P=0.0375$) and a significantly higher risk of fungal infection in the tacrolimus patients ($P<0.05$).

The one clear parallel in the evolution of the use of tacrolimus with that of cyclosporine is the progressive decrease in the dose used or prescribed with increased experience with the drug. During the initial use of cyclosporine, doses as high as 20 mg/kg per day were recommended. This resulted in impressive reductions in incidence of rejection compared to azathioprine-based therapy, but unacceptable nonimmune toxicity. The current dose of cyclosporine ranges between 4 and 6 mg/kg per day. This dose has been associated with an acceptable incidence of rejection and marked decrease in the incidence of nephrotoxicity and hypertension.

Similarly, the initial doses of tacrolimus recommended were as high as 0.3 mg/kg per day. Early trials of tacrolimus in cardiac transplantation showed an increased incidence of deaths from infection, largely due to fungal organisms. The dose has now been reduced to between 0.05 and 0.08 mg/kg per day, a dose that also achieves similar acceptable incidence of rejection, and a decrease in incidence of neurotoxicity, nephrotoxicity, and infectious complications.

In summary, the results with tacrolimus in solid organ transplantation are varied (Table 14b-1). Its use has not been associated with an increase in survival in kidney, heart, lung, or pancreas and only after five years in liver transplantation. Its use has been associated with a reduction in the incidence of acute rejection in both liver and renal multicenter trials, but not in either heart study. When used in doses that achieve similar incidence of side effects, it is at least comparable to cyclosporine-based immunosuppression. It does provide a potentially significant advantage in younger and female recipients, particularly with regard to hirsutism, which may have a significant impact on compliance. The beneficial effects on lipid metabolism and hypertension may translate to a potential beneficial impact on chronic rejection. The

observation that nearly one-half of the deaths in renal transplant patients occurs with a functioning graft largely from cardiovascular etiology may increase the importance of this drug long-term.

RECOMMENDED READING

Klintmalm G. A Review of FK506: A new immunosuppressant agent for the prevention and rescue of graft rejection. Transplant Rev. 1994;8(2):53-63.

Spencer CM, Goa KL, Gillis JC. Tacrolimus. An update of its pharmacology and clinical efficacy in the management of organ transplantation. Drugs. 1997;54(6):925-975.

Tanaka H, Kuroda A, Marusawa H, et al. Physicochemical properties of FK-506, a novel immunosuppressant isolated from streptomyces tsukubaensis. Transplant Proc. 1987;19(5 Suppl 6):11-16.

Table 14b-1. Results of Clinical Trials with Tacrolimus: Statistical Significance – Tacrolimus vs Control

	Liver	Kidney	Heart	Lung	Pancreas
Multicenter Randomized Trials	Yes	Yes	Yes	No	No
Survival	NS*,+,◊	NS*,+	NS*,+	NS	NS
Acute Rejection	↓P<.002* P=.04+	↓P<.001* P=.001+	NS*,+		P=.07++
Steroid Resistant Rejection	↓P<.01*	↓P<.001*	NS*,+		
Rescue Therapy	P=.05+ Effective	Effective			
Infection	NS*	NS* fungal+ P=.01	NS*		↑fungal P<.05 ↓bacterial P=.038
Neurotoxicity	↑headaches, ↓Sz, P<.05+	↑P<.001+ tremor*	NS*		
Nephrotoxicity	↑P<.05+	NS* P=.003+	NS*		
Hypertension	↓P=.06	NS*,+	↓P=.05* P=.02+		
GI Toxicity	P<.001*	NS* P=.005+			
Lipids		↓P=.03*	↓P<.01* P=10+		
Diabetes	↑P=.07* P<.05+	↑P=.01* P=.001+	NS+		
Chronic Rejection	↓P=.03+		?		P=.025
Steroid Use	↓P=.02+ ↓P=.05*		NS*		
Withdrawal from Study	↑P=.001*		?		
Pediatric	↓rejection				

* indicates US Trial; +, European Trial; ◊, Pediatric Trial; ++, Pitts Study; NS, not significant; ↑, increased w/Tacrolimus; ↓, decreased w/Tacrolimus

Johansson A, Moller E. Evidence that the immunosuppressive effects of FK506 and cyclosporine are identical. Transplantation. 1990;50(6):1001-1007.

Halloran PF, Miller LW. In vivo immunosuppressive mechanisms. J Heart Lung Transplant.1996;15(10): 959-971.

Halloran PF, Kung L, Noujaim J. Calcineurin and the biological effect of cyclosporine and tacrolimus. Transplant Proc. 1998;30(5):2167-2170.

Beck Y, Akiyama N. Effect of FK-506 and cyclosporine on human lymphocyte responses in vitro. Transplant Proc. 1989;21(3):3464-3467.

Halloran PF. Rethinking immunosuppression in terms of the redundant and non-redundant steps in the immune response. Transplant Proc. 1996;28(6 Suppl 1):11-18.

Halloran PF. The effect of immunosuppressive drugs on T cell signalling pathways: non-redundant steps in the T cell response. Kidney Blood Press Res. 1996;19(3-4): 174-176.

Busuttil RW, Holt CD. Tacrolimus (FK506) is superior to cyclosporine in liver transplantation. Transplant Proc. 1997;29(1-2):534-538.

The U.S. Multicenter FK506 Liver Study Group. A Comparison of tacrolimus (FK506) and cyclosporine for immunosuppression in liver transplantation. N Engl J Med. 1994;331(17):1110-1115.

European FK506 Multicentre Liver Study Group. Randomised trial comparing tacrolimus (FK506) and cyclosporin in prevention of liver allograft rejection. Lancet. 1994;344(8920):423-428.

Martinez, AJ. The neuropathology of organ transplantation: comparison and contrast in 500 patients. Path Res Prac. 1998;194(7): 473-486.

Devlin J, Williams R. Transplantation for fulminant hepatic failure: comparing tacrolimus versus cyclosporine for immunosuppression and the outcome in elective transplants. European FK506 Liver Study Group. Transplantation. 1996;62(9):1251-1255.

Vanrenterghem Y. Tacrolimus (FK506) in kidney transplantation. Transplant Proc.1998;30(5):2171-2173.

Fung JJ, Eliasziw M, Todo S, et al. The Pittsburgh randomized trial of tacrolimus compared to cyclosporine for hepatic transplantation. J Am Coll Surg.1996;183(2): 117-125.

Todo S, Fung JJ, Starzl TE, et al. Single-center experience with primary orthotopic liver transplantation with FK 506 immunosuppression. Ann Surg. 1994;220(3): 297-309.

McDiarmid SV, Busuttil RW, Ascher NL, et al. FK506 (tacrolimus) compared with cyclosporine for primary immunosuppression after pediatric liver transplantation. Transplantation.1995;59(4):530-536.

Kintmalm GB, Goldstein R, Gonwa T, et al. Use of Prograf (FK506) as rescue therapy for refractory rejection after liver transplantation. Transplant Proc. 1993;25(1 Pt 1):679.

European Tacrolimus Multicenter Renal Study Group. Multicenter randomized trial comparing tacrolimus (FK 506) and cyclosporine in the prevention of renal allograft rejection. Transplantation. 1997;64(3):436-443.

Pirsch JD, Miller J, Deierhoi MH, Vincenti F, Filo RS. A comparison of tacrolimus (FK506) and cyclosporine for immunosuppression after cadaveric renal transplantation. FK506 Kidney Transplant Study Group. Transplantation.1997;63(7):977-983.

Jensik SC. Tacrolimus in kidney transplantation: three-year survival results of the US multicenter, randomized, comparative trial. FK506 Kidney Transplant Study Group. Transplant Proc. 1998;30(4):1216-1218.

Hruban RH, Beschorner WE, Baumgartner WA, et al. Accelerated arteriosclerosis in heart transplant recipients is associated with a T-lymphocyte-mediated endothelialitis. Am J Path.1990;137(4):871-882.

Wu TC, Hruban RH, Ambinder RF, Hutchins GM. Demonstration of cytomegalovirus nucleic acids in the coronary arteries of transplanted hearts. Am J Path. 1992;140(3):739-747.

Reichart B, Meiser B, Viganò M, et al. European Multicenter Tacrolimus (FK506) Heart Pilot Study: one-year results — European Tacrolimus Multicenter Heart Study Group. J Heart Lung Transplant. 1998;17(8): 775-781.

Woodle ES, Thistlethwaite JR, Gordon JH, et al. A multicenter trial of FK506 (tacrolimus) therapy in refractory acute renal allograft rejection. Transplantation. 1996;62(5):594-599.

Neylan JF, Sullivan EM, Steinwald B, Goss, TF. Assessment of the frequency and costs of posttransplantation hospitalizations in patients receiving tacrolimus versus cyclosporine. Am J Kid Dis. 1998;32(5):770-777.

Wiesner RH. A long-term comparison of tacrolimus (FK506) versus cyclosporine in liver transplantation: a report of the United States FK506 Study Group. Transplantation. 1998;66(4):493-499.

Meiser BM, Uberfuhr P, Fuchs A, et al. Tacrolimus: a superior agent to OKT3 for treating cases of persistent rejection after intrathoracic transplantation. J Heart Lung Transplant. 1997;16(8):795-800.

Pham SM, Kormos RL, Hattler BG, et al. A prospective trial of tacrolimus (FK506) in clinical heart transplantation: intermediate term results. J Thorac Cardiovasc Surg. 1996;111(4):764-772.

Asante-Korang A, Boyle GJ, Webber SA, Miller S, Fricker FJ. Experience of FK506 immunosuppression in pediatric heart transplantation: a study of long-term adverse effects. J Heart Lung Transplant. 1996;15(4):415-422.

Gruessner RW. Tacrolimus in pancreas transplantation: a multicenter analysis. Clin Transplant. 1997;11(4):299-312.

Gruessner RW, Burke GW, Stratta R, et al. A multicenter analysis of the first experience with FK506 for induction and rescue therapy after pancreas transplantation. Transplantation. 1996;61(2):261-273.

Jordan ML, Shapiro R, Gritsch HA, et al. Long-term results of pancreas transplantation under tacrolimus immunosuppression. Transplantation. 1999;67(2):266-272.

Kennan RJ, Konishi H, Kawai A, et al. Clinical trial of tacrolimus versus cyclosporine in lung transplantation. Ann Thorac Surg. 1995;60(3):580-585.

Steinmuller TM, Graf KJ, Schleicher Jan, et al. The effect of FK506 versus cyclosporine on glucose and lipid metabolism – a randomized trial. Transplantation. 1994;58(6):669-674.

14c ACTION, EFFICACY AND TOXICITIES: MYCOPHENOLATE MOFETIL

Sita Gourishankar, MD
Philip F. Halloran, MD, PhD

Mycophenolate mofetil (MMF) ($C_{23}H_{31}NO_7$, MW of 433.50) (Figure 14c-1) was developed as an immunosuppressive drug that would have fewer effects on non-immune tissue than other agents. The principle of the drug arose from the observation that defects in de novo purine biosynthesis create immunodeficiency without affecting other tissues. Allison et al found that brain and other tissues used purine recycling, exemplified in the Lesch-Nyhan syndrome, a defect in hyoxanthine guanine phosphoribosyl transferase, which caused brain dysfunction with no immune deficit. If lymphocytes use de novo purine synthesis, and other tissues use the salvage pathway, then inhibitors of de novo synthesis should be immunosuppressive with little or no effect on other cell types.

The search for inhibitors of de novo purine synthesis led to the ancient compound mycophenolic acid (MPA), discovered first in 1896. MPA was known to be immunosuppressive, to inhibit lymphocyte DNA synthesis, and to inhibit guanine nucleotide synthesis in tumor cells. It was found to block de novo purine biosynthesis by inhibiting the key enzyme in this pathway, inosine monophosphate dehydrogenase (IMPDH) (Figure 14c-2). The structural basis of this effect is through binding to the cofactor site in the enzyme next to the substrate site, stopping the reaction and paralyzing the enzyme (Figure 14c-2). This is uncompetitive inhibition; MPA is not a purine analogue and does not compete for the IMP binding site. IMPDH converts IMP to xanthosine 5'-monophosphate (XMP), which is the rate-limiting enzyme in the de novo synthesis of guanosine monophosphate (GMP) (Figure 14c-3). GMP synthesis is pivotal in the biosynthetic pathway of purine synthesis, and de novo purine synthesis is selectively required by T and B lymphocyte proliferation, but not by other cells. Inhibition of IMPDH probably occurs in other tissues, but they can bypass the effect by the salvage pathway, whereas lymphocytes require de novo purine biosynthesis (Figure 14c-4).

Trials from the 1970s established the effectiveness of MPA in psoriasis. MMF, the morpholinoethyl ester derivative of MPA, was shown to have increased bioavailability. MMF is rapidly and completely absorbed, and is hydrolysed by esterases to yield the active drug, MPA. MMF was shown to be immunosuppressive in transplant models and was developed to replace AZA on the basis of increased potency and selectivity. MMF blocks proliferative responses of T and B lymphocytes, inhibiting antibody formation and the generation of cytotoxic T cells and the delayed-type hypersensitivity response. MPA may also inhibit the glycosylation of adhesion molecules, which is another mechanism that is dependent on guanine nucleotides.

The immunosuppressive effect of MPA and MMF is believed to be achieved primarily by limiting clonal expansion, which severely inhibits the immune response. Because of the limitation in clonal expansion, the net production of immune effector molecules such as cytokines is reduced as well. Other postulated effects include interference with lymphocyte homing, inflammation via alterations in adhesion molecules, and inhibition of smooth muscle proliferation. The significance of these mechanisms is unknown.

MPA is metabolized in a very simple fashion to the mycophenolic acid glucuronide (MPAG), which is excreted in bile and has an enterohepatic circulation (Figure 14c-5). It is metabolized by *glucuronosyl transferase*, but the reaction is potentially reversible by β-glucuronidase. The extent to which the large pool of inactive MPAG is converted back to active drug is unknown. MPA glucuronide is excreted in the urine in humans, and in the bile to a lesser extent. The dog excretes large amounts of the glucuronide in the bile, which may account for the gastrointestinal toxicity in the dog. MPA is highly protein-bound in blood.

Sita Gourishankar, MD, Nephrology Fellow, Division of Nephrology and Immunology, University of Alberta, Edmonton, Alberta, Canada

Philip F. Halloran, MD, PhD, Professor of Medicine and Immunology, Division of Nephrology and Immunology, University of Alberta, Edmonton, Alberta, Canada

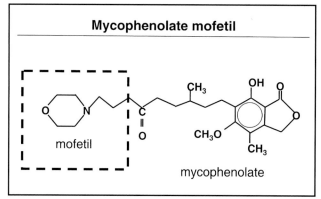

Figure 14c-1. The structure of mycophenolate mofetil, showing how mofetil moiety has been added to the mycophenolic acid compound. The active component is mycophenolate.

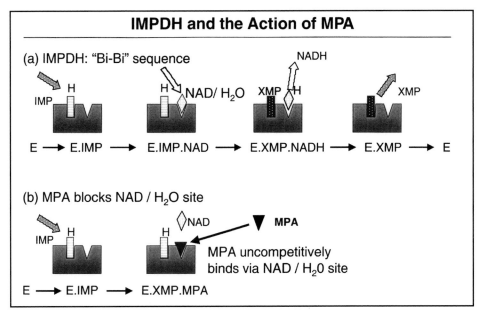

Figure 14c-2. The action of MPA on IMPDH showing (a) the action of IMPDH and (b) the effect on MPA. MPA decreases the G-to-A ratio in lymphocytes. MPA acts on IMPDH to create a blockade, which then creates a relative excess of A-to-G nucleotides, which shuts down the proximal portion of the pathways through regulatory effects on the proximal enzymes.

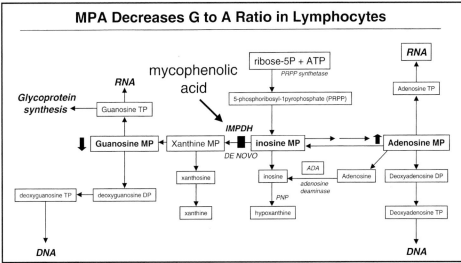

Figure 14c-3. The central role of IMPDH in de novo synthesis of GMP. IMPDH is the rate-limiting step in the pathway of de novo synthesis of XMP, which is converted to GMP. In the absence of IMPDH, de novo synthesis leads to an excess of adenosine monophosphate and its relatives. The imbalance between AMP and GMP nucleotides shuts off the proximal enzymes of the pathway.

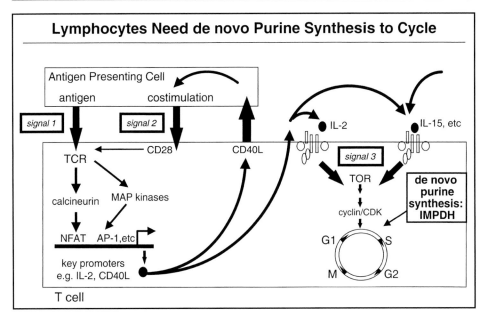

Figure 14c-4. Lymphocytes require de novo purine synthesis for successful cycling. Some evidence indicates that in the presence of an excess A-to-G ratio, lymphocytes arrest early in the S phase.

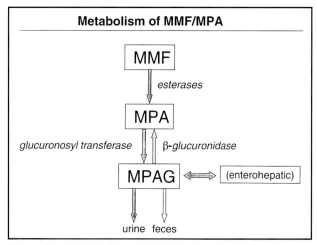

Figure 14c-5. Metabolism of MMF, showing release of esterases of the active agent, MPA, which is then rapidly glucuronylated to MPAG, most of which is excreted in urine.

The key features of MMF are:
- Moderate potency with good selectivity and few major side effects
- High oral availability with no requirement for monitoring
- No organ toxicity or lipid disorders
- Relative sparing of marrow despite immunosuppressive potency (MMF is associated with leukopenia and mild anemia)
- Simplicity of use with few drug interactions
- Some activity against pneumocystis, which may reduce the frequency of opportunistic infections

The weaknesses of MMF are:
- Gastrointestinal symptoms, chiefly diarrhea possibly related to MPAG in the gut
- Rapid metabolism means large single doses (eg, 1 g to 1.5 g) are required to achieve and sustain therapeutic levels
- Concern over the high blood levels of MPAG in renal failure. Nevertheless, no dose reduction in renal failure has been recommended

PRINCIPAL CLINICAL TRIALS

One advantage of MMF is that its characteristics have been established in randomized, controlled, double-blinded clinical trials of high validity and ability to be generalized within transplantation. In renal transplantation, three multicenter clinical trials established the efficacy of MMF plus CsA and steroid in primary prevention of renal allograft rejection in clinical renal transplantation, and a fourth study established the role of MMF in treatment of recurrent and refractory rejection. A 3-year trial of MMF plus CsA and steroid for primary prevention of rejection in heart transplantation established the role of MMF, but also established new potential endpoints for future trials.

The tricontinental study, the US trial, and the European trial were three very similar phase 3, randomized, double-blind, multicenter trials, which collectively addressed the question of efficacy of MMF in a dose of either 1 gram twice daily or 1.5 grams twice daily for primary prevention with CsA and steroid. Separately, they addressed the question of MMF vs azathioprine with no antibody induction (the tricontinental study), MMF vs azathioprine with induction (the US study), or MMF vs placebo. The primary (efficacy) endpoint in the individual trials was biopsy-proven rejection or treatment failure at six months. All demonstrated a significant reduction in acute rejection at both dose levels vs azathioprine or placebo.

A pooled analysis of clinical trials conducted in the US, Canada, Europe, and Australia was performed to further characterize the efficacy of MMF in renal allograft recipients. The three studies enrolled a total of 1,493 patients. This pooled analysis focused on graft loss, patient death, incidence and treatment of rejection episodes, and graft function (serum creatinine) at one year. The graft survival rate was 90.4% and 89.2% in the MMF 2 gram and 3 gram groups, respectively, compared with 87.6% in the placebo/azathioprine group (not statistically significant). MMF significantly reduced the incidence of rejection episodes: 40.8% for placebo and azathioprine patients vs 19.8% and 16.5% for the MMF 2 gram and MMF 3 gram groups, respectively. MMF reduced the requirement for antilymphocyte globulin or muromonab-CD3 treatment for rejection by more than 60%. Overall patient and graft survival rates were similar among the three groups, but graft loss due to rejection was reduced by MMF. Thus, MMF was superior to azathioprine or placebo as a posttransplant immunosuppressant in conjunction with CsA and steroids. MMF-treated groups showed reduced incidence and severity of rejection episodes, similar graft survival, but less loss due to rejection.

Analysis at three years has not shown any additional benefit of MMF between one and three years, similar to other immunosuppressive drugs. In organ transplantation, clinical experience has established that most patients require long-term immunosuppression, but no studies have shown that any immunosuppressive is superior after the first six to 12 months.

MMF can be used to treat acute rejection. A double-blind study evaluated the use of MMF plus steroid to prevent acute rejection requiring ALG or muromonab-CD3.

MMF is also effective in reducing graft loss in patients with refractory rejection. The treatment arm received MMF 1.5 grams twice daily while the control arm received conventional high-dose intravenous corticosteroids. Graft loss was reduced by 45% in the MMF-treated group, although the difference did not reach statistical significance, probably because the sample size calculation was not adequately powered for significance. Nevertheless, a statistically significant benefit of MMF was found for other variables, such as the incidence of later acute rejection episodes and the need for further antilymphocyte antibodies.

One of the advantages of randomized double-blind controlled trials is that one can evaluate the adverse effects of the agent objectively and control for bias and confounding. In fact, MMF in all studies gives a consistent picture of gastrointestinal side effects, most notably diarrhea, although these effects seldom require drug discontinuation. There is some leukopenia and mild normochromic normocytic anemia. The mechanism for the marrow effects is unknown because the drug was not previously believed to have marrow effects. Most encouraging is the lack of adverse effects on kidney, liver, heart, brain, or other organs, and the lack of diabetogenicity or hyperlipidemia. Most trials noted an excess of *tissue-invasive* CMV, principally on endoscopy, compared to the controls in the blinded studies. This is difficult to assess because the excess of gastrointestinal symptoms in the MMF group led to more endoscopy and thus, more biopsies. There is actually a protective effect against pneumocystis pneumonia (PCP), probably due to the direct effect of MPA on the PCP organism (perhaps due to IMPDH in the PCP organism). The use of MMF has not increased posttransplant lymphoproliferative disease significantly compared to other therapies, although there was a numerical increase in the pivotal kidney transplant studies at one year.

The results of the heart transplantation study have now been published at 1-year and presented at 3-years. The 1-year result showed a reduction in 12-month mortality or re-transplant of 46% ($P=0.031$), of rejection/re-transplant/death endpoint of 8% ($P=0.339$); of any treated rejection of 11% ($P=0.026$); of moderate or worse rejection of 15% ($P=0.055$); and of rejection needing cytolytics of 28% ($P=0.061$). Rejection with severe hemodynamic compromise was reduced by 34% ($P=0.045$). The results of the 3-year analysis indicated that the survival advantage extends to three years with 36% reduction in mortality, particularly for cardiovascular deaths. There was a modest benefit on transplant vasculopathy, with lower rates of new or progressive transplant coronary artery disease on angiography, beneficial numerical trends in ICUS endpoints, less autopsy-proven significant disease, and lower rates of heart failure and atrial arrhythmias.

The preliminary results of the randomized trial of MMF plus CsA and steroid in liver transplantation show a significant effect on acute rejection, but the detailed results await publication. Considerable experience with MMF plus tacrolimus in liver transplantation has established that this combination is effective, and the MMF

tacrolimus combination is now widely used despite the paucity of randomized trials.

CLINICAL USE OF MMF IN TRANSPLANTATION

The principal clinical role of MMF has been in combination with a calcineurin inhibitor, either CsA or tacrolimus, to prevent acute rejection in organ transplant recipients. Its initial use was for renal transplants, but its efficacy for heart transplants is now established. MMF is also used for *rescue* from refractory rejection in doses of 1 gram twice daily.

Many recipients of kidney transplants, kidney-pancreas transplants, and heart transplants now receive CsA or tacrolimus, MMF, and prednisone, with or without antibody induction therapy, at least in the first year after renal transplantation. The big drawback of MMF is the expense of using it with CsA or tacrolimus, effectively doubling the cost. Often one or two drugs are withdrawn at a specified time in stable patients (eg, steroids or MMF). Some centers change from MMF to azathioprine after one year to save expense.

MMF is not monitored but would probably be more effective if monitoring were routine. Recently it has been shown that the area-under-the-curve of the mycophenolic acid blood concentration profile is predictive of the likelihood of allograft rejection after renal transplantation in patients receiving MMF. This does not establish whether the benefits of monitoring justify the expense, however. The need for monitoring may be greater if MMF maintenance therapy with no calcineurin inhibitor is considered.

Emerging roles for MMF include:
- Use as long-term maintenance with no calcineurin inhibitor, after withdrawal of calcineurin inhibitors
- Use as primary therapy in combination with steroid and daclizumab or basiliximab or ATG with no CsA or FK
- Use with low-dose CsA
- Use with tacrolimus with increased effects because its pharmacokinetics are augmented by the tacrolimus

It has been proposed, on the basis of experimental animal studies, that the addition of MMF may slow the course of chronic rejection, but there is little clinical data to support this. An improvement in renal function will occur in any population if the dose of calcineurin inhibitor can be greatly reduced or withdrawn, which may be possible with MMF. The ability of MMF to reduce the incidence of acute rejection was also predicted to reduce chronic rejection. MMF reduces some measures of coronary vasculopathy in the heart transplant studies. However, it cannot be extrapolated from this to a general effect of chronic rejection. Current thinking on chronic rejection is that much of the disease is a complex blend of nonspecific and immune tissue deterioration, including a striking effect of tissue age. In such a model, the role of MMF would be to minimize immune injury and to reduce dependency on the nephrotoxic drugs (eg, CsA, tacrolimus).

Thus, the current role of MMF is as a maintenance agent along with a calcineurin inhibitor, but other roles, such as use as a long-term agent or with low-dose steroids, may emerge. A role in liver and lung transplantation seems possible, but this will depend on the results of ongoing clinical trials. The choice between MMF and rapamycin will be a subject of debate, since the trials have not been performed. The possibility of using rapamycin plus MMF with no calcineurin inhibitor will be evaluated in new trials.

The use of MMF has become established without a requirement for clinical monitoring of MPA blood levels. Monitoring of blood levels may improve efficacy, but whether this is worth the expense is unclear. The possibility of monitoring of IMPDH activity has been explored.

MMF is usually administered in a dose of 2 grams daily in two divided doses, (ie, 1 gram twice daily). In high-risk patients, the dose of 1.5 grams twice daily may be selected. For the heart transplant trial, the higher dose of 1.5 grams twice daily was used, but it is not clear that a lower dose of 2 grams would not suffice, since the 2 gram dose gave a superior combination of efficacy and toxicity in the renal trials.

In conclusion, MMF is now widely used as maintenance therapy of renal, heart, and possibly other types of transplants for the prevention of acute rejection. Its lack of major organ toxicity, lipid abnormalities, and requirement for monitoring are advantages. Its major side effect is diarrhea, with a tendency toward mild leukopenia and anemia. It has been associated with increased tissue-invasive CMV, but this may not be greater than for other similarly effective immunosuppressives. Its role in immunosuppression is currently in combination with CsA or tacrolimus. It is also useful for rescue from refractory rejection. Its potential role as maintenance therapy without other immunosuppressives is currently being evaluated; it remains to be established, either in combination with other agents or as the principal agent with or without steroids. If MMF is successful in this regard, it may permit reduced reliance on immunosuppressives with organ toxicity, hypertension, and lipid disorders, without sacrificing efficacy. One long-term issue to be resolved will be whether protocols containing MMF will have a reduced frequency of chronic allograft dysfunction (ie, chronic rejection).

RECOMMENDED READING

Allison AC, Hovi T, Watts RWE, Webster ADB. Immunological observations on patients with the Lesch-Nyhan syndrome, and on the role of de novo purine synthesis in lymphocyte transformation. Lancet. 1975;2(7946):1179-1183.

Danovitch GM. Mycophenolate mofetil in renal transplantation: results from the US randomized trials. Kidney Int. 1995;52:S93-S96.

European Mycophenolate Mofetil Study Group. Placebo-controlled study of mycophenolate mofetil combined with cyclosporin and corticosteroids for prevention of acute rejection. Lancet. 1995;345(8961): 1321-1325.

Franklin TJ, Cook JM. The inhibition of nucleic acid synthesis by mycophenolic acid. Biochem J. 1969;113(3): 515-524.

Franklin TJ, Cook JM. Inhibition of guanine nucleotide biosynthesis by mycophenolic acid in Yoshida ascites cells. Biochem Pharmacol. 1971;20(6):1334-8.

Giblett ER, Ammann AJ, Wara DW, Sandman R, Diamond LK. Nucleoside-phosphorylase deficiency in a child with severely defective T-cell immunity and normal B-cell immunity. Lancet. 1975;1(7914):1010-3.

Giblett ER, Anderson JE, Cohen F, Meuwissen HJ. Adenosine deaminase deficiency in two patients with severely impaired cellular immunity. Lancet. 1972; 2(7786):1067-1069.

Gomez EC, Menendez L, Frost P. Efficacy of mycophenolic acid for the treatment of psoriasis. J Am Acad Dermatol. 1979;1(6):531-537.

Hale MD, Nicholls AJ, Bullingham RE, et al. The pharmacokinetic-pharmacodynamic relationship for mycophenolate mofetil in renal transplantation. Clin Pharmacol Ther. 1998;64(6):672-683.

Halloran PF, Melk A, Barth Cl. Rethinking chronic allograft nephropathy - the concept of accelerated senescence [review]. J Am Soc Nephrol. 1999;10(1):167-181.

Kobashigawa J, Miller L, Renlund D, et al. A randomized active-controlled trial of mycophenolate mofetil in heart transplant recipients. Transplantation. 1998;66(4): 507-515.

Langman LJ, LeGatt DF, Halloran PF, Yatscoff RW. Pharmacodynamic assessment of mycophenolic acid-induced immunosuppression in renal transplant recipients. Transplantation. 1996;62(5):666-672.

Laurent AF, Dumont S, Poindron P, Muller CD. Mycophenolic acid suppresses protein N-linked glycosylation in human monocytes and their adhesion to endothelial cells and to some substrates. Exp Hematol. 1996;24(1):59-67.

Lee WA, Gu L, Miksztal AR, Chu N, Leung K, Nelson PH. Bioavailability improvement of mycophenolic acid through amino ester derivitization. Pharmacol Res. 1990;7(2):161-166.

Mitsui A, Suzuki S. Immunosuppressive effect of mycophenolic acid. J Antibiot. 1969;22(8):358-363.

Morris RE, Wang J, Blum JR, et al. Immunosuppressive effects of the morpholinoethyl ester of mycophenolic acid (RS-61443) in rat and nonhuman primate recipients of heart allografts. Transplant Proc. 1991;23(S2):19-25.

Shaw LM, Nowak I. Mycophenolic acid: measurement and relationship to pharmacologic effects. Ther Drug Monit. 1995;17(6):685-689.

Sintchak MD, Fleming MA, Futer O, et al. Structure and mechanism of inosine monophosphate dehydrogenase in complex with the immunosuppressant mycophenolic acid. Cell. 1996;85(6):921-930.

The Mycophenolate Mofetil Renal Refractory Rejection Study Group. Mycophenolate mofetil for the treatment of refractory, acute, cellular renal transplant rejection. Transplantation. 1996;61:722-729.

Tricontinental Mycophenolate Mofetil Renal Transplantation Study Group (1996). A blinded, randomized clinical trial of mycophenolate mofetil for the prevention of acute rejection in cadaveric renal transplantation. Transplantation. 1996;61:1029-1037.

US Renal Transplant Mycophenolate Mofetil Study Group, Sollinger HW. Mycophenolate mofetil for the prevention of acute rejection in primary cadaveric renal allograft recipients. Transplantation. 1995;60:225-232.

van Gelder T, Hilbrands LB, Vanrenterghem Y, et al. A randomized double-blind, multicenter plasma concentration controlled study of the safety and efficacy of oral mycophenolate mofetil for the prevention of acute rejection after kidney transplantation. Transplantation. 1999;68:261-266.

Vincenti F, Ramos E, Nashan B, et al. Preliminary results of the combined use of a humanized anti-IL-2Rα monoclonal antibody, daclizumab (DZB), and mycophenolate mofetil (MMF) without calcineurin inhibitors in renal transplantation. Transplantation. 1998;65:S190-S190 (Abstract).

Weir MR, Fink JC, Hanes DS, et al. Chronic allograft nephropathy: effect of cyclosporine reduction and addition of mycophenolate mofetil on progression of renal disease. Transplant Proc. 1999;31:1286-1287.

Zanker B, Schneeberger H, Rothenpieler U, et al. Mycophenolate mofetil-based, cyclosporine-free induction and maintenance immunosuppression. First-3-months analysis of efficacy and safety in two cohorts of renal allograft recipients. Transplantation. 1998;66:44-49.

Zucker K, Rosen A, Tsaroucha A, et al. Unexpected augmentation of mycophenolic acid pharmacokinetics in renal transplant patients receiving tacrolimus and mycophenolate mofetil in combination therapy, and analogous *in vitro* findings. Transpl Immunol. 1997;5:225-232.

14d ACTION, EFFICACY AND TOXICITIES: AZATHIOPRINE

Angelo M. de Mattos, MD

Azathioprine (AZA) was first synthesized in the 1950s as a pro-drug of 6-mercaptopurine (6-MP). It is classified as an antimetabolite agent and is used in the treatment of leukemias and other rapidly-growing malignancies. Its development is considered a significant breakthrough in science for which its developers won a Nobel prize.

CHEMISTRY

AZA (6-[(1-methyl-4-nitro-1H-imidazol-5-yl)thio]-1H-purine) is an imidazoyl derivative of 6-MP, which inhibits T and B lymphocyte proliferation by virtue of inhibiting DNA and RNA synthesis. The imidazole moiety of AZA reacts with sulfhydryl compounds such as glutathione, thus protecting 6-MP against rapid in vivo inactivation.

MECHANISM OF IMMUNOSUPPRESSIVE ACTION

There is likely a dual mechanism of action of AZA. Since the initial studies demonstrating the antiproliferative effects of purine synthesis inhibitors, these agents have also been shown to have other important effects beyond inhibiting DNA and RNA synthesis. Adenosine triphosphate (ATP) and guanosine triphosphate (GTP) play important roles in energy-requiring processes and as secondary messenger molecules. Hypoxanthine-guanine phosphorybosyl transferase (HGPRT), an enzyme of the salvage pathway of purine synthesis, plays a critical role in the activation of 6-MP. HGPRT transforms 6-MP into thioinosinic mercaptopurine (TIMP), a thiopurine nucleotide that will block phosphorybosyl pyrophosphate synthase and inosinate-monophosphate dehydrogenase, which are critical enzymes of the de novo pathway of purine synthesis. Thus, TIMP prevents the formation of building blocks for AMP and, to a lesser extent, GMP production. In addition, AZA or thiomercaptopurine inhibit inosine monophosphate dehydrogenase (IMPDH), an enzyme involved in the synthesis of GMP. Interestingly, the addition of adenine and hypoxanthine in vitro can reverse the antiproliferative effect of 6-MP but not of AZA. This finding suggests an additional role of the methylnitroimidazole moiety in inhibition of T cell and B cell lymphocytes. The methylnitroimidazole moiety of AZA tends to localize in the inner layer of the cellular membranes where it interacts with molecules that are rich in sulfhydryl and amino groups. Its exact role in membrane-associated processes such as antigen recognition, adherence, and cell-mediated cytotoxicity is currently under investigation.

ABSORPTION

AZA is rapidly absorbed following oral administration, and peak plasma concentration occurs in two hours. The absolute bioavailability (oral over intravenous concentrations) of AZA and 6-MP are approximately 20% and 40%, respectively. For the sake of simplicity, conversion on a milligram-per-milligram basis between the oral and intravenous doses has been commonly used clinically. However, acute toxicity is seen more with intravenous usage, especially with prolonged courses due to greater bioavailability. AZA's absorption is not affected by food.

DISTRIBUTION AND METABOLISM

AZA is distributed rapidly and widely throughout all body fluids. Inside the cells, it is nonenzymatically broken down by glutathione and other sulfhydryl-containing enzymes to 6-MP and a methylnitroimidazole moiety. This process occurs in vivo mainly inside red blood cells with a slow and steady release of 6-MP back into the plasma. Hypoxanthine-guanine phosphorybosyl transferase transforms 6-MP into TIMP, as described above. Before being activated by HGPRT, 6-MP can be oxidized by xanthine oxidase, producing 8-hydroxy-6-MP, or methylated by thiopurine methyltransferase, producing 6-methyl-MP. AZA can also be oxidized to 8-hydroxy-AZA. All three compounds can undergo further catabolism leading to 6-thiuric acid, the final inactive metabolite. Allopurinol, by inhibiting xanthine oxidase, and mutations of thiopurine methyltransferase, as seen in certain ethnic groups (eg, Asians), may lead to inhibition of metabolism and thus increase toxicity of AZA.

ELIMINATION

AZA, 6-MP, and its metabolites are excreted mainly in the urine. The plasma half-life of AZA and 6-MP are approximately 50 and 75 minutes, respectively. Renal impairment does not alter the kinetics of the active compounds. Thus, dose adjustment is not recommended in renal failure. In contrast, liver failure may attenuate the pharmacodynamic properties of AZA secondary to accumulation of AZA or its active metabolites.

Assistant Professor of Medicine, Division of Nephrology, Hypertension and Clinical Pharmacology, Transplantation Medicine Program, Oregon Health Sciences University, Portland, OR

ADVERSE REACTIONS TO AZATHIOPRINE

The major dose-dependent adverse drug reaction of AZA is myelosuppression. Asians and some other ethnic groups are more susceptible to this adverse reaction due to polymorphisms in the genes encoding enzymes involved in the degration of 6-MP, which lead to the accumulation of this compound and its active metabolites. Allopurinol and other xanthine oxidase inhibitors may predispose patients to excessive bone marrow suppression by a similar mechanism. No relevant clinical test has been shown to predict cytopenia. Cytopenia usually resolves five to ten days after discontinuation of AZA. The use of bone marrow-stimulating agents (ie, filgastrin, erythropoietin) is seldom necessary. Persistent leukopenia increases the risk of infection and decreases allograft survival because of the necessity to reduce AZA dose.

A wide spectrum of liver disease has been associated with AZA therapy. A rare form of idiosyncratic toxic hepatitis has been described. A rare, but irreversible and possibly fatal hepatic adverse reaction of AZA is hepatic venoocclusive disease, which is caused by obliteration of the central hepatic veins and is manifested by jaundice, hepatomegaly, and ascites. AZA has also been associated with acute pancreatitis and an increased incidence of skin cancer. AZA and 6-MP cross the placenta barrier. However, fetuses are deficient in the enzyme HGPRT, making them resistant to the toxicities of these compounds. Very small amounts of the active metabolites of AZA are incorporated into the DNA, and AZA is not likely to induce chromosomal breaks in vivo. Because AZA and its metabolites are secreted into breast milk, breast-feeding is not recommended.

CLINICAL ADMINISTRATION AND MONITORING IN TRANSPLANTATION

Plasma drug concentration monitoring of AZA or 6-MP has little clinical application, since efficacy and toxicity correlate better with tissue concentration of thiopurine nucleotide. AZA is traditionally dosed on a milligram-per-kilogram basis, with most protocols using a dose range of 1 mg/kg to 3 mg/kg of body weight. AZA is usually administered as a single daily dose, with no significant changes in bioavailability in relation to the presence or composition of meals. Conversion on a milligram-per-milligram basis between the oral and intravenous doses have been practiced extensively. However, more toxicity is seen with this approach due to the increased bioavailability of AZA and 6-MP, as explained above. Dose reduction or even discontinuation of the drug is required in the presence of cytopenia and hepatotoxicity. Efficacy as an immunosuppressive agent does not correlate with the degree of myelosuppression.

AVAILABLE PREPARATIONS

AZA is currently available in the US in 50 mg tablets (Imuran®, Faro Pharmaceutical, Inc., and in generic formulations, Roxane Laboratories, Inc.), and in 100 mg injectable vials (IV) (Imuran®, Faro Pharmaceutical, Inc., and azathioprine sodium, Bedford Laboratories).

RECOMMENDED READING

Elion GB. The pharmacology of azathioprine. Ann N Y Acad Sci. 1993;685:401-407.

Lu CY, Sicher SC, Vazquez MA. Prevention and treatment of renal allograft rejection: new therapeutic approaches and new insights into established therapies. J Am Soc Nephrol. 1993;4:1239-1256.

de Mattos AM, Olyaei AJ, Bennett WM. Pharmacology of immunosuppressive medications used in renal diseases and transplantation. Am J Kidney Dis. 1996;28(5):631-667.

14e ACTION, EFFICACY AND TOXICITIES: CORTICOSTEROIDS

David J. Cohen, MD

HISTORY

Corticosteroids have been in continuous use in the treatment of transplant recipients since the first days of solid organ transplantation in the 1950s. Corticosteroids were first developed for therapeutic use in the late 1940s, and introduced into the immunosuppressive regimen of kidney transplant recipients in the late 1950s and early 1960s, as an adjunct to irradiation. Initial doses varied from 100 mg cortisone to 300 mg prednisone. Initial indications varied from maintenance medication in the prevention of rejection, to rejection treatment in patients on azathioprine or irradiation monotherapy. Since that time, corticosteroids have remained an important element in the evolving multidrug immunosuppressive regimens used to treat solid organ transplant recipients.

Chemistry

Natural glucocorticoids are tetracyclic, terpene-based molecules that, along with mineralocorticoids and androgens, comprise the class of steroid hormones. All biologically active adrenocortical steroid compounds, whether naturally occurring or synthetic, contain a double bond in the C-4 to C-5 position, and ketone group at C-3. An 11β-OH on ring C is essential for glucocorticoid activity (Figure 14e-1).

A large number of compounds with enhanced glucocorticoid activity have been developed by modifications in chemical structure. These changes in potency may be due to altered absorption, rate of metabolism, rate of excretion, receptor affinity, protein binding and/or membrane permeability. Enhanced and longer duration glucocorticoid activity results from the introduction of an additional double bond at the C-1 to C-2 position of ring A, as seen with prednisone and prednisolone. These latter compounds are approximately fourfold more potent than hydrocortisone (cortisol). The addition of a (6α-methyl) group modestly increases the potency of prednisolone by an additional 25%. Fluorination, at the 9α position on ring B (fludrocortisone), increases glucocorticoid activity by tenfold and mineralocorticoid activity by 125-fold relative to cortisol. Fludrocortisone is effective at very low doses for mineralocorticoid replacement,

Associate Professor of Clinical Medicine; Medical Director, Renal Transplantation, Columbia University College of Physicians and Surgeons, Columbia-Presbyterian Medical Center, New York, NY

and has little glucocorticoid activity at these doses. There are several other therapeutically useful compounds derived from cortisol via other modifications, yielding topically active agents, or agents with markedly enhanced glucocorticoid activity with little to no mineralocorticoid effect (ie, dexamethasone, 16-methyl and 9α fluoro substituted).

PHARMACOLOGIC EFFECTS AND MECHANISM OF ACTION

General Mechanism of Action

Glucocorticoids exert potent immunosuppressive and antiinflammatory effects through their actions on a wide variety of leukocytes (including T and B lymphocytes, granulocytes, macrophages and monocytes), as well as on endothelial cells. They affect the concentration, distribution, and function of leukocytes. Most, if not all, corticosteroid actions are mediated by positive or negative transcriptional regulation, thereby altering expression of genes responsible for the production of factors critical in generating and maintaining immune and inflammatory responses. Unbound, circulating glucocorticoids, which are lipophilic molecules, appear to diffuse freely across cell membranes and bind with high affinity to specific cytoplasmic receptors (glucocorticoid receptors [GRs]), which contain both ligand-binding and DNA-binding domains. GR-ligand complexes act as ligand-activated transcription factors that translocate into the nucleus where they influence gene transcription by several different mechanisms. They may bind directly to specific glucocorticoid response elements (GREs) within the DNA, resulting in either positive or negative transcriptional regulation of one or more of the specific genes that encode proteins responsible for glucocorticoid action. Positive transcriptional regulation may occur by GRs binding directly a GRE sequence with promoter activity. Negative transcriptional regulation appears to occur primarily by: (1) binding to GREs that are in close proximity to positive responsive elements for other transcription factors and sterically hindering their function; (2) by promoting production of inhibitory proteins; or (3) completely preventing positive transcriptional regulators from binding. The activated GR may also down-regulate gene expression without binding to DNA, but rather by complexing with other regulatory elements, inhibiting their ability to bind to DNA. Directly repressive GREs have not been identified (Figure 14e-2).

Effects on Lymphocytes

The major effect of glucocorticoids on lymphocyte function appears to be via negative regulation of cytokine gene expression. Repression of cytokine gene transcription occurs predominantly via the inhibitory effects of glucocorticoids on the action of two important transcrip-

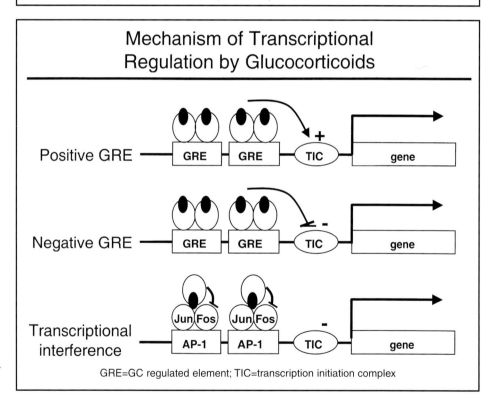

Figure 14e-1. The structures of corticosteroids.

Figure 14e-2. Mechanism of transcriptional regulation by glucocorticoids. The negative GRE is hypothetical and has not been identified.

tion factors: (1) activator protein-1 (AP-1), for which binding sites are present on target genes of glucocorticoids; and (2) nuclear factor κ-B (NF-κ-B).

In part, negative regulation of lymphocyte cytokine genes occurs via transcriptional interference between the activated GR and members of the c-Fos/c-Jun family of transcriptional regulatory proteins. Heteromeric com-

plexes of c-Fos/c-Jun family members bind to the AP-1 sites and induce the expression of several growth factors and cytokine genes, including interleukin-2 (IL-2). A direct physical interaction between AP-1 and the activated GR appears to mediate this inhibitory effect in certain genes, while the close proximity of GREs and AP-1 binding sites suggests steric hindrance in others.

NF-κ-B is an important regulator of the genes for many cytokine and cell adhesion molecules (Figure 14e-3a). Glucocorticoids repress NF-κ-B activity by: (1) the induction of I-κ-B-α production, a protein that inhibits NF-κ-B activity (Figure 14e-3b); and possibly also by (2) a direct protein-to-protein interaction between glucocorticoid-receptor complex and NF-κ-B. Both mechanisms seem to be operative in monocytes and lymphocytes, but only the former mechanism seems to be operative in endothelial cells. NF-κ-B plays a central role in the induction of a large number of immunoregulatory genes, including interleukin-1, -2, -3, and -6, interferon-γ, CD40 ligand, tumor necrosis factor (TNF-α), and GM-CSF, as well as adhesion and MHC molecules. Many of these genes are also regulated by AP-1.

Glucocorticoids may also inhibit more distal sites in the T cell activation pathway, such as the rate of degrada-

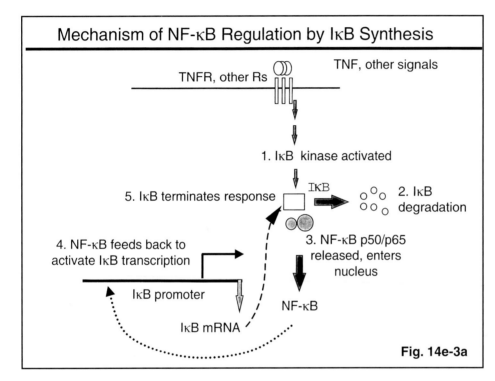

Fig. 14e-3a

Mechanism of NF-κB Regulation by IκB Synthesis

TNFR, other Rs   TNF, other signals

1. IκB kinase activated

5. IκB terminates response   IκB   2. IκB degradation

4. NF-κB feeds back to activate IκB transcription

3. NF-κB p50/p65 released, enters nucleus

IκB promoter

IκB mRNA   NF-κB

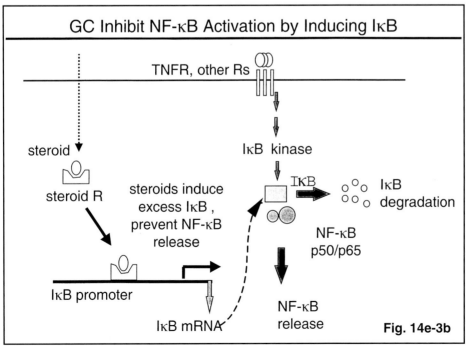

Fig. 14e-3b

GC Inhibit NF-κB Activation by Inducing IκB

TNFR, other Rs

steroid

steroid R   steroids induce excess IκB, prevent NF-κB release

IκB kinase

IκB   IκB degradation

NF-κB p50/p65

IκB promoter

IκB mRNA   NF-κB release

Figure 14e-3. The induction of NF-κB, and the effect of glucocorticoids on NF-κB release.
(a) Proinflammatory cytokine release causes degradation of the inhibitor of κB (IκB), releasing NF-κB and permitting it to enter the nucleus and activate gene transcription through NF-κB sites in promoters. This mechanism has its own feedback by induction of IκB gene transcription, which leads to inhibition of NF-κB release.
(b) Glucocorticoids act by inducing excess of IκB transcription, thereby reducing the amount of NF-κB release and therefore, the amount of NF-κB available to activate transcription of genes encoding inflammatory products.

tion of cytokine mRNAs, and the tyrosine phosphorylation of intracellular proteins.

In humans, glucocorticoids produce a substantial, but brief lymphocytopenia involving all of the lymphocyte subpopulations. This occurs due to: (1) redistribution of circulating lymphocytes to other lymphoid compartments, particularly the bone marrow; (2) changes in the expression of adhesion molecules; and (3) to a smaller extent, lysis of immature human T cells (eg, thymocytes and transformed lymphocytes) and activated T lymphocytes by programmed cell death (ie, apoptosis).

Direct B lymphocyte effects of glucocorticoids are less marked. A brief course of daily high-dose prednisone will decrease serum immunoglobulin levels with maximal suppression observed two to four weeks after treatment. This suppression is the result of an initial increase in immunoglobulin catabolism. This is followed by decreased synthesis resulting from: (1) decreased accessory or helper T cell activities through inhibition of the production of cytokines involved in immunoglobulin synthesis (IL-1 through IL-6 and interferon-γ); and/or, (2) inhibition of up-regulated CD40 ligand expression and transcription in activated T cells.

Cytotoxic T cell responses (both autoreactive and alloreactive) are inhibited by moderate to high doses of glucocorticoids, primarily because of the blockade of cytokine expression and, to a lesser extent, because of the lysis of reactive T cell clones.

Effects on Nonlymphoid Cells

Glucocorticoids alter the function of many nonlymphoid cells, inhibiting the production of vasoactive and chemoattractant factors, as well as lipolytic and proteolytic enzymes critical in generating inflammatory responses.

The major effect of glucocorticoids on neutrophils appears to be via inhibition of adhesion to endothelial cells and thus, decreased extravasation to sites of inflammation because of diminished endothelial cell adhesion molecule expression. This may also contribute to corticosteroid-induced neutrophilia. Most neutrophil functions are minimally influenced by pharmacological doses of corticosteroids.

Eosinophil and basophil counts in circulation, their accumulation in sites of allergic reactions, and the IgE-dependent release of histamine and leukotriene C4 from basophils are all decreased, as is the degranulation of mast cells.

Glucocorticoids inhibit macrophage differentiation from human monocytes. They also depress multiple functions of activated macrophages, including: (1) class II major histocompatibility antigen expression induced by interferon-γ; (2) the synthesis and release of numerous key immunomodulatory cytokines, such as IL-1, IL-6, and TNF-α; (3) the production and release of proinflammatory prostaglandins and leukotrienes; and (4) tumoricidal and microbicidal activities. The antiinflammatory effect of glucocorticoids involves synthesis of lipocortin, a protein that inhibits phospholipase A2.

Glucocorticoids also down-regulate multiple aspects of endothelial cell function, including: (1) the expression of class II MHC antigens; (2) the expression of the adhesion molecules (endothelial leukocyte adhesion molecule-1 [ELAM-1] and intercellular cell adhesion molecule-1 [ICAM-1], both of which are cell surface molecules critical to leukocyte localization); and (3) the formation of interleukin-1 and arachidonic acid metabolites (by potent inhibition of the up-regulated expression of cyclooxygenase-2). These effects limit any increase in vascular permeability at sites of tissue injury or inflammation.

ABSORPTION

Hydrocortisone, as well as its widely-used congeners – prednisone, prednisolone, and methylprednisolone – are very well-absorbed when administered orally. Water soluble esters of these drugs are commonly given intravenously when very high concentrations in various bodily fluids are necessary. These include hydrocortisone sodium succinate and methylprednisolone sodium succinate.

FATE AND EXCRETION

Corticosteroids in the blood are 70% to 90% protein bound. Transcortin (cortisol-binding globulin [CBG]) has a high affinity for steroids, but a low total binding capacity. Albumin, on the other hand, has a lower affinity, but a large total binding capacity.

Synthetic steroids with an 11-keto substituent, such as cortisone and prednisone, must be reduced by a specific hepatic 11α-hydroxy steroid dehydrogenase to the corresponding 11α-hydroxy derivative before they are biologically active. In patients with severe liver disease, where this enzymatic activity may be impaired, 11β-hydroxy steroids that do not require activation (eg, cortisol and prednisolone) may be indicated.

As noted above, all biologically active steroid compounds contain a double bond in the C-4 to C-5 position, and ketone group at C-3. Metabolism of these compounds to inactive metabolites involves the reduction of four to five double-bond, which takes place in the liver and elsewhere. Only the liver is able to reduce the C-3 ketone to a C-3-hydroxyl derivative, which can then be sulfated or glucuronidated to produce water-soluble derivatives. The primary site of excretion of these inactive water-soluble derivatives is via the urine. There is little to no biliary or fecal excretion.

Elimination half-life of prednisone and methylprednisolone is 2.6 to three hours. When orally administered before dialysis, between 7% and 17% of prednisone can be removed by dialysis.

TOXICOLOGY

There are numerous well-known and frequently adverse effects of high-dose and/or long-term glucocorticoid administration. These include: (1) cosmetic effects (eg, hirsutism, acne, easy bruising, skin fragility, moon facies, buffalo humps, weight gain, redistribution of body fat predisposing to truncal obesity); (2) metabolic effects (eg, hyperlipidemia, diabetes mellitus, salt/water retention, osteopenia, growth retardation in children); and (3) other effects (eg, gastric ulcers, emotional lability, hypertension, cataracts, poor wound healing, proximal myopathy, and enhanced risk of infection). It appears that the immunosuppressive/antiinflammatory effects, and the metabolic and other adverse effects are mediated by the same receptor.

CLINICAL APPLICATION IN TRANSPLANTATION

Steroid therapy is a standard part of every phase of immunosuppression in solid organ transplant recipients.

Induction

High-dose intravenous methylprednisolone is generally given immediately preceding, and/or during organ implantation, and continued for several days postoperatively. The details of steroid dosing protocols vary among centers, and among transplanted organs, with the total dose given on the day of transplant surgery ranging from 300 mg to 1,000 mg.

Maintenance

Following surgery, steroids are routinely tapered very rapidly to a daily dose ranging from 20 mg to 30 mg. A slower taper follows, bringing the daily maintenance dose to 10 mg within three to six months after transplantation. This dose is continued, and eventually tapered to 5 mg daily in many patients depending upon the details of the individual patient's clinical course and, upon the organ transplanted. The details of the tapering schedule may vary considerably from center to center, with little or no data available to support the specifics of any particular protocol. For long-term maintenance therapy, alternate-day administration has been used successfully, particularly in well-matched living donor renal transplant recipients, but does not enjoy widespread use elsewhere, with the exception of pediatric patients, where aggressive minimalization of steroids doses may increase the likelihood of attaining normal stature.

Because of the multitude of potential long-term side effects of corticosteroid therapy, there have been many attempts at developing a successful protocol enabling patients to discontinue steroid therapy entirely. Unfortunately, the ability to reliably identify those patients who will remain immunologically quiescent with respect to their allografts following steroid withdrawal remains rudimentary at the present time. In several large trials of steroid discontinuation in renal allograft recipients, results have been mixed, with a higher incidence of acute rejection in the short-term, and reduced allograft survival in the long-term documented in most studies. There are some data on successful steroid-free long-term success in liver and renal allograft recipients treated with tacrolimus-based immunosuppressive regimens. There is little other than anecdotal data on steroid withdrawal in heart and lung transplant recipients. The appropriate clinical setting and the appropriate combination of other immunosuppressive agents allowing for successful steroid withdrawal remain undefined.

Antirejection

High-dose corticosteroid treatment remains a mainstay of treatment for mild-moderate acute rejection. In this context, methylprednisolone is generally given intravenously for several days at doses ranging from 250 mg up to 1,000 mg. This may be given in single or divided doses, and administered for three to five days, according to local practice. Very mild rejections may be treated by oral prednisone or prednisolone at 2 to 3 mg/kg per day. The high-dose oral or intravenous antirejection doses are followed by rapid tapering back to maintenance doses within several days to weeks.

Stress

At the time of serious infection or other medical illness or surgical procedure, consideration must be given to administering "stress" dose corticosteroids in view of the possibility that the normal physiological response of increased adrenal gland steroid secretion may not occur due to adrenal suppression by the long-term use of exogenous corticosteroid immunosuppression. Standard-dose cortisol of 100 mg every six to eight hours should be sufficient in all patients to prevent Addisonian crisis.

Steroid Taper

In renal allograft recipients, if the graft has failed, immunosuppression is normally rapidly discontinued. However, corticosteroid treatment must be tapered slowly with observation for signs or symptoms of adrenal insufficiency. In addition, those patients in whom the failed allograft still remains in place, and who have discontinued all immunosuppression including corticosteroids, may experience pain in the allograft, fever, and/or gross hematuria due to episodes of ongoing immune attack in the allograft. These symptoms can frequently be treated with brief courses of oral corticosteroids (eg, prednisone 20 mg to 40 mg per day tapered over several weeks) prior to graft nephrectomy.

AVAILABLE PREPARATIONS

The commonly available preparations include prednisone, prednisolone and methylprednisolone for oral use, and the water soluble esters of hydrocortisone and methylprednisolone, such as hydrocortisone sodium succinate and methylprednisolone sodium succinate, for intravenous use.

RECOMMENDED READING

Scheinman RI, Cogswell PC, Lofquist AK, Baldwin AS Jr. Role of transcriptional activation of I kappa B alpha in mediation of immunosuppression by glucocorticoids. Science. 1995;270(5234):283-286.

Auphan N, DiDonato JA, Rosette C, Helmberg A, Karin M. Immunosuppression by glucocorticoids: inhibition of NF-kappa B activity through induction of I kappa B synthesis. Science. 1995;270(5234):286-290.

Schimmer BP, Parker KL. Adrenocorticotrophic hormone; adrenocortical steroids and their synthetic analogs; Inhibitors of the synthesis and actions of adrenocortical hormones. In: Hardman JG, Goodman Gilman A, Limbard LE, eds. Goodman & Gilman's The Pharmacological Basis of Therapeutics. 9th Ed. New York, NY: McGraw-Hill; 1996:1459-1485.

Boumpas DT, Chrousos GP, Wilder RL, Cupps TR, Balow JE. Glucocorticoid therapy for immune-mediated diseases: basic and clinical correlates. Ann Intern Med. 1993;119(12):1198-1208.

Hricik DE. Steroid withdrawal in renal transplant recipients: pro point of view. Transplant Proc. 1998;30(4):1380-1382.

Bischof F, Melms A. Glucocorticoids inhibit CD40 ligand expression of peripheral CD4+ lymphocytes. Cell Immunol. 1998;187(1):38-44.

Ray A, Sehgal PB. Cytokines and their receptors: molecular mechanisms of interleukin-6 gene repression by glucocorticoids. J Am Soc Nephrol. 1992;2(12 Suppl):S214-S221.

14f ACTION, EFFICACY AND TOXICITIES: POLYCLONAL ANTILYMPHOCYTE ANTIBODIES

Daniel C. Brennan, MD, FACP

HISTORY

Polyclonal antilymphocyte immunosuppression has the longest history of any immunosuppressive agent used in transplantation. These agents have been available since the early 1900s when they were used primarily as anti-inflammatory agents. In the 1950s and 1960s, they were shown to decrease delayed-type hypersensitivity (DTH) reactions and suppress skin graft rejection in experimental models of transplantation. Monaco showed that immunosuppression with antilymphocyte serum (ALS) alone could prolong allograft transplantation in dogs. Starzl began to use these agents for immunosuppression in human transplantation over 30 years ago, after Monaco demonstrated that rabbit anti-human ALS suppressed DTH and skin rejection in man. They have been used to prevent acute rejection in solid organ transplantation (ie, as "induction" immunosuppression), to treat rejection in solid organ transplantation, particularly "steroid-resistant rejection," and as a treatment of aplastic anemia and graft-vs-host disease.

CHEMISTRY

Polyclonal agents are called such because they are composed of several immunoglobulins that are produced by many different clones of cells. There are many similarities between the different agents; however, several important differences and distinctions must be kept in mind. Polyclonal preparations differ in the immunogen, the animal in which the immunoglobulin is generated, the purity of the preparation, the cell markers targeted, and the dose and strength of the preparation (Table 14f-1). The immunogen may be lymphocytes, thymocytes, blast cells or T cell lines. The species in which the immunoglobulin is generated is usually a horse or rabbit, although many centers have used goats or sheep, but none of these were ever commercially available. Only horse- and rabbit-derived preparations are currently available. Historically, rabbit antibodies have been felt to be more potent than horse antibodies.

Associate Professor of Medicine; Director, Transplant Nephrology, Washington University School of Medicine, Barnes-Jewish Hospital, St. Louis, MO

The initial polyclonal agents consisted of unfractionated serum obtained from animals after immunization with human lymphocytes. This was known as *antilymphocyte serum (ALS)*. When it became clear that the immunosuppressive quality of the serum was primarily contained in the immunoglobulin portion of the serum, immunoglobulin was purified and concentrated from the immunized animal's serum. This produced a more potent immunosuppressive agent on a gram-per-gram basis. Until recently, the only commercially available preparations in the US were horse-derived. These equine agents were Minnesota antilymphocyte globulin (MALG) and antithymocyte gamma globulin (Atgam®, Pharmacia & Upjohn). In Europe, a third horse preparation (Lymphoglobulin®, Pasteur Merieux) and two rabbit antilymphocyte globulins (Thymoglobulin®, Pasteur Merieux, and F-ATG®, Fresinius) were available. In 1992, the FDA prohibited the sale and distribution of MALG, and Atgam® became the only commercially available polyclonal immunosuppressive agent until 1999, when Thymoglobulin® was approved for treatment of rejection in the US.

PHARMACOLOGIC EFFECTS AND MECHANISM OF ACTION

Polyclonal agents are purified primarily monomeric anti-human gamma globulins obtained from the immunization of animals with human lymphocytes or thymocytes. The immunosuppressive effects of polyclonal antibodies are felt to result primarily from lymphocyte depletion. Within 24 hours of administration, peripheral blood lymphocyte counts drop below 100 mm to 200 mm. Lymphocyte depletion may result from complement-dependent opsonization and lysis, Fc-dependent opsonization, or Fas-mediated apoptosis, particularly at low levels of circulating polyclonal antibodies. Long-term specific depletion of the CD4+ lymphocyte subset and the preferential generation of a CD8+, CD57+ immunomodulatory subset of cells have also been postulated to explain the long-term success of polyclonal immunosuppression. In contrast to other immunosuppressive agents whose activity depends on T cell activation (eg, immunophilin ligands, corticosteroids, antimetabolites, CD25 mAbs), polyclonal agents can eliminate preactivated noncycling memory lymphocytes, which may be critical for prophylactic treatment in presensitized recipients and for treatment of steroid-resistant acute rejection.

Rejection is caused by an immunologic reaction that is a multicellular and redundant process. Conceivably, rejection may be more preventable or treatable with the polyspecific therapy of the polyclonal agents compared to the monospecific therapy provided by monoclonal antibody therapy. The polyclonal agents contain anti-

Table 14f-1. Polyclonal Comparisons

Manufacturer	Pharmacia & Upjohn	Minnesota	Pasteur Merieux	Pasteur Merieux/ Sangstatr	Fresenius
Drug	Atgam®	MALG	Lymphoglobulin®	Thymoglobulin®	F-ATG
Species	Horse	Horse	Horse	Rabbit	Rabbit
Concentration (mg/mL)	50	50	10-20	5	20
Immunogen	Thymus	Cultured lymphoblasts and thymus	Thymus	Thymus	Jurkat line
Dosage per day (mg/kg)	10-30	15-2	10	1.25 - 2.5	1-5

Reprinted and adapted with permission from Bourdage JS, Hamlin DM. Transplantation. 1995;59(8):1194-1200.

bodies to a wide variety of human T cell antigens, human B cell antigens, NK surface antigens, and adhesion or costimulatory molecules, including CD2, CD3, CD4, CD5, CD7, CD8, CD11a, CD16, CD18, CD20, CD28, CD38, CD44, CD45, CD54, CD56, CD58, the T cell receptor, CD80 (B7-1), CD86 (B7-2), CD95 (FAS), FASL, CTLA4 (CD152), CD154 (CD40L), and MHC class I and class II antigens. Recent studies have shown that early administration of antibodies directed at a variety of adhesion molecules reduces inflammation, renal insufficiency, acute rejection, and chronic rejection associated with ischemia-reperfusion injury and brain death. Intraoperative administration of polyclonal agents may reduce inflammation and prevent delayed graft function and rejection.

FATE AND EXCRETION

Polyclonal agents are immunoglobulins and may be cleared by protein degradation or antixenogenic antibodies. The half-life varies from two to nine days. Thymoglobulin has been shown to be detectable more than 90 days after the last infusion. Even at low submitogenic doses (ie, 10 mg/mL), polyclonal agents may induce apoptosis. Anti-horse or anti-rabbit antibodies may develop in up to 78% of recipients. The anti-horse antibodies persist longer than the anti-rabbit antibodies. Development of an anti-horse or anti-rabbit antibody response may not preclude retreatment, but it is recommended to assess lymphocyte counts to look for depletion.

TOXICOLOGY

Fever and chills are common, secondary to the cytokine release syndrome, although they occur less frequently and are less severe than with muromonab-CD3. Cytokine release results in "third-spacing" and the necessity of fluid resuscitation on the order of five to six liters above "dry weight" to avoid intravascular volume depletion, delayed graft function, or acute tubular necro-

sis. Hives are common with Atgam®, but not typically seen with Thymoglobulin®. Most adverse effects can be managed by stopping the infusion until the symptoms resolve, and then restarting the infusion at a reduced rate or administering steroids and antihistamines. Mild thrombocytopenia and leukopenia also may occur. Xenogenic (anti-horse or anti-rabbit) antibody formation is common and persists longer with Atgam® than with Thymoglobulin®. However, because of the polyclonal nature of these agents, this may not prevent effective retreatment. Xenogenic antibody formation may be reduced by the preferential and concomitant use of mycophenolate compared to azathioprine. Serum sickness and anaphylaxis are rare but may result, particularly if there has been prior exposure to the agent.

CLINICAL ADMINISTRATION AND MONITORING IN TRANSPLANTATION

In solid organ transplantation, polyclonal immunosuppressive agents may be used for the prevention or treatment of rejection. The only agents currently approved by the FDA for induction immunosuppression are two anti-IL-2 receptor monoclonal antibodies, basiliximab (Simulect®, Novartis Pharmaceuticals) and daclizumab (Zenapax®, Roche Laboratories). Currently, neither any polyclonal agent nor muromonab-CD3 has FDA approval for use as an induction agent. Nevertheless, polyclonal agents and muromonab-CD3 have been used widely for induction immunosuppression in kidney, kidney-pancreas, lung, heart and liver transplantation. Several recent studies have shown that induction with polyclonal or monoclonal agents is useful in reducing the incidence of rejection compared to immunosuppressive therapy that does not use induction even in low-risk, Caucasian, HLA-matched adults with low levels of panel reactive antibodies (PRA). These agents are particularly effective for children and patients with high PRA and when initiation of cyclosporine is delayed one to five days after the transplant procedure. Whether a polyclonal induction agent or a monoclonal agent is more effective is a matter of controversy. When compared to muromonab-CD3, polyclonal agents have less cytokine release and fewer side effects. There have been few direct comparisons of the two agents. To date, polyclonal therapy has not been compared directly to either of the new monoclonal anti-IL-2 receptor monoclonal antibodies.

When these agents are used for induction, the first dose should be given intraoperatively prior to anastamosis of the transplanted organ. The usual dose of Thymoglobulin® is 1.5 to 2.5 mg/kg per day and for Atgam®, 15 mg/kg per day. The duration is usually five to 14 days. Both preparations should be infused through a high-flow vein, either through a proximal central venous catheter, a peripherally inserted central catheter (PICC) line, or through a hemodialysis access over four to eight hours. A skin test is recommended prior to infusion of Atgam®, but not Thymoglobulin®, to detect prior sensitization and to prevent anaphylactoid reactions. Similar to the administration of muromonab-CD3, premedication with steroids (methylprednisolone 3 to 7 mg/kg, prednisone 1 to 2 mg/kg, or hydrocortisone 250 to 1,000 mg) and antihistamines (diphenhydramine 25 to 50 mg) is used by some programs to reduce the cytokine release syndrome and the possibility of an allergic reaction.

Polyclonal agents reduce T cells, polymorphonuclear cells, and platelets. T cell counts after the first dose should be less than 100/mm^3. If they are greater than this after the first dose, the dose should be increased by 25%. Some programs advocate further adjustment of dose based on T cell counts. However, the optimal level of T cell depletion is unknown. The dose should be decreased to half at any time for platelet counts between 50,000 to 75,000/mm^3 or white blood cell counts between 2,000 to 3,000/mm^3. The dose should be held temporarily at any time during therapy if the platelet count is less than 50,000 mm or white blood cell count less than 2,000 mm.

AVAILABLE PREPARATIONS

There are currently two polyclonal preparations available for induction in US, Thymoglobulin® and Atgam®. A recent single-center, randomized, double-blinded comparison of Thymoglobulin® vs Atgam® for induction in adult renal transplant recipients showed that use of Thymoglobulin® was associated with unprecedented prevention of rejection. At one year, Thymoglobulin® patients had fewer rejections, 4.2% vs 25% (P=0.021), less severe rejection (P=0.02), and better graft survival 98% vs 83% (P=0.02). At six months, Thymoglobulin® patients also had a lower rate of symptomatic CMV infection, 10% vs 33% (P=0.025), and no patients developed posttransplant lymphoproliferative disorder (PTLD). Only one patient in either group experienced delayed graft function requiring treatment with dialysis. The better results with Thymoglobulin® were explained in part by the more profound, and long-term lymphocyte depletion, which lasted for over one year in Thymoglobulin®-treated patients.

A recent multicenter, randomized, double-blinded comparison of Thymoglobulin® vs Atgam® for treatment of rejection in adult renal transplant recipients also showed that Thymoglobulin® reversed rejection more often than Atgam®, 88% vs 76% (P=0.028). Thymoglobulin® was also associated with a recurrent rejection rate that was half that of the Atgam® group. The availability of two polyclonal agents from two different animal species – rabbit and horse – provides additional immunosuppressive options for transplant recipients in whom polyclonal immunosuppression is desired, particularly when the recipient has had prior exposure to this form of therapy.

RECOMMENDED READING

Bonnefoy-Berard N, Revillard JP. Mechanisms of immunosuppression induced by antithymocyte globulins and OKT3. J Heart Lung Transplant. 1996;15(5):435-442.

Bourdage JS, Hamlin DM. Comparative polyclonal antithymocyte globulin and antilymphocyte/antilymphoblast globulin anti-CD antigen analysis by flow cytometry. Transplantation. 1995;59(8):1194-1200.

Brennan DC, Flavin K, Lowell JA, Howard TK, et al. A randomized, double-blinded comparison of Thymoglobulin versus ATGAM for induction immunosuppressive therapy in adult renal transplant recipients. Transplantation. 1999;67(7):1011-1018.

Brent L. Immunoregulation: The Search for the Holy Grail. In: Brent, L., ed. A History of Transplantation Immunology. San Diego, Ca: Academic Press. 1997: 230-304

Monaco AP. A new look at polyclonal antilymphocyte antibodies in clinical transplantation. Graft. 1999;2(1): S2-S5.

Szczech LA, Berlin JA, Aradhye S, Grossman RA, Feldman HI. Effect of anti-lymphocyte induction therapy on renal allograft survival: a meta-analysis. J Am Soc Nephrol. 1997;8(11):1771-1777.

14g ACTION, EFFICACY AND TOXICITIES: ANTI-CD3 MONOCLONAL ANTIBODIES

Douglas J. Norman, MD

HISTORY

The use of antibodies directed to specific molecules on lymphocytes was made possible through the development of the technique to make monoclonal antibodies. Muromonab-CD3, approved in 1986, was the first monoclonal antibody to be approved by the FDA for therapeutic use in humans. Its initial use followed the considerable previous use of the nonspecific, polyclonal antilymphocyte antibodies beginning in the 1960s. Muromonab-CD3 was originally used for treatment of rejection and eventually was also used to prevent rejection. More recently, techniques have been developed to humanize monoclonal antibodies. Several humanized anti-CD3 monoclonal antibodies have been manufactured. The one that has had the most extensive evaluation in humans is HuM291 (Protein Design Labs).

CHEMISTRY, TARGET AND MANUFACTURE

Muromonab-CD3 is a murine IgG2a monoclonal antibody that is produced by a B cell/myeloma cell hybridoma created by the technique of Kohler and Milstein. HuM291 is a genetically engineered, humanized, IgG2 monoclonal antibody that has been altered to have decreased binding to Fcγ receptors.

Target

The target of both of these antibodies is the ε chain of CD3 (Figure 14g-1), a trimeric molecule closely linked to the α-β heterodimeric T cell receptor (TcR). The three CD3 proteins are a 25 to 28 kD γ chain, a 20 kD glycosylated δ chain and a 20 kD nonglycosylated ε chain. These CD3 chains are associated, in 90% of TcR complexes, with a homodimer of 16 kD nonglycosylated ζ chains or, in 10% of complexes, with a heterodimer of a ζ chain and a 22 kD nonglycosylated ν chain. The role of CD3, ζ and ν chains, is to facilitate the expression of the TcR α and β chains on the T cell surface and to transmit a signal to the cell interior. All proteins are mutually dependent for cell surface expression. The three CD3 chains are highly

homologous and are coded for by genes on the eleventh human chromosome. They each have an N-terminal extracellular region, a short connecting peptide, a transmembrane segment, and a cytoplasmic tail. They are considered part of the Immunoglobulin (Ig) Superfamily because the extracellular part contains a single Ig-like domain. No polymorphisms of the extracellular domains have been elucidated, so it is assumed that they are not involved in antigen recognition. The cytoplasmic tails of the ζ chains are substrates of and may bind tyrosine kinases, which are activated upon binding of the TcR to a ligand. The TcR is key to the normal function of T cells. Without it, a CD4-positive T cell cannot be activated by alloantigen, nor can a CD8-positive T cell bind to a target cell and lyse it via direct cellular cytotoxicity. The target of muromonab-CD3, therefore, is a part of the key T cell activation apparatus.

Manufacture

Muromonab-CD3 was initially made by repeatedly injecting a mouse with human thymus cells, following which the mouse's splenic lymphoctyes were procured and (in the presence of polyethylene glycol) fused with mouse myeloma cells. These myeloma cells were genetically altered to prevent their own immunoglobulin production. The hybridomas formed were cloned and screened for their production of antibodies directed to T cells. A hybridoma that produced monoclonal antibodies directed to the ε chain of CD3 was chosen and a cell line from this clone was established. Seed lots from this cell line were frozen to insure a consistent and uniform product.

MUROMONAB-CD3. To manufacture muromonab-CD3, an aliquot of the seed lot, established from the original clone, is injected into the peritoneum of a pathogen-free mouse. Monoclonal antibodies harvested from ascites fluid are purified by ammonium sulfate fractionation and ion exchange chromatography, then tested for purity using gel-permeation high performance liquid chromatography (HPLC) and ion exchange HPLC. Purified muromonab-CD3 is characterized by isoelectric focusing, immunoelectrophoresis and immunodiffusion. It is then sterilized by membrane filtration and stored for use in sterile ampules.

HuM291. To manufacture HuM291, the hypervariable domain cDNA for the heavy and light chains of a murine anti-CD3 (M291) were cloned and combined with the cloned variable and constant domain cDNA of a human IgG2 in a plasmid (Figure 14g-2). The constant region (C_H2) of this humanized antibody was also mutated to reduce binding to Fcγ receptors. The plasmid containing the mouse-human immunoglobulin genes was transfected into a mouse myeloma cell line. The transfected cells were grown in serum-free medium and the anti-

Professor of Medicine; Director, Transplantation Medicine Program; Director, Laboratory of Immunogenetics and Transplantation, Oregon Health Sciences University, Portland, OR

bodies produced were purified from the cultures by protein G affinity chromatography.

PHARMACOLOGIC EFFECTS AND MECHANISM OF ACTION
Muromonab-CD3

T cells are activated by muromonab-CD3, but this activation is cofactor dependent. Soluble antibodies cannot activate T cells in the absence of monocytes. Muromonab-CD3 immobilized on polystyrene beads or plates are not monocyte dependent. This latter form of activation is dependent on the density of muromonab-CD3 on the beads or plates. Low-density antibodies can be enhanced by cofactors that also must be immobilized (anti-CD2, anti-CD11a and anti-MHC class I monoclonal antibodies) or can be soluble (anti-CD28 and anti-CD5 monoclonal antibodies). Soluble muromonab-

CD3 can also activate T cells without monocytes if either phorbol myristate acetate (PMA) or PHA/IL2 are present in the medium.

Cytokine mRNA is expressed in muromonab-CD3-activated T cells. Two hours after adding muromonab-CD3 to peripheral blood lymphocytes, mRNA for IL-1, IL-2, IL-3, TNF-α and IFN-γ can be detected in higher than baseline quantities and all remain present for at least 22 hours. mRNA for IL-6 and GM-CSF are detected after four hours, mRNA for IL-10 after seven hours, and all remain for greater than 22 hours. In contrast to all of the above, mRNA for IL-4 is expressed only transiently between four and seven hours. Within hours of adding muromonab-CD3 to PBL, CD3 is modulated (internalized) from the T cell surface. All other associated molecules, including TcR alpha and beta chains are also internalized (comodulated). The T cell becomes devoid of

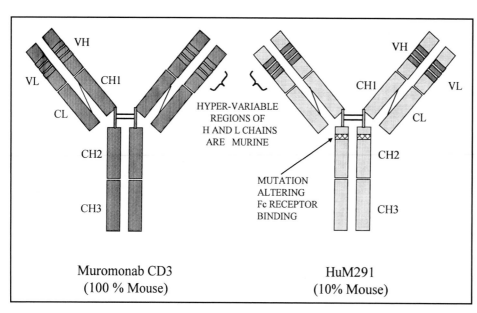

Figure 14g-1. Schematic drawing of the CD3-T cell Receptor Complex.

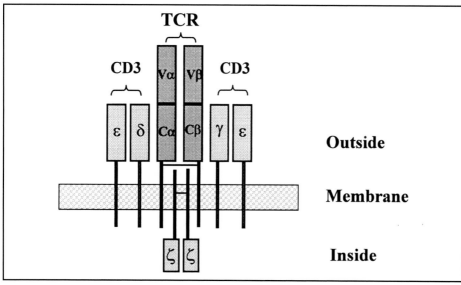

Figure 14g-2. Schematic drawing of fully murine and humanized monoclonal antibodies. Only the hypervariable regime of the humanized antibody is murine (approximately 10%).

the TcR, which renders it unable to respond to alloanti-gen in a cellular assay. Twenty-four hours after muromonab-CD3 has been removed from cells in culture, CD3/TcR complexes are re-expressed on the surface of T cells. Both T cell activation and CD3/TcR modulation are isotype dependent. Isotype switch variants of muromonab-CD3 that are directed to the same epitope on the ε chain are less able, or unable, to activate or modulate because their Fc piece cannot bind to monocyte Fc receptors.

IN VIVO ACTIVITY. Within minutes of injecting as little as 1 mg of muromonab-CD3 in vivo, T cells disappear from the circulation. This is thought to occur as a result of opsonization of T cells and their subsequent removal from the circulation by mononuclear phagocytes in the liver and spleen. Cytokines are also released following the initial injections of this antibody. During treatment with muromonab-CD3, T cells return to the circulation but, as a result of CD3/TcR modulation, these T cells express only a low-density of CD3/TcR molecules. This is believed to explain the in vivo immuno blocking effects of muromonab-CD3. Other possible mechanisms of depletion include apoptosis of activated T cells and antibody-dependent cell-mediated cytotoxicity of T cells, mediated by NK cells.

HuM291

HuM291 is significantly less able than muromonab-CD3 to activate T cells in vitro, however, when as little as 0.015 mg/kg is injected in vivo, HuM291 mediates profound T cell depletion. T cells recover fully in the absence of measurable levels of HuM291 in the serum. In the limited number of patients who have received this drug, cytokines are released by lymphocytes, but in amounts that cause few symptoms.

ABSORPTION, FATE AND EXCRETION
Muromonab-CD3

Muromonab-CD3 is injected intravenously by bolus injection over approximately one minute. The half-life of muromonab-CD3 is approximately 18 hours once a steady state is achieved. Elimination of muromonab-CD3 is related to three factors: distribution within the vascular and interstitial compartments, binding to its target, CD3 molecules and subsequent internalization into cells or phagocytosis, and immune elimination. Anti-muromonab-CD3 antibodies can greatly accelerate the elimination of muromonab-CD3.

HuM291

HuM291 is also injected intravenously by bolus injection. The half-life of HuM291 in humans has not yet been determined. HuM291 is not immunogenic in humans. Therefore, immune elimination is not a factor in its metabolism. Other factors mentioned above for muromonab-CD3 apply to HuM291.

TOXICOLOGY
Cytokine Release Syndrome

Serum levels of IL-2, IFN-γ, IL-6 and TNF-α increase significantly following the first dose of muromonab-CD3 and, to a lesser extent, HuM291. The toxicities of the anti-CD3 monoclonal antibodies are related to these cytokines, which are released from lymphocytes. These cause a syndrome (named the cytokine release syndrome) that may include fever, chills, headache, nausea, vomiting and diarrhea. The released cytokines can also cause a capillary leak syndrome leading to pulmonary edema in volume-overloaded patients, and encephalopathy. There is evidence that complement is activated following an initial dose of muromonab-CD3. It has been hypothesized that this activation leads to the observed transient drop of polymorphonuclear cells in the peripheral blood and their sequestration in the lungs. The maximal effect on polymorphonuclear cells occurs within five minutes of administering the drug and has mostly reversed by 30 minutes after injection. Sequestration of cells in the lung might be a cause of shortness of breath reported by some patients, in the absence of pulmonary edema. The use of methylprednisolone, 8 mg/kg, between one and three hours before the first dose of muromonab-CD3, significantly reduces the severity of the cytokine release syndrome. The first dose of this drug should always be given under high-dose steroid coverage. Subsequent doses should be given within three hours of the usual daily dose of prednisone to minimize the consequences of any subsequent cytokine release. Another important preventive measure is to ensure that a patient's body weight is within 3% of his or her dry weight. Pulmonary edema from a capillary leak is extremely rare in the absence of significant volume overload. Anti-TNF antibodies can block the symptoms of cytokine release. Diphenhydramine and acetaminophen are commonly used prior to the first few doses. Indomethacin can attenuate the fever that accompanies cytokine release. Orally administered pentoxifylline has not been useful.

Human Anti-Mouse Antibody Production

Muromonab-CD3 is immunogenic in humans, and approximately 50% of patients will make antibodies to it following a course of treatment. Approximately 20% of these will make a high titer (>1:1000) of human anti-mouse antibody production (HAMA). The most common consequence of HAMA is that a second course of muromonab-CD3 is ineffective. Serum sickness is very rare, possibly because of the low doses of antibody administered.

CONSEQUENCES OF OVER IMMUNOSUPPRES-SION. As detailed elsewhere, the consequences of over immunosuppression are an increased incidence of lymphoma and infections. In particular, the antilymphocyte antibodies have been implicated in causing an over immunosuppressed state. A total dose of greater than 75 mgs of muromonab-CD3 given over a period in excess of two weeks has been implicated in causing a significant increase in lymphoma incidence and, therefore, should be avoided.

CLINICAL ADMINISTRATION AND MONITORING IN TRANSPLANTATION

Muromonab-CD3 has been proven useful for both prevention and treatment of rejection. In a multicenter randomized trial in the US, the incidence of rejection was significantly lower in kidney transplant recipients who were given muromonab-CD3 for induction along with azathioprine, prednisone and the delayed (11 days) use of cyclosporine compared to triple-therapy alone. Subsets of patients in whom there was a statistically significant graft survival advantage at two years included patients without delayed graft function, patients with two HLA DR mismatches with their donors, and patients whose donor kidneys had more than 24 hours of cold ischemia time. The indication for which muromonab-CD3 has regulatory approval is treatment of first rejection episodes. In this setting, it is significantly more effective than steroids for reversing rejection. It has also been effective for reversing steroid-resistant rejections.

The usual dose of muromonab-CD3 is 5 mg, although doses as low as 2 mg have been shown to be effective for induction of immunosuppression. The usual course of therapy is ten to 14 single daily doses. Monitoring the use of muromonab-CD3 can be accomplished in two ways: measuring serum levels of the drug, or measuring the level of CD3-positive cells in the peripheral blood compartment. It is generally believed that when the serum level of muromonab-CD3 drops below 1,000 ng/mL that the desired effect of the drug on T cells may be lost. The target number of CD3-positive T cells is approximately 10 cells/mm^3 to 25 cells/mm^3 of whole blood (normal is approximately 1,000 to 1,500 CD3-positive cells/mm^3). Most hospitals are equipped to measure the number of CD3-positive cells, but not serum levels of muromonab-CD3. Since approximately 50% of patients will make antibodies to this drug, the sera of all patients who receive it should be assayed for the presence of antibodies three to four weeks after beginning a course of treatment.

AVAILABLE PREPARATIONS

Only one monoclonal anti-CD3 antibody has been approved for use in the US and Europe: Orthoclone OKT®3 (Ortho Pharmaceutical Corporation). Another antibody called ORT®3 is available in South America and a few other countries. HuM291 is still under investigation and, therefore, not yet approved by regulatory agencies.

RECOMMENDED READING

Cosimi AB, Burton RC, Colvin RB, et al. Treatment of acute renal allograft rejection with OKT3® monoclonal antibody. Transplantation. 1981;32(6):535-539.

Ortho Multicenter Transplant Study Group. A randomized clinical trial of OKT3® monoclonal antibody for acute rejection of cadaveric renal transplants. N Engl J Med. 1985;313(6):337-342.

Wilde MI, Goa KL. Muromonab CD3: a reappraisal of its pharmacology and use as prophylaxis of solid organ transplant rejection. Drugs. 1996;51(5):865-894.

Chatenoud L, Ferran C, Reuter A, et al. Systemic reaction to the anti-T cell monoclonal antibody OKT3® in relation to serum levels of tumor necrosis factor and interferon-gamma [published erratum appears in N Engl J Med. 1989;321(1):63]. N Engl J Med. 1989;320(21):1420-1421.

Kimball JA, Norman DJ, Shield CF, et al. The OKT3® Antibody Response Study: a multicentre study of human anti-mouse antibody (HAMA) production following OKT3® use in solid organ transplantation. Transpl Immunol. 1995;3(3):212-221.

Sgro C. Side effects of a monoclonal antibody, muromonab CD3/orthoclone OKT3®: bibliographic review. Toxicology. 1995;105(1):23-29.

Cole MS, Stellrecht KE, Homola M, et al. HuM291, a humanized anti-CD3 antibody, is immunosuppressive to T cells while exhibiting reduced mitogenicity in vitro. Transplantation. 1999;68(4):563-571.

Hsu D-H, Shi JD, Homola M, et al. A humanized anti-CD3 antibody, HuM291, with low mitogenic activity, mediates complete reversible T cell depletion in chimpanzees. Transplantation. 1999;68(4):545-554.

Todd PA, Brogden RN. Muromonab CD3. A review of its pharmacology and therapeutic potential. Drugs. 1989;37(6):871-899.

14h ACTION, EFFICACY AND TOXICITIES: ANTI-CD25 MONOCLONAL ANTIBODIES

Flavio Vincenti, MD

HISTORY

The recent successful introduction of two monoclonal antibodies (MAbs), daclizumab (Zenapax®, Roche Laboratories), and basiliximab (Simulect®, Ortho Biotech, Inc.), targeting the α chain of the interleukin-2 receptor (IL-2R), can be attributed to the extensive investigative efforts performed on the IL-2R in the early 1980s. The α chain was the first of the three IL-2R subchains to be fully characterized, and was initially identified as Tac (for T activation) protein. However, it soon became apparent that the 55-kD protein (also referred to as CD25), as the sole chain of the IL-2R, could not account for several observations, including the fact that an anti-Tac monoclonal antibody was shown to participate in both the high-affinity and low-affinity forms of the IL-2R, and that the IL-2R α chain had a cytoplasmic domain that was too short to transduce the receptor signals to the nucleus. Thus, it became apparent that the IL-2R represented a receptor complex that included, in addition to the α chain, the β chain and the γ chain. The IL-2R β and γ chains are required to transduce the IL-2 signal inside the cell, and addition of the α chain leads to the expression of the high-affinity IL-2R. A MAb with the ability to block the interaction between IL-2 and the α chain of the high-affinity IL-2R αβγ has the potential to block the amplification of the immune response and the prevention of rejection. In fact, in 1985, Kirkman et al showed that the administration of an anti-IL-2R α MAb prolonged allograft survival in mice. Several anti-IL-2R α MAbs were shown to be effective immunosuppression agents in experimental heart, kidney and islet cell allografts, as well as in graft-vs-host disease. Clinical trials of murine or rat MAbs followed soon thereafter, and were published in the late 1980s and early 1990s. While most of these studies were performed in renal transplant patients, some were also conducted in heart transplant, as well as in liver transplant recipients. The results from trials with the rodent MAbs, while promising, were not quite convincing. Although there may be many reasons for the uninspiring results with the rodent MAbs, the most important problem undermining their effectiveness was their immunogenecity. In all these clinical trials, a majority of patients developed a rapid immune response against the xeno-antibodies. Human anti-mouse or anti-rat antibodies accelerated the clearance of these antibodies and further reduced an already short half-life below the level necessary for clinical utility. Another potentially important factor limiting the efficacy of rodent MAbs is that they are not effective in recruiting certain human immune effector functions such as antibody-dependent cell-mediated cytotoxicity (ADCC). The chimerization and humanization of rodent antibodies resulted in more humanized constructs that had prolonged half-life and lacked immunogenecity. The successful outcome of the phase 3 trials with these more humanized MAbs provided convincing and conclusive proof that blockade of the IL-2 pathway could result in a significant reduction in acute rejection.

MECHANISM OF ACTION

The mechanism by which anti-CD25 MAbs therapy prolongs graft survival is not completely understood, but has been the object of investigations both in experimental studies and in clinical trials in humans. All effective anti-CD25 MAbs block IL-2-binding to the IL-2R α, but also interfere with IL-2-driven proliferation. MAbs that bound to the IL-2R α (ie, saturate the IL-2R) but did not also block IL-2 functions were not effective in experimental models. There is no evidence that long-term tolerance occurs with therapy with anti-CD25 MAbs. Significant depletion of T cells does not appear to play a major role in the mechanism of action of these MAbs. CD3 cell counts remain stable in patients treated with both daclizumab and basiliximab. Studies with daclizumab and basiliximab suggest that the main mechanism of action of these antibodies is through blockade of the IL-2R α. However, other mechanisms of actions may mediate the effect of these antibodies. In daclizumab-treated patients, there is approximately a 50% decrease in circulating lymphocytes staining with 7G7, which is a fluorescein-conjugated antibody that binds to an epitope distinct from the epitope on the α chain that is recognized by daclizumab. Similar results were obtained by Amlot et al in studies with basiliximab. These findings indicate that therapy with the anti-IL-2R MAbs results in a relative decrease of the expression of the α chain either from depletion of coated lymphocytes and/or modulation of the α chain, secondary to decreased expression or increased shedding. There is also recent evidence that the B chain may be modulated and down-regulated by the anti-CD25 antibody.

CLINICAL ADMINISTRATION AND MONITORING IN TRANSPLANTATION

There are currently two anti-IL-2R preparations for use in clinical transplantation. Daclizumab was approved by

Professor of Clinical Medicine, Kidney Transplant Service, University of California San Francisco, San Francisco, CA

the Food and Drug Administration (FDA) in December of 1997, and basiliximab was approved in May of 1998. Daclizumab was administered in the phase 3 trials in five doses starting immediately preoperatively, and subsequently at biweekly intervals. The dose of daclizumab used was 1 mg/kg given intravenously over 15 minutes in 50 to 100 cc solution of normal saline. This regimen was shown to result in saturation of the IL-2R α on circulating lymphocytes for up to 120 days after transplantation. Daclizumab blood concentrations of about 5 μg/mL persisted in circulation for up to 70 days after transplantation. A higher concentration of daclizumab is required to block IL-2-mediated biological responses than to saturate IL-2R. In vitro, 0.1 μg of daclizumab saturates IL-2R, while concentrations of 1 to 5 μg are required to block IL-2-mediated biological responses. The half-life of daclizumab was 20 days. In the phase 3 trials, daclizumab was used with a maintenance immunosuppression regimen that consisted of triple-therapy of cyclosporine, azathioprine and steroids, or double-therapy of cyclosporine and steroids. Subsequently, daclizumab was used with a maintenance triple-therapy regimen with mycophenolate mofetil substituting for azathioprine. These regimens were found to be safe and effective in adults as well as in pediatric patients. The combination of daclizumab and maintenance triple-therapy in pediatric patients was associated with a rejection rate at six months of approximately 6%. Pediatric patients appear to be the group that benefits the most from anti-IL-2 therapy, possibly because of their large repertoire of naive T cells. Since it has been approved by the FDA, daclizumab has been used predominately in a two dose administration, preoperatively (first dose 1 mg/kg or 2 mg/kg), and at one to two weeks posttransplant. The preliminary results with this dose regimen are promising.

In the phase 3 trials, basiliximab was administered in a fixed dose of 20 mg preoperatively and on day four after transplantation. Basiliximab is administered intravenously over 30 minutes. This regimen of basiliximab was shown in a phase 1 trial to result in a concentration of >.2 μg/mL, sufficient to saturate IL-2R on circulating lymphocytes, for 25 to 35 days after transplantation. Concentrations of basiliximab required to block IL-2-mediated biological responses are about 1 μg/mL. The half-life of basiliximab was seven days. In the phase 3 trials, basiliximab was administered with double-therapy consisting of cyclosporine and prednisone, and was shown to result in a significant reduction in acute rejection. Since its release by the FDA, basiliximab has been used in the same dose regimen, frequently with triple-therapy consisting of cyclosporine, mycophenolate mofetil and prednisone. This regimen has been shown to be safe and effective in a recently reported double-blind placebo-controlled multicenter trial.

At present, there is no marker or test to monitor the effectiveness of anti-IL-2R therapy. Saturation of α chain on circulating lymphocytes, while important as a determinant of minimal blood concentrations, is not predictive of rejection during anti-IL-2R MAb therapy. Kovarik et al analyzed the influence and duration of IL-2R blockade on the incidence of acute rejection episodes in patients who participated in the phase 3 basiliximab trials and had detailed disposition analysis of basiliximab. Serum concentrations of basiliximab exceeding 0.2 μg/mL were assumed to provide complete saturation of IL-2R. Duration of receptor blockade was similar in patients with rejection and without rejection (34± 14 days vs 37±14 days, mean±SD). A possible explanation is that those patients who reject on anti-IL-2R blockade do so through a mechanism that bypasses the IL-2 pathway. In summary, while the results from the phase 3 trials proved the anti-CD25 MAbs to be safe and effective, the optimum regimens for their use require additional studies.

RECOMMENDED READING

Waldmann TA, Goldman CK. The multichain interleukin-2 receptor: a target for immunotherapy of patients receiving allografts. Am J Kidney Dis. 1989;14(5 Suppl 2):45-53.

Taniguchi T, Minami Y. The IL-2/IL-2 receptor system: a current overview. Cell. 1993;73(1):5-8.

Hakimi J, Chizzonite R, Luke DR, et al. Reduced immunogenicity and improved pharmacokinetics of humanized anti-Tac in cynomolgus monkeys. J Immunol. 1991;147(4):1352-1359.

Amlot PL, Rawlings E, Fernando ON, et al. Prolonged action of chimeric interleukin-2 receptor (CD25) monoclonal antibody used in cadaveric renal transplantation. Transplantation. 1995;60(7):748-756.

Vincenti F, Kirkman R, Light S, et al. Interleukin-2-receptor blockade with daclizumab to prevent acute rejection in renal transplantation. New Engl J Med. 1998;338(3):161-165.

Nashan B, Light S, Hardie IR, Lin A, Johnson JR. Reduction of acute renal allograft rejection by daclizumab. Daclizumab Double Therapy Study Group. Transplantation. 1999;67(1):110-115.

Nashan B, Moore R, Amlot P, Schmidt AG, Abeywickrama K, Soulillou JP. Randomized trial of basiliximab versus placebo for control of acute cellular rejection in renal allograft recipients. CHIB 201 International Study Group. Lancet. 1997;350(9096):1193-1198.

Kahan BD, Rajagopalan PR, Hall M. Reduction of the occurrence of acute cellular rejection among renal allograft recipients treated with basiliximab, a chimeric anti-interleukin-2-receptor monoclonal antibody. United States Simulect Renal Study Group. Transplantation. 1999;67(2):276-284.

Vincenti F. Targeting the interleukin-2 receptor. Clin Ren Transpl. 1999;2:56-61.

Ettinger R, Potter D, Knechtle S, Pescovitz M, Colombani P, et al. Humanized monoclonal antiinterleukin-2 receptor (IL-2R) antibody daclizumab (Zenapax®) in pediatric (Ped) renal transplantation. JASN. 1998;9:673A.

Kovarik JM, Kahan BD, Rajagopalan PR, Bennett W, et al. Population pharmacokinetics and exposure-response relationships for basiliximab in kidney transplantation. The US Simulect Renal Transplant Study Group. Transplantation. 1999;68(9):1288-1294.

14i ACTION, EFFICACY AND TOXICITIES: RAPAMYCIN

Philip F. Halloran, MD, PhD

Rapamycin, or sirolimus, is a new immunosuppressive drug that is structurally related to tacrolimus. It is chemically a macrolide (or macrocyclic lactone) antibiotic like erythromycin and many others. It was isolated from fungi found in soil samples brought from Rapa Nui by a Canadian expedition in 1968. Its unusual immunosuppressive properties were recognized by Surin Sehgal and his coworkers. It is produced by the fermentation from the organism *Streptomyces hygroscopicus*. A second, very similar agent is also being developed, termed RAD. It is likely that its characteristics, utility, and side effects will be similar to sirolimus, but it is not yet approved for clinical use.

Along with cyclosporine and tacrolimus, rapamycin is an immunophilin-binding drug. Rapamycin enters cells freely and engages the same immunophilins that bind tacrolimus, termed FK binding proteins (FKBPs) because of the old name for tacrolimus, FK506. Unlike tacrolimus:FKBP complexes, which inhibit the phosphatase calcineurin and prevent the transcription of cytokines, the rapamycin:FKBP complex does not inhibit calcineurin or cytokine transcription, but prevents the translation of mRNAs encoding cell cycle regulators.

The rapamycin:FKBP complex binds to a protein called the target of rapamycin (TOR). TOR is a kinase that is central to a pathway by which receptors for growth factors control the cell cycle (Figure 14i-1). TOR (and possibly PP2A) controls the phosphorylation of proteins, which regulate the translation of mRNAs encoding regulators of the cell cycle, namely translation inhibitor 4E-BP1, eukaryotic translation initiator protein 4G1 (eIF4G1), and p70S6 kinase. This control may be either direct or indirect, since TOR acts at least in part by regulating phosphatase PP2A. Thus, rapamycin has led to the unraveling of a previously unknown pathway by which membrane receptors regulate the initiation of the cell cycle.

Some experimental protocols show that rapamycin may spare some tolerance mechanisms and reduce "chronic rejection," although the relevance of these systems, if any, to human transplants will need to be established. Rapamycin could theoretically be of benefit in chronic allograft dysfunction in humans by inhibiting the proliferation of smooth muscle cells, but whether this is an important element in the human disease as it is in animal models is uncertain. To date there is no evidence that long-term function of human kidney grafts is improved by rapamycin compared to other contemporary immunosuppressive protocols – indeed, as mentioned below the renal function in the pivotal trials was worse with rapamycin. The published clinical trial demonstrates the efficacy of rapamycin plus cyclosporine compared to azathioprine plus cyclosporine for reducing acute rejection in renal transplants.

Significant reduction in severe rejection (Banff grade 2 and 3) and in antibody treatment for acute rejection was also demonstrated.

The toxicity of rapamycin includes mild to moderate thrombocytopenia, serious hyperlipidemia, mouth ulcers, and impaired wound healing. Rapamycin is not nephrotoxic, but it increases the effects of cyclosporine. The rapamycin treatment group experienced significant

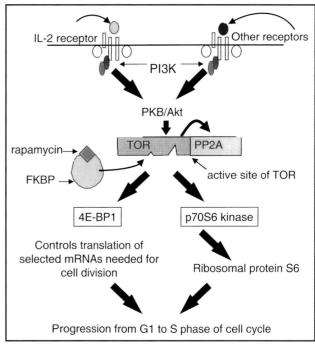

Figure 14i-1. Site of action of rapamycin. Selected cytokines (eg, IL-2) and growth factors engage receptors and activate PI3K (phosphatidyl inositol 3 kinase), which in turn activates the enzyme protein kinase B (PKB) or Akt. This in turn activates the kinase TOR, which is associated with and controls the activity of PP2A (protein phosphatase 2A). Either directly or indirectly, through PP2A, TOR controls the state of phosphorylation and activity of proteins for 4E-BP1 and p70S6 kinase. These respectively control the assembly of the translation initiation and elongation factors, and the activity of the ribosomes. The net effect is that TOR controls progression from G1 to the S phase of the cell cycle. Rapamycin combined with its binding protein FKBP engage TOR and blocks this pathway, preventing activation of translation and of ribosomal protein S6, and thus blocking the cell cycle. Other effects for rapamycin have also been reported.

Professor of Medicine and Immunology, Division of Nephrology and Immunology, University of Alberta, Edmonton, Alberta, Canada

adverse effects compared to the azathioprine controls, including impaired renal function, elevated blood pressure, and hyperlipidemia. Each of these parameters may affect long-term graft or patient survival. The reason for this is due to an incompletely understood interaction between rapamycin and cyclosporine, which may be at least partially pharmacodynamic. This also raises the possibility that some of the efficacy of rapamycin in the clinical trial may be attributable to increased exposure to cyclosporine. Indeed, the reports that rapamycin is "synergistic" with cyclosporine must now be tempered by the knowledge that rapamycin increases cyclosporine effects due to a pharmacokinetic and possibly a pharmacodynamic mechanism, making a mechanism-based synergy, if any, difficult to assess.

Rapamycin is probably best used with monitoring of blood levels, especially in patients at risk for drug interactions. It is approved for use with cyclosporine because most studies have used this combination. However, a recent randomized control trial by Kreis et al, demonstrated rapamycin in combination with MMF and steroid to be equivalent to CsA, MMF and steroids for outcomes of 12 month graft survival and patient survival. Although not statistically significant (n=78), there was a difference between the groups in the incidence of biopsy-proven rejection (rapamycin 27.5% vs CsA 18.4%). The calculated glomerular filtration rate was consistently higher in rapamycin-treated patients. Other studies of rapamycin plus steroid and rapamycin in combination with the newer anti-CD25 agents are possibilities for future study. The optimal protocol may take some time to establish. Rapamycin has drug interactions typical of immunophilin-binding drugs because of their common requirement for the cytochrome P450 enzyme IIA4 (CYP3A4) in the gut wall and liver and is a substrate for P-glycoprotein. For example, erythromycin, ketoconazole, and diltiazem increase rapamycin concentrations and anticonvulsants and rifampin decrease rapamycin concentrations.

The recommended oral dose of rapamycin is 2 mg once daily. An initial loading dose of 6 mg is recommended. It should be given four hours after a cyclosporine dose. In trials with concomitant cyclosporine, sirolimus whole blood levels, as measured by immunoassay, were 9 ng/mL for the 2 mg/day treatment group.

The pivotal studies in renal transplantation demonstrated efficacy, but suggest that the protocols used in the trials and the recommended dosing in the package insert may not be the optimal way to use the drug. Reduction of cyclosporine doses may be useful, but this will require a reevaluation of the efficacy. Some investigators have combined low dose tacrolimus with rapamycin. Rapamycin was predicted to be antagonistic to tacrolimus, because both require the same binding protein. This is true under saturating conditions but in the clinic at subsaturating conditions the two drugs can be combined

with little rejection or toxicity. This favorable experience contributed to the selection of this combination by the Canadian team who has recently reported success with islet transplants. Transplant clinicians will want to see large, long-term experience with the tacrolimus-rapamycin combination before they judge its merits. Use of rapamycin without calcineurin inhibitors, possibly in combination with mycophenolate mofetil and/or various monoclonals, will also be of interest.

RECOMMENDED READING

Gingras AC, Gygi SP, Raught B, et al. Regulation of 4E-BP1 phosphorylation: a novel two-step mechanism. Genes Dev. 1999;13(11):1422-1437.

Gregory CR, Huie P, Billingham ME, Morris RE. Rapamycin inhibits arterial intimal thickening caused by both alloimmune and mechanical injury. Its effect on cellular, growth factor, and cytokine responses in injured vessels. Transplantation. 1993;55(6):1409-1418.

Groth CG, Backman L, Morales JM, et al. Sirolimus (rapamycin)-based therapy in human renal transplantation: similar efficacy and different toxicity compared with cyclosporine. Sirolimus European Renal Transplant Study Group. Transplantation. 1999;67(7):1036-1042.

Heitman J, Movva NR, Hall MN. Targets for cell cycle arrest by the immunosuppressant rapamycin in yeast. Science. 1991;253(5022):905-909.

Kahan BD. Efficacy of sirolimus compared with azathioprine for reduction of acute renal allograft rejection: a randomised multicentre study. The Rapamune US Study Group. Lancet. 2000;356(9225):194-202.

Kreis H, Cisterne JM, Land W, et al. Sirolimus in association with mycophenolate mofetil induction for the prevention of acute graft rejection in renal allograft recipients. Transplantation. 2000;69(7):1252-1260.

Table 14i-1.

Biopsy-proven rejection at six months in the three groups in the US study were:	
The CsA aza P group CsA rap 2 P CsA rap 5 P	29.2 16.5 11.3
Biopsy proven rejection at six months in the European study were:	
CsA placebo P CsA rap 2 P CsA rap 5 pred	41.7 24.7 19.2

Li Y, Li XC, Zheng XX, Wells AD, Turka LA, Strom TB. Blocking both signal 1 and signal 2 of T-cell activation prevents apoptosis of alloreactive T cells and induction of peripheral allograft tolerance. Nat Med. 1999;5(11):1298-1302.

McAlister VC, Gao Z, Peltekian K, Domingues J, Mahalati K, MacDonald AS. Sirolimus-tacrolimus combination immunosuppression. Lancet. 2000;355(9201): 376-377.

Murphy PM. The molecular biology of leukocyte chemoattractant receptors. Ann Rev Immunol. 1994; 12:593-633.

Peterson RT, Desai BN, Hardwick JS, Schreiber SL. Protein phosphatase 2A interacts with the 70-kDa S6 kinase and is activated by inhibition of FKBP12-rapamycin-associated protein. Proc Natl Acad Sci USA. 1999;96(8):4438-4442.

Raught B, Gingras AC, Gygi SP, et al. Serum-stimulated, rapamycin-sensitive phosphorylation sites in the eukaryotic translation factor 4GI. EMBO J. 2000;19(3): 434-444.

Sehgal SN, Baker H, Vézina C. Rapamycin (AY-22,989), a new antifungal antibiotic. II. Fermentation, isolation and characterization. J Antibiot. 1975;28(10):727-732.

Shapiro AMJ, Lakey JRT, Ryan EA, et al. Islet transplantation in seven patients with Type 1 diabetes mellitus using a glucocorticoid-free immunosuppressive regimen. N Engl J Med. 2000;343(4):230-238.

Vézina C, Kudelski A, Sehgal SN. Rapamycin (AY-22,989), a new antifungal antibiotic. I. Taxonomy of the producing streptomycete and isolation of the active principle. J Antibiot. 1975;28(10):721-726.

15 NONBIOLOGICS

Jochen Klupp, MD
Randall E. Morris, MD

The first edition of this textbook, published in 1998, reviewed several new small molecular weight immunosuppressants: rapamycin, mizoribine, brequinar, leflunomide and deoxyspergualin. None of these will be reviewed in this edition, because they have been approved for use (eg, rapamycin for transplantation in the US, mizoribine and deoxyspergualin for transplantation in Japan, and leflunomide for rheumatoid arthritis in the US and Europe), or because no additional development has occurred (ie, brequinar). Leflunomide, however, will be reviewed because its active metabolite is a member of the malononitrilamide (MNA) drug class, and two new MNA analogs are being actively developed for use as immunosuppressants for transplantation.

Because there are so many new drugs currently in development, and it is impossible to predict which of them will be of clinical use (either as new primary or adjunctive therapy), this chapter has been organized based on the known mechanisms of action of these new nonbiologic immunosuppressants.

NEW INHIBITORS OF NUCLEOTIDE SYNTHESIS
VX-497

VX-497 was rationally designed based on the three-dimensional crystal structure of inositol monophosphate dehydrogenase (IMPDH). VX-497 belongs to a new class of phenyl oxazole inhibitors of IMPDH, and is structurally unrelated to other IMPDH inhibitors like mycophenolic acid (MPA) or ribavirin. In vitro, this uncompetitive and reversible inhibitor of IMPDH down-regulates proliferation of human lymphocytes dose-dependently. In vivo, VX-497 prolongs skin graft survival in mice and prolongs heterotopic heart graft survival in a Brown Norway (BN) to Lewis (LEW) heart transplant model.

The main difference between VX497 and MPA is the absence of enterohepatic circulation for VX-497. Since

Jochen Klupp, MD, Research Professor, Transplantation Immunology, Department of Cardiothoracic Surgery, Stanford University School of Medicine, Stanford, CA

Randall E. Morris, MD, Professor; Director of Transplantation Immunology, Cardiothoracic Surgery, Department of Cardiothoracic Surgery, Stanford University School of Medicine, Stanford, CA

this enterohepatic recirculation is thought to be the main reason for gastrointestinal toxicity from treatment with mycophenolate mofetil, this aspect of VX-497 may lead to an improved tolerability. In effective doses (ie, 75 mg/kg twice daily), VX-497 caused no enteritis in histopathological studies.

Although only limited data are available for VX-497, this drug offers a new perspective in drug development: using structure-based drug design to create a new molecule that inhibits a validated target (IMPDH) while simultaneously increasing safety by altering its route of excretion. Future work will be needed to determine whether VX-497 is as effective as mycophenolate mofetil, and to determine whether this new chemical entity can be used safely.

Malononitrilamides

Leflunomide (HWA 486) was first reported as a new chemical entity in 1976, but its ability to suppress immune function was not reported until 1985. Since then, the clinical, pharmacological and pharmacokinetic profiles of the drug itself and its active metabolite have become better understood. The active metabolite of leflunomide (A77 1726) has a long plasma half-life of 11 to 16 days. Therefore, changes in dose are not rapidly translated into changes in levels. This is not a problem in the treatment of rheumatoid arthritis because patients are on a fixed dose. However, if leflunomide were to be used in transplant patients, and if it were to require constant dose adjustment to maintain a narrow range of plasma levels, its long half-life would be a liability. There are no plans to develop leflunomide for transplantation, because it is at the end of its patent life.

In the last decade, more than 80 derivatives of the malononitrilamides (MNAs) have been created by systematically exchanging molecular side groups. Two compounds, MNA279 and MNA715, have been selected for further development. These are now known as FK779 and FK778. In contrast to leflunomide, FK778 and, especially, FK779 have a shorter half-life in rodents. Both have a very good oral bioavailability. Like A77 1726, both are able to bind specifically to dihydro-orotate-dehydrogenase (DHODH) and inhibit, dose-dependently, de novo pyrimidine biosynthesis. DHODH is the fourth enzyme in the de novo pathway for pyrimidine biosynthesis (Figure 15-1) and is located on the inner membrane of the mitochondria. Pyrimidine nucleotides are essential for RNA and DNA synthesis, and for membrane lipid biosynthesis and protein glycosylation. Activated T and B cells rely primarily on the de novo pathway for both purine and pyrimidine biosynthesis, whereas other cell types and resting T and B cells are able to synthesize purines and pyrimidines using the salvage pathway.

MECHANISM OF ACTION. Leflunomide and its active metabolite A77 1726 are able to inhibit T cell activation directly, T cell-independent B cell activation, IgG and IgM antibody production, and smooth muscle cell proliferation in vitro. Thus, it was expected that the MNAs would have the same mechanism of action. Data showed that FK778 inhibited human T cell activation independent of the type of the mode of stimulation. In a culture of purified human B cells, activated by the presence of BHK$_{CD40L}$ cells, FK778 effectively inhibited the proliferative response, as well as IgG and IgM synthesis. FK779 and FK778 also have an effect on monocyte function and are able to reduce oxygen-radical formation.

The primary mechanism by which MNAs inhibit cell proliferation is believed by some to be inhibition of membrane receptor-associated protein tyrosine kinase. However, later studies showed that concentrations required for inhibiting tyrosine kinase far exceed the concentration required for antiproliferative effects. It is possible that concentrations of MNAs in vivo could be high enough that inhibition of tyrosine kinase activity contributes to the antiproliferative effect of these drugs.

PRECLINICAL ANIMAL STUDIES. Prompted by their ability to suppress T and B cell proliferation, including IgG and IgM response, FK778 and FK779 were examined for treatment of graft-vs-host disease. In an acute life-threatening graft-vs-host disease model involving injection of 1×10^8 parenteral C57B1/6 spleno-cytes into B6C3F1 hybrid recipient mice, both MNAs were able to prolong survival in a dose-dependent manner (2.5 to 20 mg/kg). With high concentrations, mortality was prevented completely.

In different rodent models (ie, LEW to Fisher [F344], Dark Agouti [DA] to LEW), FK778 and FK779 were able to prolong skin allograft survival in a dose-dependent manner after oral gavage. The minimum effective dose (2.5 mg/kg) prolonged graft survival for five to ten days. Both MNAs showed similar dose response curves and an efficacy equal to cyclosporine in preventing acute skin graft rejection. For reversal of acute rejection, again, both MNAs were effective at a dose of 10 mg/kg, whereas a delayed treatment with cyclosporine (20 mg/kg) failed to rescue the skin grafts. Potentiation of efficacy was also shown between tacrolimus and MNAs for prevention and treatment of skin allograft rejection. Using a combination of ineffective doses of tacrolimus (0.2 mg/kg), and FK778 or FK779 (20 mg/kg), tolerance induction (survival >75 days) was achieved after withdrawal of immunosuppression at day 20.

After heterotopic heart transplantation between different strains of rats, oral treatment of 10 mg/kg FK778 resulted in indefinite graft survival. Even after stopping immunosuppression, more than half of the grafts survived longer than three months. Delayed treatment, from postoperative day four on, prolonged graft survival from 38 to more than 100 days. Furthermore, the

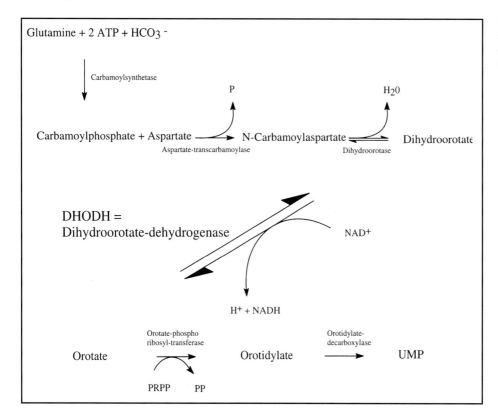

Figure 15-1. De novo pyrimidine synthesis. DHODH is the fourth enzyme in the synthesis, which is inhibited by the MNAs.

Glutamine + 2 ATP + HCO$_3$⁻

Carbamoylsynthetase

P

H$_2$0

Carbamoylphosphate + Aspartate ⟶ N-Carbamoylaspartate ⇌ Dihydroorotate

Aspartate-transcarbamoylase

Dihydroorotase

DHODH = Dihydroorotate-dehydrogenase

NAD⁺

H⁺ + NADH

Orotate-phospho ribosyl-transferase

Orotidylate-decarboxylase

Orotate ⟶ Orotidylate ⟶ UMP

PRPP   PP

MNAs potentiated the immunosuppressive effect of cyclosporine in the rat heart model.

In a life-dependent kidney transplantation trial (DA to PVG), ten days of FK779 treatment (10 mg/kg) prolongs animal survival to 36.5 ± 34.0 days vs nine days in the control group. In a dose evaluation study, 50% of the treated rats died after dosing with 15 mg/kg FK779 due to gastrointestinal side effects. At 7.5 mg/kg, no toxicity was observed and kidney allograft survival was prolonged for up to 34 days, with only slight increases in urea and creatinine.

The ability of the MNAs to prevent smooth muscle cell proliferation led to studies preventing and treating graft vascular disease and chronic rejection. It could be demonstrated that, in BN femoral allograft segments transplanted orthotopically into LEW rats, intimal thickening was reduced by MNAs at a dose of 10 mg/kg.

Blocking T cell-independent B cell activation and antibody formation is a promising mode of action for suppressing responses to xenografts. In the mouse-to-rat skin xenograft model, FK778 and FK779 prolong skin graft survival dose-dependently (10 to 20 mg/kg). Also, delayed therapy increases graft survival significantly. Xenoantibody formation was reduced at a dose of 20 mg/kg. Both cyclosporine and tacrolimus potentiate the efficacy of the MNAs, whereas single-therapy with an ineffective dose of cyclosporine (10 mg/kg) or tacrolimus (0.2 mg/kg) is not able to prolong xenograft survival.

In the hamster-to-rat cardiac xenotransplantation model, a combination of cyclosporine and MNAs results in a long-term xenograft survival. After administration of 10 mg/kg cyclosporine and 10 mg/kg of FK778, graft survival is prolonged for over 30 days.

In summary, these studies demonstrate that the MNAs are promising new immunosuppressive agents. Blocking T cell and B cell proliferation, and potentiation of the efficacy of cyclosporine or tacrolimus support ongoing development of these MNAs and other members of this class for immunosuppression. Ongoing preclinical efficacy studies in nonhuman primates and human phase 1 trials will provide the pharmacokinetic, efficacy, and safety data that will determine which of the MNAs enters phase 2 trials.

Deazaguanine Analogues

Purine nucleoside phosphorylase (PNP) is an essential enzyme of the purine salvage pathway. It has been shown that humans with an inherited deficiency of PNP have a relatively selective depletion of T cells, while B cell immunity remains intact. Most likely, this selective inhibition of T cells is secondary to an accumulation of deoxyguanosine-triphosphate (dGTP), which apparently suppresses ribonucleotide reductase activity and hence, DNA synthesis.

8-Amino-guanosine and 8-amino-9-benzyl-guanine derivatives have been developed to inhibit PNP. However, they showed high toxicity in doses required for T cell suppression. Applying crystallographic methods and structure-based design, new PNP-inhibitors (9-deazaguanine derivatives) were developed for treatment of T cell-mediated inflammatory responses, T cell leukemia, and prevention of organ rejection. BCX-34 (2-amino-1,5-dihydro-7-(3-pyridimylmethyl)-4H-pyrrolo[3,2-d]pyrimidin-4-one) is a potent 9-deazaguanine derivative, which is not only able to increase intracellular dGTP in human cells, but also to decrease intracellular guanosine-triphosphate (GTP). Decreased pools of GTP, caused by mycophenolic acid, is known to suppress T cell proliferation.

In vitro, BCX-34 inhibits human, mouse and rat red blood cell PNP with IC_{50}s of 36, 32 and 5 nmol, respectively. In a T cell culture of human leukemia cells (CCRF-CEM), BCX-34 inhibits cell proliferation in the presence, but not in the absence of deoxyguanine (dGuo). Deoxycytidine reverses the inhibition caused by BCX-34 and dGuo. The maximum inhibitory effect on human PNP and T cell proliferation is about 80%, whereas BCX-34 is not able to inhibit rat or mouse T cell proliferation. Since PNP in rodent T cells is inhibited, the reason for its lack of efficacy is explained by the fact that rodent T cells do not accumulate dGTP, but the mechanism responsible for the failure of rodent cells to accumulate dGTP is not understood.

The pharmacokinetics of BCX-34 showed a rapid disappearance after IV injection (within three hours; 1 mg/kg in rats), and a good oral bioavailability of 76%. Half-lives were not calculated in these studies, but detectable plasma levels were observed 12 hours after a 10 mg/kg oral dose of BCX-34. Toxicological data have not been published, and only neurological disorders of PNP-deficient patients suggest what the adverse effects of this drug may be.

Because BCX-34 is not able to inhibit rodent T cell proliferation, no in vivo efficacy data are available yet. Clinical trials are testing BCX-34 in dermal applications for psoriasis and T cell lymphoma. Based on its mechanism of action, its high bioavailability, and its capability to potentiate the efficacies of cyclosporine and tacrolimus, BCX-34 may be used in transplantation. Further toxicological trials and efficacy studies in nonhuman primates would have to be done to better predict its future for use in transplant patients.

NEW INHIBITORS OF SIGNAL I PATHWAY
Potassium Channel Blockers

During T cell activation, sustained elevated Ca^{2+} levels are needed to activate gene expression. After T cell receptor complex stimulation, inositol 1,4,5-trisphosphate (IP^3) formation causes Ca^{2+} release from intracellular calcium stores. Emptying of the stores triggers Ca^{2+} influx through Ca^{2+} release-activated Ca^{2+} channels, which is maintained by potassium efflux channels keeping T cell membrane polarized.

Blocking potassium channels in T lymphocytes in vitro has effects similar to calcineurin inhibitors. CD2-stimulated, CD3-stimulated or ionomycin plus PMA-stimulated T cells can be inhibited as measured by ^{3}H-thymidine proliferation and IL-2 production. This effect can be reversed by addition of exogenous IL-2. Nonselective potassium channel blockers like tetraethylammonium (TEA) and 4-aminopyridine (4-AP) show these effects in a very high, milli-molar range.

Nonspecific inhibition of potassium channels, however, would cause severe toxicity in clinical application. Further investigations showed that there are different subsets of potassium channels. For example, Kv1.3 – a voltage-gated channel, is of special interest because it is expressed abundantly in lymphocytes, compared to lower levels in fibroblasts, brain and kidney cells, and dominates the membrane potential only in T lymphocytes.

Polypeptides isolated from scorpion venoms are able to block potassium channels in the pico-molar range. Charybdotoxin inhibits Ca^{2+}-activated and voltage-gated potassium channels, and is able to inhibit T cell activation dose-dependently. Margatoxin is more specific than charybdotoxin, since margatoxin only inhibits voltage-gated channels. However, margatoxin is not specific for lymphocytes because it also inhibits Kv1.1 and Kv1.2 channels, which are expressed in brain, peripheral nerves and the heart. In vivo studies of these toxins are complicated by the fact that Kv1.3 is not expressed by rat cells or by cells of many other experimental animals. One study in mini-pigs showed that margatoxin after IV administration of 8 μg/kg per day inhibits delayed-type hypersensitivity to tuberculin, as well as an antibody response to alloantigen as effectively as 1 mg/kg per day of tacrolimus. As expected, higher doses showed neurological side effects. CP-339,818, a 1,4-dihydroquinoline compound, blocks both Kv1.3 and Kv1.4, so it is not being developed for clinical use.

Structural changes of the sea anemone toxin, ShK, generated ShK-Dap[22], which is a highly selective and potent blocker of Kv1.3 (IC_{50} of 102 pmol). ShK-Dap[22] inhibits ^{3}H-thymidine incorporation in peripheral human T cells after mitogen stimulation, with an IC_{50} below 500 pmol. When injected into mice, ShK-Dap[22] showed only minimal toxicity.

Although further studies are required on potassium channel blockers, this group of substances has the potential to inhibit signal 1 pathway specifically, and may have the potential to suppress graft rejection. Promising substances like ShK-Dap[22] need still more

development to increase its oral bioavailability and its reduced toxicity before it can be used in large animal studies or human phase 1 trials.

SP100030

SP100030, 2-Chloro-4-(trifluoromethyl)-5-N-phenyl-pyrimidine-carboxamide, is an agent that is able to inhibit NF-κB and AP-1, both known to be crucial for signal 1 transduction to induce IL-1, IL-2, IL-6, IL-8, TNF-α, and cell adhesion molecule transcription.

In a popliteal lymph node study (BALB/c - C3H mice), SP100030 dose-dependently suppresses the alloantigen-induced PLN weight. In a murine ear-heart transplant model, 15 to 20 mg/kg SP100030, administered intraperitoneally, prolongs graft survival significantly for more than 30 days. Also, adjuvant arthritis is reduced effectively in LEW rats (20 to 30 mg/kg intraperitoneally). No body weight changes or other toxicological side effects have been observed in these studies.

Although the experience with SP100030 is limited to rodent models, the results obtained show that focusing on key enzymes of signal 1 pathway should be able to produce significant immunosuppression with a good safety profile.

Tepoxalin

Another potent inhibitor of NF-κB activation is tepoxalin (5-[4-chlorophenyl]-N-hydroxy-[4-methoxyphenyl]-N-methyl-1-H-pyrazole-3-propanamide; molecular weight is 385). It was first discovered as a dual inhibitor of 5-lipoxygenase (LO) and cyclooxygenase (CO), and is effective in preventing inflammation and synovitis in several animal models. Because of its inability to inhibit gastric prostaglandin synthesis, tepoxalin does not cause gastric mucosa damage at antiinflammatory doses. Further investigations showed that naproxen and other CO inhibitors, as well as zileuton (an LO inhibitor), do not show the same antiproliferative effects as tepoxalin.

By its inhibition of NF-κB, tepoxalin also suppresses expression of the cell adhesion molecules CD62E (E-selectin), CD11b/CD18 (Mac-1), and CD106 (VCAM-1), but not CD11a/CD18 (LFA-1) and CD54 (ICAM-1). Because CD11b/CD18 and CD106 are effective in monocyte adhesion processes, tepoxalin is expected to modulate atherosclerosis and inflammation, as well as neutrophil migration. Mixed lymphocyte reaction (MLR) was suppressed with an IC_{50} of 1.3 μmol.

In vivo, tepoxalin suppresses local graft-vs-host responses by about 40% in mice. In skin transplantation (BALB/cByJ [H-2^d] to C3H/HeJ [H-2^k] mice), tepoxalin prolongs median survival time to 15 days with a 50 mg/kg dose, compared to eight days in the control group. Co-administration of suboptimal doses of tepoxalin (12.5 mg/kg) and cyclosporine (50 mg/kg) prolongs skin graft survival for more than 40 days, suggesting synergism between both drugs.

The toxicological and pharmacological profiles of tepoxalin are showing promising results. In mice and rats, LD^{50} is more than tenfold higher than immunosuppressive doses (>400 mg/kg). In healthy human volunteers, oral doses from 35 mg to 300 mg were absorbed rapidly and reached t_{max} after two to three hours of administration. No major adverse events have been recorded. Five out of 20 healthy participants reported abdominal discomfort, diarrhea or light-headedness.

In summary, by blocking NF-κB, tepoxalin is mechanistically different from cyclosporine and tacrolimus, and acts synergistically with cyclosporine. With only minor toxicity and a good pharmacological profile, transplantation studies in larger animals could be promising.

Protein Tyrosine Kinase Inhibitors

Genistein (5,7,4'-trihydroxyflavone), an isoflavanoid compound, has been shown to specifically inhibit protein tyrosine kinases (PTK). Genistein is able to reduce activated killer T lymphocyte-mediated lysis of tumor cells by 50% in a 100 μmol/L solution. Other PTK inhibitors such as herbimycin A showed a higher potency in the same experimental setting (93% inhibition by 2 μmol). Genistein (180 μmol) inhibits the induction of Fas-based cytotoxicity and is also able to inhibit PMA or PHA/anti-CD28-stimulated T cell proliferation in a 40 μmol solution. Also, IL-2R and IL-2 production are inhibited by genistein at the same concentrations needed for inhibition of proliferation.

PT 1, a synthetic derivative of genistein, was further evaluated in an in vivo study with pancreatic islet allograft transplantation; results showed that LEW rats treated with 3 mg/kg PT 1 for 15 days accepted Wistar-Furth islet allografts for almost 100 days.

Others

Other signal 1 inhibitors are listed in Table 13-1. Reports of these drugs are only anecdotal and their future importance will be seen.

NEW INHIBITORS OF SIGNAL 2 PATHWAY
Methylxanthine Derivatives

Methylxanthine derivatives are known to have some immunomodulatory effects. However, the IC_{50}s of theophylline (>400 μmol) and pentoxifylline (113 μmol) are higher than plasma levels, which can be achieved in clinical settings. By inhibition of cAMP phosphodiesterase activity, methylxanthine derivatives are able to suppress T cell proliferation to alloantigens and mitogens, and inhibit generation of cytotoxic T lymphocytes and natural killer cell-mediated cytolysis. These effects are mainly due to suppression of TH_1 function by reducing production of inflammatory cytokines, including TNF-α, IFN-γ and IL-2. Due to high plasma levels required, pentoxifylline showed no effect on the incidence of rejection episodes in renal transplant patients.

A802715 (7-propyl-1-[5-hydroxy-5 methylhexyl]-3 methylxanthin) was further developed because of its lower IC_{50} (41 μmol) in suppressing TNF-α and IFN-γ production after LPS stimulation. Additionally, A802715 enhances TH_2-driven cytokines like IL-6 and IL-10. In contrast to other methylxanthine derivatives, A802715 is able to suppress not only CD3-stimulated human T cells, but also CD28-stimulated human T cells. In vitro, a synergistic effect between A802715 and cyclosporine was shown with a high combination index (1/CI=9, where 1/CI >1 is synergistic) in MLR and cell-mediated lympholysis assays. Whereas signal I inhibition can be ascribed to cAMP elevation, the mechanism of additional signal II inhibition of A802715 is not known.

In vivo, it was also proven that minimally effective oral doses of A802715 (100 mg/kg per day) in combination with cyclosporine (7.5 mg/kg per day) for 30 days led to long-term survival of cardiac allografts in rats. In an MHC-compatible model (Wag/Rij - R/A), this combination results in donor-specific tolerance by suppressing cytotoxic T cells and persisting TH_2 cells. Tolerance could not be achieved in a MHC-incompatible model (WKAH - PVG).

Table 15-1. New Inhibitors of Signal I Pathway

Hydroquinone	Inhibits NF-κB reversibly. Plausible cause of toxicity of cigarettes.	Pyatt et al, 1998
Momordins	Reduces Jan/Fos binding to AP-1.	Lee et al, 1998
Ro 09-2210	Small molecule isolated from fungus FC2506. Able to block CD3 and CD25-induced T cell proliferation; inhibits AP-1 and selectively MEK1.	Williams et al, 1998
YM-53792	Inhibitor of NF-AT activation but not of AP-1 or NFκB. Inhibits IL-2, IL-4, IL-5 in peripheral blood.	Kuromitsu et al, 1997
Lymphostatin	Inhibits protein-tyrosine kinase p56lck dose dependently. Suppresses IL-2 production in vitro and MLR.	Aotani et al, 1997 Nagata et al, 1997

Methylxanthines may also be beneficial by decreasing cyclosporine side effects. Cyclosporine-induced nephrotoxicity may be caused by decreased cAMP levels and pentoxifylline was effective in decreasing cyclosporine-induced toxicity, probably related to an effect on endothelin release and vasoconstriction.

The combination of methylxanthine derivatives with an additional inhibitory effect on signal II, like A802715, with cyclosporine is promising not only because of its synergistic effect in immunosuppression, but also by its potential reversal of cyclosporine nephropathy.

OTHERS
FTY720

Myriocin (ISP-1) was isolated from the ascomycete *Isaria sinclairii*, which is parasitic in insects and plants. Extracts from this fungi imperfecti have been used widely in traditional Chinese medicine. However, ISP-1 produced fatal side effects in experimental animals during drug evaluation and further development was stopped. FTY720 (2-amino-2-[2-(4-octylphenyl)ethyl]-1,3-propanediol hydrochloride [$C_{19}H_{33}NO_2$–HCL], with a molecular weight of 343.94 Da) is a synthetic structural analog of ISP-1.

FTY720 has a completely new mechanism of action, which is not related to any other mechanism of action of any known immunosuppressive agent. It inhibits T cell-dependent and independent immunity, and suppresses T cell infiltration into grafted organs by depletion of peripheral lymphocytes to 3% of the original cell count within three hours after oral application. FTY720 does not effect T or B cell function in vitro in concentrations that are able to modulate immune response in vivo. Although the mechanism of action is not yet fully understood, it is likely that FTY720 acts by a combination of altered T cell traffic, but probably not by inducing apoptosis as originally thought.

MECHANISM OF ACTION. ISP-1 and related compounds inhibit allogenic mixed lymphocyte reactions (MLR) and IL-2-dependent proliferation in a mouse cell line. However, in doses up to 1,000 nmol/L, FTY720 does not inhibit MLR, IL-2 production, mRNA expression by antigen-stimulated or mitogen-stimulated T cells, cytokine-driven cell proliferation, or cytotoxic T cell generation or action. High concentrations (4×10^{-6} M) added in vitro to rat lymphocytes induce chromatin condensation, formation of apoptotic bodies, and DNA fragmentation. Two lines of evidence led to the hypothesis that FTY720 leads to apoptotic cell death. First, FTY720 (10 mg/kg) induces a marked reduction of peripheral lymphocytes in rats, and second, dead cells increased with time in spleen cells cultured with FTY720.

More recent reports, however, indicate that FTY720 acts by selectively depleting T and B cells from blood, and sequesters lymphocytes into lymph nodes and Peyer's plaques. The initial explanations for this mechanism of action were that FTY720 increases adhesion of lymphocytes to high endothelial venules in the lymphoid tissues by up-regulating LFA-1, ICAM-1, and L-selectin. Later analysis showed that FTY720 does not modulate selectins and adhesion molecule expression in lymphocytes and high endothelial venules. Since the effect of FTY720 is blocked by pertussis toxin, it has been suggested that FTY720 functions through G-protein-coupled receptors, and that an increased response of the lymphocytes to chemokines may cause the homing into lymph nodes and Peyer's plaques. Supporting the hypothesis that FTY720 is acting by increasing the homing of lymphocytes, rather than by inducing T cell death, is that FTY720 does not alter the function of the resting memory T cell pool. For example, mice immune to lymphocytic choriomeningitis virus efficiently eliminate the virus from lung, kidney, liver, spleen and blood after ending FTY720 treatment.

TOXICITY AND PHARMACOKINETICS. While ISP-1 induces severe digestive disorders at a dose of 1 mg/kg, resulting in death of the animals, the toxicologic profile of FTY720 is completely different: it was observed to have no toxic effects on rats (3 mg/kg) and monkeys (0.3 mg/kg) at doses that are immunosuppressive. LD_{50} in rats is 300 to 600 mg/kg and no deaths were reported in dogs that received a single dose of less than 200 mg/kg. Rats gained weight during 5 mg/kg treatment and showed only slightly increased levels of BUN, creatinine, and transaminase. In other toxicologic studies, no renal, pancreatic or bone marrow toxicity was observed. At high concentrations, adverse effects on the lungs have been recorded.

Oral bioavailability in rats (80%), dogs (60%), and monkeys (40%) is good, with a half-life of 12 to 29 hours in a dose range between 0.1 and 3 mg/kg. None of the identified metabolites are immunosuppressive. The metabolites are excreted in urine and feces at ratios between 20% to 50% in different species.

PRECLINICAL ANIMAL STUDIES. In autoimmune and antiinflammatory models, FTY720 inhibited hypersensitivity responses in mice (0.03 mg/kg), joint destruction in an arthritis model in rats (0.1 mg/kg), and allergic encephalomyelitis. In dose-response studies, 0.1 to 10 mg/kg FTY720 prolongs skin, heart, liver and small bowel survival in rats. Also, in graft-vs-host disease in rats, FTY720 causes unresponsiveness (0.1 to 0.3 mg/kg). In canine kidney transplantation, FTY720 given twice (5 mg/kg) before and on the day of operation resulted in a median graft survival of 21 days vs nine days in the control group. Posttransplant daily dosing (5 mg/kg) is not effective. However, FTY 720, when combined with a subtherapeutic dose of cyclosporine (10 mg/kg), prolongs graft survival significantly. Synergistic interaction with cyclosporine (CI=0.15 to 0.37) or sirolimus (CI=0.22 to 0.53) was also reported in heart, liver and small bowel transplantation in rats and with tacrolimus in heart transplantation. In a nonhuman primate kidney model, FTY720 and subtherapeutic cyclosporine prolongs graft survival in a supra-additive effect. Furthermore, FTY720 (5 mg/kg) is able to reverse ongoing rejections after heterotopic heart and orthotopic liver transplants in rats and after kidney transplantation in dogs. Together with allochimeric class I MHC antigen, FTY720 induces tolerance in a Wistar-Furth-to-ACI rat heart transplant model.

In summary, FTY720 shows promising results in different animal studies. Its different mode of action and acceptable safety profile in animals suggest this drug will have a role in clinical transplantation in combination with other drugs, or as rescue-therapy for ongoing rejections.

OUTLOOK AND FUTURE

It is hard to predict which of these drugs will be introduced into clinical trials or part of a future standard immunosuppressive regimen. Many drugs will probably fail due to unbalanced toxicity and efficacy. Others, not yet published, will therefore appear. Some of the most advanced and promising drugs of this chapter are the MNAs, BCX-34 or FTY720. They are already, or will shortly be in human trials. Additionally, the success or failure of monoclonal antibody treatment directed against signal II antigens will have a major impact on the development of future nonbiologic immunosuppressants.

RECOMMENDED READING

Silva Junior HT, Morris RE. Leflunomide and malononitrilamides. Am J Med Sci. 1997;313(5):289-301.

Schorlemmer H, Bartlett R, Kurrle R. Malononitrilamides: a new strategy of immunosuppression for allo- and xenotransplantation. Transplant Proc. 1998;30(3): 884-890.

Qi Z, Ekberg H. Malononitrilamides 715 and 279 prolong rat cardiac allograft survival, reverse ongoing rejection, inhibit allospecific antibody production and interact positively with cyclosporin. Scand J Immunol. 1998;48(4):379-388.

Gummert JF, Ikonen T, Morris RE. Newer immunosuppressive drugs: a review. J Am Soc Nephrol. 1999;10(6):1366-1380.

Schorlemmer HU, Kurrle R, Bartlett RR. The new immunosuppressants, the malononitrilamides MNA 279 and MNA 715, inhibit various graft-vs.-host diseases (GvHD) in rodents. Drugs Exp Clin Res. 1997;23(5-6):167-173.

Bantia S, Montgomery JA, Johnson HG, Walsh GM. In vivo and in vitro pharmacologic activity of the purine nucleoside phosphorylase inhibitor BCX-34: the role of GTP and dGTP. Immunopharmacology. 1996;35(1):53-63.

Conry RM, Bantia S, Turner HS, et al. Effects of a novel purine nucleoside phosphorylase inhibitor, BCX-34, on activation and proliferation of normal human lymphoid cells. Immunopharmacology. 1998;40(1):1-9.

Iwata H, Wada Y, Walsh M, et al. In vitro study of BCX-34: a new human T-lymphocyte-specific purine phosphorylase inhibitor. Transplant Proc. 1998;30(4):983-986.

Lin CS, Boltz RC, Blake JT, et al. Voltage-gated potassium channels regulate calcium-dependent pathways involved in human T lymphocyte activation. J Exp Med. 1993;177(3):637-645.

Lewis RS, Cahalan MD. Potassium and calcium channels in lymphocytes. Ann Rev Immunol. 1995;13:623-653.

Koo GC, Blake JT, Talento A, et al. Blockade of the voltage-gated potassium channel Kv1.3 inhibits immune responses in vivo. J Immunol. 1997;158(11):5120-5128.

Nguyen A, Kath JC, Hanson DC, et al. Novel nonpeptide agents potently block the C-type inactivated conformation of Kv1.3 and suppress T cell activation. Mol Pharmacol. 1996;50(6):1672-1679.

Goldman ME, Ransone LJ, Anderson DW, et al. SP100030 is a novel T-cell-specific transcription factor inhibitor that possesses immunosuppressive activity in vivo. Transplant Proc. 1996;28(6):3106-3109.

Fung-Leung WP, Pope BL, Chourmouzis E, Panakos JA, Lau CY. Tepoxalin, a novel immunomodulatory compound, synergizes with CsA in suppression of graft-vs-host reaction and allogeneic skin graft rejection. Transplantation. 1995;60(4):362-368.

Kazmi SM, Plante RK, Visconti V, Taylor GR, Zhou L, Lau CY. Suppression of NF kappa B activation and NF kappa B-dependent gene expression by tepoxalin, a dual inhibitor of cyclooxygenase and 5-lipoxygenase. J Cell Biochem. 1995;57(2):299-310.

Zhou L, Ritchie D, Wang EY, Barbone AG, Argentieri D, Lau CY. Tepoxalin, a novel immunosuppressive agent with a different mechanism of action from cyclosporin A. J Immunol. 1994;153(11):5026-5037.

Martinez-Martinez S, Gomez del Arco P, Armesilla AL, et al. Blockade of T-cell activation by dithiocarbamates involves novel mechanisms of inhibition of nuclear factor of activated T cells. Mol Cell Biol. 1997;17(11):6437-6447.

Bessho R, Matsubara K, Kubota M, et al. Pyrrolidine dithiocarbamate, a potent inhibitor of nuclear factor kappa B (NF-kappa B) activation, prevents apoptosis in human promyelocytic leukemia HL-60 cells and thymocytes. Biochem Pharmacol. 1994;48(10):1883-1889.

Lin Y, Goebels J, Rutgeerts O, et al. Use of the methylxanthine derivative A802715 in transplantation immunology: I. Strong in vitro inhibitory effects on CD28-costimulated T cell activities. Transplantation. 1997; 63(12):1813-1818.

Lin Y, Segers C, Mikhalsky D, Tjandri-Maga TB, Schonharting M, Waer M. Use of the methylxanthine derivative A802715 in transplantation immunology: II. In vivo experiments. Transplantation. 1997;63(12): 1734-1738.

Wang ME, Tejpal N, Qu X, et al. Immunosuppressive effects of FTY720 alone or in combination with cyclosporine and/or sirolimus. Transplantation. 1998;65(7): 899-905.

Suzuki S, Enosawa S, Kakefuda T, et al. A novel immuno-suppressant, FTY720, with a unique mechanism of action, induces long-term graft acceptance in rat and dog allo-transplantation. Transplantation. 1996;61(2):200-205.

Yanagawa Y, Sugahara K, Kataoka H, Kawaguchi T, Masubuchi Y, Chiba K. FTY720, a novel immunosuppressant, induces sequestration of circulating mature lymphocytes by acceleration of lymphocyte homing in rats. II. FTY720 prolongs skin allograft survival by decreasing T cell infiltration into grafts but not cytokine production in vivo. J Immunol. 1998;160(11):5493-5499.

Chiba K, Yanagawa Y, Kataoka H, Kawaguchi T, Ohtsuki M, Hoshino Y. FTY720, a novel immunosuppressant, induces sequestration of circulating lymphocytes by acceleration of lymphocyte homing. Transplant Proc. 1999;31(1-2):1230-1233.

Stepkowski SM, Wang M, Qu X, et al. Synergistic interaction of FTY720 with cyclosporine or sirolimus to prolong heart allograft survival. Transplant Proc. 1998;30(5):2214-2216.

16 INVESTIGATIONAL IMMUNOSUPPRESSIVE AGENTS: BIOLOGICALS

Susan E. Light, MD
Robert B. Ettenger, MD

Our greater understanding of the components and actions of the immune system, along with the recent progress in biotechnology, have resulted in an expanded repertoire of biological agents that are being evaluated for potential efficacy and utility in transplantation. The pace of development of such agents may not seem particularly rapid to clinicians. Nevertheless, the pace has been rapid enough to insure that much of what will be presented in this chapter will be quickly outdated.

This chapter is intended to be a snapshot in time. Various agents that have shown potential for benefit in transplantation in preclinical models will be reviewed, as well as products that are being developed for other clinical indications first, but that may also have potential usefulness in transplantation.

There are some significant impediments to bringing truly useful biological agents to the organ transplant recipient's bedside. Transplantation has been a rewarding area for the development of new biological agents. However, because of the limitations imposed by donor organ scarcity, the "market" in transplantation for drugs not given chronically may be considered limited. As a result, the biotechnology industry often moves first to develop these agents in larger, more lucrative markets. This is illustrated by the fact that two of the three humanized anti-CD3 monoclonal antibodies in development have bypassed transplantation and are being evaluated as therapy for Type I diabetes mellitus.

In addition to financial considerations, there are also scientific/medical, statistical, and regulatory considerations that impact the development of new agents in transplantation. As an example, current medical advances have dramatically decreased the rate of acute rejection in renal transplantation. The low incidence of acute rejection episodes means that any comparative trial with a new agent for acute rejection prevention must have a large number of patients for appropriate statistical power if a further decrease in acute rejection is

the desired endpoint. Studies of this size are often prohibitively expensive. In part to address this, recent trials have used a composite endpoint that includes not only the incidence of acute rejection, but also the incidences of graft loss and death. The use of such a composite endpoint increases the event rate. This helps demonstrate the desired effect of the new agent with a smaller study. Nevertheless, even with such statistical/study design modifications, the delivery to market of a potentially beneficial biological agent through Phase 3 (and often Phase 4) clinical trials is virtually always an expensive undertaking requiring international multicenter randomized studies with large numbers of patients.

Even when a biotechnology company makes a strategic decision to undertake a series of clinical trials, these trials may pose some unexpected difficulties in study design. Again, consider the example of rejection reversal. As noted above, the incidence of acute rejection episodes has been progressively decreasing with the use of newer immunosuppressive agents. The challenge for a company is that, as programs transition to newer immunosuppressive regimens and acute rejection episodes become progressively fewer, the conduct of appropriate clinical trials may be long and difficult to complete. The standard of care may change during the conduct of the study impacting on the analysis of the data. There are analogous study design issues with many of the biological agents that are in current development. The goal of achieving a state of clinical tolerance, for example, is an attractive area for clinical development. Preclinical data is promising with several biological agents. If the definition of tolerance is allogenic transplantation without long-term immunosuppression, the reality of demonstrating tolerance in a clinical trial at this time is far from a practical reality as determination of this end point is limited to only clinical observations of rejection and graft loss.

Because of these and other development costs, the therapeutic biological agents that do reach the market are usually quite expensive. These agents may be perceived by the clinician to be beneficial to his/her patient. Nevertheless, the added costs mandate that sophisticated pharmacoeconomic analysis be performed to evaluate the cost/benefit ratio. While this data generated by the corporate sponsors may be useful, data from the "real world" use of the drug in standard immunosuppressive regimens may be necessary to obtain the support of private third party payors and governments for reimbursement.

With these disclaimers, this chapter will now attempt to summarize the current spectrum and status of biological agents in development in transplantation. The arena is now primarily monoclonal antibodies, but also includes fusion proteins, and immunotoxins that are directed against a number of potential targets.

Susan E. Light, MD, Vice President, Product Development, Quark Biotech, Inc., Menlo Park, CA

Robert B. Ettenger, MD, Department of Pediatrics, UCLA Center for Health Sciences, Los Angeles, CA

ANTIBODIES

Therapeutic antibodies can mediate immunosuppressive effects through a variety of mechanisms. Once they recognize their target structure on the relevant cells, antibodies can engage the host's cytolytic effector mechanisms. These mechanisms include antibody-dependent cell-mediated cytotoxicity (ADCC) and complement-dependent cytotoxicity (CDC). Alternatively, antibodies can interrupt adhesive interactions or signaling at the cell surface by covering receptor-binding sites, or they can modulate antigens or receptors from the cell surface.

There are, as of this writing, a limited number of therapeutic antibodies that are FDA-approved and available in the field of solid organ transplantation. The first monoclonal antibody to be registered was Orthoclone OKT®3. This is a murine monoclonal antibody that modulates CD3 from the surface of T lymphocytes. It is a potent agent for both treating and preventing acute rejection. The registration of the humanized and chimeric anti-CD25 (IL2-R) antibodies for the prevention of renal allograft rejection has moved the field into a new era. The rabbit anti-lymphocyte globulin, Thymoglobulin®, approved for the treatment of allograft rejection, and Atgam®, the equine anti-lymphocyte antibody, provide other, polyclonal choices for treating physicians.

Although various rodent monoclonal antibodies are effective in experimental transplant models, the experience with rodent anti-human monoclonal antibodies has been disappointing. This disappointment has stemmed from the blocking effect of the oft-generated human anti-murine antibody (HAMA) as well as the less commonly appreciated failure of murine monoclonal antibodies to activate human complement or Fc-receptor bearing cytolytic cells to trigger target cell lysis.

In response to this disappointment with rodent anti-human monoclonal antibodies, chimeric and humanized monoclonal antibodies have been engineered. The goals of this engineering are to reduce the immunogenicity of the antibody, and in some circumstances, to attain human ADCC and/or CDC effector function. A chimeric antibody is produced by joining codons for an existing murine monoclonal antibody's variable (V) region to codons for human Fc sequences, usually employing constant (C) region sequences from a chosen IgG subclass. Humanized antibodies extend this process by further limiting the murine V region sequences to the greatest extent possible while retaining the antigen specificity and affinity of the rodent monoclonal antibody's complementarity-determining regions (CDR).

ANTI-CD3

T cell receptor proteins are expressed solely on T cells. The majority of T cells express $\alpha\beta$ heterodimers that are associated with the multichain CD3 complex. The CD3 complex consists of five non-covalently linked chains: CD3δ, CD3γ, CD3ϵ, ζ, and η. Association of the T cell receptor protein with the CD3 complex is necessary for the surface expression and function of both sets of proteins. The T cell receptor proteins are responsible for the recognition of MHC antigen complexes, and the CD3 complexes, with their intracellular domains, function to transduce activating signals to the T cell cytoplasm.

Muromonab-CD3 is a murine monoclonal antibody that binds to the CD3ϵ chain. Muromonab-CD3 has proven to be quite beneficial in clinical solid organ transplantation. However it has limitations because of both its accompanying side effects and the xenoantibody response that is often generated by its use. As the CD3 antigen on T cells is a well-defined beneficial target in transplantation, the development of an "improved" version of muromonab-CD3 is a logical move forward. There are three distinct humanized anti-CD3 antibodies that have been studied in transplantation. These include a humanized form of muromonab-CD3; an aglycosylated humanized antibody; and a humanized antibody with an additional Fc mutation. As humanized antibodies, they have longer serum half-lives than the parent murine antibody and are expected to be less immunogenic. In addition, they have fewer side effects related to the release of cytokines. The absence of cytokine release would be expected to improve both the safety and tolerability of the treatment.

The humanized form of muromonab-CD3 has been used to treat a series of patients who were experiencing acute rejection. Unlike its murine counterpart muromonab-CD3, this humanized anti-CD3 does not deplete T cells from the circulation. The dosing regimen used was designed to achieve a prospectively specified target serum concentration of the antibody. This target serum level was achieved only after multiple daily doses were administered. In this study, patients received high-dose steroid only on the first day of anti-rejection treatment. Using this antibody, the authors found that rejection was reversed in seven of nine patients and symptoms of cytokine release were minimal.

A rat anti-CD3 antibody was humanized and a single amino acid substitution in the heavy chain resulted in an aglycosylated antibody that does not bind to Fc receptors of effector cells. This antibody thus lacks the ability to activate effector cells and cause cytokine release. In a study comparable to the one with the humanized form of muromonab-CD3 described above, this aglycosylated humanized anti-CD3 antibody has also been studied in nine renal allograft recipients who were experiencing acute rejection. Seven of the nine patients experienced rejection reversal, although re-rejection was reported. The antibody was well tolerated and there was no significant cytokine release syndrome reported.

HuM291, the third humanized anti-CD3 in development, was also engineered to have less mitogenic activity than muromonab-CD3, as well as a longer half-life. HuM291 has specific mutations in the Fc domain that decrease its affinity for Fc-receptors and make it less mitogenic to human T cells. Preclinical studies also showed that the antibody had a relatively long half-life. Although the in vitro data show a dramatic decrease in T cell activation and the quantity of cytokines released, some mild to moderate symptoms of cytokine release were reported in patients receiving the antibody in the absence of high-dose steroids. HuM291 cleared CD3+ T cells from the peripheral circulation in a dose dependent and reversible manner at extremely low doses. In patients who were scheduled to undergo a living donor transplant, a single dose of 1.5 µg/kg resulted in a decrease in the peripheral CD3 to <100 cells/mm3 at six days after dosing. Recovery was rapid and complete. Treatment with higher doses resulted in a longer duration of depletion, but symptoms of cytokine release such as headache, fever, nausea, and chills were observed. Overall, the magnitude of the symptoms with HuM291 was about 30% of that reported in patients who received muromonab-CD3 with concomitant steroids. When HuM291 was given with concomitant steroids to renal allograft recipients who were experiencing acute rejection, only minimal symptoms of cytokine release were observed and cytokines were not detected in the serum.

ANTI-CD3 IMMUNOTOXIN

Linking a monoclonal antibody, with its exquisite specificity, to a cellular toxin has been a route of clinical investigation for almost two decades. Ontak® an immunotoxin that has IL-2 linked to diphtheria toxin is approved for the treatment of cutaneous T cell lymphoma, but has not been widely used outside of this area. Ricin has been coupled to anti-CD5 and was studied in both bone marrow and renal transplantation. Unfortunately, the use of this immunotoxin was associated with significant toxicity and has therefore not been approved.

Another approach has been to couple a murine anti-CD3 monoclonal antibody to diphtheria toxin. When this anti-CD3 immunotoxin is given in combination with the immunosuppressive agent deoxyspergualin to rhesus monkeys who have received mismatched renal allografts, long-term tolerance without acute or chronic rejection has been observed. Treatment with this immunotoxin results in profound T cell depletion; reconstitution of the host T cells is slow. A clinical trial is underway in renal transplant patients, but it should be noted that an intact thymus is necessary to achieve immunologic reconstitution. For this reason, older patients may be at risk for inadequate recovery and prolonged immunosuppression.

COSTIMULATORY BLOCKADE
Anti-CD40 Ligand

The complexity and redundancy of the immune system is nowhere better demonstrated than by the costimulatory pathways that are necessary for the body to generate a vigorous immune response to an antigen. Binding of the T cell receptor by the Major Histocompatibility Complex antigen is not sufficient to trigger full T cell activation. In fact, in isolation, this signal fails to stimulate the T cell to respond. The T cell may in this situation become anergic or undergo apoptosis.

Additional "costimulatory" signals are necessary for full T cell activation. In addition to adhesion antigens (see below), another set of accessory costimulatory signaling pathways involves CD28 and CTLA4 on the T cell surface. CD28, a member of the immunoglobulin superfamily, is the primary T cell costimulatory receptor. Antigen-presenting cells express B7-1 (CD80) and B7-2 (CD86). CD28 binds to, and is stimulated by B7-1 and B7-2 on the antigen-presenting cells. The binding of CD28 by B7-1/B7-2 enhances T cell proliferation, IL-2 synthesis, and expression of anti-apoptotic proteins such as bcl-x. CTLA-4 (CD152) is similar to CD28 in a number of ways. It is also a member of the immunoglobulin superfamily and shares 75% nucleotide sequence homology with CD28. The gene coding for CTLA-4 is located close to the gene for CD28. When engaged by B7-1 and B7-2, CTLA-4 generates a negative signal that down-regulates T cell activity.

CD40 and its ligand, CD154 (also known as CD40 Ligand or CD40L), comprise a second costimulatory pathway. CD40 is present on the surfaces of B cells, antigen-presenting cells and endothelial cells while CD154 is present on the surfaces of activated T cells. The interaction between CD40 and CD154 provides help for cytotoxic T cells, antibody production, and immunoglobulin class switching. Of potential importance for the field of clinical immunosuppression, the triggering of CD40 on antigen-presenting cells causes up-regulation of B7-1/B7-2, augmenting the CD28 costimulatory-signaling pathway.

The components of these pathways provide additional opportunities for immunomodulatory interventions and suggest the possibility of developing specific tolerance to the new organ. The importance of CD154 as a key component in this system has been shown by the experience in rhesus monkeys who received MHC mismatched renal allografts. Treatment with Hu5c8, a humanized anti-CD40L antibody, prevented allograft rejection in the absence of other immunosuppressants. The animals remained free of acute rejection for up to ten months after transplantation. There were no safety concerns and no depletion of peripheral lymphocytes was observed.

In human trials, a humanized anti-CD154 monoclonal antibody, 5C7, has been preliminarily evaluated in an open label study in renal allograft recipients. None of the patients received calcineurin inhibitors. In addition to a higher than expected incidence of acute rejection, there was an unacceptably high incidence of thrombosis, both venous and arterial, resulting in the cessation of the trial. Similar adverse events were reported in trials with this antibody in other indications, resulting in cessation of those trials. A different antibody directed against the same target has been studied in patients with systemic lupus erythematosus without reports of comparable thrombotic events. Based on exciting and sound immunological theory, and outstanding results in primate models, the blockade of CD154 remains highly attractive as an investigational strategy.

CTLA-4-Ig

Another key target for therapeutic intervention in T cell-mediated immune response is the CD28/ B7-1 or B7-2 interaction. CTLA-4Ig is a recombinant fusion protein that has a greater affinity for B7-1 and B7-2 than does CD28. By fusing the extracellular binding domain of CTLA-4 to the constant region of human IgG1, an effective blocking protein, CTLA-4Ig is produced. The ligation of B7-1 and B7-2 by CTLA-4Ig truncates the primary costimulatory signal, inhibiting an immune response.

In animal studies, a short course of this fusion protein administered after transplant resulted in prolonged allograft survival. The initial human trial with this antibody was conducted in psoriasis patients. While some benefit was reported, anaphylactic reactions were also observed and hence, further studies were not conducted. A new construct of this fusion protein is currently in a Phase 1 study in renal transplantation.

Anti-CD20

The first monoclonal antibody to be approved for an oncology indication is Rituximab (Rituxan®), a chimeric murine/human monoclonal antibody that has a high affinity for CD20. The CD20 antigen is found on the surface of normal pre-B and mature B lymphocytes. It is also expressed on >90% of B cell non-Hodgkin's lymphomas, but is not found on hematopoietic stem cells, pro-B cells, normal plasma cells or other normal tissues. CD20 regulates one or more early steps in the activation process for cell cycle initiation and differentiation. After administration, the Fab domain of Rituximab binds to the CD20 antigen on B cells and the Fc domain recruits effector functions to mediate B cell lysis. The antibody has also been shown to induce apoptosis in a human B cell lymphoma line. Of interest is the finding that following Rituximab administration, there is a sustained and statistically significant reduction in both IgM and IgG serum levels for five to 11 months. However, serum IgM and/or IgG levels only infrequently fall below normal ranges.

Rituximab is approved for the treatment of lowgrade or follicular CD20-positive B cell non-Hodgkin's lymphoma. In view of the challenge of treating patients with posttransplant lymphoproliferative disorders (PTLD) without losing the allograft or using toxic chemotherapy, this antibody has been used successfully to treat patients who have developed PTLD.

Because of the property of Rituximab to decrease levels of immunoglobulins, the antibody has been used to treat acute steroid-resistant rejection in highly sensitized recipients. Preliminary data suggests that this approach may be quite successful in reversing resistant rejection in patients who have high levels of circulating anti-HLA antibodies. The authors suggest that multicenter studies are appropriate to evaluate the safety and efficacy of this agent in a controlled fashion.

Anti-Adhesion Molecule Antibodies

In addition to the costimulatory molecules and pathways described above, there are a number of adhesion and/or accessory molecules that assist in cell-cell interactions and have the potential to be costimulatory molecules. Lymphocyte function-associated antigen-1 (LFA-1 or CD11a, CD18) on T lymphocytes interact with intracellular adhesion molecules-1 (ICAM-1 or CD54) and ICAM-2 (CD102) to augment adhesion and T cell receptor activation. CD2, also present on T cells, interacts with LFA-3 (CD58) on antigen-presenting cells. This interaction appears to augment T cell proliferation, although this may reflect a more direct effect upon the T cell receptor. Finally, CD5 interacts with CD72 to impart an activating costimulatory signal.

The mechanisms involved in acute rejection include a role for the migration and adhesion of immune and inflammatory cells, including T cells to the endothelium of the allograft. Ischemia to the allograft appears to up-regulate the expression adhesion molecules on the graft endothelium, and the resulting attraction of leukocytes is hypothesized to play a role in such entities as ischemia/reperfusion injury and delayed renal allograft function. For this reason, it has appeared desirable to therapeutically block cellular adhesion mechanisms. An anti-ICAM-1 (CD54) was studied as an agent for ex-vivo perfusion of the transplanted kidney prior to the creation of the vascular anastomoses. In theory, such a treatment prior to the actual transplant procedure would be expected to reduce the ability of the leukocytes to adhere to the kidney's vascular endothelium with no systemic effects. Such a protocol might be particularly beneficial if there was significant graft ischemia. Unfortunately, this protocol failed to show benefit in reducing the incidence of acute rejection or delayed graft function in a multicenter randomized trial.

A humanized antibody that targets CD11a has demonstrated clinical benefit in the treatment of psoriasis, a T cell-mediated skin disease. A study in renal transplant patients is now evaluating the potential for this agent to decrease acute rejection when administered in the peritransplant period.

OTHER PROMISING TARGETS FOR INVESTIGATIONAL BIOLOGIC AGENTS
Interleukin-15 Blockade

IL-2 was the first major T cell growth factor to be identified and for a significant period of time was thought to be the only relevant T cell growth factor. Its importance in the pathogenesis of rejection has been supported by the success in abrogating rejection of experimental and clinical measures which target IL-2 and IL-2 blockade. However, it has now been reliably demonstrated that IL-2 "knockout" mice have many intact immune functions including the ability to reject allografts. It is now well accepted that IL-2 is part of a family of cytokines that can function as T cell growth factors. The members of this family include IL-2, IL-4, IL-7, IL-9 and IL-15. Each of these cytokines uses a common gamma chain in their receptor binding.

IL-15 shares many biological properties of IL-2. Of note for this discussion, the IL-15 receptor (IL-15R) shares both the beta and gamma chains of the IL-2 receptor (IL-2R). These chains are expressed constitutively on T cells, as well as on natural killer (NK) cells, B cells, mast cells and certain nonimmune cells. When T cells are activated, the alpha chain of the IL-2R is expressed and IL-2 is bound effectively.

Both the role of IL-15 in acute rejection and the potential for decreasing acute rejection by blocking its action are being actively evaluated. Baan et al recently reported their findings in cardiac allograft recipients who received anti-CD25 monoclonal antibodies but nevertheless experienced acute rejection. Their data support the hypothesis that acute rejection occurring in the setting of IL-2 blockade may be mediated by IL-15. A soluble fragment of the murine IL-15R alpha chain has been used in mice to demonstrate that blocking IL-15 may have value in preventing allograft rejection. A ten day course of the soluble IL-15 alpha chain was able to prevent rejection in minor histoincompatible murine cardiac allografts. With major histoincompatible grafts, the soluble fragment had only a modest effect, but anti-CD4 antibody added to the treatment greatly prolonged allograft survival.

This line of research again reminds us that certain promising pivotal immune mechanisms may be specifi-

cally targeted using agents other than antibodies. The use of a soluble receptor or fragment of a receptor has been undertaken because attempts to produce an antibody to the receptor have been unsuccessful. The experience with a soluble TNF receptor for the treatment of rheumatoid arthritis suggests that this approach may be worthwhile if the binding characteristics are favorable and adequate blood levels can be attained. The half-life of a soluble receptor or a receptor fragment would be less than that of an antibody. One consequence of this is that the dosing interval is far shorter for these molecules than for a humanized antibody.

CAMPATH-1H

CAMPATH-1H is the humanized form of the rat anti-CD52 monoclonal antibody, CAMPATH-1G. CD52 is an antigen found on mature T cells and some B cells. CAMPATH-1G was found to reduce the risk of short-term rejection in kidney-pancreas transplant recipients and increases short- and long-term survival in liver transplant recipients.

As a humanized form of CAMPATH-1G, CAMPATH-1H was designed to reduce the immunogenicity and increase the efficacy and half-life of the antibody. CAMPATH-1H depletes T and B cells from peripheral blood for weeks to months. The initial clinical indication for CAMPATH-1H is patients with refractory chronic lymphocytic leukemia. As of this writing, FDA approval for this indication is pending. In addition, it has been used ex vivo for the depletion of T lymphocytes for the prevention of graft-vs-host disease in patients undergoing allogeneic bone marrow transplant. This prolonged depletion of immunologically competent cells may allow for acceptance of the graft while the lymphocyte population is recovering, but the degree and duration of cell depletion may make the patients more susceptible to opportunistic infections.

Clinical use of CAMPATH-1H for prevention of renal allograft rejection has been limited to a small number of patients, but the preliminary results of the combination of this antibody with low dose cyclosporine without corticosteroids has been encouraging. Thirty-one recipients of cadaveric allografts have been studied with a median follow-up of 21 months. Twenty-nine of the 31 patients have good renal function with an overall incidence of acute rejection of 20%. CAMPATH-1H has also been found to reverse acute rejection. It is also currently being evaluated as induction therapy in calcineurin-inhibitor-sparing protocols.

Anti-CD45 Antibodies

The CD45 complex is a family of transmembrane protein tyrosine phosphatases expressed on the surface of nucleated hematopoietic cells. CD45 appears to play a critical role in the coupling of signals from the T cell receptor to the proximal signaling apparatus. CD45 has a complex set of structures and functions. T cells bearing CD45 exist largely as two reciprocal isoforms and these populations appear somewhat functionally distinct. Murine T cells can be divided into CD45RB^{Hi} and CD45RB^{Lo} isoforms. CD4+ cells with the CD45RB^{Hi} isoform preferentially secrete IL-2, whereas those expressing CD45RB^{Lo} secrete IL-4. In humans, the analogues to these cell types are CD45RA (analogous to the CD45RB^{Hi} isoform) and CD45RO (the analogue to CD45RB^{Lo}). While it was widely held that CD45RB^{Hi} cells were intrinsically naive cells and converted to CD45RB^{Lo} memory cells after antigen exposure, it has become apparent that the two isoforms interconvert and memory cells can express the CD45RB^{Hi} isoform.

MB23G2, a murine monoclonal antibody to the RB isoform, has been shown to possess the ability to inhibit alloreactivity of lymphocytes in vitro. This antibody was evaluated in a murine renal allograft model. The mice received two doses of the antibody and experienced long-term survival with normal renal function equal to that of the isograft controls. Additional treatment with the antibody was capable of reversing acute rejection with long-term engraftment and survival. The antibody has also been evaluated in a mouse islet allograft model. When given on days -1, 0 and 5, the antibody treatment was associated with indefinite graft survival in 60% of the animals. Preliminary data with a mouse monoclonal anti-CD45RB antibody in primates also suggest that it can induce long-term engraftment, reduce rejection and allow for subsequent sustained function in primates. The mechanisms of action of anti-CD45RB antibody are not yet fully worked out, but may include alterations in T cell receptor signaling and changes in CD45 isoform expression that lead to partial anergy, immune deviation, up-regulation of CTLA4 and the generation of immuno-regulatory CD4+ cells. Unfortunately, the production on anti-mouse antibodies is common in this model. Although the exact mechanisms by which anti-CD45RB antibodies can foster long-term graft acceptance are not well understood, early data are encouraging and this appears to be a potentially fruitful line of investigation.

FUTURE DIRECTIONS

Many of the agents outlined above, as well as others not included in this discussion, show promise. Nevertheless, none of the biological agents so far studied has proven to be a "Magic Bullet" that can by itself confer long-term graft acceptance or tolerance. It is likely that combinations of these agents or others will be necessary to achieve desired goals.

The challenge of developing a new agent is compounded if the agent is believed to only be effective when used in combination with another investigational agent. This, for example, may be the case with agents that are targeting the costimulatory pathway. Clinical testing of only one antibody may be adequate to demonstrate its safety profile, but it may fail to pass the rigorous test of efficacy required for FDA registration. The combination of 2 "subtherapeutic" agents may in fact, act in either an additive or synergistic manner and provide the safe and effective blockade of the costimulatory pathway that is desired. However, the development of such a combination of agents may not be feasible in our current framework of drug development.

The use of Rituximab for the treatment of PTLD and acute rejection in the three years since it was approved provides an important example of how a drugs' true benefit may not be known until it is on the market and more widely available. The deviation of new biologics that have obvious potential in transplantation toward non-transplant indications for their first approval does not mean that these agents will not ultimately be used for transplant, only that the time to use and understanding of how to best use them may be delayed. The large number of biologics being evaluated in other indications suggests that the future for biologics to improve the life and outcome for transplant patients is quite promising.

Biotechnology advances continue to be brought forward at an astonishing rate. It is appropriate to remain optimistic that, by the time this chapter is being read, some of the investigational agents discussed herein may be in actual clinical use.

RECOMMENDED READING

Vincenti F, Kirkman R, Light S, et al for the Daclizumab Triple Therapy Study Group. Interleukin-2-receptor blockade with daclizumab to prevent acute rejection in renal transplantation. N Engl J Med. 1998;338(3): 161-165.

Nashan B, Moore R, Amlot P, Schmidt AG, Abeywickrama K, Soulillou JP. Randomised trial of basiliximab versus placebo for control of acute cellular rejection in renal transplant recipients. CHIB201 International Study Group. Lancet. 1997;350(9086):1193-1198.

Ponticelli C, Tarantino A. Promising new agents in the prevention of transplant rejection. Drugs R D. 1999;1(1):55-60.

Gaber AO, First MR, Tesi RJ, et al. Results of the double-blind, randomized, multicenter, phase III clinical trial of Thymoglobulin versus Atgam in the treatment of acute graft rejection episodes after renal transplantation. Transplantation. 1998;66(1):29-37.

Woodle ES, Xu D, Zivlin RA, et al. Phase I trial of a humanized, Fc receptor nonbinding OKT3 antibody, huOKT3gamma1(Ala-Ala) in the treatment of acute renal allograft rejection. Transplantation. 1999;68(5): 608-616.

Friend PJ, Hale G, Chatenoud L, et al. Phase I study of an engineered aglycosylated humanized CD3 antibody in renal transplant rejection. Transplantation. 1999;68(11): 1632-1637.

Norman DJ, Vincenti F, DeMattos AM, et al. Phase I trial of HuM291, a humanized anti-CD3 antibody, in patients receiving renal allografts from living donors. Transplantation. 2000;70:1707-1712.

Thomas JM, Eckhoff DE, Contreras JL, et al. Durable donor-specific T and B cell tolerance in rhesus macaques induced with peritransplantation anti-CD3 immunotoxin and deoxyspergualin: absence of chronic allograft nephropathy. Transplantation. 2000;69(12):2497-2503.

Sayegh MH, Turka LA. The role of T-cell costimualtory activation pathways in transplant rejection. N Engl J Med. 1998;338:1813-1821.

Kirk AD, Burkly LC, Batty DS, et al. Treatment with humanized monoclonal antibody against CD154 prevents acute renal allograft rejection in nonhuman primates. Nat Med. 1999;5(6):686-693.

Abrams JR, Kelley SL, Hayes E, et al. Blockade of T lymphocyte costimulation with cytotoxic T lymphocyte-associated antigen 4-immunoglobulin (CTLA4Ig) reverses the cellular pathology of psoriatic plaques, including the activation of keratinocytes, dendritic cells, and endothelial cells. J Exp Med. 2000;192(5):681-694.

Cook RC, Conners JM, Gascopyne RD, Fradet G, Levy RD. Treatment of post-transplant lymphoproliferative disease with rituximab monoclonal antibody after lung transplantation. Lancet. 1999;354(9191):1698-1699.

Salmela K, Wramner L, Ekberg H, et al. A randomized multicenter trial of the anti-ICAM-1 monoclonal antibody (enlimomab) for the prevention of acute rejection and delayed onset of graft function in cadaveric renal transplantation: a report of the European Anti-ICAM-1 Renal Transplant Study Group. Transplantation. 1999;67(5):729-736.

Gottlieb A, Krueger JG, Bright R, et al. Effects of administration of a single dose of a humanized monoclonal antibody to CD11a on the immunobiology and clinical activity of psoriasis. J Am Acad Dermatol. 2000;42(3): 428-435.

Waldmann TA, Tagaya Y. The multifaceted regulation of interleukin-15 expression and the role of this cytokine in NK cell differentiation and host response to intracellular pathogens. Annu Rev Immunol. 1999;17:19-49.

Baan CC, van Gelder T, Balk AH, et al. Functional responses of T cells blocked by anti-CD25 antibody therapy during cardiac rejection. Transplantation. 2000;69(3):331-336.

Smith XG, Bolton EM, Ruchatz H, Wei X, Liew FY, Bradley JA. Selective blockade of IL-15 by soluble IL-15 receptor alpha-chain enhances cardiac allograft survival. J Immunol. 2000;165(6):3444-3450.

Hale G, Jacobs P, Wood L, et al. CD52 antibodies for prevention of graft-versus-host disease and graft rejection following transplantation of allogeneic peripheral blood stem cells. Bone Marrow Transplant. 2000;26(1):69-76.

Calne R, Moffatt SD, Friend PJ, et al. Campath 1H allows low-dose cyclosporine monotherapy in 31 cadaveric renal allograft recipients. Transplantation. 1999;68(10): 1613-1616.

Rothstein DM, Basadonna GP. Anti-CD45: A new approach towards tolerance induction. Graft. 1999;2: 239-245.

Lazarovits AI, Poppema S, Zhang Z, et al. Prevention and reversal of renal allograft rejection by antibody against CD45RB. Nature. 1996;380(6576):717-720.

Auersvald LA, Rothstein DM, Oliveira SC, et al. Indefinite islet allograft survival in mice after a short course of treatment with anti-CD45 monoclonal antibodies. Transplantation. 1997;63(9):1355-1358.

Section III

ORGAN PROCUREMENT/ ECONOMICS

17 CADAVER DONOR MANAGEMENT

Francis L. Delmonico, MD

Since August 21, 1998, the Health Care Financing Administration (HCFA) of the Department of Health and Human Services has required every hospital in the United States to contact, in a timely manner, their local organ procurement organization (OPO) regarding individuals whose death is imminent.

ROLE OF THE OPO IN DONOR MANAGEMENT

Stratification of the subsequent OPO procedure is based upon potential clinical situations. The activities noted within each section below are exclusive and are presented in a sequential order. The importance of this paradigm is to establish a practice that is both consistent and ethical. There are two cardinal rules that should be emphasized: (1) blood sampling to determine organ donor suitability may be done after the family gives permission, in advance of death; however, (2) invasive procedures for the purpose of organ donation (eg, groin lymph node recovery) should not be performed until the patient is declared dead.

Referral for Donation by the Primary Care Team

The initial OPO Coordinator activity is to establish the criteria of donor suitability. Consultation by the OPO Coordinator with the Intensive Care Team may be given in advance of the brain death declaration, regarding discussion of the family option for donation, and a review of donation procedure.

Verbal Family Interest for Donation

Noninvasive procedures for the sole objective of donor evaluation are reasonable. Family consent for donor evaluation should be documented in the patient chart by the Intensive Care Team or the OPO Coordinator, independent of the formal consent for donation. Charges for evaluation, including clinical blood sampling, blood type and crossmatch for possible donor transfusions, urinalysis, sputum and urine cultures, chest x-ray, electrocardiogram, and echocardiogram are the responsibility of the OPO.

Professor of Surgery, Harvard Medical School; Medical Director, New England Organ Bank; Director, Renal Transplantation, Massachusetts General Hospital, Newton, MA

There should be no written orders by the OPO Coordinator until a declaration of death and written family consent are obtained.

Written Family Consent for Donation, in Advance of the Diagnosis of Death

HLA typing by peripheral blood sample should be performed if at all possible, to expedite the identification of potential recipients. However, this serologic testing may be contraindicated if RBC or platelet transfusions have been given to the donor prior to the time of death. HLA typing is then best accomplished by femoral lymph node procurement after the declaration of death. Serology testing for hepatitis and other infectious serology (see below) may also be performed, but it should not be done prior to written family consent.

Written Family Consent for Donation, Following the Declaration of Death

Once death has been declared and consent obtained, OPO orders of donor management and invasive procedures, including groin node retrieval, bronchoscopy, cardiac catheterization, and placement of a central line are permissible. Thus, HLA typing and crossmatching by lymph node sampling of the donor is indicated. However, no invasive procedures should be performed until after pronouncement of death is made. Organ and tissue procurement can then proceed following medical examiner notification.

OBTAINING CONSENT

Perhaps the most significant obstacle to increasing the number of cadaver organs available for transplantation has been obtaining consent. The lack of family consent is the most common reason why potential donors are lost. Uncoupling a family discussion of the declaration of death by the Primary Care Team from the request for organ donation by an OPO representative appears to be an approach that permits families to consider donation more favorably. The priority order of individuals who can give consent in most state jurisdictions are as follows: spouse; adult son or daughter; either parent; adult brother or sister; and then others, such as a grandparent or guardian. Family consent remains an absolute necessity for organ donation in most communities, irrespective of an individual's intention as indicated by a donor card. However, the identification of a donor card upon a deceased person can influence the decision of the family to donate, especially for minority individuals. Moreover, there are now statutes that give explicit permission to recover organs with a signed donor card, even in the absence of family consent. For example, Pennsylvania currently makes hospitals legally responsible for referring a potential donor, and mandates trained OPO personnel to accommodate the request of the family. Nevertheless, this is not akin to the presumed consent approach that is active in some European countries. In such a scenario, there is the presumption of family consent even without a signed donor card.

DIRECTED DONATION

While it is illegal in the US to restrict the donation of an organ or organs to a class of individuals (eg, by gender, race, national origin), directed donation to a specific named individual is acceptable. Ideally, this individual should be known to the family member requesting the directed donation. Since the buying and selling of human organs is also illegal, none of the care team should knowingly participate in any directed donation involving monetary exchange or other inducements to directed donation. Ideally, the nature of the relationship between the next-of-kin or donor and the individual to whom the organ is being directed should be ascertained. Unless a relationship is substantiated, the possibility of directed donation is precluded. The family should also be informed that ABO incompatibility, as well as other medical considerations, may preclude the possibility of directed donation.

DONOR IDENTIFICATION AND MANAGEMENT

Traditionally, death has been declared by an absence of cardiorespiratory function. However, as a simple and unifying concept, all death occurs when there is permanent loss of the entire function of the brain. If there is no circulation to the brain for a sustained period, the hypoxic injury to the brain is irreversible. The absence of a heartbeat during that period is a sign that there is insufficient blood flow to the brain. The consequence of this irreparable damage to the brain is death.

Ninety-nine percent of organ donors in the United States are declared dead by brain death criteria. The American Academy of Neurology (AAN) definition of brain death is "an irreversible loss of the clinical function of the brain, including the brain stem." The three cardinal findings of brain death are: coma or unresponsiveness from a known cause, absence of brain stem reflexes (ie, pupil, ocular, corneal, pharyngeal, and tracheal); and apnea.

The brain stem (responsible for spontaneous breathing and vasomotor control) has chemoreceptors that monitor the pCO_2 and ph of the CSF, which approximate changes in the plasma. An apnea test is supportive of the brain death diagnosis if the pCO_2 is greater than 60 mmHg and no respiratory movement (abdominal or chest excursion) is detected.

The clinical signs of brain death may not be reliable if a patient is hypothermic or has received medication that may alter central nervous system function. In that instance, a radionuclide isotope scan, if readily available, may reveal an absence of cerebral perfusion; and thus, the diagnosis of brain death can be ascertained conclusively. Otherwise confirmatory laboratory testing of brain death may be accomplished by either an electroencephalogram, contrast or isotope angiography, or transcranial Doppler ultrasonography. Although these tests are not mandatory for the diagnosis of brain death in adults, they are recommended in children, for whom recovery from hypoxic injury may occur more readily. Specific guidelines for the determination of brain death in children have emphasized the necessity of two clinical examinations, apnea tests, and laboratory confirmation studies 24 to 48 hours apart, depending upon the age of the child.

Neither the OPO nor the transplant team may provide any direction of care until the patient is declared brain dead. If a patient does not fulfill the criteria of brain death, and the clinical condition is unresolvable and hopeless, the primary care physician may join with the family in making a decision to withdraw care. However, the decision to withdraw life support must be rendered independently of any consideration for organ donation.

NON-HEART BEATING DONATION AFTER THE WITHDRAWAL OF CARE

Prior to the establishment of the brain death diagnosis in 1968, organs were only recovered for transplantation after a patient was declared dead by the absence of heartbeat or respiratory activity. Since then however, the number of organs obtained from non-heart beating donors (NHBD) has been limited, because the absence of cardiorespiratory function adversely affects the suitability of organs for successful transplantation. Brain dead donors (vs NHBD) are ideal because organ function is interrupted under controlled conditions that minimize ischemia. However, as a significant shortage of cadaver organs for transplantation has persisted, many have proposed that the opportunity of recovering organs from NHBD be reconsidered more broadly. With the advent of health care proxies, advance directives, and a societal reluctance for extraordinary measures of medical treatment for the terminally ill, an increasing number of NHBDs could become available for organ recovery. The continuing process of deciding to withdraw terminal care and to consenting subsequently to organ donation after death may also provide the family an important consolation at the time of bereavement.

In July 1997, a Committee on Medical and Ethical Issues in Maintaining the Viability of Organs for Transplantation was convened by the Institute of Medicine of the National Academy of Sciences. The ethical aspects of many NHBD protocols were examined. The IOM subsequently issued a supportive review affirming the following:

- That use of an NHBD is medically effective and ethically proper;
- That organ donors must be dead before organs are recovered;
- That use of NHBDs should not be an entree to euthanasia.

The most significant protocol issue to settle is the period of asystole which assures that the patient is dead. Moreover, the determination of asystole should be given consistently. The protocol definition of asystole could vary from an absence of a palpable pulse, to electro-mechanical dissociation, to a flat line tracing on the cardiac monitor. Irrespective of the method of determining asystole, the physician declaring death should not be a member of the transplant service (nor should the transplant team have any perceived consultation in the decision to withdraw care).

Some clinicians have suggested that ten minutes should elapse before the installation of organ preservation devices, so that there is a clear transition from the care of a patient, to the recovery of organs from a cadaver. However, the ten minute period of asystole likely prohibits the recovery of organs other than the kidneys. In contrast, the University of Pittsburgh protocol permits the declaration of death two minutes following the cessation of cardiorespiratory activity, providing at least an opportunity for multiple organ procurement. The IOM report has attempted to clarify this issue by stipulating that an interval of at least five minutes must elapse after complete cessation of circulatory function, before death is pronounced and organ perfusion or removal begins.

THE SUITABLE ORGAN DONOR

The age, social and medical history, and the specific organ function determine the suitability of a cadaver organ donor.

Donor Age

There are virtually no acceptable organ donors over 80. It should be noted that, depending upon the donor age, some organs might not be recoverable for transplantation. For example, infant donors under six months old generally provide only a heart allograft, since kidneys and livers from these donors are highly susceptible to thrombosis in the recipients. A donor under three years old will provide kidneys retained as an en bloc preparation for a single recipient. Donors over 60 years are not likely to permit heart or lung recovery, and kidneys that are procured from such older-aged donors are usually assessed by a post recovery frozen section biopsy for

glomerular sclerosis, vascular narrowing and interstitial fibrosis.

Medical Restrictions

A detailed social and medical history should be taken from the donor's family by the OPO representative who obtains consent for donation. Recovery surgeons should perform an appropriate examination, which might bear upon donor suitability. This includes looking for extremity lacerations that have become secondarily infected, or needle marks indicative of drug abuse, and visceral intraoperative examination.

Malignancy

The risk of transmitting a tumor from an organ donor with a known malignancy is significant, depending upon the type of malignancy. The following cancers have been transplanted to allograft recipients from organ donors: thyroid, bronchial, lung, breast, adenocarcinoma (colorectal and unknown primary), kidney, melanoma, anaplastic, prostatic, and choriocarcinoma. Donor malignancies may be detected in allograft recipients as early as hours after transplantation (noted in allograft nephrectomy and liver allograft biopsy specimens). Otherwise, metastasis may be evident within three months following transplantation (for example a choriocarcinoma metastasized to the lung of a liver allograft recipient), or they may not become evident until more than three years following transplantation (the development of melanoma on the chest, arms, and thighs of a renal allograft recipient). The tumors can also grow within the allograft and/or locally adjacent to the allograft: for example, a donor bronchial carcinoma presenting as a large mass adjacent to a renal allograft.

Extra-renal organ recipients are susceptible to the risk of donor-transmitted malignancy, even though the allograft may not be a common site of metastasis (eg, melanoma transmission to heart allograft recipients). Presumably the allograft carries the cancer cells and these cells flourish in the immunosuppressed environment of the recipient.

However, cadaver donors with primary brain tumors, a history of non-melanoma skin cancers such as basal or squamous cell, or a history of in situ carcinoma of the cervix may be acceptable organ donors.

Primary Brain Tumors

Although the spontaneous extracranial spread of a primary brain tumor is rare, presumably because of the blood brain barrier, not all brain malignancies carry the same minimal risk of metastasis. Moreover, the possibility of metastasis may be influenced by intracranial operative procedures such as a craniotomy, or the insertion of a ventricular shunt. Primary brain tumors have been transmitted from patients with a ventricular shunt; however, the absence of a shunt does not preclude the possibility of the transmission of a brain tumor to a solid organ allograft recipient. If organs are to be recovered from a donor with a primary brain tumor, the thoracic and abdominal cavities must be carefully inspected for metastases.

The type and grade of brain malignancy influence the risk of donor transmission: glioblastoma from adults and medulloblastoma from children are of higher risk.

The diagnosis of a primary brain malignancy must also be differentiated from extracranial malignancies such as melanoma, which may have metastasized to the brain. Intracerebral hemorrhage may be the presentation of not only a metastatic melanoma but also a renal cell carcinoma or a choriocarcinoma. Female potential donors with nontraumatic cerebral hemorrhage thought secondary to either a primary brain malignancy or a spontaneous subarachnoid hemorrhage should have a blood level of the human chorionic gonadotropin (hCG) determined. If a woman of reproductive age has a measurable blood hCG level, the patient should not be considered as an appropriate donor, unless there is clear evidence (postmortem) that the patient had either an intrauterine or tubal pregnancy, and the pathology of that gestation does not reveal a choriocarcinoma.

Infectious Disease Considerations

Infectious organisms transmitted by a cadaveric donor organ can result not only in a loss of the allograft, but also in death of the immunosuppressed recipient. Active viral infection in the form of encephalitis or meningitis, varicella zoster, or human immunodeficiency virus (HIV) is an absolute contraindication to organ donation. While donor screening for HIV, human T-lymphotrophic virus (HTLV), hepatitis B (HBV), hepatitis C (HCV), and cytomegalovirus (CMV) is routinely performed in the US (Table 17-1), there are no worldwide standards. The

practices among OPOs vary widely, as do the interpretation and reporting of results.

UNOS policy regarding HTLV I screening is the same as it is for HIV (organ donors are not suitable); however, not all OPOs reject a cadaver donor whose serology screening test reveals a positive anti-HTLV I donation. The risk of transmission of HTLV I by solid organ transplantation has not been clearly defined. HTLV I has been transmitted to recipients of contaminated blood transfusions. A patient infected with HTLV I by blood transfusion is at risk for the development of either adult T cell leukemia or neurologic disorders.

Hepatitis B Virus

HBsAg may be identified in the serum of an infected patient within 30 to 60 days of exposure. Hepatitis B virus (HBV) transmission has been documented to occur through organ transplantation. The serologic profile of a donor blood sample revealing an isolated anti-HBs could be observed following: the vaccination of an individual with hepatitis B vaccine; the administration of hepatitis B immune globulin (HBIG); the transfusion of a blood product from an immunized donor; or previous HBV infection. Antibody to HBsAg, unlike antibody to the HBV core antigen (anti-HBc), does not arise during the acute infection, but rather during convalescence. Thus, up to six months may elapse before anti-HBs may be detected following HBV infection. The organ donor with isolated anti-HBs is not likely to transmit HBV infection because there is no active viral replication; however, the exception is a liver allograft that can harbor the HBV indefinitely.

Anti-HBc (IgM) is the earliest antibody detected following HBV infection (ten to 14 days). The anti-HBc determination is not influenced by exposure to HBV vaccine. Recent literature reports have emphasized the importance of anti-HBc detection regardless of the anti-HBs result, especially for the liver allograft recipient. HBV may reside in the donor patient's liver. It is now well-established that HBV has been transmitted to liver allograft recipients from cadaver donors whose blood sample revealed a serologic profile of anti-HBc and anti-HBs positive (negative HBsAg); however, such HBV transmission is thought to be unusual to heart and kidney allograft recipients.

Hepatitis C Virus

The hazard of HCV transmission from a previously infected organ donor is a concern for all allograft recipients. Approximately 5% of all organ donors are anti-HCV positive. The presence of anti-HCV antibody is indicative of an HCV infection as anti-HCV antibody appears in a peripheral blood sample within two months of HCV exposure. It is also important to emphasize, however, that detecting anti-HCV in the donor serology

Table 17-1. Routine Serology Screening of the Organ Donor
HIV Antibody
HTLV I Antibody
Hepatitis B Virus Surface Antigen (HbsAg)
Hepatitis B Virus Surface Antibody (anti-HBs)
Hepatitis B Virus Core Antibody (anti-HBc)
Hepatitis C Virus Antibody (HCV)
Cytomegalovirus Antibody (CMV)
Treponemal Antigen (Syphilis)
Toxoplasma Antibody

panel is not predictive of HCV transmission. Approximately 50% of anti-HCV-positive patients have detectable hepatitis C viremia by PCR analysis of a peripheral blood specimen. All PCR-positive organ donors will transmit HCV to allograft recipients; however, the risk of HCV transmission from a PCR-negative (anti-HCV antibody-positive) donor is unclear. The consequence of receiving an organ from a donor who is anti-HCV positive is as follows: approximately 50% of the recipients have detectable anti-HCV antibody; 24% have detectable hepatitis C viremia by the PCR analysis; and 35% may develop liver disease.

Cytomegalovirus

All prospective organ donors and allograft recipients should be routinely tested for antibody to CMV. The specific CMV donor and recipient serologic status has implications for recipient prophylaxis, the highest risk group being CMV seronegative recipients of CMV seropositive donor organs. Because of successful prophylaxis and treatment of recipients, there is no contraindication to the transplantation of organs from CMV seropositive donors.

Other Viruses

Human herpesvirus 8 (HHV-8) has been transmitted through renal allografts and is a risk factor for transplantation-associated Kaposi's sarcoma.

The transmission of neurotropic viruses such as rabies and Creutzfeldt-Jakob disease has been reported from tissue donors. Thus, organ donor deaths associated with these diagnoses exclude donation. Although successful transplantation of renal allografts from donors with Reye's syndrome (encephalopathy and liver failure) has been reported, some transplant centers may be reluctant to expose their recipient to an unknown (presumed viral) etiology of donor death.

Over 95% of potential adult donors are seropositive for Epstein-Barr virus (EBV) (IgG antibody). Serological screening of organ donors for EBV has not been routinely performed, although some programs are concerned about the risk of developing posttransplant lymphoproliferative disorder (PTLD) in EBV seronegative recipients of organs from EBV seropositive donors.

Syphilis

The detection of antibody to syphilis by the rapid plasma reagin test (RPR) is not a contraindication to organ procurement. Although syphilis can be transmitted by blood transfusion, there is no recorded infection of a transplant recipient from a syphilitic donor. Moreover, a standard course of penicillin would provide sufficient antibiotic coverage to prevent syphilitic complications in an allograft recipient. This regimen has been reportedly successful in the treatment of two allograft recipients

intentionally given kidneys from a donor whose syphilis serology test was positive.

Toxoplasma

The possible transmission of the protozoan *Toxoplasma gondii*, is a concern especially for heart allograft recipients, because of the predilection of this parasite for muscle tissue. Organ procurement from seropositive donors is not contraindicated; however, the detection of seropositivity means that the recipient may be placed at high risk. Fortunately, the use of trimethoprim-sulfamethoxazole for *Pneumocystis carinii* prophylaxis prevents transmission of *T. gondii*.

Bacteriology and Donor Sepsis

OPOs now routinely evaluate donor infection on an individual basis, considering the blood culture bacteriology, the presence and duration of central lines, and the nature of the donor infection, before excluding a patient as an organ donor. The risk of bacteremia may be influenced by an extremity cellulitis (especially adjacent to external orthopedic fixatives), or a current intestinal injury or surgery. However, none of these conditions alone prohibit organ donation.

Cystitis, as manifested by a positive culture of urine obtained through a Foley catheter, is not a contraindication to donation. However, a history of pyelonephritis within three months of organ donation may increase the risk of transmission of bacteria to the recipient. Clinical judgement regarding the type of organism and verification of treatment should be exercised before recently infected kidneys are accepted for transplantation.

Patients with bacterial meningitis may be acceptable for organ donation, if the organism is identified. *Haemophilus influenza, Streptococcus pneumoniae,* and *Neisseria meningitidis* are the most common bacterial pathogens. The administration of at least a broad spectrum cephalosporin to a potential donor is indicated. However, other bacterial organisms carry a more significant hazard for blood vessel disruption following transplantation. These include: *Staphylococcus aureus, Bacteroides* species, *Klebsiella enterobacter, Escherichia coli,* and *Pseudomonas aeruginosa.*

Nevertheless, if a sufficient course of antibiotic therapy has been administered that minimizes the risk of bacterial transmission, then organ donation may be considered. In the case of donor bacteremia, if a sufficient course of antibiotic therapy has been administered that minimizes the risk of bacterial transmission, then organ donation may be considered. The New England Organ Bank has examined the outcome of recipients of solid organs from donors with bacteremia and/or fungemia at the time of organ recovery over a six year period There were 95 (5.1%) bacteremic donors from a total of 1,775, from whom 212 recipients received organs. Forty-six

(48%) of the bacteremic donors had pathogens in their blood. Among the 101 recipients of organs from these, no evidence of transmission could be documented (0% transmission rate, 95% CI 0-3). The remaining 49 donors had either *Staphylococcus epidermidis* or other unlikely pathogens recovered from the blood. Examination of the 111 recipients of organs from these donors also found no evidence for transmission (0% transmission rate, 95% CI 0-3). Of the 212 recipients, 193 (91%) received a mean of 3.8 ± 2.5 days of antibiotics postoperatively. The 30-day graft and patient survival for recipients of organs from bacteremic donors was not significantly different from recipients of organs from nonbacteremic donors (*P*=0.695 for patient survival, and *P*=0.310 for graft survival). Thus, organs transplanted from bacteremic donors may be transplanted with caution and appropriate use of donor and recipient antibiotics.

Tuberculosis

The death of a renal allograft recipient from disseminated tuberculosis transmitted through a cadaver kidney, obtained from a donor with unsuspected tuberculosis meningitis has been reported. The etiology of the meningitis only became apparent several weeks after the donor's death, when mycobacteria grew in cultures of his cerebrospinal fluid. The donor's chest radiograph was normal. As well as documenting the transmission of tuberculosis via transplanted organs, this case underscores the danger of accepting organs from individuals with a diagnosis of meningitis of unknown etiology.

Fungal infection

Candida albicans frequently colonizes the vagina and perineum of patients who are maintained on broad-spectrum antibiotics for a long period of time. Thereafter, the monilia may gain entrance to the bladder, through an indwelling Foley conduit. Wound infection and vascular disruption may follow transplantation of organs contaminated with *Candida,* especially to diabetic recipients. Because *Candida* infections are particularly hazardous to the pancreas transplant recipient, many transplant surgeons administer amphotericin B through the nasogastric tube into the donor duodenum during the recovery procedure. Fatal candidal mediastinitis has been reported in recipients of lungs from donors with a heavy growth of *Candida* in cultures from the trachea.

Histoplasma and *Cryptococcus* have been transmitted to renal allograft recipients by organs from donors who died of intracerebral pathology, without evidence of a pulmonary infection. These organisms are difficult to eradicate from the central nervous system unless a protracted course of antifungal therapy (amphotericin B) is administered. Even with careful documentation of proper therapy, however, a history of fungal infection (also including coccidioidomycosis and blastomycosis)

should exclude an individual from donation, despite the apparent absence of infection at the time of death.

Poison as a Cause of Donor Death

Accidental or suicidal poisonings through inhalation, ingestion, or injection of toxic substances result in several thousand fatalities each year. Barbiturate and benzodiazepine medications are frequently overdosed by suicide victims. Although a majority of these deaths occur following a cardiopulmonary arrest, some patients are resuscitated for a period of time, only to become brain dead. These patients may be considered for organ donation.

Each toxic exposure must be evaluated with respect to specific organ injury. Certain drugs such as acetaminophen may render the liver unsuitable for transplantation because of fulminate hepatic necrosis; but other organs may not be injured. The New England Organ Bank (NEOB) has successfully recovered a heart allograft for transplantation from a cadaver donor with acetaminophen toxicity.

Tricyclic antidepressants may cause donor liver injury, and depending upon the serum concentration of the tricyclic, adverse effects not only for donor organs, but also for recipients of organs from a donor with antidepressant medication overdose. A tricyclic contaminated liver may become the source of a recipient tricyclic blood level that is toxic to the recipient's mental status and cardiac stability. Nevertheless, the successful transplantation of kidneys has been reported from a patient who died from a trimipramine overdose.

Carbon monoxide expelled by gasoline engines is a common cause of inhalation. Accidental carbon monoxide poisoning can also occur following the exposure to solvents in paint removers, and by the release of vapors from faulty home heating systems. Death usually occurs from hypoxia prior to arrival to the emergency ward, because carbon monoxide rapidly replaces oxygen from the hemoglobin molecule. However, for those resuscitated patients who subsequently develop anoxic brain death, assessment of renal injury by urine sampling (for myoglobin, protein, and red blood cells) is useful in deciding whether to proceed with kidney procurement, as rhabdomyolysis can affect renal function. Depending upon liver function and morphology by biopsy, liver transplantation should also be considered.

Prompt identification of the toxin and treatment to minimize end-organ damage can be critical life-saving measures. However, these measures can also be consequential to successful organ salvage from patients who still succumb to the poison. For example, cyanide causes cellular anoxia within 30 minutes of ingestion or within seconds of inhalation. Decreased mitochondrial oxidative metabolism and oxygen use leads to lactic acidosis. Unless an antidote regimen of amyl nitrate inhalation, intravenous injection of sodium nitrite, and intravenous injection of sodium thiosulfate is administered promptly, irreversible CNS damage may ensue. The use of these cyanide antidotes can result in resumption of satisfactory organ function in a patient whose brain injury is beyond resolution following cyanide suicide, enabling the successful transplantation of the heart and kidneys. Liver allografts can also be successfully transplanted from donors with fatal cyanide poisoning, despite initial cyanide toxicity to the liver.

Hemodialysis and ethanol administration have been used to correct the metabolic acidosis and stabilize organ function in a patient who died following methanol ingestion, resulting in the successful transplantation of renal allografts. NEOB transplant centers have successfully transplanted the liver and both kidneys from a donor with fatal methanol toxicity.

Multiple organs have been recovered from an NEOB donor who committed suicide by the ingestion of rat poison. The active ingredient of the rat poison which caused the fatal cerebral hemorrhage was sodium warfarin. The donor's prothrombin time peaked at 200 seconds, but returned to near normal 48 hours later, enabling the successful transplantation of the kidneys, heart, lungs, and liver.

These cases demonstrate that the toxic organ injury from a fatal poisoning may be reversible. Thus, if the adverse effect of the poison to specific organ function is resolved, organ recovery and transplantation is appropriate. The function of organs transplanted from donors who have died from poisoning has not been adversely affected.

DONOR MANAGEMENT

Intensive care unit management of the brain dead potential organ donor is a complex and dynamic process directed towards maintenance of end-organ function and viability. Commonly encountered clinical problems include hypotension, polyuria, electrolyte imbalances, cardiac dysfunction, and hypothermia. Increased blood levels of cytokines occur in brain dead patients. Although interleukin-1 β (IL-1 β) and tumor necrosis factor-alpha (TNF-α) levels appear to be within normal range, interleukin-6 (IL-6) levels have been shown to be abnormal. The consequence of the IL-6 elevation is not known. However, careful monitoring, anticipation of instability and rapid treatment is required to succeed in maximizing the recovery of transplantable organs.

INITIAL MANAGEMENT GOALS

The primary donor management goals include restoration and maintenance of normothermia, normalization of blood pressure, optimization of lung function, restoration of intravascular volume, and correction of acid/base and electrolyte imbalances. Conflicting approaches to ideal management from the various transplant specialties may require the placement of a central line to assure filling pressures that avoid fluid overload but permit optimal organ perfusion. Otherwise, without this sophisticated data, the kidney team may prefer aggressive fluid administration and brisk diuresis, the liver and pancreas team may favor adequate but not excessive portal and arterial perfusion pressures, and at the same time the thoracic teams request volume contraction to minimize the development of pulmonary edema. Therefore, preliminary evaluation of organ suitability may be helpful in guiding management when one or more organs are clearly unsuitable. Subsequent management efforts can then be directed towards those organs that will likely be used.

Poikilothermia

Loss of thermoregulatory function follows hypothalamic dysfunction in brain dead patients. A shivering thermogenesis is absent. Passive heat loss may lead to progressive hypothermia, which is well known to adversely effect cellular metabolism, oxygen release, and cardiac function.

Due to the relatively high body surface area to body mass ratio in neonates and children, core temperatures may fluctuate much more rapidly than in adults. In all cases, patient temperature should be carefully monitored and hypothermia should be treated early. It is easier to prevent hypothermia than to reverse it. Nevertheless, effective treatment includes maintenance of room temperature at 75°F, keeping the body and head well-covered at all times, using warming blankets, and heating of intravenous fluids. The use of a warming blanket in the operating room is essential to counter passive heat loss and maintain normothermia. Heating humidified oxygen (to 45° C) via the ventilator, may be also of benefit; however, this is not usually necessary. Since oxygen heating may cause thermal injury to the airway, it is not employed unless the routine measures are unsuccessful.

Hypertension

Severe hypertension (systolic BP >200 mmHg) is infrequently encountered in brain dead patients. However, when hypertension is observed, it is likely related to brainstem herniation and is therefore self-limiting. The reason to treat sustained hypertension is to avoid transient rhythm disturbances. The goal of treatment should be to maintain the diastolic BP below 100 mmHg. Sodium nitroprusside (Nipride) infusion is the treatment of choice. Nipride should only be used in cases of severe, persistent hypertension, since prolonged administration may result in cyanide toxicity.

Hypotension

Alternatively, hypotension (SBP <90 mmHg) is more frequently observed in brain dead patients, especially at the time of the initial referral. The cytokine storm that occurs in association with brain death can account for donor hypotension. Since brief intervals of hypotension can influence organ function following transplantation, a central venous pressure line and an arterial line are essential to manage hypotension appropriately. The most common cause is hypovolemia. However, if a hemodynamically unstable donor persists following volume expansion, a pulmonary artery catheter should be introduced, and serial cardiac outputs and systemic vascular resistance measurements should be determined.

Hypovolemia

Excessive intravascular volume loss (eg, hemorrhage, diabetes insipidus) is common in potential organ donors, especially trauma victims. Neurogenic vasodilatation, common in brain dead individuals, may exacerbate the hemodynamic instability. Intravascular volume deficits should be corrected prior to the use of vasoactive drugs. Furthermore, severe head-injured patients may intentionally be kept volume contracted. Low-to-moderate dose dopamine hydrochloride infusion (3 to 5 μg/kg per min) may be required to maintain adequate BP during the initial period of volume repletion. Colloid (albumin) and blood products (red blood cells) may be necessary for volume expansion in combination with crystalloid solutions. Monitoring of the central venous pressure (ideally 10 to 15 mmHg) will avoid the development of pulmonary edema, especially in potential lung donors. As the blood volume is restored, vasoactive drugs should be discontinued.

DECREASED VASCULAR RESISTANCE

Despite adequate volume restoration, some donors will require additional vasoactive drug therapy because of neurogenic vasodilatation. A dopamine dosage between 5 to 10 μg/kg per min may be necessary, since the alpha-receptor of peripheral blood vessels does not respond with vasoconstriction until this dose range of dopamine is reached. However a dopamine dose that exceeds 10 μg/kg per min requires insertion of a pulmonary artery catheter for determination of cardiac filling pressures, cardiac output (CO), and systemic vascular resistance (SVR). The SVR is calculated by thermodilution cardiac output measurements. If the SVR is less than 400 dynes/sec per cm vasoconstrictor therapy is indicated; otherwise, to avoid the risk of decreased perfusion to visceral organs, vasoconstrictors (eg, levophed) should be reserved for low SVR determinations refractory to volume repletion and a dopamine dose between 5 to 10 μg/kg per min. This scenario raises the suspicion of donor sepsis.

DEPRESSED CARDIAC FUNCTION

Some donors may exhibit depressed cardiac function, not surprisingly following resuscitation from cardiopulmonary arrest, due to preexisting cardiac disease, or secondary to brainstem herniation. Brain death causes a significant loss of right and left ventricular function. These injuries are greater in the right ventricle and may contribute to early right ventricular failure after transplantation. The deterioration of myocardial performance after brain death correlates temporally with desensitization of the myocardial beta-receptor signal transduction system. Thus, these patients may be hypotensive despite adequate volume restoration. Donors with depressed cardiac function may require inotropic and chronotropic support to maintain an adequate cardiac output. If the cardiac index is less than 2.0 L/min per m², inotropic therapy is indicated, preferably with dopamine in a dose 3 to 5 μg/kg per min. The use of vasoconstrictors such as levophed may exacerbate cardiac dysfunction.

Thyroid hormone replacement therapy (triiodothyronine: maximal dose 0.6 microgram/kg) has been used to improve myocardial function, allowing the use of donor hearts that might otherwise have been considered unsuitable for transplantation; although its efficacy in this setting is controversial.

Respiratory Insufficiency

Brain dead patients require frequent pulmonary hygiene to prevent atelectasis and to maintain adequate oxygenation. In addition, brain death following head trauma may also be associated with an unexplained "neurogenic" pulmonary edema. These patients develop an abnormal capillary permeability, with movement of intravascular fluid into the pulmonary interstitium and eventually into the alveolar space, impairing gas exchange and progressively reducing the volume of ventilated lung tissue. Positive end-expiratory pressure of 5 cm H_2O ("physiologic PEEP") may be helpful to maintain alveolar expansion in these circumstances.

Ventilator settings for brain dead patients should include a tidal volume of 10 to 15 cc/kg and a respiratory rate sufficient to maintain arterial PCO_2 in the 40 to 45 mmHg range. The fraction of inspired oxygen should be kept at 40% or less in potential lung donors to prevent pulmonary oxygen toxicity. Levels of PEEP greater than 7.5 cm H_2O may impede venous return and decrease cardiac output.

Polyuria

Polyuria (urine output >500 mL/hour) is frequently seen in brain dead patients. It may be due to physiological diuresis, osmotic diuresis (eg, mannitol, hyperglycemia), diuresis caused by hypothermia, partial or complete central diabetes insipidus (DI), loop diuretics, or a combination of the above. Excessive polyuria due to osmotic diuresis or DI may lead to hypernatremia, hypokalemia, and hyperosmolality. The serum potassium should not fall below 3.5 mEq/L, to avoid arrhythmias. Urine and serum electrolyte levels and osmolality aid in the determination of the cause of polyuria.

Aggressive volume restoration may result in a physiological diuresis. No treatment is warranted, but intake and output should be monitored carefully. Prior mannitol administration or excessive glucose infusion may result in an osmotic diuresis. Glycosuria and hyperglycemia should be treated with a sliding scale of IV insulin therapy (four units of regular insulin for every 100 mg% of blood sugar above 200 mg%) to normalize blood glucose levels.

Central Diabetes Insipidus

Once the above mentioned causes for polyuria have been excluded, the diagnosis of DI can be made by evaluating the volume of urine output, urine specific gravity, urine and serum electrolyte levels, and urine and serum osmolality. When three of the following findings are noted simultaneously, the diagnosis of DI is established:

Urine output >500 mL/hour
Serum sodium >155 mEq/L
Urine specific gravity <1.005
Serum osmolality >305 mOsm/L

Treatment of DI includes aqueous pitressin IV infusion (10 U/250 mL D5W) with an initial dosage 1.2 U/hour (rate: 30 mL/hour) and subsequent titration to maintain urine output of 150 to 300 mL/hr. Aqueous pitressin should be discontinued for urine output less than 150 mL/hr to minimize the possibility of decreased visceral perfusion (especially in liver and pancreas donors). In addition to pitressin therapy, the free water deficit should be calculated and 50% of the calculated deficit should be infused as rapidly as possible, preferably with a hypotonic solution such as D5W or .5 NS. Nevertheless, a low dose pitressin infusion can decrease the plasma hyperosmolality, increase blood pressure, decrease inotrope use, and maintain cardiac output.

RECOMMENDED READINGS

Guidelines for preventing transmission of human immunodeficiency virus through transplantation of human tissue and organs. Centers for Disease Control and Prevention. MMWR 1994;43:1-17.

Alexander JW, Zola JC. Expanding the donor pool: use of marginal donors for solid organ transplantation. Clin Transplant. 1996;10(1 Pt 1):1-19.

Kauffman H, Bennett L, McBride M, Ellison M. The expanded donor. Transplant Rev. 1997;11:165-190.

Pratschke J, Wilhelm MJ, Kusaka M, et al. Brain death and its influence on donor organ quality and outcome after transplantation. Transplantation. 1999;67(3):343-348.

Colquhoun S, Robert ME, Shaked A, et al. Transmission of CNS malignancy by organ transplantation. Transplantation. 1994;57(6):970-974.

Non-Heart-Beating Organ Transplantation: Practice and Protocols. Committee on Non-Heart-Beating Transplantation II: The Scientific and Ethical Basis for Practice and Protocols, Division of Health Care Services, Institute of Medicine; Washington, DC: National Academy Press; 1999.

Pereira BJ, Wright TL, Schmid CH, et al. Screening and confirmatory testing of cadaver organ donors for hepatitis C virus infection: a U.S. National Collaborative Study. Kidney Int. 1994;46(3):886-892.

Rubin RH, Fishman JA. A consideration of potential donors with active infection—is this a way to expand the donor pool? Transplant Int. 1998;11(5):333-335.

Wachs ME, Amend WJ, Ascher NL, et al. The risk of transmission of hepatitis B from HBsAg (-), HBcAb (+), HBIgM(-) organ donors. Transplantation. 1995;59(2): 230-234.

Delmonico FL, Snydman DR. Organ donor screening for infectious diseases: review of practice and implications for transplantation. Transplantation. 1998;65(5):603-610.

18 ECONOMICS OF TRANSPLANTATION
Theodore I. Steinman, MD

Financial viability is critical for transplantation success. Unless an institution can survive economically, every program within that facility is threatened. For the 885 transplant programs currently functioning in the United States to be financially viable several objectives must be achieved:

- Appropriate expertise and transplant clinical outcomes that meet established criteria
- Positive financial outcomes because of sound management policies
- Open access to the program
- Mix of payors that facilitate patient access to the transplant program and ensure reimbursement

A transplant program must become Medicare certified as the first step towards success. While Medicare certification is not the only milestone for transplant programs, it affords the opportunity to attract other payors, in particular, managed care organizations (MCOs).

Table 18-1 defines the specific facility qualifications for Medicare certification of transplant programs. Variations by type of organ transplant are noted in the table. Of particular note is that Medicare can reimburse for kidney transplantation in the first year of a new kidney transplant program. However, in the case of extrarenal transplantation, a cumulative 24-month period of experience with a minimum volume for each 12-month period is necessary.

For the time period January 1, 1994 to September 30, 1998 the United Network for Organ Sharing (UNOS) reported how frequently Medicare was the primary source of payment for US organ transplants (Table 18-2). The importance of Medicare certifying a kidney transplant program is evident since Medicare pays for more than 50% of kidney and 40% of all organ transplants in the country. The payor mix for transplant programs continues to evolve towards two primary payor sources: Medicare and MCOs. Before an MCO will enter into a contracting arrangement with a transplant program, the MCO invariably mandates Medicare certification. The only exception to this rule involves stand-alone pediatric extra-renal transplant programs that might establish contracts without Medicare certification. Since competition among transplant programs exists in most regions of the country (rarely is there only one sole provider in

major metropolitan areas), MCOs can afford to "pick and choose" their preferred provider(s). "Centers of excellence" approach has been used by MCOs to assure high-quality patient care and containment of costs associated with transplantation. Since the health care market is dynamic and transplant programs are very competitive, achieving Medicare certification and meeting MCOs' selection criteria as a "center of excellence" are critical.

While MCOs establish specific criteria for contracting, administrative competence is also necessary for the transplant program to comply with an MCO's review, case management and communication processes. Such a support system must complement clinical competence, patient satisfaction documentation and continuous quality improvement models that are employed by the transplant program.

In summary, the MCO's minimum facility and clinical criteria for transplant programs include the following:
- UNOS approved
- Medicare certified
- Appropriate 1-year patient and graft survival statistics
- Sufficient volume of organ specific transplants
- Comprehensive/integrated services that encompass all aspects of patient care
- Appropriate patient selection criteria
- Clearly defined pretransplant and posttransplant clinical protocols

FINANCES: COST VS CHARGES

When attempting to determine resource utilization, it is important to clearly differentiate between *costs* and *charges*. While these terms are often used interchangeably, they are quite disparate. A holdover from the previous "fee for service" reimbursement method results in a confusion in terms. A charge or reimbursement for services from a third party payor would often be referred to as the cost of the service or product. In the current health care environment, reimbursement is progressively switching towards a system of capitation in one form or another. From a provider's perspective, costs and charges are two separate entities.

Charges are the amount than an institution or individual provider chooses to request for a service or good, and the charge is the price that appears on a patient's bill. Charges are invariably inflated from actual costs to include a margin for revenue. Charges vary widely among providers/institutions, and the method by which a charge is established is so highly variable as to not be comparable among providers. Charges that are established may incorporate factors such as payor mix, bad debt or regional competition for particular services. For example, one service may be "charged" at or below the actual "cost" because it is perceived to be a value added

Professor of Medicine, Harvard Medical School; Director, Dialysis Unit, Beth Israel Deaconess Medical Center, Boston, MA

service and is believed to indirectly contribute to the revenue of another program. This "charge" compared to that of a program that is breaking even or even making some profit would not be a fair economic comparison.

Even within an institution, the methods of determining charges may vary. While from the outside it may be assumed that a standard cost-to-charge ratio exists within an institution, this is often not the case.

Prices are established by the finance department in an institution, and trying to determine which products or services have, over the years, been priced differently can be an insurmountable task. Therefore, using charges in comparative economic evaluations among institutions or study groups does not provide a confident reflection of real differences in resource utilization.

In contrast to charges, *costs* are defined as the magnitude of resources consumed in producing goods or services. Cost includes an economic value for all resources consumed, but it does not include a mark-up

for revenue. Health care providers must now pay more attention than ever to determining the costs of health care in transplantation when considering the competitive environment, fixed payment by payors and new managed care contracts. Despite medicine being the third largest industry economically in the United States, many of the financial practices are run on a "mom and pop store" concept. Only recently have sophisticated cost-accounting systems been developed in institutions. These systems are the best able to estimate resource utilization.

The clarification of costs vs charges is also imperative when evaluating the literature. Actual charges should generally not be used as a substitute for costs, especially in multicenter trials. It is critical to scrutinize the economic analysis attached to any trial since a valid measure of costs may not stand critical analysis. It is clear from the literature that what were listed as "costs" were actually "charges." Therefore, it is impossible to compare one

Table 18-1. Facility Qualifications for Medicare Certification of Transplant Programs

Organ	DRG	Year of HCFA Notice of Medicare Coverage	Patient Selection Clinical Criteria	Volume per Time Period	Survival Statistics
Kidney	302	1972	End-stage renal disease	15 or more annually for unconditional status. Seven to 14 for conditional status.	Not designated
Liver	480	1991	Exclusion of hepatitis B and malignancy	12 or more per each of the two preceding 12 month periods.	1 year = 77% 2 year = 60%
Heart	103	1986	Center's written patient selection criteria	12 or more per each of the two preceding 12 month periods and at least 12 transplants prior to but since 1/1/82.	1 year = 73% 2 year = 62%
Lung / Heart-Lung	495	1995	Center's written patient selection criteria	Ten or more per each of the two preceding 12 month periods.	1 year = 69% 2 year = 62%

Source: Renal Physicians Association

Table 18-2. Percentage of Transplants Paid by Medicare as Primary Source of Payment 1997

Organ	Number of Transplants	Number Reporting Primary Payor Source	Percent Transplants Paid by Medicare
Kidney	12,323	11,848	55.4%
Liver	4,165	3,993	12.0%
Heart	2,292	2,102	21.0%
Lung / Heart-Lung	990	882	17.3%

Source: United Network for Organ Sharing reported primary source of payment for U.S. Organ Transplants: January 1, 1994 to September 30, 1998.

institution to another. For example, one recent trial reported a mean difference in cost between tacrolimus and cyclosporine arms of a trial as ranging from +$3,493 (costs higher for tacrolimus) to $51,203 (costs higher for cyclosporine). In the same trial, the average length of hospital stay in the tacrolimus-treated patients was 25 to 29 days in five of six centers while the average hospital charges varied from $82,306 to $161,123. Such large variation in the data would result in a questioning of the validity of any conclusion that can be made from this data, and also supports the assertion that charge data is not a good method to compare resource utilization. While the methods for evaluating the actual costs of health care are still evolving and there are limitations to their use, cost provides a much better representation for comparing differences in resources used than do charges, and they should be applied in economic evaluations.

THE ECONOMIC COST OF ESRD

At present, ESRD patients cannot enroll in Heath Maintenance Organizations (HMOs) under Medicare contracts, but may remain in an HMO if they develop ESRD after enrollment. The current capitation payment for such patients is state-specific but unadjusted. The Health Care Financing Administration (HCFA) now has an ongoing demonstration project to see if a monthly capitation rate for dialysis and kidney transplant patients can ultimately lower costs while maximizing care. Reimbursement schemata under the demonstration project pays a capitated amount based on 100% fee-for-service costs for dialysis patients (rather than the 95% paid by Medicare capitation outside of the demonstration project). For this additional 5% payment, HMOs have to provide additional benefits (eg, coverage for all medications, nutritional supplements, transportation costs, home health agencies, skilled nursing facilities). HCFA proposed under the Capitation Demonstration Project that kidney transplantation be reimbursed at a higher rate than for chronic dialysis care. After a three month perioperative period, the reimbursement rate would fall below the chronic dialysis rate and stay at this reduced payment level as compared to dialysis care during the 36-month ESRD benefit eligibility *period* for patients with a functioning allograft. Dialysis and post-transplant rates are adjusted for age (under 20, 20 to 64, 65+) and whether diabetes was the cause of kidney failure. It will take until 2002 before the economic analysis of this demonstration project is completed and the results published.

The United States Renal Data System (USRDS) database obtains information from the Medicare payment records and also analyzes extensive epidemiological patient histories. The financial objective is to compare and contrast Medicare reimbursements (payments) per time at risk for different modalities of renal replacement therapy and different patient characteristics. The results provide information that would be useful in the determination of "capitation" payment rates (ie, rates of spending per patient per time at risk). However, because these results do not provide simultaneous comparisons of survival and costs across treatment modalities, and are not estimated with consideration for lifetime costs, they are insufficient to determine the cost-effectiveness of different treatment modalities. Since modalities are not randomly assigned, it is likely that patients who are healthier or sicker than average systematically select different modalities.

With the above background, total Medicare payments for kidney transplantation provide the best estimates for costs associated with transplantation. Every aspect of cost must be included so a true assessment of costs can be obtained. For example, donor acquisition costs are frequently not included in the bottom-line assessment of transplantation costs, but in 1997 this cost was estimated to total $450 million for all organs. It is extremely difficult to extract the total cost for transplantation because Medicare payments to institutions include kidney acquisition costs, medical malpractice insurance and medical education costs through the Diagnosis Related Group (DRG) payment system. Medicare pays for kidney donor acquisition costs by inflating the costs of all Medicare inpatient stays (both ESRD and non-ESRD) by an amount equal to the institutional acquisition cost for all Medicare transplants and other "passed through" amounts (ie, malpractice insurance, education and capital expenditures). It is estimated that Medicare payments in 1997 for cadaver organ donation was approximately $25,000 per acquisition for the 8,000 cadaver kidney transplants. If there is a living donor, all of the donor's expenses should be charged to the recipient's insurance. Although the donor, therefore, does not incur direct medical expenses, no insurance plan currently reimburses the donor for lost wages. A recent federal statute extended the donor's medical leave from one week to one month for federal employees.

Patient Eligibility

In 1997 the Medicare Secondary Payment (MSP) was extended from 18 to 30 months under the Balanced Budget Act. In essence, this means that the patient's private insurance must pay for ESRD costs for the first 30 months of treatment if the patient is not eligible for Medicare by virtue of age or disability status at the beginning of ESRD. Medicare becomes the primary payor after 30 months of dialysis. However, transplantation is the exception. If the first ESRD service is a kidney transplant, then the entire hospital stay is covered as a Medicare cost, even if the reported day of ESRD occurs during that hospital stay. Currently, Medicare pays for all costs associated with transplantation for the first 36 months of graft function. If after three years the graft is still functioning, then the insurance coverage reverts back to the patient's primary insurer. If transplant graft function is lost during the first three years after transplantation, the patient then reverts immediately back to Medicare coverage upon the resumption of dialysis.

MEDICARE SPENDING

During the first year of transplantation (including hospitalization, organ acquisition, medication and total physician care) costs in 1999 were estimated to be approximately $120,000. About half of this amount is consumed as part of the in-hospital transplant process, which includes physician payments as well as every other aspect of care. After the first year, the costs of total care, including immunosuppressive therapy and laboratory monitoring, averages $18,000. In contrast, Medicare annual payments for dialysis average $51,000 and the total yearly cost of every aspect of care amounts to about $64,000 (the additional non-Medicare allowable expenses being covered either by secondary insurance or out-of-pocket). When analyzing the diabetic population as a separate entity, the costs increase significantly. For example, after the first year posttransplant, the total Medicare payments increase to about $25,000 per patient. As expected, age is also a cost factor. With each advancing age group, the incremental costs rise. For example, the Medicare payments rise by 20% when advancing from the age group 20 to 44 years to 45 to 64 years. An additional 20% increment is noted for the age group 65 to 74 years. Although less well-documented, costs for infants and young children tend to be high because of extended hospitalization times and requirements for corrective urologic procedures. Race adds another cost increment. Expenditures for the transplant modality of renal replacement therapy were significantly higher for African-American patients ($21,000 and $22,000 for males and females, respectively) than for Caucasian patients ($15,000 for either males or females). This difference is likely to arise from higher transplant

rejection rates among African-Americans, a cost pattern that exists among diabetic patients related to an increase in co-morbid complications.

COSTS FOR IMMUNOSUPPRESSIVE DRUGS

Access to medications, which keep transplants functioning, is a medical necessity. Current Medicare legislation limits immunosuppressive drug coverage to 36 months posttransplant. In 1986, Congress amended Medicare Part B to provide coverage for self-administered medications for one year posttransplant and Congress extended coverage to three years in the 1993 Omnibus Budget Reconciliation Act (OBRA). However, transplant recipients must take these drugs indefinitely. At the current time, legislation is being introduced that would extend or eliminate the 36 month time limitation on Medicare coverage for immunosuppressive drugs (now ranging between $11,000 and $14,000 for kidney transplant recipients, depending on the drug combination employed). The argument being made is that reimbursement policies should result in long-term benefit (indefinite payment for immunosuppressive medications) rather than putting a transplanted organ at risk for rejection. Paying for antirejection medications is far less expensive than the cost of returning to dialysis or a second transplant. Table 18-3 projects the total cost of immunosuppressive therapy coverage for all organs. It is shown that over five years the net costs for all immunosuppressive medications will be approximately $2.4 billion. This contrasts to the estimated gross cost of $300 million for heart, liver and lung transplants during the same 5-year time frame, 2000 to 2004, (Table 18-4).

To bolster the proposition that immunosuppressive medications should be covered indefinitely, Table 18-5 demonstrates the cost savings from kidney transplantation as compared to maintenance dialysis during the time frame of 2000 to 2004. It is projected that the potential cost savings would be $1.75 billion if transplantation were maximally utilized and immunosuppressive coverage was not a factor in leading to graft failure. Table 18-6

Table 18-3. Total Costs of Immunosuppressive Therapy Coverage for All Organs (millions of dollars)

Net Cost	2000	2001	2002	2003	2004	Total
Gross costs (kidney)	$603.5	$677.1	$759.7	$852.4	$956.4	$3,849.2
Gross costs (all other organs)	$ 46.5	$ 53.6	$ 60.7	$ 66.8	$ 73.2	$ 300.8
Cost savings (kidney offsets)	$134.7	$246.3	$352.0	$455.1	$558.6	$1,746.7
Net costs (gross – offsets)	$515.3	$484.5	$468.5	$464.1	$471.1	$2,403.4

Five year net costs of 2.4 billion
Source: The Lewin Group for the Renal Physicians Association

Table 18-4. Gross Cost Estimate for Heart, Liver and Lung Transplants (millions of dollars)

Gross Costs	2000	2001	2002	2003	2004	Total
Annual heart > 3 year	$1,863	$2,179	$2,506	$2,757	$3,032	NA
Annual liver > 3 year	$1,735	$2,082	$2,395	$2,634	$2,897	NA
Annual lung > 3 year	$217	$304	$395	$474	$521	NA
Total graft patient > 3 years	$5,815	$6,566	$7,297	$7,867	$8,455	NA
Cost per year of immuno	$8,000	$8,160	$8,323	$8,490	$8,659	NA
Total cost (millions)	$46.52	$53.58	$60.74	$66.79	$73.21	$300.80

Five year gross cost estimate of $0.3 billion
Source: The Lewin Group for the Renal Physicians Association

Table 18-5. Cost Savings from Kidney Transplants (millions of dollars)

Avoided Costs	2000	2001	2002	2003	2004	Total
Graft failure rate from cost pressure	2.5%	2.5%	2.5%	2.5%	2.5%	NA
Annual > 3 year failed grafts	1,886	2,075	2,282	2,510	2,761	NA
Prior number of > 3 year failed graphs	–	1,471	2,766	3,937	5,029	NA
Total > 3 year failed grafts	1,886	3,546	5,048	6,447	7,790	NA
Cost of loss	$61,057	$62,278	$63,523	$64,794	$66,090	NA
Total annual cost of removal (millions)	$115.1	$129.2	$145.0	$162.6	$182.5	$734.4
Per unit cost of dialysis	$53,042	$54,103	$55,185	$56,289	$57,415	NA
Total cost of dialysis (millions)	–	$79.6	$152.6	$221.6	$288.7	$742.6
Number re-transplanted (10% of total)	189	355	505	645	779	NA
Cost per re-transplantation	$103,607	$105,679	$107,793	$109,949	$112,147	NA
Total costs of re-transplantation (millions)	$19.5	$37.5	$54.4	$70.9	$87.4	$269.7
Total cost due to graft failure	$134.7	$246.3	$352.0	$455.10	$558.6	$1,756.7

Total five year potential cost savings of $1.75 billion
Source: The Lewin Group for the Renal Physicians Association

Table 18-6. Net Cost to Medicare of Kidney Transplant Immunosuppression Coverage (millions of dollars)

Net Cost	2000	2001	2002	2003	2004	Total
Gross costs (direct)	$603.5	$677.1	$759.7	$852.4	$956.4	$3,849.2
Cost savings (offsets)	$134.7	$246.3	$352.0	$455.1	$558.6	$1,746.7
Net costs (gross – offsets)	$468.8	$430.9	$407.8	$397.3	$397.8	$2,102.6

Five year gross cost of $3.85 billion.
Five year cost offsets of $1.75 billion.
Five year net cost of $2.1 billion.
Source: The Lewin Group for the Renal Physicians Association

summarizes the net cost to Medicare for indefinite immunosuppressive coverage for kidney transplantation. The 5-year cost of kidney transplantation (2000 to 2004) would be $3.85 billion. Cost savings of the above $1.75 billion, with maximal utilization of kidney transplants, results in a 5-year net cost of approximately $2.1 billion ($3.85 billion - $1.75 billion = $2.1 billion).

In summary, it makes economic (as well as medical) sense to maximally utilize transplantation for those who would benefit from the procedure. In addition to our obligation to provide quality care for patients, we all must become advocates for our patients by supporting legislation that maximizes appropriate medical decisions. If our legislative voices become silent, our patients will suffer. Our goal must be to modernize and strengthen the Medicare program (or some acceptable alternative). Medicare needs to become more competitive and efficient, and benefits must be focused on what is best for patients. Appropriate constraints based on cost-effective care is our mandatory obligation. There must be a long-term commitment to financing transplantation. Payment for inpatient and outpatient hospital services, medications, skilled nursing facilities, home health agencies and physician's services must be commensurate with the expert care provided by transplant physicians.

RECOMMENDED READING

United States Renal Data System, USRDS 1999 Annual Data Report, National Institutes of Health, National Institute of Diabetes and Digestive and Kidney Diseases. Bethesda, MD, April 1999.

Editorial. Medicare and managed care designation of transplant programs. Transplant Outcomes. 1999;2:2.

Steinman TI. Managed care, capitation and the future of nephrology. J Am Soc Nephrol. 1997;8(10):1618-1623.

Steinman TI. How nephrologists can understand the reimbursement system change. Nephrol News Iss. 1999;13:24-26.

Finkler SA. The distinction between cost and charges. Ann Intern Med.1982;96(1):102-109.

Eggers PW, Kucken LE. Cost issues in transplantation. Surg Clin North Am. 1994;74(5):1259-1267.

Lake JR, Gorman KJ, Esquivel CO, et al. The impact of immunosuppressive regimens on the cost of liver transplantation: results from the US FK506 multicenter trial. Transplantation. 1995;60(10):1089-1095.

Rubin RJ, Gaylin DS, Shapiro JR. End-stage renal disease, managed care, and capitation: implications for the renal community. Adv Ren Replace Ther. 1997;4(4):306-313.

Iglehart JK. The American health care system – Medicare. N Engl J Med. 1999;340(4):327-332.

Iglehart JK. The American health care system – expenditures. N Engl J Med. 1999;340(1):70-76.

Eglehart JK. Support for academic medical centers – revisiting the 1997 balanced budget act. N Engl J Med. 1999;341(4):299-304.

Section IV

MEDICAL COMPLICATIONS OF TRANSPLANTATION

19 HEART DISEASE IN NON-HEART TRANSPLANT RECIPIENTS

James B. Young, MD

Aging transplant recipients and longer allograft survival have made cardiovascular disease an important determinant of long-term patient outcome. As in the general population, the aging process affects transplant recipients with implications regarding atherosclerotic cardiovascular disease, acquired valvular heart disease, and the risk of developing cardiomyopathy. In addition, post-transplant pharmacologic stimulation (ie, steroids, calcineurin inhibitors) of hyperlipidemia and hypertension likely contribute to cardiac disease. Furthermore, immunosuppression, which fosters the presence of new and reactivated infections, may play a role in the pathogenesis of atherosclerosis, endocarditis and inflammatory cardiomyopathy. As patients are followed after transplantation, attention should be focused on three specific issues related to development of cardiac and vascular disease: (1) what is the significance of cardiovascular disease present at the time of transplantation; (2) how can development of atherosclerotic cardiovascular disease be prevented or attenuated after transplantation; and (3) what is the best way to evaluate patients suspected of having cardiac disease?

DIAGNOSTIC WORKUP OF HEART DISEASE IN NON-HEART TRANSPLANT PATIENTS

Following solid organ transplantation, patients should have a baseline electrocardiogram, chest x-ray, and lipid profile. These tests should be repeated at timed intervals. An electrocardiogram probably does not need to be repeated, unless symptoms or clinical findings suggest a newly developed cardiac ailment, or that hypertension has been longstanding. Lipid profiles, however, should be characterized, followed regularly, and used as a guide for treatment. Any complaint that could conceivably suggest an ischemic syndrome should be paid particular attention.

HISTORY, PHYSICAL EXAMINATION, AND ANCILLARY TESTS USEFUL DURING EVALUATION

Whether or not a transplant patient has, or is suspected of having, ischemic heart disease, ventricular dysfunction (heart failure), valvular heart disease, dysrhythmias,

Medical Director, Kaufman Center for Heart Failure, Department of Cardiology, The Cleveland Clinic Foundation, Cleveland, OH

pulmonary hypertension, or peripheral vascular disease, the approach to evaluation consists of obtaining the same basic information. This includes a proper history interview, physical examination, core laboratory data, general diagnostic studies, and specialized directed diagnostic tests.

Tables 19-1 and 19-2 summarize specific history and physical findings used to determine whether cardiovascular disease is present and significant. Particular attention should be paid to chest pain syndromes, angina "equivalents" (eg, short-windedness, exercise limitation, or palpitations in the absence of chest pain), and the appearance of left ventricular dysfunction. Left ventricular dysfunction can be both systolic and diastolic, with symptoms related to a variety of dyspnea syndromes, fluid retention states, or weakness and fatigue.

It should be remembered that altered cardiac performance will significantly impact transplanted lungs, kidneys or livers. Thus, exploring symptoms related to the transplanted organ system is also important. For example, in a patient with a lung transplant, pulmonary hypertension due to the insidious development of valvular heart disease or left ventricular diastolic dysfunctions, which may be due to hypertension, will contribute to dyspnea. Sudden changes in the intensity of dyspnea in some patients could reflect altered cardiac function, as well as pulmonary allograft rejection or infection. Likewise, left ventricular dysfunction causing right heart failure and elevated right atrial pressure can contribute to hepatic dysfunction following liver transplantation. Furthermore, low flow states in individuals with heart failure may decrease renal arterial perfusion and result in native or transplant kidney dysfunction. Additionally, high right heart pressures secondary to right heart failure, tricuspid insufficiency, or pulmonary hypertension cause elevated mesenteric venous pressure, which contributes to mesenteric organ hypoperfusion even when blood pressure is normal or elevated. When forward flow diminishes during an event causing hypotension, the problem worsens. Thus, symptoms sometimes attributed to hepatic or renal graft dysfunction might actually represent cardiovascular disease.

Table 19-3 summarizes common diagnostic tests for evaluating cardiac disease. Many simple and inexpensive tests, such as the chest x-ray and electrocardiogram, provide important information about disease presence, etiology and severity. Particularly important are pulmonary congestion and cardiomegaly on a chest x-ray, and ventricular hypertrophy and arrhythmias on an electrocardiogram. The most important single study to obtain in any patient suspected of having heart disease is an echocardiogram. Today's echocardiographic studies generally include M-mode, two-dimensional, and Doppler interrogations. Collectively, these images give an extraordinary and accurate assessment of cardiac chamber size, shape and function, and provide insight into valvular heart disease and architectural aberrations. Wall motion analysis can be important when done both at rest and during stress induced by exercise or pharmacologic agents, to gain insight into the presence of ischemic heart disease and its relationship to chest pain or heart failure. More sophisticated imaging techniques can be chosen for certain patients who have a need for further evaluation. First-pass radionuclide ventriculography or equilibrium radionuclide ventriculography,

magnetic resonance imaging, and computerized tomographic studies can be helpful. Table 19-4 compares echocardiographic studies with radionuclide imaging and MRI or CT scanning.

ASSESSMENT OF ISCHEMIC HEART DISEASE

Graded exercise stress testing is the cornerstone of evaluation for suspected coronary artery disease. Exercise studies can provide information even when electro-

Table 19-1. The Clinical History when Cardiac Disease is Suspected*

Cardiovascular	Pulmonary
Angina pectoris	Dyspnea on exertion
Nonspecific chest pain	Orthopnea
Fatigue	Paroxysmal nocturnal dyspnea
Weakness	Pleurisy
Orthostatic faintness	Cough
Claudication	Hemoptysis
Gastroenterologic	**Neurologic/Neuropsychiatric**
Abdominal pain	Anxiety or panic
Abdominal bloating	Depression
Constipation	Confusion
Anorexia	Decreased mental acuity
Nausea	
Vomiting	
Renal	**Systemic**
Nocturia	Edema
Oliguria	Petechiae/ecchymosis

*Ancillary history that elucidates concomitant cardiovascular and noncardiovascular illnesses is critical.

Table 19-2. Physical Examination when Cardiac Disease is Suspected*

Vital Signs	Pulmonary
Positional blood pressure	Rales
Pulse rate, rhythm, and quality	Rhonchi
Respiratory rate and pattern	Friction rubs
Temperature	Wheezes
Cardiovascular	Dullness of percussion
Neck vein distention	**Abdominal**
Abdominal-jugular neck vein reflex	Ascites
Cardiomegaly on palpitation	Hepatosplenomegaly
Chest wall pulsatile activity	Decreased bowel sounds
Gallop rhythm on auscultation	Aortic aneurysm
Heart murmurs†	**Neurologic**
Diminished S_1 or S_2	Mental status abnormalities
Friction rubs	**Systemic**
Bruits	Edema
	Cachexia

*Ancillary physical examination information that elucidates concomitant cardiovascular and noncardiovascular illnesses is critical.
†Especially mitral, tricuspid, and pulmonic insufficiency.

cardiographic changes, suggesting myocardial ischemia, are not present or cannot be used because of baseline tracing abnormalities. Stress testing inducing an adequate level of cardiac work can reliably correlate symptoms with ischemia in males with normal resting studies. Perhaps most important is risk stratification in patients known to have coronary disease. Patients who are unable to exercise for more than six minutes on the Bruce proto-col, or who demonstrate significant ischemia within this time, are at increased risk of morbid events. Additional findings of great concern include: (1) two minutes of significant ST segment depression; (2) ST segment depression lasting more than three minutes after stopping; (3) down-sloping ST depression at peak exercise; (4) ischemia developing at a low heart rate (<120 beats per minute); (5) a flat or diminished systolic blood

---

Table 19-3. Common Ancillary Diagnostic Tests when Cardiac Disease is Suspected

Chest x-ray	Echocardiography (2D/M-mode)
Cardiothoracic ratio	Chamber size and shape
Selective chamber size and shape	Valve integrity and motion
Pulmonary vascularity and congestion	Fractional shortening of ventricles
Pleural effusions	Mean circumferential fiber shortening
Mass lesions or infiltrates	Mitral E point to septal separation
Mediastinal configuration	Systolic wall thickening
Great vessel abnormality	Wall motion analysis
Electrocardiography	Estimation of wall stress
Rhythm	Endomyocardial biopsy guidance
Atrial fibrillation	Exercise and pharmacologic stress
Ventricular arrhythmias	(wall motion)
Heart rate	Tissue characterization
Evidence of hypertrophy	Pericardial effusion
Q wave presence	Pericardial restriction
P mitrale or pulmonale	**Doppler echocardiography**
Conduction disturbances	Quantification of valve stenosis / regurgitation
Drug effects	Estimation of pulmonary artery systolic pressure
Metabolic changes	Estimation of stroke volume and cardiac output
	Determination of diastolic filling characteristics
	Detection of shunts

Table 19-4. Non-Invasive Imaging Techniques in Patients with Heart Disease

Observation	M-Mode Echo	2D Echo	Doppler Echo	First-Pass RNVG	Equilibrium RNVG	MRI	CT
Anatomic Relationships	+	+++	0 / ++	+	+	++++	+++
Tissue Characterization	++	++	0	0	0	+++	+++
Wall Motion	+	++++	0	++	++++	+++	+++
Hypertrophy	+++	++++	0	0 / +	++++	+++	
Wall Thickening	+++	++++	0	0	++++	++	
Valvular Pathology	++	++++	0	0	0	+++	++
Valvular Regurgitation and Stenosis	++	++	++++	0	0	++	+
Hemodynamics	+	+	++++	0	0	0	0
Diastolic Function	++	+++	++++	++	++	+	0
Stress Exercise	++++	++++	++++	++++	++++	0	0
Pharmacologic Stress	++++	++++	++++	++++	++++	++++	+++
Lower Cost / Ease of Availability	++++	++++	+++	+++	+++	+	++

2D indicates two-dimensional; RNVG, radionuclide ventriculography; MRI, magnetic resonance imaging; CT, computed tomography; and 0/+, the relative utility of the different techniques in the authors' opinion.

pressure response at peak exercise; and (6) ventricular tachycardia (even nonsustained). Although exercise testing generally should be performed in all patients with suspected angina pectoris prior to moving toward more invasive procedures, some transplant patients are unable to exercise on a treadmill or bicycle. Thus, they often need to undergo another form of testing.

An alternative form of stress testing is generally necessary when (1) an abnormal resting electrocardiogram is present (particularly left ventricular hypertrophy); (2) there is an inability to adequately exercise; (3) more precise prognostic information is desired; (4) the physiologic significance of a stenotic or insufficient valve is questioned; or (5) when one is attempting to determine the extent of myocardial tissue viability in the presence of left ventricular dysfunction and coronary disease. Table 19-5 lists the advantages and disadvantages of stress echocardiography and myocardial perfusion scintigraphy. Pharmacologic stress echocardiography is a versatile and cost-effective tool. It does not require a license or facilities for using radioactive pharmaceuticals. Scintigraphic myocardial perfusion imaging, however, may provide a greater degree of defect-quantitation. Myocardial perfusion imaging is more sensitive, but less specific than stress echocardiographic studies. Certain patients seem to fare better with echocardiographic stress testing, including patients who are women, or who have left ventricular hypertrophy or valvular heart disease. On the other hand, nuclear imaging is favored in patients who have chronic lung disease, physiologically

significant aortic or mitral valve stenosis, or suspected multivessel coronary disease, or are on antianginal therapy. Although pharmacologic stress echocardiographic and scintigraphic studies can be done in those not capable of exercise, exercise stress testing is preferred because it: (1) evaluates exercise capacity; (2) allows correlation of symptoms to physical workload; (3) demonstrates concomitant electrocardiographic ST evaluation; (4) creates greater cardiac work loads; (5) provides specific prognostic information; and (6) may have greater sensitivity for ischemia.

False negative stress echocardiograms may be caused by inadequate exercise or pharmacologic stress, concomitant antianginal therapy, the presence of only mild coronary artery disease, poor image quality, and isolated left circumflex disease. Stress echocardiograms can be falsely positive when there is a hypertensive response in the setting of cardiomyopathy or left ventricle hypertrophy, and when abnormal septal motion at baseline is present. The latter can be seen post-open heart surgery or with left bundle branch block. Over-interpretation of images due to interpreter bias, localized basal inferior wall abnormalities and, most commonly, image quality variability are factors that limit the accuracy of stress echocardiography.

Radionuclide techniques (eg, gaited equilibrium and first-pass imaging) are used to evaluate left and right ventricular ejection fraction, left ventricular volume and regional wall motion abnormalities. Gaited radionuclide angiography uses scintigraphy to detect the course of

Table 19-5. Relative Advantages and Disadvantages of Stress Echocardiography and Myocardial Perfusion Scintigraphy: Their Effects on Patient Selection

Consideration	Stress Echocardiography Imaging	Myocardial Perfusion
Versatility	++	-
Cost	++	-
Quantitation	-	++
Sensitivity	80% to 85%	90%
Specificity	85%	70%
Prognostic value	+	++
Familiarity	++	+
LVH	++	+
Valvular heart disease	++ (provides ancillary data)	-
Left bundle branch lock	± (false positives)	+
Chronic lung disease	± (poor windows; TEE an alternative)	++
On anginal therapy	+ (requires ischemia)	++
Physiological significance of known stenosis	+ (limited sensitivity for single vessels)	++
Recognition of multivessel CAD	+	++
Localization of CAD	++	++
Ischemia within infarct zone	+	++

Adapted with permission from Marwick TH. Stress echocardiography. In: Topol ET, ed. Textbook of Cardiovascular Medicine. Lippincott-Raven; Philadelphia, PA:1998;1267-1300.

technetium pertechnetate-labeled red blood cells through the heart. Image acquisition is gaited to the electrocardiographic cycle. Gaiting allows one to distinguish systole from diastole, and assess changes in wall motion following stress. First-pass imaging allows the calculation of cardiac function by measuring counts only during the first few cardiac cycles after injecting a large bolus of radio-pharmaceutically-labeled red cells. Additionally, scintigraphic myocardial perfusion imaging allows the determination of blood flow distribution through the myocardium; abnormal flow is suggested by diminished tracer uptake in specific regions during exercise compared to a resting state. Perfusion abnormalities present at rest usually indicate areas of myocardial fibrosis caused by a prior myocardial infarction. Perfusion abnormalities occurring during stress (ie, decreased flow relative to surrounding areas) denote areas supplied by vessels that have a significant stenosis. In patients with an evolving myocardial infarction, perfusion studies can (1) measure the size of the infarcted area; (2) assess the degree of myocardial salvage in response to thrombolytic therapy or primary angioplasty; (3) provide a measurement of left ventricular ejection fraction (when simultaneous gaiting techniques are employed); (4) identify culprit arteries; (5) help triage patients with chest pain in the emergency department; and (6) give insight into myocardial viability.

The ultimate arbiter for the presence of coronary heart disease is coronary angiography. It should be stressed, however, that angiography simply provides a road map of obstructive lesions. Although anatomic configuration alone might dictate procedural intervention (eg, left main coronary lesions, multivessel disease, coronary lesions in a setting of heart failure, and proximal left anterior descending obstruction), one, more often, must correlate anatomic findings with functional studies. Each patient should be judged individually, and mechanical revascularization should be recommended only for significantly symptomatic individuals or those with large objective areas of ischemia.

Long-term ambulatory electrocardiographic monitoring can be helpful in assessing symptomatic patients with palpitations, chest pain, syncope, near syncope, and orthostatic hypotension. Rate, rhythm and ST segment changes may be evaluated by ambulatory monitoring. Recordings can be continuous over a defined period of time (24 or 48 hours) or triggered to record events when the patient is symptomatic. Obviously, if a patient faints prior to triggering the event recorder, no data will be obtained. However, the advantage of triggered event recorders is that long-term surveillance (over weeks or even months) is possible.

Interpretation of Cardiovascular Testing

Determining the appropriate test to evaluate cardiovascular disease depends upon the disease process being explored and the type of information needed. Does the clinician wish to know if coronary disease is present no matter what its severity? Does the clinician desire to know the risks of performing non-cardiac solid organ transplantation in the setting of particular cardiac disease? Does the clinician wish to diagnose a cardiovascular problem that may be producing certain symptoms or physical findings? As an example, coronary angiography is the most sensitive and specific method for detecting coronary atherosclerosis, and if just the presence of disease will modify treatments or transplant candidacy, then this is the study to perform. Conversely, if the goal of patient evaluation is to reliably determine physiologically significant coronary artery disease, then noninvasive stress testing with an 80% to 90% sensitivity and specificity should be performed. Furthermore, although angiography documents disease, unless it shows multivessel coronary disease, significant left main obstruction, or proximal left anterior descending disease, it may not give adequate information regarding the physiologic significance of the disease or risks of developing complications over the long-term. To more accurately determine the prognosis of coronary disease, other information, such as the findings during exercise testing, is needed. Additionally, radionuclide imaging or echocardiography showing a diminished ejection fraction at rest, but particularly during stress, coupled with wall motion abnormalities, denote a substantive adverse prognosis. Large areas of myocardial hypoperfusion documented by radionuclide imaging, particularly when associated with left ventricular dilation and depressed ejection fraction, are ominous.

The use of newer and more expensive tests such as positron emission tomography, magnetic resonance imaging, and computerized tomography will depend upon their availability and the specific questions to be addressed. For example, computerized tomography, magnetic resonance imaging and echocardiography all evaluate cardiac chamber size, valve integrity, and anatomic relationships (Table 19-4). In most cases, a two-dimensional, doppler echocardiogram will provide the information desired in an accurate and more cost-effective fashion.

CONSIDERING COMBINED HEART WITH OTHER ORGAN TRANSPLANTS

Combined heart-kidney, heart-liver, and heart-lung transplants have been uncommonly, but successfully, performed. The majority of experience has been with heart-lung transplantation because of the coupling of congenital cardiac abnormalities with fixed pulmonary hypertension. Heart-kidney transplantation has been performed in the patient on dialysis who develops profound, irreversible congestive heart failure and, conversely, in patients with profound congestive heart failure who subsequently develop renal failure that is unlikely to reverse following heart transplantation and exposure to nephrotoxic immunosuppressive agents. Heart-liver transplantation may be performed in the patient with premature atherosclerosis and profound congestive heart failure in a setting of dyslipidemia that arises from hepatic metabolic defects. Finally, cardiac transplantation may be sought for patients who have had prior kidney or liver allografts and develop subsequent end-stage heart failure.

Because of limited data to guide the decision for multi-organ transplantation, the best approach is careful evaluation of each individual patient. No broad recommendations can be made. It may be reasonable to consider cardiac transplant in a long-surviving abdominal organ transplant patient, provided that their renal and hepatic function, and other commonly assessed parameters, meet reasonable criteria. One could argue that these patients have already been through the rigors of immunosuppression and likely will not have additional problems after a second and different organ transplant. However, it is known that long-term function of any transplanted organ is abnormal. These issues must be taken into careful consideration.

EVALUATION OF SPECIFIC CARDIAC SYNDROMES BEFORE AND AFTER TRANSPLANTATION

Cardiovascular disease before and after solid organ transplant must be considered in the context of the clinical milieu, but usually presents with four main signs or symptoms: (1) chest discomfort, (2) heart failure, (3) syncope, and (4) palpitations or arrhythmias. Each of these problems should be evaluated specifically in the context of transplantation.

Evaluation of Patients for Non-Cardiac Surgery

When evaluating patients being considered for non-heart solid organ transplant, one must establish whether a cardiovascular disorder is present and, if so, then stratify the patient's long-term risk into low, intermediate, or high categories. Predictors of moderately increased risk for coronary artery disease include advanced age, electrocardiographic findings of left ventricular hypertrophy, left bundle branch block, nonspecific ST-T wave abnormalities, any rhythm other than sinus rhythm, and in particular, atrial fibrillation. Additional risk factors include low functional aerobic capacity such as the inability to climb one flight of stairs without halting, and a history of stroke or uncontrolled systemic hypertension. Intermediate risk is seen with mild angina pectoris, myocardial infarction by history or pathologic Q waves on

the electrocardiogram, compensated or prior congestive heart failure, and diabetes mellitus. Patients having a major risk of adverse outcome after any surgery include those with unstable coronary syndromes such as myocardial infarction with evidence of ongoing ischemia. Patients with unstable or severe angina pectoris generally manifest symptoms at rest or with minimal exercise and have a major risk for adverse outcome. Decompensated congestive heart failure and severe valvular heart disease also portend significant difficulties as do high-grade atrial ventricular block, symptomatic ventricular arrhythmias, and supraventricular arrhythmias with uncontrolled ventricular rates. A noninvasive test should be performed for patient staging. Indications for coronary angiography include those patients demonstrating high-risk results at the time of noninvasive testing, angina pectoris unresponsive to adequate medical therapy, unstable angina, and nondiagnostic or equivocal noninvasive tests in an otherwise high-risk patient. Also, many would recommend routine coronary angiography in patients recently having suffered myocardial infarction. It should be remembered, however, that coronary angiography in the perioperative evaluation should be performed only when it is likely that the test results will have a significant impact on patient selection and management.

Chest Pain

A frequent symptom that raises suspicion about cardiovascular disease is chest pain. Factors pointing toward atherosclerosis as an etiology include certain pain characteristics, location and precipitating factors. Because conditions such as esophageal reflux, peptic ulcer disease, and musculoskeletal abnormalities are common, patients may have several types of chest discomfort. Angina actually means a "choking" sensation. However, most often it is described as pressure or tightness and, sometimes, heaviness or burning. In contradistinction, patients describing a myocardial infarction more often use the word "pain." Angina is generally easy to differentiate from the profound pain associated with infarction because of the longer duration of pain, more extensive radiation, and lack of precipitating or alleviating factors seen with infarction. Because of the frightening nature of chest pain and significant implications with respect to morbidity and mortality, differentiating cardiac from noncardiac etiologies of discomfort is important. Unfortunately, complicating this issue are angina "equivalents." These are symptoms that one might not initially ascribe to cardiac ischemia. They include dyspnea, jaw or neck discomfort, shoulder, elbow or arm pain, particularly along the side of the left forearm and hand, epigastric discomfort, and interscapular pain. When evaluating chest pain, the clinician must remember that esophagitis, esophageal spasm or esophageal reflux, as well as peptic ulcer produce chest, epigastric and back discomfort. Acute gall bladder disease can mimic myocardial infarction or dissecting aneurysm. Musculoskeletal pain can arise from osteochondritis, cervical disc disease or thoracic outlet syndrome. Pulmonary embolism can result in profound chest pain, and pneumothorax, pulmonary hypertension and pneumonia also have components of chest discomfort that can mimic cardiac disease.

The predictability with which exercise or emotional stress brings on discomfort is helpful in diagnosing angina. Cold weather, rushing to activities and heavy meals are all common precipitants of angina. Alleviating factors that help to diagnose angina are pain improvement after cessation of precipitating activity or sublingual nitroglycerin. The response to nitroglycerin is not specific however, since nitroglycerin also relieves esophageal spasm. A noninvasive or invasive measure of ischemia and ventricular performance usually is key to the differentiation of cardiac vs noncardiac causes of chest pain.

Heart Failure

Historically, cardiac failure generally meant congestive heart failure. However, it is now appreciated that both systolic and diastolic left ventricular dysfunction of a wide range mandate certain treatment strategies depending on presentation (eg, asymptomatic or minimally symptomatic patients vs those with congestive states). Furthermore, patients known to have ischemic heart disease, valvular heart disease, hypertension, or diabetes mellitus are at risk of having asymptomatic left ventricular dysfunction. Still, hallmarks of heart failure are dyspnea, cough, fatigue and fluid retention. Strictly speaking, dyspnea denotes an uncomfortable awareness of breathing that is easily differentiated from normal, quiet, and unnoticed breathing. In addition to heart failure, obstructive airways disease and pulmonary embolism may also cause dyspnea. In patients with congestive heart failure, the onset of dyspnea is generally insidious and, at first, precipitated by exertion. Paroxysmal nocturnal dyspnea is a classic symptom of pulmonary edema and begins several hours after reclining. It is associated with diaphoresis, cough and sometimes wheezing. Patients awaken in a panic and find relief after getting out of the bed and sitting upright. Some patients find that they can prevent paroxysmal nocturnal dyspnea by propping their torso up and only partially reclining. This is usually done with pillows and is called orthopnea. Other symptoms of congestive heart failure are nocturia, peripheral edema, upper abdominal discomfort, anorexia and nonspecific malaise. Cough, as a symptom, is a considerably more frequent, but less specific complaint. Edematous legs after patients are upright can suggest either congestive heart failure, chronic venous insufficiency or other noncardiac causes of edema. Fatigue is a nonspecific, but common symptom that may signal poor cardiac output or result from over-diuresis or beta adrenergic blockade.

Syncope

The sudden loss of consciousness without warning characterizes cardiac syncope. Consciousness is lost due to an inadequate and usually abrupt decrement of central nervous system arterial perfusion. Arrhythmias such as ventricular fibrillation, ventricular tachycardia, advanced atrial-ventricular block, or sudden asystole are the most common serious causes of cardiac syncope. However, hemodynamically significant lesions of aortic stenosis, hypertrophic cardiomyopathy, or primary pulmonary hypertension are also important causes, generally presenting after exertion or even during prolonged standing after coughing or urinating. Still, the most common cause of syncope is vasovagal (or vasodepressor) syncope. It is mediated through the autonomic nervous system with loss of consciousness developing more slowly and associated with bradycardia, hypotension, and diaphoresis. Suspected cardiac syncope should prompt an in-depth evaluation for ischemia, valvular pathology, ventricular hypertrophy, and arrhythmias. Compared with cardiac syncope, neurologic causes often have an aura, as in the case of epilepsy, or are associated with neurologic defects characteristic of cerebral vascular ischemia, and followed by confusion.

Palpitations and Dysrhythmia

Palpitations are an unpleasant awareness of the heartbeat generally described as skipping, jumping, pounding or racing sensations. Nonetheless, some arrhythmias may not be sensed until hemodynamic instability develops and syncope or near-syncope results. A variety of rhythm disturbances should be considered, ranging from bradyarrhythmias to supraventricular or ventricular tachycardias. Palpitations alone can be remarkably common and occur simply with anxiety or during hyperventilation. When palpitations occur without exertion or with only minimal effort, heart failure, anemia, thyrotoxicosis, and atrial fibrillation should be considered. A pulse rate of 150 beats per minute generally suggests atrial flutter while faster rates suggest paroxysmal supraventricular tachycardia. Rapid rates slower than 140 beats per minute are more suggestive of sinus tachycardia, and if the rhythm is irregularly irregular, atrial fibrillation must be a consideration.

ROUTINE SURVEILLANCE TESTING FOR PATIENTS WITH ISCHEMIC HEART DISEASE

It is controversial whether routine surveillance studies for patients with known ischemic heart disease help predict changing patterns of atherosclerosis, or should dictate new therapeutic strategies. Some encourage, for example, annual exercise testing for patients either at risk for, or with known ischemic heart disease. Likewise, determining ejection fraction regularly is supported by some because of the implications of discovering asymptomatic left ventricular dysfunction. Early treatment of these patients is likely to decrease morbidity and mortality. There is general agreement, however, for routine lipid characterization so that risk factor modification can be instituted. The National Cholesterol Education Program (NCEP) recommends lipid characterization in adults at least every five years. This should probably be reduced to annually in posttransplant patients. Certainly, any change of symptoms or physical findings warrants appropriate reevaluation and therapeutic intervention.

CORRECTIVE THERAPIES FOR ISCHEMIC HEART DISEASE

In addition to preventive measures, ischemic heart disease should be addressed with pharmacotherapeutic intervention and consideration given to percutaneous or surgical revascularization procedures. The approach taken with any individual patient, however, should be dictated by the severity of symptoms and risk stratification. Patients having a higher likelihood of morbid events should be treated more aggressively.

Medical Treatment of Ischemic Heart Disease

Nitrates remain the most commonly used drugs for treatment and prevention of myocardial ischemia. Nitrates as a group reduce ventricular wall tension and subsequent oxygen demand, increase venous capacitance and diminish cardiac volume, and, therefore, myocardial wall stress. Sublingual nitroglycerin is the most frequently prescribed nitrate. Inhalent delivery systems are available, as well as transdermal preparations. Long-acting nitrates such as isosorbide dinitrate and isosorbide mononitrates have a slower onset of action but are effective for a greater period of time. When using long-acting nitrates (oral or transdermal patches), it is imperative that a nitrate-free interval ranging from eight to twelve hours be prescribed so that tolerance to the preparation does not develop.

Beta-adrenergic receptor blockers were first introduced in the late 1960s, and today are a mainstay for managing stable angina and hypertension. There is a wealth of data indicating that beta blockers substantially reduce morbidity and mortality post-infarction. Beta blockers reduce myocardial oxygen demand by decreasing heart rate at any given level of activity, and myocardial contractility. However, none of the beta blockers currently approved for the treatment of angina pectoris cause peripheral vasodilation. Labetalol and carvedilol

are beta adrenergic-blocking compounds with peripheral vasodilatory characteristics that, to date, have not been approved for use in patients with angina but are effective antihypertensive agents.

Calcium channel antagonists are a heterogenous group of compounds that have proved effective in the treatment of chronic stable angina and hypertension. Three principle pharmacologic categories are represented by (1) nifedipine, a dihydropyridine, (2) verapamil, a phenylalkylamine, and (3) diltiazem, a benzothiazipine. Verapamil, nifedipine, diltiazem, nicardipine and amlodipine have been approved for treatment of angina. These preparations may be effective on their own or, particularly when used in combination with beta blockers and nitrates. One should be cautious, however, about using a short-acting nifedipine preparation, as reflex tachycardia developing in some patients may be harmful. Calcium antagonists cause relaxation of vascular smooth muscle and inhibit the entry of calcium into myocytes producing a negative inotropic effect. In addition, verapamil and diltiazem are negative chronotropic agents. Slowing of the heart rate, in addition to vasodilation, contributes to reduced myocardial oxygen demand.

Aspirin in low doses has been shown to reduce the rate of acute coronary events for patients who have experienced myocardial infarction, and likely reduces morbidity in a wider spectrum of patients. The use of low-dose aspirin, therefore, is advocated for the medical management of coronary heart disease, but patients should be cautioned to take just one tablet daily and told of paradoxical effects noted when higher doses are used chronically.

Choosing which antianginal agent to use should be dictated largely by the presence of concomitant hypertensive heart disease, arrhythmias, and ventricular function. For example, calcium channel blockers for patients with left ventricular systolic dysfunction should largely be avoided. In addition to aspirin, beta blockers and long-acting nitrate preparations constitute the best initial approach. In view of the impressive benefits associated with beta blocker use for patients post-myocardial infarction and with heart failure, it is wise to include a drug from this class in the treatment protocol. Also intriguing is an impressive compendium of data from heart failure trials, and even from some studies of patients with normal ventricular function, demonstrating that ischemic heart and vascular disease endpoints are substantially reduced when angiotensin-converting enzyme inhibitors (ACEIs) are used. A compelling argument can be made for including this class of drugs in the protocol, as well as lipid-lowering agents if benefit can be inferred from lipoprotein profiles. This makes simplifying medical treatment regimens challenging because of the concomitant polypharmacy dictated by immunosuppressant requirements. It is important to remember that diltiazem significantly increases cyclosporine and FK506® levels, and lipid-lowering drugs from the "statin" group can predispose the cyclosporine-treated patient to rhabdomyolysis and renal failure.

Revascularization Approaches to Coronary Heart Disease

Depending on the severity of ischemia, location of obstructive coronary lesions, presence of concomitant left ventricular systolic dysfunction, and suitability of bypass or angioplasty targets, interventional procedures, in conjunction with medical management and preventive therapies, may be warranted. Generally, consideration of these approaches is recommended when there are long episodes of chest pain (>20 minutes), angina at rest, pulmonary edema related to ischemia, angina with new or worsening mitral regurgitation, angina in the presence of systolic left ventricular dysfunction, and angina accompanied by hypotension. Anatomic findings generally dictating interventions include significant left main coronary obstruction, proximal left anterior descending occlusion in a left dominant circulation, and significant double and triple vessel disease, particularly in a setting of heart failure. Finally, most would agree that residual ischemia noted in the peri-infarct period should dictate interventions. When choosing percutaneous intervention over coronary artery bypass grafting, one must remember that percutaneous procedures avoid or defer major surgery, allow rapid patient recovery, are associated with shorter initial hospitalization, result in less early morbidity with fewer post-procedural myocardial infarctions, and are less costly. On the other hand, coronary artery bypass grafting yields complete revascularization, has an excellent chance of relieving symptoms, generally results in less post-procedure anti-anginal medication use, and is associated with both fewer subsequent hospitalizations and revascularization procedures. Coronary artery bypass grafting also may result in better survival of patients with multivessel coronary artery disease or significant left ventricular systolic dysfunction.

UNUSUAL POSTTRANSPLANT INFECTIONS AFFECTING THE HEART

Endocarditis is a feared disease in any circumstance. Chronically immunosuppressed patients are likely at higher risk of developing intracardiac infections. In particular, fungal infections, aspergillosis and toxoplasmosis are all more commonly seen in immunosuppressed patients. Making the proper diagnosis is key to effectively treating endocarditis. Diseases known to mimic infective endocarditis include systemic lupus erythematosus, neoplastic diseases (carcinoid in particular), systemic vasculitis, recurrent thromboemboli, metastatic tumors

to the heart, infected peripheral aneurysms or vascular grafts, systemic sepsis without valvular involvement, and myocardial thrombus with systemic emboli. All of these conditions are more difficult to diagnose after organ transplantation. One must insure that attention is paid to the detection of anaerobic, fungal, and rickettsial organisms. An echocardiographic study should be coupled with attempts at culturing potential infectious agents. This will provide valuable information regarding the presence of vegetations, severity of valvular insufficiency, and ventricular function. It should be stressed, however, that endocarditis can certainly be present in the absence of vegetations or positive blood cultures. Explanations for "culture-negative" infective endocarditis include prior inadequate antimicrobial therapy, fastidious organisms such as peptostreptococci that are difficult to culture, and unsuspected microbes such as aspergillosis, histoplasmosis, *Legionella*, rickettsiae, chlamydiae, *Brucella*, mycobacteria, *Nocardia*, *Bartonella* and *Listeria*.

One must not tarry when the diagnosis of endocarditis is suspected. Appropriate diagnostic studies searching for infection sources must be pursued, including the biopsy and culture of all suspicious lesions. Antimicrobial coverage must be quickly begun. Indications for surgery include significant aortic or mitral regurgitation, evidence of myocardial invasion (usually indicated by heart block or new interventricular conduction defect), presence of antibiotic resistant organisms, persistent sepsis, significant congestive heart failure, and embolic events.

Perhaps the most important issue with respect to endocarditis is its prevention. Patients traditionally at the highest risk for developing endocarditis include those with previous endocarditis, prosthetic cardiac valves, systemic surgical shunts and complex cyanotic heart disease. Others at risk include those with valvular dysfunction, including mitral valve prolapse with mitral regurgitation, and hypertrophic cardiomyopathy. With respect to solid organ transplant patients, risk for endocarditis will most often be associated with valvular abnormalities, particularly those that are acquired over time (eg, sclerotic aortic or mitral valves that cause insufficiency). These patients should receive antibiotic prophylaxis prior to invasive procedures, including dental cleaning, that are likely to produce bacteremia. Patients with a low risk for infective endocarditis include cardiac transplant patients, individuals having undergone coronary artery bypass graft procedures, and patients with valvular heart disease but without significant regurgitation or stenosis. The immunosuppressed solid organ transplant patient should probably always receive antibiotic prophylaxis.

NEOPLASMS AFFECTING THE HEART

Primary cardiac tumors involving the heart may be benign or malignant; most benign tumors are left atrial myxomas. Primary cardiac neoplasms usually involve the myocardium and endocardial surfaces whereas metastatic neoplasms are more commonly noted in the pericardium. Primary cardiac malignancies are rare, even in the immunosuppressed transplant patient. Pericardial effusion and constrictive pericardial physiology are often the heralding signs of pericardial metastasis. Computerized tomography and magnetic resonance imaging are the most useful instruments for the diagnosis of cardiac tumors. Because immunosuppressive states, in general, are associated with a higher incidence of malignancy, one should always consider the possibility that the heart is involved when concomitant heart failure or unexplained cardiac events are noted after a systemic malignancy is diagnosed. Also, it is important to remember that lymphoma is the fourth most common form of metastatic neoplasm of the heart noted at necropsy. Treatment of cardiac neoplasia is, unfortunately, for the most part ineffectual.

HEART FAILURE IN THE SETTING OF TRANSPLANTED ORGAN DYSFUNCTION

Heart failure is commonly observed in patients with end-stage renal disease and can be due to uremia. Failing renal allografts can cause heart failure both by precipitating uremia and causing fluid retention. Indeed, patients with compensated systolic or diastolic left ventricular dysfunction might develop overt congestive heart failure when renal allografts fail and fluid accumulation occurs. Likewise, hepatic failure-induced fluid accumulation may predispose a marginally compensated patient to congestive failure. Treating congestive heart failure in this setting should focus on amelioration of transplant organ dysfunction, as well as optimization of cardiac hemodynamics and central volume status. Medications tailored to optimize preload and afterload should be prescribed. Particularly important in any patient with systolic left ventricular dysfunction, is keeping the blood pressure as low as tolerated, and prescribing ACEIs (for all patients) as well as beta blockers (eg, carvedilol, bisoprolol, and metoprolol for patients with mild-to-moderate heart failure). Use of ACEIs is challenging for patients with a renal graft because of the potential for potassium and creatinine elevation. Certainly, this can make diagnosing renal allograft rejection difficult. Nonetheless, because of the well-documented benefits of this drug class in heart failure, it is worth an attempt to treat patients with an ACEI, even if only a low dose, such as 2.5 mg/d of enalapril, is all that can be tolerated. Digoxin is likely to be helpful as well, and diuretics should be titrated to the degree of congestion. Recently, low-dose spironolactone (25 mg/d) has been shown to be important in class III and class IV congestive heart failure patients.

ATHEROSCLEROTIC RISK FACTOR MODIFICATION

Attenuation of risk factors is likely the most important step in the management of cardiovascular disease for patients following solid organ transplantation. This is particularly important in the setting of kidney transplantation. Indeed, the risk of cardiovascular disease for patients with chronic renal disease is far greater than that in the general population. For example, in dialysis patients, the prevalence of coronary heart disease is approximately 40% and left ventricular hypertrophy is found in almost 75%. Total deaths caused by cardiovascular disease in the dialysis population is about 9% per year, and even after stratification by age, gender, race, and presence of diabetes, cardiovascular disease mortality is ten to 20 times higher than in the general population. In fact, patients with renal failure have been considered to be one of the highest-risk groups for subsequent cardiovascular events. Furthermore, congestive heart failure is more common in chronic renal disease than in the general population (the prevalence of congestive heart failure in dialysis patients is approximately 40%), and is an independent predictor of death in these patients. The excess risk of cardiovascular disease in renal failure patients may be related to a higher incidence of conditions recognized as atherosclerosis risk factors. Hypertension, hyperlipidemia, diabetes, and physical inactivity are all examples. Other factors that may increase atherosclerosis risk in this group are hemodynamic and metabolic factors such as proteinuria, excessive extracellular fluid, electrolyte imbalance, anemia, and higher levels of thrombogenic factors and homocysteine than are found in the general population. Although renal transplantation eliminates the renal failure, certainly varying levels of kidney dysfunction remain present. Furthermore, chronic administration of steroids and, possibly, other immunosuppressants, may be independent risk factors for atherosclerosis. Additionally, most posttransplant patients are hypertensive and relatively volume-expanded. It is however, important to note that despite the high-risk status of ESRD transplant candidates, prognosis overall and, specifically, for cardiovascular disease morbidity and mortality, improves posttransplant, although it is still several-fold higher than in the general population. The incidences of hypertension and hypercholesterolemia increase post-kidney transplant and are exaggerated by the presence of the native kidneys, pretransplant hypertension, posttransplant weight gain, graft dysfunction, and steroids.

A tremendous amount of evidence is available in nontransplant settings demonstrating that blood pressure control, particularly with ACEIs and beta blockers, is valuable for attenuating cardiovascular disease mortality.

Comprehensive vascular risk reduction for noncardiac transplant patients should include: (1) complete smoking cessation; (2) lipid management when low-density lipoprotein levels are consistently above 100 mg/dL; (3) physical activity (aerobic exercise for 30 to 40 minutes three to four times weekly); (4) optimization of weight; (5) regular administration of anti-platelet agents such as aspirin; (6) maintenance of blood pressure less than 125/75 mmHg (particularly when proteinuria is present in a renal transplant patient); (7) use of ACEIs and beta blockers for heart failure (when present); and (8) postmenopausal estrogens in appropriate female patients. These recommendations have been distilled from standard approaches to nontransplant patients promulgated by the 6th Joint National Committee for Prevention, Detection, Evaluation, and Treatment of High Blood Pressure (JNC VI) and the NCEP. These approaches have also been endorsed in the clinical practice guidelines developed by the patient care and education committee of the American Society of Transplantation. Whether other approaches such as routine prescription of antioxident vitamins or folic acid is helpful awaits further study.

Table 19-6. US Multi-Organ Heart Transplants Total: 1988 to 1997

Organ Type	Number Performed	3-Year Patient Survival	3-Year Heart Graft Survival	3-Year Kidney Graft Survival
Heart-Kidney	122	76.1	73.7	73.3
Heart-Liver-Kidney	1			
Heart-Pancreas-Kidney	5			
Heart-Liver	13			
Heart-Liver-Lung	1			
Heart-Pancreas	4			

RECOMMENDED READING

Bonow RO, Carabello B, de Leon AC Jr, et al. Guidelines for the management of patients with valvular heart disease: executive summary. A report of the American College Cardiology/American Heart Association Task Force on Practice Guidelines (Committee on Management of Patients with Valvular Heart Disease). Circulation. 1998;98(18):1949-1984.

Braunwald E, Jones RH, Mark DB, et al. Diagnosing and managing unstable angina. Agency for Health Care Policy and Research. Circulation. 1994;90(1):613-622.

Danovitch GM. The epidemic of cardiovascular disease in chronic renal disease: a challenge to the transplant physician. Graft. 1999;2:S108-S112.

Joint National Committee; The sixth report of the Joint National Committee on prevention, detection, evaluation and treatment of high blood pressure. Arch Intern Med. 1997;157(21):2413-2446.

Levey AS, Beto JA, Coronado BE, et al. Controlling the epidemic of cardiovascular disease in chronic renal disease: what do we know? what do we need to learn? where do we go from here? Am J Kidney Dis. 1998;32(5):853-906.

National Cholesterol Education Program. Second Report of the Expert Panel on Detection, Evaluation, and Treatment of High Blood Cholesterol in Adults (Adult Treatment Panel II). http://pharmainfo.com/disease/cardio/atpsum.html.

Anonymous. Consensus recommendation for the management of chronic heart failure. Am J Cardiol. 1999;83(2A):1A-38A.

Paul LC, Zaltzman J. Use of angiotensin converting inhibitors in renal transplant patients. Transplant Rev. 1998;12:148-155.

Scanlon PJ, Faxon DP, Audet AM, et al. ACC/AHA guidelines for coronary angiography: executive summary and recommendations. A report of the American College of Cardiology/American Heart Association Task Force on Practice Guidelines (Committee on Coronary Angiography) developed in collaboration with the Society for Cardiac Angiography and Interventions. Circulation. 1999;99(17):2345-2357.

Simoons ML. Myocardial revascularization — bypass surgery or angioplasty? N Engl J Med. 1996;335(4):275-277.

20 PRINCIPLES OF INFECTIOUS DISEASE MANAGEMENT FOR THE ORGAN TRANSPLANT RECIPIENT

Jay A. Fishman, MD
Robert H. Rubin, MD, FACP, FCCP

Allograft rejection and infection remain the most important barriers to successful transplantation. These processes are closely linked because the immunosuppression used to prevent and treat rejection is the major determinant of the incidence and severity of infection. Furthermore, cytokines, growth factors, and other inflammatory mediators generated during rejection or infection, modulate the responses to both processes. The challenges of transplant patient care include:

- Diverse etiologies of infection, ranging from common, community acquired, bacterial and viral pathogens to uncommon opportunistic pathogens.
- Impaired inflammatory responses during microbial invasion secondary to immunosuppressive therapy, causing a decrease in symptoms, signs and radiological findings, and thus, presentation in an advanced (ie, disseminated) state. The key to a successful outcome is early recognition, diagnosis and treatment of infection in the face of muted inflammatory responses.
- Complex antimicrobial treatments related to the urgency of empiric therapy, the frequency of drug toxicity and drug interactions, and the need for prolonged courses of therapy.
- Increasing antimicrobial resistance in bacterial, fungal, and viral pathogens.
- Altered posttransplant anatomy contributing to the risk of nosocomially-acquired infection may alter the physical signs of infection; surgery is generally needed to cure localized infections.
- The inability to individualize immunosuppressive regimens based upon measurement of specific immune function relevant to allograft rejection rather than monitoring immunosuppressive drug levels.
- The contribution of infections to both direct tissue injury (eg, pneumonia, hepatitis) and to "indirect effects" including the pathogenesis of the "net state of immunosuppression," allograft injury, and certain forms of malignancy (eg, papillomavirus and squamous cell cancer, Epstein-Barr virus [EBV]-associated posttransplant lymphoproliferative disease [PTLD]).

RISK OF INFECTION

The risk of infection in the transplant recipient is largely determined by the interaction between two factors: the patient's net state of immunosuppression and the epidemiologic exposures that are encountered. The relationship between these two factors can be described as being semi-quantitative.

Net State of Immunosuppression

The net state of immunosuppression is determined by the interaction of the following factors: (1) dose, duration and temporal sequence in which immunosuppressive drugs are deployed; (2) underlying diseases (eg, systemic lupus) or comorbid conditions (eg, congestive heart failure); (3) foreign bodies (eg, catheters, drains, stents), or injuries to the primary mucocutaneous barrier to infection (eg, the presence of devitalized tissues, hematomas, effusions, or strictures); (4) immunomodulating conditions such as neutropenia and metabolic disorders (eg, diabetes); and (5) infection with immunomodulating viruses (eg, herpes group viruses, hepatitis B and C).

The sum of congenital, metabolic, operative, and transplant-related factors is the patient's "net state of immunosuppression."

Generally, more than one factor is present in each host, and the identification and correction of the relevant factors is essential in the prevention and treatment of infection. Clearly, the prime determinant of the net state of immunosuppression is the nature of the immunosuppressive therapy. However, it is important to recognize that most major opportunistic infections occur in individuals who have preexisting viral infections or who have suffered from a technical mishap related to surgical care. Indeed, the occurrence of opportunistic infection in the absence of one of these factors is an important clue to the presence of an excessive epidemiologic exposure.

Epidemiologic Exposures

Epidemiologic exposures include a variety of microbiologic contacts including those that are relatively remote. Epidemiologic exposures of importance can be divided

Jay A. Fishman, MD, Associate Professor of Medicine, Clinical Director, Transplant Infectious Disease, Massachusetts General Hospital, Harvard Medical School, Boston, MA

Robert H. Rubin, MD, FACP, FCCP, Gordon and Marjorie Osborne Professor of Health Sciences and Technology, Professor of Medicine, Harvard Medical School; Chief of Surgical and Transplant Infectious Disease, Massachusetts General Hospital; Director, Center for Experimental Pharmacology and Therapeutics, Harvard-M.I.T. Division of Health and Technology, Cambridge, MA

into two general categories: those occurring within the community and those occurring within the hospital.

COMMUNITY-ACQUIRED INFECTION. Within the community, common acute infectious exposures have a greater impact on transplant recipients than on the general population, and occur via the respiratory route, or exposures to contaminated water or foods. These include *Salmonella, Mycoplasma, Legionella,* influenza virus, parainfluenza virus, respiratory syncytial virus, *Streptococcus pneumoniae,* and *Listeria monocytogenes.* Common viral agents may also include herpes simplex virus (HSV), cytomegalovirus (CMV), influenza, and hepatitis B and C viruses. While specific infectious exposures within the community will vary based on such factors as geography and socioeconomic status, the general dictum, "common things occur commonly," applies. In the case of enteric bacterial infections, nontyphoidal *Salmonella* infection is a particular problem, as it is associated with more prolonged and severe gastrointestinal disease, and a higher rate of bacteremia and metastatic spread than in the general population. Patients must be educated to avoid potential exposures, as vaccine prevention is not an option for most infections, and the efficacy of the few available vaccines (eg, *S pneumoniae,* influenza) is attenuated by immunosuppression.

More distant exposures may include geographically-restricted systemic mycoses (eg, *Histoplasma, Coccidioides, Blastomyces*), *Mycobacterium tuberculosis, Toxoplasma gondii, Strongyloides stercoralis,* or *Toxoplasma cruzi.* In this latter group of organisms, the mycobacterial and systemic mycotic infections generally have one of three epidemiologic patterns: reactivation of latent infection with secondary dissemination; progressive primary infection with systemic dissemination; or, occasionally, reinfection of a formerly immune individual. Clinically, all three epidemiologic patterns of infection are associated with pulmonary disease, metastatic infection, which may be the presenting manifestation, or fever of unknown origin. In the case of strongyloidiasis, the unique autoinfection cycle of this parasite can maintain asymptomatic gastrointestinal carriage for decades after the individual has left endemic areas of infection. With the initiation of immunosuppressive therapy, there is reactivation and amplification of *Strongyloides,* resulting in the hyperinfection syndrome characterized by hemorrhagic and obstructive pneumonia and/or hemorrhagic enterocolitis. With disseminated strongyloidiasis, parasites migrate, often accompanied by gut flora leading to gram-negative sepsis or meningitis unresponsive to otherwise appropriate antibacterial therapy.

NOSOCOMIAL INFECTIONS. Within the hospital, especially in the patient with a prolonged hospitalization or intubation as a complication of primary illness or transplant surgery (eg, hemorrhage, ascites, renal or hepatic dysfunction, and congestive heart failure), common nosocomial pathogens include *Aspergillus* species and azole-resistant yeasts, *Legionella* species, gram-negative bacilli, vancomycin-resistant enterococcus, methicillin-resistant *Staphylococcus aureus,* and *clostridium difficile.* When the air, food, equipment, or potable water supplies either in the hospital or the domicile are contaminated with pathogens such as *Aspergillus* species, *Legionella* species, *Pseudomonas aeruginosa,* or other gram-negative bacilli, outbreaks of infection will be observed. The acquisition of nosocomial infection occurs in two patterns: domiciliary, on the hospital ward, or nondomiciliary, in-hospital procedure suites. Infections of importance that can exhibit both epidemiologic patterns are those due to *Aspergillus* species, *Legionella* species, and *Pseudomonas aeruginosa,* and other gram-negative bacilli. In addition, staff-to-patient spread can occur with such organisms as methicillin-resistant *Staphylococcus aureus* (MRSA), vancomycin-resistant enterococci (VRE), and *Clostridium difficile.*

TIMETABLE OF INFECTION POSTTRANSPLANT

Failure to prevent disease in the transplant recipient results in unacceptable morbidity and mortality. Thus, identification of risk factors (above) and pretransplant screening efforts (below) are coupled to a variety of preventive strategies in the posttransplant period. As immunosuppressive regimens for organ transplantation have become reasonably standardized, it has been recognized that different infectious processes occur at different points in the posttransplant course. A timetable outlining these infectious events (Figure 20-1) can assist with the following: (1) development of a microbiologic differential diagnosis in the individual patient with a clinical infectious disease syndrome; (2) recognition of excessive immunosuppression, or too many infections of excessive severity; (3) recognition of an excessive epidemiologic hazard for organisms causing infection at the wrong time (these excess hazards may be nosocomial [eg, *Aspergillus,* MRSA, VRE], technical [eg, anastomotic leaks, lines], community-based [eg, influenza, respiratory syncytial virus, *Legionella*], or individual [eg, gardening, travel]); and (4) design and implementation of targeted preventive antimicrobial strategies. While this timetable is generally applicable, it must be recognized that modification of the immunosuppressive regimen and the presence of various infections themselves will alter host susceptibility and thus, the paradigm for the expected pathogens to which the patient is considered most susceptible (Table 20-1).

It is useful to divide the posttransplant course into three time periods: the first month posttransplant, the

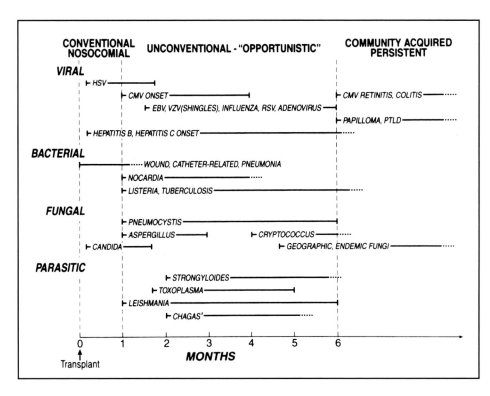

Figure 20-1. Timetable for the occurrence of infection following organ transplantation. Exception to the usual sequence for infections following transplantation suggests the presence of unusual epidemiologic exposure or excessive immunosuppression. HSV indicates herpes simplex virus; CMV, cytomegalovirus; EBV, Epstein-Barr virus; VZV, varicella-zoster virus; RSV, respiratory syncytial virus; and PTLD, posttransplant lymphoproliferative disease. (Reprinted with permission from Fishman JA and Rubin RH. Infection in organ transplant recipients. New Engl J Med. 1998;338(24):1741-1751.)

period one to six months posttransplant, and the period after six months posttransplant. In the first month posttransplant, there are two major causes of infection in all forms of organ transplantation. The first cause is recurrence of infection that was present in the donor (ie, contamination of the graft) or the recipient prior to transplantation but that was unrecognized or incompletely treated. Such infections include underlying diseases related to the transplant (eg, bacterial or fungal colonization, hepatitis B [HBV] or hepatitis C [HCV] infection), and nosocomial pathogens acquired during pretransplant in-hospital management. Postoperative complications such as aspiration pneumonitis, wound

infection, "line sepsis," urinary tract infection, and infection of devitalized tissues, anastomotic suture lines, and fluid collections (eg, hematomas, lymphoceles, pleural effusions, urinomas) are the second cause. Particular risk of nosocomial infection is experienced by the patient requiring prolonged ventilatory support, and those with diminished lung function, persistent ascites, stents of the urinary tract or biliary ducts, cholesterol emboli, or poorly revascularized graft tissue.

The infection profile changes one to six months posttransplant when traditional "opportunistic infections" emerge. These include latent infections, particularly *Pneumocystis carinii* and protozoa (eg, *Toxoplasma gondii, Leishmania,* Chagas' disease), the geographic fungal infections (eg, histoplasmosis, coccidioidomycosis, and blastomycosis), and viral pathogens, particularly herpes group viruses. Viruses, especially CMV, serve as an important cofactor to many other infections.

The potential effects of viral infection are diverse and apply not only to CMV but also to HBV, HCV, EBV, and probably to other common viruses as well (eg, respiratory syncytial virus [RSV], human herpes virus 6 [HHV-6], and adenovirus). These viruses contribute to: (1) direct allograft injury (eg, endothelialitis, epithelial cell invasion, myositis) and native tissue injury including retinitis, hepatitis, pneumonia, vasculitis, nephritis, pancreatitis, enteritis and encephalitis; (2) indirect cellular effects (eg, upregulation of histocompatibility antigens or adhesion proteins) or systemic inflammation which, via mediators TNF-α and Nfkβ, contribute to the immunologic graft rejection and necessitate increased immuno-

Table 20-1. Infections and Conditions Possibly Associated with Specific Immunosuppressive Regimens

Corticosteroids: *Pneumocystis, Aspergillus*, hepatitis B and C
Cyclosporine and Tacrolimus: Increased viral replication, intracellular pathogens, gingival disease
Azathioprine: Neutropenia, papillomavirus
Mycophenolate Mofetil: Early bacterial infections, late CMV, neutropenia
Antilymphocyte Globulins: Activation of latent virus
Costimulatory Blockade (IL-2 receptor): Unknown
Plasmapheresis: Encapsulated bacteria

suppression with increased risk of opportunistic infection; and (3) enhanced systemic immunosuppression, increasing the risk for infections (eg, *Pneumocystis carinii, Aspergillus* species, *Nocardia asteroides*) in the absence of an unusual epidemiologic exposure. Thus, CMV prevention and early identification of significant CMV infection by antigenemia assays, polymerase chain reaction (PCR) assays, and shell vial cultures with early antigen detection may deter several posttransplant complications.

The spectrum of viral infection has widened as new viruses are discovered (Table 20-2). Recently, BK virus, or polyomavirus, has been associated with infection of renal allografts causing hemorrhagic cystitis, ureteric obstruction, and rising creatinine values. Diagnosis is made by

Table 20-2. The Growing Family of Viral Pathogens in Transplantation

Herpes Simplex	Hepatitis B and C
Varicella-Zoster	Papillomavirus
Epstein-Barr Virus	Polyomavirus BK
Cytomegalovirus	Adenovirus
HHV-6 (role with CMV)	Influenza (A and B)
HHV-7	Respiratory Syncytial Virus
HHV-8 (Kaposi's)	HIV
	New Viruses

Table 20-3. The Pretransplantation Epidemiologic Evaluation

	All Patients	Patients in Endemic Area
Serologies		
CMV	X	
HSV	X	
VZV	X	
EBV	X	
HIV	X	
HBV: HBsAg	X	
HCV	X	
Treponema pallidum	X	
Toxoplasma gondii	X	
Strongyloides stercoralis		X
Leishmania spp		X
Histoplasma capsulatum		X
Coccidioides immitis		X
Cultures		
Urinalysis and culture	X	
Skin Test: PPD	X	
Chest x-ray	X	
Stool or urine ova and parasites		X

urine cytology or PCR testing of urine, and by electron microscopy of renal biopsy samples. In the absence of specific therapy, reduction of immunosuppression is necessitated despite the fact that the early clinical presentation mimics graft rejection. Adenovirus may cause a similar hemorrhagic nephritis or cystitis picture diagnosed by culture or antigen detection by immunofluorescence. Human herpes viruses 6 (HHV-6), 7 (HHV-7), and 8 (Kaposi's sarcoma-associated virus) have also been identified in transplant recipients. HHV-6 has been implicated as a cofactor to CMV infection (and vice versa), or may cause leukopenia and fever as part of a viral syndrome. The role of HHV-7 remains to be clarified. EBV and HSV are often activated during this early period. EBV is associated with the development of B cell lymphoma, particularly in the EBV-seronegative recipients of EBV-seropositive organs. Parvovirus (B19) may also present with anemia in this time period. Influenza and RSV remain important community-acquired pathogens, particularly in the lung transplant recipient, predisposing patients to bacterial infections and graft rejection.

There is significant geographic and institutional variation in the occurrence of opportunistic infections during the first six months posttransplantation. At centers with a fixed, high incidence of infections including *Pneumocystis, Toxoplasma,* or *Nocardia* (rates of 5% to 10% percent or higher), low-dose trimethoprim-sulfamethoxazole (TMP-SMX) prophylaxis effectively prevents disease. Similarly, in programs with a fixed, high incidence of *Aspergillus, Histoplasma,* or azole-resistant yeasts (eg, in liver transplant recipients), both epidemiologic protection (eg, high efficiency particulate air [HEPA] filtered air supply within the hospital) and fungal prophylaxis, appropriate to the common isolates, may be used.

More than six months posttransplant, most patients are receiving stable and relatively modest levels of immunosuppression. These patients are subject to community-acquired pneumococcal and respiratory virus infection, particularly influenza or RSV. Chronic manifestations of other common infections (eg, papillomavirus) are also seen. The remaining patients who have less satisfactory graft function requiring more intensive immunosuppressive therapies, the "chronic n'er do wells," remain at the highest risk for severe community-acquired and opportunistic infection. For this subgroup of patients, prolonged (lifelong) antimicrobial prophylaxis is indicated.

THE PRETRANSPLANTATION EVALUATION

Given the importance of the prevention of infection in the transplant recipient, a pretransplant determination of unusual risks is essential (Table 20-3). This includes:

- Identification and eradication, prior to transplantation, of all known infections.
- Recognition that allografts or transfusion may transmit *T gondii, Trypanosoma cruzi* (Chagas' disease), *Leishmania spp,* Acanthamoeba, Naegleria, *Strongyloides stercoralis,* Taenia or *Echinococcus* species with exacerbation of infection by immunosuppression.
- Identification of patients with chronic or recurrent infections (eg, cystic fibrosis) and antimicrobial exposures. These patients often carry resistant bacteria (especially *Pseudomonas,* Burkholderia, Stenotrophomonas, and *Staphylococcus species*), or are colonized with *Candida* or *Aspergillus.* These patients require radiographic evaluation (CT of infected area), and often surgical drainage to eradicate infection to the degree possible before transplantation.
- Notation of the ineffectiveness of vaccination in the setting of immunosuppression and uremia, following surgery, and after splenectomy. Vaccinations against common community-acquired illnesses (eg, *S pneumoniae, Haemophilus influenzae,* influenza, hepatitis B) are recommended pretransplant; influenza and pneumococcal vaccines are maintained posttransplant. Those at risk for specific infections (eg, hepatitis A, meningococcemia, cholera) should receive appropriate vaccination.
- Consideration of the risks of highly immunogenic vaccines (eg, tetanus toxoid) or attenuated live virus vaccines (eg, varicella). In the case of polio, family members and transplant patients should only receive inactivated vaccine (eg, not the oral "Sabin vaccine"), as central nervous system disease can develop in these patients. In the case of varicella vaccination, pretransplant vaccination is recommended for seronegative individuals and, particularly, children. Some pediatric transplant recipients have developed a chickenpox-like illness after varicella vaccination requiring administration of acyclovir. The exact incidence of varicella infection and the efficacy of this vaccine in organ transplant patients remain to be defined. Use of tetanus toxoid should be reserved for tetanus-prone wounds.
- Pretransplant therapy for those with exposures to tuberculosis, *Strongyloides,* or syphilis.
- Screening of potential donors and recipients for human immunodeficiency virus (HIV) 1 and 2, human T cell leukemia virus (HTLV1), hepatitis A, HBV, HCV, CMV, EBV, HSV, varicella-zoster virus (VZV), syphilis and *gondii.* The results of serologic screening for HSV, VZV, CMV, and EBV are used as guides for the development of pro-

phylactic strategies after transplantation. Donor seropositivity for herpes group viruses is not a contraindication to donation. Routine screening for human herpes viruses 6, 7, and 8 may soon be advised.
- Special attention to clearance of donor infection with organisms that tend to infect anastomotic sites (eg, *Salmonella, S pneumoniae, enterococci,* and *Aspergillus* species).

Transplantation of an allograft from an HIV-positive or HBsAg-positive donor has a transmission efficiency of approximately 100%, and should be avoided. Fortunately, current serologic techniques are sufficiently sensitive and specific to provide virtually complete protection against these infections, provided an appropriate blood specimen from the donor is tested. Appropriate donor specimens are those taken prior to massive blood transfusion to avoid false-negative testing.

The appropriate approach to the anti-HCV-positive donor remains controversial. HCV will be transmitted to up to 50% of recipients of extrahepatic organs from anti-HCV-positive donors, and to a greater fraction from donors who carry circulating virus in the blood documented by mRNA PCR. Recipients who themselves are anti-HCV-positive appear not to be protected against this new viral exposure. Short-term (<5 years) follow-up of patients infected with HCV at the time of transplant appears to be satisfactory but, over time, progressive liver disease is likely to develop in a subset of individuals. Thus, in the absence of more effective antiviral therapies, it seems reasonable to restrict the use of organs from anti-HCV-positive donors to patients on life-support (ie, awaiting heart or liver allografts), the elderly, or the highly sensitized. HCV-infected organs are being used in HCV-seropositive recipients at a number of centers, especially for critically ill or highly sensitized patients. Limited data suggest that outcomes are generally comparable to those of noninfected donors. The use of these organs must be avoided in children and young adults.

The determination of donor and recipient CMV, toxoplasmosis, and EBV-seropositivity is used to connote risk of recipient infection after transplant, and directs posttransplant antimicrobial strategies. In the case of CMV, three levels of risk can be determined on the basis of the serologic data:

- Primary Infection: When the donor is seropositive and the recipient is seronegative (D+R-, approximately 10% of transplants), the risk that CMV disease will occur posttransplant is approximately 60% to 75%.
- Reactivation Infection: When the donor is seronegative and the recipient is seropositive (D-R+, 25% to 50% of transplants), the risk of CMV disease is less than 20% due to reactiva-

tion of endogenous virus. Additionally, asymptomatic viremia is common and CMV reactivation is enhanced by the use of antilymphocyte antibodies.

- Superinfection: When the donor and recipient are seropositive (D+R+, 25% to 50% of transplants), CMV disease occurs in 20% to 35%, and the reactivated virus is generally from the donor.

Each of these groups requires a different level of prophylaxis to prevent symptomatic disease, with effective regimens now available for the latter two categories, but not yet defined for primary infection. Firm recommendations regarding prophylaxis are not yet possible. In general, oral ganciclovir is given for ten weeks after courses of intravenous ganciclovir for patients at risk for primary disease (D+R-), or in those (D+ or R+) receiving antilymphocyte preparations. Otherwise, patients at lesser risk for CMV infection may be routinely monitored for viral activation by antigenemia or PCR assays. Lung and liver recipients require special attention. New antiviral programs are under study.

Strongyloides stercoralis should be eradicated prior to transplant, using ivermectin or thiabendazole, given the risk of the life-threatening syndromes associated with reactivation posttransplant. Serologies and immunofluorescent stool exams are used to guide preemptive therapy of patients from endemic regions.

EBV-seronegative allograft recipients who are primarily children (>95% of adults are EBV-seropositive), are at high risk for primary EBV infection, and for the development of EBV-related PTLD. Such individuals require reduced immunosuppression and lifelong antiviral prophylaxis. This includes oral acyclovir, or ganciclovir if at risk for CMV infection, and intravenous therapy during treatment for acute rejection.

Tuberculin testing of recipients is advised. However, patients with end-stage organ failure, particularly uremia, may be anergic even though they harbor *M tuberculosis*. It is apparent that tuberculin-positive individuals without other risk factors are at low-risk for developing active tuberculosis, and probably are best managed with close surveillance.

Toxoplasmosis is primarily an issue in cardiac transplantation. If the donor is seropositive and the recipient seronegative for *T gondii*, then there is a high risk of myocarditis and disseminated infection posttransplant. Accordingly, cardiac allograft recipients who are D+R- for toxoplasmosis require antitoxoplasmosis therapy for at least four to six months posttransplant (eg, pyrimethamine and sulfonamide), generally with TMP-SMX thereafter. Recipients of extra-cardiac organs or seropositive heart recipients reactivate infrequently and require no special intervention.

GENERAL PRINCIPLES IN MANAGEMENT OF INFECTION IN THE TRANSPLANT RECIPIENT

Given the inability of immunosuppressed individuals to clear infection spontaneously, a number of concepts merit consideration.

Diminished manifestations of infection are seen in symptoms, physical signs, and in radiologic studies. The use of the CT scan (or MRI of the neuraxis) is essential for assessing the presence and nature of infectious and malignant processes. Thus, CT scans performed, despite normal chest or abdominal radiographs, may reveal diffuse interstitial disease in *Pneumocystis pneumonia*, or unexpected focal disease due to *Aspergillus*, *Nocardia* or lymphoma.

The "gold standard" for diagnosis is tissue histology with microbiology. No radiologic finding is sufficiently diagnostic to obviate the need for tissue, as the diagnosis is often in question and multiple simultaneous infections are common.

Serologic tests are useful in the pretransplant setting but rarely of use after transplantation. Tests that detect proteins (ELISA, direct immunofluorescence for influenza, RSV) or nucleic acids (PCR for HCV) should be used.

Antimicrobial resistance can be acquired during therapy (eg, inducible B-lactamases) and resistant organisms acquired during hospitalization. Sites at risk for infection (eg, ascites, blood clots, drains, lungs) must be sampled routinely to guide empiric therapy at times of clinical deterioration.

Antimicrobial agents are of little use in the presence of undrained fluid collections, blood, or devitalized tissues. Early and aggressive surgical debridement of such collections is essential.

Successful treatment of major infections and EBV-associated PTLD may require an improvement in a host's immune response. Reductions in exogenous immunosuppression, correction of neutropenia with growth factors, or treatment of simultaneous infections that predispose to superinfection (RSV, CMV) may be needed.

Principles of Antimicrobial Use in the Organ Transplant Recipient

There are three different modes in which antimicrobial drugs can be prescribed for the prevention and treatment of infectious diseases in the transplant patient:

- Therapeutic: The administration of antimicrobial agents to eradicate clinically overt infection.
- Prophylactic: The administration of an antimicrobial regimen to an entire population before an event to prevent infection. One such prophylactic strategy is the administration of low-dose

TMP-SMX, which effectively eliminates the risk of *Pneumocystis carinii* pneumonia and *Toxoplasma gondii,* and reduces the incidence of nocardiosis, listeriosis, and urosepsis.

- Preemptive: The administration of an antimicrobial regimen to a subgroup of patients at particularly high-risk of clinical disease as determined by a predictive clinical or laboratory marker.

Drug Toxicity

Complications of drug therapy may include: TMP-SMX-induced pneumonitis, meningitis, hepatitis, or Stevens-Johnson Syndrome; ganciclovir-related renal dysfunction and neutropenia; interferon-induced flu-like illnesses or pulmonary edema; antibody and blood product-stimulated serum sickness, immune responses, renal dysfunction, and pulmonary infiltrates; and cyclosporine and tacrolimus-related renal dysfunction, hepatitis, neuropathy, hyperglycemia, hypertension, and hemolytic-uremic syndrome. Antimicrobial agents also increase the incidence of thrush, noninfectious diarrhea, and *C difficile* colitis. However, drug toxicity in the transplant recipient is more often due to drug interactions rather than individual adverse drug effects.

Because cyclosporine or tacrolimus are used in the majority of transplant recipients, interactions with these agents are of unique importance. Some of the important antimicrobial drug interactions with cyclosporine and tacrolimus are outlined in Table 20-4. Agents that increase or decrease the serum levels of cyclosporine and tacrolimus, or that enhance the toxicity of these agents are common and must be carefully monitored. Based on these potential toxicities, therapeutic compromises are often made. The loss of renal function due to the use of antimicrobial agents significantly hinders patient management. However, it is unacceptable to allow, for example, the progression of fungal infection while on inadequate doses of amphotericin, or while using second-line agents (eg, itraconazole for primary therapy of *Aspergillus* infection in the compromised host) or agents to which microbial resistance is likely. Lastly, drug toxicity may be increased in the allograft recipient because longer courses of antimicrobial therapy are needed to clear infections than in the immunocompetent individual.

INFECTIONS AND INFECTIOUS SYNDROMES OF SPECIAL IMPORTANCE IN TRANSPLANTATION

Cytomegalovirus

Cytomegalovirus (CMV) is among the most important causes of infectious disease morbidity and mortality in transplant patients. Evidence of active viral replication is found in 50% to 75% of transplant recipients. Clinically significant disease can be seen at anytime after transplantation, but is most common one to four months posttransplant. Two common exceptions to this pattern may be observed: (1) a CMV-seronegative recipient can develop primary CMV disease due to acquisition of the virus in the community following intimate contact; and (2) a seropositive patient with an ongoing inflammatory process such as urosepsis can develop viral reactivation and CMV disease three to four weeks later, probably due to inflammatory cytokines. Allograft rejection is also a major stimulus to CMV activation. The general pattern of CMV disease is similar in all forms of organ transplantation. However, it appears that allografts are more vulnerable than native organs, possibly due to the role of rejection in viral activation, preexisting injury, or to the careful monitoring of allograft function.

The range of effects produced by CMV is broad. Asymptomatic viral shedding, especially in patients with reactivation infection, is common in pulmonary secretions and in the urine, and rarely merits therapy. The most common clinical manifestation of CMV infec-

Table 20-4. Common Antimicrobial Interactions with Cyclosporine and Tacrolimus*

Increased Absorption	Decreased Absorption	Increased Metabolism	Decreased Metabolism	Enhanced Nephrotoxicity
Macrolides†	Rifampin	Nafcillin Rifampin Imipenem Isoniazid	Macrolides† Azole-antifungals† Quinolones Dapsone	TMP-SMX (iv) Aminoglycosides Vancomycin Acyclovir Amphotericin B Ganciclovir Quinolones‡

* Many non-antimicrobial agents will alter the absorption and metabolism of cyclosporine and tacrolimus.

† Individual members of each class of antimicrobial agents will alter cyclosporine and tacrolimus levels to different degrees; the effect in individual patients will also vary. (Terbinafine may reduce cyclosporine levels.)

‡ Fluoroquinolone antimicrobials at higher doses may cause nephrotoxicity in the setting of cyclosporine or tacrolimus administration.

tion is termed the CMV syndrome, a prolonged episode of otherwise unexplained fever associated with constitutional symptoms and such laboratory abnormalities as leukopenia, thrombocytopenia, a mild lymphocytosis, and mild transient hepatitis. Severe, progressive CMV disease may cause persistent leukopenia, thrombocytopenia, pneumonia, gastrointestinal ulceration, hepatitis (common), myocarditis with conduction abnormalities in heart transplant recipients, elevated creatinine levels in renal transplants, and pancreatitis. Not infrequently, opportunistic superinfection will further complicate the course of severe CMV infection. CMV chorioretinitis is a late manifestation of systemic CMV infection, usually presenting four months or more posttransplantation. Chorioretinitis may follow earlier clinical manifestations of CMV infection or be the first manifestation of CMV disease.

There is increasing evidence that CMV contributes to the pathogenesis of allograft injury. CMV infection has been particularly linked to accelerated coronary artery atherosclerosis in cardiac allograft recipients; to bronchiolitis obliterans in lung transplant recipients; to certain forms of hepatic injury in liver transplant patients; to an unusual glomerulopathy in renal transplant patients; as well as to more conventional patterns of rejection. Each of these lesions has also been observed in the absence of viral infection, particularly in graft rejection. Direct viral injury and immunologic mimicry (eg, sequence homology and immunologic crossreactivity between a portion of the immediate early antigen of CMV and the HLA-DR β chain, and the production by CMV-infected cells of a glycoprotein homologous to MHC class I antigens) have been described. Cytokines elaborated in the course of CMV infection, and other processes, affect the display of histocompatibility antigens, thus, modulating intragraft immune responses. Furthermore, in a small series, patients with late renal allograft dysfunction have been successfully treated with ganciclovir without increased immunosuppression.

The most valuable diagnostic test for managing clinical CMV disease is the demonstration of viremia. While tissue biopsies are more specific, disease is often patchy and viral inclusions are not always seen. Viremia is usually present as early as five to seven days prior to the onset of clinical disease. Demonstration of "shed"virus in respiratory secretions and urine correlates poorly with clinical events. Similarly, measurements of rising antibody titers are generally too delayed to be useful clinically. The major use of antibody testing is to characterize donor and recipient at the time of transplant in an effort to guide preventive strategies. The "gold standard" for virus detection is cell culture, which may require up to six weeks for definitive results. The centrifuged shell vial technique is more rapid, but has a sensitivity of less than 50%. CMV neutrophil antigenemia

assay (CMV early antigen pp65), and quantitative serum DNA PCR are the diagnostic tests of choice, with less than 90% sensitivity and high specificity.

Intravenous ganciclovir, at a dose of 5 mg/kg twice daily, with dosage correction during renal dysfunction, for two to three weeks usually cures symptomatic disease. Relapse may occur, and prolonged therapy with oral or intravenous ganciclovir is often recommended, particularly for those with primary infection. At some centers, oral ganciclovir at a dose of 2 to 3 g/d is added for ten weeks after an intravenous course of therapy for those with active, primary CMV disease. Many clinicians add anti-CMV hyperimmune globulin to the treatment program for seronegative patients with active disease or for prophylaxis. Ganciclovir-resistant CMV remains uncommon in organ transplant patients. Resistence is a major problem in this population, as foscarnet and cidofovir are significantly more toxic and difficult to manage (eg, magnesium wasting, nephrotoxicity).

The optimal regimen for the prevention of CMV disease is not yet determined. Patients must be stratified as to relative risk for disease. The limited bioavailability of oral ganciclovir and limited efficacy of acyclovir for CMV infection have been demonstrated in multiple studies. In such studies, oral ganciclovir appears to reduce the severity of disease, but fails to prevent viremia in patients at risk for primary infection. For patients at greatest risk (CMV D+R-), preemptive treatment during antilymphocyte therapy is combined with routine monitoring for viremia using antigenemia or PCR assays.

Fever and Pneumonitis

Pulmonary infection is the most common form of tissue-invasive infection observed in organ transplant patients. Early diagnosis and specific therapy remain the cornerstones of cure and justify the use of invasive diagnostic techniques, which provide rapid pathogen identification and tissue histology.

The depressed inflammatory response of the immunocompromised transplant patient modifies and/or delays the appearance of pulmonary lesions on radiographs. In particular, fungal infection, which excites a less exuberant inflammatory response than does bacterial invasion, may be difficult to detect. Even so, the presentation and evolution of the chest radiograph provide clues to the differential diagnosis and diagnostic work-up (Table 20-5). Focal or multifocal consolidation of acute onset is likely caused by bacterial infection. Similar multifocal lesions with subacute to chronic progression are more likely secondary to fungal, tuberculous, or nocardial infections. Large nodules usually signify fungal or nocardial infection, particularly when subacute to chronic in onset. Subacute disease with diffuse abnormalities, either of the peribronchovascular type or miliary micronodules, are usually caused by viruses

Table 20-5. Pulmonary Infections in Organ Transplant Recipients: Differential Diagnosis Based on Progression of Chest Radiograph

Abnormality	Acute (<24 hours)*	Subacute and chronic †
Consolidation	Bacterial (Legionella) Hemorrhage Thromboembolic Pulmonary edema	Fungus, Nocardia Tumor, Tuberculosis Pneumocystis, Viral Drug-induced, Radiation
Peribronchovascular	Pulmonary edema Leukoagglutinin reaction Bacteria Viral (influenza, RSV)	Viral, PCP, Radiation Drug-induced (Nocardia, tumor Fungus, tuberculosis)
Nodular Infiltrate ‡	Bacterial Legionella Pulmonary edema Tuberculosis, PCP	Fungus, Nocardia

* An acute illness is one that develops and requires medical attention in a matter of relatively few hours (<24).

†A subacute and chronic process develops over several days to weeks.

‡A nodular infiltrate is defined as one or more focal defects of >1 cm² on chest radiography with well-defined borders, surrounded by aerated lung. Multiple tiny nodules of smaller size are seen in a wide variety of disorders (eg, CMV or varicella-zoster virus) and are not included. (Modified from Rubin and Green).

(especially CMV) or *Pneumocystis carinii* or, in the lung transplant patient, rejection. Additional clues can be found by examining the pulmonary lesion for the development of cavitation. Cavitation suggests necrotizing infections such as those caused by fungi, *Nocardia*, and certain gram-negative bacilli (eg, *Klebsiella pneumoniae, Pseudomonas aeruginosa*).

CT scan of the chest is particularly useful when the chest radiograph is negative despite a high index of clinical suspicion, or when the radiographic findings are subtle or nonspecific. CT scan is also needed to define the extent of the disease process and to aid in the selection of the optimal diagnostic technique. Particularly with fungal and nocardial infection, precise knowledge of the extent of the infection at diagnosis, and the response of all sites to therapy, will lead to the best therapeutic outcome; therapy is continued until all evidence of infection is eliminated. The morphology of the abnormalities found on CT scan can also assist in outlining a differential diagnosis. Atypical CT scan findings may suggest the presence of dual or sequential infections of the lungs. For example, in a patient with *Pneumocystis* infection, the appearance of acinar, macronodular, or cavitary lesions is suggestive of secondary *Aspergillus* invasion of lung tissue compromised by the primary process.

The techniques available for specific diagnosis include immunologic techniques (eg, serologic assays, skin testing), antigen detection systems, and molecular assays (eg, hybrid capture, PCR), coupled with sputum examination and invasive techniques including bronchoscopy, aspirational needle biopsy, thoracoscopic

biopsy, and open lung biopsy. Immunologic techniques are generally of little use in the diagnosis of active infection in the transplant recipient. In these hosts, immune responses to microbial invasion may be greatly attenuated or delayed, positive immunologic tests are present in the absence of clinical disease, and appropriate serologic or skin tests are not available for many of the disease processes that should be considered.

BACTERIAL PNEUMONIA. Bacterial pneumonia is particularly common postoperatively in lung transplant patients because the lower respiratory tracts are frequently colonized with gram-negative organisms, and the devascularized bronchial anastamoses are vulnerable to infection and disruption. Transplanted lungs, which have been physically traumatized, as well as subjected to possible immunologic injury, are far more susceptible to invasive infection than are lungs of other organ transplant recipients.

Nocardia **and Tuberculosis.** Nocardial infection is usually prevented by low-dose TMP-SMX prophylaxis. Patients with nocardial infection or tuberculosis should be assumed to have disseminated infection at the time of diagnosis. Cranial CT scan, sampling of the cerebrospinal fluid, and careful bone examination (eg, bone scan) are mandatory for the detection of metastatic nocardial infection and assessing the efficacy of therapy. The prevention of active tuberculosis is more challenging. Routine tuberculin skin testing is essential. Purified protein definitive (PPD) skin tests should probably be interpreted as for other immunocompromised hosts (eg, AIDS). The key issue is the management of the patient with a known positive tuberculin test posttransplant. Because the mainstays of antituberculous therapy, isoniazid and rifampin, are both hepatotoxic and interact with cyclosporine and tacrolimus metabolism, there is controversy regarding optimal management of PPD-positive patients. Isoniazid prophylaxis is recommended for transplant patients with positive tuberculin tests and at least one additional risk factor. Risk factors of importance include non-Caucasian racial status; the presence of other immunosuppressing conditions; the presence of protein-calorie malnutrition; history of active tuberculosis; the presence of a significant abnormality on chest x-ray; or the presence of tuberculous infection in the organ being transplanted. Such patients merit nine to 12 months of isoniazid prophylaxis, ideally prior to transplant, but otherwise in the posttransplant setting. For patients without these risk factors, and who are reliable in terms of follow-up, close observation may be the best approach. In endemic regions, new combination therapies for prophylaxis and therapy, with at least three bactericidal agents, possibly including a fluoroquinolone, are under study. Mycobacterial resistance remains a concern; active disease must be excluded before initiating prophylaxis.

VIRAL PNEUMONIA. Most pulmonary viral infections begin insidiously with constitutional symptoms. About a third of patients will also develop a dry, nonproductive cough, and varying degrees of tachypnea and dyspnea and hypoxemia. CMV, often in association with other organisms, is among the most important causes of viral pneumonia in the transplant patient. CMV pneumonitis usually occurs one to four months posttransplant, is most common in patients at risk for primary CMV infection, and develops in those most intensively immunosuppressed. The attack rate and severity of pneumonia is greater in recipients of lung allografts than of other organs. Radiographically, CMV presents most commonly as a bilateral, symmetrical, peribronchovascular and alveolar process affecting predominantly the lower lobes. Less often, CMV appears as a focal consolidation more suggestive of bacterial or fungal infection or a solitary nodule. Mixed patterns may suggest dual infection of which CMV and *P carinii* are the most commonly associated. Other viral agents generally cause more subtle radiographic findings.

The transplant patient is also at increased risk for community-acquired pneumonia compared with normal hosts. Influenza, RSV, and adenovirus infection are of special importance. Severe bacterial pneumonias are common due to superinfection of previous respiratory viral infections. The clinical history is key in determining the possibility of bacterial or other superinfection. Gross hypoxemia should suggest *P carinii* or other coinfection.

FUNGAL PNEUMONIA. The three most important causes of fungal pulmonary infection are *Pneumocystis carinii, Aspergillus* species (especially *A fumigatus*), and *Cryptococcus neoformans.*

Pneumocystis Carinii. The risk of infection with *Pneumocystis* is greatest in the first six months after transplantation and during periods of increased immunosuppression. Aerosol transmission of infection has been demonstrated by a number of investigators. Activation of latent infection remains a significant factor in the incidence of disease in immunocompromised hosts. In the solid organ transplant recipient, chronic immunosuppression that includes corticosteroids is most often associated with pneumocystosis. Bolus corticosteroids and cyclosporine may also contribute to the risk for *Pneumocystis* pneumonia. In patients not receiving TMP-SMX (or alternative drugs) as prophylaxis, most transplant centers report an incidence of *Pneumocystis carinii* pneumonia of approximately 10% in the first six months posttransplant, with a continuing risk in the "chronic n'er do well" patient. In unprophylaxed lung transplant recipients, two-thirds carry asymptomatic *P carinii* on lung lavage. Of these, up to half are expected to develop symptomatic disease without prophylaxis. The occurrence of *Pneumocystis* infection is associated with CMV infection. The importance of preventing *Pneumocystis* infection cannot be overemphasized. While low-dose TMP-SMX or other prophylactic agents are well tolerated in this patient population, treatment doses of TMP-SMX or pentamidine are associated with a high rate of toxicity, particularly renal and hepatic. Extrapulmonary disease is uncommon.

The expected mortality due to *Pneumocystis* pneumonia is increased in patients on cyclosporine when compared to other immunocompromised hosts. The hallmark of infection due to *P carinii* is the presence of marked hypoxemia, dyspnea, and cough with a paucity of physical or radiologic findings. In the transplant recipient, *Pneumocystis* pneumonia is generally acute to subacute in development. The chest radiograph may be entirely normal or develop the classical pattern of perihilar and interstitial ground glass infiltrates. Microabscesses, nodules, small effusions, lymphadenopathy, asymmetry, and linear bands are common. Chest CT scans will be more sensitive to the diffuse interstitial and nodular pattern than routine radiographs. The nodularity seen in transplanted lungs due to *Pneumocystis* may be mimicked by rejection. The clinical and radiologic manifestations of *P carinii* pneumonia are virtually identical to those of CMV.

Aspergillus. Invasive pulmonary aspergillosis may present as a primary, usually nosocomially-acquired, infection or as an invader of tissues (tracheal anastomosis or parenchyma) damaged by surgery or prior illness. Primary infection is usually focal and macronodular on radiograph. The picture in secondary cases can be obscured by the manifestations of the underlying parenchymal process, but should be suspected when evidence of new, focal nodular disease develops. The risk of invasive pulmonary aspergillosis approaches 50% when the respiratory tract, including the sinuses or trachea, is colonized. "Preemptive" antifungal therapy, usually with intravenous amphotericin B three to six weeks prior to surgery, may be indicated for such colonization. The clinical presentation is usually one of fever and systemic toxicity, with the variable occurrence of cough, dyspnea, tachypnea and pleurisy. The clinical course includes necrotizing bronchopneumonia with vascular invasion producing infarction, hemorrhage and metastasis. Most patients have metastatic disease at the time of diagnosis, notably to brain and skin. Amphotericin B remains the cornerstone of therapy, with the roles of liposomal amphotericin, itraconazole, voriconazole and other newer agents as yet undefined.

Cryptococcus Neoformans. Cryptococcal infection of the lungs in transplant patients is usually asymptomatic or minimally symptomatic. It commonly presents as an asymptomatic pulmonary nodule on routine chest x-rays. Infection disseminates from the lung, particularly to the central nervous system. Thus, asymptomatic pulmonary nodules must be aggressively pursued, with preemptive fluconazole or amphotericin therapy administered to prevent dissemination.

Significant pulmonary infection due to *Candida* species is uncommon although candidal isolation from sputum cultures is common. Such culture results should not, by themselves, be treated. The one exception to this rule is protection of the bronchial anastomotic suture line in the fresh lung transplant in whom candidal colonization of the respiratory tract is aggressively investigated and treated.

Epstein-Barr Virus and Posttransplantation Lymphoproliferative Disorders

Active Epstein-Barr Virus (EBV) replication is present in a greater percentage of organ transplant patients on maintenance immunosuppression than the general population. The critical impact of EBV is as a cofactor in the development of Posttransplantation Lymphoproliferative Disorder (PTLD). PTLD is usually a B cell lymphoproliferative process (see Chapter 8). Both antilymphocyte antibodies and cyclosporine or tacrolimus contribute to the pathogenesis of PTLD by the reactivation of latent EBV and, most likely, the loss of immune surveillance against EBV-immortalized B cells. Other risk factors for PTLD include primary EBV infection, the level of virus replicating in the oropharynx, and preceding CMV dis-

ease (by threefold to tenfold). It is not clear whether antiviral agents or reduction of immunosuppression will interrupt the pathogenesis of PTLD, either directly through effects on EBV replication, or indirectly through effects on CMV.

Hepatitis Viruses

Both HBV and HCV have significant effects on transplant patients. Chronic infection is the rule with the replication of both viruses being upregulated by immunosuppressive therapy posttransplant. Both viruses appear to contribute to the net state of immunosuppression. The rate of progression of the liver disease appears to be accelerated posttransplant. By ten years after transplant, patients with HBV infection have a less than 50% incidence of either end-stage liver disease or hepatocellular carcinoma. The prognosis for HCV infection is somewhat better, with a 15% to 20% incidence of end-stage liver disease after ten years (See Chapters 22 and 29).

Central Nervous System Infection in Transplantation

The presentation of fever and headache or other signs of central nervous system (CNS) infection in organ transplant recipients is a medical emergency. The presentation of such infection differs from that of the normal patient as immunosuppressive therapy may obscure signs of meningeal inflammation, and changes in the level of consciousness may be subtle. A differential diagnosis is developed based on the neurologic deficits, brain imaging studies, and the temporal development of disease (Table 20-6). In addition, the likelihood of certain pathogens is determined by prior antimicrobial prophylaxis, unusual exposures, the risk of viral infection, and the recent use of intensive immunosuppression for graft rejection.

Four distinct patterns of CNS infection are recognized: (1) acute meningitis, usually caused by *Listeria monocytogenes;* (2) subacute to chronic meningitis (eg, fever and headaches evolving over several days to weeks, sometimes with altered state of consciousness), usually due to *Cryptococcus neoformans,* although also with systemic infection with *M tuberculosis, Listeria, Histoplasma capsulatum, Nocardia asteroides, Strongyloides stercoralis, Coccidioides immitis,* HSV; (3) focal brain infection, presenting with seizures or focal neurologic abnormalities, most commonly due to metastatic *Aspergillus* or other invasive fungal infection (often with lung infection), but also caused by *L monocytogenes, T gondii,* or *N asteroides,* occasionally nodular vasculitis infarction due to CMV or VZV, and occasionally with EBV-associated PTLD; and (4) progressive dementia (± focal processes) related to progressive multifocal leukoencephalopathy (PML) (JC virus), or with other viral infections or the toxic effects of cyclosporine or tacrolimus.

Table 20-6. Neurologic Infectious Syndromes in Transplant Recipients

Presentation	Common Pathogens	Other Considerations
Acute Meningitis	*Listeria*	Pneumococcus, Meningococcus, Bleed
Subacute and chronic Meningitis	*Cryptococcus*	TB, Cancer (PTLD), HSV, *Nocardia, Histoplasma, Coccidiodes*, Brain Abscess
Focal Neurologic Deficit Seizure/Cerebritis	*Aspergillus*	*Nocardia*, Cancer (EBV-PTLD), Bacterial Brain Abscess, Bleed/Ischemic, *Toxoplasma*, Vasculitis
Dementia	PML (JC Virus)	Toxic Drug Effects, Demyelination, HSV, CMV

RECOMMENDED READING

Fishman JA, Rubin RH. Infection in organ transplant recipients. N Engl J Med. 1998;338(4):1741-1751.

Rubin RH. Infection in the organ transplant recipient. In: Rubin RH, Young LS, eds. Clinical Approach to Infection in the Compromised Host. 3rd ed. New York, NY: Plenum Press; 1994:629-705.

Winston DJ, Emmanouilides C, Busuttil RW. Infection in liver transplant recipients. Clin Infect Dis. 1995;21(5):1077-1089.

Paya CV, Herman PE, Wiesner RH, et al. Cytomegalovirus hepatitis in liver transplantation: prospective analysis of 93 consecutive orthotopic liver transplantations. J Infect Dis. 1989;160(5):752-758.

van den Berg AP, Klompmaker IJ, Haagsma EB, et al. Evidence for an increased rate of bacterial infections in liver transplant patients with cytomegalovirus infection. Clin Transplant. 1996;10(2):224-231.

Erice A, Holm MA, Gill PC, et al. Cytomegalovirus (CMV) antigenemia assay is more sensitive than shell vial cultures for rapid detection of CMV in polymorphonuclear blood leukocytes. J Clin Microbiol. 1992;30(11):2822-2825.

Reinke P, Fietze E, Ode-Hakim S, et al. Late-acute renal allograft rejection and symptomless cytomegalovirus infection. Lancet. 1994;344:1737-1738.

Snydman DR, Werner BG, Dougherty NN, et al. Cytomegalovirus immune globulin prophylaxis in liver transplantation. A randomized, double-blind, placebo-controlled trial. The Boston Center for Liver Transplantation CMVIG Study Group. Ann Intern Med. 1993;119(10):984-991.

Arnow PM, Furmaga K, Flaherty JP, George D. Microbiological efficacy and pharmacokinetics of prophylactic antibiotics in liver transplant patients. Antimicrob Agents Chemother. 1992;36(10):2125-2130.

George MJ, Snydman DR, Werner BG, et al. The independent role of cytomegalovirus as a risk factor for invasive fungal disease in orthotopic liver transplant recipients. Am J Med. 1997;103(2):106-113.

Paya CV. Fungal infections in solid-organ transplantation. Clin Infect Dis. 1993;16(5):677-688.

Fishman JA. Pneumocystis carinii and parasitic infections in transplantation. Infect Dis Clin North Amer. 1995;9(4):1005-1044.

Fishman JA. Prevention of infection due to Pneumocystis carinii). Antimicrob Agents Chemother. 1998;42(5):995-1004.

Fishman JA. Treatment of infection due to Pneumocystis carinii. Antimicrob Agents Chemother. 1998;42(6):1300-1314.

Rubin RH, Greene R. Clinical approach to the compromised host with fever and pulmonary infiltrates. In: Rubin RH, Young LS, eds. Clinical Approach to Infection in the Compromised Host. 3rd ed. New York, NY: Plenum Press; 1994:121-161.

Lake KD. Drug interactions in transplant patients. In: RW Emery, LM Miller, eds. Handbook of Cardiac Transplantation. Philadelphia, Pa: Hanley and Belfus; 1995:173-200.

Preiksaitis JK, Diaz-Mitoma F, Mirzayans F, Roberts S, Tyrrell DL. Quantitative oropharyngeal Epstein-Barr virus shedding in renal and cardiac transplant recipients: relationship to immunosuppressive therapy, serologic responses, and the risk of posttransplant lymphoproliferative disorder. J Infect Dis. 1992;166(5):986-994.

Riddler SA, Breinig MC, McKnight JL. Increased levels of circulating Epstein-Barr virus (EBV)-infected lymphocytes and decreased EBV nuclear antigen antibody responses are associated with the development of posttransplant lymphoproliferative disease in solid-organ transplant recipients. Blood. 1994;84(3):972-984.

21 KIDNEY DISEASE IN NONRENAL TRANSPLANTATION

Thomas A. Gonwa, MD, FACP

Transplant physicians are often confronted with the evaluation of renal disease or dysfunction in nonrenal transplant candidates (heart or liver). Several questions, which will be addressed in this chapter, must be asked during this evaluation. These are:

- Is the renal function adequate to withstand the proposed transplant?
- Is the renal dysfunction secondary to the underlying disease process and reversible posttransplant or is it fixed and irreversible?
- If there is underlying renal dysfunction, what is its impact on posttransplant morbidity and mortality?
- Is it severe enough to preclude transplantation?
- Under which conditions is combined transplant (liver-kidney or heart-kidney) justifiable and necessary?
- What is the impact of sustained immunosuppressive therapy on renal function in heart and liver recipients?

PRETRANSPLANT EVALUATION OF RENAL FUNCTION

Evaluation of renal status in liver transplant candidates is complicated by the lack of correlation between the usual marker of renal function, serum creatinine, and the true glomerular filtration rate (GFR) in advanced liver disease. High serum bilirubin levels may interfere with measurement of serum creatinine. Severe nutritional depletion and deranged protein metabolism associated with advanced liver disease produce a low serum creatinine, which may reflect decreased protein stores and not renal dysfunction. The true level of renal function must be established by determining the clearance of other agents such as inulin, radioactive-labeled tracers (eg, iothalamate, technicium-labeled DTPA [diethylenetriamine pentaacetic acid] and EDTA [ethylenediamine tetraacetic acid], or iohexol.) If a patient has a low GFR, a urine sample should be obtained and evaluated for protein excretion, fractional excretion of sodium, and the presence of red cells, white cells and casts. A renal ultrasound should be performed to determine renal size,

Thomas A. Gonwa, MD, FACP, Associate Director, Transplant Services; Professor of Transplant Medicine, Baylor University Medical Center; Clinical Associate Professor of Medicine, University of Texas, Southwestern Medical School

detect structural abnormalities, and evaluate the collecting system. Alternatively, similar information can be obtained if MRI or CT scans are part of the workup and as long as the entire abdomen is included in these studies. These tests help differentiate between renal dysfunction due to: (1) functional renal disease seen in liver disease, Hepatorenal syndrome (HRS) being the extreme manifestation; and (2) native kidney disease. Further workup to identify the underlying renal disease should proceed as it normally would. Of note, glomerular abnormalities have been reported frequently in cirrhotics with immune deposition recorded in 50% to 100%. Also, some underlying liver diseases have associated renal diseases, such as hepatitis C and cryoglobulinemia with membranoproliferative glomerulonephritis. Functional renal impairment secondary to liver failure may result in the overestimation of the severity of primary renal disease. The differentiation between functional and structural renal disease is important as it may determine if concomitant kidney-liver transplant is to be performed. If questions remain, a kidney biopsy should be performed preoperatively, if possible, or intraoperatively.

As is true for liver candidates, heart failure patients may be malnourished and thus, the serum creatinine may underestimate true GFR. Furthermore, heart failure patients require high doses of vasopressors and inotropes, the use of angiotensin-converting enzyme inhibitors, and diuretics. These agents, plus heart failure itself, can adversely affect renal circulation leading to functional depression of the GFR. Therefore, a true measurement of GFR should be obtained. A low GFR must be evaluated, as in the liver candidate, to uncover coexisting structural renal disease such as amyloidosis, diabetic glomerulopathy, or atheroembolic disease. Functional renal disease often reverses following left ventricular assist device placement or successful cardiac transplant.

IMPACT OF RENAL FUNCTION ON POSTOPERATIVE MORBIDITY AND MORTALITY
Liver Transplantation

Once evaluation of renal function is complete, one must determine if transplantation may proceed. The question often arises as to whether underlying renal dysfunction is a prognostic indicator of long-term outcome following nonrenal transplantation. Some reports on liver transplant recipients have indicated that renal dysfunction has a negative impact on posttransplant survival by increasing infectious and bleeding complications. Patients with renal dysfunction were reportedly more likely to have extended intensive care unit (ICU) stays, and prolonged hospitalization, and to require greater resources to achieve successful outcomes. However, this finding may apply more to the patient with acute fulminate hepatic failure as opposed to those with chronic liver disease. Analysis of the United Network for Organ Sharing (UNOS) database for liver transplants, performed between 1988 and 1995, demonstrated that patients undergoing liver transplant with a preoperative serum creatinine greater than 2 mg/dL had a 5-year actuarial patient survival rate of only 50.4% compared to a 5-year patient survival rate of all liver transplant recipients of 72.4%. More recent publications from a single center have questioned this finding. In a study at Baylor University Medical Center (BUMC) of over 600 patients, preoperative renal function (other than HRS) had no impact on short-term (one month) or long-term (five years) patient survival. Tailoring the immunosuppressive therapy to the patient's renal function helped to achieve these results and preserved function. A subsequent study of larger patient numbers demonstrated no difference in patient survival following liver transplantation in patients with a preoperative serum creatinine greater than 2 mg/dL (including HRS patients) compared to those with preoperative serum creatinine less than 2 mg/dL (5-year actuarial patient survival of 66.1% vs 70.1%). However, in patients presenting with a serum creatinine greater than 2 mg/dL, postoperative dialysis predicted worse 5-year survival (75.7%, no dialysis vs 55.7%, dialysis). Unfortunately, there was no preoperative variable that predicted a long-term need for dialysis or renal transplantation. A study from the University of Pittsburgh evaluated risk factors associated with mortality and infectious complications following liver transplant in high-risk patients. Ninety-eight percent of these patients were hospitalized at the time of transplant. Although preoperative renal dysfunction requiring dialysis was associated with increased risk of death in a univariate analysis, only posttransplant dialysis, along with donor age, major infection, additional immunosuppression, and subsequent transplantation, was a significant independent predictor of mortality in a multivariate analysis. Thus, the literature is mixed. Overall, it appears that patients with preoperative renal dysfunction may have increased morbidity and mortality following liver transplantation, although this risk may only occur in patients with acute hepatic failure rather than chronic liver disease. However, centers with more extensive experience in caring for these patients may achieve excellent results despite poor preoperative renal function.

The aforementioned studies were performed in patients undergoing primary liver transplantation. A different situation may exist in patients undergoing liver re-transplantation. Markmann and colleagues at the University of California, Los Angeles have developed a simple model to estimate survival after re-transplantation of the liver. They studied their population of 150 liver re-transplant recipients and constructed a Cox multivariate regression model and a simple scoring system. Five variables predicted postoperative mortality: ischemic time, mechanical ventilation, total bilirubin, serum creatinine, and recipient age. A serum creatinine greater than 1.6 mg/dL was a poor prognostic indicator. This model has been validated using data from patients transplanted at BUMC and the UNOS database.

HEPATORENAL SYNDROME. Patients presenting with Hepatorenal Syndrome (HRS) represent a different challenge. This syndrome represents the extreme manifestation of the functional abnormalities of renal function that occur in response to cirrhosis. Once the diagnosis of HRS is made in the liver transplant candidate, two questions are invariably asked: (1) is this patient still a candidate for liver transplant, and (2) should a combined liver-kidney transplant be performed? HRS is clearly a reversible condition. Renal function improves following a successful liver transplant, and kidneys from patients with HRS function well when used for cadaveric renal transplantation. Despite these landmark findings, many centers are reluctant to transplant patients with HRS, and instead perform combined liver-kidney transplantation. In recent analysis of data from BUMC, patients with HRS (n=79) had a 5-year actuarial patient survival of 67.1% compared to 70.1% in patients without HRS, but did have longer ICU stays (17.4 days vs 6.4 days), prolonged hospitalization (42 days vs 27 days), and a greater need for postoperative dialysis (35% vs 5%). Thus, more resources are required to care for these patients. Most patients recovered renal function, however 8.9% of HRS patients developed subsequent end-stage renal disease (ESRD), compared to 2% in non-HRS patients. By comparison, a study by Fisher et al from Birmingham found an incidence of ESRD of 4% in 883 consecutive patients undergoing liver transplant between 1982 and 1996. The BUMC studies could not identify a preoperative factor (even dialysis) that could predict subsequent development of ESRD in patients with end-stage liver disease (ESLD). However, early postoperative risk factors identified by both Birmingham and BUMC, that predict ESRD include postoperative need for dialysis, older recipient age, CMV disease, and re-transplant. Current recommendations are that patients with well-documented HRS undergo liver transplantation only. A summary of the effect of renal function on postoperative outcome in liver transplant is presented in Table 21-1.

Heart Transplantation

The situation in heart transplantation is less clear. A report from the Transplant Cardiologists Research Database in 1993 examined pretransplant risk factors for death after heart transplantation in 911 patients transplanted over an 18 month period. Preoperative risk factors for death were examined in a multivariate analysis. Abnormal renal function was a weak predictive factor with a *P*-value of only 0.1. This registry has grown into the International Society for Heart and Lung Transplantation (ISHLT) Registry representing data on over 45,993 heart transplants worldwide. In their most recent report, no mention of abnormal renal function as a risk factor was made after a multivariate logistic regression analysis of the data. Single-center studies from Italy and Spain have supported these conclusions. To the contrary, Smith et al specifically examined results of heart re-transplantation over a 25 year period at a single center. In a group of 66 patients, renal dysfunction (serum creatinine >2 mg/dL) was significantly associated with the need for postoperative dialysis (63%) or death (67%) in the first 12 months. Unfortunately, all these studies use different criteria for abnormal renal function, varying from a serum creatinine greater than 2 mg/dL to oliguria (<300 cc/24 h). Furthermore, it must be noted that published data on heart transplant outcome from patients with preoperative renal dysfunction is limited, as most centers considered a serum creatinine greater than 2 mg/dL or a creatinine clearance of less than 50 mL/min to be a contraindication to heart transplant. To address this and other pretransplant issues, the American Society of Transplantation recently held a consensus conference on listing criteria for cardiac transplant candidates. At the conference, it was recognized that many of the drugs candidates needs (ie, angiotensin-converting enzyme inhibitors and diuretics) may cause decreased renal function in the absence of intrinsic renal disease. The majority opinion was that a benign urine sediment, absence of significant proteinuria, and presence of two normal kidneys by ultrasound may be adequate evidence of reversibility of renal dysfunction. Most conference attendees, however, believed that a serum creatinine of greater than 3 mg/dL should be considered a relative contraindication to transplant. Instead, some centers perform combined heart-kidney transplantation in candidates with compromised renal function.

Table 21-1. Effects of Pretransplant Renal Function on Posttransplant Mortality

Condition	5-Year Actuarial Patient Survival	Time
OLTX (UNOS, n=20,063)	72.3%	10/87-12/95
OLTX with creatinine >2 mg/dL (UNOS, n=2,442)	50.4%	10/87-12/95
OLTX with creatinine >2 mg/dL (BUMC, n=123)*	66.1%	5/85-12/96
OLTX only in patients with HRS (BUMC, n=79)*	67.1%	5/85-12/96
OLTX with creatinine <2 mg/dL (BUMC, n=1,003)*	70.1%	5/85-12/96

UNOS indicates United Network for Organ Sharing; BUMC, Baylor University Medical Center; and OLTX, orthotopic liver translant.

Reprinted with permission from Gonwa TA, Klintmalm GB, Levy M, et al. Impact of pretransplant renal function on survival after liver transplantation. Transplantation. 1995;59:361-365.

1998 OPTN/SR AR 1988-1997. HHS/HRSA/OSP/DOT;UNOS.

Table 21-2. Combined Transplantation in the US: 1988-1998

Year	Total Liver	Liver-Kidney	(%)	Total Heart	Heart-Kidney	(%)
1988	1,713	23	-1.3	1,676	3	-0.2
1989	2,151	30	-1.4	1,698	5	-0.3
1990	2,631	46	-1.7	2,095	12	-0.6
1991	2,895	43	-1.5	2,121	5	-0.2
1992	2,989	57	-1.9	2,160	9	-0.4
1993	3,367	49	-1.5	2,277	16	-0.7
1994	3,549	85	-2.4	2,321	19	-0.8
1995	3,818	82	-2.1	2,344	12	-0.5
1996	3,916	111	-2.8	2,319	21	-0.9
1997	4,001	116	-2.9	2,266	20	-0.9
1998	4,339	94	-2.2	2,307	35	-1.5
Total	35,369	736		23,584	157	

UNOS Scientific Registry Data as of September, 1999.

COMBINED TRANSPLANTATION OF THE KIDNEY WITH EITHER LIVER OR HEART

Liver-Kidney Transplantation

When a thorough evaluation of renal status in a patient being evaluated for liver disease reveals fixed irreversible renal disease, or when a patient with ESRD develops ESLD, combined transplantation of the liver and kidney can be considered. Patients with certain metabolic diseases, such as hyperoxaluria, are also considered for combined transplantation. For the patient not on dialysis, one must decide at what level of renal function to consider combined transplant. It is known that renal function can deteriorate posttransplant due to long-term exposure to immunosuppressive agents. On the other hand, it is also known that renal function can improve following successful liver transplant in patients with HRS or functional deterioration of renal function due to cirrhosis. The histology of the native kidney, obtained by biopsy pretransplant or at the time of liver transplant, and the GFR are both important. Patients with a GFR of less than 25 cc/min with histological findings of fixed renal disease, and the ESRD patient on dialysis requiring liver transplant, undergo combined transplant of the liver and kidney. In cases in which this is not clear-cut, both organs are procured, intraoperative kidney biopsy is performed at the start of liver transplantation, then reviewed, and finally, a decision whether or not to proceed with kidney transplantation is made. Others have recommended a GFR of 35 cc/min or less as the cutoff. An examination of the UNOS database demonstrated that the number of combined transplants in the US is increasing, and that perhaps up to 33% were being performed in patients with HRS. Table 21-2 lists the combined transplants done in the US from 1988 through September 1998.

Patients undergoing a combined liver-kidney transplant generally do well. The liver transplant is performed first, followed by the kidney. Five-year actuarial survival, according to the UNOS database for patients undergoing combined liver-kidney transplant in the US (1988-1995), was 62.2%, compared to 50.4% in patients with preoperative serum creatinine greater than 2 mg dL (Table 21-1). At BUMC, 37 combined transplants have been performed with a 5-year actuarial survival of 56.7%. Compared to 67.1% in HRS patients undergoing liver transplant only (Table 21-1). Generally, the combined transplant recipients have prolonged ICU and hospital stays compared to liver-only patients, 5% to 20% require postoperative dialysis, and renal function is excellent at one year. Death in combined transplant recipients is usually due to the underlying morbidity related to the liver disease, such as recurrence of hepatitis C or liver graft failure. Initial reports suggest that combined transplants of the liver and kidney protected the kidney from rejection. In fact, several centers have reported that combined transplants can be performed in the face of a positive crossmatch and hyperacute rejection of the kidney does not occur. However, Katznelson and Cecka reviewed 248 combined liver-kidney transplants in the UNOS database, and compared rejection rates and graft survival to a control group comprised of 206 contralateral kidneys from the same donors transplanted as kidneys only. They found no difference in rejection or graft survival, suggesting that a liver does not protect the kidney. Thus, each organ must be monitored separately, as rejection may occur in one organ without occurring in the other. Results of combined transplantation in the US are summarized in Table 21-3.

Heart-Kidney Transplantation

The number of combined heart-kidney transplants done in the US from 1988 through September 1997 is shown in Table 21-2. Although fewer in number and percentage of transplants as compared to combined liver-kidney transplants, the incidence appears to be increasing. Narula et al recently reviewed the entire US experience with combined transplants from October 1987 through May of 1995. There were 84 combined transplants done

Table 21-3. Results of Combined Transplantation in the US

Organ	Number	Time	Actuarial 2-Year Survival
Heart Patient	14,340	10/87 - 5/95	78.6%
Heart-Kidney Patient	84	10/87 - 5/95	66.5%
Cadaveric Kidney Patient	72,914	10/87 - 12/96	90.8%
Cadaveric Kidney Graft	72,914	10/87 - 12/96	76.9%
Organ	Number	Time	Actuarial 5-Year Survival
Liver Patient	20,063	10/87 - 12/95	72.3%
Liver-Kidney Patient	414	10/87 - 12/95	62.2%
Cadaveric Kidney Patient	68,652	10/87 - 12/95	81.4%
Cadaveric Kidney Graft	68,652	10/87 - 12/95	61.9%

during that time period. No significant difference in 24-month survival rate was found for these patients when compared to patients receiving a heart transplant only. The combined transplant patients had a 24-month survival of 66.5% compared to 78.6% in the heart-only recipients (P=.2) (Table 21-3). Although rejection of both heart and kidney have been reported to be lower than in recipients of single organs, rejection may be discordant and occur in either transplant alone. Therefore, independent surveillance of each organ is necessary. The indications for kidney transplantation include a variety of intrinsic renal diseases exacerbated by end-stage heart failure. At least 90% of the detailed published cases report a renal diagnosis that is appropriate for renal transplant. However, the literature does not clarify the level of renal function that one should use to consider a combined transplant. As for the liver transplant candidate, it is often difficult to sort out the contribution of heart failure to the severity of the observed renal dysfunction. This decision is complicated by the knowledge that one must use a calcineurin inhibitor postoperatively. The first report of cyclosporine nephrotoxicity in non-renal transplantation was in cardiac recipients. Myers clearly demonstrated that in patients transplanted at Stanford University, a depressed GFR was present at the time of transplant. In those patients treated without cyclosporine, the GFR improved to nearly normal with successful transplantation. In those patients treated with cyclosporine, GFR did not increase and in most cases, declined.

Thus, it is difficult to decide which patients should be offered a combined heart-kidney transplant vs a heart transplant alone. When confronted with the patient presenting with heart failure and renal dysfunction, one must consider all the above points. As there is no clear-cut evidence of the effect of renal dysfunction on long-term outcome in primary heart transplant, each center must set their own standards. As referenced earlier in this chapter, a serum creatinine greater than 2 mg/dL in a heart re-transplant candidate has been shown to be a harbinger of poor outcome. Those authors recommend combined transplant in that setting.

One may also be presented with the patient who is already on dialysis and who presents with severe congestive heart failure or is found to have poor cardiac function during evaluation for renal transplantation. Should these patients be considered for combined transplant? Burt et al reported on four ESRD patients with New York Heart Association class III or IV heart failure referred to their institution. All received a renal transplant only, and all had marked improvement of cardiac function following successful renal transplant. BUMC observed similar findings in its population of patients, and recommended a period of intense dialysis to determine if there is a component of fluid overload, systolic

dysfunction, or uremic toxicity contributing to the observed heart failure in these patients before considering combined transplantation.

POSTTRANSPLANT RENAL FUNCTION

As clearly delineated in Section II, Chapters 14a and 14b, the calcineurin inhibitors cyclosporine and tacrolimus are both nephrotoxic. In addition to one of these two drugs, liver transplant recipients are exposed to a variety of other potential nephrotoxins such as IV contrast and antibiotics. Management of these nephrotoxins is no different than in other patients with renal dysfunction. In addition to nephrotoxins, there are many perioperative and postoperative renal considerations in the liver transplant recipient. These include attention to the electrolyte (eg, citrate, lactate, calcium, potassium), acid base and fluid changes that occur during the operation itself, the anhepatic phase, and the immediate postoperative period. In the patient with HRS or compromised renal function in the immediate postoperative period, calcineurin inhibitors should be avoided. Induction therapy is used at this point with mycophenolate mofetil, steroids, and muromonab-CD3 or another antithymocyte preparation. There is little experience with anti-IL-2 receptor antibodies in liver transplantation. In patients with HRS or severe renal dysfunction immediately postoperative, mycophenolate mofetil and steroids are started immediately. Antibody induction therapy is initiated if renal function has not improved by 48 to 72 hours. This protocol has allowed BUMC to successfully transplant patients with HRS without the addition of a kidney transplant.

After the initial postoperative period, patients are placed on a nephrotoxic calcineurin inhibitor long-term. An average of 40% reduction in GFR is seen in liver transplant recipients postoperatively. However, this is variable. By carefully following renal function with not only serum creatinine, but also GFR measurements, long-term immunosuppression can be individually tailored to the patient's renal function. By decreasing the calcineurin inhibitor and optimizing therapy with either azathioprine or mycophenolate mofetil, renal function can be preserved even in those patients with a low pretransplant GFR. This will not lead to either increased rejection or decreased patient survival. Thus, patients presenting for transplant at BUMC with an average GFR of 47 mL/min (n=109) had a 1-year GFR of 45 mL/min and a 5-year actuarial survival of 69%, compared to a 1-year GFR of 68 mL/min and 5-year survival of 73% in patients presenting with an average pretransplant GFR of 140 mL/min (n=114). Although the majority of published work on the nephrotoxicity of calcineurin inhibitors is with cyclosporine, tacrolimus gives similar results. Results from the US multicenter trial of tacrolimus vs cyclosporine in liver transplant recipients demonstrated an equivalent fall in GFR posttransplant. GFR in the cyclosporine group fell from 89 + 37 mL/min pretransplant to 63 + 28 mL/min at 12 months. In the tacrolimus group, GFR fell from 85 + 28 mL/min pretransplant to 59 + 22 mL/min at one year. Management of these patients consists of decreasing the calcineurin inhibitor and adding or increasing a third immunosuppressive drug such as azathioprine or mycophenolate mofetil. Caution must be urged, however, if one considers withdrawing the calcineurin inhibitor. In a study from the Mayo Clinic, 12 consecutive stable patients were withdrawn from cyclosporine for nephrotoxicity. Sustained improvement of renal function was minimal and 50% of patients developed rejection and three of six developed chronic rejection. Lastly, HCV infection may specifically influence post-liver transplant renal function by increasing the occurrence of proteinuria and membranoproliferative glomerulonephritis (MPGN), as well as the development of diabetes.

Long-term renal function in cardiac recipients is similar to that in liver recipients. There appears to be an initial decline in renal function of between 15% to 25% during the first six months in patients treated with cyclosporine. However, several studies of patient cohorts from different centers have demonstrated a stabilization of function at time points out to five years. The ISHLT registry reported that 10.4% of patients have renal dysfunction and 7.7% have a serum creatinine greater than 2.5 mg/dL. Tinawi et al studied 133 consecutive patients who had survived more than five years. Mean serum creatinine rose from 1.3 mg/dL at one to two months posttransplant to 1.66 mg/dL at 50 months. During the time period of six to 60 months posttransplant, 12% to 17% of patients had a serum creatinine of greater than 2 mg/dL. At all time points, patients with a serum creatinine greater than 2 mg/dL had lower cyclosporine dosage reflecting a judicious decrease in an attempt to preserve renal function. No patients in their series progressed to ESRD. Thus, as with the liver recipients, careful management of heart recipients may preserve renal function over the long term.

END-STAGE RENAL DISEASE, DIALYSIS AND RENAL TRANSPLANT IN HEART AND LIVER RECIPIENTS
Liver Transplantation
Despite efforts to reduce nephrotoxicity, some patients with liver and cardiac transplants will progress to ESRD. As noted above, patients at BUMC who had HRS had an 8.9% incidence of ESRD compared to 2% in patients without HRS. ESRD developed anywhere from one month to seven years posttransplant. Twenty-one patients were treated with or are on dialysis, and seven

of those have died. Their management is similar to other dialysis patients with the additional need for immunosuppressive therapy monitoring. Seventeen patients have received 18 kidney transplants. In the first 14 transplanted patients, the 2-year patient survival was only 67% compared to 93% in primary kidney allograft recipients. Two-year graft survival was only 49% compared to 83% in primary kidney allografts. Of patient deaths, two were due to sepsis, two due to cardiac causes and one due to aspiration. However, the three patients most recently transplanted are all doing well six to 18 months posttransplant. A series from Birmingham, England reported an incidence of ESRD of 2% in a series of 883 liver recipients with a mortality of 44%. It appears that liver transplant recipients developing ESRD have increased mortality regardless of the renal replacement modality chosen, although this may be due to the pre-existing liver disease or problems with the liver transplant itself. Further study is needed to determine the optimal therapy.

Heart Transplantation
Heart recipients have also been reported to develop ESRD. The ISHLT registry reported that in patients undergoing heart transplant, ESRD developed in 1% at three years. Single-center studies have reported rates from 3% at ten years (Stanford University) up to 8% at ten years (Rotterdam). Hornberger et al studied the risk of development of ESRD in 2,088 Medicare beneficiaries who received cardiac transplants between 1989 and 1994. They found a risk of 0.37% in the first year posttransplant, which rose to 4.49% by the sixth posttransplant year. They made no estimate of the mortality in this cohort of patients. Frimat et al reported on 16 patients who developed ESRD following heart transplant. Eight underwent renal transplant and were doing well. Of the eight staying on dialysis, 1-, 2-, and 23-month survival was 100%, 78%, and 60%, respectively, similar to dialysis survival reported in Europe. This was, however, inferior to survival in cardiac recipients without ESRD. At the University of Pittsburgh, 12 patients developing ESRD after heart transplant were treated with renal replacement therapy, four with hemodialysis and eight with peritoneal dialysis. Survival rates were significantly worse compared to other dialysis patients. Stanford University reported on eight patients undergoing renal transplant following development of ESRD post-heart transplant. Patient and graft survivals were 89% at both 1- and 3-years posttransplant, and rejection rates were lower. From these few series, it appears that transplantation is preferred over dialysis for the heart recipient developing ESRD. However, further studies are needed.

RECOMMENDED READING

Distant DA, Gonwa TA. The kidney in liver transplantation. J Am Soc Nephrol. 1993;4(2):129-136.

Baliga P, Merion RM, Turcotte JG, et al. Preoperative risk factor assessment in liver transplantation. Surgery. 1992;112(4):704-711.

Brown RS Jr, Lombardero M, Lake JR. Outcome of patients with renal insufficiency undergoing liver or liver-kidney transplantation. Transplantation. 1996;62(12):1788-1793.

Jeyarajah DR, Gonwa TA, McBride M, et al. Hepatorenal syndrome: combined liver kidney transplants versus isolated liver transplant. Transplantation. 1997;64(12):1760-1765.

Gonwa TA, Klintmalm GB, Levy M, Jennings LS, Goldstein RM, Husberg BS. Impact of pretransplant renal function on survival after liver transplantation. Transplantation. 1995;59(3):361-365.

Gayowski T, Marino IR, Singh N, et al. Orthotopic liver transplantation in high-risk patients: risk factors associated with mortality and infectious morbidity. Transplantation. 1998;65(4):499-504.

Markmann JF, Gornbein J, Markowitz JS, et al. A simple model to estimate survival after retransplantation of the liver. Transplantation. 1999;67(3):422-430.

Fisher NC, Nightingale PG, Gunson BK, Lipkin GW, Neuberger JM. Chronic renal failure following liver transplantation: a retrospective analysis. Transplantation. 1998;66(1):59-66.

Hosenpud JD, Bennett LE, Keck BM, Fiol B, Boucek MM, Novick RJ. The registry of the International Society for Heart and Lung Transplantation: fifteenth official report — 1998. J Heart Lung Transplant. 1998;17(7):656-668.

Miller LW. Listing criteria for cardiac transplantation: results of an American Society of Transplant Physicians - National Institutes of Health conference. Transplantation. 1998;66(7):947-951.

Smith JA, Ribakove GH, Hunt SA, et al. Heart retransplantation: the 25-year experience at a single institution. J Heart Lung Transplant. 1995;14(5):832-839.

Jeyarajah DR, McBride M, Klintmalm GB, Gonwa TA. Combined liver-kidney transplantation: what are the indications? Transplantation. 1997;64(8):1091-1096.

Katznelson S, Cecka JM. The liver neither protects the kidney from rejection nor improves kidney graft survival after combined liver and kidney transplantation from the same donor. Transplantation. 1946;61:1403-1405.

Narula J, Bennett LE, DiSalvo T, Hosenpud JD, Semigran MJ, Dec GW. Outcomes in recipients of combined heart-kidney transplantation: multiorgan, same-donor transplant study of the International Society of Heart and Lung Transplantation/United Network for Organ Sharing Scientific Registry. Transplantation. 1997;63(3):861-867.

Burt RK, Gupta-Burt S, Suki W, Barcenas CG, Ferguson JJ, VanBuren CT. Reversal of left ventricular dysfunction after renal transplantation. Ann Intern Med. 1989;111(8):635-640.

Sandborn WJ, Hay JE, Porayko MK, et al. Cyclosporine withdrawal for nephrotoxicity in liver transplant recipients does not result in sustained improvement in kidney function and causes cellular and ductopenic rejection. Hepatology. 1994;19(4):925-932.

Tinawi M, Miller L, Bastani B. Renal function in cardiac transplant recipients: retrospective analysis of 133 consecutive patients in a single center. Clin Transplant. 1997;11(1):1-8.

Hornberger J, Best J, Geppert J, McClellan M. Risks and cost of end-stage renal disease after heart transplantation. Transplantation. 1998;66(12):1763-1770.

Frimat L, Villemot JP, Cormier L, et al. Treatment of end-stage renal failure after heart transplantation. Nephrol Dial Transplant. 1998;13(4):2905-2908.

Bernardini J, Piraino B, Kormas RL. Patient survival with renal replacement therapy in heart transplantation patients. ASAIO J. 1998;44(5):M546-M548.

Kuo PC, Luikart H, Busse-Henry S, et al. Clinical outcome of interval cadaveric renal transplantation in cardiac allograft recipients. Clin Transplant. 1995;9(2):92-97.

22 LIVER DISEASE IN NON-LIVER TRANSPLANT PATIENTS

Hugo R. Rosen, MD

In the current era of extreme organ scarcity, it is of paramount importance to identify factors that impact outcome following organ transplantation. Clearly, liver diseases are an important cause of morbidity and mortality in this setting. This chapter will review the appropriate workup and evaluation of liver disease in the prospective transplant recipient, the impact of liver disease, particularly related to viral hepatitis, and the hepatotoxicity of immunosuppressive agents.

EVALUATION OF UNDERLYING LIVER DISEASE IN THE PROSPECTIVE ORGAN RECIPIENT

There is a broad array of biochemical tests used to provide indirect evidence of hepatobiliary disease. The term *liver function tests* (LFTs) is firmly entrenched in routine medical usage, although it has been criticized because the tests most commonly used in the evaluation of liver disease (ie, the serum aminotransferase and alkaline phosphatase levels) assess hepatocyte integrity rather than a known synthetic function. In fact, it might be argued that *liver injury tests* would be the more appropriate term. Patients with abnormal liver tests and obvious signs and symptoms of liver disease usually do not represent diagnostic challenges, while the asymptomatic individual who is found to have a mild elevation of one or more liver enzymes may. Screening biochemical tests of healthy, asymptomatic populations has revealed that up to 6% have abnormal LFTs, although the prevalence of liver disease in the general population is significantly lower at approximately 1%. Although comparable data do not exist for prospective organ recipients, it is imperative to consider limitations to the use of LFTs, including sensitivity and specificity. For example, cirrhotic patients may have minimally abnormal or even normal LFTs. Problems with specificity (ie, the patient with elevated serum aminotransferase levels of cardiac origin) also need to be considered. Even measures of specific hepatic functions, such as the serum albumin concentration, bilirubin concentration, and prothrombin time, can be

Associate Professor of Medicine, Molecular Microbiology, and Immunology, Division of Gastroenterology/Hepatology; Medical Director, Liver Transplantation Program, Oregon Health Sciences University, Portland Veterans Affairs Medical Center, Portland, OR

affected by extrahepatic factors such as nutritional state, hemolysis, and antibiotic use (Table 22-1).

Tests that Reflect Hepatobiliary Injury

AMINOTRANSFERASES. Aminotransferases are the most frequently used and most specific indicators of hepatic injury, and represent markers of hepatocellular necrosis. These enzymes, aspartate aminotransferase (AST, formerly serum glutamic oxaloacetic transaminase) and alanine aminotransferase (ALT, formerly serum glutamic pyruvic transaminase), catalyze the transfer of the alpha-amino groups of aspartate and alanine, respectively, to the alpha-keto group of ketoglutaric acid.

Whereas ALT is primarily localized to the liver, AST is present in a wide variety of tissues including heart, skeletal muscle, kidney, brain, and liver. AST is present in both the mitochondria and cytosol of hepatocytes, however, ALT is found only in the cytosol. In an asymptomatic individual with an isolated elevation of AST or ALT, diagnostic clues can be garnered from the degree of elevation.

Serum levels of AST and ALT are elevated to some extent in almost all liver diseases. Mild elevations are typically found in patients with fatty liver, nonalcoholic steatosis (NASH), and chronic viral hepatitis. The highest elevations (eg, more than 20-fold) occur in acute viral hepatitis, drug-induced (ie, acetaminophen) or toxin-induced hepatic necrosis, and ischemic hepatitis related to circulatory shock. The height of the elevation of aminotransferases does not appear to correlate with the extent of necrosis on liver biopsy specimens, and therefore has no prognostic value. In fact, rapidly declining aminotransferase levels may reflect decreased viable hepatocytes and indicate a poor prognosis. Moderately elevated levels (threefold to 20-fold) are typical of acute or chronic hepatitis including alcoholic hepatitis. A characteristic feature of chronic hepatitis C infection is an episodic, fluctuating pattern of serum ALT levels; periods of elevated enzyme activity alternate with periods of normal or near normal ALT. In patients with extrahepatic biliary tract obstruction, serum levels of AST and ALT may become elevated to greater than 300 U/L, usually declining rapidly after peaking within the first 24 to 48 hours after obstruction.

Although elevations in aminotransferases may be the first clue to liver disease, and screening has proved useful for detecting subclinical liver disease in asymptomatic persons, prospective organ recipients with normal levels may have significant liver damage. For instance, recent studies have demonstrated that asymptomatic hepatitis C (HCV) carriers may have evidence of chronic hepatitis on liver biopsy despite repeatedly normal LFTs. This appears to be a frequent finding in patients maintained on hemodialysis, with more than one-third of

Table 22-1. Nonhepatic Causes of Abnormal Liver Function Tests

Test	Nonhepatic Causes	Discriminating Tests
Albumin	Protein-losing enteropathy Nephrotic syndrome Malnutrition Congestive heart failure	Serum globulins, α_1 antitrypsin clearance Urinalysis, 24 hour urinary protein Clinical Setting Clinical Setting
Alkaline phosphatase	Bone disease	GGTP, SLAP, 5'-NT
	Pregnancy	GGTP, 5'-NT
	Malignancy	Alkaline phosphatase electrophoresis
Serum AST	Myocardial Infarction	MB-CPK
Bilirubin	Hemolysis	Reticulocyte count, peripheral smear, urine bilirubin
	Sepsis	Clinical setting, cultures
	Ineffective erythropoiesis	Peripheral smear, urine bilirubin, hemoglobin electrophoresis, bone marrow examination
	Shunt hyperbilirubinemia	Clinical setting
Prothrombin time	Antibiotic and anticoagulant use, steatorrhea, dietary deficiency of vitamin K (rare)	Response to vitamin K, clinical setting

GGTP indicates Gamma-glutamyl transpeptidase; SLAP, serum leucine aminopeptidase; 5'-NT, 5'-nucleotidase; AST, aspartate aminotransferase. Adapted from Moseley FH: Approach to the patient with abnormal liver chemistries. In Yamada T (ed): Textbook of Gastroenterology, ed 2. Philadelphia, JB Lippincott, 1996, p 919; with permission.

HCV-infected patients demonstrating persistently normal LFTs, although the underlying mechanisms are unknown. Yasuda et al have recently suggested that the upper normal limits of AST and ALT in patients undergoing dialysis should be reduced considerably, and that values greater than 20 U/L are definitely abnormal and possibly indicative of liver disease.

ALKALINE PHOSPHATASE, GAMMA-GLUTA-MYLTRANSFERASE AND BILIRUBIN.

The usual markers to identify cholestasis are alkaline phosphatase (ALP) and gamma-glutamyltransferase (GGT). Serum alkaline phosphatase is the name applied to a group of enzymes that catalyze the hydrolysis of phosphate esters at an alkaline pH. The enzymes are widely distributed and may originate from bone, liver, intestine or placenta. In children and adolescents, where bone growth is active, the serum alkaline phosphatase may increase up to threefold. In patients with hepatobiliary disorders, increased ALP results from increased hepatic production with leakage into the serum, rather than failure to clear or excrete circulating ALP. Markedly elevated levels of ALP suggest the possibility of disorders such as extrahepatic biliary obstruction, primary biliary cirrhosis, drug-induced cholestasis, primary sclerosing cholangitis, and infiltrative processes such as amyloid, granulomatous disease and neoplasms. The degree of elevation does not differentiate extrahepatic and intrahepatic cholestasis. Depressed serum levels of ALP have been

associated with congenital hypophosphatasia, hypothyroidism, pernicious anemia, and zinc deficiency.

GGT is useful to confirm whether an elevated ALP is secondary to hepatobiliary disease or of extrahepatic origin. Unfortunately, because the enzyme is ubiquitous, an elevated GGT has poor specificity, and indeed may be due to induction by alcohol or medications (eg, phenytoin). It has been suggested that GGT be used as a marker for surreptitious alcohol ingestion, but the lack of sensitivity and specificity of GGT levels limits its usefulness. 5'-Nucleotidase, on the other hand, is very specific for liver disease, and its measurement is particularly helpful in diagnosing liver disease in children and during pregnancy, settings in which ALP is elevated physiologically, but 5'-nucleotidase is not.

Bilirubin is an endogenous organic anion derived primarily from the degradation of hemoglobin released from red blood cells. Hyperbilirubinemia is classified as either unconjugated or conjugated. In patients with hyperbilirubinemia due to hepatocellular dysfunction or cholestasis, the serum bilirubin is predominantly conjugated and hence, water soluble, allowing easy renal excretion. Extreme hyperbilirubinemia (ie, >25 mg/dL) usually signifies severe liver disease in association with another cause of "unconjugated hyperbilirubinemia" (ie, hemolysis).

The level of serum bilirubin has been used to predict survival and natural history of specific liver diseases. The level of hyperbilirubinemia has prognostic significance in patients with primary biliary cirrhosis, fulminant hepatic failure, and acute alcoholic hepatitis. Moreover, recent studies have suggested that a subset of virally infected solid organ transplant recipients develop marked hyperbilirubinemia and hepatic failure, and have a high rate of mortality. Initially described following hepatitis B (HBV) recurrence in liver allograft recipients, recent reports in heart and renal transplantation recipients infected with HCV have shown extremely high viral levels in serum and tissue in patients with severe cholestasis, suggesting a direct cytopathic effect.

Assessment of Extent of Liver Injury

Laboratory abnormalities may provide information about severity of liver damage and thus, prognosis. Originally developed to predict survival of cirrhotic patients after portosystemic shunt surgery, the Childs-Turcotte-Pugh Score (Table 22-2) provides an estimate of liver dysfunction in patients with cirrhosis. Moreover, a number of sophisticated imaging modalities are now available to assess the hepatic parenchyma, vasculature, including evidence of portal hypertension, and biliary tree. The choice of initial and subsequent imaging studies should be determined by the clinical scenario in consultation with a radiologist. Liver biopsy remains the definitive test before and following organ transplantation to confirm the diagnosis of specific liver disease and assess prognosis in many forms of parenchymal liver disease, particularly chronic viral hepatitis.

CHRONIC VIRAL HEPATITIS

Solid organ recipients represent a special group of patients for the study of infectious agents and their associated diseases because of the highly immunocompromised state required to prevent allograft rejection. A number of critical issues pertaining to viral hepatitis are of significance in clinical transplantation (Table 22-3). These include: (1) transmission by infected donor tissue;

(2) viral reactivation by immunosuppression and allogeneic stimulation; (3) acceleration of underlying liver disease (ie, more rapid natural history as compared to non-transplant controls); (4) extrahepatic manifestations of viral hepatitis (eg, glomerulonephritis, impact on rejection); and (5) therapeutic management. Although new viral hepatitides (eg, hepatitis G and TT-V) are being identified at a relatively rapid pace, this section will focus on infection with HBV and HCV.

Transmission

Is it safe to use organs from donors with serologically, biochemically and clinically-resolved HBV infection? The answer appears to depend on the organ being transplanted. A study from the University of California, San Francisco showed that three of six (50%) orthotopic liver transplant (OLT) recipients, only one of 42 (2.4%) renal transplantation (RT) recipients, and none of seven heart transplantation (HT) recipients of HBcAb(+) and HBsAg(-) organs became HBsAg(+) following transplantation. Therefore, the reluctance to use organs from HBcAb-positive donors does not appear to be justified for organs that do not support replication of HBV.

Table 22-3. Viral Hepatitis in the Solid Organ Recipient: Critical Issues
Transmission
Reactivation (immunosuppression, allogeneic stimulation)
Liver disease (recurrent disease in the liver allograft recipient; progression in others)
Extrahepatic manifestations (effects on cellular immune response, glomerulonephritis)
Treatment (antivirals, immunoprophylaxis, modulation in immunosuppression)

Table 22-2. Childs-Turcotte-Pugh (CTP) Scoring System to Assess Severity of Liver Disease

Points Assigned	1	2	3
Encephalopathy	None	1 to 2	3 to 4
Ascites	Absent	Slight or controlled by diuretics	At least moderate despite diuretic treatment
Albumin (g/dL)	>3.5	2.8 to 3.5	<2.8
PT (seconds prolonged)	<4	4 to 6	>6
or INR	<1.7	1.7 to 2.3	>2.3
Bilirubin (mg/dL)	<2	2 to 3	>3
For PBC, PSC, or other cholestatic liver diseases			
Bilirubin (mg/dL)	<4	4 to 10	>10

Transmission of HCV by infected donor tissue has been demonstrated in kidney, heart, and liver transplantation. The ability of the transplanted organ to sustain viral replication, the size of the inoculum, degree of HLA match or mismatch, and immunosuppression regimens are all likely to have an impact on the risk of transmission and clinical disease. In an early study, stored sera from 716 consecutive cadaver organ donors between 1986 and 1990 (prior to the availability of anti-HCV testing) were screened with first-generation enzyme-linked immunosorbent assay. Thirteen (1.8%) HCV-seropositive donors were identified. Of the 29 organ recipients from these 13 donors, 14 (48%) developed clinical hepatitis within a mean follow-up of 20 months, and two patients developing subfulminant hepatic failure. An additional study by Pereira et al of 70 recipients of organs from 42 donors who were seropositive for anti-HCV by second-generation enzyme immunoassay (EIA) testing emphasizes the importance of viremia as a predictor of HCV transmission by organ transplantation. Liver dysfunction developed in 22 of 47 (47%) organ recipients from viremic donors, in contrast to five of 23 (22%) recipients of anti-HCV-seropositive donor organs that were negative for HCV RNA by polymerase chain reaction testing. Therefore, exclusion of viremic donors would decrease, but not eliminate, de novo HCV transmission by donor organs. Studies based on antibody testing, rather than HCV RNA assessment, likely underestimated the true prevalence of acquired infection, due to the lower sensitivity of antibody testing in the posttransplant, immunosuppressed population. A long-term follow-up analysis of RT recipients who acquired HCV at the time of transplantation failed to show any difference with regard to mortality or graft loss as compared to patients who did not acquire HCV infection. In contrast, RT recipients who had HCV prior to transplantation demonstrated significantly increased relative risk of death due to sepsis, graft loss, and overall mortality. A number of analyses have demonstrated that transplantation confers a survival advantage in the HCV-positive patients with end-stage renal disease (ie, as compared to patients maintained on hemodialysis).

Viral-Related Liver Disease Following Solid Organ Transplantation

The hepatitis B genome contains a glucocorticoid-responsive element that, when activated, may increase the transcription of HBV genes. Dusheiko et al and others have demonstrated reappearance or increase in serum HBV DNA levels and HBeAg, as well as reappearance of serum HBsAg following apparent clearance of previous HBV infection. Accordingly, the spontaneous clearance of HBsAg and HBeAg, and repeated negativity for HBV DNA are significantly diminished following RT as compared to a control nontransplant population of HBV-infected individuals.

Reports from the early 1970s suggested that HBsAg seropositivity was associated with severe hepatic dysfunction in RT recipients. Parfrey et al demonstrated progression of liver disease in their prospective analysis of 22 HBV-infected RT recipients. Cirrhosis developed in 12 of 20 (60%) patients who did not have cirrhosis on initial biopsy. In contrast, HBV-infected contemporary controls maintained on hemodialysis experienced no evidence of progressive hepatic dysfunction. Similarly, Harnett and colleagues studied 31 HBV-infected patients who underwent RT. Eight of 14 (57%) deaths were attributable to liver disease, whereas only one of the 12 deaths in the dialysis group were related to liver disease. In another study of 41 HBV-infected RT recipients, 15 (36.6%) died of liver failure and four developed hepatocellular carcinoma. HCV infection was a synergistic factor, as almost two-thirds of the cirrhotic patients were co-infected with HBV, compared with 34% of noncirrhotic patients. In summary, these studies support an accelerated natural history of underlying liver disease related to HBV following RT.

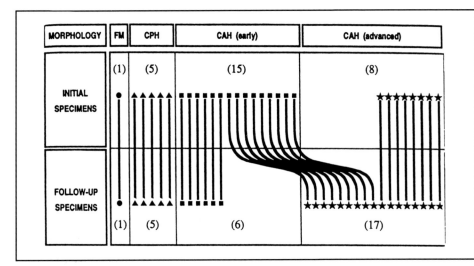

Figure 22-1. Relationship between the pretransplant histologic diagnosis and subsequent progression of chronic liver disease in renal allograft recipients. FM indicates fatty metamorphosis; CPH (solid triangles), chronic (mild) persistent hepatitis; CAH (solid squares), early (moderate) chronic active hepatitis; and CAH (solid stars), advanced chronic active hepatitis (with bridging fibrosis). Reprinted with permission from Rao et al. Value of liver biopsy in the evaluation and management of chronic liver disease in renal transplant recipients. Am J Med. 1993;94(3):241-250.

The underlying liver disease prior to RT is likely an important predictor of histologic progression post-RT. In a seminal study by Rao and colleagues from Minneapolis of RT recipients infected with either HBV, or non-A/non-B hepatitis (the majority of whom were likely HCV-seropositive), approximately one-third of patients with early chronic active hepatitis and nearly two-thirds with advanced chronic active hepatitis experienced clinical deterioration with the development of cirrhosis and death due to liver disease following RT (Figure 22-1). Specifically, nine of 15 (60%) patients with advanced chronic active hepatitis died of hepatic failure as compared to none of the 28 patients with only chronic persistent hepatitis or hepatic steatosis.

A recent large study of HBV-infected HT recipients demonstrates that 56% of infected patients developed severe fibrosis or cirrhosis within a mean of 7.4 years, and HBV-related liver failure was the cause of death in 18% of deceased patients. However, the clinical course was highly variable. Seventeen percent of patients with de novo infection had spontaneous seroconversion from HBeAg to anti-HBe and HBV-DNA clearance. Although survival for the first ten years was comparable between the infected and noninfected recipients, patient survival was significantly diminished in the HBV-infected patients with longer follow-up.

The prevalence of HCV infection in heart or lung transplant recipients ranges from 8% to 16%. In a recent survey, it appeared that only 16% of programs screen for and exclude anti-HCV-positive candidates. Nearly 70% of programs will accept organs from anti-HCV-positive donors, at least for some patients. A preliminary analysis from the cardiac transplantation registry demonstrates a significant increase in mortality in HCV-seropositive recipients, with liver failure accounting for a quarter of the deaths.

The prevalence of HCV infection averages 10% in chronic hemodialysis (HD) patients, with some units reporting rates greater than 60%. The annual incidence of de novo HCV acquisition in the HD setting in the absence of parenteral risk factors has been estimated to be 0.73% to 3% per year. In patients receiving a kidney transplant, chronic liver disease leads to enhanced morbidity and mortality, and since the advent of routine HBV vaccination, the majority of hepatic disease in RT recipients is related to HCV infection. A recent multivariate analysis of 834 RT recipients, of whom 216 were anti-HCV-positive, demonstrated that at ten years following transplantation, the presence of HCV antibodies (P=.02) and biopsy-proven cirrhosis prior to RT (P=.02) are independently associated with patient survival. Furthermore, to improve the comparison between HCV-infected and HCV-uninfected recipients, a case control analysis was performed using age, sex, year of transplantation, and immunosuppressive regimen as matching variables. Again, HCV-infected patients had significantly diminished long-term survival (Figure 22-2).

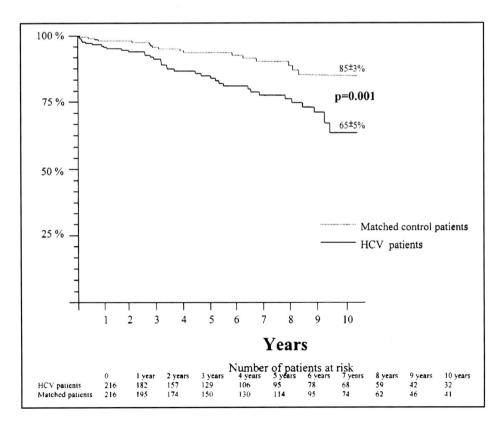

Figure 22-2. Patient survivals at 10 years in anti-HCV(+) renal transplant recipients compared to matched control HCV-uninfected RT recipients. The controls were matched for age, sex, year of transplantation, and immunosuppressive regimen. Reprinted with permission from, Marthurin et al. Impact of hepatitis B and C virus on kidney transplantation outcome. Hepatology. 1999;29(1):257-263.

Number of patients at risk

	0	1 year	2 years	3 years	4 years	5 years	6 years	7 years	8 years	9 years	10 years
HCV patients	216	182	157	129	106	95	78	68	59	42	32
Matched patients	216	195	174	150	130	114	95	74	62	46	41

Extrahepatic Manifestations of HBV and HCV Infection in the Solid Organ Recipient

Many extrahepatic manifestations in immunocompetent individuals infected with either HBV or HCV have been reported (eg, autoantibodies, leukocytoclastic vasculitis, cryoglobulinemia, membranous glomerulonephritis). De novo membranoproliferative glomerulonephritis (MPGN) has been confirmed in HCV(+) RT recipients and following OLT in HCV-infected patients, prompting the search for viral-related glomerular disease in solid organ recipients with significant proteinuria. In a longitudinal analysis of OLT recipients from the University of Washington, a greater proportion of HCV(+) patients excreted greater than 2 g protein per day after transplantation and had renal biopsies showing MPGN than did HCV(-) recipients (four of ten infected patients vs zero of seven noninfected patients). Moreover, treatment of HCV-related MPGN with interferon-alpha-2b appeared to stabilize proteinuria and renal function, but did not reverse renal dysfunction or cause liver allograft rejection.

The indirect effect of viral hepatitis on cell-mediated immunity remains far from elucidated. London et al paradoxically found that HBsAg positivity prior to RT was associated with a higher rate of allograft survival and a lower rate of rejection, presumably the result of depression of cell-mediated immunity in the chronically infected recipient. Similarly, other investigators have come to the same paradoxical conclusions regarding the effect of HCV. In a study by La Quiglia, as compared to noninfected RT recipients, those infected with HCV had an increased rate of graft survival, and this trend has been confirmed by more recent analyses. These findings have obvious clinical implications. Although unproven, it has been speculated that the increased allograft survival rate in the subset of virally infected recipients suggests that they could tolerate reduction in immunosuppression without undue graft loss, but this remains to be addressed in a controlled manner.

Without leading to a significant decrease in patient or graft survival, recurrent HCV post-OLT has been associated with an increased incidence of infections, which is likely a reflection of depressed cell-mediated immunity. Moreover, a recent large analysis demonstrated that HCV(+) patients undergoing liver re-transplantation had significantly diminished survival as compared to uninfected patients, and extrahepatic sepsis was the leading cause of death.

Treatment of Chronic Viral Hepatitis in the Solid Organ Recipient

Interferon treatment of viral hepatitis following solid organ transplantation has lacked convincing efficacy, with concern about an increased incidence of rejection associated with its use. Antiviral therapy should be considered prior to transplantation of other solid organs, and preliminary data, for example, suggests that response rates in hemodialysis patients are comparable to other study groups. However, whether preemptive antiviral treatment prior to transplantation changes the natural history after transplantation remains undefined. New antivirals have dramatically changed our approach to the HBV-infected individual. For example, liver transplantation in the HBV-infected patient who is HBeAg-positive, until recently a controversial issue, is now common with lamivudine and/or HBIg prophylaxis. The significance of lamivudine-induced HBV mutations in this setting, however, remains to be fully defined, and many reports have failed to demonstrate clinically significant liver disease. Lamivudine, an oral nucleoside analogue, interferes with the reverse transcriptase activity of both the HIV and HBV virus, and has recently been shown to be effective and safe in renal and heart transplant recipients. It is possible that in the future, patients with HBV-related cirrhosis awaiting organ transplantation will be considered appropriate candidates if viral replication can be eliminated by lamivudine, but prospective studies are required. Clearly, because therapy for hepatitis C is less efficacious, improved identification prior to transplantation of the subset of patients likely to develop progressive HCV-related liver disease is needed.

HEPATOTOXICITY OF MEDICATIONS
Transplant Immunosuppressive Agents

Hepatotoxicity associated with the use of standard immunosuppressive agents (eg, corticosteroids, cyclosporine, tacrolimus, mycophenolate mofetil) is remarkably uncommon, but does occur. Although cholestasis and other types of liver damage (eg, peliosis hepatis) have been described with estrogens and androgenic steroids, glucocorticoids are rarely classified as hepatotoxic. Corticosteroids may cause fatty metamorphosis in hepatocytes, but hepatic dysfunction from this mechanism has not been recognized in the setting of organ transplantation.

Cyclosporine is metabolized by the liver and excreted in bile, and cholestasis of any cause results in accumulation of cyclosporine metabolites in plasma. Most of the reports of cyclosporine hepatotoxicity have been characterized as cholestasis with hyperbilirubinemia with or without associated mild elevation of hepatocellular enzymes. In one report from the National Institutes of Health of nontransplant patients receiving cyclosporine for uveitis, 19 of 59 (32%) patients had persistent LFT abnormalities, predominantly of the cholestatic pattern. Lorber et al described liver test abnormalities in 228 of 466 (49%) renal transplant recipients, with serum total bilirubin, ALT, and lactate dehydrogenase being the most frequently abnormal tests, usually noted in the first 90 days posttransplant. Pharmacokinetic data revealed that patients with hepatotoxicity had increased cyclosporine bioavailability and decreased clearance. Of note, there appears to be no characteristic histologic description of cyclosporine-induced cholestasis, which makes it difficult to justify discontinuation of cyclosporine without further supportive evidence. An additional study of RT recipients suggested an interaction between HCV infection, cyclosporine, and LFT abnormalities. Three of eight patients with substantially elevated liver tests were HCV-infected, and all three demonstrated normal parent drug levels but an abnormally high concentration of metabolites. Small series of heart transplant recipients have suggested that cholestasis related to cyclosporine can occur, particularly in recipients with preoperative evidence of hepatic congestion. Moreover, the inhibitory effects of cyclosporine on normal biliary function may increase the risk of biliary calculus disease in organ transplant recipients. For example, it has been demonstrated that up to a third of diabetic patients with pancreas and kidney transplants develop cholelithiasis, and it has been speculated that a combination of cyclosporine and gallbladder hypomotility account for these findings.

A broad spectrum of histopathologic hepatic lesions have been attributed to azathioprine (Table 22-4), with the central mechanism presumed to be damage to endothelial cells in terminal hepatic venules and sinusoids. Solid organ recipients who develop nodular regenerative hyperplasia (NRH) are at great risk of developing portal hypertension (eg, ascites, variceal hemorrhage), and therefore, early histologic evidence of NRH should prompt discontinuation of azathioprine.

Table 22-4. Hepatotoxic Reactions Attributed to Azathioprine
Cholestasis
Asymptomatic elevation of LFTs
Hepatic sinusoidal congestion and dilation
Centrilobular dilation or necrosis
Peliosis hepatis
Hepatic veno-occlusive Disease
Fibrosis or stenosis of hepatic veins
Nodular regenerative hyperplasia (NRH)
Clinical signs of portal hypertension

Tacrolimus appears to be associated with minimal, if any hepatotoxicity in the clinical setting, although experimental data suggest similar effects as cyclosporine on biliary secretion, as well as possible induction of hepatic fibrogenesis in experimental models.

Other Medications

Drug-induced liver injury must always be considered in the solid organ recipient who develops signs or symptoms of liver disease. Potential mechanisms include disruption of metabolic processes, toxic destruction of hepatocytes, exacerbation of underlying liver disease, and carcinogenesis. Table 22-5 outlines drugs used for other medical issues, which may lead to hepatic abnormalities.

RECOMMENDATIONS AND SUMMARY

In the current era of extreme organ scarcity, it is of paramount importance to determine factors that might impact outcome. Liver diseases have a significant influence on morbidity and mortality following solid organ transplantation. Active HBV vaccination is mandatory for all organ transplant candidates prior to undergoing transplantation. Further research is required to define the role of preemptive antiviral therapy prior to solid organ transplantation. The differential diagnosis of hepatic disease following transplantation includes chronic viral hepatitis and medications. Although cyclosporine may cause cholestasis following organ transplantation, sulfonamides (used for prophylaxis of *Pneumocystis carinii*) and azathioprine may be more common causes of drug-induced cholestasis.

In reviewing the literature, a number of common themes arise. Assays for HCV RNA should be considered a screening test for the detection of HCV infection in the population of solid organ recipients and in hemodialysis patients because of the significant rate of impaired serologic response. HCV infection posttransplantation appears to have a more indolent course than HBV, although a subset of patients develop rapidly progressive HCV-related liver failure following organ transplantation. In patients without clear-cut evidence of advanced hepatic disease, liver biopsy prior to organ transplantation is the only objective method to stage the degree of injury. In general, patients with cirrhosis should be precluded from consideration of non-liver transplantation. Considerable work needs to be done to define the optimal immunosuppression regimen in the virally-infected patient, particularly to determine how these regimens should be modulated once significant liver disease is identified.

Table 22-5. Potential Hepatotoxic Drugs According to Medical Indications

Medical Indication	Drug
Diabetic Agents	Sulfonylureas Metformin Rezulin
Antimicrobials	Carbenicillin Oxacillin (cholestaic hepatitis) Ceftriazone (biliary sludge) Amoxicillin-clavulanic acid Sufonamides (usually necroinflammatory) Ketoconazole Fluconazole Isoniazid (incidence increases with age) Zidovudine Ganciclovir
Neurologic and antipsychotic Agents	Chlorpromazine Carbamazepine (22% patients develop ↑LFTs) Phenytoin Valproic acid Tricyclic antidepressants
Cardiovascular Agents	Amiodarone (40% patients develop ↑LFTs) Alpha-methlydopa (most commonly hepatocellular pattern) Angotensin-converting enzyme inhibitors (unusual; mixed patterns) Calcium channel blockers (verapamil and nifedipine)
Hormonal Agents and Antihypertensives	Oral contraceptives (cholestasis, adenomas) Anabolic and androgenic steroids (peliosis hepatitis, hepatocellular carcinoma) Flutamide Niacin HMG CoA reductase inhibitors (lovastatin, simvastatin)
Pain Management Agents	Tylenol (dose-dependent, predictable hepatoxicity) Nonsteroidal anti-inflammatory agents (NSAIDs; idiosyncratic) Diclofenac (more common in older women) Sulindac (high incidence of hepatoxicity) Feldene Aspirin (mild and reversible)

RECOMMENDED READING

Rosen HR, Keeffe E. Laboratory evaluation of the patient with signs and symptoms of liver disease. In: Brandt LJ, ed. Clinical Practice of Gastroenterology. Vol. 2. Philadelphia, Pa; Churchill Livingstone; 1998:812-820.

Healey CJ, Chapman RAG, Fleming KA. Liver histology in hepatitis C infection: a comparison between patients with persistently normal or abnormal transaminases. Gut. 1995;37(2):274-278.

Davies S, Portmann BC, O'Grady JG, et al. Hepatic histological findings after transplantation for chronic hepatitis B virus infection, including a unique pattern of fibrosing cholestatic hepatitis. Hepatology. 1991;13(1):150-157.

Lim HL, Lau GKK, Davis GL, Dolson DJ, Lau JY. Cholestatic hepatitis leading to hepatitic failure in a patient with organ-transmitted hepatitis C virus infection. Gastroenterology. 1994;106(1):248-251.

Booth JCL, Goldin RD, Brown JL, Karayiannis P, Thomas HC. Fibrosing cholestatic hepatitis in a renal transplant recipient associated with the hepatitis B virus precore mutant. J Hepatol. 1995;22(4):500-503.

Wachs ME, Amend WJ, Ascher NL, et al. The risk of transmission of hepatitis B from HBsAg(-), HBcAb(+), HBIgM(-) organ donors. Transplantation. 1995;59(2):230-234.

Pereira BJG, Milford EL, Kirkman RL, et al. Transmission of hepatitis C virus by organ transplantation. New Engl J Med. 1991;325(7):454-460.

Lau JYN, Davis GL, Brunson ME, et al. Hepatitis C virus infection in kidney transplant recipients. Hepatology. 1993;18(5):1027-1031.

Pereira BJG, Milford EL, Kirkman RL, et al. Prevalence of hepatitis C virus RNA in organ donors positive for hepatitis C antibody and in the recipients of their organs. N Engl J Med. 1991;327(13):910-915.

Pereira BJG, Wright TL, Schmid CH, et al. Screening and confirmatory testing of cadaver organ donors for hepatitis C virus infection: a US National Collaborative Study. Kid Intl. 1994;46(3):886-892.

Rosen HR, Friedman LS, Martin P. Hepatitis C and the renal transplant patient. Semin Dial. 1996;9:39-47.

Farza H, Salmon AM, Hadchouel M, et al. Hepatitis B surface antigen gene expression is regulated by sex steroids and glucocorticoids in transgenic mice. Proc Natl Acad Sci. 1987;84(5):1187-1191.

Dusheiko G, Song E, Bowyer S, et al. Natural history of hepatitis B virus infection in renal transplant recipients — a fifteen-year follow-up. Hepatology. 1983;3(3):330-336.

Nagington J. Reactivation of hepatitis B after transplantation operations. Lancet. 1977;1(8011):558-560.

Parfrey PS, Forbes RDC, Hutchison TA, et al. The impact of renal transplantation on the course of hepatitis B liver disease. Transplantation. 1985;39(6):610-615.

Wedemeyer H, Pethig K, Wagner D, et al. Long-term outcome of chronic hepatitis B in heart transplant recipients. Transplantation. 1998;66(10):1347-1353.

Fagouli S, Cooper DKC, Zhudi N. Hepatitis C status of heart transplant recipients. Clin Transplantation. 1998;12(1):5-10.

Zein NN, McGreger CG, Wendt NK, et al. Prevalence and outcome of hepatitis C infection among heart transplant recipients. J Heart Lung Transplant. 1995; 14(5):865-869.

Milfred SK, Lake KD, Anderson DJ, et al. Practices of cardiothoracic transplant centers regarding hepatitis C-seropositive candidates and donors. Transplantation. 1994;57(4):568-572.

Marthurin P, Mouquet C, Poynard T, et al. Impact of hepatitis B and C virus on kidney transplantation outcome. Hepatology. 1999;29(1):257-263.

LaQuaglia MP, Tolkoff-Rubin NE, Dienstag JL. Impact of hepatitis on renal transplantation. Transplantation. 1981;32(6):504-507.

Rao KV, Ma J. Chronic viral hepatitis enhances the risk of infection but not acute rejection in renal transplant recipients. Transplantation. 1996;62(12):1765-1769.

Singh M, Gayowski T, Wagener MM, Marino IR. Increased infections in liver transplant recipients with recurrent hepatitis C virus hepatitis. Transplantation. 1996;61(3):402-406.

Rosen HR, Martin P. Hepatitis C virus infection in patients undergoing liver retransplantation. Transplantation. 1998;66(12):1612-1616.

Izopet J, Rostaing L, Moussion F, et al. High rate of hepatitis C virus clearance in hemodialysis patients after interfero-alpha therapy. J Infect Dis. 1997;176(6):1614-1617.

Markowitz JS, Martin P, Conrad AJ, et al. Prophylaxis against hepatitis B recurrence following liver transplantation using combination lamivudine and hepatitis B immune globulin. Hepatology. 1998;28(2):585-589.

Kowdley KV, Keeffe EB. Hepatoxicity of transplant immunosuppressive agents. Gastroenterol Clin North Am. 1995;24(4):991-1001.

Lorber MI, Van Buren CT, Flechner SM, Williams C, Kahan BD. Hepatobiliary and pancreatic complications of cyclosporine therapy in 466 renal transplant recipients. Transplantation. 1987;43(1):35-40.

Horina JH, Wirnsberger GH, Kenner L, Holzer H, Kregs GJ. Increased susceptibility for CsA-induced hepatotoxicity in kidney graft recipients with chronic viral hepatitis C. Transplantation. 1993;56(5):1091-1094.

23 LUNG DISEASE IN NON-LUNG TRANSPLANT PATIENTS

David D. Ralph, MD

INTRODUCTION

The major role of the lungs is to translocate oxygen into and carbon dioxide out of the body. These processes cannot be interrupted for more than a few minutes before permanent damage results to other organs. During conditions that increase demands for oxygen and carbon dioxide exchange, such as strenuous exercise, the volume of oxygen exchanged increases tenfold. Even during daily activities, the exchange rate has to increase by threefold. Additionally, the lungs have a dominant role in acid-base homeostasis since carbon dioxide exchange is the major means of acid elimination.

The lungs also perform non-gas exchange functions. They filter nearly the entire cardiac output every minute and metabolize several circulating substances. Additionally, they are constantly exposed to particulates, bacteria, viruses, and gas pollutants from the outside world, which requires maintenance of self-protective mechanisms.

PRETRANSPLANT PULMONARY DISORDERS

Many transplant candidates have common pulmonary disorders that are unrelated to the disease necessitating transplantation and may require pretransplant pulmonary evaluation (Table 23-1). Asthma occurs in approximately 5% of the population. Chronic obstructive pulmonary disease (COPD) is common in long-term smokers. Patients with chronic heart, liver, renal or pancreatic disease may have episodes of pneumonia, pulmonary embolism or pulmonary damage from aspirated gastric acid or oral secretions. In addition, other pulmonary disorders occur with increased frequency in patients with nonpulmonary end-stage organ disease.

Pleural Effusions

Pleural effusions are usually first detected on chest x-ray. If the effusion is small, the patient will likely be asymptomatic. Occasionally, removal of a relatively small amount of a moderate-sized effusion may relieve dyspnea, not by improving hypoxemia, but instead, by improving diaphragmatic motion. Thoracentesis is indicated when there is suspicion of infection, malignancy, or pulmonary embolism. Therapeutic thoracentesis is indicated for significant dyspnea or hypoxemia. Empyema requires chest tube drainage.

In heart transplant candidates, effusions are most often transudative due to elevated left ventricular filling pressures. These effusions are often bilateral, but may be unilateral, usually on the left. Thoracentesis is not necessary if the effusion improves with treatment of the congestive heart failure. Effusions due to hemothorax have occurred after endomyocardial biopsy.

In liver transplant candidates, transudative right-sided or bilateral effusions are common in patients who have ascites. In the absence of signs of empyema or severe interference with gas exchange, thoracentesis is not required. Chest tube drainage should be avoided as the fluid will continue to form and drain, and thus interfere with nutrition due to an ongoing protein loss.

In renal transplant candidates, effusions form most commonly due to volume overload and respond to intensive dialysis. Uremic patients may also develop uremic pleuritis.

Pulmonary Infiltrates

Pulmonary infiltrates can develop rapidly with pneumonia, aspiration, pulmonary edema, or embolic infarction. Pneumonia is reviewed in Chapter 20.

In heart failure patients, the infiltrates due to cardiogenic pulmonary edema may start with an interstitial chest x-ray pattern before progressing to an alveolar chest x-ray pattern. Sarcoidosis is a cause of both cardiomyopathy and pulmonary infiltrates. Amiodarone can cause severe pulmonary fibrosis.

Patients with renal failure can have infiltrates due to edema associated with volume overload, or to pleuro-pericarditis or interstitial fibrosis. Primary pulmonary-renal diseases that cause infiltrates include Goodpasture's syndrome and Wegener's granulomatosis.

Patients with Sjögren's syndrome associated with primary biliary cirrhosis may have lymphocytic interstitial lung disease.

Associate Professor of Medicine, Pulmonary and Critical Care Medicine, University of Washington, University of Washington Medical Center, Seattle, WA

Table 23-1. Indications for Pretransplant Pulmonary Consultation
History of previous or active lung disease
History of dyspnea, cough, wheezing, chest pain
Abnormal chest radiograph
Abnormal pulmonary function test results
Hepatopulmonary syndrome
Diagnosis of pulmonary hypertension by echocardiography
Indications to measure oxygen consumption

Pulmonary Nodules

Pulmonary nodules always raise suspicion for tumor, especially in current or former smokers. Patients with hepatopulmonary syndrome may have basilar lung nodules. Pulmonary calcification has been observed in renal failure patients.

Hepatopulmonary Syndrome

Mild hypoxemia in liver transplant candidates can be caused by atelectasis secondary to pleural effusions or ascites, by basilar airway closure associated with the pressure of ascites on the diaphragms or by the hepatopulmonary syndrome. The hypoxemia due to basilar airway closure can be overcome by several deep breaths. The hypoxemia of atelectasis may also improve after deep breaths as atelectatic regions are pulled open by pulmonary interdependence.

Hypoxemia due to hepatopulmonary syndrome is seen in approximately ten percent of patients and is caused by shunting of intrapulmonary blood flow through intrapulmonary vascular dilations. Shunting may be demonstrated by lung scan or echocardiography. Measurement of the right-to-left shunt fraction is performed by injection of macroaggregated albumin during a perfusion lung scan. The shunt is calculated from the percentage of radioactivity that travels through the pulmonary circulation into the systemic circulation (Figure 23-1). Bubbles injected into the right side of the heart during echocardiography monitoring will traverse the shunts and appear three to five beats later in the left heart. With deep breaths, the hypoxemia due to hepatopulmonary syndrome may actually worsen as additional blood flows through the shunt passages. Fortunately, hepatopulmonary syndrome may improve after transplantation. Thus, it is no longer considered a contraindication to transplant and may in fact be an indication for transplant in patients even when other aspects of the liver failure are not yet severe.

Pulmonary Hypertension

Pulmonary hypertension occurs in 2% to 4% of patients with chronic portal hypertension. Hypoxemia from pulmonary hypertension is usually mild unless the foramen ovale has stretched open from high right-heart pressures secondary to pulmonary hypertension. Evaluation should include screening with echocardiography and confirmation of abnormal pulmonary pressures detected by echocardiography by right-heart catheterization. There is no contraindication to transplant in patients who have the high cardiac output common in chronic hepatic failure and associated mild pulmonary hypertension, but a normal pulmonary vascular resistance. However, patients with truly elevated pulmonary vascular resistance are at risk of dying from right-heart failure and systemic hypotension in the intraoperative and postoperative periods. Due to the scarcity of data, clear-cut guidelines for when pulmonary hypertension is a contraindication to transplant do not exist. One approach is to first treat pulmonary hypertension with medications such as epoprostenol. If the mean pulmonary artery pressure decreases to below 40 torr the patients may proceed to liver transplant. If not, simultaneous lung transplantation should be considered.

Patients with left-heart failure who secondarily develop pulmonary hypertension are at high risk for heart failure at the time of implantation of a new heart. They are usually rejected for cardiac transplantation if their pulmonary vascular resistance cannot be reduced to less than two to three times normal with medications, but still could be considered for combined heart-lung transplantation.

INDICATIONS FOR COMBINING LUNG TRANSPLANTATION WITH OTHER ORGAN TRANSPLANTATION
Combined Liver-Lung Transplantation

Combined liver-lung transplantation could be considered in patients with advanced pulmonary disease from α-1-antitrypsin deficiency. However, the liver and

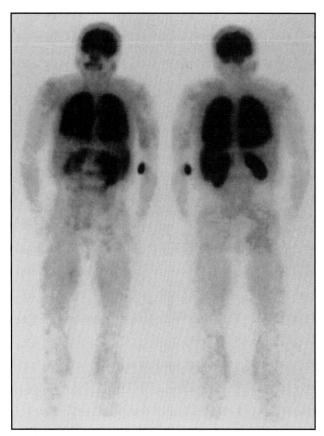

Figure 23-1. Hepatopulmonary syndrome: macroaggregated albumin perfusion scan in a hypoxemic patient with 51% intrapulmonary shunt. Note that much of the tracer has passed through the lungs and lodged in the systemic circulation including the brain, kidneys and liver.

pulmonary consequences of α-1-antitrypsin do not usually advance in concert to simultaneous end-organ failure. Lung transplant would also need to be considered in addition to liver transplant in any patient with noninfected end-stage lung disease. According to the United Network for Organ Sharing (UNOS) data, only six simultaneous liver-lung transplantations were performed from 1995 through 1998.

Combined Heart-Lung Transplantation

Combined heart-lung transplantation is no longer necessary for most patients with primary pulmonary hypertension, as most patients do well with only lung transplantation. Current indications for combined heart-lung transplant mainly include patients with pulmonary hypertension secondary to surgically uncorrectable congenital cardiac lesions. Six hundred twenty-three simultaneous heart-lung transplantations were reported to UNOS from 1986 through 1998.

Combined Kidney-Lung Transplantation

Combined kidney-lung transplantation is unusual. Renal failure from Goodpasture's syndrome can be treated with renal transplantation alone. Lung involvement may still occur after renal transplantation, but is treatable without lung transplantation. UNOS recorded only four simultaneous kidney-lung transplantations from 1995 through 1998.

Combined Pancreas-Lung Transplantation

Combined pancreas-lung transplantation could be indicated in type I diabetics with unrelated types of lung disease or patients with combined organ failure from cystic fibrosis.

LUNG DISEASE FOLLOWING TRANSPLANTATION (Table 23-2)
General Problems

HYPOXEMIA. Any disorder that primarily or secondarily affects the respiratory drive, respiratory musculature, airways, or pulmonary parenchyma may cause hypoxemia after transplantation. Most of the disorders are transient and common to other postoperative conditions.

DYSPNEA. Just as in the pretransplant stage, there are numerous causes of posttransplant dyspnea. Edema, effusions, infiltrates and diaphragm dysfunction are common causes of dyspnea. Patients with a bladder-drained pancreas transplant promptly develop a metabolic acidosis due to bicarbonate loss. To maintain a normal pH, ventilation must increase (decreasing the PCO_2) by 20% to 30%. In patients with normal ventilatory reserve, this is easily accomplished, but patients with limited reserve may become dyspneic or be unable to fully compensate for the metabolic acidosis. In the immediate postoperative period, the use of narcotics may blunt the dyspnea and compensatory hyperventilation leading to substantial tissue acidosis.

Specific Problems

BRONCHOSPASM. Wheezing and bronchospasm are common in intubated asthmatics. The mainstays of treatment are aggressive administration of inhaled beta-agonist bronchodilators plus early extubation to remove the bronchospastic stimulation caused by the endotracheal tube irritation of the trachea. Bronchospasm can also be caused by volume overload leading to bronchial cuffing by interstitial fluid.

ATELECTASIS. Atelectasis is most common in the postoperative period in patients who have had thoracic (heart transplant) or upper abdominal (liver transplant) surgery, and is less common with lower abdominal surgery (pancreas or renal transplant). Hypoxemia and dyspnea may result. Treatment includes positioning the atelectatic lung upwards, using periodic deep inspirations, and adequately treating chest wall pain. Large pleural effusions may need

Table 23-2. Pulmonary Disorders after Transplantation

Disorders in the early postoperative period
Pulmonary edema
ARDS
Aspiration pneumonia
Atelectasis
Pleural effusions
Bronchospasm
Diaphragmatic dysfunction
Pulmonary hypertension
Pulmonary contusion

Disorders in the later postoperative period
Pneumonia
Pulmonary embolism

Disorders appearing or persisting after the postoperative period
Pneumonia
Hepatopulmonary syndrome
Pulmonary hypertension
Pulmonary calcification
Diaphragmatic dysfunction
Posttransplant lymphoproliferative disorder
Drug-related pulmonary fibrosis
Drug-related eosinophilic pneumonia
Pulmonary vasculitis (Goodpasture's, Wegener's, hepatitis C)

to be drained. Routine bronchoscopy for removal of secretions is not needed, but bronchoscopy may be useful if there are mucus plugs or lobar atelectasis.

PLEURAL EFFUSIONS. Volume overload is a common cause of postoperative effusions after any transplant. Effusions are frequent after cardiac transplantation, especially on the left side but do not need removal unless they are large and interfering with gas exchange. Similarly, the right-sided effusions associated with liver transplantation only occasionally need drainage. Pleural effusions have also been reported in the presence of posttransplant lymphoproliferative disease (PTLD) or in relation to perirenal allograft lymphocele.

PULMONARY INFILTRATES. Edema, aspiration and infection are the most common causes of postoperative pulmonary infiltrates. Adult respiratory distress syndrome can occur after any organ transplant. Treatment of adult respiratory distress syndrome (ARDS) includes attention to ventilator management, positive end-expiratory pressure, and avoidance of volume overload. The pulmonary edema that sometimes results from administration of monoclonal antibodies against CD3 can be severe, and requires immediate volume reduction and temporary discontinuation of such therapy until the infiltrates resolve. Goodpasture's syndrome and Wegener's granulomatosis have both recurred in the lungs after successful renal transplantation.

PULMONARY CALCIFICATION. Pulmonary calcification has been observed in both renal transplant patients and liver transplant patients who have renal insufficiency after transplant.

DIAPHRAGM DYSFUNCTION. During heart replacement the left diaphragm and phrenic nerve may be damaged due to traction and injury. Weaning mechanical ventilation may be difficult and delayed, but most patients can ventilate adequately with one functionally intact hemidiaphragm. This complication may resolve in the first six months after transplant or be permanent. Similar injury to the right hemidiaphragm and phrenic nerve may occur during liver transplantation.

PULMONARY EMBOLISM . The most common symptom of pulmonary embolism is dyspnea. Hemoptysis occurs in a minority of patients who have pulmonary embolism. The clinical suspicion for pulmonary embolism increases if the patient has risk factors (eg, previous venous thrombo embolism, stasis, inherited or transient hypercoagulable states), has no other good explanation for the dyspnea, and has tachypnea on examination. Unfortunately, ventilation-perfusion (V/Q) scanning can only lead to definitive decisions regarding

anticoagulation treatment in about a third of patients. Patients with normal perfusion scans and patients with a low clinical suspicion and a low-probability V/Q scan do not need further testing for pulmonary embolism. Patients felt clinically to have a high or intermediate probability of pulmonary embolism who have high-probability scans may be anticoagulated without proceeding to arteriography. All other patients suspected of pulmonary embolism need further testing, but various protocols have been proposed for evaluation of these patients. Anticoagulation is indicated for those patients in whom duplex evaluation of the lower extremities reveals acute deep venous thrombosis (DVT). For those in whom a properly performed D-dimer assay is negative, anticoagulation is not needed. In the remaining patients, some clinicians would perform pulmonary angiography or C-angiogram while others would perform serial duplex examinations over the next ten to 14 days. The literature on pulmonary embolism is complex and evolving, so decisions regarding diagnostic work-up are best made by clinicians experienced in the disease.

Although liver transplant patients have low platelet counts and abnormal clotting factor levels in the postoperative period, they still are at risk for pulmonary emboli. The risk of embolization in renal transplant candidates is lower than might be expected although clotting may occur on indwelling vascular catheters. Following transplant however, venous thrombosis may be noted in up to 4.5% of kidney only, and 18% of kidney-pancreas recipients with pulmonary emboli recorded in up to 1.7% and 4.7%, respectively.

PULMONARY HYPERTENSION. Pulmonary hypertension associated with liver failure may cause severe hemodynamic instability at the time of the transplant operation and in the early postoperative phase. Epoprostenol and nitric oxide have been helpful in postoperative management of the pulmonary hypertension. After successful transplant, the pulmonary hypertension often recedes over a period of many months.

Pulmonary hypertension associated with chronic cardiac failure may similarly lead to acute failure of the newly-implanted heart. Treatment with pulmonary vasodilators such as nitric oxide may be necessary until cardiac function stabilizes.

HEPATOPULMONARY SYNDROME. The hypoxemia from hepatopulmonary syndrome may lead to a complicated postoperative course. Hypoxemia may become more marked as the protective elevated cardiac output present pretransplant normalizes after transplant. However, the hepatopulmonary syndrome usually stabilizes or slowly improves over the long-term as the intravascular dilations regress after a successful liver transplant.

PULMONARY TOXICITY OF DRUGS USED FOR TRANSPLANTATION

Fortunately, pulmonary toxicity is unusual from most of the chronic immunosuppressive and prophylactic medications used after transplantation. The dominant pulmonary adverse effect occurs through the increased risk of pulmonary infections.

The first few doses of muromonab-CD3 (Orthoclone OKT®3) frequently cause a diffuse capillary leak syndrome that occurs several hours after administration and is manifested in the lungs as pulmonary edema. Subsequent doses should be delayed and volume administration restricted until infiltrates clear. Pretreatment with corticosteroids and possibly antihistamines one to four hours before dosing with Orthoclone OKT®3 lessens the cytokine release and pulmonary edema.

Corticosteroid-containing medications have no direct adverse effects on normal lung tissue. Diaphragmatic weakness has been occasionally described as part of the acute or chronic myopathy that may accompany use of steroids. Prolonged neuromuscular weakness is most likely to occur in patients treated simultaneously with paralytic medications.

Cyclosporine and tacrolimus have no reported pulmonary toxicity except for rare reports of a possible association with ARDS and interstitial fibrosis.

Azathioprine and mycophenolate have been associated with interstitial pneumonitis and pulmonary fibrosis in rare case reports.

Trimethoprim-sulfamethoxazole used for infection prophylaxis can cause eosinophilic pneumonia, interstitial lung disease, or pleural effusions. Dapsone can cause an eosinophilic pneumonia.

EFFECTS OF PROLONGED INTUBATION FOLLOWING TRANSPLANTATION

The greatest danger in those patients who require prolonged intubation after transplantation is acute sinopulmonary infection. The risk of acute sinusitis occurs with both nasal and oral intubation and rises after three days of intubation. The presence of an endotracheal tube or tracheostomy convert the normally sterile distal trachea into a colonized region. This increases the risk of subsequent pneumonia. Tracheostomy decreases the risk, but many centers are reluctant to perform tracheostomy in patients treated with immunosuppressants.

Mechanical irritation or erosion of tissues occurs at points of contact between the endotracheal tube and the upper airway. Erosions may occur in the naso-oropharynx, the vocal cords, or the trachea. The greatest danger of serious bleeding is from erosion into the innominate artery as it passes anterior to the trachea.

Sentinel bleeding often precedes major bleeding from innominate erosions.

Vocal cord paralysis occurs after nasotracheal, orotracheal, and tracheostomy intubations. Vocal cord paralysis may resolve after periods as long as six months after extubation. With the use of modern low-pressure endotracheal tube cuffs, tracheal stenosis has become an uncommon complication even after prolonged intubation. Prolonged intubation has little or no effect on eventual recovery of full diaphragmatic strength.

RISK FACTOR MANAGEMENT PRECEDING AND FOLLOWING TRANSPLANTATION

α-1 Antitrypsin Deficiency

α-1 Antitrypsin deficiency is associated with liver failure in both children and adults. The pulmonary damage from the disease takes many years to become significant, progresses much faster in smokers, and has a variable rate of progression among individuals. Unfortunately, early damage is difficult to detect and, by the time the FEV_1-to-FVC ratio or diffusion capacity decline, there has already been significant damage to the lungs. The most important factor in treating the pulmonary status of A1AT patients is avoidance or cessation of smoking. Patients with A1AT deficiency who do not smoke may live to an advanced age without clinical limitations.

Intravenous A1AT replacement therapy has now been available for over a decade. The National Heart Lung and Blood Institute-sponsored registry followed pulmonary function in nonrandomized patients treated with or without replacement therapy for up to six years. With replacement therapy, a decrease in mortality and slower rate of deterioration in FEV_1 and FVC were demonstrated in the subgroup of patients who had an initial FEV_1 of 35% to 50% of predicted. There is little data to show an advantage to replacement therapy in patients with little or mild pulmonary dysfunction. Thus, it is reasonable to recommend replacement therapy to patients with FEV_1-to-FVC ratios less than 50%, and to follow other patients with yearly pulmonary function tests to determine if they will need replacement therapy.

Occupational Hazards

Pulmonary disorders caused or worsened by occupational exposure fall into the categories of occupational asthma, hypersensitivity pneumonitis, and pneumoconiosis. There are myriad causes of occupational asthma. Some exposures may cause the de novo development of asthma in patients with no history of lung disease. Exposure to toluene diisocyanate, Western Red Cedar, and crab processing is associated with a high rate of development of asthma. Exposure to these agents should be avoided, especially by those with underlying asthma.

Hypersensitivity pneumonitis is caused by exposure to organic protein antigens in substances such as moldy hay, bird feathers, etc. Its presentation is usually one of subacute or chronic dyspnea and cough, sometimes accompanied by fever. Chest x-ray shows diffuse interstitial infiltrates. Thoracoscopic lung biopsy specimens will show lymphocytic alveolar infiltration with occasional granulomas. The treatment is use of glucocorticoids and avoidance of the offending substance. Pneumoconioses are interstitial lung diseases caused by exposure to inorganic substances such as silica, asbestos and coal. Risk for these exposures can usually be identified easily from the patient's work and hobby history. Treatment is removal from the exposure. There is no response of the scarring process to corticosteroid therapy.

Some occupations are associated with a potential risk of fungal infection. *Aspergillus* grows in bird droppings, organic debris and at construction sites, posing a potential infectious risk to patients employed in construction, forestry, farming, and garbage collection.

Travel After Transplantation

Tuberculosis is a worldwide infection, especially prevalent in developing countries. Pneumococcal infections are also widespread. Avoidance of infected populations is the best prophylaxis for these infections. Prophylaxis with fluconazole should be considered to prevent acquisition of invasive coccidioidomycosis infection in travelers to the Lower Sonoran life zone including the southwestern United States and neighboring Mexico.

Paracoccidioidomycosis is endemic in South America and causes cutaneous and pulmonary infection. Histoplasmosis usually results from reactivation but can newly arise in spelunkers. Travel to southeast Asia and southern China can result in pneumonia from the fungus *Penicillium marneffei.*

Smoking

Smoking is associated with chronic bronchitis, increased susceptibility to respiratory infections, chronic obstructive pulmonary disease (COPD), and lung cancer. In the general population, the main risk of smoking is the doubling of the risk of coronary artery disease. Thus, avoidance of smoking and smoking cessation are a vital part of pretransplant and posttransplant care. The problem should be addressed if possible before transplantation to optimize preoperative pulmonary function. The risk of postoperative pulmonary complications is reduced after two months of cigarette cessation. Within one year of smoking cessation, there is a decreased risk of coronary artery disease, a return to the normal rate of pulmonary function decline, and a decreased occurrence of bronchitis. The risk of lung cancer decreases gradually over several years.

Marijuana smoke is even more toxic to the lungs than cigarette smoke, and presents the additional danger of invasive infection from *Aspergillus* that grows on the marijuana.

Continuation of smoking is based on both a pharmacologic addiction and on psychological patterns and habits. Smoking cessation is best approached by medical and behavioral methods. Cessation rates increase in patients who are individually encouraged to stop smoking by their physicians. Cessation rates improve when nicotine addiction and withdrawal is managed with nicotine replacement therapy (eg, gum, patch, nasal spray, inhaler). The more difficult aspect of therapy is psychological and behavioral support. Patients who also participate in some form of group support have higher rates of sustained abstention than do patients who are only treated with pharmacologic methods. Methods vary, but most include education, recognition and avoidance of situations where the patient feels the need for a cigarette, and positive reinforcement for smoking cessation. It is difficult for an individual physician to provide this behavioral support, so patients should usually be referred to an effective local program for this aspect of treatment.

RECOMMENDED READING

Anonymous. Dyspnea. Mechanisms, assessment, and management: a consensus statement. American Thoracic Society. Am J Respir Crit Care Med. 1999;159(1):321-340.

Ettinger NA, Trulock EP. Pulmonary considerations of organ transplantation. Part 1. Am Rev Respir Dis. 1991;144(6):1386-1405.

Ettinger NA, Trulock EP. Pulmonary considerations of organ transplantation. Part 3. Am Rev Respir Dis. 1991;144(2):433-451.

Smetna GW. Preoperative pulmonary evaluation. N Engl J Med. 1999;340(12):937-944.

Krowka MJ, Porayko MK, Plevak DJ, et al. Hepatopulmonary syndrome with progressive hypoxemia as an indication for liver transplantation: case reports and literature review. Mayo Clin Proc. 1997;72(1):44-53.

Kuo P, Plotkin JS, Gaine S, et al. Portopulmonary hypertension and the liver transplant candidate. Transplantation. 1999;67(8):1087-1093.

Costard-Jackle A, Fowler MB. Influence of preoperative pulmonary artery pressure on mortality after heart transplantation: testing of potential reversibility of pulmonary hypertension with nitroprusside is useful in defining a high risk group. JACC. 1992;19(1):48-54.

Chang SW, Ohara N. The lung in liver disease. Clin Chest Med. 1996;17:1-169.

Hunt SA. Pulmonary hypertension in severe congestive heart failure: how important is it? J Heart and Lung Transpl. 1997;16(1):S13-S15.

Judson MA, Sahn SA. The pleural space and organ transplantation. Am J Resp Crit Care Med. 1996;153(3):1153-1165.

Hyers TM. Venous thromboembolism. Am J Respir Crit Care Med. 1998;159(1):1-14.

Maurer JR, Frost AE, Estenne M, Higgenbottam T, Glaville AR. International guidelines for the selection of lung transplant candidates. Transplantation. 1998;66(7):951-956.

Hain A, Khanna A, Molmenti EP, Rishi N, Fung JJ. Immunosuppressive therapy. Surg Clin N Amer. 1999;79(1):59-76.

Dekhuijzen PN, Decramer M. Steroid-induced myopathy and its significance to respiratory disease: a known disease rediscovered. Eur Resp J. 1992;5(8):997-1003.

The alpha-1-antitrypsin deficiency registry study group. Survival and FEV1 decline in individuals with severe deficiency of alpha 1-antitrypsin. Am J Respir Crit Care Med. 1998;158(1):49-59.

Raw M, McNeill A, West R. Smoking cessation: evidence based recommendations for the healthcare system. BMJ. 1999;318(7177):182-185.

Mileno MD, Bia FJ. The compromised traveler. Infect Dis Clin N Am. 1998;12(2):369-412.

24   METABOLIC COMPLICATIONS
Fuad S. Shihab, MD

Metabolic disorders presenting posttransplantation result from a complex interaction between such factors as genetic susceptibility, medications, and physiologic changes related to ischemic, immunologic, vascular and mechanical injury. This chapter focuses on the pathogenesis, diagnosis, and management of the most commonly encountered metabolic abnormalities.

DISORDERS OF POTASSIUM METABOLISM
Hypokalemia
Hypokalemia can result from potassium shifts and gastrointestinal or renal potassium losses (Table 24-1). Potassium shifts result from alkalosis or insulin administration. The use of antacids, sodium bicarbonate and corticosteroids increases serum alkalinity. Extracellular alkalinity promotes the intracellular accumulation of potassium by stimulating the Na^+/H^+ and the Na^+K^+ adenosine triphospatase (ATPase) exchangers. Insulin administration stimulates the same transporters.

Gastrointestinal potassium losses occur frequently after transplantation. However, since potassium concentration in gastrointestinal secretions is low (5 to 15 mEq/L), massive fluid losses are required to significantly lower potassium stores. In fact, it is hypovolemia developing during gastrointestinal fluid losses that stimulates the renin-aldosterone axis and tubular potassium excretion responsible for hypokalemia. Primary renal potassium losses usually result from diuretic therapy but can also occur with renal tubular acidosis (RTA), posttransplant renal artery stenosis (RAS), corticosteroid use, and glycosuria. Diuretic use is frequently necessary to treat hypertension caused by calcineurin inhibitor-induced volume expansion. On the other hand, renal tubular acidification defects are usually short-lived and do not contribute considerably to posttransplant hypokalemia. If RAS develops in the renal allograft, the initial aldosterone increase becomes quickly suppressed by volume expansion; as a result, hypokalemia is uncommon in this setting. Finally, the supraphysiologic glucocorticoid levels attained following transplantation overwhelm the enzymatic action of 11β-hydroxysteroid dehydrogenase, which cleaves glucocorticoids into metabolites that lack mineralocorticoid receptor binding. Thus, glucocorticoid

Associate Professor of Medicine, Division of Nephrology and Hypertension; Medical Director, Kidney Transplantation Program, University of Utah Medical Center, Salt Lake City, UT

binding to type I mineralocorticoid receptors in the distal nephron increases, resulting in increased urinary potassium excretion. Additionally, high doses of corticosteroids may promote the development of glycosuria increasing urinary flow rates, distal substrate delivery, and urinary potassium losses. Other possible mechanisms include glucocorticoid-induced increases in proximal convoluted tubule and medullary thick-limb Na-K-ATPase activity, as well as an augmentation of the glomerular filtration rate (GFR).

Correction of hypokalemia is generally most safely accomplished via the oral route. Potassium chloride is the preparation of choice and promotes rapid correction of hypokalemia and metabolic alkalosis. Potassium bicarbonate and citrate are more appropriate for hypokalemia associated with diarrhea or RTA.

Hyperkalemia
Hyperkalemia occurs frequently during the first three months after transplant, especially in the presence of cyclosporine or tacrolimus use. Hyperkalemia results from increased potassium intake, redistribution, and decreased renal excretion (Table 24-1). It should be kept in mind that, despite increased distal sodium delivery, tubular potassium secretion is particularly impaired in the first 48 hours after kidney transplantation. Contributors to the development of hyperkalemia may include potassium-rich organ preservation solutions (eg, Collins solution contains 141 mEq/L K^+) if the organ is incompletely flushed prior to placement. Newer preservation solutions (eg, University of Wisconsin's solution) however, contain minimal amounts of potassium and do not carry a similar threat. Redistributional hyperkalemia results from hyperglycemia with insulin deficiency and/or the use of beta blockers for hypertension. Hyperkalemia may also be the first sign of allograft infarction due to the cellular release of potassium. Impaired distal renal tubular potassium secretion is seen with cyclosporine and tacrolimus use, and is associated with a mild hyperchloremic metabolic acidosis (type IV RTA). The afferent arteriolar vasoconstrictor properties of cyclosporine decrease GFR and lead to enhanced proximal tubular reabsorption of sodium and water. Extracellular volume expands and renin levels decrease. In addition, studies in heart transplant recipients suggest that cyclosporine decreases the conversion of prorenin to renin and impairs renin release. Furthermore, there is evidence to suggest that calcineurin inhibitors impair aldosterone production, impair renal response to aldosterone, and inhibit cortical collecting duct potassium secretory channels. Alternatively, enhanced chloride absorption by the loop and distal nephron has been postulated to explain the volume expansion, hypertension, low renin, relatively low aldosterone levels, and decreased potassium excretion.

Table 24-1. Causes of Posttransplant Potassium Disorders

Hypokalemia		Hyperkalemia	
Redistribution	Alkalosis Insulin therapy	Redistribution	Hyperglycemia Beta blockers Allograft infarction
Gastrointestinal losses	Vomiting Diarrhea Bladder drainage of pancreas Ileal conduit	Decreased renal exretion	Delayed renal graft function Acute renal rejection Obstructive uropathy Hypoaldosteronism Cyclosporine, tacrolimus NSAIDs ACE inhibitors Heparin
Renal losses	Polyuria Diuretics Renal tubular acidosis Renal artery stenosis Corticosteroids Hyperglycemia Hypomagnesemia	Increased intake	High [K+] preservation solutions K+ administration

Hyperkalemia is rarely dangerous as long as the patient is nonoliguric with a serum potassium less than 6 mEq/L. However, if the serum potassium exceeds 6 mEq/L, restriction of potassium intake to less than 70 mEq/d becomes warranted. Since cyclosporine and tacrolimus can inhibit the renin-aldosterone system, aldosterone supplementation with fludrocortisone acetate should be considered. However, its use is limited by the frequent development of volume expansion and hypertension. While dialysis may be required for patients with oliguria, other therapies involve cation-exchange resins (eg, sodium polystyrene sulfonate) and diuretics. Care should be taken when administering drugs that may exaggerate hyperkalemia such as angiotensin-converting enzyme (ACE) inhibitors, beta blockers, potassium-containing phosphate supplements, and nonsteroidal antiinflammatory drugs.

DISORDERS OF ACID-BASE METABOLISM
Metabolic Alkalosis
Despite the common use of antacids (bicarbonate gain) to prevent corticosteroid-induced gastric diseases, metabolic alkalosis is rarely observed following transplantation. Gastric hydrogen losses (eg, nasogastric suction, postoperative ileus or diabetic gastroparesis-induced emesis), corticosteroids, and diuretics are common causes of metabolic alkalosis in transplant recipients with concomitant volume depletion often responsible

for maintenance of alkalemia. Bladder-drained pancreas recipients receiving oral bicarbonate may develop metabolic alkalosis if the oral bicarbonate intake exceeds the pancreatic exocrine bicarbonate output.

Metabolic Acidosis
Although high anion gap metabolic acidosis can develop (eg, diabetic ketoacidosis, lactic acidosis due to sepsis or cardiovascular instability after antibody administration), hyperchloremic metabolic acidosis is the more common type of metabolic acidosis following transplantation. Extrarenal forms of normal anion gap acidosis may occur in the presence of diarrhea and urinary diversions. If the kidney transplant ureter is anastomosed to an ileal conduit instead of the bladder, the Cl^- to HCO_3^- anion exchanger in the ileal luminal mucosa leads to chloride absorption and bicarbonate secretion; potassium is excreted to preserve electroneutrality, and a hyperchloremic-hypokalemic metabolic acidosis develops. In the case of the pancreas allograft, bladder drainage of pancreatic exocrine secretions causes excess sodium and bicarbonate losses and results in a hyperchloremic metabolic acidosis. If bicarbonate supplements are not used, severe metabolic acidosis follows.

Type I and II RTA may also develop posttransplantation but rarely require therapeutic intervention. Proximal RTA (type II) is a form of bicarbonate wastage that develops in 19% of renal recipients in the early posttransplantation period, and is the result of parathyroid hormone (PTH)-induced reduction in proximal tubular bicarbonate reabsorption. If it develops in the late posttransplantation period, it may indicate the development of allograft rejection or monoclonal gammopathy. Distal RTA (type I) occurs frequently (43%), may present early, and can last many years. It is usually associated with chronic renal allograft rejection and is thought to result from a hydrogen secretory abnormality, possibly immune-mediated. Type IV RTA is now fairly common since the introduction of cyclosporine and tacrolimus, and occurs particularly in diabetic patients. Its pathogenesis is related to decreased distal sodium delivery, suppression of the renin-aldosterone system, and impairment in tubular aldosterone responsiveness or perhaps the enhanced distal absorption of chloride.

DISORDERS OF MAGNESIUM METABOLISM
Hypomagnesemia

Hypomagnesemia occurs commonly following transplantation. Prior to cyclosporine, it was attributed to increased urinary losses due to hypercalcemia, hypophosphatemia, RTA, diuretics and post-renal transplantation diuresis. Since the introduction of cyclosporine, an inverse correlation between cyclosporine and magnesium levels has been established. Urinary magnesium excretion is increased by cyclosporine and tacrolimus, and remains high despite low magnesium blood levels. The cause of magnesuria is not well characterized but an attractive explanation is decreased tubular magnesium reabsorption as a result of volume expansion. Sirolimus also may increase magnesium losses, however, hypomagnesemia is not as frequently reported. Other drugs that can cause magnesium wasting include aminoglycosides, amphoteracin B, cisplatin, pentamidine, foscarnet and diuretics. Unlike the aforementioned

medications, cyclosporine-induced hypomagnesemia is not accompanied by hypokalemia and hypocalcemia.

Hypomagnesemia is usually asymptomatic except for occasional muscle cramps. Hypomagnesemia however, may predispose to seizures following transplantation especially in the setting of cyclosporine treatment. Magnesium replacement is usually initiated when the plasma levels fall below 1.5 mg/dL. Dietary magnesium replacement is inadequate, necessitating the use of magnesium supplements. The effectiveness of such supplements is not well-studied. Magnesium can be replaced intravenously (magnesium oxide) or orally. Some available oral supplements are Mag-Ox 400® (19.86 mEq elemental Mg^{2+} as magnesium oxide), Uro-Mag® (6.93 mEq elemental Mg^{2+} as magnesium oxide), and MagTab®SR (7 mEq Mg^{2+} as magnesium lactate). Oral magnesium replacement is complicated by dose-dependent diarrhea.

Hypermagnesemia

Hypermagnesemia is an unusual complication after transplantation and usually results from the administration of magnesium-containing antacids or laxatives when the renal function is compromised.

DISORDERS OF PHOSPHORUS METABOLISM
Hypophosphatemia

Hypophosphatemia is the most common divalent ion abnormality following kidney transplantation and is caused by renal or gastrointestinal phosphate losses (Figure 24-1). Profound hypophosphatemia develops in the first few weeks, particularly if allograft function is excellent, typically in living-related donor recipients who experience a prompt diuresis, and may persist in 20% to 35% of well-functioning renal allograft recipients. Renal phosphate losses can be either PTH-dependent or inde-

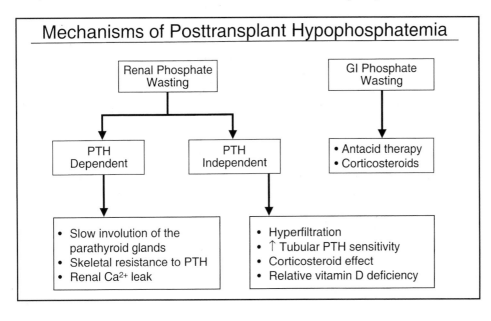

Mechanisms of Posttransplant Hypophosphatemia

Renal Phosphate Wasting

GI Phosphate Wasting

PTH Dependent

PTH Independent

• Antacid therapy
• Corticosteroids

• Slow involution of the parathyroid glands
• Skeletal resistance to PTH
• Renal Ca^{2+} leak

• Hyperfiltration
• ↑ Tubular PTH sensitivity
• Corticosteroid effect
• Relative vitamin D deficiency

Figure 24-1. Mechanisms of Posttransplant Hypophosphatemia. Adapted from Rubin MF, Badalamenti J, Bennett WM. Kidney transplantation: associated physiologic, fluid, electrolyte, and acid-base abnormalities. In: Narins RG, ed. Clinical Disorders Fluid Electrolyte Metab, 5th Ed. New York, NY: McGraw-Hill; 1994:1379-1406.

pendent. PTH inhibits proximal tubular reabsorption of phosphate resulting in phosphaturia. Serum PTH levels initially decrease rapidly after transplantation but may take many months or years (if ever) to normalize. A persistently high PTH level may be the result of the slow involution of hyperplastic parathyroid glands, skeletal resistance to PTH action, and persistence of a negative calcium balance. A PTH-independent tubular phosphate leak is also observed following transplantation and may be partially explained by corticosteroid-induced phosphaturia. In addition, metabolic alkalosis and glucosuria are associated with urinary phosphate losses. Gastrointestinal losses of phosphorus commonly result from the inadvertent use of phosphate-binding antacids.

Phosphate repletion is necessary if the serum phosphate falls below 2.0 mg/dL. Treatment of hypophosphatemia should be based upon the underlying pathogenesis. Gastrointestinal losses can be reduced by substituting antacids with H^2 blockers or hydrogen pump inhibitors. Patients with persistent hyperparathyroidism should undergo a parathyroidectomy. Patients with a renal phosphate leak should receive a trial of 1,25-dihydroxy (1,25-OH_2) vitamin D therapy. Skim milk (1 gram of elemental phosphorus per liter) is the most cost-effective way of replacing phosphorus (whole milk is best avoided because of its large fat content). Some available phosphorus supplements are shown in Table 24-2.

Hyperphosphatemia

Following renal transplantation, hyperphosphatemia can be a brief laboratory finding. However, it may persist if the renal graft function is poor or if phosphate is given injudiciously (eg, Fleet® enema). Its appearance in the late posttransplant period is usually the result of renal allograft dysfunction (eg, chronic renal rejection) although it may also be seen in association with rhabdomyolysis or other causes of acute renal failure. Rhabdomyolysis may occur when cyclosporine is used in combination with an HMG-CoA reductase inhibitor. Hyperphosphatemia may be seen in other allograft recipients, usually in the face of renal failure or massive tissue injury. Treatment of hyperphosphatemia includes phosphate-binding antacids, modification of phosphorus intake to less than 1 gram per day or, in the setting of severe renal failure, dialysis.

DISORDERS OF CALCIUM METABOLISM
Hypocalcemia

Hypocalcemia results from increased calcium losses (eg, tissue deposition, urinary losses) or from decreased calcium entry into the circulation (eg, malabsorption, decreased bone resorption) (Table 24-3). The major determinants of serum calcium are the serum phosphate acutely, and serum PTH and vitamin D levels chronically. When approaching a patient with hypocalcemia, it is important to measure the serum albumin. Since 40% of the circulating calcium is bound to albumin, hypoalbuminemia lowers plasma calcium concentration by 0.8 mg/dL for every 1.0 g/dL reduction in plasma albumin without affecting the ionized calcium.

Infusion of large amounts of blood that contain citrate or EDTA result in hypocalcemia by chelating serum calcium. This is particularly frequent during liver transplantation when large volumes of blood products are infused and citrate metabolism is impaired due to hepatic and, occasionally, renal failure. Treatment of refractory cytomegalovirus infection with foscarnet, which complexes ionized calcium, may also lead to symptomatic hypocalcemia.

Pretransplant parathyroidectomy resulting in hypoparathyroidism may predispose patients to severe

Table 24-2. Phosphate Preparations for Oral and Parenteral Use

	Preparations	Phosphorus	Sodium	Potassium
Oral	Skim milk	1 mg/mL	0.022 mEq/mL	0.036 mEq/mL
	Neutra-Phos (Willen)	250 mg/capsule	7 mEq/capsule	7 mEq/capsule
	Neutra-Phos-K (Willen)	250 mg/capsule		14 mEq/capsule
	K-Phos® original (Beach)	114 mg/tablet		3.68 mEq/tablet
	K-Phos® Neutral (Beach)	250 mg/tablet	13 mEq/tablet	1 mEq/tablet
	Fleet® Phospho®-Soda (CB fleet)	149 mg/mL	6 mEq/mL	
Parenteral	Sodium phosphate (Abbott)	93 mg/mL	4 mEq/mL	
	Potassium phosphate (Abbott)	93 mg/mL		4 mEq/mL
	Hyper-Phos-K (Hoyt)	67 mg/mL		3.3 mEq/mL
	In-Phos (Hoyt)	25 mg/mL	1.6 mEq/mL	0.2 mEq/mL

posttransplant hypocalcemia due to decreased PTH-dependent bone resorption, decreased tubular calcium reabsorption and decreased intestinal calcium absorption. Decreased 1,25-dihydroxy vitamin D levels also contribute. Decreased vitamin D levels are a consequence of decreased production because stimulation of 1α-hydroxylase is impaired in the face of PTH deficiency. Posttransplant hyperphosphatemia causes hypocalcemia by decreasing calcitriol production, inhibiting bone resorption, enhancing bone formation and precipitating calcium phosphate in soft tissues. Posttransplant hypomagnesemia induces hypocalcemia, which is refractory to calcium and vitamin D therapy. Posttransplant proximal RTA may only rarely be associated with hypocalcemia due to impaired 1α-hydroxylation of vitamin D. Liver disease (eg, viral or toxic hepatitis, allograft liver dysfunction) causes hypocalcemia by impairing 25-hydroxylation of vitamin D, by limiting bile salt formation and thus vitamin D absorption, and by limiting vitamin D-binding protein production. Pancreatitis may cause hypocalcemia by precipitating calcium soaps. In addition, sepsis causes hypocalcemia, not only because of hypoalbuminemia, but also as a result of impaired secretion of PTH and calcitriol, and resistance to PTH action.

Symptomatic hypocalcemia (neuromuscular irritability) generally responds promptly to intravenous 10% calcium gluconate (90 mg elemental calcium) or 10% calcium chloride (360 mg Ca^{2+}). In patients with chronic hypocalcemia, treatment with oral calcium should be instituted. The commonly used preparations are: (1) calcium lactate (60 mg Ca^{2+}), (2) chewable calcium gluconate 1 g (90 mg Ca^{2+}); and (3) calcium carbonate (250 mg Ca^{2+}). In patients who fail to respond to oral calcium, vitamin D is added. Patients with associated hypomagnesemia respond poorly to calcium supplementation unless the hypomagnesemia is corrected. In patients with renal failure, calcium levels increase after reducing elevated serum phosphorus levels.

Hypercalcemia

Hypercalcemia is a frequent electrolyte abnormality after kidney transplantation and results from persistent secondary hyperparathyroidism, resorption of extraskeletal calcifications, phosphate deficiency, abnormalities in vitamin D metabolism, and posttransplant elevations in serum albumin (no effect on ionized calcium) (Table 24-3). Persistent hypercalcemia (ie, elevated calcium levels for more than one year) occurs in as many as 66% of renal transplant recipients, and is observed mostly in those who start with very high PTH levels.

Secondary hyperparathyroidism is the most common cause of posttransplant hypercalcemia. It correlates with duration of dialysis and severity of the pretransplant renal osteodystrophy. High serum PTH levels are found in 35% to 70% of recipients during the first six months following transplantation. Levels remain elevated indefinitely in half of these patients as a result of obligatory PTH secretion due to glandular hyperplasia. Although parathyroid glands tend to involute after transplantation, the process takes from months to several years. In addition, failure to achieve a positive calcium balance because of poor gastrointestinal calcium absorption or a renal tubular calcium leak contributes to persistent PTH stimulation.

Mobilization of extraskeletal calcifications results in hypercalcemia mostly in recipients with clinical evidence of pretransplant metastatic calcifications. Hypophosphatemia, by stimulating renal 1α-hydroxylase, increases $1,25-OH_2$ vitamin D and results in bone resorption and increased gastrointestinal calcium absorption. In patients with hypercalcemia and normal or low PTH levels, a thorough search for neoplasia and granulomatous disease is warranted. Less common causes of hypercalcemia such as Addison's disease, thiazide use, calcium carbonate use, hyperthyroidism, and vitamin A or D intoxication should also be considered.

The treatment of hypercalcemia should be directed at the underlying disorder. With the exception of severe hypercalcemia ($Ca^{2+}>13$ mg/dL), milder increases in serum calcium do not carry an adverse effect on the allograft function or the bone. As a result, the management of mild to moderate hypercalcemia should be conservative and phosphate supplementation alone is usually adequate. On the other hand, severe hypercalcemia has an increased morbidity (eg, allograft dysfunction, calciphylaxis, peptic ulcer, pancreatitis) and acute therapy is warranted. The mainstay of therapy in patients with

Table 24-3. Causes of Posttransplant Calcium Disorders

Hypocalcemia	Hypercalcemia
Calcium chelation	High PTH level
Citrate or EDTA Foscarnet	Hyperparathyroidism Mobilization of metastatic calcifications
Low PTH level	Renal tubular calcium leak GI calcium malabsorption
Hypoparathyroidism Hypomagnesemia	Normal / low PTH level
High PTH level	Immobilization Vitamin A excess Vitamin D excess Malignancy Granuloma Addison's disease Thiazides Calcium carbonate
Renal tubular acidosis Renal dysfunction Liver disease Pancreatitis Sepsis Hyperphosphatemia Hypovitaminosis D	

reasonable cardiac and renal function is intravenous saline at rates as high as 200 to 250 mL/h, which promotes renal calcium excretion. Furosemide is also calciuric and is often used with saline infusions. Biphosphonates may also be used to lower the serum calcium. Etidronate (7.5 mg/kg per day) infused intravenously for three days or pamidronate (60 to 90 mg/d) given over three to four hours lowers the serum calcium in a few days. Care should be taken to limit the rate of infusion as rapid infusion of biphosphonates has been associated with acute renal insufficiency. Parathyroidectomy should be considered in severe hyperparathyroidism, and if serum calcium remains elevated one year following transplantation, particularly if associated with symptoms or organ damage (occurs in 4% to 10%).

DISORDERS OF URIC ACID METABOLISM

Uric acid excretion drops after transplantation and may result in hyperuricemia and, in some cases, gouty arthritis. In the cyclosporine era, the frequency of hyperuricemia has increased from a range of 25% to 55%, to 56% to 84%, and gout from less than 1% to 5%, to 28%. Uric acid values greater than 14 mg/dL have been reported only in association with cyclosporine administration. The majority of hyperuricemic patients have uric acid values between eight and 14 mg/dL. Hyperuricemia commonly develops in the first three months after transplantation and is more frequent in patients taking diuretics and in those with renal insufficiency.

The main mechanism of cyclosporine-induced hyperuricemia is increased proximal uric acid absorption, especially in the presence of volume depletion associated with diuretic use; however, tubular damage may also contribute by impairing urate secretion. Cyclosporine-induced hyperuricemia is not restricted to renal transplant recipients but is common in other transplant recipients.

While hyperuricemia is associated with an increased risk of symptomatic gout, the incidence of gouty arthritis bears little relationship to the degree of hyperuricemia. Gouty attacks generally begin 17 to 24 months after transplantation and are more common in recipients with a history of gouty attacks. Gouty attacks are more common in recipients who are males, are on diuretics, and have advanced renal dysfunction. The spectrum of gouty arthritis extends from the typical single acutely inflamed joint to the development of extensive incapacitating tophaceous gout. The differential diagnosis of acute gout includes cellulitis, septic arthritis, serum sickness (about ten days) after ALG or ATG, pseudogout (calcium pyrophosphate), stress fracture, avascular necrosis, and lupus relapse. A review of the manifestations and treatment of gout can be found in Chapter 30.

POSTTRANSPLANT GLUCOSE INTOLERANCE

As transplant recipients survive longer, posttransplant diabetes mellitus (PTDM) has emerged as a major adverse effect of immunosuppressants and its secondary complications have assumed greater importance. Depending upon the definition and duration of follow-up, the estimated incidence of PTDM varies widely from 4% to 20%, but the true prevalence is thought to be higher. The onset may be within three weeks of transplantation to more than 20 years later. The abnormalities in glucose homeostasis range from transient glucosuria to mild hyperglycemia to severe elevations leading to hyperosmolar nonketotic coma. About 40% of those who develop PTDM will require insulin therapy.

Pathogenesis and Risk Factors for Posttransplant Diabetes Mellitus

The risk factors for the development of PTDM include higher corticosteroid doses, surgical stress and hyperalimentation, older age (>45 years), positive family history of diabetes, race (African-Americans and Hispanics), obesity, cadaveric transplant, and the development of infections. Unexplained new-onset hyperglycemia is frequently associated with sepsis. One consequence of hyperglycemia is the development of an osmotic diuresis and volume depletion, which can raise the serum creatinine. The diagnosis of PTDM is of extreme clinical importance because of the associated microvascular complications. PTDM has also been shown to result in a higher incidence of sepsis and poorer patient and graft survival. The three major immunosuppressants (ie, corticosteroids, cyclosporine, tacrolimus) are diabetogenic. The purine antagonists azathioprine and mycophenolate mofetil do not appear to be diabetogenic. The information on sirolimus is inconclusive.

Corticosteroids

The major effect of corticosteroids is induction of insulin resistance. Other mechanisms include modified insulin receptor activity, impaired peripheral glucose uptake in muscles, impaired insulin release, and activation of the glucose-free fatty acid cycle. An increased rate of leucine oxidation may be critical in corticosteroid-induced PTDM and may partly explain the associated protein wasting. PTDM usually occurs within the first three months of transplantation when the highest doses of corticosteroids are used and, often when the dose is increased to treat acute rejection. Although there is no relationship between the total dose or duration of corticosteroid therapy and the development of PTDM, centers with a low incidence of PTDM generally use lower doses of corticosteroids. Typically, the onset of PTDM is mild, without associated ketoacidosis, and resolves upon reducing or withdrawing the corticosteroids. However, Ost observed that renal transplant patients developed a Cushingoid appearance despite using low corticosteroids doses when cyclosporine was administered concomitantly. Cyclosporine may potentiate the effect of corticosteroids by reducing the clearance of the latter through competitive inhibition since both drugs are metabolized by the same cytochrome P450 enzyme.

Cyclosporine and Tacrolimus

The incidence of PTDM in the cyclosporine and tacrolimus era has remained between 4% to 20% despite an overall reduction in the doses of corticosteroids. Both cyclosporine and tacrolimus contribute to PTDM by a number of mechanisms including inhibition of insulin secretion from islet cells, impairing beta cell insulin production, and induction of peripheral insulin resistance. Cyclosporine impairs insulin synthesis to a greater degree than insulin release. The molecular mechanism of impaired insulin synthesis may be related to cyclosporine-induced inhibition of calcineurin phosphatase activity, which inhibits the phosphorylation and translocation of nuclear transcription factors (cAMP response element-binding protein) blocking the activation of insulin transcription normally initiated by islet membrane depolarization. A calmodulin inhibitor has been shown to restore the insulin secretory capacity of islet cells suppressed by cyclosporine. Clinically, glucose tolerance curves and insulin output have been shown to improve after stopping cyclosporine. However, although some centers have found a correlation between hyperglycemia and high cyclosporine levels, this observation has not been consistent. Of note, the acinar portion of the pancreas does not appear to be affected by calcineurin inhibitors.

The diabetogenic mechanisms of tacrolimus are similar to cyclosporine. In addition, the selective localization of FK binding protein-12 and calcineurin in the islets vs acinar tissue may partially explain the toxic effect of tacrolimus. Tacrolimus causes dose-dependent islet cell toxicity; upon withdrawal of tacrolimus, there is some recovery of function although it is not complete.

Clinically, tacrolimus may be more diabetogenic than cyclosporine. A systematic review of the effect of tacrolimus on the development of diabetes was performed in the US trial of tacrolimus vs cyclosporine in renal transplantation. A threefold to fourfold increase in the incidence of PTDM was shown in tacrolimus compared with cyclosporine-treated patients. Within the first year, 25% of tacrolimus-treated patients required insulin vs only 5% of patients receiving cyclosporine. In another multicenter trial where tacrolimus was used to treat refractory renal allograft rejection, the incidence of PTDM was 8%. In liver transplantation however, neither the European nor the US tacrolimus trials showed a

higher frequency of PTDM compared to cyclosporine. Yet again, the lower corticosteroids doses in tacrolimus-treated patients did not translate into a lower incidence of PTDM, thus supporting the theory that tacrolimus is more diabetogenic than cyclosporine. In heart transplantation, tacrolimus was associated with a 13.4% incidence of PTDM, which is comparable with liver recipients but lower than renal recipients.

Diagnosis of Posttransplant Diabetes Mellitus

A diagnosis of PTDM can be made using the newly established WHO criteria; fasting plasma glucose ($\geq$) 126 mg/dL, or a random glucose value (or 2-hour value in an oral glucose tolerance test) ($\geq$) 200 mg/dL. The majority of transplant recipients with PTDM produce insulin, but not in amounts adequate to overcome their insulin resistance, similar to type II diabetic patients. Transplant recipients with PTDM may have a normal fasting blood glucose but will have an abnormal postprandial or post-glucose challenge blood values. Aggressive treatment and preventive measures are indicated because the development of posttransplant diabetes has been associated with the onset of diabetic complications including decreased survival due to infection and cardiovascular disease. Furthermore, de novo diabetic nephropathy can develop as early as six years after the onset of PTDM with biopsy findings ranging from mesangial changes to nodular glomerulosclerosis.

Treatment of Posttransplant Diabetes Mellitus

Once PTDM is diagnosed, the patient should be referred for nutritional counseling. Weight loss is encouraged because obesity worsens insulin resistance. However, very few patients can be managed with diet alone. If the patient has moderate hyperglycemia (fasting glucose <250 mg/dL or normal fasting glucose with postprandial hyperglycemia), an oral hypoglycemic agent can be used. Sulfonylureas act primarily by stimulating the release of insulin from islet cells. Short-acting oral hypoglycemics (eg, glypizide) are preferred if the renal function is impaired in order to avoid hypoglycemia because insulin half-life is prolonged due to decreased renal catabolism. Hypoglycemia occurs less frequently with oral agents than with insulin but, when it occurs, it tends to be severe and prolonged. Metformin is a biguanide that may be prescribed as monotherapy in obese diabetics but is usually added as an adjunctive agent in patients whose disease is not controlled by maximal doses of sulfonylureas. The primary action of metformin is inhibition of hepatic gluconeogenesis; it also enhances glucose disposal in muscle and adipose tissue. Metformin does not cause hypoglycemia but can induce severe lactic acidosis. To avoid this complication, the drug should not be given to patients with impaired renal function and should be stopped at once if volume depletion develops. Thiazolidine derivatives such as rosiglitazone lower blood glucose, free fatty acids and triglycerides, and reduce insulin resistance by increasing insulin-receptor kinase activity. Hepatic function tests must be monitored during thiazolidine administration.

Although diet, exercise and oral hypoglycemic agents are helpful, studies have shown that this regimen is not adequate in controlling blood glucose in 40% to 50% of transplant recipients. Insulin is needed in these patients and its amount and dose should be individualized. The help of a nurse educator trained in diabetic teaching is invaluable. Routine posttransplant measurement of HbA_1C levels, preferably quarterly, gives an estimate of diabetic control for the preceding three months and is useful for monitoring treatment compliance. On average, nondiabetic subjects have HbA_1C values less than 6%, while levels in patients with poorly controlled diabetes may be considerably above 10%. HbA_1C levels have also been shown to predict some of the microvascular complications associated with diabetes mellitus.

POSTTRANSPLANT HYPERLIPIDEMIA

Hyperlipidemia is an important concern because of the established correlation with atherosclerosis. In addition, there is emerging evidence in transplant recipients linking elevated lipid levels to chronic allograft vasculopathy. Hyperlipidemia is reported in 50% to 80% of renal and heart recipients, and in 45% of liver recipients. The lipid abnormalities after transplantation consist of increased total cholesterol, LDL (low-density lipoprotein) cholesterol, VLDL (very low-density lipoprotein) cholesterol, and apolipoprotein B levels. HDL (high-density lipoprotein) cholesterol levels may be low, normal, or slightly elevated, and lipoprotein (a) (Lp[a]) levels may be normal or high. While hypertriglyceridemia is present early posttransplant, hypercholesterolemia develops gradually, reaches a plateau at six months, and tends to persist. In heart transplant recipients, increases in total and LDL cholesterol, apolipoprotein B and triglyceride levels develop three to eight months following transplant, and thereafter, may decline. The natural history of HDLC levels is variable. Interestingly, Lp(a) levels have been found to decrease by 40% after cardiac transplantation. Of note, an elevated HDL cholesterol in solid organ transplant recipients may not be protective because it is abnormally enriched in triglycerides and cholesterol, and the HDL cholesterol-to-apoprotein A ratio is elevated. In addition to abnormal lipid levels, the lipoprotein particles in transplant recipients are also more atherogenic due to increased oxidation. Transplant recipients have also been found to have lower antioxidant levels. The evaluation

and management of posttransplant hyperlipidemia are reviewed in further detail in Chapters 1 and 12.

Causes of Posttransplant Hyperlipidemia

The presence of posttransplant hyperlipidemia is associated with immunosuppressive agents, older age, male gender, diet, obesity, genetic predisposition, hyperglycemia, hyperinsulinemia, renal dysfunction, proteinuria, and the use of diuretics and beta blockers. There is a close correlation between pretransplant and post-transplant lipid levels suggesting that genetic predisposition is a dominant factor. Also, many recipients tend to gain weight after a successful transplantation. Of the commonly used immunosuppressive drugs, azathioprine and mycophenolate mofetil likely do not affect lipid metabolism. However, corticosteroids and cyclosporine independently, and perhaps synergistically, generate hyperlipidemia (Figure 24-2). Tacrolimus seems to have a less prominent effect while sirolimus has a more pronounced effect. The lipid abnormalities may improve somewhat after three to six months of transplantation as the doses of immunosuppressive agents decrease.

Corticosteroids

Corticosteroids enhance lipogenesis by increasing the activity of acetyl-coenzyme A carboxylase and free fatty acid synthetase, increasing hepatic synthesis of VLDL, down-regulating LDL receptor activity and increasing the activity of 3-hydroxy-3-methylglutaryl coenzyme A reductase. Insulin resistance also results in decreased action of the lipoprotein lipase responsible for the clearance of triglycerides available to the liver for the synthesis of VLDL. The corticosteroid-induced decrease in ACTH release may contribute to the lipid abnormalities since ACTH upregulates LDL receptor activity. A correlation between cholesterol blood levels and the cumulative corticosteroids dose has been clearly observed. However, corticosteroid withdrawal may not benefit lipid metabolism. After withdrawal, although the total cholesterol falls, there is a proportionate or even greater reduction in HDL cholesterol leading to no change or even an undesirable elevation in the total-to-HDL cholesterol ratio.

Cyclosporine

Cyclosporine binds to the LDL receptor, which results in increased serum LDL cholesterol levels. Cyclosporine increases hepatic lipase activity and decreases lipoprotein lipase activity resulting in impaired clearance of VLDL and LDL cholesterol, and may also raise serum Lp(a). It is not completely understood how these lipid changes occur, but cyclosporine is lipophilic and transported in the blood in the core of low-density and high-density lipoprotein particles. It is possible that cyclosporine-induced alterations in LDL interfere with its removal from the circulation. Cyclosporine also

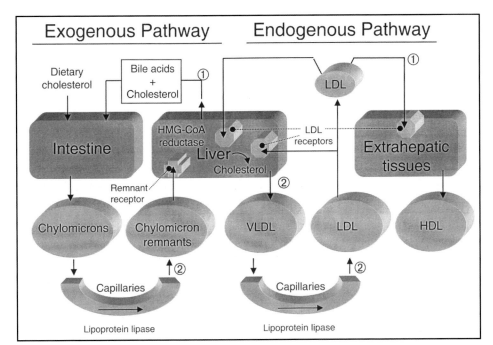

Figure 24-2. Effect of immuno-suppressive agents on lipid metabolism. The potential effect of cyclosporine is designated as "1." The potential effect of corti-costeroids is designated as "2." Adapted from Kobashigawa JA, Kasiske BL. Hyperlipidemia in solid organ transplantation. Transplantation. 1997;63(3):331-338.

impairs cholesterol removal by decreasing bile acid synthesis by interfering with cholesterol conversion to bile acids. Additionally, cyclosporine, like corticosteroids, may induce peripheral insulin resistance, hyper-insulinemia and hyperlipidemia. The effect of cyclosporine seems to be dose-dependent, and there is a correlation between cyclosporine levels and degree of hypercholesterolemia.

Tacrolimus

The effect of tacrolimus on lipid metabolism is similar to that of cyclosporine. In one study, total cholesterol, HDL cholesterol and triglycerides were similar in cyclosporine and tacrolimus-treated renal transplant recipients. However, LDL cholesterol, Lp(a) and fibrinogen levels were lower with tacrolimus. Other studies have reported lower total serum cholesterol levels in tacrolimus-treated recipients when compared to cyclosporine-treated recipients. In addition, the substitution of tacrolimus for cyclosporine has been shown to improve the lipid profile of stable renal transplant patients by reducing total and LDL cholesterol without a change in renal function or glycemic control; however, no patient was able to discontinue lipid lowering agents. In liver transplantation, many studies have found a significantly higher total and LDL cholesterol in cyclosporine-treated patients compared to tacrolimus-treated patients.

Sirolimus

There is a growing body of evidence that sirolimus has deleterious effects on the lipid profile. The early trials with this drug have consistently shown markedly elevated triglyceride levels and, although to a lesser extent, high cholesterol levels. The mechanisms of sirolimus-induced hyperlipidemia have not been completely elucidated.

Clinical Importance of Posttransplant Hyperlipidemia

There may be two important reasons for aggressive therapy of hyperlipidemia in transplant recipients: prevention of atherosclerosis progression and slowing the development of transplant vasculopathy. There is increasing evidence linking hyperlipidemia with cardiovascular disease in transplant recipients. There is also growing evidence linking hyperlipidemia to chronic allograft vasculopathy, which is characterized by intimal fibroplasia reminiscent of atherosclerosis. For instance, the total and LDL cholesterol levels are significantly higher in renal transplant recipients with chronic rejection than in patients with stable renal function. Likewise, effective lipid-lowering therapy has been shown to improve renal graft outcome as judged by both functional and histological parameters. However, proteinuria, which is present with renal transplant rejection, may explain the lipid abnormalities, and thus, the contribution of lipid abnormalities to renal allograft rejection requires further investigation. Hyperlipidemia may also play a role in coronary transplant vasculopathy. Pravastatin therapy in heart transplant recipients has been shown to result in a lower incidence of transplant vasculopathy, lower intimal thickness and index, less rejection episodes, and a higher survival rate. However, the association of lipid levels with vasculopathy is not rigorous. Additionally, the benefits of pravastatin may be mediated through influences on the immune system (eg, up-regulation of the vasculoprotective gene of hemoxygenase-1 and inhibition of the protooncogene product p21^{r}as rather than through changes in serum lipid levels. It has yet to be determined whether hyperlipidemia is associated with the vanishing bile duct syndrome and bronchiolitis obliterans.

RECOMMENDED READING

Arnadottir M, Berg AL. Treatment of hyperlipidemia in renal transplant recipients. Transplantation. 1997;63(3):339-345.

Barton CH, Vaziri ND, Martin DC, Choi S, Alikhani S. Hypomagnesemia and renal magnesium wasting in renal transplant recipients receiving cyclosporine. Am J Med. 1987;83(4):693-699.

Chatterjee SN, Friedler RM, Berne TV, Oldham SB, Singer FR, Massry SG. Persistent hypercalcemia after successful renal transplantation. Nephron. 1976;17(1):1-7.

Ekstrand AV, Eriksson JG, Gronhagen-Riska C, Ahonen PJ, Groop LC. Insulin resistance and insulin deficiency in the pathogenesis of posttransplantation diabetes in man. Transplantation. 1992;53(3):563-569.

Garvin PJ, Castaneda M, Linderer R, Dickhans M. Management of hypercalcemic hyperparathyroidism after renal transplantation. Arch Surg. 1985;120(5):578-583.

Hricik DE. Posttransplant hyperlipidemia: the treatment dilemma. Am J Kidney Dis. 1994;23(5):766-771.

Jindal RM. Posttransplant diabetes mellitus — a review. Transplantation. 1994;58(12):1289-1298.

Jindal RM, Sidner RA, Milgrom ML. Post-transplant diabetes mellitus: the role of immunosuppression. Drug Saf. 1997;16(4):242-257.

Kamel KS, Ethier JH, Quaggin S, Levin A, Albert S, Carlisle EJ, Halperin ML. Studies to determine the basis for hyperkalemia in recipients of a renal transplant who are treated with cyclosporine. J Am Soc Nephrol. 1992;2(8):1279-1284.

Kasiske BL, Guijarro C, Massy ZA, Wiederkehr MR, Ma JZ. Cardiovascular disease after renal transplantation. J Am Soc Nephrol. 1996;7(1):158-165.

Kobashigawa JA, Katznelson S, Laks H, et al. Effect of pravastatin on outcomes after cardiac transplantation. N Engl J Med. 1995;333(10):621-627.

Kobashigawa JA, Kasiske BL. Hyperlipidemia in solid organ transplantation. Transplantation. 1997;63(3):331-338.

Lin HY, Rocher LL, McQuillan MA, Schmaltz S, Palella TD, Fox IH. Cyclosporine-induced hyperuricemia and gout. N Engl J Med. 1989;321(5):287-292.

Markell MS, Armenti V, Danovitch G, Sumrani N. Hyperlipidemia and glucose intolerance in the postrenal transplant patient. J Am Soc Nephrol. 1994;4(8 Suppl):S37-S47.

Massy ZA, Kasiske BL. Post-transplant hyperlipidemia: mechanisms and management. J Am Soc Nephrol. 1996;7(7):971-977.

Noordzij TC, Leunissen KM, Van Hooff JP. Renal handling of urate and the incidence of gouty arthritis during cyclosporine and diuretic use. Transplantation. 1991;52(1):64-67.

Pirsch JD, D'Alessandro AM, Sollinger JW, et al. Hyperlipidemia and transplantation: eiologic factors and therapy. J Am Soc Nephrol. 1992;2(12 Suppl)S238-S242.

Rubin MF, Badalamenti J, Bennett WM. Kidney transplantation: associated physiologic, fluid, electrolyte, and acid-base abnormalities. In: Narins RG, ed. Clinical Disorders Fluid Electrolyte Metab. 5th Ed. New York, NY: McGraw-Hill; 1994:1379-1406.

Sakhaee K, Brinker K, Helderman JH, et al. Disturbances in mineral metabolism after successful renal transplantation. Miner Electrolyte Metab. 1985;11(3):167-172.

Wilson DR, Siddiqui AA. Renal tubular acidosis after kidney transplantation. Natural history and significance. Ann Intern Med. 1973;79(3):352-361.

25 BONE DISEASE FOLLOWING TRANSPLANTATION

Susan M. Ott, MD

Skeletal complications of transplantation include loss of bone mass, fractures, avascular necrosis and bone pain. Metabolic bone disease may begin prior to transplant in patients with failure of the kidney, pancreas, or liver, and be partially ameliorated by the new allograft. Those with heart and lung disease may have secondary osteoporosis, but the bone disease is unlikely to improve with transplantation.

This chapter will review the diagnostic evaluation of bone disease, risk factors common to all transplant recipients, and the pathophysiology of bone disease specific to each type of allograft. Prevention and treatment strategies will be presented, with the caveat that much of the data is preliminary, and treatment must be individualized. Bone disease unrelated to transplantation will not be reviewed, but coexisting risks for osteomalacia, osteoporosis, or abnormal calcium metabolism may also be present in transplant recipients.

DIAGNOSTIC EVALUATION OF BONE DISEASE
Radiographs

Radiographs are still the basic method used to determine the presence of fractures. Vertebral compression fractures are usually defined as a decrease in the anterior height of the vertebral body greater than 20%. These fractures are often asymptomatic and their presence in women with postmenopausal osteoporosis increases the risk of a new fracture fourfold compared to women of the same age and bone density. The presence of a fracture is a risk factor for future fractures in transplant recipients as well.

Some fractures, on the other hand, may be symptomatic but not seen on standard radiographs. Detection of stress fractures of the foot, leg, hip or pelvis may require radionucleotide bone scanning and sequential radiographs. Transplant patients are at such a high risk for fractures that bone pain should not be ignored or ascribed to a soft-tissue sprain without full evaluation.

Imaging Tests for Avascular Necrosis

Avascular necrosis (AVN) commonly affects the hip, shoulder, knee, or wrist. The most sensitive test for AVN is magnetic resonance imaging (MRI). Surveillance MRI examinations have shown that early AVN is asymptomatic. Bone scans may also detect AVN. Patients with a positive MRI but negative bone scan may recover without specific therapy except advice to limit vigorous activity. By the time AVN is seen on a plain film, it is in the later stages.

Bone Densitometry

Currently, most of the data about bone density changes in transplant patients have come from dual energy x-ray absorptiometry (DEXA). DEXA causes no medical risk, has become widely available and is well-tolerated by patients. Bone density is measured at the proximal femur and the lumbar spine. Other locations can be measured, but are not as clinically useful. Of note, density results obtained from equipment manufactured by different companies may vary by 6% to 12%. Equations are now available to convert these measurements into standardized values.

The World Health Organization (WHO) uses bone density to define degrees of osteoporosis (Figure 25-1). These definitions are based on standard deviations (SD) below the mean of young adults (T score). For the total hip, the cutoff values for these definitions (using a national cohort of white women) are: normal, greater than 833 mg/cm^2; osteopenia, 648 to 833 mg/cm^2; and osteoporosis, less than 648 mg/cm^2. These correspond to T scores of -1 and -2.5. Those with fragility fractures are defined as "established" or "severe" osteoporosis. The WHO criteria were not defined for men, but recent studies suggest that the risk of hip fracture according to absolute bone density is the same in men and women.

Bone density is age, race and gender-dependent. By definition, 16% of young white women in the US have osteopenia. By the age of 65, only 50% have normal bone density, and by age 85, fewer than 10% are normal. The risk of fractures depends on both age and bone density.

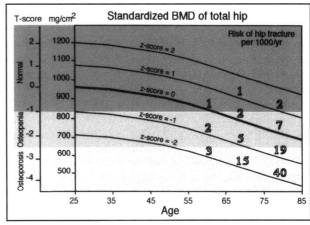

Figure 25-1. Bone density changes with age in white women. Shading shows the definition of degrees of osteoporosis. Risk of hip fracture is shown in outlined numbers.

Associate Professor, Department of Medicine, University of Washington, Seattle, WA

Epidemiological studies report the risk of fracture relative to the SD from age-matched and sex-matched controls (Z scores). In the general population, the relative risk of a hip fracture approximately doubles for each SD below the mean (Figure 25-1). Since both Z scores and T scores are standard deviations, they are commonly confused.

It is important to avoid over-interpretation of bone density changes in individual patients due to dual-energy x-ray absorptiometry (DEXA) intratest variability. For example, when the hip is measured twice on the same day, the second measurement is within 2% of the first measurement in 80% of subjects, but the range is ± 6%. A real loss of 3% in one year is cause for concern, although a measured loss of 3% is expected in 10% of patients who are actually stable.

In transplant recipients, the relationship between fracture and bone density is different than in the general population, and many patients develop fractures with a normal or only modestly low bone density. This is because the bone strength also depends on unmeasureable factors such as trabecular architecture, blood flow, and ability to repair microdamage.

Biochemical Markers of Bone Formation and Resorption

Urine or serum levels of collagen crosslinking molecules reflect bone resorption. After collagen is deposited in bone, covalent crosslinks in a ring structure (pyridinoline) are formed at the N-terminal or C-terminal regions to stabilize the fibrils. When bone is resorbed, the collagen is digested and the fragments containing the crosslinks are released into the circulation and excreted in the urine. These can be measured by various assays including the pyridinoline, the N-telopeptide (NTX), or the C-telopeptide (ICTP). These levels show large variations with growth and thus, must be age-adjusted for children. Additionally, they are cleared by the kidney and are difficult to interpret in renal failure patients.

Biochemical markers of bone formation are enzymes or structural proteins made by active osteoblasts, including alkaline phosphatase, bone-specific alkaline phosphatase, osteocalcin and the carboxy-terminal propeptide of type I procollagen (PICP). These markers are elevated when there is increased production of the matrix, but they do not measure mineralization, so that increased markers will also be seen in osteomalacia. In patients with renal insufficiency, the bone-specific alkaline phosphatase is a more reliable indicator of bone formation.

Vitamin D is formed in the skin and absorbed from the diet. It is hydroxylated in the liver to 25-hydroxyvitamin D (25(OH)D), and again in the kidney to the active form, 1,25-dihydroxyvitamin D (1,25(OH)$_2$D). Although the active form, dihydroxyvitamin D is difficult to measure and the levels obtained do not accurately reflect vitamin D status. For example, in patients with moderate vitamin D deficiency, parathyroid hormone increases and drives the renal 1-alpha-hydroxylase, increasing 1,25(OH)^{2}D levels. 25(OH)D levels, however, should be checked in transplant recipients with bone disease. These levels are reproducible and accurately reflect vitamin D status. The optimal values of 25(OH)D (20 to 50 ng/mL or 50 to 125 nmol/L) are higher than the ranges usually used for reference. In cases of renal insufficiency, the 1,25(OH)^{2}D levels may be decreased even with normal levels of 25(OH)D.

RISK FACTORS COMMON TO ALL ORGAN TRANSPLANTS
Corticosteroids

Table 25-1 lists effects of corticosteroids on bone. This medication is the single most important risk factor in posttransplant bone disease. The most important effect of corticosteroids is thought to be inhibition of osteoblasts. Corticosteroids are also associated with elevated parathyroid hormone in some studies, but not others. Most investigators have concluded that vitamin D metabolism is not affected by corticosteroids.

Cyclosporine

Cyclosporine causes increased bone resorption in animal models. Isolating the effects of cyclosporine on human bones, however, has been difficult since most human studies have been performed in clinical situations in which corticosteroids were also used. Not withstanding, the bone formation and resorption rates in transplant patients (assessed by osteocalcin, collagen crosslinks, and a limited number of bone biopsies) are higher than generally seen in patients treated with prednisone alone. Thus, it appears that cyclosporine increases bone turnover and enhances bone loss.

Inactivity

Most patients with end-stage disease requiring transplant are unable to maintain physical, weight-bearing activity. A sedentary life style is a minor risk factor for osteoporosis, but complete bed rest causes substantial bone loss.

Table 25-1. Corticosteroid Effects on Bone
Inhibits osteoblasts
Enhances bone resorption
Decreases intestinal calcium absorption
Increases urine calcium loss
Inhibits gonadotropins (central effect)
Increases size of marrow fat cells leading to AVN
Causes apoptosis of osteocytes

Other Factors

Cytokines in the bone marrow, especially interleukins 1, 6 and 11, increase osteoclast formation and activity. Many patients who receive transplants have associated infections or inflammation that increase cytokines that may contribute to bone loss. Nitric oxide (NO) is a newly discovered vasodilator that may increase with inflammation or infection. NO also has been shown to enhance bone resorption. Further research is needed to determine the role of NO in the development of osteoporosis in transplant recipients.

BONE DISEASE IN ORGAN FAILURE BEFORE AND AFTER TRANSPLANTATION
Kidney

RENAL OSTEODYSTROPHY. Renal osteodystrophy is a complex, multifactorial metabolic bone disease (Figure 25-2). Variable exposure to the multitude of factors involved in renal failure-related bone disease results in a spectrum of histological changes. Types of renal osteodystrophy are based on the bone formation rate, presence of fibrosis or increased osteoid, and the amount of aluminum staining. These types do not necessarily correspond to the bone density or the risk of fracture. Low bone density may be associated with either low bone formation rates or, in the presence of secondary hyperparathyroidism, with high bone formation rates. Furthermore, hyperparathyroidism increases trabecular bone volume while decreasing cortical bone volume, so

that the effects on bone density depend on the site that is measured. Estrogen protects the bone from the resorbing effects of PTH, so that hyperparathyroidism may particularly enhance bone loss in women with estrogen deficiency. Figure 25-3 shows that women, in general, lose more bone mass than men.

Most investigators who study renal osteodystrophy consider low bone formation to be undesirable, and suggest that parathyroid hormone should be allowed to increase to maintain a high to normal bone formation rate. This approach has not been validated by studies with fracture endpoints, nor has it been shown to increase bone density. Investigators who study osteoporosis, on the other hand, strive to reduce high bone turnover with medications that result in bone formation rates that would be called "adynamic bone disease" by nephrologists. The ideal bone formation rate for either situation has not yet been determined.

CHANGES AFTER KIDNEY TRANSPLANT. Although many aspects of renal osteodystrophy improve following renal transplant, the bone density and strength may worsen due to the adverse effects of immunosuppressive drugs.

Fracture Rates. Symptomatic fractures are reported in 4% to 11% of kidney transplant patients, with the first fracture noted on average two to five years after transplantation. A large retrospective survey showed 33 of 432 (7.6%) renal allograft recipients had a symptomatic fracture. Fractures of the feet accounted for 40% of the

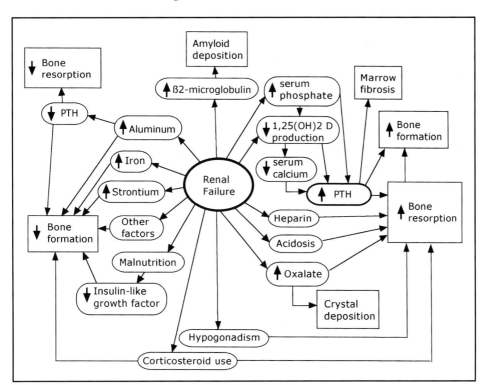

Figure 25-2. Pathophysiology of renal osteodystrophy.

fractures. The average time from transplant to fracture was 20 months. Prospective studies have generally not identified symptomatic fractures during the first year after transplant, however, sequential radiographs have not been performed to determine the frequency of occurrence of asymptomatic fractures.

Bone Density. Bone density decreases most significantly within the first year after renal transplant, but

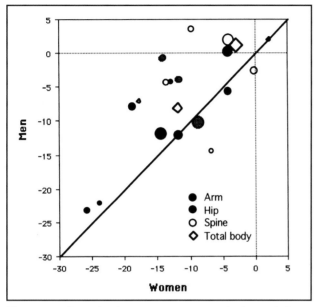

Figure 25-3. Bone density as percent age-matched normals in patients with end-stage renal failure. Values above the 45° line are studies in which men had better BMD than women. Size of the point is proportional to number of subjects.

after several years the rate of loss is about 1% to 2% per year. There is significant variation among studies, however, in the reported rates of bone loss. These differences in the bone density readings are likely caused by differences in renal osteodystrophy histology that predated transplantation (Figure 25-4). For instance, the spine BMD z-score has been reported to be -0.4 with abnormal histology, and +0.8 in those with normal histology.

Bone Histology. Bone biopsies frequently show abnormalities after kidney transplantation. The findings are variable, which is not surprising because there is such a wide spectrum of abnormalities before transplantation. In clinical practice, biopsies are only performed for the evaluation of complex cases and in research studies. Bone biopsies, which directly measure bone formation rates using tetracycline labeling and estimate resorption rates from the number of osteoclasts and eroded surfaces, show that formation and resorption are often very high before transplantation. Following transplantation, bone formation and resorption usually decrease but are often still higher than normal. However, osteoid mineralization is usually normal, indicating that osteomalacia is rare after transplantation, even in cases of hypophosphatemia. Of note, the osteoid surface is slightly higher in those taking cyclosporine.

Hyperparathyroidism. Hyperparathyroidism usually improves after transplantation, since the new kidney can excrete phosphate and produce 1,25-dihydroxyvitamin D in appropriate amounts. About one-third of patients

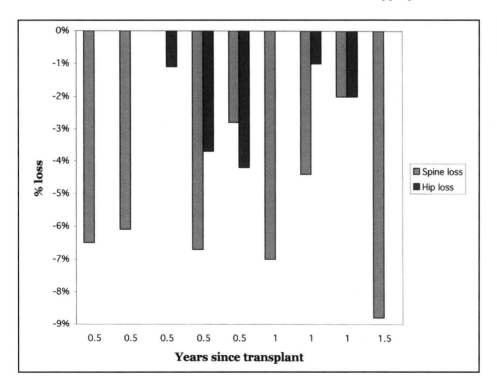

Figure 25-4. Prospective studies of bone loss after kidney transplantation.

develop hypercalcemia after transplant; this persists in 7% and requires parathyroid surgery in about 2%. PTH levels may continue to gradually decrease for seven years after surgery.

Higher pretransplant PTH and longer time on dialysis predict higher posttransplant PTH. The persistence of high PTH is related to the size of the parathyroid glands. Each parathyroid cell secretes a basal level of PTH. If the total number of cells is increased, even with maximal metabolic inhibition, total PTH secretion may be markedly elevated. The number of cells must decrease to return the PTH level to normal. The number of cells and PTH level may decrease after several years, but some patients with hypercalcemia require partial parathyroidectomy. Late increases in PTH following transplant may be related to corticosteroid use, which may cause secondary hyperparathyroidism. Osteitis fibrosis may persist in the bone, but in other cases it may resolve. Radiographic studies of hyperparathyroidism also may improve after transplantation. In some of the larger studies, PTH levels are directly correlated to decreases in bone density.

Aluminum Deposition. Aluminum intoxication is rare in dialysis patients now that aluminum content in water used for dialysate is monitored and oral aluminum intake is limited. Older studies reported exacerbation of aluminum-associated dementia after kidney transplant. This was probably related to the stress of surgery, use of corticosteroids, and postoperative bedrest, which increased bone resorption with subsequent aluminum release that worsened the neurological disease. In more moderate cases, aluminum toxicity was shown to reverse rather than increase following transplantation, because aluminum is easily cleared by the new kidney.

Bone aluminum content also has been shown to decrease following successful transplantation. One study reported that the mean stainable aluminum decreased from 48% to 11% of the bone surface within two years, and in another, the content decreased from 63 to 36 mcg/kg. Furthermore, aluminum may be found within the cement lines after transplant, indicating that new bone formation buries the aluminum, reducing the toxicity.

Oxalate Removed by the Kidney. Oxalate accumulates in all dialysis patients, but it is unusual to see crystal deposition in the bone. When seen, oxylate crystals are surrounded by giant multinuclear cells, which are resorbing the adjacent bone. Whether small amounts of oxalate increase bone resorption is not known. After transplantation, oxalate is cleared. Normal oxalate metabolism may be a factor in the recovery of renal osteodystrophy following successful transplantation.

Amyloidosis. Patients receiving long-term hemodialysis accumulate β2 microglobulin, which can aggregate into amyloid deposits in the bones and joints. After transplantation the pain associated with these deposits improves quickly, but the cysts and subchondral bone erosions remain. After four years the cysts persist, but no enlargement or new cysts develop. The pain relief may be due to steroid use, suggesting an inflammatory component to amyloid bone disease.

Gonadal Steroids. Estradiol levels measured prospectively following transplantation may not increase, likely as a consequence of corticosteroid use. However, in many women, menses return and fertility is restored. Testosterone remains low in approximately half the males.

Avascular Necrosis. Avascular necrosis (AVN) is seen in 1% to 30% of renal allograft recipients an average of three years after transplantation. Variation in the reported incidence is partially due to different anti-rejection regimens: higher prednisone doses are associated with a higher incidence of AVN. The incidence is also higher in those studies that report asymptomatic findings on radiographic studies. Abnormal changes seen on MRI surveys can resolve spontaneously in half the cases in which the bone scan is normal. Most patients with abnormalities on both a bone scan and MRI have symptoms, and 80% of symptomatic patients require hip replacement within five years to manage the pain.

Treatment. There are little data on treatment of bone disease in patients after kidney transplantation. One reason is that the spectrum of posttransplant disease reflects the complexity of renal osteodystrophy, and many aspects of bone physiology improve with no specific management.

Commonly used antiresorbing medications such as alendronate or calcitonin could worsen hyperparathyroidism. This is frequently a problem in patients following kidney transplant, which is not seen in patients after other transplantation. Although clinical data are lacking, it makes physiological sense to be sure PTH is controlled before starting such treatment. Patients may still require calcitriol, but doses would be lower than in dialysis patients, as hypercalciuria and hypercalcemia could occur with too much calcitriol.

Kidney-Pancreas

Because this is a relatively new procedure, there is little information about the bone disease in these patients. However, available studies have shown fracture rates of 15% to 45%, and bone density is frequently low. Diabetes itself may contribute to low bone formation rates, but patients who have high body mass index tend to have high bone density. After transplantation, acidosis may complicate the bone disease. Also, diabetic neuropathy enhances the likelihood of stress fractures in the feet and ankles, which account for a large proportion of the fractures in this group of patients.

Liver

HEPATIC OSTEODYSTROPHY. Patients with end-stage liver failure, like those with renal failure, have multifactorial metabolic bone disease (Table 25-2). Sera from patients with cirrhosis inhibit osteoblast function; one study showed that bilirubin was responsible for much of

Table 25-2. Factors That Contribute to Hepatic Osteodystrophy

Factor	Bone Effect
Bilirubin excess	↓ bone formation
↓ vitamin D hydroxylation	Osteomalacia
Malnutrition	↓ bone formation
Acidosis	↑ bone resorption
Hypogonadism	↑ bone resorption

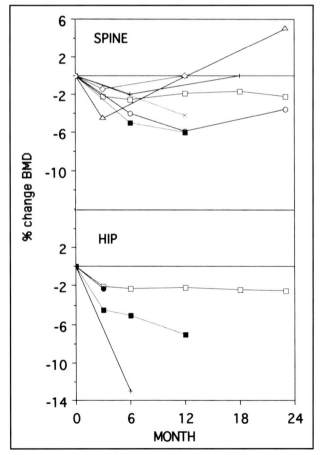

Figure 25-5. Prospective studies of bone density changes after liver transplantation. Each line represents data from a different study.

the inhibition. Other metabolites that accumulate in cirrhosis may also be detrimental to osteoblast vigor.

The liver metabolizes vitamin D, and in some cases patients may develop osteomalacia due to deficiency of 25-OH-vitamin D. This is generally seen only in severe cases of hepatic failure.

Poor nutrition, inactivity, and use of corticosteroids also contribute to bone loss in these patients. Estrogen deficiency is not necessarily seen with liver failure, but may result from general ill health. Most physicians are reluctant to prescribe estrogen to these patients, because it may, in some cases, have hepatic toxicity. Transdermal estrogen does not have a first-pass through the liver and may be safer in this population.

CHANGES AFTER LIVER TRANSPLANTATION. Bone density decreases during the first six to twelve months after the transplant. Thereafter, in patients with a successful transplant whose prednisone dose is decreased, the bone density increases and may exceed the pretransplant levels (Figure 25-5).

Fractures. Prospective studies have shown fracture rates of 20% to 30% within the first year after transplant. Those with preexisting fractures were more likely to develop new fractures. Longer-term follow-up shows that 31% of patients had vertebral fractures after three years (Figure 25-6).

Markers. Osteocalcin decreases during the first couple of months after transplantation, then increases to values higher than normal. The high levels persist as long as immunosuppressive medications are continued. Women with primary biliary cirrhosis have low osteo-

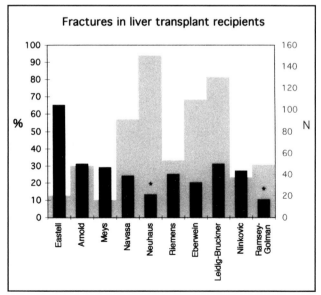

Figure 25-6. Fractures in liver transplant recipients. Gray shading indicates number of patients each study (* indicates asymptomatic).

calcin levels, which increase with cyclosporine therapy even without a transplant. Twenty-five or 1,25 vitamin D levels are not characteristically decreased following liver transplantation.

Bone Biopsies. Posttransplant biopsies show increased bone formation rates; other abnormalities are not significant. However, patients with primary biliary cirrhosis show low bone formation before transplant and variable rates after transplantation.

Other Complications. AVN was seen in 8% of patients in one series. Most studies have not reported this complication, but have not followed patients longer than two years.

Treatment. In one study, etidronate or calcitonin was given to subjects with low bone density, who were one to seven years posttransplant. Spine bone marrow density (BMD) increased 6% to 8% with either treatment.

In a study of intravenous pamidronate every three months, 13 patients did not develop symptomatic fractures. However, there was no control group. In an observational study of subjects who were six months posttransplant, fluoride increased BMD by 25% in spine and 19% in hip, and calcitriol increased BMD 13% in spine and 10% in hip.

Heart

PRE-HEART TRANSPLANT. Table 25-3 shows factors that lead to secondary osteoporosis in heart or lung transplant candidates. Lumbar spine BMD shows that, on average, women have osteopenia and men have normal density, but at the hip, osteopenia is seen in men and women. Many patients are taking loop diuretics and not receiving calcium supplementation or vitamins.

POSTTRANSPLANT

Bone Density Following Transplantation. Bone density decreases after heart transplantation are shown in Figure 25-7. The most rapid loss is seen in the first six months. The rate of loss at the spine lessens after six months, but continues at the hip for the first year.

Fractures. Fracture rates are shown in Figure 25-8. Vertebral compression fractures are the most common. The incidence of symptomatic fractures varies with the study protocol and how symptoms are elicited. The fracture rates continue to increase with time after transplant.

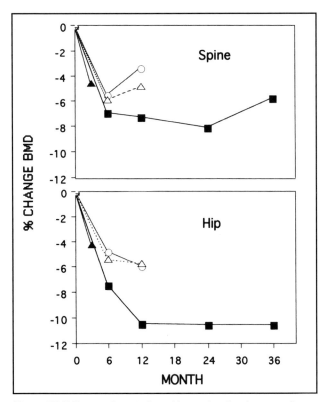

Figure 25-7. Prospective studies of bone density changes after heart transplantation. Each line represents data from a different study.

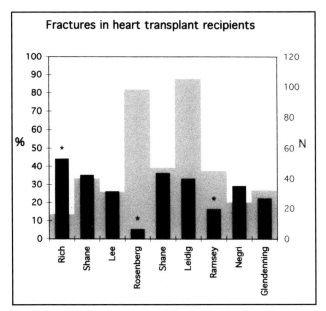

Figure 25-8. Fractures in heart transplant recipients. Gray shading indicates number of patients each study (* = asymptomatic).

Table 25-3. Factors That Contribute to Osteoporosis in Lung or Heart Transplant Candidates
Cigarette smoking
Lack of weight bearing activity
Corticosteroid use
Furosemide use
Malnutrition
Hypogonadism

Bone density is generally lower in patients who fracture, but some patients fracture despite normal bone density. Older patients and women are more likely to fracture.

Markers. Osteocalcin levels decrease during the first three months after transplantation and then increase to levels higher than normal. The collagen crosslinks also increase.

Magnesium. A recent study has shown that magnesium intake was inversely associated with bone loss in heart transplant recipients. This is possibly related to PTH, which may be lower in the patients who took less magnesium.

Treatment. Several small or uncontrolled studies have been performed in patients after heart transplantation, but the results are not uniform. Agents used have included calcitonin, calcidiol, calcitriol, etidronate, pamidronate, or alendronate. Hypercalcemia has been reported after vitamin D treatment. The bisphosphonates have decreased bone loss in some studies but not in others. No obvious side effects or interactions with cyclosporine have been described in these studies during the first year of treatment.

Lung

Lung transplantation is a new procedure and although few studies of bone problems in these patients have been performed, the skeletal complications reported are serious. Figure 25-9 shows an x-ray of a man who developed seven vertebral compression fractures in the first year after his lung transplant; before surgery he had normal bone density and no fractures.

Bone density is markedly reduced in lung transplant recipients; on average they are two standard deviations below age-matched reference ranges. One prospective study showed loss of 4% in the first six months. The fracture rate is also high; in a prospective study, 10% developed fractures in the first year. Patients continue to fracture for several years, and observational studies show a 26%, 35%, and 42% incidence of vertebral compression fractures. Markers of bone metabolism in lung transplant recipients include elevated osteocalcin levels, variably elevated PTH levels, and variable vitamin D levels.

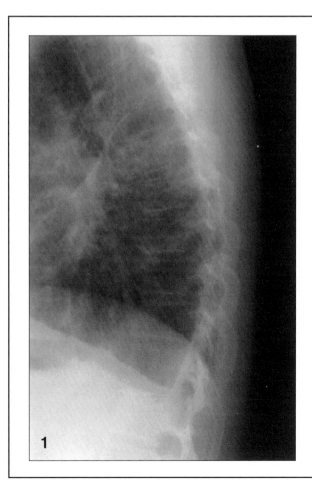
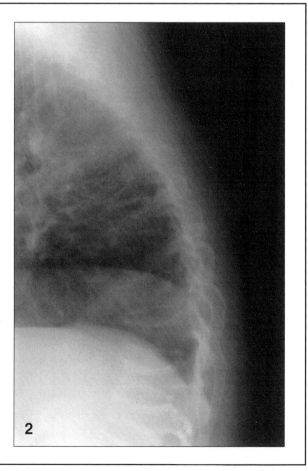

Figure 25-9. Lateral chest radiographs in a patient after lung transplantation. The first film was one month after the transplant and the second was five months later, showing multiple vertebral compression fractures.

PRETRANSPLANT EVALUATION

Table 25-4 lists some basic tests recommended for pretransplant evaluation of bone disease. Patients with bone density below 1.5 SD from age-matched controls, or those with preexisting fragility fractures, should also have a more thorough work-up for other causes of metabolic bone disease by a specialist in metabolic bone disease.

POSTTRANSPLANT SURVEILLANCE

Research studies to determine the most effective therapy and follow-up are needed. Because the rate of bone loss and the incidence of fractures are so high in transplant recipients, it is reasonable to recommend annual bone density measurements and lateral chest or spine x-rays. Patients who have normal bone density after several years and have not experienced transplant rejection are at lower risk and may not require regular surveillance.

Patients with normal gonadal function prior to transplant may become hypogonadal afterwards. Testosterone in men and history of menses in women should be checked three to six months following transplant. Those treated with active metabolites of vitamin D should have measurements of 24-hour urine calcium every six to twelve months while on treatment. PTH and 25 (OH) vitamin D may increase or decrease after transplant, and so should be measured six months following surgery. If they are normal, further surveillance is necessary only if serum calcium is abnormal. Patients who report pain in the hip, shoulder, knees or wrists should have either a bone scan or MRI to determine the presence of AVN.

PREVENTION AND TREATMENT
General Prevention

NUTRITION. Nutritional support is essential in transplant recipients. In addition to general protein-calorie nutrition, patients require an adequate calcium intake of 1,000 to 1,500 mg/d. Dietary sources should be supplemented if necessary with chewable calcium carbonate (taken with meals) or calcium citrate.

Magnesium wasting is often seen in patients taking cyclosporine, so many of these patients are given supplements. In view of the recent study showing an inverse relationship between magnesium supplementation and bone density, patients should be given only enough magnesium to prevent deficiency.

VITAMIN D. Vitamin D stores should be adequate. Recommended amounts are 800 units/d of cholecalciferol. The more active metabolites such as calcitriol may be necessary in patients who have secondary hyperparathyroidism or hypocalciuria. Calcitriol can overcome the steroid-induced decrease in calcium absorption. If used, the urine and serum calcium must be monitored closely, because hypercalcemia or hypercalciuria can occur.

ACTIVITY. Exercise is beneficial to the bone. Active individuals are also less likely to fall or to sustain a serious injury if they do fall, because they have better balance and muscle mass. Walking is a good exercise that should be encouraged.

Table 25-4. Basic Pretransplant Bone Evaluation

Bone density of hip and spine

Radiographs, lateral spine

History of fractures

History of oligomenorrhea

Nutritional evaluation, including estimation of calcium intake

Comprehensive chemistry panel and serum phosphate (includes calcium, alkaline phophatase, creatinine, bicarbonate, albumin)

Thyroid function

Complete blood count

Liver function tests

In patients with low bone density or history of fragility fractures:

Parathyroid hormone

25-OH-vitamin D

Testosterone

24-hour urine calcium (except in renal failure or furosemide use)

If appropriate, serum and urine protein electrophoresis

Consider bone biochemical markers

Refer to bone metabolism specialist

GONADAL HORMONES. Although data from clinical trials in transplant recipients are lacking, it makes physiological sense to treat hypogonadism with testosterone in males and estrogen in females. The route of delivery does not seem to alter bone effects, but the transdermal medicines are preferred in patients with liver allografts to avoid high "first-pass" concentrations in the liver.

In females, regular menstrual periods suggest adequate estrogen; irregular menses are essentially a bioassay for insufficient estrogen. Depot-medroxyprogesterone acetate contraception, which has recently been shown to decrease bone density, should be avoided. Women with a history of breast cancer, hypertriglyceridemia or pulmonary emboli should not be given estrogen.

In males, testosterone should be routinely measured, because it may be low without obvious clinical signs. Hypogonadal males may have smaller prostate size than expected, and with testosterone therapy the prostate may enlarge to the usual size for normal age-matched men. In older men this may cause obstructive symptoms and limit its use.

Antiresorptive Agents

Most transplant recipients require corticosteroids to prevent rejection, although physicians try to limit exposure. Although several new medications have been studied in nontransplant patients with steroid-induced osteoporosis, the experience in transplant recipients is much more limited. Drugs that block bone resorption (bisphosphonates and calcitonin) have been studied most carefully. Pilot studies of drugs thought to enhance bone formation (eg, fluoride, growth hormone, PTH) have shown interesting results but are not consistent enough to allow recommendation.

Bisphosphonates are potent antiresorbing agents that increase the bone density and reduce fracture risk in postmenopausal women with established osteoporosis. In women with low bone density but without fragility fractures, 4.2 years of alendronate therapy increased bone density but did not change the risk of clinical fractures. Bisphosphonates also increase bone density in steroid-treated patients, but the increase is not as great as in patients with postmenopausal osteoporosis. Studies in steroid-treated patients have not had adequate power to assess fracture prevention.

Physicians should not automatically prescribe bisphosphonates for low bone density, just as they should not give iron to treat every case of anemia. The decision to treat with bisphosphonates should be made individually, weighing the immediate benefit with the known risks and, because these are new drugs, with the potential future risks. The most serious side effect seen with amino-bisphosphonates is esophageal erosion.

Patients who are at bed rest should not be given these medications orally. Serious hypocalcemia is also seen in patients treated with bisphosphonates; this is not surprising since these drugs block bone resorption, which may be maintaining the serum calcium level. In patients with secondary hyperparathyroidism caused by malabsorption or renal failure, bisphosphonates worsen the hyperparathyroidism. Theoretically, osteomalacia would become worse with bisphosphonates, but this has been documented only with etidronate, which has an independent adverse effect on mineralization. Bisphosphonates are excreted by the kidney, and thus should be used cautiously in patients with renal insufficiency; elevated creatinine is listed on the label as a contraindication. Effects during pregnancy have only been studied in animals, in which fetal calcium metabolism may be severely altered. Thus, these drugs should be avoided in women who may become pregnant. Acutely, intravenous bisphosphonates decrease the white blood cell count and produce a febrile reaction. Thus, they should not be given to transplant recipients if there is a question about ongoing infection. Fractures appear to heal in animals treated with bisphosphonates, although it takes longer to remodel the callus.

There are no data about the long-term effects of amino-bisphosphonates. The half-life in the bone is longer than ten years. Subtle white blood cell abnormalities are seen in vitro, but the consequences of this are unknown. Preliminary data suggest that coronary artery calcifications might worsen; this requires more study. The bisphosphonates cause marked suppression of bone formation, which leads to increased bone

Table 25-5. Prevention/Treatment of Bone Disease in Transplant Recipients
Calcium supplements (adjust for dietary intake, urine calcium, and PTH)
Vitamin D (Active metabolites in cases of malabsorption and secondary hyperparathyroidism, otherwise 800 units/day cholecalciferol)
Exercise (walking)
Nutrition (adequate calories and protein)
Avoid excess magnesium supplementation
Treat hypogonadism (unless contraindicated)
Use thiazides instead of loop diuretics if possible
Consider bone specific medications:
Calcitonin
Bisphosphonates (alendronate, pamidronate, risedronate)

density in the first few years of use, but over-suppression could theoretically weaken the bone over the long term.

Calcitonin has been used for prolonged time periods with a good safety profile. The results on bone density in steroid-treated patients or transplant recipients is not as consistent as with bisphosphonates. Calcitonin is an antiresorptive medication and thus could worsen hyperparathyroidism. Calcitonin appears to be a gentler, safer drug than bisphosphonates, and is a good choice for transplant recipients with a relatively low risk of fractures.

Treatment of Avascular Necrosis

In early cases, AVN sometimes resolves with restriction of vigorous activity. There is controversy about whether core decompression will prevent progression of AVN of the femoral head in mild to moderate cases. There is no other specific therapy, and if pain becomes persistent, hip replacement is indicated.

Treatment of Posttransplant Bone Pain

A syndrome of leg pain occurring days-to-weeks after transplantation has been described. These patients do not have thrombi or claudication, but they have altered vascularity caused by cyclosporine. This pain resolves rapidly with calcium channel blockers.

RECOMMENDED READING

Aringer M, Kiener HP, Koeller MD, et al. High turnover bone disease following lung transplantation. Bone. 1998;23(5):485-488.

Aris RM, Neuringer IP, Weiner MA, Egan TM, Ontjes D. Severe osteoporosis before and after lung transplantation. Chest. 1996;109(5):1176-1183.

Barbosa LM, Gauthier VJ, Davis CL. Bone pain that responds to calcium channel blockers. A retrospective and prospective study of transplant recipients. Transplantation. 1995;59(4):541-544.

Boncimino K, McMahon DJ, Addesso V, Bilezikian JP, Shane E. Magnesium deficiency and bone loss after cardiac transplantation. J Bone Miner Res. 1999;14(2):295-303.

Crosbie OM, Freaney R, McKenna MJ, Curry MP, Hegarty JE. Predicting bone loss following orthotopic liver transplantation. Gut. 1999;44(3):430-434.

Cueto-Manzano AM, Konel S, Hutchison AJ, et al. Bone loss in long-term renal transplantation: histopathology and densitometry analysis. Kidney Int. 1999;55(5):2021-2029.

Davenport A, Goel S, Mackenzie JC. Treatment of hypercalcemia with pamidronate in patients with end stage renal failure. Scand J Urol Nephrol. 1993;27(4):447-451.

Epstein S. Post-transplantation bone disease: the role of immunosuppressive agents and the skeleton. J Bone Miner Res. 1996;11(1):1-7.

Glendenning P, Kent GN, Adler BD, et al. High prevalence of osteoporosis in cardiac transplant recipients and discordance between biochemical turnover markers and bone histomorphometry. Clin Endocrinol. 1999;50(3):347-355.

Grotz WH, Rump LC, Niessen A, et al. Treatment of osteopenia and osteoporosis after kidney transplantation. Transplantation. 1998;66(8):1004-1008.

Guo CY, Johnson A, Locke TJ, Eastell R. Mechanisms of bone loss after cardiac transplantation. Bone. 1998;22(3):267-271.

Massari PU. Disorders of bone and mineral metabolism after renal transplantation. Kidney Int. 1997;52(5):1412-1421.

Messa P, Sindici C, Cannella G, et al. Persistent secondary hyperparathyroidism after renal transplantation. Kidney Int. 1998;54(5):1704-1713.

Meys E, Fontanges E, Fourcade N, Thomasson A, Pouyet M, Delmas PD. Bone loss after orthotopic liver transplantation. Am J Med. 1994;97(5):445-450.

Ramsey-Goldman R, Dunn JE, Dunlop DD, et al. Increased risk of fracture in patients receiving solid organ transplants. J Bone Miner Res. 1999;14(3):456-463.

Rodino MA, Shane E. Osteoporosis after organ transplantation. Am J Med. 1998;104(5):459-469.

Shane E, Rivas M, Staron RB, et al. Fracture after cardiac transplantation: a prospective longitudinal study. J Clin Endocrinol Metab. 1996;81(5):1740-1746.

Siddiqui AR, Kopecky KK, Wellman HN, et al. Prospective study of magnetic resonance imaging and SPECT bone scans in renal allograft recipients: evidence for a self-limited subclinical abnormality of the hip. J Nucl Med. 1993;34(3):381-386.

Smets YF, van der Pijl JW, de Fijter JW, Ringers J, Lemkes HH, Hamdy NA. Low bone mass and high incidence of fractures after successful simultaneous pancreas-kidney transplantation. Nephrol Dial Transplant. 1998;13(5):1250-1255.

26 NEOPLASIA FOLLOWING TRANSPLANTATION

Israel Penn, MD

The largest database in the world on posttransplant malignancies is the Cincinnati Transplant Tumor Registry (CTTR). This chapter emphasizes the findings of the CTTR and supplements these with data with pertinent recent publications.

PRETRANSPLANT SCREENING

Transplant candidates aged 45 years and over should be routinely screened for cancers common to the general population (eg, carcinomas of the skin, breast, bronchus, prostate, colon, and uterus). In particular, individuals who have had prolonged exposure to carcinogens such as sunlight, smoking, alcohol or occupational chemicals should be evaluated. Other groups to be screened are those in whom underlying diseases may predispose them to malignancies. These include analgesic abuse or acquired cystic disease of the kidney, which predispose renal failure patients to urinary tract, particularly renal, malignancies; or liver allograft candidates who have long standing ulcerative colitis, and who are at increased risk for colon carcinomas and cholangiocarcinomas.

POSTTRANSPLANT MALIGNANCY
Incidence of de novo Cancers

Overall, there is a threefold to fivefold increased incidence of cancers in transplant patients compared with age- and sex-matched controls in the general population.

Age and Sex of Patients

Neoplasms occur in relatively young patients following transplantation. Those with cancers are on average 43 years old at transplantation (range is eight days to 80 years) with 40% being younger than 40. Patients are on average 48 years old at the time of diagnosis of their cancers. Of these, 66% are male and 34% female, in keeping with the 2:1 ratio of male-to-female patients who undergo renal or cardiac transplantation.

Types of Recipients

The group of 11,101 recipients with posttransplant cancers is comprised of 8,926 who received kidney, 1,185 heart, 567 liver, 217 bone marrow, 110 pancreas, 52 lung,

University of Cincinnati Medical Center, Department of Surgery, Cincinnati Veterans Affairs Medical Center, Cincinnati, OH

38 combined heart-lung, four upper-abdominal organ "cluster," and two small bowel transplants.

Time of Appearance After Transplantation

The incidence of neoplasms increases with the length of posttransplant follow-up. An Australian study of 6,596 patients showed that the percent probability of developing a tumor following renal transplantation from cadaver donors 24 years postoperatively was 66% for skin malignancies, 27% for non-skin cancers, and 72% for any type of neoplasm. These exceptional figures must be treated with caution as most tumors were skin cancers, which are very common in Australia, and the number of 24-year survivors was small. Nevertheless, they emphasize the need for indefinite surveillance.

Review of the CTTR database shows that malignancies occur a relatively short time posttransplant, with Kaposi's sarcoma (KS) appearing at an average of 21 (median 13) months after transplant, posttransplant lymphoproliferative disease (PTLD) at an average of 34 (median 13) months; skin cancers at an average of 66 (median 51) months; and anogenital carcinomas at an average of 115 (median 114) months. Considering all cancers, the average time of appearance was 63 (median 47) months.

NEOPLASIAS THAT ARE GREATLY INCREASED IN TRANSPLANT PATIENTS

A consistent finding in the CTTR is the predominance of certain malignancies. There has been no increase in the incidence of tumors that are commonly seen in the general population (eg, carcinomas of the lung, breast, prostate, and colon, and invasive uterine cervical carcinomas). Up until March 1999, the CTTR had data on 11,820 malignancies that occurred in 11,101 patients. These are listed in Table 26-1.

These above findings are consistent with several epidemiologic studies that showed a fourfold to 21-fold increased incidence of skin cancers; 28-fold to 49-fold increased incidence of PTLD; 29-fold increase in lip carcinomas; 400-fold to 500-fold increase in KS compared with controls of the same ethnic origin; 100-fold increased incidence of vulvar and anal carcinomas; 20-fold to 38-fold increased incidence of hepatocellular carcinomas; and 14-fold to 16-fold increased incidence of in situ uterine cervical carcinomas.

Cancers of the Skin and Lip

Skin tumors are the most common cancers in organ allograft recipients comprising 38% of all malignancies. The incidence of skin cancer increases with the length of follow-up after transplantation as shown by an

Type of Tumor	Number of Tumors
Table 26-1. Most Common De Novo Malignancies*	
Cancers of skin and lips	4467
Posttransplant lymphoproliferative disease	1977
Carcinomas of the lung	663
Kaposi's sarcoma	475
Carcinomas of uterus (cervix, 358; body, 69; unknown, 4)	431
Carcinomas of the kidney (host kidney, 352; allograft kidney, 45; both, 1; unknown, 21)	419
Carcinomas of colon and rectum	397
Carcinomas of the breast	365
Carcinomas of the head and neck (excluding thyroid, parathyroid and eye)	331
Carcinomas of the vulva, perineum, penis, scrotum	292
Carcinomas of urinary bladder	254
Carcinomas of prostate gland	230
Metastatic carcinoma (primary site unknown)	226
Leukemias	213
Hepatobiliary carcinomas	191
Sarcomas (excluding Kaposi's sarcoma)	149

*There were 11,101 patients of whom 674 (6%) had two or more distinct tumor types involving different organ systems. Of these, 43 patients each had three separate types of cancer and one had four.

Australian study of 6,596 cadaveric renal transplant recipients who experienced a linear increase in the incidence of cutaneous cancers reaching 66% at 24 years posttransplant. Similarly, a Dutch study showed a 10% incidence of nonmelanoma skin cancers in kidney recipients at ten years posttransplant, rising to 40% after 40. The time of appearance after transplantation increased in higher latitude regions: 86 months in Canada vs 33 months in Australia. The interval was also shorter in older individuals.

Skin cancers affect sun-exposed areas, mainly of the head, neck and upper limbs. They occur especially in light-skinned individuals with blue eyes and blond or red hair. Most lesions, in patients transplanted after the age of 40 years, occur on the head, whereas lesions in individuals transplanted at a younger age appear mainly on the dorsum of the hands, forearms and chest.

The patterns of skin cancer in transplant patients differ in several ways from those seen in the general population. Basal cell carcinomas (BCCs) outnumber squamous cell carcinomas (SCCs) in the general population by 5:1, but the reverse occurs in transplant patients in whom SCCs outnumber BCCs by 1.8:1. The SCC-to-BCC ratio is much higher (nearly 5:1) in children than in adults. SCC is calculated to occur at a frequency between 40 and 250 times higher than in the general population, and BCC at ten times higher, and malignant melanoma

five times more frequently than expected. Malignant melanomas comprise 5.1% of cutaneous tumors in the CTTR in contrast with an incidence of 2.7% in the general population of the US. In the general population, SCCs usually occur in persons in their 60s and 70s, but the average age of transplant patients is 30 years younger. In addition, the incidence of multiple skin cancers is remarkably high (at least 43%). Some patients have had more than 100 skin tumors. Apparently, some patients have a widespread cutaneous abnormality with areas of unstable epithelium that contain multifocal premalignant and malignant lesions.

The behavior of skin tumors in transplant patients differs markedly from that in the general population, in whom they cause only 1% to 2% of all cancer deaths, the great majority of which are from malignant melanoma. In contrast, SCCs were much more aggressive in transplant patients than in the general population, and account for the majority of lymph node metastases and deaths from skin cancer. In the CTTR, 5.7% of patients with skin cancers have had lymph node metastases of which 73% were from SCCs, 18% from malignant melanomas, and the remainder mainly from Merkel's cell tumors. Similarly, 5% of patients died of their skin cancers, of which 60% were from SCCs, 30% from malignant melanomas, 8% from Merkel's cell tumors, and 2% from BCCs. Aggressive SCCs occur particularly where there is heavy sun exposure, in older individuals, in patients with multiple lesions, in lesions located on the head, and in histologically thick tumors that involve the subcutaneous tissues. Patients with skin cancer are also more likely to develop other more fulminant types of malignancy than are allograft recipients without skin cancer.

Lymphoproliferative Disorders

Lymphoproliferative tumors, known nonspecifically as PTLD, are second only to skin cancers in their frequency in transplant patients. PTLD covers a very wide spectrum of diseases ranging from benign hyperplasias at one end of the spectrum to frankly malignant lymphomas at the other. Of 1,977 cases of PTLD in the CTTR, only 3% are Hodgkin's disease, which comprises 10% of lymphomas in the general population. Similarly, plasmacytoma and myeloma comprise less than 4% of PTLDs in the CTTR, whereas in the general population they comprise 19% of lymphomas. Of the PTLDs in the CTTR that were studied immunologically, 85% were of B cell origin, 15% were of T cell origin, and rare cases were of null cell origin or were combined B and T cell lymphomas.

RISK FACTORS. There are several risk factors for the development of PTLD. Intense immunosuppression is a major factor. Often three, four or even five immunosuppressive agents are administered over a short time period. Whenever a new immunosuppressive agent is introduced, there is a "learning curve" while physicians discover how to use it in appropriate doses, especially when it is added to combinations of other immunosuppressive medications. An increased frequency of PTLD was observed after the introduction of antilymphocyte globulin, then cyclosporine, then muromonab-CD3, and with limited experience gained thus far, tacrolimus and mycophenolate mofetil.

Nonrenal allograft recipients are much more prone to develop PTLD than are renal recipients. Heavy immunosuppressive therapy is often used in the former group to reverse rejection in order to save their lives, whereas with severe rejection of kidney allografts, physicians have the option to discontinue immunosuppression and return the patients to dialysis. Thus, when 2,246 neoplasms in recipients of non-renal organs in the CTTR were compared with 9,574 malignancies in renal allograft recipients, lymphomas comprised 40% of tumors in the former group compared with only 11% in the latter. These findings are reinforced by reports that, whereas PTLD occurs in less than 1% of renal recipients, it involves 3% of heart, 3% of liver, 8% of lung, and 19% of intestinal recipients. The risk of PTLD in bone marrow recipients is less than 2% at four years posttransplant, but may reach levels as high as 24% in recipients of HLA-mismatched T cell-depleted marrow.

More than 90% of PTLDs are positive for Epstein-Barr virus (EBV), including some T cell PTLDs. A risk factor for development of PTLD is seronegative status at the time of transplant. In one study, 11% of seronegative pediatric and 5% of seronegative adult recipients developed PTLD, whereas the corresponding figures in their seropositive counterparts were 0% and 2%, respectively. Some studies suggest that high viral loads of EBV in the peripheral blood predict development of PTLD.

The CTTR data show that pediatric organ transplant recipients have a disproportionately high incidence of PTLD compared with adults. When 447 tumors in pediatric allograft recipients were compared with 8,673 tumors in adults, PTLDs comprised 53% of malignancies in the former group and 15% in the latter. Primary EBV infections are more common in childhood than in adulthood, and children have more lymphoid tissue, which may undergo neoplastic change when exposed to the appropriate stimuli. Furthermore, 61% of pediatric patients who developed PTLDs received nonrenal organ allografts and thus, more intense immunosuppressive therapy.

PRESENTATION. Almost any organ may be involved by PTLD, so the disorder may present in many different ways. Of the PTLDs in the CTTR, 53% involved multiple organs or sites, and 47% were localized to a single organ or site. Whereas lymphomas in the general population frequently involve lymph nodes, 70% of PTLDs occur in extranodal locations. The most common extranodal sites are the liver (24%), lungs (21%), central nervous system (CNS) (20%), kidneys (18%), intestines (17%), and spleen (12%). CNS disease usually involves the brain and frequently is multicentric in distribution. Spinal cord involvement is rare. Another notable feature is that in 54% of patients with CNS disease the lesions are confined to this site, whereas in the general population cerebral lymphomas are frequently associated with lesions in other organs, with only 1% of lymphomas confined to the CNS.

Macroscopic or microscopic involvement of the allograft occurs in 23% of patients with PTLD. In some recipients of renal, cardiac or hepatic allografts, the lymphomatous infiltrate has been misdiagnosed as rejection on biopsies performed for allograft dysfunction. Because of this, intensified rather than decreased immunosuppressive therapy has been incorrectly given.

The clinical presentation of PTLD is extremely variable. Some patients are completely asymptomatic or present with a picture resembling infectious mononucleosis. Other presenting features include fever, night sweats, upper respiratory infection, weight loss, diarrhea, abdominal pain, lymphadenopathy and tonsillitis. Tonsillar enlargement is sometimes so severe that emergency tracheostomy is necessary. As the gastrointestinal tract is frequently involved, patients may present with intestinal perforation and peritonitis. Less commonly, gastrointestinal bleeding or intestinal obstruction is the presenting feature. Patients may also present with lung lesions or other visceral masses. Occasionally, the presentation imitates allograft rejection. And some patients present with a confusing picture of disseminated sepsis and multiple organ failure.

A CNS lymphoma should be suspected whenever a transplant patient develops neurologic symptoms. A thorough workup is necessary and may include examination of the cerebrospinal fluid, computerized axial tomography, magnetic resonance imaging, and single-photon emission computed tomography (SPECT). Such tests help to exclude other causes of neurologic symptoms such as hypertensive encephalopathy, meningitis, brain abscess or intracranial bleeding.

TREATMENT. Several treatment options are available for PTLD. Localized disease may be successfully excised or treated with radiation therapy. However, multi-modality therapy is used often. A significant proportion of lesions regress, partially or completely, after reduction or cessation of immunosuppressive therapy. In particular, in recipients with widespread, extensive, or potentially life-threatening PTLD, all immunosuppression should be stopped except for a minimal dose of prednisone, until all evidence of tumor has disappeared. Allograft rejection may not occur or may develop slowly in chronic fashion, as many of these patients have been very heavily immunosuppressed and a long time may elapse before they regain immunocompetence. Nevertheless, the risk of rejection is very real. For example, in a series of 14 renal recipients whose PTLD was treated by reduction or cessation of immunosuppression (among other methods), eight of 12 survivors lost their allografts. Once PTLD has regressed, immunosuppressive therapy should be resumed in small doses and then gradually increased to maintenance levels which, however, should be lower than those given before the appearance of PTLD.

Acyclovir, ganciclovir or related antiviral agents are often used to treat an associated EBV infection. INF-α may be used for its antiviral and antineoplastic effects. However, it is an immunostimulant, and in large doses may cause rejection. Chemotherapy may be successfully used to treat widespread PTLD using combinations such as CHOP or ProMACE-CytaBOM. In one series, administration of anti-B cell monoclonal antibodies caused complete remissions in 58% of patients, but not in those with CNS disease. However, PTLD was reversed in two such cases when the antibodies were administered directly into the CNS via an Ommaya reservoir. Anti-EBV cytotoxic T cells, obtained from the original donor, have been used successfully to treat donor cell-derived PTLDs in bone marrow allograft recipients. In one case, use of third-party HLA-matched T cells was effective against a CNS PTLD. Lymphokine-activated killer (LAK) cells, derived from the patients' own peripheral blood mononuclear cells, have been successful in several cases as a type of cellular immunotherapy. Other treatments that have been used include administration of IgG anti-CD22 immunotoxin.

Survival outcomes were studied in 1,391 patients with PTLD in the CTTR. Of these, 226 patients (16%) had no treatment and the tumor was discovered at autopsy in 106 (7%). No data regarding therapy were available in 63 (5%) other patients. Treatment was given to 1,102 patients of whom 418 (38%) had complete remissions. Of the 1,391 patients, both treated and untreated, 495 (36%) died of PTLD, 222 (16%) died of other causes (but PTLD may have contributed to some of the deaths), and 674 patients (48%) are currently alive.

Recurrence of PTLD occurs in less than 5% of cases, and may either be a true recurrence of the original tumor or the emergence of a neoplasm of different clonal composition. Of 33 patients who underwent re-transplantation, three (9%) had recurrence or persistence of PTLD after re-transplantation. Two recurrences were in patients requiring re-transplantation after removal of an allograft (one kidney, one liver) affected by PTLD, and one recurrence occurred in a liver allograft recipient who required re-transplantation for rejection 3.5 months after treatment of PTLD. If at all possible, re-transplantation should be delayed for at least one year after complete remission of PTLD.

Kaposi's Sarcoma

The frequency of Kaposi's sarcoma (KS) is borne out by the fact that the total number of cases reported to the CTTR exceeded those of each of three tumors that are common in the general population, namely carcinomas of the colon, breast and prostate (Table 26-1). The average age at presentation of KS reported to the CRRT is 43 (range is 4.5 to 67) years. The disease is uncommon in pediatric transplant recipients. The male-to-female ratio is nearly 3:1, whereas it is as high as 17:1 in classical KS. KS is observed mainly in kidney allograft recipients with a much smaller number occurring in other solid organ or bone marrow recipients. Results of tests for human immunodeficiency virus in most patients have been negative. The majority of tumors (46%) appear within one year of transplant. When patients' racial or ethnic backgrounds are noted, the majority are of Arabic, African-American, Italian, Jewish, Greek or Turkish origin. KS was reported in 1.6% of 820 Italian renal transplant recipients who were followed for more than six months. It is the most common cancer in renal transplant recipients in Saudi Arabia, affecting approximately 5% of renal transplant recipients, whereas in the general population of Saudi Arabia, the incidence of KS is 0.2% to 0.38%.

Fifty-eight percent of patients reported to the CTTR have had nonvisceral KS confined to the skin, conjunctiva, or oropharyngeal mucosa, and 42% have had visceral disease that involved mainly the gastrointestinal tract, lungs and lymph nodes, but other organs have also been affected. The majority (98%) of patients with nonvisceral disease have had skin lesions and 2% involvement of the mouth or oropharynx. Diagnosis is difficult in patients who present without typical skin lesions. Thus, 23% of patients who have visceral disease have no skin involvement, but 4% have oral lesions, which provide easy access for biopsy and diagnosis.

A clinician should suspect KS whenever a transplant patient, particularly one belonging to the ethnic groups described above, presents with reddish-blue macules or plaques in the skin or oropharyngeal mucosa, or apparently infected granulomas that fail to heal. If the diagnosis is confirmed, a thorough workup, including CT scans of the chest and abdomen and upper and lower gastrointestinal endoscopy, is needed to exclude any internal visceral involvement. Diagnostic confusion may occur when the initial presentation of KS is as a diffuse pulmonary infiltrate.

Many of the treatments used for PTLD, including reduced immunosuppression, interferon, surgery, chemotherapy and radiation, are also applicable to KS. In the CTTR study, 44% of patients with KS had complete remissions following various treatments, and 42% of these followed reduction or cessation of immunosuppressive therapy. Patients with nonvisceral disease had a higher remission rate (55%) than did those with visceral disease (30%). However, such therapy does have a price, as 54% of renal recipients in whom it was successful lost their allografts or had impaired function. Impressive results were reported in one study, in which 8 of 13 patients (61%) had complete remissions, following reduction of immunosuppressive therapy, and 69% of the patients did not lose their grafts, even many months after reduction or withdrawal of immunosuppression.

The importance of the immunosuppressed state in perpetuating the disease is borne out by a multicenter study of eight renal allograft recipients. Seven patients with posttransplant KS had been successfully treated by reduction or cessation of immunosuppressive therapy (combined with excision and radiation therapy in one patient), but developed recurrences, either when regular dosage of immunosuppressive therapy was resumed or when a second transplant was performed. KS regressed once more when immunosuppression was again reduced or discontinued, but at least four patients lost their allografts to rejection. The eighth patient had KS successfully treated many years before transplantation and developed a recurrence six months after transplantation.

Mortality from KS may be high. In the CTTR study, 54% of patients with visceral disease died, and 75% of those deaths were attributable to KS. In contrast, only 23% of patients with nonvisceral KS died, most commonly from infection or rejection, or from both causes, but only rarely from KS.

Cancers of the Perineal Areas

Females outnumber males by 2.6:1 in the occurrence of carcinomas of the vulva, perineum, scrotum, penis, perianal skin or anus. For most other posttransplant cancers, males outnumber females by more than 2:1. One-third of patients have in situ lesions. A disturbing feature is that patients with invasive lesions have been much younger (average age is 42 years) than their counterparts in the general population, whose average age is usually between 50 and 70 years. More than 40% of transplant patients with these malignancies have a history of condyloma acuminatum. Frequently, female patients exhibit a "field effect" with cancerous involvement not only of the vulva, but also the vagina or uterine cervix.

LESS COMMON CANCERS
Renal Carcinoma

An important finding of the CTTR is that 24% of renal carcinomas are discovered incidentally during workup for other disorders, at nephrectomy for hypertension or other reasons, during operation for some other disease, or at autopsy examination. Most cancers in renal recipients develop in their own diseased kidneys, although 11% appear in renal allografts, from two to 258 (average is 85) months after transplantation. Of these tumors, 20% are diagnosed within two years of transplantation. It is possible these tumors may have been present in the allograft at the time of transplant but were sufficiently small to escape notice. Only a few renal cell carcinomas have been reported in nonrenal transplant recipients. Two predisposing causes of renal carcinomas have been identified. Analgesic nephropathy was the underlying indication for transplantation in 8% of transplant patients with carcinomas of their native kidneys. Analgesic abuse may cause cancers, mostly transitional cell carcinomas, in various parts of the urinary tract. This is borne out by the CTTR series in which 59% of patients with analgesia-related renal carcinomas had similar tumors elsewhere in the urinary tract. Another predisposing cause of cancer in renal transplant recipients is acquired cystic disease (ACD). ACD of the native kidneys occurs in 30% to 95% of patients receiving long-term hemodialysis, and is complicated by renal adenocarcinoma, which is increased 30-fold to 40-fold over its incidence in the general population. With a successfully functioning renal allograft, ACD tends to regress, theoretically decreasing the risk of developing carcinoma. However, cases of persistence of ACD and development of renal cell carcinoma have been reported in patients with successfully functioning transplants. The precise incidence of ACD-related carcinomas in renal transplant recipients is not known, but the CTTR has data on at least 17 patients with renal carcinomas associated with ACD.

Carcinomas of the Cervix

Carcinomas of the cervix occur in 10% of the women with posttransplant malignancies. In situ lesions comprise at least 70% of cases. As two epidemiologic studies indicate a 14-fold to 16-fold increased incidence of in situ cervical carcinoma, the small numbers of cases reported to the CTTR suggest that many cases are being missed or are not reported because it is a known association.

Hepatobiliary Tumors

Most cases (70%) in the CTTR are hepatomas, and in a substantial number there is a history of hepatitis B infection. Since hepatitis C screening became available, increasing numbers of hepatomas, related to chronic hepatitis C infection, are being reported.

Sarcomas Excluding Kaposi's Sarcoma

The majority of sarcomas involve the soft tissues or visceral organs, whereas cartilage or bone involvement is uncommon. The most common types are fibrous histiocytoma, leiomyosarcoma, fibrosarcoma, rhabdomyosarcoma, hemangiosarcoma and mesothelioma.

Other Malignancies

The Nordic Transplant Registry and the Australian and New Zealand Transplant Registry have reported an increased incidence of a variety of other malignancies than those described above. These may represent regional variations in cancer incidence. However, some of the calculated increases are based on very small numbers of patients. Whether or not there is an increased incidence of other neoplasms will require epidemiologic studies of large numbers of transplant recipients.

BIOLOGICAL BEHAVIOR OF TUMORS

When treating malignancies in organ allograft recipients, one must emphasize that some tumors demonstrate more aggressive behavior than do similar cancers in nontransplant patients. Early tumors are curable with local therapy provided that their growth has not given them adequate vascular access. Once this has been obtained, the host's depressed immune system is believed to permit greater than normal survival of cancer cells in the bloodstream. The result is more rapid tumor dissemination and demise of the host than would be expected in a setting of immunocompetence.

A decreased peritumoral lymphocytic infiltrate may also contribute to the aggressiveness of some cutaneous SCCs and melanomas.

Pathophysiology of Increased Risk of Neoplasia in Organ Transplant Recipients

Posttransplant neoplasms probably result from a complex interplay of multiple factors. Severely depressed immunity may impair the body's ability to eliminate malignant cells induced by various carcinogens. Chronic antigenic stimulation by the foreign antigens of transplanted organs, by repeated infections, or by transfusions of blood or blood borne products may overstimulate a partially depressed immune system and lead to PTLD. Alternatively, defective feedback mechanisms may fail to control the extent of immune reactions and lead to unrestrained lymphoid proliferation and PTLD. Furthermore, once this loss of regulation occurs, the defensive ability of the immune system is undermined and other nonlymphoid malignancies may appear. Host-donor microchimerism may also be an overlooked factor in the development of PTLD.

The activation of oncogenic viruses in some immunosuppressed patients is highly likely. EBV is strongly implicated in causing lymphomas in patients with primary immunodeficiency diseases, AIDS, and organ transplants. Also, it may play a role in the development of some posttransplant smooth muscle tumors, and in some cases of Hodgkin's disease. Certain papillomaviruses play a role in the etiology of carcinomas of the vulva, perineum, uterine cervix, and anus. The role of human papillomavirus in causing skin cancers in transplant patients is the subject of much disagreement. Hepatitis B and C viruses are known to give rise to hepatomas. Human herpesvirus 8 (HHV-8), also known as Kaposi's sarcoma-associated virus, may play a key role in the development of KS.

Some immunosuppressive agents such as azathioprine, cyclophosphamide, and cyclosporine may directly damage DNA and cause neoplasms. Immunosuppressive agents may enhance the effects of other carcinogens, such as sunlight, in causing carcinomas of the skin or papillomavirus in causing carcinomas of the uterine cervix. Genetic factors may affect susceptibility to cancer by affecting carcinogen metabolism, level of interferon secretion, response to viral infections, or regulation of the immune response by the major histocompatibility system. For example, HLA antigens play an important role in host defense against the development and spread of tumors, especially in virus-induced neoplasia. Thus, in renal transplant recipients, HLA A11 may have protected patients against skin cancers, whereas HLA B27 and HLA DR7 are associated with an increased risk of these neoplasms.

PROPHYLACTIC MEASURES

Measures to avoid the development of malignancies include minimizing immunosuppressive therapy to a level that is compatible with good allograft functions while at all times realizing the consequences of a failed vital organ transplant from too little immunosuppressive therapy. Additionally, hepatitis B vaccination in non-immune individuals may prevent HBV-related hepatocellular cancers. Avoidance of excess sun exposure, wearing protective clothing and using sunscreen may prevent skin tumors. Use of barrier methods of contraception may prevent the development of condyloma acuminatum, which may decrease the occurrence of carcinomas of the vulva, perineum and uterine cervix. And finally, although the currently available antiviral agents are virustatic and not virucidal, and act only on linear EBV and not the circular (latent) virus, peritransplant or perirejection administration of ganciclovir or acyclovir may decrease the development of PTLD. A recent study showed that ganciclovir or acyclovir given preemptively, during administration of antilymphocyte agents, reduced the incidence of PTLD to one in 198 consecutive recipients, compared with an historic control group in which seven of 179 recipients developed this disorder. Antiviral prophylaxis is especially important when transplanting organs from EBV-positive donors into EBV-negative recipients, most of whom are children.

TREATMENT OF CANCERS

The treatment of PTLD and KS has been mentioned above. Treatment of skin cancers is discussed in Chapter 28. Cancers other than those mentioned above should be treated by standard surgical, radiation, or chemotherapeutic modalities.

In patients requiring systemic chemotherapy of widespread malignancies, one must remember that most agents depress the bone marrow. It is, therefore, prudent to stop or reduce the administration of azathioprine, cyclophosphamide or mycophenolate mofetil dosage during such treatment to avoid severe bone marrow depression. Reduction of overall immunosuppressive dosage may be advisable to prevent over-immunosuppression. As most chemotherapeutic agents have immunosuppressive side effects, satisfactory allograft function may persist for prolonged periods. Treatment with prednisone may be continued as it is an important component of many cancer chemotherapy protocols. As many transplant patients are already heavily immunosuppressed, chemotherapeutic agents should be used with caution as some patients have died of overwhelming infections following their use. Prophylactic antimicrobials and granulocyte colony stimulating factors may be helpful. When using cytotoxic therapy in renal transplant recipients, or in non-kidney recipients who have impaired renal function, one should avoid, if possible, the use of nephrotoxic agents such as cisplatin. Similarly, cardiotoxic agents such as doxorubicin should be avoided if possible in cardiac allograft recipients.

INF-α has been used to treat some patients with KS or PTLD or other malignancies. Interferon is a potent immune modulator that increases membrane expression of class I antigens of the major histocompatibility complex, T cell-mediated cytotoxicity, and natural killer cell function. Thus, it may stimulate rejection. However, conflicting findings have been reported following its use in renal allograft recipients. A review of the literature suggests that small doses may be safe but large doses may precipitate rejection.

ROUTINE SURVEILLANCE TESTING

As the incidence of cancer increases with the length of follow-up, it is important that patients are seen at regular intervals and any premalignant lesions are treated or any untoward symptoms are investigated. For example, patients who have a history of, or will experience, prolonged sun exposure should be seen on a regular basis by a dermatologist. Any suspicious lesion should be immediately biopsied. Renal transplant patients whose original disease was analgesic nephropathy should have ultrasound or CT examinations of the urinary tract on a regular basis, as well as repeated urinary cytology. Any suspicious lesion should be promptly removed. Similarly, liver allograft recipients whose underlying disease was chronic ulcerative colitis should undergo regular colonoscopies to detect areas suspicious of colonic carcinoma at an early and readily treatable stage. They should also be kept under surveillance for the possible development of cholangiocarcinoma.

As papillomavirus infections (suspected as causes of carcinoma of the cervix, vulva and anal area) are sexually transmitted, patients should be advised to use condoms. All postadolescent females should undergo regular pelvic examinations and cervical smears. All premalignant lesions such as condyloma acuminatum or uterine cervical dysplasia should be treated at an early stage in the hopes of preventing progression to in situ or frankly invasive cancers.

ACKNOWLEDGMENT

The author thanks his many colleagues throughout the world who have generously contributed data concerning their patients to the CTTR.

RECOMMENDED READING

Birkeland SA, Storm HH, Lamm LU, et al. Cancer Risk after renal transplantation in the Nordic countries 1964-1986. Intl J Cancer. 1995;60(2):183-189.

Bouwes Bavinck JN. Epidemiological aspects of immunosuppression: role of exposure to sunlight and human papillomavirus on the development of skin cancer. Hum Exp Toxicol. 1995;14(1):98.

Davis CL, Wood BL, Sabath DE, Joseph JS, Stehman-Breen C, Broudy VC. Interferon-alpha treatment of post-transplant lymphoproliferative disorder in recipients of solid organ transplants. Transplantation. 1998;66(12): 1770-1779.

Euvrard S, Kanitakis J, Pouteil-Noble C, Claudy, A, Touraine JL. Skin cancers in organ transplant recipients. Ann Transplant. 1997;2(4):28-32.

Green M, Reyes J, Rowe D. New strategies in the prevention and management of Epstein-Barr virus infection and posttransplant lymphoproliferative disease following solid organ transplantation. Curr Opin Transplant. 1998;3:143-147.

Hanto DW. Classification of Epstein-Barr virus-associated posttransplant lymphoproliferative diseases: implications for understanding their pathogenesis and developing rational treatment strategies. Annu Rev Med. 1995;46:381-394.

McDiarmid SV, Jordon S, Kim GS, et al. Prevention and preemptive therapy of posttransplant lymphoproliferative disease in pediatric liver recipients. Transplantation. 1998;66(12):1604-1611.

Montagnino G, Bencini PL, Tarantino A, Caputo R, Ponticelli C. Clinical features and course of Kaposi's sarcoma in kidney transplant patients: report of 13 cases. Am J Nephrol. 1994;14(2):12l-126.

Nalesnik MA. Clinicopathologic features of posttransplant lymphoproliferative disorders. Ann Transplant. 1997;2(4);33-40.

Nalesnik MA, Rao AS, Furukawa H, et al. Autologous lymphokine-activated killer cell therapy of Epstein-Barr virus-positive and -negative lymphoproliferative disorders arising in organ transplant recipients. Transplantation. 1997;63(9):1200-1205.

Penn I. Why do immunosuppressed patients develop cancer? In: Pimentel E, ed. CRC Critic Reviews in Oncogenesis. Boca Raton, Fla: CRC; 1989:27-52.

Penn I. The problem of cancer in organ transplant recipients: an overview. Transplant Sci. 1994;4(1):23-32.

Penn I. Kaposi's sarcoma in transplant recipients. Transplantation. 1997;64(5):669-673.

Penn I. De novo cancers in organ allograft recipients. Curr Opinion Org Transplant. 1998;3:188-196.

Penn I. Posttransplant malignancies. Transplant Proc. 1999;31(1-2):1260-1262.

Penn I. De novo malignant lesions of the central nervous system in organ allograft recipients. In Wijdicks EFM, Ed. Neurologic complications in organ transplant recipients. Boston, Mass: Butterworth - Heinemann; 1999:217-227.

Rowe DT, Qu L, Reyes J, et al. Use of quantitative competitive PCR to measure Epstein-Barr virus genome load in the peripheral blood of pediatric transplant patients with lymphoproliferative disorders. J Clin Microbiol. 1997;35(6):1612-1615.

Sheil AG, Disney AP, Mathew TH, Amiss N. De novo malignancy emerges as a major cause of morbidity and late failure in renal transplantation. Transplant Proc. 1993;25(1 Pt 2):1383-1384.

Sheil AG. Skin cancer in renal transplant recipients. Transplant Sci. 1994;4(1):42-45.

Starzl TE, Nalesnik MA, Porter KA, et al. Reversibility of lymphomas and lymphoproliferative lesions developing under cyclosporin-steroid therapy. Lancet. 1984;1(8377): 583-587.

27 TRANSPLANTATION AND REPRODUCTIVE HEALTH

Thomas R. Easterling, MD
Darcy Carr, MD

Procreation is a central event of human experience. The physiological and psychological impact of chronic, debilitating disease weakens sexual identity and reproductive function. While diminished child-bearing potential may be grieved as deeply as a lost child, this grief may be displaced by the patient and go unnoticed by the health care practitioner in the midst of a life-threatening illness. Successful organ transplantation frequently improves the sense of self and corrects physiological barriers to reproductive function. The desire to reproduce, an affirmation of renewed personal potential, is consequently aroused. Given an expected ambivalence between the desire to reproduce and fear of graft compromise, reproductive counseling prior to transplantation may be beneficial for many patients and their partners.

GYNECOLOGICAL CARE
Birth Control
Ovulatory function and menstrual regularity should return after kidney and liver transplants. Conception shortly after transplant has been reported. Pregnancy in the context of early rejection will bode poorly for the pregnancy and the graft. Table 27-1 summarizes available methods of birth control. Failure rates are reported as pregnancies in the first year of use. Natural methods, based on timing of ovulation, require menstrual regularity and attention to detail. They are generally not appropriate in the context of the need to absolutely prevent pregnancy and are not practical while recovering regular menstrual function. Barrier methods do not provide an absolute level of pregnancy prevention for many couples.

Low-dose mixed estrogen/progestational oral contraceptives, ($\leq$35 μg ethinyl estradiol), are very effective and safe for many women. Estrogen-containing pills are contraindicated in women with a history of thrombosis, worsening migraine headaches, worsening antihypertensive control and in women who are over 35 years old and continue to smoke. Specific information on

Thomas R. Easterling, MD, Associate Professor, Department of Obstetrics and Gynecology, University of Washington Medical Center, Seattle, WA

Darcy Carr, MD, Acting Instructor, Department of Obstetrics and Gynecology, University of Washington Medical Center, Seattle, WA

the use of these pills in female transplant patients is not available, although many recipients have safely received mixed oral contraceptives.

Progestin-only oral contraceptive pills (OCPs), (ie, the mini-pill), avoid the thrombotic risks of estrogen-containing pills. They are used frequently in patients with clotting disorders, diabetes, or cardiovascular disease. They are somewhat less effective than mixed OCPs and require careful attention to compliance and should be taken at the same time every day. These limitations are probably less of a problem for transplant patients. Over time, the lack of estrogen influence on the endometrium may result in breakthrough bleeding. While not usually heavy, bleeding can be persistent and inconvenient. Periodic short courses of estrogen may mitigate the problem.

Parenteral progestins offer certain advantages. They are not associated with medical complications; they do not require daily compliance. Depo Provera requires an IM injection every three months. Fertility may not return for six to nine months after the last injection. Norplant achieves its effectiveness through the tonic release of a very low dose of progestational agent, norethindrone. The effective dose of hormone is much lower than with Depo Provera. Norplant requires a minor surgical procedure to insert five silastic rods and a second procedure to remove them. A single insertion is effective for five years. Both Depo Provera and Norplant provide a progestational dominant effect on the endometrium and therefore may be associated with irregular bleeding. Although there is no published data on the safety and efficacy of these agents in transplant recipients, they are used quite frequently with few recorded side effects.

Intrauterine devices are very effective and do not require daily compliance. In healthy women, a risk of pelvic inflammatory disease exists but has been overstated. While clinical trials do not exist in transplanted patients, the presence of a foreign body in the face of immunosuppression is probably an unacceptable risk. In addition, immunosuppression may reduce the associated inflammatory response and therefore reduce contraceptive effectiveness.

Sterilization by tubal ligation or vasectomy are good options for couples who are certain that they want no more children. Given the complexity of decision making and the stress surrounding transplant, care must be exercised in performing sterilization at or around the time of transplant.

Fertility
Transplantation is usually associated with improved fertility. The exception is bone marrow transplantation. High-dose chemotherapy with or without total body irradiation frequently results in ovarian failure or azoospermia. Oophoropexy to shield the ovaries from

Table 27-1. Methods of Birth Control

	Failure Rate (in first 12 mo.)	Major Complications	Minor Complications	Benefits
Ovulation Prediction	20%	pregnancy	—	—
Barrier • condoms • diaphragm • cervical cap	10-20%	pregnancy	UTI's with diaphragm	STD protection
Combined oral contraceptive pills (≤μg ethinyl estradiol)	3%	thrombosis (RR 2.2) Stroke (RR 3.1) Hypertension (5%) MI (smokers > 35 yo)	migraine	protection from PID, ovarian and endometrial cancer, Fe deficiency
Progestin oral contraceptive pills	2%	none	irregular bleeding	protection from PID and endometrial cancer
Intrauterine device	3%	pelvic infection	dysmenorrhea	none
Parenteral • Depo provera • Norplant	<1%	none	irregular bleeding, removal, delayed return to ovulation	improved compliance
RR indicates relative risk				

radiation has not been effective. Pharmacological down-regulation of gonadal function prior to treatment has had limited success. Men can easily store semen prior to treatment. Embryos after hyperstimulation and in vitro fertilization (IVF) can also be stored. Women without a partner can store embryos from IVF with donor semen or conceive with donor oocytes through IVF after successful transplantation. Oocyte preservation has not been successful. Preservation of ovarian tissue with reimplantation is potentially feasible in the future.

Spontaneous pregnancies after bone marrow transplant, although uncommon, have been reported. Elevated gonadotropins indicative of menopausal ovarian function seen often in bone marrow recipients do not insure against subsequent recovery of function. Recovery of ovarian function is frequently delayed by as much as five to six years. Patients not wishing to be pregnant should receive contraceptive counseling and possible sterilization despite loss of ovarian function.

Cancer

Cyclosporine-based maintenance immunosuppression increases the risk for cervical cancer by as much as ninefold. Regular gynecological care and annual PAP smears are critical.

PREGNANCY

Pregnancy is not a disease state, but it is a state of significant physiological stress, especially in the context of abnormal maternal physiology. Pregnancy frequently requires subjugation of maternal needs in favor of the needs of the developing fetus. Table 27-2 lists important considerations for medical practitioners interacting with woman who are considering pregnancy. The decision to become pregnant represents the balance of two forces: (1) the risk of the pregnancy to the mother and to the fetus itself, and (2) the value of the pregnancy, the potential child, to the woman herself. The objective medical risk may be consistently defined from patient to patient based on our growing experience. The subjective value of the pregnancy will vary widely between patients and is therefore usually the critical driver of the final decision. Table 27-3 summarizes the physiological changes associated with pregnancy.

Hemodynamic Physiology in Pregnancy

Hemodynamic changes in pregnancy are described in Figure 27-1. Mean arterial pressure falls sharply in the first half of pregnancy and rises to near nonpregnant levels by the end of the third trimester. Cardiac output rises early in pregnancy and steadily into the third trimester. Commensurate with the rise in cardiac output, plasma volume increases by approximately 40%. Vascular resistance falls in the first trimester and rises toward term as blood pressure increases to near nonpregnant levels. After midpregnancy, pregnant women are vulnerable to supine hypotension due to a reduction in venous return due to compression of the vena cava by the gravid

---

Table 27-2. Counseling Medically Complicated Patients Regarding Pregnancy

- The inherent value of one's child is immeasurable and not rationally based.
- All women accept some risk to their health and life when undertaking a pregnancy.
- The specific value of a pregnancy, a potential child, will be different from woman to woman.
- The specific value of a pregnancy will be different in the same woman at different points in her life.
- The inherent value of a pregnancy, of reproducing, is frequently enhanced rather than diminished by a serious medical condition.
- Personal values directing choices regarding pregnancy are patient-specific.
- The goal of counseling should be to achieve concordance between partners. However, the counseling should focus on the partner assuming risk with a pregancy, the woman.
- The physician's role counseling a medically complicated patient regarding pregnancy involves:
  - educating the patient regarding risks.
  - admitting to the variability and unpredictability of risk.
  - assisting the integration of risk into the context of the patient's value system to form a decision.
  - supporting the patient in carrying out her decisions.

---

uterus. Sedated or anesthetized pregnant women can become profoundly hypotensive if left supine. Rotating the pregnant woman as little as 15 to 20 degrees out of the supine position will prevent hypotension. While rotation to the left side is usually recommended, rotation to the right is usually as effective.

Most cardiac disease, with the notable exception of pulmonary hypertension, can be effectively managed through pregnancy. Intercurrent events such as febrile infections or hemorrhage may result in rapid decompensation. Appropriate management of the patient's volume status with diuretics and heart rate control are the cornerstones of antepartum management.

Renal Physiology in Pregnancy

Glomerular filtration rate is elevated as soon as pregnancy can be detected and rises to 40% above nonpregnant norms by the end of the first trimester. Increased filtration is mediated primarily by a commensurate rise in renal blood flow. Adjustment in dosage of medications that are renally cleared is therefore required. Under the influence of progesterone, ureters relax during pregnancy creating a dilated collecting system and substantial dead space. If untreated, as many as 20% of women with asymptomatic bacteriuria in pregnancy will develop febrile pyelonephritis.

Renal insufficiency of modest degree increases the risk for new hypertension during pregnancy, exacerbation of preexisting hypertension or for the development of preeclampsia. Women with a serum creatinine at or over 2.5 mg/dL can expect to hasten the course to dialysis by carrying a pregnancy. Women with serum creatinine at or under 1.5 mg/dL can be expected to have an outcome similar to a cohort of analogous women who did not get pregnant. The fetuses of women with renal disease are at risk for preterm delivery, fetal growth restriction, and fetal demise.

Table 27-3. Physiology of Pregnancy

- Hemodynamic
  - 40% increase in plasma volume
  - reduced colloid osmotic pressure
  - 40% increase in cardiac output
  - cardiac output driven by heart rate in third trimester
  - stroke work index unchanged
- Renal
  - 40% increase in GFR
  - dilated collecting system
- Pulmonary
  - increased O_2 consumption
  - 40% increase in minute ventilation
  - normal pCO_2 - 30 mmHg
  - normal HCO_3 - 22 mEq/L
  - increased severity of respiratory infections
- Gastrointestinal
  - increased esophageal reflux
  - increased constipation
  - gastroparesis tolerated poorly
- Diabetes
  - increased insulin resistance
  - 1st trimester hyperglycemia associated with birth defects
  - late hyperglycemia associated with neonatal complications
- Hematological
  - need for increased hematopoiesis
  - increased risk for thrombosis

Respiratory Physiology in Pregnancy

Oxygen consumption in pregnancy is increased by 15% to 20%. Due to the effects of progesterone, minute ventilation is increased by 40%, reducing pCO_2 to approximately 30 mmHg. Renal compensation results in an HCO_3 of approximately 22 mEq/L and a pH that is slightly elevated, 7.42. Tidal volume increases from 500 to 700 mL without change in respiratory rate. Additionally, it is important to note that expansion of total body albumin lags the expansion of plasma volume. Thus, in normal pregnancy, colloid osmotic pressure (COP) can be expected to fall to 20 to 22 mmHg facilitating the development of pulmonary edema.

Chronic pulmonary disease is usually well-tolerated in pregnancy. In general, asthma is unaffected by pregnancy and women with a vital capacity of greater-than-or-equal-to 30% of expected tolerate pregnancy well. However, although women with limited reserve may be well saturated at rest they may desaturate with minimal activity. Oxygen supplementation may be indicated to maintain adequate oxygen delivery to the fetus. Furthermore, pulmonary infections are tolerated poorly in pregnancy. While inherent immunosuppression may be in part responsible, reduced colloid osmotic pressure and an increased tendency for loss of capillary integrity predispose for loss of fluid into alveolar spaces.

Gastrointestinal Physiology in Pregnancy

Progesterone relaxes smooth muscle. While beneficial to uterine function, loss of tone complicates gastrointestinal function. Esophageal reflux associated with loss of tone in the lower esophageal sphincter is common and may present with classic "heartburn" symptoms, or with persistent nausea. Conservative measures such as antacid use or elevation of the head of the bed will be sufficient for some women. Others will require the use of H_2 blockers. Constipation due to decreased colonic transit time is common and is usually managed with bulk agents. Women with gastroparesis due to diabetes can be difficult to manage during pregnancy.

Hepatic function is generally unaltered in pregnancy. Clinical liver function tests are unchanged except for an elevated level of alkaline phosphatase due to placental isoenzyme. Intrahepatic cholestasis, characterized by intense itching, responds poorly to therapy and may be associated with fetal distress and fetal demise near term. Elevations of liver function tests may occur in association with preeclampsia and may precede the onset of hypertension. Acute fatty liver, also unique to pregnancy, is characterized by moderate elevations in liver function tests, increased serum bilirubin, profound coagulopathy and hypoglycemia which, if not treated aggressively, can be fatal.

Diabetes in Pregnancy

Pregnancy is a state of increasing insulin resistance. Women who are insulin resistant but euglycemic when not pregnant may become hyperglycemic when pregnant and require diet and/or insulin therapy. Women with established diabetes will require as much as twofold to threefold increases in insulin dosing by term. Medications such as prednisone, especially at higher doses, and tacrolimus will increase the tendency to be hyperglycemic. Poor glycemic control in the first trimester is associated with marked increase in risk for

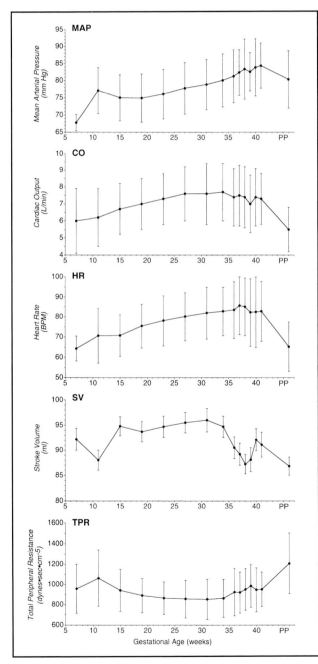

Figure 27-1. Hemodynamic changes in normotensive pregnant women.

birth defects and miscarriage. Later in pregnancy, poor control is associated with fetal macrosomia, increased neonatal complications, fetal demise, and potentially maternal hypertension. Euglycemia, (glucose $\leq$ 90 to 105 mg/dL and postprandial glucose $\leq$ 120 mg/dL), is the goal for diabetic management in pregnancy. Screening should be repeated with advancing gestation due to increasing insulin resistance. Usually, insulin injections at breakfast, dinner and bedtime or management with a pump are required to maintain euglycemia.

Hematological Physiology in Pregnancy

Expansion of red cell mass usually lags the expansion of plasma volume resulting in physiologic anemia. Blunted erythropoiesis due to a maternal shortage of substrate (eg, iron), immunosuppressive agent toxicity (eg, azathioprine), or chronic disease can result in significant anemia. When clinically indicated, erythropoietin therapy can be used in pregnancy.

Pregnant women have an increased tendency for clot formation associated with marked increases in the levels of fibrinogen and factor VIII and lesser elevations in factors VII, IX, and X. Acquired or inherited coagulopathies are frequently first diagnosed during pregnancy. Women with known coagulopathy or a history of a significant thrombosis are usually anticoagulated with heparin for all or part of their pregnancies.

Labor

Labor is a physiological stress unique to a pregnancy. Uterine contractions are associated with an abrupt return of 400 to 500 mL of blood to the central circulation. Heart rate, stroke volume, cardiac output, and pulmonary artery pressure increase with contractions. Pain augments the physiological stress. Pushing in the second state of labor further increases maternal work. Women with limited cardiac or pulmonary reserve may tolerate an unmedicated birth poorly. With careful fluid management, sometimes directed with invasive hemodynamic monitoring, careful pain control with regional anesthesia, and limited or no pushing, most women with medical complications can deliver vaginally. Cesarean section is usually reserved for obstetrical indications. Postpartum, most women mobilize extravascular fluid and diurese spontaneously. Women with pregnancies complicated by heart disease, renal disease, or hypertension frequently benefit from augmented diuresis.

Hypertension and Preeclampsia

Hypertension remains a significant cause of maternal and fetal morbidity and mortality. Preeclampsia is characterized by the rapid onset of hypertension and proteinuria. With increasing severity, preeclampsia is associated with deteriorating renal function, abnormal liver function tests, and thrombocytopenia. Cerebral edema, pulmonary edema or hepatic subcapsular hematoma represent life-threatening complications. The pathophysiology of preeclampsia is poorly understood, and therefore efforts to cure or prevent preeclampsia have had limited success. Endothelial activation and/or injury and the loss of endothelial functions associated with blood pressure regulation, vessel wall integrity, and regulation of thrombosis are central features to our current, but limited, understanding of the disease. Neither low-dose aspirin therapy nor calcium supplementation have been found to prevent preeclampsia. Diverse maternal conditions associated with the development of preeclampsia include: nulliparity, chronic hypertension, renal insufficiency, diabetes, hyperthyroidism, collagen vascular disease, multiple gestation, and molar pregnancy. Many preexisting medical conditions associated with preeclampsia are associated with microvascular injury and endothelial activation outside pregnancy. Aggressive preconceptual management of associated medical conditions may decrease the risk for subsequent preeclampsia.

Near term, preeclampsia is managed with delivery of the fetus. Intrapartum, magnesium sulfate is used for seizure prophylaxis and maternal blood pressure is controlled with antihypertensive agents. A further exacerbation in hypertension can be expected for several days after delivery. Near term preeclampsia requires careful management of the maternal and fetal condition but is rarely a complication of significant magnitude to dissuade women from carrying a pregnancy. Complete recovery to prepregnant baseline is expected.

The development of preterm preeclampsia requires more complicated decision making. The most prudent course for maternal health continues to be delivery of the fetus. However, as described below, preterm delivery carries significant short-term and long-term risks to the neonate. In general, preterm preeclampsia is managed with the following priorities: (1) protection of the mother from life-threatening complications; (2) prolongation of the pregnancy to achieve a more mature fetus at birth; and (3) support of fetal growth in utero. The maternal condition is protected with control of hypertension and careful observation for advancing disease. Angiotensin-converting enzyme inhibitors and receptor blockers are avoided in the second and third trimesters due to associated risks of oligohydramnios, pulmonary hypoplasia and neonatal renal failure. While alpha methyldopa is frequently cited as the first drug of choice, it is rarely used in patients with serious hypertension. Beta blockers and diuretics when used in excess are associated with poor fetal growth. Vasodilators used alone may not be effective in controlling hypertension. No specific antihypertensive regimen is clearly favored in pregnancy. From our experience using noninvasive hemodynamics to direct antihypertensive therapy, we have found that hypertension characterized by elevated cardiac output can be managed effectively with a beta blocker. Hypertension mediated by increased resistance can be treated with vasodilators such as hydralazine or clonidine and low-dose beta blockade.

Prematurity

High-risk pregnancies are managed understanding the relative impact of different degrees of prematurity on the fetus. The rates of mortality and long-term serious complications associated with preterm delivery are described in Figure 27-2. Fetuses delivered prior to 24 weeks' gestation rarely survive. The survivors between 24 and 26 weeks gestation will experience very prolonged hospitalization and high rates of long-term handicaps such as cerebral palsy, blindness, and learning disabilities. At 28 weeks, survival exceeds 90% and severe long-term handicaps are less than 10%. Births at 34 weeks and beyond will have outcomes close to infants born at term. Premature infants born at less than the tenth percentile for gestational age will have a more complicated course than those at the same gestational age but normally grown.

Congenital Infections

Certain maternal infections can be transmitted to the fetus. Syphilis, rubella, toxoplasmosis, varicella and cytomegalovirus (CMV), can be transmitted transplacentally resulting in congential infections, neonatal mortality and long-term morbidity. Human immunodeficiency virus (HIV), can be transmitted transplacentally or at delivery. Aggressive maternal antiviral therapy will reduce transmission. Human parvovirus can be transmitted transplacentally resulting in a transient but potentially lethal fetal aplastic anemia that can be successfully treated with intrauterine transfusion. Viral

hepatitis, herpes simplex, and human papilloma virus can be transmitted at delivery. Perinatal transmission of hepatitis B can be reduced with neonatal treatment with immune globulin and subsequent immunization.

CMV infection is of particular concern for immunosuppressed transplant patients. CMV can be transmitted with primary infection or with reactivation. Between 0.5% and 2.5% of newborns are infected during pregnancy. Primary maternal CMV infections acquired at or before 20 weeks gestation are more likely to result in symptomatic infection. Adverse neonatal outcomes such as low birth weight, microcephaly, or chorioretinitis, are more likely with disease that is symptomatic at birth and with primary maternal disease. Long-term prognosis is poor. Survivors are likely to suffer hearing loss, mental retardation, psychomotor delay, seizures and learning disabilities. Congenital infection with CMV can be suspected in the presence of fetal hydrops, echogenic fetal bowel, and intracerebral calcifications detected on antenatal ultrasound. The diagnosis can be confirmed with culture of amniotic fluid or CMV-PCR. Congenital CMV infection has been reported in mothers carrying pregnancies after kidney and liver transplant. Mothers with primary infection after transplant are clearly at risk for transplacental infection but neonatal infection following CMV reactivation in the mother has also been reported. At this time there is little systematic information available about CMV disease in pregnant transplant recipients; thus the necessity for CMV surveillance, especially in CMV-positive recipients, is not known.

TRANSPLANTATION AND PREGNANCY

Pregnancy after renal transplantation, (from an identical twin), was first reported in 1963. Since that time, a large experience with pregnancy after renal transplantation has developed. The reported experience after liver and heart transplantation, although not as large, is substantial. Reports of pregnancy after pancreas transplant are less common and are usually in the context of a kidney transplant. Experience after lung transplant is very limited and has frequently been in conjunction with a heart transplant. Although the data collected to date on posttransplant pregnancy is limited in scope and is from varied sources with different definitions of disease categories and outcome, some reasonable conclusions can be drawn.

Graft Survival

Increased renal blood flow and GFR associated with pregnancy could potentially mediate deterioration of renal function. Renal transplant recipients with modest renal insufficiency, (serum creatinine ≤1.5 mg/dL), augment renal function early in pregnancy causing a fall in

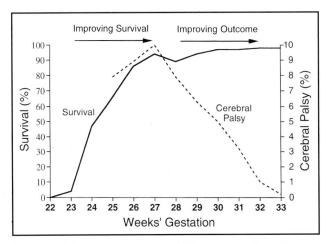

Figure 27-2. Long-term severe morbidity and mortality associated with preterm delivery. Long-term severe morbidity includes cerebral palsy, blindness and deafness. Mortality includes death prior to hospital discharge.

the serum creatinine. If pregnancy-induced hypertension or preeclampsia develop in these patients, the ensuing renal deterioration can be expected to resolve weeks to months after delivery. Long-term graft survival in renal transplant patients with good renal function at conception has not been shown to be adversely affected by the pregnancy. Several studies have evaluated the graft survival and function of women carrying pregnancies compared to men with similar renal function or to comparable women who did not carry a pregnancy. Survival and function have been shown to be the same at four, 15, and 12 years.

Long-term outcomes for transplant recipients carrying pregnancies with more severe renal insufficiency are not available. However, reasonable generalizations from women with renal insufficiency not associated with renal allografts can be made. Women with a serum creatinine of or more than 2.5 mg/dL can expect to lose renal function associated with pregnancy and move more quickly to the need for dialysis. Women with a serum creatinine between 1.5 and 2.5 mg/dL can expect mixed results; some will experience a loss in function while others will not.

Systematic reports of graft loss associated with other transplanted organs is lacking. To date, 168 pregnancies in liver allograft recipients have been recorded with each of the following reported once: graft dysfunction, graft loss in the second trimester, and re-transplant postpartum. These outcomes are probably not different than expected outside pregnancy. In 34 reports of pregnancy associated with pancreas transplant, graft dysfunction is not reported, although rejection soon after delivery has been reported. Despite the challenge of insulin resistance associated with pregnancy, glucose intolerance requiring insulin has not been documented. In 29 pregnancies reported in cardiac recipients, significant cardiac dysfunction has not occurred. In ten cases of lung transplantation, two women deteriorated in the third trimester and died within 24 months of delivery. While these outcomes may suggest concern, the numbers are small and may fall within the expected outcome of patients with lung transplant outside pregnancy. In general, pregnancy does not seem to impact graft survival. Rejection is certainly not more common in pregnancy.

Liver transplantation has been performed during pregnancy. The coagulopathy associated with liver failure makes termination of pregnancy prior to transplant more dangerous than proceeding with transplantation while continuing the pregnancy. Of six reviewed cases, four fetuses survived to viability. Two of these had a preterm delivery; one of the infants born preterm was severely growth-restricted.

Neonatal Outcomes

Potential causes of adverse neonatal outcomes are congenital malformations, premature delivery, fetal growth restriction, and fetal demise. Congenital malformations will be discussed in the context of medications. The risk for fetal demise is managed through the use of maternal fetal movement counts, electronic fetal monitoring, (nonstress tests or contraction stress tests), and the use of ultrasound to assess fetal growth, amniotic fluid volume and biophysical profile. Ultrasound Doppler measurements of flow velocity in the umbilical cord and uterine arteries can be used to predict fetal growth restriction. A complimentary set of tests is usually used with increasing frequency towards term to predict the risk for fetal demise.

Fetal growth restriction and preterm birth are the most common neonatal complications associated with transplantation. Spontaneous preterm labor or rupture of membranes, fetal distress, or severe hypertension prior to term are responsible for preterm births. Table 27-4 lists complication rates associated with different organ transplants. These estimates of risk are subject to the limitations of the data previously discussed. Patients with renal transplants seem to have higher rates of neonatal complications than do patients with heart, liver, or pancreas transplants. The increased complication rates are consistent with those in patients with renal insufficiency and therefore more likely to be due to impaired renal function than transplantation itself. Lung transplantation, however, may be associated with even greater risks, but the data is limited by small numbers and the significant possibility of reporting bias.

Medications

Medications used in pregnancy can be associated with adverse outcomes due to teratogenicity or to physiological effects throughout pregnancy. The potential for teratogenicity is limited to the period of organogenesis,

Table 27-4. Transplant Complications in Pregnancy

	Cases	Preterm Delivery	Fetal Growth Restriction
Kidney	1556	50%	40%
Pancreas	34	15%	14%
Liver	168	8%	10%
Heart	29	14%	14%
Lung	10	50%	40%

Pregnancies included that completed at least 20 weeks' gestation.

*Preterm delivery reported as <34 weeks gestation at delivery except in renal transplant where data is summarized in large series (<37 weeks).

Cases with pancreas/kidney transplants are classifed as pancreas transplant. Cases with heart/lung transplant are classified as lung transplants.

15 to 60 days after conception corresponding roughly to four to 11 weeks from the last menstrual period. Despite legitimate, serious concerns due to the adverse reproductive experience with drugs such as thalidomide, a very limited number of drugs are known to be teratogens.

PREDNISONE. Prednisone has been used extensively in pregnancy. Prednisone and prednisolone are actively metabolized by the placenta resulting in minimal passage to the fetus. When treatment of the fetus with glucocorticoids is desirable, (eg, induction of pulmonary maturity, congenital adrenal hyperplasia), treatment with betamethasone or dexamethasone is required. While some animal studies have suggested teratogenicity associated with glucocorticoids, the association has not been confirmed in human pregnancy.

The use of glucocorticoids in pregnancy is associated with the development of glucose intolerance. Hyperglycemia in the first trimester is clearly teratogenic. In the second and third trimesters, it is associated with the development of fetal macrosomia and neonatal complications. All pregnant women on glucocorticoids should be regularly screened for hyperglycemia.

Treatment with prednisone during pregnancy is also associated with an increased risk for preterm premature rupture of membranes. The mechanism of action may be an alteration in the maternal immune response and resulting change in the vaginal bacterial ecology.

Alternatively, prednisone might have a direct effect on the strength of the connective tissue in the amnion and chorion. Women on prednisone should have their vaginal flora screened and treatment initiated for evidence of bacterial vaginosis.

The impact of prednisone in pregnancy is dependent on the dose and length of therapy. Immunosuppression at the lowest dose possible is desirable. A short course of high-dose steroids is relatively benign and is frequently used in anticipation of a premature delivery to improve pulmonary maturity.

AZATHIOPRINE. Azathioprine has been used extensively in pregnancy. Small series have reported anomaly rates from 0% to as high as 9% but without consistent patterns of malformation. Use of azathioprine with other medications and in the face of azotemia complicate interpretation of reported cases. Based on "poor to fair" data, the Teris Data Base suggests that the risk for malformations is "minimal to small." Increased rates of fetal growth restriction are reported in patients treated with azathioprine. Serious neonatal anemia, thrombocytopenia, and lymphopenia have been reported. A single case of de novo constitutional chromosomal anomalies has been reported in a fetus of a treated mother. If this case represents a risk of azathioprine during gametogenesis, the risk is small.

Adequate expansion of maternal red cell mass to match the increase in plasma volume associated with

Table 27-5. Transplant Medications in Pregnancy

	Experience in Pregnancy	Teratogenicity	Placental Transfer	Physiological Impact	Breast Feeding
prednisone	extensive	unlikely	limited	glucose intolerance risk for premature rupture of membranes	no restriction
azathioprine	extensive	minimal to small	yes	anemia, leukopenia thrombocytopenia maternal and fetal	limited secretion complications not reported
cyclosporine	large	minimal	yes	hypertension	not recommended neonatal levels undetectable
tacrolimus	limited	(-) animal data	yes	hypertension hyperglycemia	not recommended
mycophenolate mofetil	very limited	(+) animal data resorbtion and malformation at 4.5mg/kg/day	—	—	secreted in milk of rats
muromonab-CD3	very limited	unlikely	yes	cytokine activation	unlikely secretion
acyclovir	extensive	none	yes	none	no restriction

pregnancy may not occur while being treated with azathioprine. After other causes of maternal anemia are ruled out, discontinuation of the drug can be considered based on the perceived need in the individual patient.

CYCLOSPORINE. Cyclosporine has been used extensively in pregnancy. All women treated have had serious medical problems and have usually received other concurrent medications. Case reports and small series of treated patients do occasionally report significant malformations. However, these reports do not suggest a pattern of malformation nor a rate of malformation inconsistent from baseline. Based on "fair" data, the Teris Data Base suggests that the risk for malformations is "minimal".

Fetal growth restriction is common among women treated with cyclosporine and is in part due to their diagnoses requiring treatment. However, cyclosporine treatment itself is associated with a uniquely vasoconstrictive form of hypertension. Vasoconstrictive hypertension poses a particular risk for fetal growth restriction. Supporting a plausible physiological basis is the report in 1994 from the National Transplant Registry. While women treated with a cyclosporine based regimen had comparable rates of prematurity with those treated with regimens of prednisone and azathioprine alone, they were at greater risk for small babies. Fifty percent of pregnancies exposed to cyclosporine resulted in babies less than 2,500 grams compared to 31% of those managed without cyclosporine. Eighteen percent of pregnancies exposed resulted in births less than 1,500 grams compared to 8% in those not exposed. Again, based on only "fair" data, the risk for fetal growth restriction associated with cyclosporine seems to be "small to moderate." Since the vasoconstrictive effects of cyclosporine may be dose-dependent, drug levels should be maintained in a narrow therapeutic window.

Treatment with cyclosporine has not been associated with fetal renal toxicity. Transient neonatal thrombocytopenia, neutropenia and lymphopenia have been reported, as have fetal infection with cytomegalovirus.

Breast-feeding while taking cyclosporine has been discouraged by the American Academy of Pediatrics. These recommendations are based on breast milk-to-serum ratios of .28 to .40. However, breast milk concentrations are in ng/mL concentrations. Based on average milk consumption and equally poor absorption in the neonate compared to adults, unmeasurable levels would be expected. Undetectable levels of cyclosporine have been reported in a small series of breast-feeding women. Given the uncertain impact of even modest exposure to cyclosporine, the decision to breast-feed must be an individualized informed decision balancing small unknown risks against the potential benefits of breast-feeding.

TACROLIMUS. Tacrolimus has been used in pregnancy, but the total reported literature is too small at this time to be conclusive. Reports to date have not suggested problems beyond those already described for cyclosporine. Given a lower incidence of hypertensive complications with tacrolimus outside pregnancy, there may be cause to hope that rates of fetal growth restriction will be lower. Patients treated with tacrolimus should be expected to be at increased risk for gestational diabetes.

OTHERS. The current experience with mycophenolate in pregnancy is too limited to draw meaningful conclusions. Animal data suggest that fetal malformations and resorbtions occur at doses higher than used for immunosuppression. Experience with muromonab-CD3 in pregnancy is also limited. Like all IgG, it is actively transported across the placenta. As noted above, pregnant women are more prone to pulmonary edema and tolerate capillary leak poorly. Activated cytokine pathways are probably central in the pathophysiology of premature labor and preeclampsia. Muromonab-CD3 should therefore be used carefully in pregnancy with vigilant surveillance undertaken for the development of pulmonary edema, preeclampsia or premature labor.

MANAGEMENT DURING PREGNANCY
Timing of Pregnancy
Most young women receiving a transplant have been avoiding pregnancy but will be anxious to have a child some time following surgery. Recommendations regarding a delay in pregnancy have ranged from six months to two years. Postponing pregnancy beyond the first six months after transplant when graft loss is the highest will reduce the risk of acute rejection superimposed on pregnancy. Additionally, primary CMV infection may be more easily cleared while on maintenance immunosuppression (beyond six months) thus avoiding primary CMV in utero exposure.

The "ideal" transplant patient should be on a stable regimen of immunosuppression without evidence of rejection for six to 12 months prior to conception. The necessary prednisone dose should be at or under 15 mg/d. Renal function should be minimally impaired with a serum creatinine less than 1.5 mg/dL. Proteinuria should be minimal. Hypertension should be absent or well-controlled for six to 12 months. Blood sugar should be normalized with insulin if necessary. Many patients who choose to attempt pregnancy will not meet all of these criteria. To the extent that they do not, more complicated pregnancies and worse perinatal outcomes should be expected.

After an individual patient achieves their "optimal" condition, a decision should be made to proceed with conception or to avoid pregnancy based on the individual's medical circumstances and the value associated with pregnancy. Significant delay increases the chance that the patient develops worsening renal insufficiency and vasoconstrictive hypertension associated with the use of cyclosporine or tacrolimus.

Hypertension

Hypertension is the most common complication experienced by pregnant women with a transplant. Women with a kidney transplant are at risk, as are all women with renal insufficiency. Acute cyclosporine nephrotoxicity, mediated by afferent arteriolar vasoconstriction, is typically associated with hypertension and systemic vasoconstriction. Vasoconstrictive hypertension is difficult to treat in pregnancy while maintaining adequate fetal perfusion.

Clear standards do not exist for the pharmacological management of hypertension in pregnancy. Early treatment may prevent maternal hypertensive crisis but can further impair fetal growth. Based on the impact of hypertension on the clinical course of renal disease outside pregnancy, hypertension in pregnancy should be aggressively managed. The choice of therapy is frequently a compromise between maximal maternal benefit and preservation of placental perfusion. Our management is based on the following principles: (1) Endothelial activation and injury are central to the pathophysiology of preeclampsia. Women entering pregnancy with activated endothelium will be more likely to develop preeclampsia and to develop it at an earlier gestational age. Therefore, aggressive antihypertensive control preconceptually is recommended, frequently with an ACE inhibitor in conjunction with a beta blocker or diuretic. ACE inhibitors are not teratogenic and therefore do not require discontinuation prior to conception. They should be stopped in the first trimester. (2) Antihypertensive therapy is directed by noninvasive measurements of maternal hemodynamics with the goal of normalizing cardiac output and vascular resistance. Some women can be treated with a single agent such as atenolol. Many, particularly those with more advanced hypertension such as that due to cyclosporine, will require the addition of a vasodilator. These patients may be treated with 25 to 50 mg of atenolol and 100 to 200 mg of hydralazine per day. Clonidine is usually a second line vasodilator. Alternatively, other groups have found success with the combined alpha and beta effects of labetalol. (3) The threshold to initiate antihypertensive therapy with small doses of medication should be low. (4) Postpartum, fluid that has been accumulated peripherally throughout pregnancy is mobilized rapidly. The magnitude of the intrinsic volume loading is frequently not appreciated and therefore not treated. We routinely initiate and maintain diuresis early in the postpartum period to prevent and treat worsening hypertension.

Cytomegalovirus

Congenitally acquired CMV infections are devastating to the fetus. Once fetal disease is clinically evident, fetal damage has occurred and intervention should not be expected to be successful. Ganciclovir treatment after diagnosis of fetal infection has been attempted, but without success. Delaying pregnancy (particularly when the patient is CMV negative with a CMV positive transplant) until an antibody response is achieved and viremia has resolved will reduce the chance of serious fetal infection. Where the risk of primary CMV infection is high, surveillance for plasma viremia with CMV-PCR and treatment of early viremia with ganciclovir, while untested, could potentially ameliorate fetal complications. Therapy for maternal disease should not be withheld due to concerns for the pregnancy. When congenital CMV infection is diagnosed antenatally, mothers should be counseled regarding prognosis and potential choices regarding continuation of the pregnancy.

Immunosuppression

Immunosuppression should be maintained at levels consistent with nonpregnant management. The effector of pregnancy on cyclosporine pharmacokinetics is inconsistent. Adjustments in dosing should be individualized based on regular monitoring of serum levels.

Organ-Specific Considerations

Heart transplant patients who are well-compensated prior to conception usually tolerate pregnancy without difficulty. Neither failure of a transplanted heart nor accelerated atherosclerosis has been reported in pregnancy. Heart rate control with a beta blocker is appropriate as is management of fluid retention with judicious use of diuretics. Normal pregnancy is characterized by afterload reduction. Preeclampsia can be associated with a rapid transition from a vasodilated condition to one of intense vasoconstriction. Heart transplant recipients with accelerating hypertension should therefore be monitored intensively and treated early. Noninvasive measurements of maternal hemodynamics may be useful in detecting and initiating early treatment of vasoconstriction.

Although patients with a pancreas transplant should remain euglycemic in pregnancy, many exhibited end-stage diabetic complications prior to transplant. Autonomic neuropathy and gastroparesis, if present prior to transplantation, will persist. Gastroparesis in pregnancy can be very difficult to treat and at times requires prolonged parenteral nutrition. Adequate bowel motility frequently returns early in the postpartum period. If the exocrine pancreas is drained into the bladder, urine pregnancy tests will be falsely negative due to the enzymatic digestion of hCG, a polypeptide.

RECOMMENDED READING

Barrou BR, Gruessner AC, Sutherland DE, Gruessner RW. Pregnancy after pancreas transplantation in the cyclosporine era: report from the Internaltional Pancreas Transplant Registry. Transplantation. 1998;65(4):524-527.

Casele HL, Laifer SA. Pregnancy after liver transplantation. Semin Perinatol. 1998;22(2):149-155.

Dabney BJ, Ed. REPROTEXT® System (Edition expired 6/99). CD-Rom deliverable by MICROMEDEX, Inc., Englewood, CO. http://www.micromedex.com/products/pd-reprorisk.htm

Davison JM. Renal transplantation and pregnancy. Am J Kidney Dis. 1987;9(4):374-380.

Ghandour FZ, Knaus TC, Hricik DE. Immunosuppressive drugs in pregnancy. Adv Ren Replace Ther. 1998;5(1):31-37.

Gulati SC, Van Poznak C. Pregnancy after bone marrow transplantation. J Clin Oncol. 1998;16(5):1978-1985.

Jungers P, Chauveau D. Pregnancy in renal disease. Kidney Int. 1997;52(4):871-885.

Laifer SA, Ehrlich GD, Huff DS, Balsan MJ, Scantlebury VP. Congenital cytomegalovirus infection in offspring of liver transplant recipients. Clin Infect Dis. 1995; 20(1):52-55.

Little BB. Immunosuppressant therapy during gestation. Semin Perinatol. 1997;21(2):143-148.

Morini A, Spina V, Aleandri V, Cantonetti G, Lambiasi A, Papalia U. Pregnancy after heart transplant: update and case report. Hum Reprod. 1998;13(3);749-757.

Nyberg G, Haljamae U, Frisenette-Fich C, Wennergren M, Kjellemr I. Breast-feeding during treatment with cyclosporin. Transplantation. 1998;65(2):253-255.

Parry D, Hextall A, Banner N, Robinson V, Yacoub M. Pregnancy following lung transplantation. Transplant Proc. 1997;291-2):629.

Patapis P, Irani S, Mirza D, et al. Outcome of graft function and pregnancy following liver transplantation. Transplant Proc. 1997;29(1-2):1565-1566.

Radomski JS, Moritz MJ, Monoz SJ, Cater JR, Jarrell BE, Armenti VT. National transplantation pregnancy registry: analysis of pregnancy outcomes in female liver transplant recipients. Liver. Transplant Surg. 1995:1(5):281-284.

Rayes N, Neuhaus R, David M, Steinmuller T, Bechstein W, Neuhaus P. Pregnancies following liver transplantation–how safe are they? A report of 19 cases under cyclosporine A and tracrolimus. Clin Transplant. 1998;12(5):396-400.

Scott JR, Wagoner LE, Olsen SL, Taylor DO, Renlund DG. Pregnancy in heart transplant recipients: management and outcome. Obstet Gynecol. 1993;82(3):324-327.

Troche V, Ville Y, Fernandez H. Pregnancy after heart or heart-lung transplantation: a series of ten pregnancies. Br J Obstet Gynaecol. 1998;105(4):454-458.

Ville Y, Fernandez H, Samuel D, Bismuth H, Frydman R. Pregnancy in liver transplant recipients: course and outcome in 19 cases. Am J Obstet Gynecol. 1993:168 (3 Pt 1):896-902.

28 DISEASES OF THE SKIN FOLLOWING TRANSPLANTATION

Thomas Stasko, MD
Mark A. Russell, MD

Because the vast majority of transplant recipients will develop clinically significant skin problems in the post-transplant period, it is important that transplant physicians be familiar with the most common conditions. Transplant medications and the resulting chronic immunosuppression can lead to a multitude of cutaneous problems ranging from cosmetic defects such as hypertrichosis, increased skin fragility, and easy bruising, to more serious problems such as cutaneous infections and malignancies (Table 28-1).

SKIN CANCER
Basal Cell Carcinoma and Squamous Cell Carcinoma

There is a marked increased incidence of premalignant and malignant lesions in organ transplant recipients. A moderate increase in basal cell carcinoma (BCC) is seen while there is a dramatic increase in squamous cell carcinoma (SCC) and its precursor lesions, dysplastic keratoses. These lesions are similar to actinic keratoses and develop in sun-exposed areas, most often the face, exposed scalp, neck, upper trunk, and the upper extremities. Early lesions, like actinic keratoses, are poorly circumscribed macules or papules with an overlying rough, hyperkeratotic scale, which may be minimal or quite protuberant as a cutaneous horn. The lesions vary from a few millimeters to a centimeter or more in diameter. The scale is usually adherent, and mechanical removal will result in bleeding. These keratoses may be flesh colored, pigmented or erythematous. If inflamed, the base may be indurated. In the nonimmunosuppressed population, sporadic lesions tend to occur most commonly on the face, followed by the dorsal forearms and hands in an approximately 9:1 ratio. In organ transplant patients, lesions occur more commonly on the hands and forearms (a 4:1 ratio, extremities-to-face). Lesions on the forearms and hands may become so numerous that,

Thomas Stasko, MD, Assistant Professor of Medicine, Department of Dermatology, Vanderbilt University Medical Center, Nashville, TN

Mark A. Russell, MD, Instructor in Medicine, Department of Dermatology, Vanderbilt University Medical Center, Nashville, TN

combined with warts and SCCs, which may also be present, only small islands of clinically normal skin may be visible. This condition has been termed *transplant hand* (Figure 28-1). Additionally, leukoplakia with histologic dysplasia and SCC appears with increased frequency on the lower lip of transplant recipients (Figure 28-2).

In the nonimmunosuppressed population, a small percentage of actinic keratoses develops into SCC. In

Table 28-1. Cutaneous Side Effects of Common Immunosuppressive Drugs

Azathioprine	Mycophenolate Mofetil
Skin Cancer	Skin Cancer
Infections	Infections
Hair Loss	
Cyclosporine	**Prednisone**
Skin Cancer	Infections
Infections	Acne
Acne	Sebaceous Hyperplasia
Hypertrichosis	Striae
Sebaceous Hyperplasia	Easy Bruising
Gingival Hyperplasia	
Tacrolimus	
Skin Cancer	
Infections	
Hair Loss	

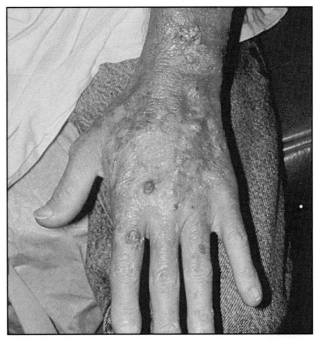

Figure 28-1. Numerous scars, warts, premalignant dyskeratotic lesions and squamous cell carcinomas on the dorsal hand and forearm of a renal transplant recipient.

287

immunosuppressed patients, the number of dysplastic keratoses is directly related to the risk of developing SCC. Unfortunately, both clinically and histologically, it may be difficult to distinguish premalignant dysplastic keratoses and hypertrophic warts from SCC in situ or invasive SCC. SCC in situ, also termed *Bowen's disease,* or invasive SCC may appear as a hyperkeratotic macule or papule similar to a dysplastic keratosis, or as a larger plaque of erythema, and scale up to several centimeters in diameter. SCC may grow rapidly in size and thickness. The resulting nodule may have an overlying thick scale or ulceration with marked hyperkeratosis. The tumor may palpate deeply into the dermis or the subcutaneous fat. Extensive lesions may invade deeper structures such as muscle fascia, cartilage or bone. A particular type of SCC often seen in transplant patients, keratoacanthoma, presents as a rapidly growing, well-circumscribed, dome-shaped nodule with a central keratin-filled crater (Figure 28-3).

Ultraviolet radiation is carcinogenic in animal models, and strongly implicated in the development of cutaneous malignancy in man. In transplant patients, the relative risk and the mean time to the development of premalignant lesions and SCC varies with the geographic latitude of the transplant center and the skin type of the population. The vast majority of non-melanoma skin cancers develop in fair-skinned individuals on sun-exposed skin. Intense sun exposure both before and after transplantation, a history of skin cancer, advancing age, and length of time since transplantation are associated with an increased risk for the development of skin cancer. The age of initial onset of skin cancer is markedly decreased (perhaps by 50%) in transplant patients. Although most centers report an overall skin cancer incidence in transplant patients of less than 15%, studies from transplant centers with high geographic and ethnic risk have reported skin cancer rates of almost 70% in long-term transplant recipients. Most significantly, rates for SCC have been reported to be 65 times that of the general population. Transplant patients also develop more tumors, with studies reporting the average number of tumors per affected patient to be as high as 15. SCC is generally more aggressive in immunosuppressed patients with higher recurrence rates after treatment and an increased risk of mortality. In Australian heart transplant recipients, 27% of the deaths occurring four or more years after transplantation were due to skin cancer, and over half of those deaths were due to SCC. In dark-skinned populations, the risk of skin cancer is increased over normal controls, but still negligible.

In the general population, BCC outnumbers SCC approximately 5:1. Although the ratio in transplant recipients is reversed to approximately 1:2, the risk of BCC is still slightly increased. BCC has many clinical presentations. The most frequent form, nodular BCC, presents as a translucent to erythematous papule or nodule with peripheral telangiectasia (Figure 28-4). Lesions may have pigment, especially at the borders. Larger lesions may have central ulceration and a spreading border with a rolled appearance. The frequent ulceration led to the term *rodent ulcer.* Sclerosing BCC has a scar-like appearance. There may be atrophy and telangiectasia. Superficial BCC presents as a slowly

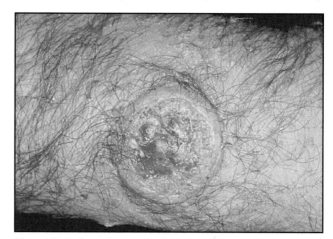

Figure 28-3. Large keratoacanthoma-type squamous cell carcinoma.

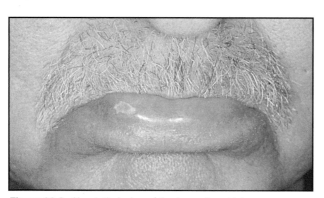

Figure 28-2. Keratotic lesion of the lower lip, which was squamous cell carcinoma on biopsy.

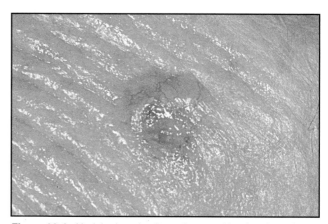

Figure 28-4. Nodular basal cell carcinoma with telangiectasia and a rolled border.

enlarging erythematous plaque or patch with fine scale and telangiectasia. It occurs most commonly on the sun-exposed portions of the trunk and extremities and may be confused with SCC in situ. The natural history of all BCCs is relatively slow, relentless growth with possible invasion and destruction of underlying structures.

The exact role of immunosuppression in the development of skin cancer is unclear. Studies have suggested that the incidence of skin cancer increases with the level of immunosuppression being higher in patients on triple-drug therapy (ie, cyclosporine/azathioprine/prednisone) than on double-drug therapy. Although there is evidence that azathioprine, unlike other immunosuppressives, may act as a direct carcinogen, studies do not show a conclusive advantage of immunosuppression with cyclosporine over azathioprine. In isolated patients, cessation or diminution of immunosuppression has been associated with an improved response to therapy and the development of fewer new lesions. However, this response has been quite variable and may lag the cessation of drug therapy by a year or longer.

Human papilloma virus (HPV) has also been implicated in the development of cutaneous malignancies. There are marked histologic similarities between SCC and verrucae. Specific HPV types have been linked to SCC of the cervix, SCC of the head and neck, and SCC in patients with epidermodysplasia verruciformis. As transplant recipients are very susceptible to HPV infection, a link in this setting has also been proposed. Several studies have found evidence of oncogenic HPV types in cutaneous malignancies in transplant patients. This strong circumstantial evidence is clouded by the lack of association of SCC with HPV in some studies, the frequent isolation of the same oncogenic HPV types from noninvolved skin in some transplant patients, and the identification of other viral infections (eg, Epstein-Barr virus, Kaposi's sarcoma-associated herpes-like DNA) in some SCC and BCC lesions. Additionally, it has been postulated that the E6 oncoproteins of oncogenic HPV types bind to and promote the degradation of p53 tumor suppressor gene product, allowing the development of malignancies. However, the overall role of p53 suppressor gene products and mutations is unclear, and the rate of p53 mutation in cutaneous malignancies is similar in transplant patients and the general population. Finally, comparing multiple studies, there has been no consistent link between HLA type or HLA transplant mismatch and the development of cutaneous malignancies.

Treatment of cutaneous premalignant lesions and malignancies should begin with prevention. Ideally, prospective transplant patients should be examined and counseled prior to transplantation. Although prior sun exposure cannot be corrected, the patient should be instructed on vigorous daily sun protection. Protection should begin with avoiding sun exposure, especially during the mid-day (approximately 10:00 am to 3:00 pm). Protective clothing, to include broad-brimmed hats and tight-weave garments should be worn to cover as much body surface as is practical. Patients should also apply broad-spectrum sunscreens, which cover both UVA and UVB with an SPF of 15 or higher, daily to all areas exposed to the sun. Tanning booths should be avoided. Education on sun protection should be reinforced at subsequent visits as studies have shown initial poor adherence to the advice given.

Both warts and dysplastic keratoses should be treated at their first appearance. The development of premalignant lesions should alert the patient and the physician to the need for close surveillance for the development of skin cancers. The patient should be instructed on self-examination and a periodic follow-up schedule should be established. Lesions are best treated when early and small. Individual premalignant lesions can be treated with cryosurgery, electrodesiccation and curettage or surgical excision. Diffuse actinic damage with multiple premalignant lesions may also be treated with topical fluorouracil, chemical peels, dermabrasion or CO_2 laser ablation. Regular application of topical retinoic acid or alpha hydroxy acids may be beneficial in decreasing the number of new premalignant hyperkeratotic lesions. Because of the difficulty in distinguishing premalignant lesions from malignant lesions, any suspicious or treatment-resistant lesions should be biopsied. Small, early SCC and BCC may be treated with cryosurgery, electrodesiccation and curettage or excision. Larger lesions, rapidly-growing lesions, recurrent lesions, and lesions in difficult anatomic locations should be treated with the histologic margin control available with Mohs micrographic surgery. Advanced transplant hand has been successfully treated with excision of the skin from the entire dorsal hand and forearm, and replacement with split-thickness skin grafts. Because most patients develop multiple lesions, radiation therapy is only appropriate for advanced aggressive tumors. It is extremely important that the patient be routinely examined for evidence of lymph node metastasis. No effective systemic chemotherapy exists for extensive primary or metastatic disease. The oral retinoids, isotretinoin, etretinate and acitretin have shown some success in decreasing the rate of development of new lesions. Unfortunately, these drugs must be used at dosages that have significant side effects ranging from dry skin and headaches to elevated lipid levels and bony changes of the spine. As a result, many patients cannot tolerate long-term therapy. The effect of the retinoids is not persistent after cessation of therapy. The rate of development of new lesions rapidly returns to the pretreatment level.

Melanoma

The risk of developing malignant melanoma in the adult transplant population is estimated to be three to four times that of the general population. Because these rates are much lower than those for BCC or SCC, the problem is only seen with one-tenth to one-thirtieth the frequency of BCC and SCC. However, the poorer prognosis associated with melanoma requires careful observation for the disease. Although both melanoma and SCC or BCC are felt to be induced by UV radiation, acute, intense exposure (ie, sunburn) may be more important in melanoma, whereas chronic exposure may be more important in SCC and BCC. Patients who have shown little tendency to develop dysplastic keratoses or SCC or BCC, but who have a large number of nevi may still be at risk for the development of melanoma.

Careful attention should be paid to all pigmented lesions, with changes in size, color or texture of a pre-existing nevus prompting consideration of melanoma. The following *ABCD* guideline has been published to aid in the evaluation of pigmented lesions, and characteristics such as these are suspicious for melanoma: (A) asymmetry; (B) borders notched or irregular; (C) color that varies from light to dark or areas of dark black to blue-black pigmentation are suspicious for melanoma ("red, white and blue"); and (D) diameter greater than 0.6 cm (pencil eraser) is suspicious for melanoma (Figure 28-5). As the prognosis and treatment of melanoma is dependent on tumor depth (Breslow measurement), a biopsy should be taken full-thickness into the subcutaneous fat. Superficial shave biopsy should be avoided.

Treatment of melanoma is based on staging, which largely relies on tumor thickness and evidence of metastasis. In almost all cases, excision of the tumor is required with margins dependent on tumor depth. Thin melanomas (0.75 mm) have a high cure rate (>95%) with excision alone. Five-year survival declines to less than 50% for lesions greater than 4.0 mm in depth. The value of elective lymph node dissection in intermediate depth

tumors is controversial. Recently, sentinel lymph node biopsy based on lymph node mapping with dye or lymphoscintigraphy has been used to further evaluate nodal involvement and the need for nodal dissection. Although early results indicate a high degree of accuracy with such procedures, the effect on long-term survival has not been established. Adjuvant therapy for high-risk tumors is centered on modulation of the immune system. Interferon-α-2b has been approved for general use in high-risk melanoma patients. Experimental protocols have involved the use of adoptive immunotherapy and vaccines. The effect of such therapies in immunosuppressed transplant patients is unclear.

Kaposi's Sarcoma

Kaposi's sarcoma (KS) is seen with increased frequency in renal transplant recipients with rates in some studies as high as 5.3%. KS usually appears first on the skin of the lower extremities, but may affect any cutaneous surface. Lesions may be macular or palpable, are red to purple in color, and may vary in size from a few millimeters to several centimeters (Figure 28-6). With progression, nodules may develop; lymph node involvement and visceral lesions are not uncommon.

Human herpesvirus 8 (HHV8) has now been detected in KS lesions from both immunocompromised and immunocompetent patients. The immunosuppression associated with transplantation may allow expression of HHV8 in previously infected transplant patients. A recent rise in the incidence of KS at one transplant center was at least temporally associated with the introduction of mycophenolate mofetil to the immunosuppressive regimen. There is also evidence that in some patients the HHV8 infection originated in the donor tissue.

Some transplant patients with KS, even widespread disease, respond well to reduction or withdrawal of immunosuppression. Conventional therapy for KS includes the treatment of individual lesions with cryotherapy, laser therapy, excision, radiation therapy,

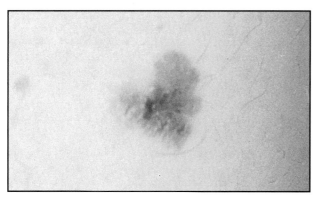

Figure 28-5. Melanoma with irregularities of color, border and symmetry.

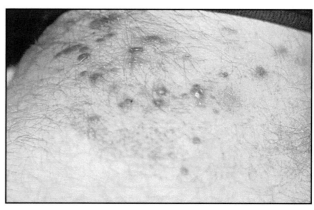

Figure 28-6. Kaposi's sarcoma.

topical retinoids and intralesional injection of antineo-plastic chemotherapeutic agents or interferon. Systemic therapy has included cytotoxic chemotherapy, interferon and zidovudine, either as monotherapy or in combination. Most transplant patients with KS respond to a combination of reduced immunosuppression and conventional therapies.

INFECTIONS

Infectious agents are a common cause of skin lesions in transplant patients. Cutaneous lesions may represent the primary site of infection or signify disseminated disease from systemic sources of infection such as the lungs (Table 28-2). The risk of infection by bacteria, fungi, and viruses is highest during periods of maximal immunosuppression and with increasing length of immunosuppression.

Viral Infections

HUMAN PAPILLOMAVIRUS. Warts caused by human papillomavirus (HPV) occur frequently in immunosuppressed patients. HPV infection correlates with the length of immunosuppression and up to 90% of transplant patients have warts after five years. Common warts (verruca vulgaris) are flesh-colored hyperkeratotic papules or plaques, often with visible dark thrombosed capillaries ("seeds"). Flat warts (verruca plana) appear as slightly elevated, flesh-colored to mildly erythematous flat-topped papules with little or no scale. Warts may occur anywhere on immunosuppressed patients but have a predisposition for the hands, feet and genitalia. The lesions may be solitary or multiple. Warts in transplant patients may be particularly resistant to treatment, which consists of topical keratolytics and destructive modalities such as liquid nitrogen, electrodessication, and laser therapy. Immune modulating therapies such as oral cimetidine and intralesional interferon have demon-strated some effectiveness in treating recalcitrant warts, but the appropriateness of such therapies in the transplant population has not been established.

HERPES VIRUS. Cutaneous manifestations of infection with herpes simplex virus (HSV), varicella-zoster virus (VZV), and cytomegalovirus (CMV) are relatively common after transplantation. Another member of the Herpesviridae family, the Epstein-Barr virus (EBV), also causes infection but rarely has cutaneous manifestations beyond a transient maculopapular or morbilliform eruption of the trunk and upper extremities.

HSV infections may be associated with prolonged viral shedding, decreased healing time, and increased incidence of viral dissemination in the immunocompromised host. Although primary infection can occur, most cutaneous lesions of HSV represent reactivation of latent infection. The most common presentation of HSV1 is grouped vesicles on an erythematous base, at the vermilion border of the lip, but lesions also occur on the face and buccal mucosa. Infections with HSV2 typically occur in the anogenital region and consist of painful grouped vesicles on an erythematous base, which may coalesce and ulcerate. The most reliable way to diagnose HSV infection is to culture a vesicular lesion. The virus usually grows in tissue culture within 48 to 72 hours. A skin biopsy and Tzanck preparation will also support the diagnosis by revealing the characteristic multinucleated giant cells. Acyclovir, famciclovir and valacyclovir are effective for treatment and chronic suppression. Foscarnet may be used for acyclovir-resistant HSV. Primary infection with VZV results in varicella (chickenpox), while reactivation of latent infection results in herpes zoster (shingles). The incidence of herpes zoster in immunosuppressed individuals is increased 20 to 100 times that of immunocompetent patients, and up to 22% of transplant patients may experience clinically apparent

Table 28-2. Reported Infectious Causes of Cutaneous Lesions in Transplant Patients

Bacterial	Fungal	Virus
Atypical mycobacteria	*Aspergillus*	Cytomegalovirus
Nocardia	*Candida*	Epstein-Barr virus
Pseudomonas aeruginosa	*Coccidiodes immitis*	Herpes simplex
Staphylococcus aureus	*Cryptococcus neoformans*	Varicella-zoster
Rochalimaea henselae	*Exophiala jeanselmei*	Human herpesvirus-8
(bacillary angiomatosis)	*Histoplasma capsulatum*	Human papilloma virus
	Malassezia furfur	
	Mucor	
	Pseudallescharia boydii	
	Rhizopus	
	Trichophyton rubrum	
	Trichosporon beigelli	

disease. The severity and duration of disease (up to 27 weeks), as well as the incidence of post-herpetic neuralgia is increased. The cutaneous appearance of VZV infection is characterized by erythematous macules and papules, which progress to form vesicles and pustules, and eventually crust over (Figure 28-7). In herpes zoster, the lesions are usually localized to a single unilateral dermatome, which does not cross the midline. In disseminated zoster, the lesions usually begin in a dermatomal distribution and spread to other skin sites. Visceral involvement, particularly of the lungs, liver and brain may occur. Transplant recipients can be particularly susceptible to severe infections with VZV if they have no established immunity. Varicella vaccine should be given to susceptible patients prior to transplantation and varicella-zoster immunoglobulin is recommended for the nonimmune transplant patient within 96 hours of significant exposure. The same diagnostic techniques used for HSV can be used for VZV. Acyclovir, famciclovir, and valacyclovir can decrease viral shedding, accelerate healing, and decrease post-herpetic neuralgia.

Cutaneous manifestations of cytomegalovirus (CMV) infection can be quite variable. The most specific cutaneous manifestations of CMV infection are ulcerations in the perineal area, buttocks, and oral mucosa. Other less specific lesions include vesicobullous lesions, papules, plaques, purpura and morbilliform eruptions. Biopsy of a lesion reveals the characteristic intranuclear and intracytoplasmic inclusions of endothelial cells. Leukocytoclastic vasculitis may also be present.

MOLLUSCUM CONTAGIOSUM. Molluscum contagiosum consists of discrete, firm, umbilicated white to erythematous papules caused by a DNA-containing poxvirus (Figure 28-8). Lesions have a predilection for the face, trunk and anogenital area. The virus is spread by fomites, close contact, or autoinoculation. Molluscum contagiosum has been described in organ transplant patients, but the incidence and extent of involvement appear to be greater in AIDS patients. Infection may

resemble disseminated fungal infection such as *Cryptococcus,* histoplasmosis, coccidioidomycosis, or penicillinosis, and biopsy confirmation is warranted. Intracytoplasmic inclusion bodies (Henderson-Patterson bodies) are apparent on stained smears of the expressed core or on biopsy. Treatments include tretinoin, cantharidin, liquid nitrogen, electrodessication, curettage, topical fluorouracil, cimetidine, oral isotretinoin, and 30% trichloroacetic acid peel.

Fungal Infections

Fungal disease involving the skin may be caused by a primary infection or disseminated from a systemic source. Following transplantation, there is an increased probability that the causative agent may be an opportunistic organism such as *Aspergillus, Candida,* and *Cryptococcus.* Infection with primary pathogens such as *Coccidioides* and *Histoplasma* also occur. Superficial mycoses such as dermatophytosis and pityriasis versicolor are common and appear to be especially prominent in tropical and subtropical environments.

CANDIDA. Disseminated candidiasis caused by *C albicans* and, less frequently, *C tropicalis* occurs in transplant patients. Fever and diffuse muscle tenderness accompany infection. Skin lesions occur in 10% to 13% of patients via hematogenous spread from the oropharynx, gastrointestinal tract, or contaminated intravenous catheters. Clinical appearance is variable but lesions may present as erythematous maculopapules or papulonodules, which may develop hemorrhagic or necrotic centers. The demonstration of organisms on biopsy or culture of affected tissue will help substantiate the diagnosis. Disseminated infection is treated with intravenous amphotericin and/or fluconazole. Primary cutaneous infection may also occur and present as cutaneous candidiasis, onychomycosis or paronychia. Treatment of primary cutaneous infection includes topical nystatin, imidazoles, fluconazole and itraconazole.

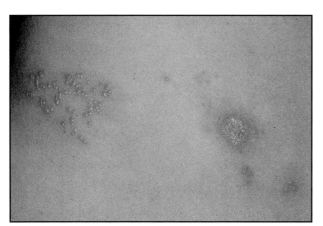

Figure 28-7. Varicella-zoster infection with vesicles and crusting.

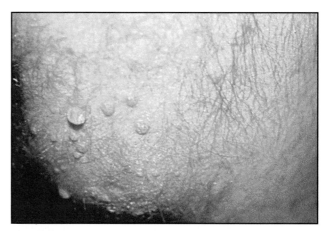

Figure 28-8. Molluscum contagiosum: multiple large umbilicated papules in an immunosuppressed patient.

ASPERGILLOSIS. Aspergillus species are ubiquitous in nature and commonly found in soil or other organic matter. Hospital air ducts, especially during construction or renovation, can be the source of *Aspergillus* isolates. Infection is most commonly caused by *A fumigatus, A flavus,* and *A niger,* and usually disseminates from a pulmonary focus, but may present as a primary cutaneous infection. Early lesions present as discrete erythematous papules that become pustular, and develop into ulcerative necrotic lesions covered with black eschar. The diagnosis can be confirmed by culture, and biopsy reveals septate hyphae with acute angle branching. Treatment includes amphotericin and itraconazole.

CRYPTOCOCCUS. Cryptococcus neoformans is found throughout the world and is commonly found in soil contaminated with pigeon droppings. A primary pulmonary infection disseminates hematogenously to the skin in approximately 15% of patients. Cutaneous manifestations are variable and may present as erythematous papules, plaques, nodules, abcesses, and vesicles, and occasionally resemble bacterial cellulitis. Infection is treated with amphotericin B and fluconazole.

MISCELLANEOUS FUNGAL INFECTIONS.

Pseudallescharia boydii (Scedosporium apiospermum), Trichosporon beigleii, and *Exophiala jeanselmei* have all been reported to cause cutaneous nodules in transplant patients. Pityriasis versicolor and pityrosporum folliculitis are superficial dermatomycoses caused by the fungi *Malassezia furfur,* and are frequently encountered in transplant patients. Pityriasis versicolor presents as discrete and confluent white to tan patches with fine scale, usually on the upper trunk and upper arms. Pityrosporum folliculitis is characterized by pruritic follicular papules and pustules on the chest, back, and occasion-

ally the face (Figure 28-9). A potassium hydroxide (KOH) preparation reveals budding yeast and short hyphal elements. Treatment includes selenium sulfide, imidazoles, itraconazole, and fluconazole. Dermatophyte infections involving the skin and/or nails appear to be more frequent with increasing length of immunosuppression. *Trichophyton rubrum* is the predominant pathogen and infection with this organism has caused tinea unguium and tinea corporis, as well as resulted in atypical invasion of the skin presenting as subcutaneous nodules in transplant patients (Figure 28-10). Treatment may require prolonged administration of oral itraconazole, fluconazole or terbidifine.

Bacteria

The most common cutaneous manifestations of bacterial infections are folliculitis, cellulitis and furunculosis. Ecthyma gangrenosum resulting from pseudomonas sepsis has been described in organ transplant recipients. Opportunistic bacterial pathogens including nontuberculous mycobacterium and *Nocardia* species occur more frequently in immunosuppressed patients. Bacillary angiomatosis, caused by *Rochalimaea henselae,* may present on the skin of profoundly immunosuppressed patients. The cutaneous lesions are erythematous, vascular papules or nodules, which may resemble Kaposi's sarcoma.

Mycobacteria

Mycobacterial infections occur 32 times more frequently in renal transplant patients than in the general population. Skin infections may result from direct inoculation from an exogenous source, contiguous spread from an endogenous source (eg, osteomyelitis), or hematogenous dissemination. *M chelonae* and *M hemophilia* are commonly identified sources of infection in transplant

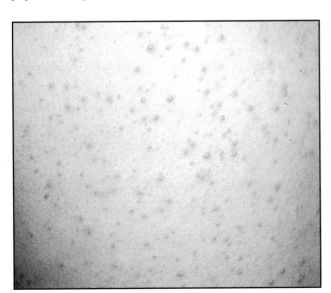

Figure 28-9. Pityrosporum folliculitis-papules and pustules.

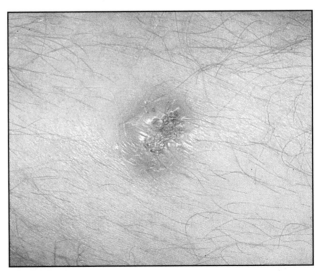

Figure 28-10. Cutaneous nodule caused by dermatophyte infection.

patients. Cutaneous lesions, usually found on the extremities, present as papules, erythematous plaques and nodules, with or without pain. Abscess formation may occur and sporotrichoid spread with nodules in an ascending pattern on the extremities has been reported. Treatment of mycobacterial infections in transplant patients should be guided by the results of antimicrobial susceptibility testing.

Nocardia

Nocardia are aerobic, Gram-positive filamentous rods found in the soil. Nocardiosis is usually acquired by inhalation of airborne spores, which may be followed by hematogenous dissemination. Primary percutaneous inoculation is also possible, but rare. Up to 13% of transplant patients may have nocardiosis. Of the patients with nocardiosis, 20% have cutaneous lesions. Skin lesions consist of nodules, abscesses and sinus tracts. Sulfonamides are the drug of choice for treating nocardiosis.

DRUG-RELATED SKIN FINDINGS

Cutaneous manifestations associated with transplantation and immunosuppressive therapy are quite common, affecting most patients. Many patients complain of episodes of scalp hair loss and diffuse thinning after transplantation. Increased hair loss has been attributed to azathioprine and tacrolimus. A more common complaint is the hypertrichosis associated with cyclosporine therapy. This hair growth is not confined to the androgen-specific areas, but is often found on the trunk and extremities (Figure 28-11).

Acne due to corticosteroids occurs on the face, upper trunk and upper extremities. Papules and pustules without comedones usually appear in the same stage of development. Acne shows a declining prevalence as the transplant interval increases, and is more common and more severe in younger patients. This condition usually responds to topical benzoyl peroxide, tretinoin or antibiotics. Oral antibiotics or isotretinoin may be necessary for more severe involvement. The most commonly used antibiotics for acne are tetracycline and erythromycin, while secondary drugs include doxycycline, trimethoprim-sulfa or cephalexin.

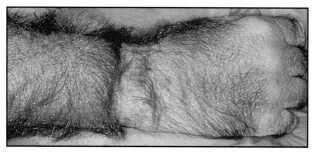

Figure 28-11. Hypertrichosis of the forearm.

Sebaceous hyperplasia secondary to corticosteroids or cyclosporine presents as cream-colored or yellow umbilicated papules on the forehead, temples and cheeks. Other cutaneous manifestations of corticosteroids include striae, skin atrophy, ecchymoses, and telangiectasias. Striae appear as violaceous linear bands especially prominent in the axilla, groin, and back. Ecchymoses tend to occur in areas of sun exposure and minor trauma such as the dorsal forearms and hands. Telangiectasias are commonly found on the face. Atrophy and xerosis are more prevalent with increasing duration of immunosuppression. Many patients with dry, fragile skin will benefit from the use of moisturizers containing alpha hydroxy acids or ammonium lactate.

SKIN EXAMINATIONS

Because skin problems in transplant recipients are so common, patients should become accustomed to performing monthly skin checks and consult a physician for any unusual or changing lesions. Cutaneous lesions in immunosuppressed transplant patients warrant a high level of suspicion, and appropriate biopsy and culture should be performed on all atypical lesions to evaluate for infection or malignancy.

RECOMMENDED READING

Abel EA. Cutaneous manifestations of immunosuppression in organ transplant recipients. J Am Acad Dermatol. 1989;21(2 Pt 1):167-179.

Bavinck JN, Tieben LM, Van der Woude FJ, et al. Prevention of skin cancer and reduction of keratotic skin lesions during acitretin therapy in renal transplant recipients: a double-blind, placebo-controlled study. J Clin Oncol. 1995;13(8):9133-9138.

Blohme I, Larko O. Skin lesions in renal transplant patients after 10-23 years of immunosuppressive therapy. Acta Derm Venereol. 1990;70(6):491-494.

Bouwes Bavinck JN, Hardie DR, Green A, et al. The risk of skin cancer in renal transplant recipients in Queensland, Australia. A follow-up study. Transplantation. 1996;61(5):715-721.

DiGiovanna JJ. Posttransplantation skin cancer: scope of the problem, management, and role for systemic retinoid chemoprevention. Transplant Proc. 1998;30(6):2771-2778.

Eberhard OK, Kliem V, Brunkhorst R. Five cases of Kaposi's sarcoma in kidney graft recipients: possible influence of the immunosuppressive therapy. Transplantation. 1999;67(1):180-184.

Espana A, Redondo P, Fernandez AL, et al. Skin cancer in heart transplant recipients. [Review]. J Am Acad Dermatol. 1995;32(3):458-465.

Gentry LO, Zeluff B, Kielhofner MA. Dermatologic manifestations of infectious diseases in cardiac transplant patients. Infect Dis Clin North Am. 1994;8(3):637-654.

Jensen P, Clausen OP, Geirna O, et al. Cutaneous complications in heart transplant recipients in Norway 1983-1993. Acta Derm Venereol. 1995;75(5):400-403.

Jensen P, Hansen S, Moller B, et al. Skin cancer in kidney and heart transplant recipients and different long-term immunosuppressive therapy regimens. J Am Acad Dermatol. 1999;40(2 Pt 1):177-186.

Khorshid SM, Glover MT, Churchill LM, McGregor JM, Proby CM. p53 Immunoreactivity in non-melanoma skin cancer from immunosuppressed and immunocompetent individuals: a comparative study of 246 tumours. J Cutan Pathol. 1996;23(3):229-233.

Leigh IM, Glover MT. Cutaneous warts and tumours in immunosuppressed patients. J R Soc Med. 1995;88(2):61-62.

Lugo-Janer G, Sanchez JL, Santiago-Delphin E. Prevalence and clinical spectrum of skin diseases in kidney transplant recipients. J Am Acad Dermatol. 1991;24(3):410-414.

Ong CS, Keogh AM, Kossard S, Macdonald PS, Spratt PM. Skin cancer in Australian heart transplant recipients. J Am Acad Dermatol. 1999;40(1):27-34.

Regamey N, Tamm M, Wernli M, et al. Transmission of human herpesvirus 8 infection from renal-transplant donors to recipients. N Engl J Med. 1998;339(19):1358-1363.

Seckin D, Gulec TO, Demirag A, Bilgin N. Renal transplantation and skin diseases. Transplant Proc. 1998;30(3):802-804.

Seukernan DC, Newstead CG, Cunliffe WJ. The compliance of renal transplant recipients with advice about sun protection measures. Br J Bermatol. 1998;138(2):301-303.

Severson JL, Tyring SK. Viral disease update. Curr Probl Dermatol. 1999;11(2):37-72.

Taylor AE, Shuster S. Skin cancer after renal transplantation: the causal role of azathioprine. Acta Derm Venereol. 1992;72(2):115-119.

van Zuuren EJ, Posma AN, Scholtens REM, Vermeer BJ, van der Woude FJ, Bavinck JN. Resurfacing the back of the hand as treatment and prevention of multiple skin cancers in kidney transplant recipients. J Am Acad Dermatol. 1994;31(5 Pt 1):760-764.

29 OCULAR COMPLICATIONS IN TRANSPLANT PATIENTS

Saad Shaikh, MD
Steven Sanislo, MD

Ocular complications are increasingly seen in the ever-enlarging number of long-term survivors of transplantation. The ophthalmic findings in transplant patients can be broadly divided into three categories: (1) complications resulting from opportunistic pathogens in immunocompromised hosts; (2) direct involvement of the eye in graft-vs-host disease; and (3) ocular side effects of chemotherapeutic and radiation regimens.

OCULAR COMPLICATIONS IN THE IMMUNOCOMPROMISED HOST

Opportunistic infections of the eye present with higher frequency in immunocompromised patients, including transplant patients. Even then, severe opportunistic infections of the eye, such as herpes group viral infections and fungal endophthalmitis, tend to be found in transplant patients at a frequency of only 2%. The implications of these infections on visual morbidity and as a marker of the severity of underlying disease, however, are profound.

Cytomegalovirus Retinitis

Cytomegalovirus (CMV) retinitis is most frequently seen in cardiac allograft patients, at an incidence as high as 15% in a recently reported series. Early symptoms include a painless, sometimes bilateral decrease in vision associated with floaters. Funduscopic examination reveals widely-distributed yellow/white patches representing areas of retinal necrosis that frequently develop along the vascular arcades (Figure 29-1). The lesions often start in the mid-periphery of the retina and extend toward the macula with bleeding along the advancing edge of the lesion, known as a brushfire response. The healed areas in its wake are characterized histopathologically by marked atrophy and gliosis of all layers of the retina, including the retinal pigment epithelium and choroid. This results in irreversible loss of vision corresponding to the areas of retina involved. The advancing edge of the lesions in the retina is important for manage-

Saad Shaikh, MD, Resident Physician, Department of Ophthalmology, Stanford University School of Medicine, Stanford, CA

Steven Sanislo, MD, Assistant Professor, Department of Ophthalmology, Stanford University School of Medicine, Stanford, CA

ment and follow-up in these individuals. Prompt diagnosis of CMV retinitis is critical if the retinitis is to be stopped before the macula is affected. Intravenous ganciclovir or foscarnet remain the primary antiviral agents of choice for treatment. Intravitreal injections or intraocular ganciclovir implants may also be required. Retinal detachment commonly occurs in areas of extensive necrosis and is treated with pars plana vitrectomy and silicone oil tamponade. CMV retinitis tends to occur most frequently during the second year after transplantation. Given that recurrence is rare and the retinitis resolves through normal immune responses as the host's immune status returns to normal, treatment should be maintained until the lesions are quiescent.

Herpes Zoster Ophthalmicus

Herpes zoster ophthalmicus (HZO) occurs when the ophthalmic division of the trigeminal nerve becomes involved after reactivation of latent virus in the trigeminal ganglia. Immunocompromised hosts manifest HZO in much higher frequencies than the normal population and develop more severe visual sequelae. Patients notice progressive neuralgic pain on the involved side, followed by a vesicular rash with areas of ulceration and subsequent scarring, which may involve the eyelids (Figure 29-2). A blepharoconjunctivitis often occurs even without direct ocular involvement and is treated by topical antibiotics. Corneal dysesthesia, punctate epithelial keratitis, and dendritiform keratopathy commonly develop but tend to be self-limited. Zoster dendrites are treated with lubricants to promote epithelial healing, as well as with topical antibiotics to prevent bacterial superinfections. Topical antivirals are contraindicated because they are ineffective and toxic to the corneal epithelium. Corneal complications, such as recurrent neurotrophic ulcers and stromal keratitis with corneal neovascularization and lipid deposition, may require

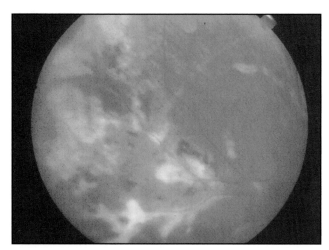

Figure 29-1. CMV Retinitis. The characteristic finding of yellowish CMV retinitis lesions with secondary hemorrhages are observed in this immunocompromised patient after heart transplantation.

corneal transplantation. Adequate lubrication remains the mainstay of preventative therapy.

Treatment of active varicella infections includes oral acyclovir (800 mg five times a day for seven to ten days). Administration within seven days of presentation, and especially within 72 hours, has been found to speed resolution of skin lesions, reduce viral shedding, decrease the incidence of dendritic and stromal keratitis, as well as anterior uveitis. Oral acyclovir generally is not recommended for the treatment of corneal lesions as these tend to be self-limited. Acyclovir may be used for extended durations as an adjunct to topical steroids in severe cases of zoster keratouveitis.

Varicella-zoster retinitis is the most severe complication of HZO. Reported cases have presented with varying degrees of severity but often with great similarity to the progressive outer retinal necrosis syndrome, a clinical variant of necrotizing herpetic retinopathy in patients with acquired immunodeficiency syndrome (AIDS). Symptoms include blurred vision and pain in both eyes. Early disease is characterized by multifocal deep retinal opacities. Lesions rapidly coalesce and often progress to total retinal necrosis over a short period of time with irreversible loss of vision in the affected areas. Less severe cases have responded to oral acyclovir or oral bromovinyldeoxyuridine, but often the prognosis is poor with a weak response to intravenous antiviral drugs. Disease progression within days to weeks to involve the posterior pole and optic disk is common, as is total retinal detachment. Like CMV retinitis, pars plana vitrectomy with silicone oil tamponade may be necessary to salvage any remaining vision.

Fungal Endophthalmitis

Endogenous fungal endophthalmitis, a relatively uncommon disease in the normal population, is sometimes seen in the transplant host as a complication of immunosuppressive therapy. The most common species responsible are *Candida albicans* and *Candida tropicalis.* Infection is usually indolent elsewhere in the body and spreads hematogenously to the eye. Presenting symptoms are minimal or nonexistent initially, but if the organism affects the macula, diminished vision is the primary complaint. Fundus examination reveals white fluffy chorioretinal lesions with overlying vitreous and anterior chamber inflammation (Figure 29-3). Staining and culture of intraocular vitreous aspirates reveal fungal organisms. Mild cases can be treated initially with systemic antifungal therapy (IV amphotericin B or oral fluconazole). In cases with progression despite systemic therapy, or when the lesions threaten the macula, intravitreal injection of amphotericin B or fluconazole is considered. When there is clear progression of disease despite initial therapy with appropriate systemic and intravitreal antifungal agents, pars plana vitrectomy is required. *Aspergillus fumigatus* (Figure 29-4) has also been reported as a cause of fungal endophthalmitis in liver, lung and bone marrow transplant patients, and merits similar diagnostic and treatment measures. Fungal endophthalmitis generally occurs as an early complica-

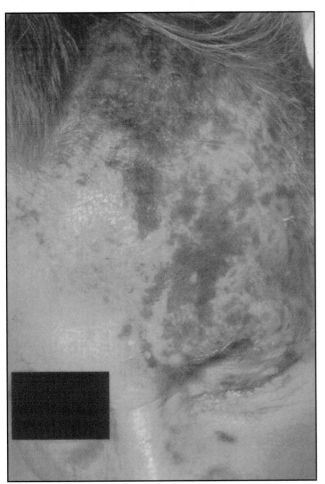

Figure 29-2. Zoster Ophthalmicus. Vesicular skin eruptions involving the first division of the fifth cranial nerve.

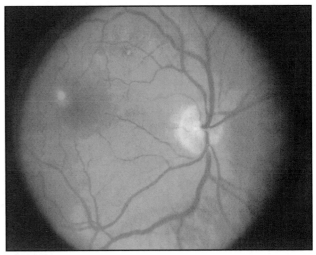

Figure 29-3. Candidal Endophthalmitis. A paramacular candidal puffball is observed in this immunocompromised patient.

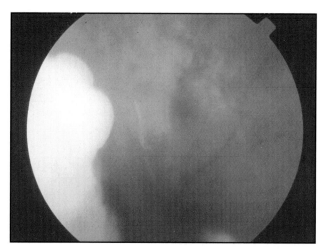

Figure 29-4. *Aspergillus* Endophthalmitis. A large chorioretinal lesion with associated retinal hemorrhages and vitreous inflammation is noted in the peripheral retina of this patient.

tion, usually within the first four months after transplantation, in contrast to viral infections with herpes zoster or cytomegalovirus, which tend to present later. Nonetheless, prompt therapy following early diagnosis significantly reduces visual loss in all forms of fungal endophthalmitis and, hence, it has been recommended that all transplant patients undergo ophthalmic screening three to four months after transplantation with repeat examinations yearly or as ocular symptoms occur.

Toxoplasma Retinitis

Toxoplasma gondii presents as a fulminant retinochoroiditis in transplant patients and should, therefore, be considered along with fungi and viruses in the differential diagnosis of necrotizing retinitides in immunocompromised patients. The aggressive presentation parallels that which has been previously reported to occur in AIDS and other forms of immunosuppression. This is in contrast to the reactivated congenital retinochoroiditis that occurs in immunocompetent patients, which presents with minimal symptoms and is self-limited. Symptomatic reactivation of ocular toxoplasmosis has been observed in transplant patients with a history of toxoplasma retinochoroiditis, as documented by formal ophthalmologic examination in the early posttransplant period. Therapy with sulfadiazine, pyrimethamine and prednisone ultimately leads to resolution in these patients. It remains speculative to what extent cases represent primary disease or reactivation of congenital disease given the aggressive necrotizing presentation, which prevents identification of congenital scars. Thus, transplant patients who are seropositive for *Toxoplasma gondii* antibody, and have findings consistent with previous toxoplasma retinochoroiditis on pretransplant ophthalmologic examination, appear to be at risk for reactivation of ocular toxoplasmosis in the early post-

transplant period and may warrant preventive chemoprophylaxis.

Skin Cancer

The high incidence, up to 15%, of skin cancer in solid organ transplant recipients as a result of immunosuppression is well-recognized. These lesions tend to present between two and three years after transplantation and may involve the eyelid and globe as well. Although not as commonly reported in the literature, eyelid neoplasms presenting after transplantation include keratoacanthoma, squamous cell carcinoma, basal cell carcinoma, papillomas, and to a much lesser degree, malignant melanoma of the periocular tissue. Additionally, intraocular melanoma has also been reported after transplantation. These cases represent de novo tumor formation, metastasis from donor organs, as well as recurrence of host disease. Risk factors for the development of skin cancer include immunosuppression, increased exposure to ultraviolet radiation, and skin type. In addition to regular skin cancer screening examinations and photoprotection, treating physicians must be alert to the occurrence of eyelid tumors so that prompt referral of these patients may facilitate diagnosis and treatment.

DIRECT OCULAR COMPLICATIONS OF TRANSPLANTATION
Graft-vs-Host Disease

Although not as commonly observed as in bone marrow transplantation, graft-vs-host disease (GVHD) has been reported as a complication in various solid organ transplant recipients as well. Ocular manifestations develop in 60% to 90% of patients with GVHD. The key to management is the appropriate treatment of the underlying GVHD.

Perhaps the most frequent ocular complication after bone marrow transplant is the dry eye syndrome or keratoconjunctivitis sicca occurring in up to 76% of patients in a reported series. The syndrome is characterized by subjective symptoms such as pain, foreign body sensation, and blurring of vision. Clinical signs include markedly decreased tear production and superficial punctate keratopathy. These can be diagnosed by Schirmer's testing and fluorescein dye staining, respectively. Histopathologic studies have shown the presence of periodic acid-Schiff-positive mucopolysaccharide material in the acini and ductules of lacrimal glands in GVHD patients, causing luminal obliteration and ductal distention similar to the cholestasis of hepatic GVHD. In addition, immunological abnormalities in the tears of GVHD patients probably also contribute to the dry eye syndrome. The primary mode of treatment includes lubricants and punctal occlusion.

The most characteristic ocular finding of GVHD is a hemorrhagic pseudomembranous conjunctivitis, which presents in up to 17% of patients commonly within the first 90 days after transplantation. Histopathologic analysis of biopsy specimens reveals an immunologic response directed against the conjunctiva. Accordingly, a staging classification by severity has been proposed. Patients may initially present with conjunctival hyperemia (stage 1) or conjunctival chemosis, which may be associated with a serosanguinous exudate (stage 2) (Figure 29-5). A pseudomembrane may form (stage 3) and, in most severe cases, corneal epithelial sloughing occurs (stage 4). Ulceration of the lids and a cicatrizing conjunctivitis (scarring of the conjunctiva) may also occur. The severity of the conjunctivitis has been shown to correlate with the severity of GVHD. Healing is promoted by appropriate local measures (such as lubricants and patching) and treatment of the systemic GVHD. Topical cyclosporine may be an appropriate adjunct in managing ocular surface abnormalities in patients with ocular GVHD after conventional modalities have failed. Corneal involvement may result in corneal epithelial sloughing, peripheral corneal neovascularization, keratitis, keratinization, and corneal scarring or perforation. In these cases tarsorrhaphy (temporarily suturing the eye lids closed), bandage contact lenses, tissue adhesives, or conjunctival flaps may be indicated. As a result of the compromised integrity of the cornea and the host's poor immunity, bacterial infection and reactivation of herpes simplex keratitis are often secondary complications. These patients benefit from timely diagnosis and appropriate antimicrobial therapy.

Other ocular complications of GVHD have been reported and include cotton wool spots (localized ischemia of the nerve fiber layer from retinal capillary nonperfusion), optic disc edema, optic neuropathies, reactivation of toxoplasma retinitis and other opportunistic infections. However, these are likely manifestations of underlying systemic abnormalities, side effects of cytotoxic medications, and the susceptibility of the immunocompromised host, and probably should not be attributed directly to GVHD.

OCULAR COMPLICATIONS OF TRANSPLANT THERAPY

Ocular toxicity induced by transplant therapy is not uncommon and, given the number of emerging regimens and new agents, one can expect an increased frequency of resulting ocular complications. In most cases the pathogenesis of ocular toxicity is not well understood and complications are generally not preventable. Hence, clinicians must be aware of their potential vision-threatening side effects so that timely consultation with an ophthalmologist can lead to early detection and appropriate management.

Corticosteroids

Ocular toxicity to steroids is relatively common and well-established. The most common ocular complication is the development of posterior subcapsular cataracts (Figure 29-6). The overall incidence of cataract formation ranges from 10% to 40%, with up to 20% of patients developing symptomatic visual impairment. However, the prognosis for normal vision in these patients with modern cataract and intraocular lens surgery is excellent. Observational studies and animal models of steroid-induced cataractogenesis suggest that multivitamin supplements, especially vitamin E, may protect lenses against oxidative damage and prevent cataract formation. Hence, routine multivitamin supplementation in patients posttransplantation may be beneficial in this regard. Additionally, an elevation in intraocular pressure with subsequent secondary open angle glaucoma may occur with topical corticosteroid therapy, although oral steroids are less likely to cause an intraocular pressure elevation. Rapid tapering or discontinuation of long-term steroid therapy has been associated with the development of pseudotumor cerebri manifesting with papilledema, resulting in decreased visual acuity, headaches, vomiting and occasional sixth nerve palsy.

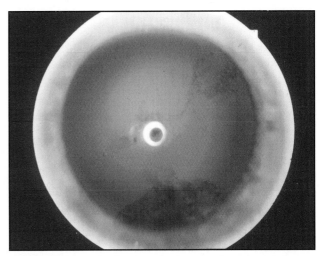

Figure 29-6. Posterior Subcapsular Cataract. Posterior subcapsular cataract seen in retroillumination in a 40-year old patient receiving corticosteroids after transplantation.

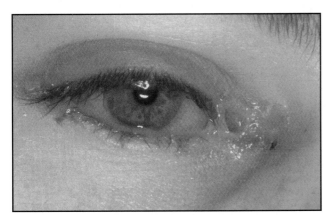

Figure 29-5. Graft-vs-Host Disease. Conjunctival injection and chemosis associated with exudates in this patient with pseudomembranous conjunctivitis associated with graft-vs-host disease.

Cyclosporine

Immunosuppressive-associated posterior leukoencephalopathy is a unique and potentially reversible complication of cyclosporine therapy in solid organ transplant patients that can usually be diagnosed on the basis of its distinctive time of onset, and clinical and neuroimaging characteristics. Median time to onset is approximately one month with 82% of cases occurring within 90 days of transplantation. Lesions occur earlier and more frequently in liver transplant recipients than in other solid organ transplant recipients. Clinical symptoms generally result from involvement of the posterior cerebral cortex and include visual abnormalities ranging from loss of central vision to complete cortical blindness as well as seizures and altered mental status. Characteristic posterior signal changes are present on CT and MRI. Both the clinical and neuroradiologic abnormalities are reversible on cessation or reduction of cyclosporine in most but not all cases.

Decreased visual acuity with optic disc edema has been reported in up to 3% of transplant patients receiving cyclosporine. The etiology is unclear and may represent a direct toxic effect of the drug, an idiosyncratic response, papilledema due to increased intracranial pressure, or some combination of these mechanisms. Discontinuation of cyclosporine and treatment with corticosteroids is generally followed by recovery of visual acuity. In addition, cotton wool spots have been associated with cyclosporine therapy, but the causal relationship is confounded by the presence of other factors including total body irradiation and chemotherapy.

Cyclophosphamide

Cyclophosphamide has been associated with ocular toxicity in the form of blurred vision, keratoconjunctivitis sicca, blepharoconjunctivitis, and pinpoint pupils. Reversible blurred vision without ophthalmoscopic findings sometimes occurs within 24 hours after administration with episodes lasting from 60 minutes to two weeks.

Total Body Irradiation

Total body irradiation (TBI), though used less often as an adjunct in solid organ than bone marrow transplantation, has also been associated with ocular complications including posterior subcapsular cataracts, keratoconjunctivitis sicca and superficial punctate keratopathy. The relationship between irradiation and the development of ocular disease depends not only on total dose, but rate of administration and coexistent risk factors including systemic immunosuppressive therapy.

Radiation retinopathy occurs as a result of retinal vascular damage and has been reported in a recent series in 60% of patients after as little as 1,200 cGy of total body irradiation. The posterior segment signs seen with radiation retinopathy include cotton wool spots (Figure 29-7), retinal hemorrhages, macular edema, hard exudates, retinal pigment epithelial changes, and neovascularization of the optic disc or retina. The development of radiation retinopathy after such low doses of teletherapy suggests that patients receiving high-dose chemotherapy and those with preexisting microangiopathies are at increased risk for the development of retinopathy at otherwise safe radiation doses. The mean time for onset of radiation retinopathy is 18 months, and management includes focal laser treatment for visual loss secondary to macular edema and panretinal photocoagulation when neovascularization develops.

Hemorrhagic Complications

Transient anemia and thrombocytopenia are often encountered as side effects of systemic medications or in the postoperative course of transplant patients. Reported intraocular hemorrhagic complications include subconjunctival hemorrhage, intraretinal hemorrhage, and

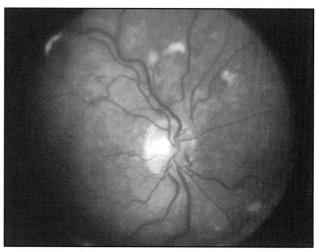

Figure 29-7. Radiation retinopathy occurring after external beam irradiation manifested by peripapillary cotton wool spots.

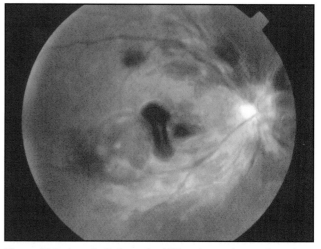

Figure 29-8. Anemic Retinopathy. Diffuse hemorrhages throughout all layers of the retina in this anemic patient presenting with decreased visual acuity after transplantation.

vitreous hemorrhage. An anemic retinopathy may also present with markedly decreased vision and hemorrhages at all levels of the retina extending into the macula (Figure 29-8). Fortunately, symptoms improve with treatment of the underlying anemia and thrombocytopenia.

CONCLUSION

Physicians involved in the care of transplant patients should be aware of the ocular side effects of immunosuppressive and therapeutic regimens, as well as ophthalmic involvement in GVHD, since complications are often severe. Generally, patients should be examined before transplantation to determine whether preventive chemoprophylaxis is indicated, and then reexamined three to four months postoperatively, and subsequently on a yearly basis or as symptoms develop so that prompt treatment can minimize the severity and duration of vision-threatening side effects. Although studies indicate a relatively low incidence of sight-threatening complications after transplantation, early referral and timely management of patients with visual symptoms can lead to early detection, proper diagnosis, and appropriate therapeutic measures.

RECOMMENDED READING

al-Tweigeri T, Nabholtz JM, Mackey JR. Ocular toxicity and cancer chemotherapy: a review. Cancer. 1996;78(7):1359-1373.

Brown GC, Shields JA, Sanborn G, Augsburger JJ, Savino PJ, Schatz NJ. Radiation retinopathy. Ophthalmology. 1982;(12):1494-1501.

Coskuncan NM, Jabs DA, Dunn JP, et al. The eye in bone marrow transplantation. VI. Retinal complications. Arch Ophthalmol. 1994;112(3):372-379.

Diepgen TL, Eysenbach G, et al. Dermatology Online Atlas. Published online at: http://www.derma.med.uni-erlangen.de/bilddb/.

Dullaert H, Maudgal PC, Leys A, Dralands L, Clerq E. Bromovinyldeoxyurdine treatment of outer retinal necrosis due to varicella-zoster virus: a case-report. Bull Soc Belge Ophthalmol. 1996;262:107-113.

Fishburne BC, Mitrani AA, Davis JL. Cytomegalovirus retinitis after cardiac transplantation. Am J Ophthalmol. 1998;125(1):104-106.

Holland GN. The progressive outer retinal necrosis syndrome. Int Ophthalmol. 1994;18(3):163-165.

Jabs DA, Hirst LW, Green WR, Tutschka PJ, Santos GW, Beschorner WE. The eye in bone marrow transplantation. II. Histopathology. Arch Ophthalmol. 1983;101(4):585-590.

Johnson DA, Jabs DA. The ocular manifestations of graft-versus-host disease. Int Ophthalmol Clin. 1997;37(2):119-133.

Kende G, Sirkin SR, Thomas PR, Freeman AI. Blurring of vision: a previously undescribed complication of cyclophosphamide therapy. Cancer. 1979;44(1):69-71.

Kiang E, Tesavibul N, Yee R, Kellaway J, Przepiorka D. The use of topical cyclosporin A in ocular graft-vs-host disease. Bone Marrow Transplant. 1998;22(2):147-151.

Lopez PF, Sternberg P Jr, Dabbs CK, Vogler WR, Crocker I, Kalin NS. Bone marrow transplant retinopathy. Am J Ophthalmol. 1991;112(6):635-646.

Meyers JD. Chemoprophylaxis of viral infection in immunocompromised patients. Eur J Cancer. 1989;25(9):1369-1374.

Ng P, McCluskey P, McCaughan G, Glanville A, MacDonald P, Keogh A. Ocular complications of heart, lung, and liver transplantation. Br J Ophthalmol. 1998;82(4):423-428.

Ohta Y, Okada H, Majima Y, Ishiguro I. Anticataract action of Vitamin E: its estimation using an in vitro steroid cataract model. Ophthalmic Res. 1996;28(2):16-25.

Papanicolaou GA, Meyers BR, Fuchs WS, et al. Infectious ocular complications in orthotopic liver transplant patients. Clin Infect Dis. 1997;24(6):1172-1177.

Peacock JE Jr, Greven CM, Cruz JM, Hurd DD. Reactivation toxoplasmic retinochoroiditis in patients undergoing bone marrow transplantation: is there a role for chemoprophylaxis? Bone Marrow Transplant. 1995;15(6):983-987.

Spees EK Jr, Kramer KK, Light JA, Oakes DD, Zimmerman LE. Reactivation of ocular malignant melanoma after renal transplantation. Transplantation. 1980;29(5):421-424.

Singh N, Bonham A, Fukui M. Immunosuppressive-associated leukoencephalopathy in organ transplant recipients. Transplantation. 2000;69(4):467-472

Stewart WB, Nicholson DH, Hamilton G, Tenzel RR, Spencer WH. Eyelid tumors and renal transplantation. Arch Ophthalmol. 1980;98(10):1771-1772.

30 LONG-TERM MANAGEMENT OF THE TRANSPLANTED PATIENT: HEALTH MAINTENANCE ISSUES

Alan Wilkinson, MD, FRCP

The early struggle to prevent the rejection of transplanted organs led to an understandable focus on early patient and graft survival. Today, however, the success of transplantation must be measured by more than this. Current goals of transplantation include not only preventing loss of life due to organ failure, but minimizing complications of immunosuppressive medications and the accelerated progression of common medical conditions. Focus is therefore needed on preventive strategies capable of limiting the onset and progression of conditions such as cardiovascular disease. Other impediments to long-term quality of life are organ-specific. All physicians caring for transplant patients should pay attention to the prevention of the general and organ-specific conditions discussed below. For many areas of preventive medicine, routine surveillance and immunizations, the website of the National Guideline Clearinghouse (www.guideline.gov/index.asp) is an excellent resource for physicians and other healthcare providers.

LIFESTYLE MODIFICATIONS

Education about healthy lifestyle options should be a part of every posttransplant medical visit. Lifestyle modifications, as recommended in the Sixth Report of the Joint National Committee on the Prevention, Detection, Evaluation and Treatment of Hypertension (JNC VI) are applicable to all transplant patients. If followed, they would considerably reduce the risk of complications from cardiovascular disease, the main source of morbidity for transplanted patients. All patients should be encouraged to increase their physical activity, preferably in a structured exercise program, and to limit their intake to a low-fat but balanced diet. Exercise and weight control are beneficial in reducing blood pressure, improving diabetic blood glucose control, and minimizing the effects of the immunosuppressive medications on bone density. Transplant patients who exercise have increased peak heart rates and peak levels of VO_2, which are measures of overall aerobic fitness. Kobashigawa has concluded from a study of the effects of exercise on heart transplant recipients that exercise training should be considered as part of standard care.

Professor of Medicine; Director, Kidney and Pancreas Transplantation, UCLA School of Medicine, Los Angeles, CA

An alcohol intake history should be obtained regularly and patients should be advised on how much they can safely consume. Women, who absorb alcohol more readily than do men, and lighter weight patients should be advised to drink less than larger men. Other dietary advice includes limiting sodium and fat intake. Lowering sodium in the diet should reduce blood pressure. It is also important to stress the adequate intake of potassium, calcium and magnesium. The DASH diet (Dietary Approaches to Stop Hypertension), which is rich in fruits, vegetables and low fat dairy foods, and low in saturated and total fat, is a sound foundation for posttransplant meals. Additionally, patients who continue to smoke not only markedly increase their cardiovascular risks, but also reduce the effectiveness of their antihypertensive therapy. Discontinuation of smoking is imperative and can be assisted by cessation aids and counseling.

STRATEGIES FOR THE PREVENTION OF CARDIOVASCULAR DISEASE

By the start of the second year after transplantation, cardiovascular disease becomes the leading cause of death. Early steps need to be taken, even prior to transplantation, to prevent its onset and progression. For example, cardiovascular disease is the major cause of death in end-stage renal disease (ESRD) as emphasized by the report of the National Kidney Foundation Task Force on Cardiovascular Disease. The mortality for patients on dialysis is 9% per year, about 30 times the risk in the general population. Factors with a high prevalence in the ESRD population and an association with cardiovascular disease are: (1) hypertension; (2) LDL cholesterol; (3) elevated homocysteine levels; (4) preexisting coronary artery disease; and (5) left ventricular hypertrophy. In diabetic dialysis patients, cardiovascular disease is even more common and may be masked by the relative lack of anginal pain.

The most significant risk factors for posttransplant cardiovascular disease in all organ recipients are pretransplant hypertension, elevated LDL cholesterol and diabetes. Statistical analysis has shown that other important factors are age, gender, nicotine use, and the cumulative dose of corticosteroids. Thus, while patients are awaiting transplantation, every effort should be made to minimize the risk factors for vascular disease. Hyperlipidemia should be treated aggressively to bring the total cholesterol, and particularly the low-density lipoprotein levels, down to the levels recommended for the prevention of the progression of vascular disease. In high-risk groups, the target LDL level is defined as at or under 100 mg/dL. This same approach must continue in the years after transplantation. In liver transplant candidates, cholesterol levels are often low so that lipid lowering therapy is not needed until after transplantation. Elevated homocysteine levels in ESRD and transplant patients are thought to increase the risk of cardiovascular disease, and treatment with folic acid and B vitamins is recommended to reduce this risk. It is also important to encourage changes in life style such as stopping cigarette smoking, weight reduction and exercise.

Hyperlipidemia Following Transplantation

Within three months of transplantation, about half the patients have an elevated serum cholesterol, with or without hypertriglyceridemia. This elevation persists in studies of long-term transplant recipients with 15% having a serum cholesterol level greater than 7.7 mmol/L (300 mg/dL) at two years. The levels of all forms of cholesterol are increased. Low-density lipoproteins (LDL) and the very low-density lipoproteins (VLDL) are usually the most affected. Although high-density lipoprotein (HDL) levels may be high, the HDL in this patient group may not be as protective as in the general population since it is unusually rich in cholesterol and triglycerides. Triglyceride levels are high in the first few months following transplantation, but thereafter tend to decline steadily for the next three years. Hyperlipidemia is strongly associated with the morbid complications of diabetic patients.

There are a number of factors that correlate with the presence of posttransplant hyperlipidemia including diabetes mellitus, renal dysfunction, age, beta blocker treatment, marked weight gain, diuretic use, and if present, heavy proteinuria. However, posttransplant immunosuppressive agents have been credited with the greatest influence on posttransplant lipid levels.

In some studies, but not all, patients treated with cyclosporine (CsA) have had elevated lipoprotein(a) [Lp(a)] levels suggesting that CsA may elevate Lp(a). An elevated Lp(a) level is an independent risk factor for the development of coronary artery disease. CsA is lipophilic and binds to LDL receptors. This may result in abnormal cholesterol synthesis. CsA, in addition, increases glucose intolerance and impairs bile acid synthesis by inhibition of 26-hydroxylase activity.

Corticosteroid therapy appears to be the most important factor in posttransplant hyperlipidemia and peripheral insulin resistance. The cumulative steroid dose and the daily steroid dose both correlate with hypertriglyceridemia and hypercholesterolemia. There is evidence that the insulin resistance is caused by an increase in the activity of the enzymes acetyl-coenzyme A carboxylase and free fatty acid synthetase. Corticosteroids can inhibit lipoprotein lipase, resulting in increased triglyceride levels and decreased HDL levels.

Sirolimus use is associated with increased cholesterol and triglyceride levels. This elevation usually decreases with time, and these abnormalities respond to

treatment with 3-hydroxy-3-methylglutaryl coenzyme A [HMG CoA] inhibitors. Those that reduce both the cholesterol and triglyceride levels, such as atorvastatin, are most beneficial in this group of patients. None of the clinical studies of this drug have shown a difference in coronary or cerebro-vascular disease during the relatively short periods the patients have been treated with the drug. If the hyperlipidemia does not respond adequately to treatment, another immunosuppressant should be substituted.

Treatment of Hyperlipidemia

NONPHARMACOLOGICAL TREATMENT. Diet, exercise and weight control are important parts of the plan to help transplant recipients limit the onset and progression of vascular disease. Patients should be encouraged to enter exercise rehabilitation programs. Exercise training is worthwhile for its effect on a patient's sense of well-being, blood pressure and overall rehabilitation, but it is not yet proven that this will prevent the progression of preexisting vascular disease. In dialysis patients, the correction of anemia by erythropoietin will allow them to exercise more regularly and more vigorously. Nutritional counseling should be provided to encourage patients to adopt a modified low-cholesterol diet.

REDUCTION IN CORTICOSTEROID DOSE. Reduction in the corticosteroid dose may improve the ease of weight loss, muscle strength and cosmesis making adherence to exercise programs easier. Additionally, in those patients who discontinue steroids, there is a significant reduction in total cholesterol and LDL. However, HDL levels also fall, and there is not yet conclusive data indicating that this strategy will diminish posttransplant vascular morbidity.

PHARMACOLOGICAL TREATMENT OF HYPERLIPIDEMIA. The National Cholesterol Education Program guidelines for treatment of nontransplant patients can be used to guide therapy in transplant recipients. These guidelines emphasize the use of the cardiovascular risk profile. Transplant patients usually have a number of risk factors in addition to an elevated LDL cholesterol. The positive risk factors are: (1) age, 45 in men and 55 in women; (2) a family history of cardiovascular disease; (3) smoking; (4) hypertension; (5) HDL cholesterol over 0.9 mmol/L (35 mg/dL); and (6) diabetes mellitus. An outline of the treatment of hyperlipidemia is shown in Table 30-1.

Lipid-reducing agents have been intensely studied in transplant recipients. Whereas almost all of the approved agents will reduce lipid levels, each is associated with a number of potential problems. The

Table 30-1. Treatment of Hyperlipidemia

Transplant patients should be considered high-risk for treatment stratification
Target LDL Cholesterol ≤100 mg/dL
Threshold for diet therapy: LDL cholesterol ≥100 mg/dL
Threshold for drug therapy: LDL cholesterol ≥130 mg/dL
Diet: Step I and Step II NCEP
Drug: HMG CoA RIs, starting at low doses in patients on calcineurin inhibitors
Isolated elevations in serum triglycerides, or a low HDL cholesterol (<35 mg/dL): Diet and exercise, treat an LDL cholesterol >130 mg/dL

HMG -CoA reductase inhibitors (HMG CoA RI), or "statins," are probably tolerated best, and effectively lower lipid levels. Additionally, there is accumulating evidence that the beneficial effects of these drugs are only partly a consequence of the reduction in cholesterol levels. In studies where the patients have been stratified according to their cholesterol levels, there is a reduction in vascular events in patients on HMG CoA RI as compared to patients with similar cholesterol levels in the control population. Initial concern that transplant patients would develop an unacceptably high incidence of myositis or rhabdomyolysis when HMG CoA RI were used with CsA has not been confirmed by their continued use. These early reports of elevated creatinine phosphokinase (CPK) levels and rhabdomyolysis were in patients treated with higher doses of lovastatin than are currently recommended. Myositis also occurred when lovastatin was used in combination with gemfibrozil or niacin, two agents that raise the serum levels of HMG CoA RI. Although the current risk of myositis is low, CPK levels must be measured in patients who complain of muscle pain while taking HMG CoA RI.

Pravastatin and simvastatin have gained wide acceptance in heart and kidney transplant patients. However, atorvastatin use is increasing as it appears to be the most effective at lowering both the cholesterol and triglyceride levels, and appears to cause myolysis less frequently than do some of the older agents. Currently, the most common toxicity of HMG CoA IR use is hepatotoxicity. When patients develop elevated transaminase levels, HMG CoA RI treatment should be discontinued.

Hypertriglyceridemia may be treated by the addition of a fibric acid derivative, such as clofibrate or gemfibrozil. The fibric acid derivatives have also been associated with myositis in CsA treated patients and care must be taken to monitor CPK levels. Bile acid sequestrants, cholestyramine and colestipol, may bind both cyclosporine and tacrolimus, thus decreasing absorption and necessitating increased drug level monitoring. Nicotinic acid can cause flushing and gastric toxicity. Some of these symptoms may be alleviated by the addition of low-dose aspirin therapy. Nicotinic acid may also be hepatotoxic in some patients.

Treatment with angiotensin-converting enzyme inhibitors (ACEI) has been shown, in the Heart Outcomes Prevention Evaluation study, to reduce mortality and vascular complications significantly in patients with preexisting vascular disease. Treatment with ACEI should be considered even in normotensive patients. Monitoring serum creatinine and potassium levels is necessary during ACEI treatment.

Table 30-2. Oral Agents for the Treatment of Posttransplant Diabetes Mellitus

Sulfonylureas (second generation). These are preferred to first generation sulfonylureas and are synergistic when used with metformin, or troglitazone.
   - Glipizide (Preferred in patients with impaired renal function.)
   - Glyburide
   - Glimepiride

Biguanides. Synergistic with troglitazone in lowering blood glucose.   - Metformin. Not recommended in patients with impaired renal or hepatic function.

Thiazolidinediones
   - Troglitazone. Should be used with caution because of potential hepatotoxicity.
   - Rosiglitazone

Meglitinides   - Repaglinide
Nateglinide (still investigational)
Alpha-glucosidase inhibitor   - Acarbose

POSTTRANSPLANT DIABETES MELLITUS

Steroid-induced diabetes mellitus has long been recognized as a risk for transplant patients, and the introduction of tacrolimus has further increased the incidence of this complication. Elevated blood glucose levels, although most common in the first months after transplantation, may persist even after the steroid dose has been reduced. Many patients with adult onset diabetes will become normoglycemic when they reach ESRD, and it is important to warn them of the likely need for insulin therapy after transplantation.

Treatment of posttransplant diabetes starts with dietary guidelines and exercise. In fact, exercise should be emphasized in all transplant candidates as well as recipients in order to improve glucose utilization. Oral agents are the primary medication therapy of posttransplant diabetes. The introduction of drugs that increase insulin sensitivity has markedly improved glucose control (Table 30-2). Metformin use, however, must still be carefully governed by renal function, and occasionally some patients will require insulin. Unless there is a contraindication, aspirin should be prescribed for diabetic patients to reduce their risk of vascular complication.

STRATEGIES FOR LIVER SURVEILLANCE

Recipients of non-liver transplants who have hepatitis are at an increased risk of progressive liver disease when they are immunosuppressed. Patients with hepatitis B infection should receive prophylactic lamivudine therapy. A number of drugs used commonly after transplantation may cause a mild hepatitis with elevated transaminases.

STRATEGIES FOR PREVENTION AND SURVEILLANCE OF INFECTIOUS DISEASES

Please refer to Chapter 20.

ROUTINE VACCINATION

Patients often inquire about the safety of immunizations. As a rule, patients should not receive live vaccines; exceptions may include the measles, mumps, and rubella and varicella vaccines, although there is no consensus about the safety of their use in immunocompromised hosts. In addition to the concern about a rampant viral syndrome from live vaccines, there is also concern that immunizations, by stimulating the immune system, may precipitate acute rejection episodes. Thus, it has been felt prudent to wait at least six months following transplantation before giving immunizations. Additionally, during this early period the intense immunosuppression may reduce the response to immunization. Vaccines that are acceptable in transplant recipients and those that should be avoided are listed in Table 30-3. Tetanus and inactivated polio virus vaccinations are tolerated and patients develop protective antibody levels. Diphtheria vaccination is less effective, and within one year after vaccination the level of antibody may no longer be protective. The influenza vaccine should be offered to all transplant patients beyond six months from transplantation, particularly to those at highest risk including those over age 65, and those with chronic cardiopulmonary or metabolic diseases. It is given as a single dose of 0.5 cc intramuscularly, annually in October or November. Pneumococcal vaccination is recommended for all patients, and pneumococcal vaccine (0.5 cc IM) should be given to those patients that have not received it in the previous five years. It is particularly important that patients who have undergone splenectomy receive this vaccine.

Hepatitis B vaccination should be completed while patients are waiting for transplantation. An HB_sA level should be checked in patients that have received a prior vaccination series and, if the level has fallen below 10(SI) a booster should be administered. Hepatitis A vaccination should be given before transplantation and repeated if patients are at high risk of infection or if they travel to areas where the disease is endemic.

Table 30-3. Vaccinations for Immunocompromised Patients

Contraindicated Live Vaccination
 - BCG
 - Oral polio vaccine
 - Oral typhoid vaccine (ty21a)
   Varicella Zoster vaccine
   Yellow Fever vaccine

Acceptable Live Vaccination - Measles-mumps-rubella vaccine (indications and   use as for immunocompetent adults)

Acceptable Vaccination
 - Pneumococcal polysaccharide vaccine
   (recommended for all patients)
 - Influenza vaccine (after six months posttransplant)
 - Hepatitis B vaccine
 - Hepatitis A vaccine
 - Tetanus-diphtheria
 - Enhanced potency inactivated Polio vaccine (eIPV)
 - Inactivated (parenteral) typhoid vaccine or Typhoid
   Vi polysaccharide vaccine
 - Japanese B encephalitis vaccine

TRAVEL

Adventurous transplant recipients have demonstrated the safety of traveling to exotic locations. In addition, transplantation is now practiced in most parts of the world and there are usually local experts to whom travelers can turn if they become ill while away from home. Before traveling, patients should be referred to a travel clinic to receive counseling, and appropriate vaccinations and prophylaxis for diseases they are likely to encounter. Refer to Table 30-3 for acceptable and contraindicated vaccines.

PETS AT HOME

Many transplant programs have advised against household pets after transplantation. This is particularly true for patients who keep birds, because of a concern about

Table 30-4. Animal Infections Transmitted to Humans

Type of Illness	Etiologic Agent	Common Pet Carrier
Skin	Bartonella henselae (cat-scratch/bacillary angiomatosis)	Cat
	Sarcoptes scabei (scabies)	Dog/Cat-occasional
	Pasteurella multocida	Dog/Cat
	Staphylococcus aureus	Dog/Cat
	Streptococcus spp.	Dog/Cat
	Microsporum gypseum (Tinea capitus)	Dog/Cat
	Trichophyton mentagrophytes (Ringworm)	Dog/Cat
	Ancylostoma braziliense (Cutaneous larvae migrans) (intestinal nematode/hookworm)	Dog/Cat
	Mycobacterium marinum (swimming pool granuloma)	Tropical fish
	Sporothrix schenckii	Pet fur—Cats
	Basidiobolus ranarum (phycomycosis)	Frog/Toad/Lizard
Systemic from Bite/Scratch	Bartonella henselae (cat-scratch)	Cat
	Streptobacillus moniliformis (rat bite fever)	Rat
	Spirillum minus (rat bite fever)	Rat
	Capnocytophaga canimorsus	Dog
Diarrhea/GI	Campylobacter spp	Cat/Puppy
	Salmonella, Campylobacter	Turtle/Iguana/Lizard/ Alligator/Bird/Monkey
	Edwardsiella	Turtle/Snake
	Plesiomonas	Snake
	Yersinia	Dog
	Dipyllidium canum (tapeworm)	Dog/Cat – Fleas
	Echinococcus granulosus (tapeworm)	Dog
Respiratory	Chlamydia psittaci	Bird
	Dirofilaria immitis (canine heartworm)	Dog – Mosquito
	Beta-hemolytic streptococci	Dog/Cat
	Rhodococcus equi	Horse/Cow/Pig
	Atypical mycobacterium	Monkey/Cattle/ Reptiles/Bird/all
Multisystem Illness	Toxoplasma gondi	Cat
	Toxocara canis/cati (roundworm)	Dog/Cat
	Leptospira (leptospirosis)	Dog/Rat
	Brucella	Dog/Cow/Pig/Goat
	Lymphocytic choriomeningitis Virus	Hamster (Rodents)
	Cryptococcosis neoformans	Bird/Cat/Dog
	Histoplasma capsulatum	Bird
	Aeromonas hydrophila	Reptiles
	Eastern & Western encephalitis	Reptiles
	Mucor sp.	Reptiles
	Aspergillus	Reptiles
	Fusarium	Reptiles
	Penicillium sp.	Reptiles
	Trichinosis	Swine (Pot-bellied pigs)

psittacosis. However, the loss of a pet may be a significant emotional burden; provided pets are screened and treated for infections, it is safe for patients to continue to have household pets. The pets and their cages and bedding should be kept clean; it is prudent for someone other than the patient to deal with litter boxes and the cleaning of bird cages, at least for the first six months after transplantation. Most pets can remain in the household. It is only reptiles that are contraindicated as pets. Reptiles can carry untreatable infections such as salmonellosis. Infections that are carried by domesticated animals are listed in Table 30-4.

CHILD CARE AND OTHER OCCUPATIONAL EXPOSURE TO INFECTIONS

Patients will frequently ask about the risk of contracting illnesses from children. Other patients may look after young children as care givers or teachers and will be exposed to the many illnesses from which young children suffer. In general, provided sensible precautions such as avoiding direct close contact and regular hand washing are followed, there is no significant risk. Patients exposed to a person with a varicella-zoster virus or other herpes viral infections should receive prophylactic gammaglobulin and acyclovir therapy. Patients who work as nurses or physicians can return to work, as can others exposed to sick people. Patients who work outside or with wood in occupations that expose them to fungal spores should wear masks and gloves and minimize dust exposure wherever possible. This is also true for recreational gardeners.

PSYCHIATRIC COMPLICATIONS

Depression is quite common in patients with chronic illnesses and may be exacerbated by immunosuppressive medications. Awareness and treatment of this commonly overlooked disorder are important functions of the transplant center. Depression is known to adversely impact medication compliance. The selective serotonin re-uptake inhibitors are widely used. However, as they inhibit the cytochrome P-450 enzyme system, they may affect the metabolism of immunosuppressive medications. Nefazodone may increase CsA levels by as much as 70%. Of all the newer antidepressant medications, nefazodone and fluvoxamine are associated with the greatest risk of inhibiting CsA metabolism and inducing toxicity.

ROUTINE CANCER SURVEILLANCE
Breast, Cervical and Prostate Cancer Screening

Female patients over the age of 40 should have an annual breast examination in conjunction with mammography screening, as well as an annual pelvic examination and Pap smear. Male patients should have an annual digital rectal examination after the age of 40, and an annual prostate-specific antigen test after the age of 50.

Skin Cancer

Please see Chapter 28.

Colorectal Cancer Screening

Cancer screening should include a rectal examination every two years from the age of 40 to 59, and thereafter annually. Fecal occult blood testing should be done annually, and a flexible sigmoidoscopy should be done periodically, approximately every five years, after the age of 50. Alternatively, patients may have a total colon examination by either colonoscopy every ten years, or double-contrast barium enema every five to ten years.

DENTAL CARE

Dental hygiene, with regular brushing and flossing, should be emphasized to prevent gum disease and tooth loss, and to reduce CsA and calcium antagonist-induced gum hypertrophy. Patients should visit their dentist regularly, and most transplant centers recommend the use of antibiotic prophylaxis prior to dental work. If attention to oral hygiene and periodontal surgery do not prevent significant gum overgrowth in patients on CsA, calcium antagonists should be replaced with other antihypertensive medications and the dose of CsA reduced as far as is compatible with adequate immunosuppression. If gum overgrowth still persists, patients should be converted from CsA to tacrolimus, or potentially sirolimus. This usually results in resolution of this complication.

ADHERENCE TO PRESCRIBED MEDICATIONS

Nonadherence to immunosuppressive medications impacts long-term allograft survival. There are a number of recent studies examining this problem and the extent to which it is possible to predict those patients most likely to become noncompliant. The study by Greenstein and Siegal included 2,500 patients from 56 transplant centers in the US. They identified three groups: (1) accidental noncompliers, (2) invulnerables, and (3) decisive noncompliers. Age was positively associated with compliance. Other significant predictors are education, employment and occupation. A longer time since transplant increased the likelihood of noncompliance, as did receiving a living-related donor allograft.

MUSCULOSKELETAL DISEASE
Diseases of the Bone

All transplant patients suffer from bone disease. Liver disease is associated with bone disease, and many patients with heart disease have reduced bone mineral density from reduced physical activity. Renal transplant patients are at particular risk as the majority already have quite significant renal osteodystrophy. Additionally, the incidence of osteonecrosis, particularly of the femoral neck, occurs in as many as 6% to 8% of patients in the first few years after transplantation. For an in-depth review, please refer to Chapter 25.

Nonspecific Musculoskeletal Pain

Bone and joint pain has been described in patients receiving CsA. As this frequently affects the lower femur, it is often confused with arthritis of the knee. Studies have suggested that CsA can cause ischemia of the distal femur. This often occurs at night and may respond to treatment with calcium channel blockers. It is postulated that these agents reverse CsA-induced vasoconstriction. During or following high-dose corticosteroid therapy, particularly when the dose is reduced rapidly, a few patients complain of joint pain and myalgias.

Corticosteroid use may cause a proximal myopathy. Treatment includes physical therapy and a reduction in steroid dose. It is another reason to encourage fitness training in patients waiting for transplantation. Care should be taken however, when starting a posttransplant exercise program as both the muscles and tendons are at increased risk of rupture. Ciprofloxacin administration, used frequently to treat urinary tract infections, has been implicated in the development of tendinitis and rupture of the Achilles and other tendons. Patients on CsA and statin therapy for hypercholesterolemia are at risk of myolysis and may complain of muscle fatigue and pain. When this occurs the statin should be discontinued and they should be tested for an elevation in creatine phosphokinase (CPK) levels.

Gout

Gout is a fairly common complication and may present as a polyarticular arthritis. Long-term treatment is usually with allopurinol, adjusted for renal function. However, in patients already on azathioprine, care should be taken not to induce significant leucopenia as a result of more pronounced bone marrow suppression. Colchicine should be used for acute attacks of gout and allopurinol for long-term prevention. Short courses of oral steroids may be used in those who do not tolerate colchicine or allopurinol. Care should be taken when giving nonsteroidal medications as they increase the risk for renal dysfunction and inhibit the effects of some antihypertensive medications.

SEXUAL AND REPRODUCTIVE FUNCTION

Men

In approximately half to two-thirds of male patients, libido, sexual activity and fertility will improve after transplantation. Sex hormone profiles normalize with an increase in plasma testosterone and follicle-stimulating hormone levels with correction of end-organ disease. In patients with end-stage renal disease, high-luteinizing hormone levels fall to normal or low levels.

Immunosuppressive medications may affect libido and reproduction. For instance, CsA may affect testosterone production by direct damage to Leydig cells and germinal cells, and impairment of the hypothalamic-pituitary-gonadal axis. However, neonatal malformations are not increased in pregnancies fathered by men immunosuppressed with CsA, corticosteroids and azathioprine. There is as yet little data on the outcome of pregnancies fathered by men on newer immunosuppressives such as mycophenolate and sirolimus.

The underlying disease, as in diabetic patients with autonomic neuropathy, may also affect sexual function. Vascular disease may reduce penile arterial flow and impair erectile function. The use of Viagra®, and potentially CsA, may improve sexual function, but before prescribing Viagra® the potential cardiac risks should be reviewed. It is possible that Viagra® may affect CsA levels as it is a weak inhibitor of the cytochrome P-450 enzyme system. Antihypertensive medications are frequently an etiologic factor in impaired sexual function and in a lack of improvement following transplantation. Antihypertensive therapy should be reviewed to minimize their deleterious effect.

Women

Please refer to Chapter 27.

INSOMNIA

Insomnia is a common complaint, especially in the first months after transplantation. Prednisone in particular, and some of the other routinely used medications may exacerbate it. The possibility of underlying conditions such as esophageal reflux, sleep apnea and depression should be investigated when there is sufficient clinical suspicion. Additionally, inquiring about the number of naps taken during the day and the amount of exercise may help outline treatment plans. Other therapies include relaxation techniques and the use of Ambien® or a drug such as clonazepam. Shorter-acting benzodiazepines should be avoided, as these can cause significant symptoms of withdrawal. Melatonin has been used in the treatment of sleep disorders in the elderly. Provided patients understand that the preparations available are not approved or monitored by the FDA, and may contain unknown additives, it is acceptable for them to use melatonin for a short period. Kava, described below, has some relaxing and sedative properties.

USE OF NATUROPATHIC MEDICATIONS

Many patients who suffer from chronic illnesses are interested in alternative remedies that may be effective in alleviating some of their symptoms without adding significantly to the burden of side effects and complications. Patients must be warned that the data on most of these remedies are insufficient for physicians to give advice on safety and the potential risk of interactions with the standard medications used in this population. Herbal remedies for which there is more substantial laboratory and clinical testing are known as phytopharmaceuticals. Some of the more popular herbal medications available for general use and about which patients may ask questions are described below. For most of them there is little documentation of their toxicities, and none about possible interactions with the drugs used routinely after transplantation. Only the regulatory authorities in Germany have published data on the use of some of these preparations.

Echinacea is used for the treatment of colds, flu and infection. It is prepared from the root of the Purple Coneflower, *Rudbeckia purpurea*; its actions are believed to include antimicrobial and immunomodulating properties; it is anticatarrhal; and it has been used in combination with Yarrow or Bearberry to treat cystitis.

Gingko biloba is a Chinese tree from which the herb *Gingko* is extracted. This herbal remedy has been in use for thousands of years and the seeds were used originally in traditional Chinese medicine to strengthen the kidneys, improve digestion and to hasten recovery from illness. *Gingko* leaves are used in modern herbal preparations that are believed to improve the circulation to the legs and brain in older people. There is some evidence that it may improve memory even in patients with Alzheimer's disease. Care must be taken when patients are on anticoagulants or aspirin as some extracts of *Gingko* may have anticoagulant properties.

Kava is the popular name for the remedies extracted from the plant *Piper methysticum* Forst, a member of the pepper family indigenous to the South Sea islands. Kava is prepared from the roots and rhizomes. It is a mild sedative and anxiolytic and is used as a relaxant. Studies suggest it may be as useful as benzodiazepines in relieving anxiety. There has been one report of profound sedation when kava and alprazolam were used at the same time.

St. John's Wort, derived from the plant *Hypericum perforatum* L, has been used for its properties since at least the time of the Ancient Greeks. It was used widely as a folk remedy to heal wounds, remedy kidney troubles, and alleviate nervous disorders. It may be useful in the treatment of depression, and has been used in conjunction with monoamine oxidase (MAO) and selective serotonin reuptake inhibitors, such as Zoloft. Some studies have demonstrated that extracts have antibacterial and wound healing qualities. Photosensitization is possible in lighter skinned individuals. However, experimental and clinical evidence has shown that St. John's Wort affects the activity of the Cytochrome P450 (CYP3A4 isoenzyme) system, and by increasing CsA metabolism will decrease patients' exposure to CsA unless an adjustment is made in dosing. For this reason it is best to avoid this herbal preparation and it should not be used without consultation with a transplant physician.

Garlic has been used widely in Ayurveda (traditional Indian medical system), traditional Chinese medicine and European herbal medicine. Enthusiasts for its use claim that it may reduce blood pressure, blood cholesterol levels and reduce fungal overgrowth of, for example, *Candida albicans.*

Ginseng is believed to reduce stress and increase energy. Chinese practitioners believe it increases longevity and general health, appetite and memory.

Phytoestrogens, obtained in plants rich in isoflavones, may reduce menopausal symptoms, but there is insufficient evidence to know whether they reduce heart disease and osteoporosis. They can be obtained in herbal preparations or in soy, linseed and redclover.

Saw palmetto, from the plant Serenoa *repens*, is claimed to reduce the symptoms of prostatic hypertrophy. It inhibits the conversion of testosterone to dihydrotestosterone (DHT) and inhibits the binding of DHT to receptor sites on the prostate.

RECOMMENDED READING

American Association of Clinical Endocrinologists Clinical Practice Guidelines for the Management of Diabetes Mellitus, ©1995, AACE, developed by The American Association of Clinical Endo urologists and The American College of Endocrinology.
http://www.aace.com/clin/guides/diabetes_2000.pdf

National Guideline Clearinghouse®. A public world wide web resource for evidence-based clinical practice guidelines produced by the Agency for Healthcare Research and Quality, in partnership with the American Medical association and the American Association of Health Plans.
http://www.guidelines.gov/index.asp

Pharmaceutical Information Network, a world wide web high-volume pharmaceutical information resource.
http://www.pharminfo.com

Healthfinder®, a public world wide web gateway to reliable consumer health and human services information developed by the US Department of Health and Human Services. http://www.healthfinder.com

The National Center for Complementary and Alternative Medicine, a public information clearinghouse of the NIH, facilitates the evaluation of alternative medicinal treatment modalities to determine their effectiveness. http://nccam.nih.gov

Health Net® a California health care company that provides information and advice on alternative medicine. http://www.healthnet.com

NOAH, New York Online Access to Health®, a world wide web service providing full-text health information and resources for multilingual and latino web communication. http://www.noah.cuny.edu

The National Heart, Lung, and Blood Institute Clinical Guidelines on the Identification, Evaluation and treatment of Overweight and Obesity in Adults. http://www.nhlbi.nih.gov/guidelines/obesity/ob_home.htm

Greenstein S, Siegal B. Compliance and non-compliance in patients with a functioning renal transplant: a multicenter study. Transplantation. 1998;66:1718-1726.

Levey AS. Controlling the epidemic of cardiovascular disease in chronic renal disease: What do we know? What do we need to learn? Where do we go from here? Special Report of the National Kidney Foundation Task Force on Cardiovascular Disease. Am J Kid Dis. 1998;32(5) Suppl 3:S1-S199.

Willett WC, Dietz WH, Colditz GA. Guidelines for healthy weight. N Engl J Med. 1999;341(6):427-434.

Joint National Committee on Detection, Evaluation, and Treatment of High Blood Pressure (JNC VI): The Sixth Report of the Joint National Committee on Prevention, Detection, Evaluation and Treatment of High Blood Pressure. Arch Intern Med. 1997;157(21):2413-2446.

Appel LJ, Moore TJ, Obarzanek E, et al. A clinical trial of the effects of dietary patterns on blood pressure. DASH Collaborative Research Group. N Engl J Med. 1997;336(16):1117-1124.

Stempfle HU, Werner C, Echtler S, et al. Prevention of osteoporosis after cardiac transplantation: a prospective, longitudinal, randomized, double-blind trial with calcitriol. Transplantation. 1999;68(4):523-530.

Painter P. Exercise after renal transplantation. Adv Ren Replace Ther. 1999;6(2):159-164.

Poulter N. Coronary Heart Disease is a multifactorial disease. Am J Hypertens. 1999;12(10 Pt 2):92S-95S.

Beilin LJ, Puddey IB, Burke V. Lifestyle and Hypertension. Am J Hypertens. 1999;12(9 Pt 1):934-945.

31 SPECIAL ISSUES IN PEDIATRIC ORGAN TRANSPLANTATION

William E. Harmon, MD

Children with end-stage organ failure generally have different underlying diseases, different immune responses, different medical and surgical complications of organ transplantation and different treatment end-points than do adults. Thus, those who provide transplant care for children should be aware of these differences and experienced in dealing with them. These issues can be categorized under four major headings: (1) Primary disease leading to end-stage organ failure in children; (2) Pediatric-specific responses; (3) Pediatric end-points; and, (4) Pediatric complications posttransplantation.

PRIMARY DISEASES LEADING TO END-STAGE ORGAN FAILURE IN CHILDREN

In general, the incidence of end-stage organ failure in children is low. The etiology of organ failure is typically different in children and adults. For example, Table 31-1 compares the causes of end-stage renal disease (ESRD) in children (derived from the North American Pediatric Renal Transplant Collaborative Study [NAPRTCS] registry) and in adults (derived from the United States Renal Disease Study [USRDS] report). Adults develop ESRD because of acquired diseases (eg, hypertension, diabetes, glomerulonephritis), whereas children have congenital or hereditary causes (eg, renal dysplasia, urologic abnormalities, polycystic renal disease). Importantly, the pediatric causes of ESRD are not consistent in all age groups, with acquired diseases becoming more common in older children (Figure 31-1). Similar patterns of causes of end-stage heart and liver disease have been described.

The Burden of Congenital and Inherited Diseases

Children with congenital heart, liver, kidney and lung diseases generally have been burdened by their disease for their entire lives. Their growth and development are hampered by abnormal metabolism, perfusion or oxygenation. Furthermore, since many of these diseases are structural, such as hypoplastic left heart syndrome,

Associate Professor of Pediatrics, Harvard Medical School; Director, Pediatric Nephrology, Children's Hospital Boston, Boston, MA

biliary atresia and obstructive uropathy, these children require many operations to attempt to preserve function or to correct abnormalities prior to transplantation. In these circumstances, the children are frequently growth and developmentally retarded and their social, emotional and educational skills are also quite underdeveloped. Preparation prior to and rehabilitation after transplantation must be undertaken with these additional problems in perspective.

Recurrence of Disease Posttransplantation

Most congenital structural diseases, such as biliary atresia, reflux nephropathy and hypoplastic left heart syndrome will not recur after transplantation. The recipients, however, may have complications related to surgery performed prior to transplantation. Children, therefore, may have some minor advantage over adults who may have other chronic disease, such as diabetes, hepatitis or atherosclerosis, that may affect the outcome of the transplant. One notable exception is focal segmental glomerulosclerosis (FSGS) in children. Recurrence rates of FSGS in children, especially young children, are 30% to 50% and may occur immediately after transplantation, often with devastating consequences.

PEDIATRIC-SPECIFIC RESPONSES
Pediatric Immune Responsiveness

There are conflicting data about whether infants and small children have a "heightened" immune response and an increased incidence of acute rejection episodes. Very young infants may have low levels of immunoglobulins, may be particularly susceptible to certain types of bacterial infections and may not respond to immunizations to certain antigens, leading to a delay of immunizations until after the first birthday. All of these data suggest that the infant younger than one year may have an immature immune response. On the other hand, indirect evidence suggests a vigorous immune response in young children between one and five years of age. These data include increased numbers of lymphocytes in

Table 31-1. Etiology of End-Stage Renal Disease in Children and in Adults

Etiology	Child	Adult
Dysplasia	17%	3%
Urologic	26%	4%
Other Congenital	15%	5%
FSGS	11%	2%
Other GN	14%	17%
Hypertension	0%	22%
Diabetes	0%	40%

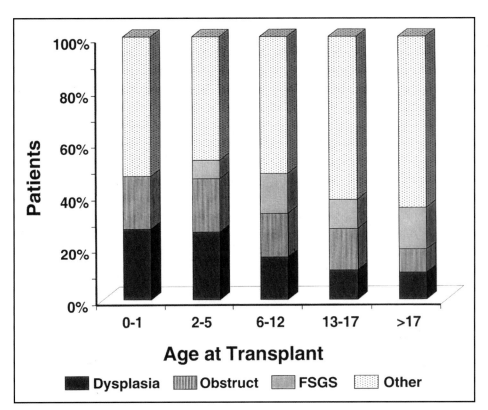

peripheral blood and blastogenesis responses to mitogens and allergens. Also, data from the United Network of Organ Sharing (UNOS) registry suggest a higher rate of acute rejections in young children after kidney, liver and heart transplantation, although adolescents have been noted to have a higher rate of late acute rejections, especially following kidney transplantation.

In contrast to these reports, single center data from large pediatric liver and kidney transplant programs have demonstrated that infants younger than one or two years may have a lower rate of acute rejection and better graft survival rates than older children and adults. Also, data from surveillance kidney transplant biopsies suggest equivalent intragraft cytokine gene expression in all age groups of kidney transplant recipients. Finally, long-term UNOS data demonstrate that although very young kidney transplant recipients may have relatively poor 1-year graft survival rates, those whose grafts survive the first year have the longest graft half-lives of any age group, including adults. This observation has been corroborated by results from a large pediatric renal transplant center that found the longest half-lives in infant recipients who had not had any acute rejection episodes. Whether this finding is related to a relatively large renal reserve from adult kidneys in young recipients, or to the likelihood of developing relative tolerance in these recipients is not clear. In either case, these outcomes do not support an enhanced immune response in young children compared to young adults. On the other hand,

elderly adults have substantially lower rates of rejection than younger adults, so it might be more appropriate to characterize older adults as having a diminished immune response, rather than suggesting that young children have a heightened response. Furthermore, data from the most recent UNOS annual report demonstrate substantially better 5-year patient survival in children than in older adults. Children six to ten years old have 97.4% 5-year patient survival following live donor transplants, compared to 90.3% for 35 to 49 year-olds and 81.9% for 50 to 64 year-olds. On balance, therefore, children generally make excellent candidates for organ transplantation.

Pharmacokinetics/Pharmacodynamics in Pediatric Transplant Recipients

Since there is a substantial variation in the size of pediatric organ transplant recipients, it should be obvious that the doses of immunosuppressive and other medications must be adjusted appropriately for their size. Thus, doses are typically administered on a "per kg" or a "per M2" basis. In addition to having adjustments of the dose for their size, the pediatric patient frequently needs different doses because of differences in metabolism. Unfortunately, until recently, pediatric patients were not included in preclinical studies of immunosuppressive medications, and these differences were discovered only on the basis of trial and error observations. For example, early use of cyclosporine in young children resulted in suboptimal blood levels with usual dosing, and subsequent pharmacokinetic profiling uncovered enhanced metabolism of the drug. Thus, typically children under six must receive the drug three times per day rather than twice. Very similar observations are now being reported with the early use of rapamycin. Recent data demonstrate wide intersubject variability in concentration and AUCs (area-under-the-curve) of mycophenolate mofetil in children and very probably variation among different age groups. Overall, it is extremely important to perform frequent determinations of drug levels in children, to perform pharmacokinetic analyses if drug levels are erratic and to adjust the doses and intervals appropriately.

PEDIATRIC END-POINTS
Growth Posttransplantation

A major distinguishing feature of pediatric from adult recipients is the need for children to grow. Growth failure is common in children with chronic organ failure and is frequently related to malnutrition. This growth failure is frequently most pronounced in children with chronic renal insufficiency in which the etiology is multifactorial; however, the most important causes are malnutrition and the reduced response to endogenous growth hormone. Growth failure often begins insidiously early in the course of chronic renal insufficiency. In a NAPRTCS analysis of 1,768 children with chronic renal insufficiency (glomerular filtration rate <75/mL per min/m2), over one-third had a height deficit of more than two standard deviations (SDS) from the mean. It has been amply demonstrated that chronic renal insufficiency beginning in infancy leads to permanent reduction in growth potential. Growth retardation continues in children on a dialysis regimen, whether the mode of dialysis is peritoneal or hemodialysis.

For several years it has been suggested that a functioning transplant would enable a child to achieve catch-up growth. Long-term data from registry studies, however, has shown a more disappointing outcome. NAPRTCS has tracked growth posttransplantation longitudinally, using the same cohort for at least five years. In these studies height data was analyzed at two years, again at three years, and repeated at 54 months posttransplantation. The height deficit was -2.41 in the first study, -2.46 in the second evaluation, and -2.29 at the end of the third study period. Children in the first study had an improvement in height SDS of +0.18, of +0.16 in the second period, and of +0.11 in the third period. When improvement in height deficit was evaluated by donor source, no differences were noted between living-related and cadaver donor recipients. Analysis of height SDS by race revealed that, whereas for Caucasian children a steady improvement was noted during the second and third periods, there was an actual deceleration of growth

for African-American and Hispanic children. Only the initial height deficit and recipient age are independent predictors of improved height posttransplantation. Catch-up growth, defined as an improvement of one SDS, was seen only in children birth to one year. Overall catch-up growth was seen in only 47% of children between the ages of two and five years. For children over the age of five, who form 72% of the study cohort, little catch-up growth was noted. Children with heart transplants frequently grow well, especially after steroids are withdrawn from their immunosuppression regimen after two to three years. However, as with kidney transplant recipients, the best growth response is seen in the youngest patients and the worst in the adolescents. Similar patterns are described after liver transplantation. Younger recipients grow better than older recipients. Children with more severe growth retardation at the time of transplantation may have more pronounced catch-up growth, but their final adult height is less. Poor growth is seen in pediatric liver recipients with chronic rejection and posttransplant complications. Cumulative steroid dose varies inversely with long-term growth.

Overall, therefore, final adult height after organ transplantation in children is generally affected by complications and growth failure prior to transplantation, and by the cumulative steroid dose, graft function and complications after transplantation.

The studies on long-term growth posttransplantation are disappointing; however they do focus on mechanisms that prevent growth despite a milieu with normal organ function. Individual center studies have adopted a variety of techniques, such as discontinuation of corticosteroids, alternate-day steroid therapy, or the use of recombinant human growth hormone. It has been known for several years that steroids used for immunosuppressive therapy will inhibit growth. It has also been demonstrated that steroids affect growth hormone secretion. Measurements of pulsatile and pharmacologically-stimulated hormone release reveal that steroids play an inhibitory role. Conversion of children to alternate-day steroid therapy has shown improvement in growth; however, the best catch-up growth is seen in patients completely withdrawn from steroids. Numerous uncontrolled studies have shown that steroids can be withdrawn from children posttransplantation for all organ transplants; however, acute rejection tends to occur shortly afterwards in many of these patients, especially kidney transplant recipients. There is not yet a reliable immune marker that can identify individual patients who are hyporesponsive and can safely undergo steroid withdrawal. An alternative method of attaining catch-up growth posttransplantation would be the use of growth hormone. Recombinant human growth hormone is not approved for use in children posttransplantation, however, numerous uncontrolled studies have shown its ability to accelerate growth in this setting. Several complications of the use of rhGH posttransplantation have been suggested, including immunostimulation or enhancement of fibrosis in recipients with chronic rejection. Thus, the proper use of rhGH posttransplantation has yet to be defined.

Development

Although less obvious than growth retardation, developmental delay is frequently just as common as growth retardation in pediatric organ transplant recipients. The toll of chronic disease prior to transplantation leads to a substantial need for hospitalizations, operations, medications and other treatments, which interferes with normal socialization and educational activities. In addition, growth retardation, limitations on physical activity and cosmetic changes related to immunosuppressive medications often set these children apart from their peers. One of the major hallmarks of adolescence is to establish independence from parents and other supports. Children with chronic diseases are generally unable to accomplish this important landmark and, thus, frequently are undergoing developmental changes at far older ages than their peers.

Children with chronic organ insufficiency may have poor intellectual functioning and school performance. School function studies in children with chronic renal insufficiency, for example, have demonstrated global dysfunction, with worsening scores and even decreases in IQ testing correlating with diminishing renal function. The worst scores were recorded in children who were receiving chronic dialysis treatments. Even school attendance is adversely impacted by repeated testing and treatments for organ dysfunction. Importantly, school function and even IQ scores have improved following successful kidney transplantation.

Virtually all pediatric transplant recipients have delayed puberty, but most will complete pubertal development if the graft function is satisfactory. Many of these children will have a diminished pubertal growth spurt. However, their epiphyses generally close at a later age, and they may continue to grow until a much later age, even into their 20s, permitting an improved final adult height. Thus, it is important to assure a minimal steroid dose at the critical interval during and immediately following puberty.

PEDIATRIC COMPLICATIONS
Graft Thrombosis

Graft thrombosis is an almost unique complication of pediatric kidney and liver transplantation. Although usually a major cause of immediate graft nonfunction, it can be seen later on in the course, and has been recorded to occur as late as one month posttransplant

following initial engraftment and function. Graft thrombosis is the third most common cause of graft failure in pediatric renal transplantation. The critical nature of this complication can be appreciated from the fact that it accounts for 12% of graft failure in index transplantation and 20% in repeat transplants in the NAPRTCS registry. A dreaded event, this condition is irreversible in most cases and necessitates removal of the graft. Graft thrombosis should be suspected in cases in which there has been immediate function followed by the development of oligoanuria. The diagnosis is established by a radionuclide scan using diethylenetriamine pentaacetic acid (DTPA) or Tc-mercaptoacetythiglycine (MAG3), which reveals a photopenic defect with no uptake by the transplant kidney. Since the outcome of graft thrombosis is uniformly dismal, numerous studies have been conducted in an attempt to understand and anticipate this complication. The etiology of graft thrombosis is multifactorial, but it is more commonly seen in young recipients. In a special study of 2,060 living donor and 2,334 cadaver donor kidneys, the NAPRTCS has shown that having had a prior transplant increases the risk, whereas increasing recipient age has a protective effect for living donor kidneys. The prophylactic use of antilymphocyte antibody also decreases the risk. For cadaver source kidneys, a cold ischemia time longer than 24 hours increases the risk of thrombosis. The use of antibody induction therapy, the use of donors over five years old, and increasing recipient age are factors that decrease the risk of thrombosis. A more recent analysis has demonstrated that renal graft thrombosis is more common in programs that have less experience in transplanting pediatric recipients than in larger pediatric programs.

Thrombosis of the portal vein or hepatic artery is also a devastating problem in pediatric liver transplantation. Similarly, the risk of thrombosis is increased in very young recipients, in transplants in which there is extended time between recovery and transplantation and in programs with less experience. Appropriate preparation of the recipient, intraoperative and postoperative anticoagulation and the use of innovative operative techniques have been successful in reducing the incidence of graft thrombosis.

Infections and Immunizations

In contrast to other immunosuppressed states (such as congenital deficiencies), the posttransplantation setting introduces a unique set of additional factors that must be taken into consideration in the pathogenesis, evaluation and treatment of infections. The currently used immunosuppressive agents are nonspecific and suppress multiple components of the immune system. Thus, patients are at risk for a wide variety of infections, including bacterial, viral and fungal infections. These agents have multiple portals of entry, including the allograft itself, as described below. Children pose a special risk group due to the lower incidence of prior immunity to many opportunistic infectious agents, such as EBV (Epstein-Barr virus), CMV (cytomegalovirus) and *Pneumocystis carinii.* Currently, many organs transplanted into children originate from adults and are more likely to be positive for these organisms. The transplantation of seropositive donor organs into seronegative recipients introduces the possibility of primary infection after immunosuppression has been initiated. Primary infection is generally more severe than reactivation or reinfection. For example the risk for PTLD is greatest when primary infection with EBV is present. Additionally, children have longer postoperative stays in the hospital than adult transplant recipients. The duration of hospitalization is inversely related to the age of the child. The duration of instrumentation is longer and places them at greater risk for infections that originate from a portal of entry (eg, urinary catheter and UTIs, endotracheal tubes and lung infections). Many children lack a fully competent immune system even prior to transplant. Children with uremia (especially those on dialysis) are partially immune deficient and are unable to mount a serological response to many vaccines. Similarly, patients with liver failure cannot synthesize the immunoglobulin proteins of the immune system. Malnutrition may be more prevalent in a large percentage of these children, which also contributes to the impaired immune response. Also, infants tend to be more susceptible to certain types of infections, such as *H influenzae* and do not respond satisfactorily to some kinds of vaccinations until after their first birthday. Paradoxically, infections may also enhance the immune response to the allograft. Thus, pyelonephritis in the kidney or systemic CMV infection can lead to up-regulation of MHC class II molecules in nonprofessional antigen-presenting cells. These molecules then present foreign peptide to T cells, which can then mount a rejection response. Thus, the overall magnitude of risk for infection in children posttransplant is subject to a very large number of factors, some unique to the transplant setting and some unique to pediatric transplantation.

Pediatric recipients should complete their routine immunizations before the transplant, as per the schedule in their country. Some recipients lose their protective antibodies at an accelerated rate posttransplant and, thus, monitoring of titers could be useful if they are exposed to specific infectious agents posttransplant. Repeat immunization is recommended with some vaccines posttransplant if titers are low. The use of varicella vaccine prior to transplant has been shown to reduce the incidence and severity of varicella posttransplant. Pneumococcal vaccine is also recommended for all patients pretransplant. Live microbial vaccines have been generally avoided posttransplant, although recent studies have reported that they may be safe to use post-

transplant. Modification of immunosuppression has not been necessary. Influenza vaccine has variable seroconversion posttransplant but has been documented to be efficacious even with concomitant immunosuppression and should be considered annually.

Since immunosuppression for organ transplantation remains nonspecific, infections are a major cause of morbidity and mortality for transplant recipients. Perhaps the most successful method of managing infections is to prevent them through vaccination. Indeed, many serious and potentially fatal diseases such as smallpox and poliomyelitis have been virtually eradicated by mandatory immunization programs. Within the past decade, the introduction of the *H influenzae* vaccine has eliminated what once used to be a major source of epiglottitis and meningitis in young children. The hepatitis B vaccine has similarly been responsible for ending the epidemics of hepatitis that were previously common in dialysis units. Thus, it is somewhat surprising that there are so few well-established recommendations for immunizing potential transplant recipients prior to transplantation and even less information about what to do following transplantation.

It is generally accepted that all potential transplant recipients should have their immunizations brought up to date prior to transplantation if at all possible. Children should receive a series of immunizations of diphtheria and tetanus toxoids and acellular pertussis and a booster of diphtheria-tetanus should be administered to everyone every ten years. Children should also receive the combination live-virus measles, mumps and rubella (MMR) vaccine and nonimmune individuals born before 1957 should receive a two-dose vaccination. Infants should also receive inactivated *H influenzae* B vaccine, and although adults are not typically affected by this bacteria, some (such as those who are asplenic) may be susceptible to infection with encapsulated organisms and should be immunized. Because the risk of poliomyelitis in the Western Hemisphere is now very low, vaccination with inactivated poliovirus vaccine (IPV) is generally recommended over the use of oral poliovirus vaccine (OPV) because of a reduced risk of vaccine-related polio. Varicella zoster virus (VZV) vaccine has been available in Europe for many years but was only recently approved for general use in the United States. Varicella-zoster infections in transplant recipients are common, with one study showing a 45% incidence in unimmunized children and adolescents after transplantation. These infections can be severe and even fatal. Pretransplant immunization has been shown to be effective in lowering the incidence and severity of these infections. Thus, it would seem intuitive that the administration of the vaccine prior to transplantation unquestionably would be beneficial. However, a recent report from the Laboratory of DNA Viruses of the FDA concerning varicella vaccination in healthy children raises interesting speculation as to the long-term safety of this procedure. Previous studies had shown that mean serum anti–VZV levels in some individuals continue to increase after vaccination, perhaps related to postimmunization exposure to wild-type VZV virus. The authors explored an alternative explanation, and found that titers were most likely to rise in individuals with initially low titers and that the frequency substantially exceeded the expected rate of exposure to wild type virus. They concluded that the attenuated virus persisted in vivo and reactivated as serum antibody titers fell. Thus, the vaccination seems to be "auto-boosting" through this reactivation process. Although this phenomenon might be beneficial to the otherwise healthy population because it results in increased antibody levels in these individuals, its effect on the immunosuppressed transplant recipient is unpredictable and possibly morbid. Indeed, chronically ill individuals receiving the vaccine pretransplantation might be expected to have the weakest response, making them more susceptible to reactivation. The result of the reactivation posttransplantation remains speculative. Certainly, every patient undergoing transplantation should receive the hepatitis B vaccine and should receive additional doses if necessary to raise antibody titers. Pneumococcal infections have been reported to affect up to 1% of transplant recipients annually, so pneumococcal vaccine is also generally recommended. Finally, influenza can be especially serious or even fatal in transplant recipients, so vaccination seems worthwhile. However, annual revaccination is generally indicated, suggesting that posttransplantation vaccination is necessary.

In general, although there are very few studies addressing the issue of posttransplant vaccination practices, most programs support the practice, at least for vaccines that do not contain live viruses. A survey of centers NAPRTCS to which there was a 62% response rate, found that 86% of centers recommended standard inactive vaccines, but that few administered live virus vaccines. Diphtheria and tetanus vaccines appear to be safe and effective when administered after renal transplantation, as does *H influenzae* vaccine. Inactive polio virus vaccine has been studied in adult renal transplant recipients and has been without serious complications. Hepatitis B vaccine, however, is less effective posttransplantation than before immunosuppression is started. Indeed, antibody response rate following transplantation is between 9% and 36%. Guidelines for revaccination are lacking. Similarly, influenza vaccine response rates are generally worse in immunosuppressed transplant recipients than in healthy controls, but most studies report responses in greater than 50% of recipients. Importantly, no study has shown any increased incidence of rejection episodes or other adverse events. Pneumococcal vaccine has been shown to be safe and effective in kidney, heart

and liver transplant recipients. There are very few studies of live virus vaccines in transplant recipients. One series examined the efficacy of varicella vaccine in a small number of pediatric renal transplant recipients and showed no serious side effects. A subsequent larger prospective study is ongoing.

Certainly, pretransplant vaccination must be considered routine practice today. Despite concerns about nonspecific immune stimulation in immunosuppressed transplant recipients and about the diminished antibody responses to the vaccines, most programs have found routine immunizations, at least with inactive vaccines, to be safe and reasonably effective. Concerns, however, about live virus vaccines that might permit reactivation in transplant recipients require ongoing study.

Posttransplant Lymphoproliferative Disease

Perhaps the greatest change in the epidemiology of infectious complications has occurred in the spectrum of EBV infections. EBV is a member of the herpes virus family of DNA viruses. It is ubiquitously present. Most adults have detectable antibodies to EBV, but young children, particularly in developed countries, may not have acquired antibodies at the time of transplant. This carries great significance for the development of posttransplant lymphoproliferative disease (PTLD). Generally, initial entry of the virus is believed to be through infected saliva. The virus remains latent in the hosts' B cells and oropharyngeal epithelium. The clinical disorders that can be seen posttransplant include an infectious mononucleosis syndrome, hepatitis syndrome and PTLD. Unlike normal children, the infectious mononucleosis syndrome in transplant recipients may be severe and can be fatal. The hepatitis syndrome is indistinguishable from that of CMV described above. Primary EBV infections posttransplant are generally more severe than reactivation. The diagnosis may be based on serological tests or detection of viral antigen. Evidence of recent EBV seroconversion, such as EBV Viral Capsid Antigen IgM, in the presence of febrile illness, would strongly suggest primary EBV infection. Similarly, elevation in EBV IgG titers might suggest reactivation.

PTLD is a perplexing and frequently devastating complication of pediatric solid organ transplantation. Its consequences include both high mortality (33% to 58%) and high rates of allograft loss, up to 60%. The incidence of PTLD varies with the type of solid organ transplanted. The highest incidence is seen in hepatic (4% to 20%), cardiac (4% to 10%) and intestinal transplantation (up to 30%). Pediatric renal transplant recipients appear to have a lower incidence of PTLD (approximately 1%), though this may vary by center, as some centers report higher incidences, up to 10%. However, the incidence of PTLD seems to be increasing, as evident from NAPRTCS data and other reports. In the NAPRTCS database, the incidence of PTLD has risen from 254 cases/100,000 posttransplant years of follow-up from 1987 to 1991, up to 395 cases/100,000 years posttransplant follow-up from 1992 onwards.

PTLD is believed to arise most commonly from EBV virus infection of B lymphocytes. There is a strong association with EBV infection, particularly with primary EBV infection posttransplant. The incidence of PTLD in EBV seronegative recipients ranges from 23% to 50%, as compared to 0.7% to 1.9% for EBV seropositive recipients. The incidence rate for seronegative recipients is 24 times higher than that for seropositive recipients. Evidence of active EBV infection is found in up to 66% to 90% of patients at the time of diagnosis of PTLD. CMV disease has also been shown to be associated with an increased risk of PTLD. This risk is synergistic with EBV infection. CMV disease posttransplant increases the relative risk of PTLD to 7.3. CMV seronegative recipients of a CMV positive allograft have fourfold to sixfold higher risk of PTLD and the risk is multiplied in association with EBV seronegativity in the recipients. Data from a NAPRTCS special study indicates that CMV disease has been diagnosed posttransplant in 44% of PTLD patients. It is currently believed that the role of young age is secondary to the increased likelihood of being EBV seronegative.

Newer immunosuppressive agents have also been implicated in the development of PTLD. The use of muromonab-CD3 independently increases the risk of PTLD fourfold to sixfold. In combination with the risk factors of EBV seronegative recipient and concurrent CMV disease, the incidence rate increases by a factor of 529. Pediatric liver transplant recipients receiving FK506 have a higher incidence of PTLD (13% to 20%) vs those receiving cyclosporine (2% to 3%). The combined use of muromonab-CD3 and FK506 also appears to be synergistic, with the incidence of PTLD increasing to 28% from 6%. In the NAPRTCS registry, the use of tacrolimus in the induction regime increases the incidence of PTLD to 11.5%, compared to 1.1% in patients who receive CsA.

The diagnosis of PTLD may often be complicated. Histopathologic diagnosis remains the "gold standard". Other methods include semiquantitative PCR techniques to detect EBV viral DNA from the peripheral blood lymphocytes and detection of IgM monoclonal proteins in serum and urine. A high index of suspicion should be maintained for PTLD in high-risk patients, particularly when diagnosing late rejection. The use of ganciclovir and acyclovir for prophylaxis against EBV and CMV is now gaining acceptance. Recently published protocols in pediatric liver transplant centers have used IV ganciclovir in high-risk cases and oral ganciclovir or acyclovir in low-risk cases. The incidence of PTLD has reportedly dropped from 4% to 10% to 0.5% to 2.5% in

association with these treatments. High risk is determined by EBV serotesting at the time of transplant; seropositive organs into seronegative recipients is graded as the highest risk.

Treatment of primary EBV depends on the severity of the presentation. For mononucleosis-like syndromes, partial reduction in immunosuppression and ganciclovir therapy (ie, first IV, then oral) is probably adequate. For PTLD, complete cessation of immunosuppression may be needed, along with longer courses of ganciclovir. More disseminated or malignant forms of PTLD require the above, plus interferon and occasionally chemotherapy. Data on the use of anti-B cell antibodies are promising, but scanty, at present and multicenter studies are in progress.

Complications Associated with Adult Donor Organs for Pediatric Recipients

Living donors comprise more than 50% of the donors for pediatric kidney transplantation and an increasing percentage of the donors for pediatric liver transplantation. Since living donors are generally restricted to those who can personally give permission, virtually all pediatric organ transplant programs will only accept donors older than 18 years. Furthermore, pediatric kidney transplant programs generally prefer to use kidneys from adult donors rather than from young child cadaver donors. Thus, it is very likely that the donor for pediatric kidney and liver transplantation is an adult. As noted above, the adult donors are more likely to have been exposed to multiple viral pathogens than the pediatric recipients, leading to a higher incidence and severity of transmitted viral diseases in pediatric recipients.

Furthermore, pediatric kidney transplant recipients are often required to perfuse a much larger organ than their native kidneys. The discrepancy between the adult kidney and the pediatric cardiovascular system has recently been described. The infant recipient of an adult kidney may be required to double his cardiac output to perfuse the adult organ adequately. Failure to do so may lead to graft thrombosis in the immediate posttransplant period or to relative hypoperfusion and graft dysfunction in the later period. For pediatric liver transplant recipients, lobes, "splits" or reduced-size grafts have been used frequently. In this setting, the possibility of vascular thrombosis or technical complications is similarly increased. Transplantation at sites with substantial experience is generally related to decreased risk of these complications.

Recurrence of Original Disease in Pediatric Organ Transplant Recipients

As noted above, children with developmental or structural organ abnormalities are generally at reduced risk of recurrence than are those with acquired disorders.

However, some pediatric diseases are associated with a heightened risk of recurrence after transplantation. Recurrence of hepatitis C or autoimmune hepatitis in pediatric recipients may occur at about the same rate seen in adults, although the incidence is low because of the young age of the recipients. Recurrence of original disease in pediatric heart or lung disease is rare in children.

Focal segmental glomerulosclerosis is the most common acquired cause of end-stage renal disease in children. Unfortunately, this disorder recurs in the graft frequently. It may recur immediately and generally leads to severe nephrotic syndrome and accelerated loss of graft function. Treatment of recurrence with enhanced immunosuppression is sometimes successful, albeit with increase risk of infection and other complications.

CONCLUSION

Pediatric organ transplantation is highly successful. Although early reports indicated worse outcome in children than in adults, improvements in surgical techniques, donor selection, knowledge of pediatric pharmacokinetics and pharmacodynamics and the development of specialized pediatric transplant teams have resulted in outcomes for children that are at least on a par with those of adults.

Although the pediatric immune response is vigorous and likely more active than elderly adults, appropriate immunosuppression can be used successfully and outstanding long-term outcomes can be achieved, especially in infants. Children, however, must be treated by providers with special experience and expertise, so that their unique needs and end-points may be addressed. Importantly, unique complications seen in children require unique research perspectives for successful resolution.

RECOMMENDED READING

Tejani A, Harmon WE, Fine RN, eds. Pediatric Solid Organ Transplantation. Copenhagen, Denmark: Munksgaard; 2000.

Boucek MM, Faro A, Novick RJ, et al. The Registry of the International Society of Heart and Lung Transplantation: Third Official Pediatric Report – 1999. J Heart Lung Transplant. 1999;18(12):1151-1172.

Benfield MR, McDonald R, Sullivan EK, Stablein DM, Tejani A. The 1997 Annual Renal Transplantation in Children. Report of the North American Pediatric Renal Transplant Cooperative Study (NAPRTCS). Pediatr Transplant. 1999;3(2):152-167.

Tejani A and Harmon WE. Pediatric Renal Transplantation. In: Dialysis and Transplantation. Owen WF, Pereira BJG, Sayegh MH, eds. Philadelphia, Pa: WB Saunders; 2000:653-660.

Alonso MH, Ryckman FC. Current concepts in pediatric liver transplant. Sem Liv Dis. 1998;18(3):295-307.

Section V

HEART TRANSPLANTATION

32 HISTORICAL OVERVIEW OF HEART TRANSPLANTATION

Sharon A. Hunt, MD

The development of cardiac transplantation, which has culminated in its currently widespread acceptance as the "ultimate" therapy for end-stage heart disease, is truly a remarkable saga. The first work in the field around the beginning of the 20th century was no doubt considered "fantastical" or even preposterous by some. By the end of the same century, however, cardiac and other solid organ transplantation have become "staples" of clinical practice in the developed world. By the end of the 20th century, well over 50,000 patients had undergone heart transplantation. This is not to say that the widespread acceptance and practice of this procedure have not been attended by controversy and debate at many levels, or that it currently is free of controversy or debate. This chapter attempts to outline the major ideas and technical developments that were pivotal to the evolution of the field of cardiac transplantation in the 20th century.

In the early 1960s, the concept of pharmacologic immunosuppression was being introduced along with the field of kidney transplantation. Support for the patient with end-stage renal disease with the "artificial kidney" or hemodialysis had become widespread and it was most logical that the first organ transplants should be performed with an organ for which there was a "backup" system such as dialysis. In 1964, James Hardy in Jackson, Mississippi felt that the state of clinical organ transplantation "…justified a planned approach directed toward eventual heart transplantation in man." Unfortunately, this "planned approach" did not include the concept of brain death of the donor and it was felt that "… for a homotransplant to succeed, the donor and recipient must 'die' at almost the same time." When Hardy's patient, a 68 year-old comatose recipient with lower extremity gangrene, was already on cardiopulmonary bypass and the donor's heart was still beating, they elected to use the heart of a chimpanzee, which they had available for experimental kidney transplantation. The transplant was technically satisfactory, but the graft was never able to maintain the circulation and the patient was declared dead one hour after discontinuing cardiopulmonary bypass. Presumably, hyperacute rejection had occurred in this early xenograft.

Professor, Cardiovascular Medicine, Cardiac Transplant Program, Stanford University Medical Center, Stanford, CA

Attempts at clinical heart transplantation remained in abeyance for another three years after Hardy's failed xenotransplant, but by the late 1960s a number of centers were preparing to begin clinical heart transplantation. The first human-to-human heart transplant was performed on December 3, 1967 by Christian Barnard, who had spent time with Richard Lower in Virginia observing orthotopic heart transplantation prior to returning to Capetown, at the Groote Schuur Hospital in Capetown, South Africa. The recipient was a 54 year-old diabetic man with end-stage ischemic heart disease and *Pseudomonas* cellulitis of his legs. The donor, a victim of head trauma, was declared dead five minutes after cessation of heartbeat and spontaneous respiration, and was then placed on cardiopulmonary bypass to resuscitate the heart. The allograft functioned well, but the patient died of *Pseudomonas* pneumonia 18 days after transplant.

The first successful heart transplant in the US was performed just weeks later by the Shumway team at Stanford on January 6, 1968 on a 54 year-old recipient who lived just 15 days after the procedure. These experiences were widely covered in the public press and seemed to stimulate an extremely active period in heart transplantation with 101 transplants performed worldwide in the next 12 months by 64 surgical teams in 24 countries. Most of these teams were unprepared and untrained; the patients died rapidly and most of the teams quickly discontinued their programs. By the end of 1969, only a small number of centers continued to pursue clinical programs in heart transplantation, primarily Stanford, Cape Town, University of Virginia, and La Pitie in Paris.

Several related and important advances were introduced at Stanford during the mid-1970s. In 1972, Philip Caves, a trainee from Papworth in Great Britain, developed the use of biopsy forceps for right ventricular endomyocardial biopsy. The forceps were modified from an original design by Sakakibara and Konno. The technique was introduced into the clinical program in late 1972 and demonstrated to be safe and repeatable, and of major clinical importance to assess the degree of graft rejection as well as the adequacy of response to therapy. Simultaneously, Billingham developed a histologic grading scale, which stood the test of time and was adapted for international use in 1990. At about the same period of time, rabbit antithymocyte globulin was developed and introduced for enhanced treatment of acute graft rejection. With the introduction of these two clinical modalities, 1-year post-heart transplant survival rates increased from 42% to 62% after 1974 in the Stanford program.

During the 1970s, lack of societal acceptance of brain death as the criteria for organ donation eligibility continued to limit the availability of donor organs. As early as 1968, the "Report of the Ad Hoc Committee of the Harvard Medical School to Examine the Definition of

Brain Death" had promoted the acceptance of brain death criteria, which were critical for effective organ donation. It was not until the mid-1970s that legal recognition of the concept of brain death became widespread. This acceptance, along with the introduction of distant heart procurement, led to a marked increase in the number of available donors. Procurement of the heart at the donor hospital with the attendant longer ischemic times was shown to be safe in the laboratory and was introduced clinically in 1977 using single-dose cold potassium cardioplegia followed by topical cooling in 4°C saline. The subsequent lack of need to transport the brain dead donor to the transplant center satisfied more donor families who did not want their loved one moved, and satisfied local legal authorities who often wished to perform autopsies on the donors.

The next major landmark in the field of clinical heart transplantation was the one that ushered in a worldwide renewed interest in the field and resurgence of clinical program activity after 1980. In 1973 Jacques Borel discovered that the fungal metabolite cyclosporine had potent immunosuppressive properties. Cyclosporine was introduced in clinical renal transplantation in Cambridge in 1977 by Calne, who reported 86% 1-year patient survival with the use of cyclosporine alone, a result clearly superior to his historical controls. Cyclosporine was first used in clinical heart transplantation at Stanford in December 1980, and by 1983, the group was able to report an 80% 1-year survival rate, again an obvious improvement over the historical "controls" of the 1974 to 1980 era, which had a roughly 60% 1-year survival. Data published by the Registry of the International Society for Heart and Lung Transplantation have shown a maintenance of 80% to 85% 1-year survival rates even as larger numbers of less experienced programs have entered the field. Cyclosporine has never been, and undoubtedly will never be, subjected to prospective or randomized controlled studies. Since it was so overtly an improvement over prior methods of immunosuppression it became rapidly and widely accepted, leading to the resurgence of clinical program activity in the mid-1980s noted above. Only 90 heart transplants were performed worldwide in 1980, but the number rose to 440 in 1984, and to nearly 2,500 by 1988, and reached a plateau at roughly 3,000 per year worldwide in the 1990s, a plateau now dictated strictly by donor availability.

RECOMMENDED READING

Barnard CN. The operation. A human cardiac transplant: an interim report of a successful operation performed at Groote Schuur Hospital, Cape Town. S Afr Med J. 1967;41(48):1271-1274.

Billingham ME, Cary NR, Hammond ME, et al. A working formulation for the standardization of nomenclature in the diagnosis of heart and lung rejection: Heart Rejection Study Group. The International Society for Heart Transplantation. J Heart Transplant. 1990;9(6): 587-593.

Beecher HK, Adams RD, Burger AC, et al. A definition of irreversible coma: a report of the Ad Hoc Committee of the Harvard Medical School to examine the definition of brain death. JAMA. 1968;205:337-340.

Hosenpud JD, Bennett LE, Keck BM, Fiol B, Boucek MM, Novick RJ. The Registry of the International Society for Heart and Lung Transplantation: Fifteenth Official Report-1998. J Heart Lung Transplant. 1998;17(7): 656-668.

33 EVALUATION AND MANAGEMENT OF PROSPECTIVE HEART RECIPIENTS

Daniel P. Fishbein, MD

Heart failure is an increasingly common syndrome that effects approximately five million people in the US. Each year, 400 thousand to 700 thousand patients develop congestive heart failure. Both the incidence and prevalence are expected to continue to increase over the next decade. Heart failure is the principle cause of 40 thousand deaths, and a contributing factor in 250 thousand deaths annually. The syndrome is responsible for more than 3.5 million patient days of hospitalization per year.

Continuing advances in medical therapy have improved symptoms and survival in patients with heart failure. Treatment with angiotensin-converting enzyme (ACE) inhibitors have been shown to reduce mortality and morbidity. More recently, beta blockers have been shown to significantly reduce mortality in patients with mild and moderate heart failure. Despite these advances, the 1-year mortality is 5% to 10% for patients with mild heart failure, and 30% to 40% for patients with severe heart failure. Patients with severe heart failure unresponsive to medical therapy have a 1-year mortality of more than 50%.

Over the last 15 years, heart transplantation has become an accepted and successful treatment for patients with advanced heart failure. Survival following transplantation has significantly improved as a result of advances in rejection prophylaxis, surgical technique and treatment of infectious diseases. Adult transplant recipients can now be expected to have a 1-year survival of 85% to 90%, and a 5-year survival of approximately 70%. At one year after transplantation, 85% of patients are physically active and have no limiting cardiovascular symptoms.

The success of heart transplantation combined with the increase in the number of patients with heart failure has resulted in an increasing demand for donor organs. Since 1992, approximately 3,800 new patients have been listed for cardiac transplantation annually. During the same period, however, the number of organs transplanted has remained constant at approximately 2,300 per year. The increased demand for donor organs has resulted in an increase in the waiting time from listing to transplantation, and an increase in the acuity of patients being transplanted. The median waiting time from listing

to transplantation for patients listed and transplanted as United Network for Organ Sharing (UNOS) Status 1 (ie, patients dependent on parenteral inotropes or mechanical support) has increased from 29 days in 1991, to 58 days in 1996. During the same time period, the median waiting time for patients listed as UNOS Status 2 (ie, not dependent on inotropes or mechanical support) has increased from 237 days to 382 days. Between 1991 and 1998, the percent of patients transplanted who were UNOS Status 1 increased from 55.4% to 72.8%.

These observations underscore the critical shortage of donor organs available for heart transplantation. This shortage necessitates that the candidate selection process identify patients who will have the greatest benefit from the procedure with respect to improvement in survival and quality of life. In general, heart transplantation should be considered in patients who: (1) have severe symptoms despite an aggressive and appropriate medical regimen; (2) have a poor 1-year to 2-year prognosis; (3) are not candidates for other accepted surgical alternatives to transplantation; and (4) do not have comorbid conditions that could have a negative impact on postoperative recovery and long-term survival.

INDICATIONS FOR HEART TRANSPLANTATION

Generally accepted indications for transplantation include advanced heart failure, New York Heart Association (NYHA) Function Class (FC) III-IV, refractory angina, and recurrent life-threatening ventricular arrhythmias.

Advanced Heart Failure

Patients who are evaluated for heart transplantation because of advanced heart failure generally have systolic dysfunction due to underlying coronary artery disease or idiopathic dilated cardiomyopathy. Other underlying causes of heart failure include valvular cardiomyopathy, congenital heart disease, restrictive cardiomyopathy, and hypertrophic cardiomyopathy. Table 33-1 summarizes the underlying heart disease in patients who were transplanted from 1988 to 1997.

Patients with heart failure who are dependent on parenteral inotropic medication or mechanical support are clearly ill enough to be listed as candidates for heart transplantation. In 1997, 35% of patients listed for heart transplantation were dependent on parenteral inotropic or mechanical support at the time of listing. It is important to emphasize that the short-term need of parenteral inotropic support is not an indication for heart transplantation. Many patients hospitalized for decompensated heart failure are treated with inotropes but can be discharged from the hospital on conventional oral heart failure medications and remain well compensated. Patients should not be considered to be inotrope-

Division of Cardiology, Heart Failure/Cardiac Transplantation Service, University of Washington Medical Center, Seattle, WA

Table 33-1. Heart Transplant Recipient Characteristics: 1988-1997

	1988	1989	1990	1991	1992	1993	1994	1995	1996	1997
# of Transplants	1676	1705	2107	2126	2171	2297	2341	2361	2344	2292
Male (%)	79.3	79.8	78.6	77.2	76.8	78.5	76.3	76.8	76.5	74.8
Status 1 (%)*				55.4	56.6	60	60.9	66.1	68	69.4
Diagnosis (%)										
Cardiomyopathy	36.8	38.3	36.9	41.9	43.9	42	45.7	42.6	41.8	41.6
Coronary artery disease	50.4	47.6	49.1	41.1	41	42.6	42	45.4	45.5	44.8
Congenital	4	6.2	6.9	8.9	7.4	8.4	6.6	6.6	6.5	7.5
Valvular	5.4	4.4	4	3.4	3	2.7	2.6	1.9	2.6	2.2
Re-transplantation	2.7	2.4	2.6	2.9	2.9	3	2.2	2.8	2.7	2.8
1-Yr Survival %	82.6	83.3	84.4	82.7	82.9	83.3	85.3	85.5	86.2	

1998 UNOS Annual Report

*Medical urgency Status 1 includes patients who: (a) require mechanical support (total artificial heart, left and/or right ventricular assist system, intra-aortic balloon pump, ventilator); (b) require inotropic support and are in an ICU; or (c) are under six. Medical urgency status criteria for heart transplantation were changed in January 1999.

dependent until an attempt has been made to wean inotropes after diuretic and vasodilator therapy have been optimized with the help of continuous hemodynamic monitoring. Some patients who are initially dependent on inotropes may be able to be weaned after several months of parenteral therapy.

Four ventricular assist devices have been approved by the FDA for long-term use to "bridge" patients to transplantation. These devices include the HeartMate® Implantable Pneumatic Left Ventricular Assist System (LVAS), the HeartMate® Vented Electric (VE) LVAS, the Novacor LVAS, and Thoratec® VAS. The HeartMate® VE and Novacor devices are designed to enable patients to be discharged to home to wait for transplantation. The Thoratec® device can be used for both right and left ventricular support while the other devices can be used for left ventricular support only. In general, left ventricular assist devices are implanted in transplant candidates who have persistent decompensated heart failure despite aggressive treatment with vasodilators, diuretics, and inotropic infusion.

Most patients referred for transplant evaluation are ambulatory and have significant symptoms of heart failure (NYHA FC III-IV) due to underlying severe left ventricular systolic dysfunction. In light of the increasing shortage of donors on the one hand, and improvements in the pharmacologic treatment of heart failure on the other, there has been an effort to use reliable predictors of survival to identify patients who have the greatest need for heart transplantation. A number of clinical variables have been found on univariate analysis to predict survival, including left ventricular ejection fraction, NYHA FC, pulmonary capillary wedge pressure, serum sodium concentration, and peak oxygen consumption (VO_2 max). VO_2 max has been found to be a powerful independent predictor of 1-year and 2-year survival and has emerged as the most useful predictor of survival in ambulatory patients referred for heart transplantation. VO_2 max is measured during maximal exercise testing with respiratory gas analysis. It is primarily a function of cardiac output and provides a reliable, reproducible, and objective assessment of functional impairment and cardiovascular reserve in patients with heart failure.

In a study by Mancini et al, exercise testing was performed prospectively on all ambulatory patients referred to the University of Pennsylvania for heart transplantation. Based on the results of exercise testing, 116 patients were divided into three groups. Group 1 included patients with a VO_2 max under 14 mL/kg per minute who were accepted as candidates for transplantation. Group 2 included patients who had a VO_2 max greater than 14 mL/kg per minute who were considered too well for heart transplantation. Group 3 included patients who had a VO_2 max less than 14 mL/kg per minute who were not listed for cardiac transplantation because they had significant contraindications to the procedure. Age, left ventricular ejection fraction and resting hemodynamic parameters were similar in all three groups. The 1-year survival rate for patients having a VO_2 max over 14 mL/kg per minute (Group 2) was 94%. In the groups of patients with VO_2 max less than 14 mL/kg per minute, the 1-year survival rate was 70% in those patients listed for transplantation (Group 1), and 47% in those patients with contraindications to transplantation (Group 3). It was also observed that patients having a VO_2 max less than 10 mL/kg per minute had the worst survival. Multiple subsequent studies have confirmed an important independent relationship between VO_2 max and survival.

There is uniform consensus regarding the prognostic significance of both severely reduced and significantly preserved exercise capacity. Patients who have a marked reduction in exercise capacity (ie, VO_2 max <10 mL/kg per minute) have a poor prognosis and should be listed for transplantation. Patients with preserved exercise capacity (ie, VO_2 >18 mL/kg per minute) have a good prognosis and do not need to be listed for transplantation.

Between 10 mL/kg per minute to 18 mL/kg per minute, VO_2 max functions as a continuous rather than a discreet variable in its relation to survival. In this range, survival worsens with decreasing VO_2, but there is not a precise threshold at which survival precipitously worsens. There is, however, general consensus that patients with NYHA FC III-IV symptoms and a VO_2 less than 14 mL/kg per minute are ill enough to warrant being listed for heart transplantation.

Although VO_2 max is a powerful predictor of survival, it needs to be interpreted with an understanding of the limitations of the measurement and in the context of the total pretransplant evaluation. Factors other than cardiac reserve that may effect VO_2 include age, gender, muscle mass, deconditioning, or pulmonary limitation. Selection of transplant candidates based solely on VO_2 is inappropriate. Other factors including clinical stability, NYHA FC, quality of life, history of recurrent hospitalization, underlying coronary anatomy, and evidence of rapidly worsening heart failure need to be considered.

Refractory Angina

Recurrent or refractory angina not controlled by maximum medical therapy and not amenable to appropriate surgical or catheter-based revascularization is an accepted indication for transplantation. Many patients who are evaluated for this indication also have significant left ventricular systolic dysfunction and may have undergone previous revascularization procedures.

Recurrent Symptomatic Arrhythmias

Patients who have recurrent ventricular tachycardia or fibrillation despite correction of underlying pro-arrhythmic factors and treatment with optimal anti-arrhythmic therapy may be candidates for cardiac transplantation. Most of these patients have severe underlying ventricular dysfunction and have been treated with amiodarone and implantation of a pacemaker cardioverter defibrillator.

Table 33-2 summarizes the currently accepted indications for heart transplantation. This table is based largely on a report of the 24th Bethesda Conference of the American College of Cardiology, held in November 1992; a report from a consensus conference held before the meeting of the International Society of Heart and Lung Transplantation held in 1993, and the American Heart Association Medical/Scientific Statement of Selection and Treatment of Candidates for Heart Transplantation published in 1995.

CONTRAINDICATIONS TO HEART TRANSPLANTATION

A number of comorbid conditions and psychosocial factors have been identified that have a negative impact on outcome after heart transplantation (Table 33-3). Many of these factors are continuous rather than discreet variables, and need to be considered in the context of the severity of the patient's heart disease and the presence of other comorbidities. The difficulty of assessing the importance of these factors on transplant candidacy is illustrated by the different approach of transplant centers to different comorbidities. This difficulty is compounded by the lack of substantial data concerning the impact of many of these comorbidities on long-term outcome.

Coexistent Systemic Illness

Any coexistent systemic disease that affects prognosis may be a contraindication to transplantation. Illnesses may cause recurrent disease in the transplanted organ, decrease survival independent of heart function, or cause persistent limitation despite improvement in cardiac function. Examples of such diseases include systemic lupus, primary amyloidosis, HIV infection, muscular dystrophies, and sarcoidosis. The severity of the underlying disease at the time of transplant evaluation and the anticipated natural history of the disease after transplantation need to be considered when patients with a systemic disease are evaluated.

Pulmonary Vascular Hypertension

Patients with long-standing heart failure may develop pulmonary vascular hypertension in response to chronically elevated left atrial pressure. Pulmonary hypertension may be reversible or irreversible, depending on the duration and severity of heart failure. Multiple studies have shown that pulmonary vascular hypertension is associated with an increase in perioperative mortality. Patients with pulmonary vascular hypertension are at risk for perioperative right heart failure and death because the unconditioned donor right ventricle may be unable to function adequately in the setting of increased resistance to pulmonary blood flow. It is, therefore, important to perform a right heart catheterization in potential transplant candidates to evaluate whether pulmonary hypertension is present and, if so, whether it is reversible. Two measures of pulmonary vascular hypertension have been used to assess perioperative risk: transpulmonary gradient (TPG) and pulmonary vascular resistance (PVR). TPG is calculated by subtracting the mean pulmonary capillary wedge pressure (PCWP) from the mean pulmonary artery pressure. PVR is calculated by dividing TPG by cardiac output. Both TPG and PVR act as continuous rather than discreet variables in relation to postoperative mortality. While it is not clear that there is a specific PVR or TPG at which the risk of transplant becomes prohibitive, there is consensus that a PVR greater than 5 Wood Units or a TPG greater than 15 mmHg unresponsive to short-term and long-term treatment are associated with a significant increase in postoperative mortality and are, at least, relative contraindications to cardiac transplantation.

Lung Disease

Chronic obstructive pulmonary disease may increase the risk of pulmonary infection and make it more difficult to wean ventilatory support after heart transplantation. In addition, patients with lung disease may not have a significant improvement in functional capacity after transplantation because of persistent pulmonary limitation. Maximal exercise testing with respiratory gas analysis

---

Table 33-2. Indications for Heart Transplantation

Patients should be evaluated for heart transplantation for the following indications:
  Heart failure with significant functional limitation (NYHA FC III-IV) despite optimal medical therapy
  Refractory angina
  Recurrent life-threatening arrhythmias
  Surgical alternatives to transplantation have been excluded
Specific Indications
  Definite
    Dependence on mechanical support or parenteral inotropic therapy
    VO_2 max <10 mL/kg per minute
    NYHA FC IV
    Recurrent hospitalization for heart failure
    Recurrent ischemia limiting routine activity not amenable to bypass surgery or catheter-based intervention
    Recurrent symptomatic ventricular arrhythmias refractory to all appropriate therapeutic modalities
  Probable
    VO_2 max <14 mL/kg per minute
    NYHA FC III-IV

Table 33-3. Conditions that may Increase Morbidity and Mortality after Heart Transplantation

Coexistence of systemic illness with a poor prognosis
Irreversible pulmonary parenchymal disease (FEV_1<1L or <50% of predicted; FEV_1/FVC <40% to 50% of predicted)
Irreversible pulmonary hypertension (transpulmonary gradient >15 mmHg; pulmonary vascular resistance >5 Wood Units despite treatment with vasodilators)
Severe peripheral or cerebrovascular disease
Active infection
Irreversible hepatic dysfunction
Coexisting neoplasm
Irreversible renal dysfunction
Active peptic ulcer disease
Acute pulmonary embolism, especially with pulmonary infarction
Active diverticulitis
Severe osteoporosis
Severe obesity
Protein malnutrition
Diabetes mellitus with significant end-organ damage
Demonstrated noncompliance with medical regimen
Current substance abuse: tobacco, alcohol and/or drugs
Psychosocial instability
NYHA FC III-IV

can be helpful in determining whether functional limitation is primarily due to heart or lung disease and in predicting whether a patient with heart failure and lung disease will have an improvement in functional capacity after heart transplantation.

Because severe heart failure can worsen pulmonary function, resting pulmonary function and exercise testing should be performed after heart failure medications have been optimized at a time when pulmonary capillary wedge pressure is not elevated.

There is some consensus that an FEV_1 less than 1 liter, an FEV_1 less than 50% of predicted, and an FEV_1/FVC less than 40% to 50% of predicted are significant contraindications to cardiac transplantation.

Renal Dysfunction

Moderate elevations in BUN and creatinine are common in severe heart failure and may be due to heart failure, intrinsic kidney disease or both. Kidney dysfunction from heart failure generally improves after heart transplantation. Dysfunction from intrinsic kidney disease generally does not improve and may progress to chronic renal failure especially in the setting of long-term treatment with cyclosporine or tacrolimus.

Patients who have a creatinine over 2.0 mg/dL to 2.5 mg/dL, or a creatinine clearance of under 40 to 50 mL/min should be evaluated for intrinsic renal disease. Findings that suggest that renal insufficiency is due to heart failure rather than intrinsic renal disease include absence of noncardiac risk factors for kidney disease (eg, diabetes, hypertension), normal-size kidneys on renal ultrasound, normal urinary sediment, absence of significant proteinuria on 24-hour urine collection, and improvement in BUN and creatinine with parenteral inotropic therapy.

"Significant" renal dysfunction is considered to be a relative contraindication to transplantation. However, there is little uniformity among transplant centers with respect to a specific creatinine above which, or creatinine clearance below which transplantation is contraindicated. This issue has been made more complex by the relative success of heart-kidney transplantation. A study based on UNOS Scientific Registry data compared the outcome of 84 patients who underwent heart-kidney transplantation with that of patients who underwent isolated heart transplantation. Combined heart-kidney recipients had 1-year and 2-year actuarial survivals of 76% and 67%, respectively, compared with 83% and 79% in the isolated heart group.

Liver Disease

Liver function test (LFT) abnormalities are common in patients with decompensated heart failure and hepatic congestion. Patients who have persistent LFT abnormalities, despite normalization of systemic venous pressure, need further evaluation to exclude cirrhosis or underlying progressive liver disease that may increase the risk of bleeding during surgery or limit posttransplant survival because of progressive liver failure. In some patients, percutaneous liver biopsy is indicated.

Controversy exists about whether patients with positive hepatitis C serologies should undergo heart transplantation. In immunocompetent patients, hepatitis C causes slowly progressive liver disease. The natural history of hepatitis C in heart transplant recipients is less well-defined. Preliminary data suggests that short-term survival is not decreased in recipients who are seropositive at the time of transplantation. A survey of US transplant centers performed in 1995 found that 45 of 72 (63%) centers that responded listed patients with positive hepatitis C serologies for transplantation.

Diabetes

Diabetes has been considered a contraindication to heart transplantation in the past because of concern about corticosteroid-induced complications in diabetic patients. However, current immunosuppressive regimens allow rapid tapering of corticosteroids. Several studies have shown comparable outcomes in diabetic and nondiabetic transplant recipients. Most insulin-dependent patients will have a significant increase in insulin requirements after transplantation. Similarly, most noninsulin-dependent patients will require insulin after transplantation.

Diabetic end-organ complications remain relative contraindications to heart transplantation. However, the total "end-organ burden," the anticipated natural history of end-organ complications, and the impact of these complications on overall health and quality of life need to be considered when determining transplant candidacy.

Malignancy

Active or recently treated malignancy is a contraindication to heart transplantation. However, patients with a remote history of malignancy have been successfully transplanted. Patients with a history of malignancy may be referred for transplant evaluation because of doxorubicin-induced cardiomyopathy or heart disease unrelated to prior malignancy. Patients should have a comprehensive evaluation to insure freedom from malignancy at the time of transplant or to assess the probability of malignancy recurrence after heart transplantation. Evaluating patients with a history of malignancy is difficult because of the uncertainty about the effect of chronic immunosuppression on disease recurrence.

Pretransplant screening for malignancy should include a rectal exam and stool occult blood; a pelvic, pap smear, breast exam, and mammography for women; and a prostate-specific antigen for men.

Psychosocial Issues

Psychosocial factors that compromise medical compliance or overall health represent significant contraindications to transplantation. Most transplant programs consider demonstrated medical noncompliance or continuing substance abuse of alcohol, drugs or tobacco to be absolute contraindications to transplantation. Determining transplant candidacy in patients with underlying psychiatric disorders, cognitive impairment, or unstable social or living situations can be difficult and needs to be individualized.

Pretransplant Evaluation

Potential transplant candidates should be evaluated by a multidisciplinary team that has expertise in the evaluation and management of patients with advanced heart

---

Table 33-4. Heart Transplant Candidate Evaluation

General Data
 Comprehensive history and physical examination
 Blood chemistry, renal and liver function panels, lipid panel
 Complete blood count, differential, platelet count, prothrombin time, partial thromboplastin time, fibrinogen
 Thyroid function tests (TSH, T4)
 Urinalysis
 Chest x-ray
 Twenty-four hour urine for creatinine clearance and total protein
 Stool guaiac examination
 Mammography
 Papanicolaou smear*
 Prostate-specific antigen*
 Pulmonary function tests
 Carotid and lower extremity noninvasive arterial studies*
 Ultrasound of gallbladder*
Specialty Consultation
 Psychosocial evaluation (psychiatry, psychology and/or social work)
 Dental exam
 Nutritional evaluation
 Financial services
Cardiovascular Data
 Electrocardiogram
 Echocardiogram
 Exercise test with determination of peak oxygen consumption
 Coronary angiography
 Thallium scintigraphy or positron emission tomography to determine viability (if indicated)
 Right heart catheterization with determination of transpulmonary gradient and pulmonary vascular resistance
 Endomyocardial biopsy*
Immunologic Data
 Blood group
 Human leukocyte antigen (HLA) typing
 Panel of reactive antibodies screen (% PRA)
Infectious Disease Screening
 Serology for:
 Hepatitis B (HBsAg, HBsAb, HBcAb)
 Hepatitis C
 Human immunodeficiency virus
 Cytomegalovirus (IgM, IgG)
 Toxoplasmosis
 Varicella and rubella titers
 Epstein-Barr virus (IgM, IgG)
 Histoplasmosis and coccidiomycosis complement fixing antibodies
 VDRL
 Stool for ova and parasites x 3*
 Skin testing for PPD with control for mumps, dermatophytin, histoplasmosis and coccidiomycosis

*Only if appropriate

failure. The goals of the pretransplant evaluation are to: (1) identify reversible factors that may contribute to heart failure decompensation; (2) ensure that the patient is being treated with an optimal heart failure regimen; (3) identify appropriate surgical alternatives to transplantation; (4) assess functional limitation and prognosis; and (5) identify comorbidities that may have a negative impact on posttransplant morbidity and mortality. Table 33-4 summarizes the recommended evaluation for patients referred for consideration of heart transplantation.

Optimization of Heart Failure Medications

Optimization of heart failure medications is an essential part of the evaluation and management of patients referred for transplantation. Patients on an inadequate heart failure regimen may improve to the point where they do not need to be transplanted. For this reason, adjustment of medication should begin at the time of the initial evaluation. If possible, the decision to list a patient for heart transplantation should be delayed until medical therapy has been optimized. All patients should be treated with an ACE inhibitor unless they exhibit intolerance secondary to angioedema, intolerable cough, or severe renal insufficiency. In general, ACE inhibitors should be up-titrated to the maximum tolerated dose (eg, enalapril 20 mg PO bid, captopril 100 mg PO tid) provided patients do not have symptomatic hypotension, significantly worsening renal function, or refractory hyperkalemia. Diuretics should be used to control symptoms of pulmonary and systemic venous congestion. Patients with advanced heart failure are commonly diuretic-resistant and may need high doses of a loop diuretic. Patients who are unresponsive to increasing doses of diuretics may benefit from intravenous diuretic therapy or

from the addition of a thiazide diuretic or metolazone. Digoxin is useful in improving symptoms in patients with severe heart failure and should be used in all patients who have persistent NYHA FC III-IV symptoms.

Patients may benefit from the addition of hydralazine and nitrates, especially if they remain symptomatic and their systolic blood pressure remains greater than 90 mmHg despite high-dose ACE inhibitor therapy. Some patients with advanced heart failure develop significant worsening renal function in response to up-titration of ACE inhibitors. Treatment with hydralazine and nitrates may be particularly helpful in this group of patients.

Patients who have refractory heart failure, despite attempts to optimize their medical regimen in the outpatient setting, may benefit from hospitalization and treatment with parenteral followed by oral vasodilators and diuretics guided by continuous hemodynamic monitoring.

Beta blockers have been shown to decrease hospitalization and improve clinical status, ejection fraction, and survival in patients with mild and moderate heart failure. Experience using beta blockers in patients with advanced (NYHA FC IIIB-IV) heart failure is limited. The data available suggest that these patients may develop worsening heart failure with beta blocker initiation but may have significant clinical improvement if drug initiation is tolerated. Beta blocker initiation is contraindicated in acutely ill patients with decompensated heart failure.

Factors that may Contribute to Heart Failure Decompensation

Table 33-5 lists reversible factors that may contribute to heart failure decompensation. Excessive alcohol intake is a common and frequently unrecognized cause of cardio-

---

Table 33-5. Potentially Reversible Factors that may Contribute to Heart Failure

Myocardial ischemia
Excessive alcohol intake
Excessive salt and water intake
Poor compliance with medical regimen
Atrial fibrillation
Intercurrent infection
Inadequate diuretic prescription
Medications: Nonsteroidal antiinflammatory agents, beta blockers*, calcium channel blockers (except amlodipine), antiarrhythmic agents (disopyramide, flecainide, sotolol, propafenone)
Cardiovascular deconditioning
Inadequate control of hypertension
Hyperthyroidism/hypothyroidism
Sleep apnea
Worsening intrinsic renal disease

*Although used to treat heart failure, beta blockers may contribute to decompensation in patients with advanced heart failure.

myopathy. Abstinence from alcohol may result in a significant improvement in symptoms and ventricular function. Development of atrial fibrillation frequently leads to heart failure decompensation, which may reverse with reestablishment of normal sinus rhythm. Intercurrent infection may also worsen heart failure symptoms. Patients with heart failure should be vaccinated for pneumococcal pneumonia and influenza.

A number of medications may make heart failure worse. Many calcium channel blockers increase the risk of worsening heart failure and death. However, there is strong evidence that the use of amlodipine is safe in patients with systolic dysfunction. Class I anti-arrhythmic agents increase the risk of sudden death in patients with systolic dysfunction. Many of these drugs are also negative inotropes and worsen heart failure symptoms.

Excessive thirst may be a vexing problem for patients with advanced heart failure and contributes to recurrent volume overload. Treatment with ACE inhibitors, careful adjustment of diuretics, dietary counseling, performance of daily weights, and ongoing patient education and support can help patients control their volume status.

Evaluation for Coronary Artery Disease

Coronary artery disease is the major underlying cause of heart failure in patients referred for cardiac transplantation. A number of reports suggest that carefully selected patients with ischemic cardiomyopathy, low ejection fraction, and predominant symptoms of heart failure can undergo revascularization with acceptable perioperative risk and long-term improvement in symptoms, functional class, and ventricular function. This response to revascularization is thought to be due to improvement in contractile function in areas of dysfunctional but viable (either hibernating or repetitively stunned) myocardium following restoration of blood flow to these areas. Improvement after revascularization is predicted by the presence of suitable target vessels and the amount of viable myocardium demonstrated by thallium scintigraphy or positron emission tomography (PET).

In light of these considerations, transplant candidates should undergo coronary angiography. If significant coronary artery disease is present, thallium scintigraphy and/or PET imaging should be performed to assess myocardial viability. Patients with suitable target vessels and significant areas of underperfused but viable myocardium should be considered for coronary revascularization.

Cardiopulmonary Exercise Testing

All patients should undergo maximal exercise testing with expired gas analysis after heart failure therapy has been optimized. To insure that exercise is truly maximal,

an anaerobic threshold, which indicates the onset of lactate production, should be reached at 50% to 70% of VO_2 max. Anaerobic threshold may not be achieved because of exercise-induced ischemia or arrhythmia, severe deconditioning, inadequate effort, or pulmonary limitation.

Hemodynamic Evaluation for Pulmonary Vascular Hypertension

All candidates should undergo right heart catheterization to determine whether pulmonary vascular hypertension is present and whether it is reversible. In general, patients are considered to have pulmonary vascular hypertension if the transpulmonary gradient is greater than 10 mmHg to 15 mmHg, or the pulmonary vascular resistance is greater than two to three Wood Units. Transplant programs differ in their approach to demonstrating reversibility. Some programs will try to demonstrate reversibility by giving pulmonary vasodilators at the time of the initial catheterization. Drugs that have been used to test reversibility include sodium nitroprusside, nitroglycerin, milrinone, intravenous or inhaled prostacyclin, and inhaled nitric oxide. Pulmonary hypertension that does not respond to drug testing in the catheterization laboratory may reverse after long-term normalization of pulmonary capillary wedge pressure. For this reason, some programs do not perform vasodilator testing, but rather repeat right heart catheterization after up-titrating oral vasodilators and diuretics in the outpatient setting.

Psychosocial Evaluation

A complete social and psychologic evaluation should be performed to evaluate whether patients are at risk for noncompliance after transplantation. This evaluation may be performed by the transplant physician, nurse coordinator, social worker, psychologist, or psychiatrist. Candidates should be evaluated for a history of Axis I or II psychiatric disorder, substance abuse, criminal history, and medical noncompliance. Details concerning employment, marital history, social support, and living conditions (eg, phone, permanent address) should be sought. In patients with cognitive impairment, specific information about social support, reading level and ability to live independently, take medications, and manage financial affairs should be obtained. Neuropsychiatric testing may be helpful in evaluating some patients, but is not routine.

Financial Evaluation

The cost of heart transplantation is substantial. Furthermore, patients continue to need subspecialty care and expensive medications after transplantation to insure good long-term outcome. Many patients are medically disabled at the time of transplantation and only one-third of patients return to full-time employment after transplantation. In light of these considerations, all potential transplant candidates should undergo a financial evaluation to assess the adequacy of insurance coverage with respect to the cost of the procedure, long-term care, and long-term pharmacy expenses. Financial counseling should help patients anticipate their short-term and long-term out-of-pocket expenses. It is essential to insure that patients will be able to receive appropriate medical care and medication after transplantation.

Approval for Transplantation

Figure 33-1 summarizes the transplant candidate evaluation process. Once this process has been completed, patient information is presented to a selection committee for final approval. This committee is generally made-up of cardiologists, transplant surgeons, nurse coordinators, a social worker and/or psychiatrist, and a financial specialist.

It is important to emphasize that transplant candidacy may change over time. Patients may improve to a point where they no longer have indications for heart transplantation, or they may develop comorbidities that preclude heart transplantation. Alternatively, patients who remain good candidates for heart transplantation may elect not to proceed with transplantation and remove themselves from the transplant waiting list.

REEVALUATION

Patients listed for heart transplantation are at risk for sudden cardiac death, hemodynamic decompensation, and development of end-organ dysfunction. Many patients awaiting heart transplantation require a complex regimen of diuretics and vasodilators that need to be modified on a frequent basis. Furthermore, transplant candidates are at risk of developing end-organ dysfunction that could preclude heart transplantation. Patients should be seen by a transplant cardiologist at least every two months at which time heart failure symptoms, functional capacity, drug side effects, kidney function, volume status, symptoms of arrhythmia, nutritional status, and medical compliance should be assessed. In general, liver function tests, CBC, coagulation profile, chemistry panel and creatinine clearance should be rechecked every six months. Most programs repeat a panel reactive antibody (PRA) determination (Section II, Chapter 14g) every three to six months depending upon the patient's history of sensitization. Serial right heart catheterization should be performed every six months or every three months in patients with a history of significant pulmonary vascular hypertension.

A patient's clinical condition may improve after they are listed as a candidate for heart transplantation. Patients should undergo cardiopulmonary exercise testing with a determination of VO_2 max every six months. Programs differ in their approach to patients who

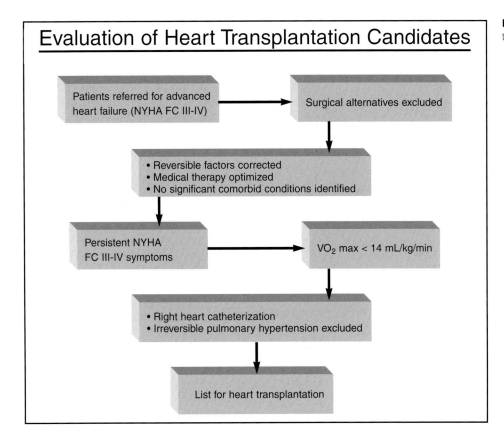

Figure 33-1. Evaluation of heart transplantation candidates.

Evaluation of Heart Transplantation Candidates

Patients referred for advanced heart failure (NYHA FC III-IV)

Surgical alternatives excluded

• Reversible factors corrected
• Medical therapy optimized
• No significant comorbid conditions identified

Persistent NYHA FC III-IV symptoms

VO_2 max < 14 mL/kg/min

• Right heart catheterization
• Irreversible pulmonary hypertension excluded

List for heart transplantation

improve maximum oxygen consumption to more than 15 mL/kg per minute. Some programs will inactivate these patients if they are otherwise clinically stable. Other programs will repeat a cardiopulmonary exercise test in three to six months and inactivate patients only if they are clinically stable and have a sustained improvement in VO_2 max demonstrated on repeat cardiopulmonary testing.

RECOMMENDED READING

Anonymous. Guidelines for the evaluation and management of heart failure. Report of the American College of Cardiology/American Heart Association Task Force on Practice Guidelines (Committee on Evaluation and Management of Heart Failure). J Am Coll Cardiol. 1995;26(5):1376-1398.

Beniaminovitz A, Mancini D. The role of exercise-based prognosticating algorithms in the selection of patients for heart transplantation. Curr Opin Cardiol. 1999; 14(2):114-120.

Bourge RC, Naftel DC, Costanzo-Nordin MR, et al. Pretransplantation risk factors for death after heart transplantation: a multiinstitutional study. J Heart Lung Transplant. 1993;12(4):549-562.

Brann WM, Bennett LE, Keck BM, Hosenpud JD. Morbidity, functional status, and immunosuppressive therapy after heart transplantation: an analysis of the Joint International Society for Heart and Lung Transplantation/United Network for Organ Sharing Thoracic Registry. J Heart Lung Transplant. 1998;17(4):374-382.

Costanzo MR, Augustine S, Bourge R, et al. Selection and treatment of candidates for heart transplantation. A statement for health professionals from the Committee on Heart Failure and Cardiac Transplantation of the Council on Clinical Cardiology, American Heart Association. Circulation. 1995;92(12):3593-3612.

Hunt SA, Frazier OH. Mechanical circulatory support and cardiac transplantation. Circulation. 1998;97(20): 2079-2090.

Keck BM, Bennett LE, Fiol BS, Daily OP, Novick RJ, Hosenpud JD. Worldwide thoracic organ transplantation: a report from the UNOS/ISHLT International Registry for Thoracic Organ Transplantation. Clin Transpl. 1997;3:29-43.

Mancini DM, Eisen H, Kussmaul W, Mull R, Edmunds LH Jr., Wilson JR. Value of peak exercise oxygen consumption for optimal timing of cardiac transplantation in ambulatory patients with heart failure. Circulation. 1991;83(3):778-786.

Miller LW, Kubo SH, Young JB, Stevenson LW, Loh E, Costanzo MR. Report of the Consensus Conference on Candidate Selection for Heart Transplantation-1993. J Heart Lung Transplant. 1995;14(3):562-571.

Mudge GH, Goldstein S, Addonizio LJ, et al. 24th Bethesda conference: Cardiac transplantation: Task Force 3: recipient guidelines/prioritization. J Am Coll Cardiol. 1993;22(1):21-31.

Myers J, Gullestad L. The role of exercise testing and gas-exchange measurement in the prognostic assessment of patients with heart failure. Cur Opin Cardiol. 1998; 13(3):145-155.

O'Connell JB, Bourge RC, Costanzo-Nordin MR, et al. Cardiac transplantation: recipient selection, donor procurement, and medical follow-up. A statement for health professionals from the Committee on Cardiac Transplantation of the Council on Clinical Cardiology, American Heart Association. Circulation. 1992;86(3): 1061-1079.

Anonymous. Consensus recommendations for the management of chronic heart failure. On behalf of the membership of the Advisory Council to Improve Outcomes Nationwide in Heart Failure. Am J Cardiol. 1999; 83(2A):1A-38A.

Pina IL. Optimal candidates for heart transplantation: is 14 the magic number? J Am Coll Cardiol. 1995; 26(2):436-437.

34 LIVING HEART DONORS – DOMINO HEART TRANSPLANTATION

Jayan Parameshwar,
MBBS, MD, M.phil, FRCP

Heart-lung transplantation was used initially as a treatment for patients with pulmonary vascular disease (primary and secondary), but rapidly became the procedure of choice for patients with bilateral lung disease in several centers around the world. Concurrently, cardiac transplantation had become an established form of therapy with excellent results and it was apparent that applicability of the technique was limited mainly by availability of donor organs. In domino heart transplantation, the normal heart of a heart-lung transplant recipient is transplanted into another recipient with end-stage cardiac failure, thus allowing for optimal organ utilization.

The first report of heart transplantation from a living donor, the so-called domino procedure, was in 1988 from the Harefield group in the United Kingdom (UK). It was introduced into the US soon after, but the procedure has subsequently been far more popular in the UK and Australia than in the US. Several factors have contributed to this: (1) the difficulty in getting access to heart-lung blocks in the US because of organ allocation policies; (2) the increasing use of bilateral lung transplants; (3) the difficulty in transporting the "domino heart" long distances; and (4) the large number of centers that perform heart transplants but do not have the expertise to perform heart-lung transplants.

ADVANTAGES AND DISADVANTAGES OF DOMINO HEART TRANSPLANTATION

Several theoretical advantages of the domino procedure over conventional cadaveric transplants have been suggested:
- In experienced hands, heart-lung transplantation results in excellent short-term and long-term outcomes and largely avoids the airway anastomotic complications associated with bilateral lung transplantation.
- The domino heart has not been exposed to the potentially noxious environment of brain stem death and its accompanying catecholamine surge.

Transplant Cardiologist, Transplant Unit, Papworth Hospital, Cambridge, UK

- When both operations can be carried out in the same center, it is possible to minimize ischemic time.
- Patients on the heart transplant waiting list with high titers of cytotoxic antibodies can have suitable "donors" identified on the heart-lung waiting list, thus avoiding the need for a pretransplant crossmatch on the night of the operation.
- It was thought that the right ventricle in the heart-lung recipient with pulmonary hypertension would be "conditioned" and perhaps be suitable for the patient with heart failure and a high pulmonary vascular resistance.

Those centers opposed to the use of the domino procedure have marshaled the following arguments against its use:
- The use of heart-lung transplantation in a patient with bilateral lung disease unnecessarily exposes that individual to the risks of an allograft heart, principally cardiac allograft vasculopathy.
- It is difficult to be certain that hearts from patients with long-standing lung disease are indeed normal, particularly if they have been exposed to significant pulmonary hypertension.
- Because significant numbers of heart-lung transplants are now carried out in relatively few centers, the expertise required is not widely available. In centers without adequate experience, the results of heart-lung transplantation are inferior to bilateral lung transplantation.

The evaluation and outcomes of potential domino donors are described from the experience at a single large center (Papworth Hospital) and by a literature review of reports from other institutions.

EVALUATION OF POTENTIAL DOMINO DONORS

All potential domino heart donors undergo echocardiography to assess left and right ventricular dimensions and function. The patients give consent for heart-lung and lung transplantation and permission is sought for use of their hearts in the domino procedure. Patients over 40 also undergo coronary angiography and those with evidence of coronary artery disease are not accepted as domino donors. Right heart catheterization is not routinely performed but is restricted to patients where it is indicated for their clinical care. In the UK all domino donors have to be registered with the Unrelated Living Transplant Regulatory Authority (ULTRA).

THE RIGHT VENTRICLE

In contrast to the early years of the program, Papworth Hospital does not currently use hearts from patients with primary pulmonary hypertension (PPH) for heart transplantation. Some centers have reported early pulmonary edema in recipients of such hearts and, in the Papworth Hospital experience, most patients with PPH have dilated, poorly-functioning right ventricles by the time they come to transplantation. Right ventricular dysfunction has not been a problem in other domino donors. Domino hearts have not been used to transplant recipients with a high pulmonary vascular resistance who would not otherwise have qualified for selection.

OUTCOME

Between March 1989 and August 1988, 101 domino hearts were retrieved by Papworth Hospital. The diagnoses of the domino donors include cystic fibrosis (62 patients); bronchiectasis (17 patients); emphysema (11 patients); primary pulmonary hypertension (five patients); and miscellaneous (six patients). Sixty-eight (68%) of these were transplanted into recipients at Papworth, while 33 were exported to other centers within the UK. The mean age of the domino donors was 31 (+13.1 years). The 68 patients who received domino hearts at Papworth comprised 55 males and thirteen females, mean age 49 (+9.5 years). The preoperative diagnosis in these patients was ischemic heart disease in 36 (57%), dilated cardiomyopathy in 24 (35%), and other diagnoses in five (7%).

During the same nine year period, 364 heart transplants were performed using organs from cadaveric donors. The mean age of these donors was 33.3 (+12.4 years) (ie, not significantly different from the domino donors). The etiology of heart failure in the recipients of these hearts was similar to the domino recipients. There was no difference between groups in pretransplant transpulmonary pressure gradient, endotracheal incubation period, stay in the critical care unit, hospital stay, or frequency of acute rejection episodes. The ischemic time in the domino organs was significantly shorter than in the cadaveric group, 135.6 minutes vs 195.4 minutes ($P<0.01$). The actuarial survival of the recipients of cadaveric hearts was 81.1%, 75.6% and 70% at one, three and five years, respectively, from transplantation (Figure 34-1), while that of domino recipients in Papworth was 83.5%, 78.6% and 76.7% at one, three and five years (no significant difference). Survival of the recipients of the 33 exported hearts was similar (83.6%, 71.5% and 61.6%, respectively). There was a trend toward better survival in recipients of hearts from domino donors who had cystic fibrosis; the 5-year survival in this group was 82.9%. Thirty-day mortality in the domino group was 5.8% compared to 10.3% in the cadaveric group, an interesting difference although not statistically significant. The incidence of permanent pacemaker implantation was no different from the rest of the transplant population (4%).

CARDIAC ALLOGRAFT VASCULOPATHY

Only one recipient of a domino heart has died of cardiac allograft vasculopathy (CAV) to date (seven years posttransplant). There is no significant difference in the prevalence of angiographic CAV between the groups at four years. Intravascular ultrasound studies have not

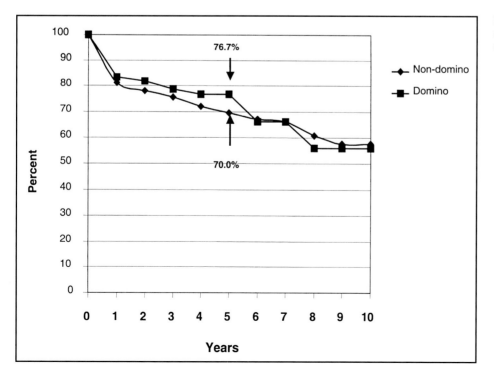

Figure 34-1. Actuarial survival of domino heart transplantation (Papworth) vs non-domino group.

been performed in these patients. Further follow-up is required to assess any potential difference in the frequency of CAV in this population.

While CAV undoubtedly occurs in the recipients of heart-lung transplants, several studies have suggested that its prevalence is less than that in recipients of heart transplants. In Papworth Hospital's experience, CAV is extremely rare in the absence of obliterative bronchiolitis (OB) in the lungs, and in the vast majority of patients it is the latter that leads to functional impairment in the heart-lung recipient. Nevertheless, CAV has contributed to or been the cause of death in seven of the series of 254 heart-lung recipients (with 144 deaths). Of these seven, only three had primary lung disease as their pretransplant pathology, and could therefore have been offered bilateral lung transplants.

REPORTS FROM OTHER CENTERS

Lowell et al reported data obtained from the United Network for Organ Sharing (UNOS) on patients transplanted between October 1987 and June 1996. Twenty-three domino transplants were identified and a significant decrease in survival in these domino recipients reported compared to 17,076 cadaveric recipients transplanted in the same period. No detail is provided about the etiology of the domino donors, or cause of death in the recipients. The Stanford group reported their early experience with domino transplantation in seven patients; at a mean follow-up of 20 months, graft and patient survival were 100%. Five of the seven domino donors had cystic fibrosis, and there was no difference in infection or rejection rates when domino heart recipients were compared to the rest of the heart transplant population.

Right ventricular function and size either improved or remained unchanged in all patients after transplantation.

Smith et al reported their experience from Melbourne, Australia: 14 domino transplants had been carried out with an actuarial 2-year survival of 86%. Yacoub et al reported on the initial Harefield experience with 20 domino transplants (from heart-lung recipients with cystic fibrosis), 1-year survival was 75%. Twelve of these patients underwent coronary angiography at 1-year and none had evidence of CAV.

In conclusion, recipients who receive "domino" hearts have an excellent initial and long-term outcome, which is at least as good as other heart transplant recipients. The issue of whether it is ethically justifiable to perform a heart-lung transplant in a patient with lung disease and a normal heart remains unresolved. Centers performing relatively large numbers of heart-lung transplants report results as good as those for bilateral lung transplants without the morbidity associated with bronchial anastomoses. While obliterative bronchiolitis remains the most important problem in this population, the risk of cardiac allograft vasculopathy cannot be ignored. Nevertheless, in centers where heart-lung transplantation continues to be performed for lung disease, the use of the domino procedure offers a chance to maximize the utilization of donor organs.

RECOMMENDED READING

Yacoub MH, Banner NR, Khaghani A, et al. Heart-lung transplantation for cystic fibrosis and subsequent domino heart transplantation. J Heart Transplant. 1990;9(5):459-467.

Baumgartner WA, Traill TA, Cameron DE, Fonger JD, Birenbaum IB, Reitz BA. Unique aspects of heart and lung transplantation exhibited in the "domino-donor" operation. JAMA. 1989;261(21):3121-3125.

Cooper JD. Dominoes-pragmatism or piracy? Transpl Int. 1991;4(1):1-2.

Smith JA, Roberts M, McNeil K, et al. Excellent outcome of cardiac transplantation using domino donor hearts. Eur J Cariothorac Surg. 1996;10(8):628-633.

Lowell JA, Taranto SE, Singer GG, et al. Transplant recipients as organ donors: the domino transplant. Transplant Proc. 1997;29(8):3392-3393.

Kells CM, Marshall S, Kramer M, et al. Cardiac function after domino-donor transplantation. Am J Cardiol. 1992;69(1):113-116.

Smith JA, Williams TJ, Rabinov M, et al. Combined heart-lung transplantation including the "domino" donor procedure in the single lung transplant era. Transplant Proc. 1992;24(5):2264-2266.

35 CADAVER HEART DONOR SELECTION CRITERIA

Jonah Odim, MD, PhD
Daniel Marelli, MD
Hillel Laks, MD

The success of a cardiac transplantation program demands careful scrutiny and selection of potential cadaver donors. The growing divergence in donor supply relative to burgeoning recipient demand requires a screening process tailored to specific recipient needs. This flexible clinical approach spurs efficient use of donor organs with minimal wastage of a scarce commodity and widens the potential therapeutic benefit.

Potential allografts must pass through the medicolegal bottleneck of specific brain death criteria and family or next-of-kin permission for organ donation. In certain instances the coroner must consent to release the body for organ donation. Only then can regional organ procurement organizations (OPOs) activate the allocation system based on recipient urgency status, donor/recipient proximity and time logged on the waiting list. The Uniform Anatomic Gift Act of 1968 established the voluntary basis of organ donation. The Uniform Brain Death (1978) and Uniform Determination of Death (1980) Acts laid down the legislative matrix upon which the diagnosis of brain death is established. The United Network for Organ Sharing (UNOS) was established in 1984 to facilitate organ sharing. Thus, formal declaration of brain death and confirmation of written informed consent must be documented in the patient's medical record prior to organ donation. Hospitals are now required to report all deaths to the OPO in an effort to maximize the recovery of transplantable organs to meet escalating demand. Other countries have enacted presumed consent legislation enabling organ procurement to automatically proceed in brain dead individuals if wishes to the contrary were not in existence prior to death.

Jonah Odim, MD, PhD, Clinical Instructor, Division of Cardiothoracic Surgery, UCLA Medical Center, Los Angeles, CA

Daniel Marelli, MD, Assistant Clinical Professor, Division of Cardiothoracic Surgery, UCLA Medical Center, Los Angeles, CA

Hillel Laks, MD, Chairman, Division of Cardiothoracic Surgery, UCLA Medical Center, Los Angeles, CA

DONOR SELECTION

There are three phases of donor selection. The primary screening is performed by the OPO. Pertinent demographic information is collected about the potential donor including age, height, weight, gender, ABO blood group, mechanism of death, hospital course and routine laboratory and serologic data. After verification of brain death and informed consent, potential recipients are identified through an extensive computerized database.

Secondary screening involves the notification of the recipient hospital team of nurse specialist, cardiac surgeon or cardiologist who scrutinize the potential donor by examining medical history, clinical and hemodynamic status, complete blood counts, Gram stains and cultures, arterial blood gas analysis, chest roentgenogram, electrocardiogram, echocardiogram (resting or under dobutamine stress) and cine-angiogram. This team identifies potential contraindications (absolute or relative) to transplantation and coordinates the clinical management of the donor (see Table 35-1). Assessment of any adverse issues is always considered in relation to the clinical needs of the potential recipient. A team may be dispatched to the donor hospital to complete this formal evaluation and stabilize a complicated patient.

The final phase or definitive screening occurs at the time of organ retrieval. Upon arrival at the donor hospital the cardiothoracic surgeon examines the donor and reviews the medical record, chest roentgenogram, electrocardiogram, echocardiogram and cine-angiogram. Once in the operating theater the surgeon inspects the heart directly looking for signs of myocardial contusion, infarction and ventricular dysfunction. The great arteries are palpated for thrills and signs of valvular dysfunction or intracardiac shunts. The coronary arteries are palpated for plaques and gross calcifications – a potential harbinger of underlying atherosclerotic occlusive disease. A mini-catheterization can be obtained by direct measurement of cardiac chamber, aortic and main pulmonary artery pressures. If necessary, oximetry occasionally can be performed to evaluate intracardiac shunts. The recipi-

---

Table 35-1. Criteria for Excluding a Potential Donor Allograft

Systemic sepsis or endocarditis
Positive serology for HIV, HBV or HCV infection
Active malignancy (extracranial)
Important coronary artery disease (requiring extensive revascularization)
Previous myocardial infarction
Irreversible ventricular dysfunction
Intractable ventricular arrhythmias (prolonged QT interval)
Important structural cardiac abnormalities (requiring extensive repair/reconstruction)

ent hospital is notified of the findings in the field and procurement can proceed if indicated (see Table 35-2). This is usually a multi-organ retrieval with several surgical teams from different hospitals. The cardiothoracic surgeon coordinates the operative management of the patient and the sequence of organ retrieval.

LEGAL CRITERIA FOR BRAIN DEATH

The criteria for brain death – absent cortical and brainstem function – must be reached according to accepted medical standards and in the absence of clinical states that might temporarily alter these findings. These comatose states include systemic hypothermia (<32.2 (C), drug overdose (eg, barbiturate), shock, metabolic and endocrinologic derangements and electrolyte and acid-base disorders. If definitive diagnosis is difficult to reach on clinical grounds, confirmation of brain death with electro-encephalography, cerebral angiography or radionuclide cortical blood flow studies is useful. A periodic challenge to the current definition of brain death and a stimulus of debate and controversy involves the use of anencephalic newborns as organ donors. Anencephalic newborns represent a relatively small cohort of potential donors for neonatal cardiac recipients and their inclusion would negligibly impact donor organ supply.

Cause of Death

The mechanism of brain death for patients serving as cardiac donors in urban USA is usually the end result of penetrating and blunt head trauma. A majority of these deaths are secondary to motor vehicle accidents, gunshot wounds to the head and closed head trauma. Intracranial bleeding and sundry other etiologies including drug poisonings, asphyxia, intracranial neoplasms and cold water drowning round out the list.

ABO MATCHING

A minimum prerequisite for allograft survival is ABO compatibility. Crossing this biologic barrier results in lethal hyperacute rejection secondary to preformed,

donor-specific antibodies in the recipient. Recipients at risk for hyperacute rejection due to anti-HLA antibodies are patients with a history of exposure to multiple transfusions, multiparous women and infants with congenital heart disease and multiple operations. Prospective cross-matching is advised when a recipient has preformed anti-HLA antibodies. The use of flow cytometry to define the risk for hyperacute rejection and need for plasmapheresis therapy in the peri-transplantation period has improved the management of these high-risk recipients. To date, the limited organ preservation window has prohibited prospective HLA matching associated with better long-term allograft survival in other solid organ transplants.

SPECIFIC CONCERNS
Age

Over the 30-year history of heart transplantation there has been a gradual relaxation of strict age criteria for the donor. The use of coronary angiography permits transplantation teams to identify important coronary artery occlusive disease and in certain isolated instances to perform surgical or catheter-based revascularization perioperatively. So far, this strategy is promising in the early and intermediate follow-up. The physiologic age of an allograft has proven more worthy than the chronologic age. Hearts from all donors are considered on a case by case basis depending on the age and medical needs of the potential recipients. In the UCLA Medical Center program there is no chronologic age criteria for donor cardiac allografts. While a recent analysis from the multi-institutional database of the International Society for Heart and Lung Transplantation (ISHLT) found higher mortality and graft failure in recipients of allografts older than 40, this outcome has not borne out in large single institutional experiences.

Malignancy

The presence of active extracranial malignancy in brain dead donors is an absolute contraindication to donation

---

Table 35-2. Criteria for Accepting a Potential Donor Allograft

Compatible donor/recipient blood types
Medical record: verification of brain death and consent for organ donation
Age <45 years OR Male >45 years with acceptable coronary angiography
Male >40 years at risk for coronary artery disease with acceptable coronary angiography
Female >50 years with acceptable coronary angiography
Female >45 years at risk for coronary artery disease with acceptable coronary angiography

Stable hemodynamics without high-dose hemodynamic support
Donor/recipient size match within 20% (height and weight) (pediatric patients flexible)
Projected ischemic time <8 hours
Functionally normal heart upon visual inspection at time of recovery

because of the potential for accelerated replication of transferred malignant cells in the immunosuppressed host. Recipients of donor hearts from patients with primary brain malignancies that have very low metastatic potential have done well after transplantation. However, these donor hearts should not be used if existing ventriculostomies or other decompressive or extirpative procedures have breached the brain-blood barrier and increased the potential for systemic seeding. Cardiac allografts from individuals deemed cured (> 5-year survival without clinical or laboratory evidence of residual or recurrent disease) from a previously treated malignancy may be cautiously considered for transplantation on a case by case basis.

Infection

Organ transplantation is a very efficient means of transmitting certain diseases; therefore a critical evaluation of a potential donor is essential to prevent the transmission of a life-threatening infection with the cardiac allograft. One can divide the infections into these groups: (1) active viral infection (eg, HIV, hepatitis B and hepatitis C viruses); (2) latent infection with CMV and toxoplasma that are capable of being reactivated after transplantation; (3) active infection of the allograft with bacteria, fungi and certain viruses due to terminal illness or preceding clinical illness.

HIV INFECTION. The rate of transmission of HIV infection from solid organ transplantation approaches 100% resulting uniformly in death of the recipients. Thus, organs from donors with a positive antibody screening to HIV are declined unless subsequent confirmation deems a false-positive initial screening test. A confirmatory Western blot is realistically only feasible in living organ donors at the present time.

HEPATITIS B VIRUS. Hepatitis B virus (HBV) transmission is documented to occur in heart transplant recipients. Within 30 to 60 days of exposure hepatitis B surface antigen (HbsAg) may be detected in the sera of inoculated patients. Hemolysis of the donor blood sample may lead to false positive HbsAg screening. Heart recipients who are anti-HBs positive (secondary to immunization or natural immunity) are considered candidates for such a donor at some transplantation centers.

HEPATITIS C VIRUS. About one-half of anti-HCV-positive patients have detectable hepatitis C viremia by polymerase chain reaction (PCR) analysis of the blood. All PCR-positive donors will transmit HCV to allograft recipients. The risk of HCV transmission from an anti-HCV antibody-positive donor (PCR-negative) is indeterminate. PCR testing is usually performed retrospectively for heart donors given the short preservation

window. In short, about 50% of recipients of anti-HCV antibody-positive cardiac allografts will have detectable anti-HCV antibody. And half of these (25%) have detectable hepatitis C viremia by PCR analysis. Overall, in time, 35% of recipients receiving a heart from a donor who is anti-HCV antibody-positive may develop liver disease.

BACTERIOLOGY AND SEPSIS. Donor infection is evaluated in the setting of blood culture bacteriology, the presence and duration of catheters and intravenous lines, and the nature of the infection, prior to decisions about acceptability for transplantation. The removal of the offending foreign body and administration of appropriate antibiotics may suffice to ensure suitability for organ donation. Donors with bacterial meningitis (usual offenders include *H influenzae, S pneumoniae* and *N meningitidis*) may be acceptable for organ donation following systemic administration of a broad-spectrum cephalosporin. Donor infection with Gram negative organisms as *Klebsiella, Enterobacter, E coli* and *P aeruginosa* portend an important risk for the development of anastomotic rupture and generally disqualify a cardiac allograft. This has also been reported for infections with *S aureus* and *Bacteroides* species. Similarly, the presence of important donor fungal infection automatically prohibits cardiac organ donation. In the case of donor heart endocarditis, the extent of local disease, bacteremia (ie, bacteriology and antibiotic sensitivities) and urgency status of the recipient weigh on the decision to transplant the graft. Appropriate donor and recipient perioperative antibiotics may prevent inoculation and adverse infectious sequelae. The basic tenet not to transplant an already infected organ, or an organ obtained from a patient with ongoing bacteremia or fungemia is a safe one. However, indiscriminate adherence to this premise leads to wastage of some potentially usable grafts. Certain donors are at higher risk for occult sepsis including victims of drowning, burns and ventilator dependency with indwelling lines and catheters for over a week duration.

Ischemia Time

The upper cold ischemia limit of the heart has historically been set at four to six hours. Present day organ preservation techniques have extended heart preservation from six to eight hours. This biologic constraint has limited the geographic area from which donor hearts can be obtained for specific transplant centers and any potential benefits that may accrue from prospective crossmatching potential donor hearts for transplantation. The successful preservation of other solid organs for up to two days by flushing the organs with University of Wisconsin (UW) solution and storage at hypothermia (0° to 5°C) has led to the use of UW solution for heart preservation as well.

Cellular impermeable agents (ie, lactobionic acid, raffinose and hydroxyethyl starch) prevent cell swelling during cold ischemic storage. The addition of glutathione and adenosine may promote organ recovery by combating the reperfusion injury due to oxygen free radicals and stimulating high-energy phosphate replenishment. A standard donor cardiectomy is performed following diastolic arrest and flush cooling of the empty heart with cold UW solution (10 to 12 cc/kg), at a mean aortic root pressure of 60 to 70 mmHg for four to six minutes, and topical saline slush. The excised allograft is rinsed in cold UW solution to remove blood and submerged in cold UW solution and placed in sterile bowel bags for transportation in a chest of ice. At the recipient hospital, orthotopic transplantation of the donor heart is performed using a bicaval technique with continuous topical endocardial cold plasmalyte solution infusion. All allografts are reperfused with leukocyte-depleted aspartate-glutamate-enriched warm blood cardioplegia for four minutes followed by four minutes of leukocyte-depleted warm blood prior to releasing the aortic crossclamp. The use of UW solution and leukocyte-depleted perfusion has reduced the incidence of allograft failure associated with long donor ischemia times (>5 H).

Size Match

A guideline established from the Stanford experience is that heart transplantation is safely performed when donor/recipient size mismatch is greater than 0.8 in the setting of normal recipient pulmonary vascular resistance and transpulmonary gradient. A donor is considered marginal if mismatch is less than 0.7 or if body surface area of donor and recipient differ by more than 30%. Before accepting an undersized donor heart, other variables in both donor and recipient should be considered, such as duration of donor ischemic time, lean body mass, recipient's pulmonary artery pressures, donor heart hypertrophy and gender mismatch, particularly when considering implanting an undersized female heart into a male recipient. The goal is to match the donor myocardial mass to the circulatory demands of the recipient. In this context an estimation of lean body mass is more relevant than absolute weight, particularly in obese donors. Most patients suffering from end-stage heart failure have cardiomegaly and can accept a larger donor heart. This is particularly true for the neonatal and infant recipients for whom congruent size-matched donor organs are more difficult to find. A greater discrepancy in size match is generally tolerated, but may require removal of recipient costal cartilages to enlarge the mediastinal domain for an oversized allograft. Undersizing should be avoided whenever possible, particularly in patients with elevated pulmonary vascular resistance and reoperative sternotomy (higher likelihood for blood transfusion).

Ventricular Dysfunction

Ventricular dysfunction has usually been defined as a subnormal ejection fraction by echocardiography, the need for high doses of inotropic agents and hemodynamic abnormalities. A donor heart with a history of cardiac arrest and prolonged ventricular resuscitation or death by asphyxia was previously considered unacceptable for transplantation. A more recent experience suggests that it is possible to use donor hearts after arrest if this event predates procurement by a few days, the heart is optimally resuscitated and the recipient size is smaller than that of the donor. The function of donor hearts requiring high-dose inotropic support can often be optimized. Fluid replacement to match urine or blood losses and blood transfusion to optimize myocardial oxygen delivery can improve donor heart function. Thyroid hormone replacement with Triiodothyronine is useful and may permit reducing pressor support. Despite careful management, the ejection fraction by echocardiography may still remain below 45%. Such a heart could be used for a smaller recipient with normal pulmonary artery pressures who is listed Status I. A shorter donor ischemic time is preferred for such a heart.

Left Ventricular Hypertrophy

The diastolic dysfunction of the hypertrophied heart has presented particular concerns. Donor allografts with left ventricular hypertrophy (LVH) may be used selectively, particularly if there are no electrocardiographic criteria of hypertrophy and the graft ischemia time is short. Caution is advised if the donor has a documented history of hypertension. Precise measurement of LV wall thickness by echocardiography is warranted in all potential donor allografts to estimate severity and compliment ECG interpretation.

SUMMARY

The factor most responsible for restricting the widespread application of heart transplantation to patients with terminal congestive heart failure is the dearth of donor organs. Judicious matching and scrutiny of all potential donors with patients on the growing rolls awaiting heart transplantation will optimize the utility of this preciously scarce resource.

RECOMMENDED READING

Bennett LE, Edwards EB, Hosenpud JD. Transplantation with older donor hearts for presumed "stable" recipients: an analysis of the Joint International Society for Heart and Lung Transplantation/United Network for Organ Sharing Thoracic Registry. J Heart Lung Transplant. 1998;17(9):901-905.

Coll P, Montserrat I, Ballester M, et al. Epidemiologic evidence of transmission of donor-related bacterial infection through a transplanted heart. J Heart Lung Transplant. 1997;16(4):464-467.

Delmonico FL, Snydman DR. Organ donor screening for infectious diseases: review of practice and implications for transplantation. Transplantation. 1998;65(5):603-610.

Jeevanandam V, Furkawa S, Prendergast TW, Todd BA, Eisen HJ, McClurken JB. Standard criteria for an acceptable donor heart are restricting heart transplantation. Ann Thorac Surg. 1996;62(5):1268-1275.

Kobashigawa JA, Laks H, Marelli D, et al. The University of California at Los Angeles experience in heart transplantation. Clin Transpl. 1998:303-310.

Koerner MM, Tenderich G, Minami K, et al. Extended donor criteria: use of cardiac allografts after carbon monoxide poisoning. Transplantation. 1998;63(9):1358-1360.

Marelli D, Laks H, Fazio D, Moore S, Moriguchi J, Kobashigawa J. The use of donor hearts with left ventricular hypertrophy. J Heart Lung Transplant. 2000;19(5):496-503.

Novitzky D. Selection and management of cardiac allograft donors. Curr Opin Cardiology. 1996;11(2):174-182.

Southard JH, Belzer FO. Organ preservation. Ann Rev Med. 1995;46:235-247.

Wheeldon DR, Potter CD, Oduro A, Wallwork J, Large SR. Transforming the "unacceptable" donor: outcomes from the adoption of a standardized donor management technique. J Heart Lung Transplant. 1995;14(4):734-742.

Young JB, Naftel DC, Bourge RC, et al. Matching the heart donor and heart transplant recipient. Clues for successful expansion of the donor pool: a multivariable, multiinstitutional report. The Cardiac Transplant Research Database Group. J Heart Lung Transplant. 1994;13(3):353-365.

36 THE CONTINUING EVOLUTION OF DONOR HEART ALLOCATION

Lynne Warner Stevenson, MD

When cardiac transplantation was an experiment performed by a few lone pioneers, the selection and distribution of donor hearts was not an issue of national resource allocation. Indeed, in the first Bethesda conference on cardiac transplantation in 1968, it was estimated that the number of potential recipients would be ten to 50,000 and the supply of potential donors would ultimately be the same as the need. The investigators selected, from among many, those recipients and those donor hearts most likely to demonstrate the success of the controversial procedure. When a donor heart became available, difficult choices were made within an institution regarding the best use of that organ. The severity of recipient illness, risks for postoperative complications, and characteristics of the donor heart were all considered, but the geographic separation of the first programs meant that there was little need to consider the possible urgency of unknown candidates at other institutions.

Once cardiac transplantation was accepted and supported as "best therapy" for patients meeting defined inclusion and exclusion criteria, the number of active heart transplant centers rapidly increased to the current number of 153, often with several in the same city, until virtually every candidate was in competition with multiple patients listed at his own program and at other programs in the same region for a scarce supply of donor hearts. Fundamental principles of triage dictated that the patients with the most urgent need would receive the highest priority for donor hearts, and initial efforts were made to define multiple characteristics that could be applied across programs to define urgency on the basis of intensity of support, hospitalization, and activity levels such as employment for patients waiting at home. While logical for patients in one care system, there were inevitable differences in management style such that patients classified at a given level might have very different clinical profiles in different programs. These differences were widened by the recognition that patients in jeopardy would have greater chance of surviving to transplant from higher priority levels with shorter waiting times. A physician acting primarily as a patient's advocate might escalate the patient's apparent need.

Director, Cardiomyopathy and Heart Failure Program, Cardiovascular Division, Brigham and Women's Hospital, Harvard Medical School, Boston, MA

To simplify the priority scheme and allow some objective means of standardizing acuity of illness, a simple two-tiered system was introduced. Status I was given to patients who required mechanical assist devices (including ventilator or intra-aortic balloon pump) or patients who were in an intensive care unit requiring intravenous inotropic agents to maintain adequate cardiac output (or infants younger than six months old). All other patients, regardless of hospitalization or functional limitation, were Status II. By 1990-1991, between 15% and 25% of patients listed for transplantation were initially listed as Status I. Because they received priority, approximately 46% of donor hearts were going to Status I patients, who comprised about 5% of the patients on the list at any given time.

As this trend was increasingly recognized, concern arose that the systematic allocation of hearts to the sickest recipients would compromise the outcome of transplantation. This concern simultaneously reflected both the growing allegiance to a national "transplant community" responsible for optimal allocation of an increasingly limited resource, and reaction to institutional pressures to demonstrate good local survival statistics for patient recruitment and reimbursement.

The fundamental goal of transplantation is clearly to maximize the benefit from the procedure, the difference between survival and function with transplantation compared to survival and function without transplantation. Although the postoperative survival rate itself is more easily measured and compared, it is obviously less relevant, as it would be maximized by restricting transplantation to healthy normal subjects who would derive no benefit.

When designing an allocation strategy, the impact of decisions should be considered for the entire candidate population, not just those transplanted. In addition to transplantation, outcomes for transplant candidates include sudden death while waiting, deterioration to a higher status from which death may occur, and continued survival without transplantation. The decision to award priority to the patients with the most critical need should maximize the chances of survival even for a patient initially listed without urgent status, who may subsequently deteriorate. From population modeling using a Markov model and observed pretransplantation and posttransplantation transition rates from 1990 to 1991, the advantage of this general priority system is predicted to persist even if the preoperative sudden death rate doubled and the postoperative mortality for urgent patients increased to 28%. In fact, both of these event rates are decreasing. The outpatient risk of sudden death, estimated at 0.02 monthly before 1990, has since decreased to 0.008 from 1992 to 1995. The analysis from the Cardiac Transplant Research Database indicates that survival for patients transplanted as Status I was equivalent to that for Status II patients.

As the proportion of donor hearts used for critical patients increases, the waiting time for regular status patients continues to increase. The event rates for deterioration and death from heart failure are highest in the first three to six months after listing, following which deterioration occurs at a slower rate. Risk of sudden death is less dependent on time after listing. When defined as the risk of 1-year mortality without transplant minus the risk of 1-year mortality with transplantation, the first-year benefit of transplantation is highest for outpatients early after listing, with declining first-year benefit thereafter, until by approximately nine months, the anticipated 1-year survival is 88% for patients still able to wait at home whether or not transplantation is performed. The average waiting time for outpatients is currently 385 days as of 1998. This waiting list maturation has led to reconsideration of some patients who have survived their period of early risk, during which clinical improvement may also occur due to delayed effects of redesigned medical regimens and in some cases to spontaneous resolution of unrecognized reversible factors. Periodic reevaluation is now recommended every three to six months to identify patients in whom transplantation can be deferred. For ambulatory candidates, criteria for clinical stability include improvement in peak oxygen consumption, absence of congestion, and freedom from severe angina or arrhythmias. Up to 30% of patients reevaluated may meet such criteria for "de-listing", with 2-year survival of 80% to 90% without transplantation. Such reevaluation is essential in order to distill the waiting list to those candidates with the great-est need for imminent transplantation. It is critical to note, however, that good outcomes for patients listed and "de-listed" depend on close surveillance and rapid response to any evidence of deterioration that would warrant more urgent transplantation.

The majority of our information regarding baseline characteristics and changes in priority on the waiting list has been derived from the Pretransplant Research Database, formed in conjunction with the Cardiac Transplant Research Database. Twelve centers participated from 1992 to 1995, providing extensive baseline and follow-up information on 1,340 patients listed for transplantation. Of 366 patients initially listed as Status I, 70% underwent transplantation as Status I, 23% died, and 6% were removed from the list due to spontaneous improvement. Complete extended follow-up of patients initially listed as Status II indicated that 13% of patients died out of the hospital as Status II, 32% underwent transplantation as Status II, 29% of patients deteriorated to Status I, of whom 10% (3% of total Status II) died without transplant and the remainder underwent transplantation as Status I (from II). The survival for patients transplanted as Status I from II during this period was equivalent to that for patients listed and transplanted as Status II. This experience highlights the dynamic nature of the waiting list for heart transplant candidates (Figure 36-1).

During the two-status period, over half of the national regions had variances in place, often defining an intermediate status agreed upon by all heart transplant programs within the region. The Pretransplant Research Database was used to analyze outcomes for

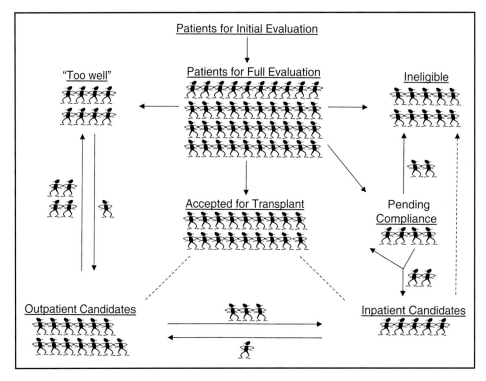

Figure 36-1. Diagram illustrating flow through the evaluation process both before and after listing for transplantation. Omitted for clarity are the occasional patients waiting at home who develop contraindications to transplantation.

those 164 patients (17% of all Status II patients) who were not in an intensive care unit but required continued hospitalization or received intravenous inotropic infusions at the time of listing, either in hospital or at home. These patients had a rate of death and deterioration to urgent transplantation higher than that of Status II patients out of the hospital without intravenous inotropic infusions, and a death rate lower than Status I patients (Figure 36-2).

Another trend developing during this period was the establishment of a population enjoying hemodynamic stability and increased mobility on implantable left ventricular assist devices. When the previous status system was designed, the mechanical support devices available could be used only for a brief time before severe problems developed with the coagulation system, infection, and often multiorgan failure. As patients began to rehabilitate on more robust assist devices prior to transplantation, they continued to receive the highest priority for transplantation, although no longer at the same level of risk as other Status I patients. The period of highest risk after placement of these devices occurs during the first three weeks. During this time, most patients are not on the active list for transplantation, but are recovering from the initial operation and from the compromised organ function resulting from previous hypoperfusion and congestion. Following that time, as indicated for 284 patients undergoing implantation during the investigational experience with the Heartmate® ventricular assist device, the weekly risk for death declines to a level intermediate between that of the other Status I patients and that of the Status II patients, comparable to that for the patients on intravenous inotropic infusions (Figure 36-2).

As the period of support prior to transplantation continues to be extended beyond the early rehabilitation period, infections and occasional device malfunctions can develop such that patients return to a higher risk group.

These considerations were incorporated into the most recent allocation system for heart transplantation, instituted on January 15, 1999 (Table 36-1). The IA status is similar to the previous Status I with the exceptions that patients with left ventricular assist devices are Status I only for the first 30 days after implantation or subsequently if they are in hospital with objective evidence of impending device failure or life-threatening complications. Patients with continued support from a mechanical ventilator, total artificial heart, intra-aortic balloon pump, or extra-corporeal membrane oxygenation can retain Status IA indefinitely. Other patients can be Status IA for seven days, renewable once, on inotropic infusions if they have an indwelling pulmonary artery catheter and require inotropic support comparable to 7.5 mcg/kg per minute of dobutamine. An additional category is included for other hospitalized patients with critical cardiac compromise and life expectancy less than seven days, requiring narrative justification and retroactive approval by a local review board. It is anticipated that this category will be employed for patients with severe compromise on intravenous inotropic support in whom the infectious risk of continued central hemodynamic monitoring is not warranted.

Transplantation represents a unique example of the challenges presented for rational distribution of a fixed resource. As with other natural resources, effective use requires a sense of community beyond individual institutions. For donor hearts, the most appropriate

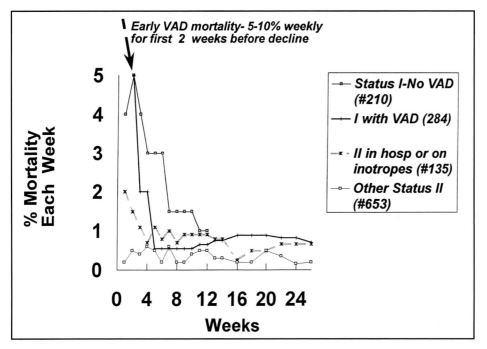

Figure 36-2. Graph of weekly hazard for patients according to severity of clinical status while on the list for transplantation (adapted from Stevenson, et al., J Am Coll Cardiol.1998;31A;251A). Data for survival without mechanical assistance derived from the Pre-Transplant Research Database and data for survival on left ventricular assist devices is derived from the investigational period of the HeartMate® experience (courtesy Krauskopf, TCI).

Table 36-1. Listing for Heart Transplantation – 1999
Status IA. A patient is hospitalized at the listing transplant center with at least one of the following:

a) Mechanical circulatory support for acute hemodynamic decompensation with at least one of the following:
        Left and/or right ventricular assist device for ≤30 days
        Total artificial heart
        Intra-aortic balloon pump
        Extracorporeal membrane oxygenator
   b) Mechanical circulatory support for > 30 days with objective medical evidence of significant device-related complications (narrative form required).
   c) Mechanical ventilation
   d) Continuous infusion of single high-dose inotropic infusion or multiple intravenous inotropes, in addition to continuous hemodynamic monitoring of left ventricular filling pressures (valid for seven days with one time seven day renewal). Patient without any of the above criteria who is hospitalized at the transplant center with life expectancy under seven days (full narrative form required and reviewed by regional and national boards).

Status IB. A patient at home or in the hospital has at least one of the following:
a) Left and/or right ventricular assist device longer than 30 days   b) Continuous infusion of intravenous inotropes.
Status 2 includes all patients not meeting criteria for Status IA or Status IB..
Status 7 applies to patients considered temporarily unsuitable to receive a heart transplant.

community is regional. The size of this community is most obviously defined by the correlation between organ donation and the public perception of local needs, then by the constraints of ischemic time. The less obvious but equally profound virtues of regional organization are the standards of collegial accountability for fair practices of initial candidate selection and the designation of appropriate support/priority while on the waiting list.

RECOMMENDED READING

Stevenson LW, Warner SL, Hamilton MA, et al. Modeling distribution of donor hearts to maximize early candidate survival. Circulation. 1992;86(5 Suppl):II225-II230.

Bourge RC, Naftel DC, Constanzo-Nordin MR, et al. Pretransplantation risk factors for death after heart transplantation: a multiinstitutional study. J Heart Lung Trans. 1993;12(4):549-562.

Stevenson LW, Bourge RC, Naftel DC, et al. Deterioration and death on the current waiting list: a multicenter study of patients awaiting heart transplantation. Cardiac Transplant Research Database Group. Circulation. 1995;92:1-124.

Rodeheffer RJ, Naftel DC, Stevenson LW, et al. Secular trends in cardiac transplant recipient and donor management in the United States 1990-1994; a multi-institutional study. Cardiac Transplant Research Database Group. Circulation. 1996;94(11):2883-2889.

Stevenson LW, Hamilton MA, Tillisch JH, et al. Decreasing survival benefit from cardiac transplantation for outpatients as the waiting list lengthens. J Am Coll Cardiol. 1991;18(4):919-925.

Mudge GH, Goldstein S, Addonizio LJ, et al. Cardiac transplantation. Task Force 3: Recipient guidelines/prioritization. J Am Coll Cardiol. 1993;22(1):21-31.

Stevenson LW, Steimle AE, Fonarow G, et al. Improvement in exercise capacity of candidates awaiting heart transplantation. J Am Coll Cardiol. 1995;25(1):163-170.

Stevenson LW, Bourge RC, Naftel DC, et al. Weekly risk of death while awaiting transplantation: relationship to support required. Cardiac Transplant Research Database. J Am Coll Cardiology. 1998;31A;251A.

37 HEART TRANSPLANTATION: TECHNICAL TIPS TO THE SURGICAL PROCEDURE

Robert E. Michler, MD
Eric W. Schneeberger, MD

Improved drug therapy and experienced management protocols have made heart transplantation the best treatment for patients with end-stage cardiac disease. Between 3,000 and 4,000 heart transplants are performed worldwide annually, which bears witness to both the reproducibility of the procedure and the severe shortage of available donor organs. Experience has also shown that cardiac transplantation is a viable proposition for pediatric patients with complex congenital abnormalities. This chapter reviews the technical details involved in the performance of orthotopic heart transplantation. The suggestions and tips for this procedure are delivered with the recognition that there are certainly alternative perspectives, but that the opinions rendered are those from a personal heart transplant experience that presently exceeds 400 procedures.

DONOR CARDIECTOMY

The success of every transplant procedure begins with the preoperative hemodynamic management of the donor and the skill with which the donor organ is harvested. Experienced surgeons recognize subtle changes in hemodynamics, cardiac contractility and cardiac chamber size, all of which may signal impending circulatory collapse or arrhythmia. Organ procurement generally occurs at night, when donor institutions have completed the elective operative schedule and when the donor team may be tired from a heavy workload in their home institution. Notwithstanding, the donor team must be prepared to carefully and thoroughly review all clinical information first-hand to confirm all information that has previously been communicated by telephone. In addition, the cardiac surgeon must be constantly vigilant and observant of all clinical changes with the donor during multiple organ procurement. Inadvertent bleeding, compression of the heart, bowel contamination, and respiratory insufficiency

Robert E. Michler, MD, Professor and Chief, Cardiothoracic Surgery and Thoracic Transplantation; Director, Heart Hospital, Ohio State University Medical Center, Columbus, OH

Eric W. Schneeberger, MD, Fellow, Cardiothoracic Surgery, Ohio State University Medical Center, Columbus, OH

are all events that may necessitate urgent action by the cardiac surgeon. Heart procurement is usually part of multi-organ retrieval and requires thoughtful and thorough communication between the surgical teams to ensure that all organs are procured in excellent condition.

The donor is brought into the operating room and a standard mid-line incision is made from the sternal notch to the symphysis pubis. After opening the sternum and pericardium, the heart is inspected for signs of external damage and the coronary arteries are palpated. The vigor of ventricular contraction is noted, as well as any evidence of distension of the atrial or ventricular chambers and any unsuspected abnormalities (eg, a left superior vena cava).

The ascending aorta is dissected from the pulmonary artery to permit application of a cross-clamp. The superior vena cava (SVC) is mobilized to above the level of the azygos vein, where it can be divided well clear of the sinoatrial node and incorporate the azygos vein. The inferior vena cava (IVC) is encircled. A cardioplegia infusion cannula is inserted into the ascending aorta just proximal to the fatty fold in the midportion of the aorta. This location permits subsequent doses of cardioplegia to be administered by the recipient team without having to reinsert or move the cannula. The team procuring the abdominal organs is then given time to prepare for procurement of the abdominal organs.

When all teams have completed preparations, the donor is administered heparin in a dose of 1 to 3 mg/kg. When all of the surgical teams are ready, the SVC is ligated cephalad above the level of the azygos vein. The azygos vein itself may be double ligated. The fate of the SVC depends on the planned technique of transplant anastomosis; bicaval or atrial. The IVC is divided at the level of the diaphragm or slightly higher if the liver transplant surgeons require additional length. This maneuver decompresses the right side of the heart. A suction catheter may be introduced into the abdominal IVC in order to aspirate blood. Alternatively, the IVC blood may be drained into the abdominal cavity or right pleural space. This prevents warm blood from washing out of the liver and into the pericardial cavity, rewarming the heart. One of the inferior pulmonary veins (usually the left inferior pulmonary vein) is then incised in order to decompress the left heart. If the lungs are to be procured, the left atrial appendage is incised instead, so as not to damage a pulmonary vein.

Naturally, decompression of the heart by incising the IVC and pulmonary veins is accomplished in rapid sequence in order to prevent distension of the heart. Only at this stage, when the heart is completely decompressed, is the aortic cross-clamp applied and cardioplegia delivered. Most authors recommend a minimum of one liter of ice cold (4° C) cardioplegic solution into the root of the aorta. This is usually done by attaching a pressure bag to the vaculiter of cardioplegia and inflating it to 300 mmHg. This results in a root pressure of approximately 100 mmHg and should be confirmed with digital palpation by the surgeon. In cases where the donor heart has evidence of left ventricular hypertrophy, an additional liter of cold cardioplegia is administered, taking care not to introduce air into the system during the changing of cardioplegia bags.

One to two liters of ice cold saline slush are also poured over the heart to help cool it rapidly. All of the saline and cardioplegia are aspirated from the pericardial cavity, and the four pulmonary veins are then divided at the point of entry into the pericardial cavity. If, however, lung transplantation is planned, the pulmonary veins are divided with a cuff of the left atrium. The aorta is then divided just proximal to the innominate artery, and the pulmonary artery is divided at the level of the bifurcation. Naturally, the donor team must be familiar with the anatomy of the intended recipient. This permits the procurement of any additional length of great arteries or atria as required by the particular recipient. The heart is then lifted gently from the pericardial cavity and placed in a basin of cold cardioplegia solution for inspection and preparation.

PREPARATION OF THE DONOR HEART

At this stage, the cardiac valves must be inspected for any signs of damage or disease. In addition, the coronary arteries are palpated for signs of atheroma or calcification.

Communication between donor and recipient teams is cruicial to successful outcomes in transplantation. A message must be relayed to the recipient team advising them that a suitable donor heart has been procured and an estimate should be given of the anticipated arrival time in the recipient operating room. The donor heart is then placed in a sterile plastic bag in one liter of cold saline solution or cardioplegia solution. This bag is then placed into a second bag with a liter of cold saline. These bags are then placed into an ice cooler containing crushed ice.

RECIPIENT PREPARATION AND CARDIECTOMY

Once word has been received that a suitable donor heart is available, a calculation should be made as to how long it will take for the heart to be transported to the recipient hospital. Generally, one hour is set aside for the anaesthesia and insertion of monitoring lines. If no previous cardiac surgery has occurred in the patient, then it usually only takes 15 to 30 minutes to open the sternum and prepare the patient for cardiopulmonary bypass. However, if there has been previous cardiac surgery, approximately an hour is required, in addition to the anaesthetic time, to prepare the patient for surgery. Acute hemodynamic fail-

ure or ventricular arrhythmia during the procedure should lead immediately to the initiation of cardiopulmonary bypass. In complex reoperative situations such as multiple sternotomies, prior congenital surgery with right ventricular distension or any potential for cardiac adherence to the sternum, exposure of the groin and even the initiation of cardiopulmonary bypass prior to the sternotomy is recommended.

Once cardiopulmonary bypass has been successfully established and the donor heart is in the operating room, excision of the recipient heart is performed. First, the recipient aorta is cross-clamped just proximal to the aortic cannula and a needle is inserted into the ascending aorta through which cardioplegia may be delivered if the heart is to be used for IRB research. The aorta and pulmonary artery are transected close to the commisural tips of the valves. The angle of division of each great vessel is different, in that transection of the aorta at this precise level requires a slight upward anterior/posterior angulation of the scissors, while that of the pulmonary artery requires a slight downward anterior/posterior angulation. This is most important for the pulmonary artery, for it leaves most of the recipient main pulmonary artery intact. The aorta and pulmonary artery are pulled forward, exposing the roof of the left atrium.

By grasping the tip of the left atrial appendage, one can incise into the left atrium at the base of the appendage (Figure 37-1). Doing so will prevent incising too close to the left pulmonary veins. This incision is then carried forward to the base of the transected aorta and to the juncture of the right atrium (Figure 37-2).

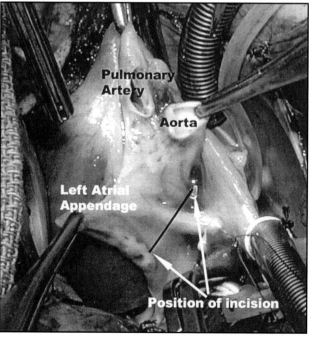

Figure 37-1. The tip of the left atrial appendage is grasped, to allow the incision into the left atrium at the base of the appendage.

Incising the right atrial free wall in the atrial portion of the right atrioventricular groove and extending this incision inferiorly to the coronary sinus permits a good cuff to be created, but also exposes the fossa ovalis. Extending the right atrial incision superiorly over the appendage and then down toward the base of the aorta places this incision opposite the previously-created incision in the left atrium. The angle of the incision to join these two opposing areas is very important in order to leave adequate septal tissue for subsequent anastomosis to the donor heart (Figure 37-3). The surgeon should now scan the area of the base of the aorta, the open left and right atria and the fossa ovalis.

One now joins these atrial incisions by cutting directly behind the aorta and angling the incision toward the base of the heart so as to leave a generous ridge of atrial septal tissue along the fossa ovalis (Figure 37-4). (Note: At the time of implant it is preferable not to suture directly to the fossa ovalis since this tissue can be quite thin and may hold suture poorly.)

The incision continues inferiorly to the coronary sinus. The coronary sinus is excised along with the recipient heart by cutting along the free wall of the left atrium in an inferior/posterior, then cephalad direction.

Importantly, the presence of a left SVC necessitates leaving the coronary sinus intact as part of the remaining left atrial cuff to serve as a conduit for blood drainage from the left SVC. Remember, the coronary sinus serves to channel the left SVC into the right atrium. The middle cardiac vein must be oversewn to prevent later bleeding from this site (Figure 37-5).

The recipient heart is now free for removal from the pericardial cavity.

RECIPIENT OPERATION

Two very different operations have been described for heart transplantation. The first is the orthotopic heart

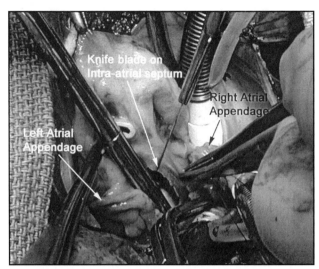

Figure 37-3. Incising the right atrial free wall in the atrial portion of the right atrioventricular groove. This incision is extended inferiorly to the coronary sinus, permitting a good cuff to be created and exposing the fossa ovalis. Extending the right atrial incision superiorly over the appendage and then down toward the base of the aorta places this incision opposite the previously-created incision in the left atrium. Note the angle of the incision to join these two opposing areas. This angle will leave adequate septal tissue for subsequent anastomosis to the donor heart, and therefore, is critical.

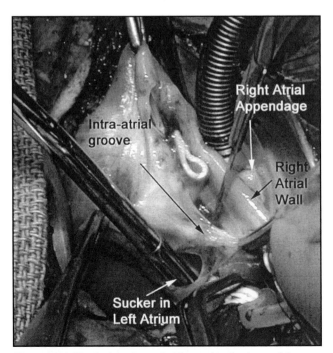

Figure 37-2. The incision is carried forward to the base of the transected aorta and to the juncture of the right atrium.

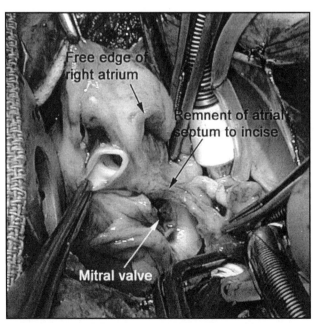

Figure 37-4. The atrial incisions are joined by cutting directly behind the aorta, angling toward the base of the heart, leaving a generous ridge of atrial septal tissue along the fossa ovalis.

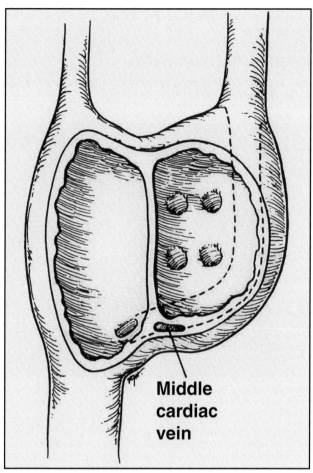

Middle cardiac vein

Figure 37-5. The middle cardiac vein must be oversewn to prevent later bleeding from this site.

cava. He believed this incision avoided the area of the sinoatrial node.

In 1989, Yacoub and Banner reported modifications to the standard technique by removing both native atria and performing anastomoses directly to the pulmonary veins and vena cava. In 1990, Reitz used the heart of a patient undergoing a heart-lung transplantation. At the time he performed a bicaval anastomoses with end-to-end anastomoses of both superior and inferior vena cavae. In 1991, the total orthotopic heart transplant technique was reported by Dreyfus and Carpentier.

The order of the anastomoses for implantation of the donor heart may vary from institution to institution. However, the left atrial/pulmonary vein anastomosis is generally performed first since it is the most posterior anatomic structure. If the "standard" technique is being used, the heart is placed in the pericardial cavity and rotated to the left so that the posterior aspect of the donor heart is facing upward. This aligns the free edge of the lateral aspect of the left atrial cuff of the donor with that of the recipient. Generally, the suture line begins at the base of the donor left atrial appendage and corresponds to the recipient left atrial cuff at a point just above the recipient left pulmonary vein. This suture line can be sewn forehand down to the point where the free edge of the left atrium turns to become the interatrial septum. At this juncture, the opposite end of the suture may be taken and used to sew forehand the dome of the left atrium followed by the interatrial septum, eventually reaching the inferior aspect of the atrial septum where the previous suture ended.

Remember that the extra tissue left on the recipient interatrial septum at the time of recipient cardiectomy is the edge to which one will suture, thus avoiding the fossa ovalis, which is composed of relatively thin tissue that may tear, resulting in an atrial septal defect. In addition, this ridge of tissue also forms part of the right atrial suture line and it is important to have sufficient tissue for this suture line. A single 3-0 monofilament (54 inches) is generally used to secure this anastomosis.

Once the left atrial suture line is completed a dose of cardioplegia is administered. Various methods have been employed for myocardial preservation. Many surgeons wrap the heart in an iced cold laparotomy pad and run an ice cold saline solution onto it. Others introduce catheters though the left atrial appendage, and irrigate the inside of the left heart with ice cold saline. Still other surgeons will insert a retrograde cardioplegic cannula into the coronary sinus and administer continuous cold cardioplegia. Near the completion of the implantation procedure this may be converted to warm blood cardioplegia.

If pulmonary venous anastomoses will be performed, the bridge of tissue between the superior and inferior pulmonary veins on the left and separately on

transplant in which the recipient heart is removed and replaced by the donor heart in the correct anatomical position. The second is the heterotopic heart transplant, in which the donor heart is placed in the right chest beside the recipient heart, and anastomosed in such a way as to allow blood to pass through both hearts, essentially using the donor heart as an assist device. Both procedures have undergone various modifications over the years. This chapter will focus on orthotopic heart transplantation.

The standard technique of orthotopic heart transplantation was developed in research laboratories in the late 1950s and early 1960s. Lower and Shumway (1960) described the operation using an atrial technique in which the incision in the right atrium extended from the inferior vena cava to the superior vena cava. This incision was posterior to the sinoatrial node and created a large cuff for the anastomosis. In 1968, Barnard described a modification to the operative technique by changing the direction of the right atrial incision of the donor heart. He extended the incision from the postero-lateral aspect of the inferior vena cava to the base of the right atrial appendage instead of the superior vena

the right are resected, creating a single left and single right-sided pulmonary venous orifice. These orifices should be at least as wide as the mitral annulus to avoid restriction following anastomoses. With this technique, the recipient heart is excised in standard fashion but then trimmed to create separate pulmonary venous cuffs. This requires that the right atrium be divided at the level of each vena cava leaving a large residual cuff of atrial tissue surrounding each vena cava. The central portion of the recipient right atrium contains the recipient interatrial septum. The free wall of this segment of atrium may be excised, leaving the septal portion intact, for it becomes the roof of the right pulmonary veins and the right lateral suture line for the right pulmonary venous orifice.

Usually, the left-sided anastomoses is performed first. A single monofilament suture of 4-0 is used to sew this anastomoses. The heart is then rotated to the left and suturing begun on the medial aspect of the right pulmonary venous orifice.

Generally, the right atrial anastomoses is performed next. One practice is to doubly ligate the donor SVC and incise from IVC upward to the SVC, stopping at a point corresponding to the approximate diameter of the recipient right atrium. This incision is posterior to the sinoatrial node, and by directing the incision in this manner, one avoids splaying the right atrium over the recipient right atrial orifice, which, it is believed, leads to a higher incidence of tricuspid valve regurgitation (Figure 37-6a and 37-6b).

On occasion, the recipient right atrium is very large and redundant. If a standard anastomosis is to be performed instead of a bicaval anastomosis, the cephalad aspect of the recipient right atrial orifice may be oversewn. This acts to reduce the orifice size of the recipient right atrium and essentially lengthens the recipient SVC (Figure 37-7).

The septal portion of the right atrial suture line is performed first, beginning at the superior aspect of the

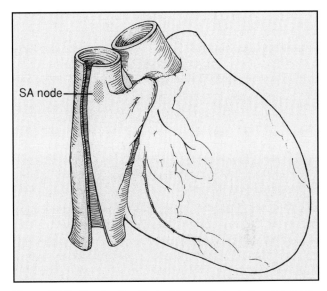

Figure 37-6b. By directing the incision posterior to the sino-atrial node one avoids splaying the right atrium over the recipient right atrial orifice.

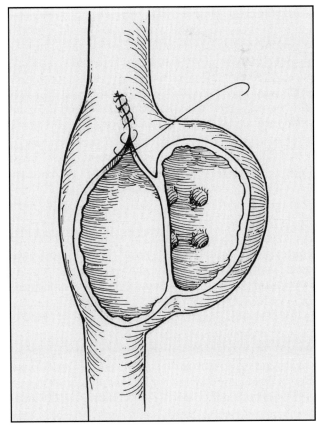

Figure 37-7. The cephalad aspect of the recipient right atrial orifice may be oversewn to reduce the orifice size of the recipient right atrium and lengthen the recipient SVC.

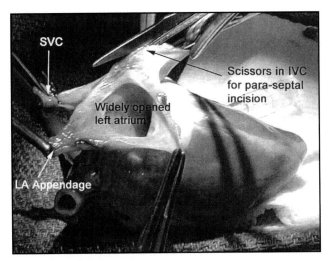

Figure 37-6a. To begin the right atrial anastomosis, the donor SVC is doubly ligated and the IVC is incised upward to the SVC stopping at a point corresponding to the approximate diameter of the recipient right atrium.

newly created atrial septum. While the suture line is constructed, the donor coronary sinus is carefully avoided. Once the posterior aspect of the suture line has been completed, the Swan Ganz catheter is introduced through the tricuspid valve into the right ventricle and out of the donor pulmonary artery. If bicaval technique is employed, the IVC anastomosis is usually performed first using a running 4-0 polypropylene suture. The SVC anastomosis can be performed next or alternatively (if one wishes to limit the cross-clamp time), it can be performed as the last anastomosis.

The next anastomosis to be performed is the pulmonary artery. The donor and recipient pulmonary arteries are trimmed, with the suture line being approximately 1 cm above the pulmonary valve. Care should be taken not to leave the pulmonary artery too long, as this will lead to kinking of the pulmonary artery after the anastomoses. This can be avoided by transecting each vessel at approximately the same point during the respective cardiectomy procedures. A continuous 5-0 polypropylene suture is used for the pulmonary artery anastomosis.

The aorta is first trimmed. The position of transection of the recipient aorta depends largely on the quality, length, and whether the patient has had previous aortic or coronary artery surgery with grafts. The anastomosis is usually made with a continuous 4-0 polypropylene suture. In cases where the cross-clamp time is expected to be long, the aortic suture line can be created prior to the pulmonary suture line. In fact, it is possible to reduce the cross-clamp time significantly by performing the left atrial anastomosis first followed by the aorta. This will limit the ischemic time and requires that the heart be vented via either the right superior pulmonary vein or atrial appendage to avoid distension of the left ventricle. It also requires considerable technical aptitude in retracting the aorta during the performance of the pulmonary artery anastomosis as well as careful retraction and suctioning of blood during the performance of the right atrial anastomosis.

With the cross-clamp still applied, air is thoroughly aspirated from the heart by employing suction on a needle vent in the root of the aorta while digitally manipulating the heart and ventilating the lungs. If all the anastomoses have been completed, then the caval snares can be released and volume added to the heart in an effort to displace air from the left side of the heart. It is routine to elevate the apex of the heart and place an 18 gauge needle in the left ventricular apex to aspirate air. A renal dose of Dopamine and infusion of Isoproterenol at a dose of 0.05 μg/kg-1/min-1 is generally started about ten minutes before the cross-clamp is removed. Atrial and ventricular epicardial pacing wires are inserted at this stage.

Separation from cardiopulmonary bypass requires careful coordination between the anesthesiologist and surgeon. Most importantly, transesophageal echocardiography has become an invaluable tool in the ability to know when the heart has recovered from the ischemic period and whether both left and right ventricular function are sufficient for discontinuation from cardiopulmonary bypass. Ideally, the patient should be in normal sinus rhythm or A-V sequentially paced. Bleeding must be carefully assessed along each suture line and with sufficient volume in the patient to test each suture line under pressure. One practice is to routinely use either Aprotinin or Amicar® to aid in the control of bleeding.

Some of the most difficult patients to manage are those with elevation of pulmonary vascular resistance. Administering nitric oxide after intubation may help precondition the pulmonary vascular bed prior to the initiation of cardiopulmonary bypass. This is stopped while the patient is not being ventilated and then restarted as early as possible following the completion of the technical portion of the operation. A general practice is to combine this regimen with a phosphodiesterase inhibitor, renal dose dopamine and, if necessary, an alpha agonist such as levophed (0.1-1 μg/kg per min). In patients with long-standing heart failure and receptor desensitization, levophed may not be effective and in such cases vasopressin (10 to 15 units/hr) can be used.

RECOMMENDED READING

Barnard CN. The Operation. A human cardiac transplant: an interim report of a successful operation performed at Groote Schuur Hospital, Cape Town. S Afr Med J. 1967;41(48):1271-1274.

Blanche C, Valenza M, Czer LS, et al. Orthotopic heart transplantation with bicaval and pulmonary venous anastomoses. Ann Thorac Surg. 1994;58(5):1505-1509.

Carrier M, Leung TK, Solymoss BC, Cartier R, Lecerc Y, Pelletier LC. Clinical trial of retrograde warm blood reperfusion versus standard cold topical irrigation of transplanted hearts. Ann Thorac Surg. 1996;61(5):1310-1315.

Cooper DKC, Miller LW, Patterson GA. The Transplantation and Replacement of Thoracic Organs. London, England: Kluwer Academic Publishers; 1996.

Doring V, Marcsek P. Atrial flap anastomosis: an alternative technique for orthotopic heart transplantation. Ann Thorac Surg. 1998;65(4):1163-1164.

Doty, DB. Cardiac Surgery: A Loose Leaf Workbook and Update Service. Chicago, Il: Yearbook Medical Publishers, Inc.; 1985.

Dreyfus G, Jebara V, Mihaileanu S, Carpentier AF. Total orthotopic heart transplantation: an alternative to the standard technique. Ann Thorac Surg. 1991;52(5):1181-1184.

Kahan BD. Cyclosporin A: A new advance in transplantation. Tex Heart Inst J. 1982;9:253-66.

Kapoor AS, Laks H. Atlas of Heart-Lung Transplantation. San Francisco, Ca: McGraw-Hill; 1994.

Novitzky D, Cooper DK, Barnard CN. The surgical technique of heterotopic heart transplantation. Ann Thorac Surg. 1983;36(4):476-82.

Peteiro J, Redondo F, Calvino R, Cuenca J, Pradas G, Castro Beiras A. Differences in heart transplant physiology according to surgical technique. J Thorac Cardiovasc Surg. 1996;112(3):584-589.

Shumway SJ, Shumway NE. Thoracic Transplantation. Cambridge, Ma: Blackwell Science; 1995.

Chen JM, Michler RE. The problem of pulmonary hypertension in the potential cardiac transplant recipient. In: Cooper DKC, Miller LW, Patterson GA, eds. The Transplantation and Replacement of Thoracic Organs. 2nd ed. Lancaster, U.K. Kluwer Academic Publishers. 1997.

38 IMMEDIATE POSTOPERATIVE MANAGEMENT OF THE HEART TRANSPLANT RECIPIENT

James K. Kirklin, MD

The ultimate goal of cardiac transplantation is to provide high-quality, long-term survival for patients with end-stage heart disease. The probability of such an outcome is determined in a major way during the hospital admission for the transplant procedure. This chapter reviews the major areas of recipient management during the immediate posttransplant period.

MAINTENANCE OF GRAFT FUNCTION

The ability of the transplanted heart to generate adequate cardiac output in the early hours and days following cardiac transplantation is the primary determinant of posttransplant survival. The donor heart can sustain injury in the donor during trauma leading to death (myocardial contusion), in the process of brain death, and during implantation and subsequent reperfusion, all of which may contribute to initial systolic and/or diastolic dysfunction. Some degree of initial donor heart dysfunction occurs in 30% to 50% of transplanted hearts, but fortunately, with current methods of preservation, less than 3% of patients die from early graft failure. Most forms of early graft dysfunction are reversible, resulting in normal donor heart function if the heart is properly supported during its recovery phase.

Hemodynamic Monitoring

The assessment and management of function of the transplanted heart begins in the operating room during the final phases and discontinuation of cardiopulmonary bypass. Systolic function may be directly assessed with transesophageal echocardiogram, which is also useful to assure effective de-airing of the heart. Left atrial pressure is directly measured and monitored for 12 to 24 hours following transplantation. Central venous pressure is monitored and the relationship between right and left atrial pressure is observed for signs of isolated right or left ventricular dysfunction. If depressed cardiac performance is detected, a pulmonary artery catheter, with continuous cardiac output and continuous mixed venous oxygen saturation monitoring, can be placed in the intensive care unit and provides excellent continuous

Professor of Surgery, University of Alabama at Birmingham, Birmingham, AL

assessment of cardiac performance and evaluation of the response to pharmacologic interventions.

Left Ventricular Systolic Dysfunction

When catecholamine support is required early after cardiac transplantation, dopamine, dobutamine, amrinone, and milrinone are effective in augmenting cardiac output without the deleterious severe alpha-adrenergic effects seen with epinephrine and norepinephrine. The pharmacologic effects and doses of various inotropic agents are listed in Tables 38-1 and 38-2. Isoproterenol was often used in the past for its chronotropic effects, but currently is rarely needed with the availability of temporary postoperative atrial pacing. Occasionally, systemic vascular resistance is very low following cardiac transplantation with low mean and systolic arterial pressure despite adequate cardiac output. In that setting, neo-synephrine and/or norepinephrine are useful agents to increase peripheral vascular resistance. Vasopressin infusion (0.04 to 0.1 units/min) may also increase systemic resistance. If cardiac function is otherwise good, the low systemic resistance usually normalizes within six to 12 hours, and these agents can be gradually discontinued. When more than moderate doses of combined inotropic agents are required, circulatory assistance with an intra-aortic balloon pump (IABP) is recommended. Under rare circumstances, the depression of left ventricular function may be so profound that mechanical circulatory support is necessary as a life-sustaining maneuver.

Left Ventricular Diastolic Dysfunction

The hallmark of isolated left ventricular diastolic dysfunction is an elevated left atrial (and left ventricular end diastolic) pressure required to produce adequate cardiac output in the presence of normal or near-normal systolic function. Temporary diastolic dysfunction of either right or left ventricle occurs commonly after cardiac transplantation, usually secondary to reversible myocardial injury associated with ischemia and reperfusion. Acquired diastolic dysfunction may also result from an "oversized" heart placed in a smaller pericardial space (usually after previous cardiac operations), or accumulation of blood in the mediastinum after transplantation with resultant tamponade.

Treatment of diastolic dysfunction in the operating room usually begins with intravenous nitroglycerin, usually at a dose of one-half to two micrograms per kilogram per minute. Attention must be paid to the total volume infused with a nitroglycerin drip, since standard concentration often requires 30 or more mL/min of fluid administration. Further concentration of the nitroglycerin preparation may be advisable when urine output is not robust. Diuretic therapy and intravenous fluid restriction may also be useful. When calculated systemic vascular resistance is increased, further afterload reduction with nitroprusside in the first 24 to 48 hours and subsequently with oral afterload reducing agents is indicated. Inotropic agents such as milrinone may also favorably impact peripheral vascular resistance and diastolic relaxation while increasing cardiac output. The sudden appearance of apparent right or left ventricular dysfunction during the first several postoperative days may indicate cardiac tamponade from blood accumulation in the mediastinum. A transthoracic echocardiogram (echo) may indicate retained blood that, if accompanied by altered hemodynamics, should prompt surgical evacuation of retained hematoma. In any case, an echo should be routinely obtained prior to hospital discharge to evaluate heart function and identify any pericardial effusion that, if large, should be surgically drained.

Right Ventricular Dysfunction

The thin-walled right ventricle is particularly susceptible to injury during the period of ischemia and reperfusion, and also compensates poorly for an increase in afterload (pulmonary vascular resistance), which is typically elevated to some degree due to long-standing elevation of left atrial pressure in patients with heart failure. The management of right ventricular dysfunction is summarized in Table 38-3.

A rare but treatable cause of right ventricular dysfunction is obstruction at the pulmonary artery anastomosis, secondary to torsion or redundancy of the donor or recipient pulmonary artery. Thus, right ventricular pressure and pulmonary artery pressure should always be measured in the operating room when any signs of right

Table 38-1. Adrenergic Receptor Activity and Other Properties of Sympathomimetic Amines

	Alpha (peripheral vasoconstriction)	Beta$_1$ (cardiac contractility)	Beta$_2$ (peripheral vasodilation)	Chromotropic Effect	Arrhythmia Risk
Norepinephrine	++++	++++	0	+	+
Epinephrine	++++	++++	+	++	+++
Dopamine*	+++	+++	+	+	+
Dobutamine	+	+++	++	+	+
Isoproterenol	0	++++	+++	++++	++++
Neo-synephrine	++++	0	0	0	0

*Causes renal arteriolar dilation at low doses by stimulating dopaminergic receptors, moderate diuretic effect.

Table 38-2. Standard Inotropic Doses

Drug	Starting Dose	Dosing Range
Dopamine	2.5 mg/kg per min	2.5-20 mg/kg per min
Dobutamine	2.5 mg/kg per min	2.5-20 mg/kg per min
Milrinone	0.2-0.3 mg/kg per min	0.2-1.0 mg/kg per min
Epinephrine	0.025 mg/kg per min	0.025 - 0.1 mg/kg per min
Norepinephrine	0.025 mg/kg per min	0.025 - 0.1 mg/kg per min
Isoproterenol	0.025 mg/kg per min	0.025 - 0.1 mg/kg per min

Table 38-3. Management of Right Ventricular Dysfunction

Evaluate pulmonary artery (PA) anastomosis for possible obstruction (measure right ventricular (RV) and PA pressures); surgical revision if systolic gradient ≥10 mmHg
If PA pressure normal or near normal, add inotropic support for RV contractility and adjust RV reload.
If PA pressure and transpulmonary gradient are elevated, add vasodilator agents (via central venous pressure line) and alpha-adrenergic agents (via left atrial catheter) as necessary to support systemic perfusion pressure ± intra-aortic balloon pump.
If PA systolic pressure elevation persists (≥45 mmHg) with important RV dysfunction, initiate inhaled nitric oxide.
RV assist device if above measures fail.

ventricular dysfunction occur; an important systolic gradient (≥10 mmHg) indicates the need for surgical revision.

If no mechanical cause is identified, pharmacologic intervention is dictated by the degree of pulmonary hypertension and the severity of right ventricular dysfunction. Mild right ventricular dysfunction is quite common after cardiac transplantation and generally responds well to a vasodilating agent such as nitroglycerin and inotropic support with a phosphodiesterase inhibitor such as milrinone plus dobutamine. If vasodilator therapy results in systemic arterial hypotension, a second left atrial catheter can be placed so that inotropic agents with alpha-adrenergic effects such as neosynephrine, higher-dose dopamine or norepinephrine, can be infused through the left atrial catheter to maintain systemic perfusion pressure while infusing vasodilator agents through the central venous catheter.

If more than moderate alpha-adrenergic support is required to offset the vasodilator effects of nitroglycerin and milrinone on systemic perfusion pressure, an intra-aortic balloon pump is a useful intervention to maintain coronary perfusion pressure while treating right ventricular dysfunction with higher-dose vasodilator agents.

When right ventricular dysfunction is accompanied by marked pulmonary hypertension (ie, pulmonary artery systolic pressure exceeding about 50 mmHg), primary attention must focus on reducing the pulmonary pressure. Although intravenous infusion of nitroprusside, aminophylline, and nitroglycerin are useful in reducing elevations of pulmonary artery pressure, intravenous prostaglandin E_1 (0.01 to 0.1 mg/kg per minute) and prostacyclin are more effective. Inhaled nitric oxide is the agent with the most specific and pronounced effect on lowering pulmonary vascular resistance without affecting systemic resistance. The dose is usually 20 to 60 parts per million, with monitoring of methemoglobin levels, reducing the dose if levels exceed 4/dL.

Disturbances of Cardiac Rate and Rhythm

The majority of transplanted hearts exhibit normal sinus rhythm in the operating room soon after reperfusion, and clinically important arrhythmias are uncommon in the first few weeks following transplantation. However, electrophysiologic studies have established that asymptomatic rhythm disturbances are common, the most prevalent being sinus node dysfunction, occurring in 25% to 50% of patients during the first several weeks. When sinus node dysfunction is manifested as important sinus bradycardia (ie, less than about eighty beats per minute) therapy early after transplantation is easily initiated by atrial pacing through the temporary atrial wires placed at time of transplantation. If important bradycardia persists after four or five days, beta-adrenergic agonists such as aminophylline or terbutaline may be effective at augmenting heart rate.

The indications for early pacemaker implantation remain controversial, particularly in view of the favorable natural history of early sinus node dysfunction. However, pacemaker implantation is probably advisable for patients with persistent symptomatic bradycardia associated with depressed cardiac output or symptoms despite beta-adrenergic agonist therapy, and possibly those with persistent junctional escape rhythms or intermittent bradycardia of less than 50 beats per minute despite beta-adrenergic agonist treatment during 24-hour Holter monitoring two to three weeks after transplantation.

Asymptomatic atrial and ventricular arrhythmias are very common following cardiac transplantation, with transient atrial arrhythmias occurring in about one-fourth and ventricular arrhythmias in about two-thirds of patients during the transplant hospitalization.

Atrial fibrillation and atrial flutter are unusual early after cardiac transplantation and may herald the onset of acute allograft rejection. In the setting of rejection, atrial fibrillation or flutter is frequently responsive to antirejection therapy. Atrial flutter can be managed with rapid atrial pacing if the temporary atrial pacing wires are in place. In the absence of rejection, atrial fibrillation or flutter with a rapid ventricular response rate can be managed with intravenous diltiazem or a short-acting beta-blocking agent such as esmolol if the hemodynamics are good. Otherwise, cardioversion should be considered. Digoxin is relatively ineffective in reducing the rate of ventricular response in atrial fibrillation in the denervated heart.

Maintenance of Renal Function

Renal reserves may be impaired prior to transplantation secondary to prolonged low cardiac output and chronic high-dose diuretic therapy. In such a state, kidney function is particularly vulnerable following transplantation due to the combination of abnormal renal perfusion during cardiopulmonary bypass, the potential for early graft dysfunction and associated low cardiac output, and the nephrotoxic effects of cyclosporine.

The primary determinant of effective renal function early posttransplant is robust cardiac performance. Appropriate support of the cardiovascular subsystem will minimize the probability of important renal dysfunction. In the presence of oliguria or rising creatinine, particularly if greater than about 1.7 mg/dL, initiation of cyclosporine therapy should be delayed until renal function normalizes. If more than 48 hours elapse posttransplant before cyclosporine therapy can be initiated, it is advisable to begin cytolytic therapy with an antilymphocyte antibody. If early renal dysfunction is reversed, there is generally no deleterious effect on long-term posttransplant renal function.

Dopamine may be routinely employed after cardiac transplantation in a "renal dose" of 2.5 mg/kg per minute to maximize renal blood flow. The use of diuretic therapy in the first few days after transplantation is controversial. There is a known tendency for patients receiving high-dose diuretics prior to transplantation to exhibit relative oliguria if diuretic therapy is suddenly stopped. Therefore, diuretic therapy may require re-initiation in order to maintain adequate urine output in such patients. When oliguria (ie, urine output <50 mL/h) is present early after transplantation, preload is augmented with volume administration to increase the central venous pressure or left atrial pressure to 12 mmHg to 13 mmHg. Cardiac output should be measured and optimized as discussed in the preceding section. If a cyclosporine infusion has been initiated, it should be stopped. If urine output remains low, furosemide may be administered at an initial dose of 20 to 40 mg (or 1 mg/kg in pediatric patients). If blood urea nitrogen (BUN) and creatinine are elevated (BUN >40 mg/dL and/or creatinine >1.6 mg%), special care is required to maintain intravascular volume while administering diuretics. If a brisk diuresis occurs after diuretic administration, it may be useful to perform "urine output replacement" in which hourly urine output is matched with an infusion of normal or half-normal saline up to a maximum left atrial or central venous pressure of 13 or 14 mmHg. If renal dysfunction is severe and refractory to other measures, dialysis or continuous hemofiltration is usually well-tolerated if the cardiac performance is robust.

PULMONARY SUBSYSTEM

Ventilator management, weaning, and extubation criteria following cardiac transplantation follow the same general protocols used for cardiac operations employing cardiopulmonary bypass, with the exception that eight to 12 hours are usually necessary to assess adequacy of graft function prior to extubation. Management of persistent pulmonary hypertension should include mechanical hyperventilation with pCO_2 maintained at 25 mmHg to 35 mmHg, and oxygen saturation in excess of 97% if possible, to minimize the tendency for pulmonary vasoconstriction. When prolonged mechanical ventilation is required (longer than four or five days), early consideration for tracheostomy facilitates patient mobilization, comfort and gradual weaning.

Special considerations in pulmonary management are necessary for patients receiving chronic administration of amiodarone therapy pretransplant for life-threatening ventricular arrhythmias. Although it remains controversial whether amiodarone use is a risk factor for early mortality following cardiac transplantation, patients on chronic amiodarone are at increased risk for serious and potentially fatal postoperative pulmonary dysfunction. The mechanism of this acute lung injury is unknown, but may relate to the generation of oxygen-free radicals, which could be potentiated with high inspired oxygen concentration during the transplant procedure. The clinical manifestation is the acute onset of dyspnea, often requiring re-intubation two to five days following cardiac transplantation. There is radiographic evidence of acute pulmonary edema in the absence of left atrial hypertension. Such patients are likely prone to superimposed pulmonary infection. The only recognized (though not proven) preventive measures against amiodarone-induced pulmonary toxicity following cardiac transplantation are: (1) maintenance of the lowest possible amiodarone dose that prevents ventricular tachycardia prior to transplantation (about 200 mg daily if possible), and (2) strict avoidance of high inspired oxygen fraction during and after the transplant procedure. Whenever possible, the inspired oxygen fraction should be maintained at 40% or lower.

PREVENTION OF EARLY INFECTION

Infection remains a major cause of morbidity and mortality early after cardiac transplantation, with approximately 25% of patients experiencing one or more major infections within the first two months. Bacterial infections predominate during the initial transplant hospitalization, with a peak risk during the first posttransplant week.

Successful prevention of infection contributes immensely to the reduction of long-term morbidity and increased patient survival. Strict surgical aseptic technique and proper care of indwelling lines and devices postoperatively is of obvious importance. Strict hand-washing before and after examining the postoperative transplant patient is routinely recommended. Protective isolation has not proved beneficial in reducing infection incidence or mortality, and is not currently recommended unless severe bone marrow suppression is present.

Prophylactic Antimicrobial Therapy

Perioperative prophylactic antibiotics (eg, vancomycin and ceftazidime) are routinely employed. In order to provide effective circulating levels prior to skin incision, the preoperative dose of each antibiotic (15 mg/kg) is administered one hour before operation. Vancomycin (10 mg/kg) is readministered at the conclusion of cardiopulmonary bypass (CPB) to overcome the dilutional effects of CPB. Prophylactic antibiotics are routinely discontinued 48 hours after operation.

Several additional prophylactic regimens are recommended after cardiac transplantation. Prophylactic ganciclovir against cytomegalovirus (CMV) is recommended for patients who have CMV-negative serology and receive a heart from a CMV-positive donor, and for patients who receive prophylactic muromonab-CD3 or ATG® therapy, in view of their known association with subsequent CMV infection. In patients not receiving ganciclovir, oral acyclovir prophylaxis against herpetic infections is recommended, beginning in the hospital and continued for six to 12 months. Sulfamethoxazole trimethoprim is routinely initiated for prophylaxis against pneumocystis. Nystatin is administered prophylactically to retard *Candida* infections. Patients with a negative serology for toxoplasmosis who receive a heart from a donor with a positive toxoplasmosis serology should receive prophylactic therapy for four to six months. A standard oral regimen in adults includes pyrimethamine 50 mg/d and leucovorin 5 mg/d.

Management of the Surgical Wound

The same surgical concepts of strict asepsis, hemostasis, and secure wound closure are applied during closure of the sternum and superficial incisions after cardiac transplantation as for routine cardiac surgery. Irrigation of the mediastinum and superficial wounds with dilute vancomycin is employed by some groups to decrease colony counts of Gram-positive skin organisms. The surgical dressing is left in place for 48 hours to allow sealing of the skin edges unless bleeding under the dressing necessitates earlier wound examination. The wound is painted with an iodine-containing solution such as Betadine® twice daily for several days.

Because the pericardial space is frequently large in the transplant recipient with previous heart failure and marked cardiomegaly, there is frequently excess "dead space" following implantation of the donor heart. In addition to standard angled and straight Argyle® chest tubes, a useful maneuver to decrease the incidence of postoperative pericardial effusions is placement of a soft surgical drainage catheter (Blake®) in the posterior pericardial space connected to a drainage bulb that can be compressed to induce negative pressure. Such drains can be left in place for three to four days, following removal of standard chest tubes, to allow evacuation of fluid collecting in the posterior mediastinal space. They are generally removed when the total drainage is less than about 40 mL in a 24 hour period.

ADDITIONAL POSTOPERATIVE CONSIDERATIONS

Fluid Management

Because of the tendency for extravascular fluid accumulation during cardiopulmonary bypass and the obligatory associated weight gain, maintenance intervenous fluid administration, in addition to the fluid requirements for monitoring devices and intravenous medications, is unnecessary for the first 24 to 48 hours. Colloid and packed red blood cells for maintenance of a desired hemoglobulin level are administered as needed to maintain the desired level of cardiac preload indicated by left and right atrial pressures.

Transfusions

Although undesirable because of the potential for sensitization development of anti-HLA antibodies and transmission of transfusion-related infections, transfusion of packed red cells, platelets, and fresh-frozen plasma may be necessary to correct clotting abnormalities following cardiopulmonary bypass and to maintain the desired level of hemoglobulin and hematocrit. Because of the known risks of transmitting CMV in transfused red blood cells and platelets, all platelet transfusions should be administered through a leukocyte filter and packed red cells should be leuko-reduced when possible or infused through a leukocyte filter, since the CMV virus is carried within leukocytes that accompany red cells and platelets in standard transfusions.

Pain Relief and Sedation

The standard agent for pain relief after cardiac surgery and cardiac transplantation is morphine sulfate in intravenous (iv) doses of 1 mg to 3 mg (0.05 mg/kg in pediatric patients). Additional sedation with diazepam in 1 mg to 2 mg iv doses (0.05 mg/kg in pediatric patients) or midazolam hydrochloride at doses of 1 mg to 1.5 mg as needed every two to three hours is useful while the patient is intubated. A continuous fentanyl infusion provides effective analgesia and sedation in patients who are hemodynamically unstable or unusually agitated.

Physical Activity

Early ambulation and physical therapy are of great importance following extubation. As soon as the patient is physically able, convalescence is expedited by a program of progressive ambulation and physical therapy. More intensive physical therapy programs are necessary for patients who are severely physically deconditioned or who have been largely bed-ridden from severe heart failure requiring inotropic support.

RECOMMENDED READING

Armitage JM, Hardesty RL, Griffith BP. Prostaglandin E1: an effective treatment of right heart failure after orthotopic heart transplantation. J Heart Transplant. 1987;6(6):348-351.

Vereckei A, Blazovics A, Gyorgy I, et al. The role of free radicals in the pathogenesis of amiodarone toxicity. J Cardiovasc Electrophysiol. 1993;4(2):161-177.

Bhatia SJ, Kirshenbaum JM, Shemin RJ, et al. Time course of resolution of pulmonary hypertension and right ventricular remodeling after orthotopic cardiac transplantation. Circulation. 1987;76(4):819-826.

Colucci WS, Wright RF, Braunwald E. New positive inotropic agents in the treatment of congestive heart failure. N Engl J Med. 1986;314(6):349-358.

Ellenbogen KA, Szentpetery S, Katz MR. Reversibility of prolonged chronotropic dysfunction with theophylline following orthotopic heart transplantation. Am Heart J. 1988;116(1 Pt 1):202-206.

Heinz G, Hirschl M, Buxbaum P, Laufer G, Gasic S, Laczkovics A. Sinus node dysfunction after orthotopic cardiac transplantation: postoperative incidence and long-term implications. PACE. 1992;15(5):731-737.

Hines RL. Management of acute right ventricular failure. J Card Surg. 1990;5(3 Suppl):285-287.

Kay GN, Epstein AE, Kirklin JK, Diethelm AG, Graybar G, Plumb VJ. Fatal postoperative amiodarone pulmonary toxicity. Am J Cardiol. 1988;62(7):490-492.

Kieler-Jensen N, Lundin S, Ricksten SE. Vasodilator therapy after heart transplantation: effects of inhaled nitric oxide and intravenous prostacyclin, prostaglandin E1, and sodium nitroprusside. J Heart Lung Transplant. 1995;14(3):436-443.

Little RE, Kay GN, Epstein AE, et al. Arrhythmias after orthotopic cardiac transplantation. Prevalence and determinants during initial hospitalization and late follow-up. Circulation. 1989;80(5 Pt 2):III140-III146.

Lokhandwala MF, Amenta F. Anatomical distribution and function of dopamine receptors in the kidney. FASEB J. 1991;5(15):3023-3030.

Miller LW, Naftel DC, Bourge RC, et al. Infection after heart transplantation: a multi-institutional study. Cardiac Transplant Research Database Group. J Heart Lung Transplant. 1994;13(3):381-393.

39 PHYSIOLOGY OF THE TRANSPLANTED HEART

Jon A. Kobashigawa, MD

Cardiac transplantation is the therapy of choice for end-stage heart disease. Despite major advances in organ preservation and immunosuppression, the function of the cardiac allograft is not normal. The donor heart is denervated and has altered physiology, which has significant effects on exercise tolerance. The physiologic components of the denervated heart include ventricular loading conditions, circulating catecholamine levels, myocardial contractile capabilities, and donor/recipient size mismatch. These components may be responsible for abnormal hemodynamics including restrictive physiology early and late after transplantation and increased resting heart rate. Denervation of the cardiac allograft also leads to impaired renin-angiotensin-aldosterone regulation and impedes normal vasoregulatory response to changes in intracardiac filling pressures. These physiologic factors and many others (Table 39-1) affect exercise tolerance in the heart transplant recipient and are reviewed in this section.

CARDIAC DENERVATION

Cardiac transplantation involves removing the diseased heart and leaving an atrial cuff, which results in the complete denervation of the donor heart with loss of both afferent and efferent nerve connections. Therefore, the donor heart rate will not respond to vagolytic muscle relaxants, anticholinergics, anticholinesterases, digoxin, nifedipine, phenylephrine, or nitroprusside. Afferent denervation alters cardiovascular homeostasis by: (1) impairing renin-angiotensin-aldosterone regulation; (2) impeding the normal vasoregulatory response to changing cardiac filling pressures; (3) eliminating the normal diurnal variation in blood pressure; and (4) eliminating the subjective experience of angina. Efferent denervation results in loss of sympathetic and parasympathetic nervous system effects. These include: (1) increasing the resting heart rate; (2) eliminating the influence on the heart of vagal signaling from the central nervous system; and (3) blunting the usual rapid changes in heart rate and contractility during exercise, hypovolemia or vasodilation.

Clinical Professor of Medicine, Division of Cardiology, University of California, Los Angeles School of Medicine; Medical Director, UCLA Heart Transplant Program, UCLA Medical Center, Los Angeles, CA

Cardiac reinnervation has been demonstrated, but this phenomenon appears to be both delayed and incomplete. Recent studies suggest that reinnervation can produce physiologically meaningful changes in left ventricular function and coronary artery tone.

ELECTROPHYSIOLOGY

The midatrial cuff transplant surgical technique allows for the presence of two P waves on the electrocardiogram. The P wave from the remnant of the recipient atria does not transmit past the anastomosis suture lines, which accounts for one P wave being asynchronous. Two P waves are not seen in the more recent bicaval surgical technique. The resting heart rate of the denervated heart is usually between 90 and 110 beats per minute due to the loss of vagal tone. There appears to be little autonomic nervous system influence on the atrioventricular and His-Purkinje conduction systems in the resting denervated heart. Clinically significant atrial and ventricular arrhythmias are infrequent following cardiac transplantation, although atrial arrhythmias are associated with cardiac rejection. Prolonged bradyarrhythmias (>24 hours) are seen, especially if patients were taking amiodarone just prior to transplant. Fewer than 5% of these patients require a permanent pacemaker and the majority return to normal sinus rhythm within one year.

NEUROENDOCRINE RESPONSE

Various studies have suggested an increased sensitivity to the effects of β-adrenergic agonists, particularly with respect to chronotropic actions as a means to compensate for the lack of innervation. The mechanisms for this increased sensitivity appear to involve increased β-2-receptors and/or presynaptic lack of neuronal uptake of catecholamines. While plasma catecholamine levels are markedly elevated in patients with severe congestive heart failure, normalization of plasma levels of norepinephrine occurs at about two weeks following heart transplant. Norepinephrine levels are markedly elevated with exercise, as compared with healthy subjects, but are not chronically elevated at rest. Similarly, the hypersecretion of vasopressin and plasma renin activity is observed during exercise. This is believed to be a result of ablation of the cardiac mechanoreceptor afferents.

Plasma volume generally increases about 15% in cyclosporine-treated transplant patients. This is linked to cyclosporine and corticosteroid-mediated renal fluid retention and to an abnormal cardiorenal neuroendocrine reflex, which together contribute to an increase in intracardiac filling pressures and to a diluted hematocrit. Atrial natriuretic peptide is reportedly increased in heart transplant patients. However, the kidneys appear refractory to its effects and the mechanism is not clear.

MYOCARDIAL FUNCTION AT REST

The denervated heart requires mechanisms other than neural to function normally in daily activities. The Frank-Starling mechanism remains a major factor in the transplanted heart, and thus, cardiac transplant patients are often referred to as preload-dependent. In the presence of hypotension or hypovolemia, the denervated heart cannot respond with a reflex tachycardia, but rather responds primarily with an increase in stroke volume. Increases in venous return with a subsequent increase in left ventricular end-diastolic volume results in an increase in stroke volume, and thus, ejection fraction by means of the Frank-Starling mechanism. Therefore, assurance of adequate preload is especially important in the heart transplant patient prior to the administration of anesthesia.

Hemodynamics in heart transplant patients may be abnormal immediately after transplant due to inadequate preservation, acute withdrawal of sympathetic myocardial support, or afterload mismatch. However, ventricular function quickly recovers, and the resting cardiac output is usually normal or low. Since the resting heart rate is usually elevated, the resting stroke volume is therefore small. Systolic and diastolic hypertension are seen in up to 90% of posttransplant patients as a result of cyclosporine therapy. Left ventricular wall mass may be increased, possibly due to compensation for hypertension or to the effects of cyclosporine, or as a result of no lymphatic drainage in the donor heart. Up to one-third of the patients may exhibit an elevated pulmonary capillary wedge pressure, most likely due to a combination of depressed systolic function, decreased compliance, and hypervolemia. However, the majority of cardiac transplant patients have stable hemodynamics long-term after transplant. The midatrial anastomosis between donor and recipient heart is reported to have an effect on cardiac function. Since the native and donor atria do not contract synchronously, less than the expected 15% to 20% of the normal atrial contribution to the net stroke volume is seen; however, the clinical impact is not known.

Table 39-1. Factors Affecting Function of the Transplanted Heart

Hemodynamic

    Donor-to-recipient body size relation
    Donor-to-recipient atrial asynchrony
    Early postoperative restrictive physiology
    Late postoperative restrictive physiology

Denervation

    Afferent denervation
        Altered reflex control of peripheral vasoconstriction and vasodilation
        Altered Na^+/H_2O regulation via central nervous system - dependent vasopressin, renin, angiotensin,
            aldosterone secretion
    Efferent denervation
        Absent vagal nerve control
        Rapid heart rate at rest
        Attenuated heart rate response to exercise
    Hypersensitivity to circulating catecholamines

Altered hormonal milieu

    Atrial natriuretic peptide secretion changed
    Elevated exercise-induced circulating catecholamines

Myocardial injury/maladaptation

    Organ preservation/recovery injury
    Intraoperative complications
    Rejection
    Ventricular hypertrophy
    Hypertension (increased ventricular wall stress)
    Allograft arteriopathy (ischemia)

From Young JB, Winters WL Jr, Bourge R, Uretsky BF. 24th Bethesda conference: Cardiac transplantation. Task Force 4: Function of the heart transplant recipient. J Am Coll Cardiol. 1993;22(1):31-41.

A restrictive hemodynamic pattern has been documented early postoperatively that resolves within days or weeks. A subclinical, latent restrictive hemodynamic state may persist for much longer. In approximately 10% to 15% of patients, a persistently impaired ventricular filling late after transplant may occur, usually due to graft rejection. Donor heart/recipient heart size mismatch may also affect resting hemodynamics. At three months after transplant, there is a reported negative linear relationship between resting heart rate, right atrial pressure, pulmonary capillary wedge pressure, and the donor-to-recipient body weight ratio. However, by one year after transplant, the effect was not significant.

MYOCARDIAL FUNCTION DURING EXERCISE

The manner in which the denervated heart responds to exercise is similar to the normal heart except for the sequence of physiologic mechanisms used. In the transplanted heart, the initial response to exercise is an increased stroke volume secondary to the increased venous return, which is due to a combination of muscle and thoracic pumping and to decreased peripheral vascular resistance. Through this mechanism, stroke volume can be increased by up to 20%, thus increasing cardiac output via the Frank-Starling mechanism. If exercise is more vigorous, further increases of cardiac output are mediated by chronotropic and inotropic responses to circulating catecholamines. This contrasts to the normal heart in which increased stroke volume and heart rate occur simultaneously rather than sequentially.

The response to exercise is abnormal in heart transplant patients but appears adequate to enable the patients to perform the activities of daily life. Table 39-2 summarizes the abnormal exercise physiology in heart transplant patients. Initiating physical activities is slower for heart transplant patients, who require six to ten minutes of steady work to increase heart rate compared to two to three minutes in subjects without a denervated heart. During the first year after transplant, myocardial function in response to exercise improves, probably as a result of increasing β-2-receptor density of the denervated donor heart. However, even with this β-adrenergic supersensitivity to the action of plasma adrenaline, the chronotropic response at the peak of effort is reduced.

The peak heart rate, cardiac output, and ventricular ejection fraction are subnormal when compared to healthy controls. Because there is a normal or elevated rise in circulating catecholamines at peak exercise, and the responsiveness of the sinoatrial node to β-adrenergic stimulation is normal or increased, the most likely reason for the attenuated peak heart rate response to exercise after transplant is lack of direct innervation of the sinoatrial node.

Hemodynamics in response to exercise are dependent on loading conditions. During exercise, intracardiac filling pressures (ie, right atrium, pulmonary artery, pulmonary capillary wedge pressures) are elevated. Elevation of intracardiac pressures during mild to moderate exercise, associated with a slightly lower cardiac output elevation, can unmask a latent persistent pulmonary hypertension, limiting exercise stroke volume adaptation. This may be responsible for mild pulmonary congestion during exercise and, while stimulating pulmonary J-receptors, may lead to the restrictive breathing pattern documented at exercise among some heart transplant recipients.

Table 39-2. Abnormal Exercise Physiology in Heart Transplant Patients

Increased resting heart rate
Delayed heart rate increase at onset of exercise
Delayed return to resting heart rate after cessation of exercise
Decreased resting left ventricular ejection fraction
Decreased exercise right and left ventricular ejection fractions
Reduced exercise cardiac output
Increased exercise arterial-mixed venous oxygen difference
Decreased maximal oxygen uptake
Reduced maximal power output
Slower oxygen uptake kinetics during exercise
Reduced anaerobic threshold
Increased exercise ventilatory equivalents for oxygen and carbon dioxide
Increased exercise left ventricular end-diastolic pressure
Increased exercise pulmonary artery, pulmonary capillary wedge, and right atrial pressures
Increased exercise left ventricular end-systolic and diastolic volume indices

From Squires RW. Exercise training after cardiac transplantation. Med Sci Sports Exerc. 1991;23(6):686-694.

It has been reported that oxygen uptake during exercise training is low at one month and one year after transplant compared with expected values of 42% and 58% of predicted values, respectively. The immediate functional consequence of the low peak oxygen consumption in transplant patients is that exercise is quickly halted by fatigue. It has also been reported that anaerobic metabolism is used at a lower power output in heart transplant recipients compared to normal volunteers. Lactate production is increased relative to normal controls with a resultant increase in ventilation and ventilatory equivalent for oxygen. However, the oxygen consumption at anaerobic threshold is substantially lower relative to both normal subjects and to age-matched general surgery patients. It is noteworthy that approximately 57% of heart transplant patients are still functional NYHA Class II-IV at one year after transplant.

Isometric exercise in cardiac transplant patients results in no increase in cardiac output due to the denervated heart; however, there is the expected increase in blood pressure. This pressor response is most likely due to an increase in α-adrenergic tone mediated by the central nervous system, and not from increased circulating catecholamines.

OTHER FACTORS AFFECTING CARDIAC PERFORMANCE

Early after heart transplantation, skeletal muscle atrophy may affect exercise, which may limit exercise capabilities. In the immediate postoperative period, the transplant patient has a 10% to 50% reduction in lean body mass due to prolonged preoperative physical inactivity, together with high corticosteroid administration. Consequently, maximal work output is reduced, and maximal oxygen uptake is only two-thirds of the normal age-matched population. Therefore, in early exercise testing of transplant patients, anaerobic metabolism is common before peak exercise levels are reached. Many of these exercise parameters improve later after transplant once muscle mass and physical condition is restored.

Acute rejection may affect both systolic and diastolic function. The diastolic dysfunction associated with acute rejection is similar to that observed in restrictive cardiomyopathy, with reduced end-diastolic volume and peak filling. It has been reported that decreased coronary flow reserve in heart transplant patients experiencing acute rejection occurs, but returns to baseline levels after successful antirejection therapy. This would imply that, in the presence of acute rejection, there may be impairment of ventricular function during exercise. The development of transplant coronary artery disease, which is observed in up to 50% of all heart transplant patients by five years after transplant, may affect both systolic and diastolic function. As the donor heart is denervated,

angina is usually not experienced and silent myocardial infarctions may occur.

More recently, the bicaval anastomosis technique has been used in performing heart transplantation. This differs from the standard midatrial anastomosis by keeping both atria intact and performing anastomoses in both cava and pulmonary veins. This avoids desynchronized atrial contractions and may improve cardiac performance by contributing more blood flow to the ventricles.

EXERCISE TRAINING

The role of physical exercise training for cardiac transplant patients has not been established. A randomized trial in cardiac transplant patients has been conducted to assess the effects of physical exercise training on exercise capacity early after transplantation. Twenty-seven heart transplant patients discharged within two weeks after transplantation were randomized to receive a structured cardiac rehabilitation program (exercise group, n=14) or unstructured home therapy (control group, n=13). A 6-month, individualized physical exercise program of muscular strength and aerobic training was provided by a physical therapist to exercise study patients, while control patients received no formal supervised exercise sessions. Cardiopulmonary stress testing was performed at baseline (within one month after heart transplantation) and repeated six months later. Compared to the control group, the exercise group had significantly greater increases in peak oxygen consumption (+4.4 [+49%] v +1.9 [+18%] cc/kg per min, $P= 0.01$), workload (+35 [+59%] vs +12 [+18%] watts, $P=0.01$), and reduced ventilatory equivalent for carbon dioxide (-13 [-20%)] vs –6 [-11%], $P=0.02$). Mean prednisone dose, number of antihypertensive medications, average rejection and infection episodes during the study period, and weight gain were not significantly different between groups. It was concluded that, after cardiac transplantation, early initiation of physical exercise training increases physical work capacity levels and should be part of standard postoperative care.

SUMMARY

Experience and success with heart transplantation has led to the understanding of the pathophysiology of the denervated heart. Understanding the importance of preload, the electrophysiology of the denervated heart, the altered response to exercise, and the potential complications after transplant will be necessary to provide appropriate care for the heart transplant patient. Finally, the finding that the donor heart does not respond normally to exercise should elicit an appreciation for the functional limitations of many heart transplant patients and, perhaps, suggest therapy that may improve their functional state.

RECOMMENDED READING

Young JB, Winters WL Jr, Bourge R, Uretsky BF. 24th Bethesda conference: Cardiac transplantation. Task Force 4: Function of the heart transplant recipient. J Am Coll Cardiol. 1993;22(1):31-41.

Squires RW. Exercise training after cardiac transplantation. Med Sci Sports Exerc. 1991;23(6):686-694.

Bextonn RS, Nathan AW, Hellestrand KJ, et al. The electrophysiologic characteristics of the transplanted human heart. Am Heart J. 1984;107(1):1-7.

Braith RW, Wood CE, Limacher MC, et al. Abnormal neuroendocrine responses during exercise in heart transplant recipients. Circulation. 1992;86(5):1453-1463.

Stover EP, Siegel LC. Physiology of the transplanted heart. Int Anesthesiol Clin. 1995;33(2):11-20.

Niset G, Hermans L, Depelchin P. Exercise and heart transplantation. A review. Sports Med. 1991;12(6):359-379.

Kavanagh T, Yacoub M, Mertens DJ, Kennedy J, Campbell RB, Sawyer P. Cardiorespiratory responses to exercise training after orthotopic cardiac transplantation. Circulation. 1988;77(1):162-171.

Kobashigawa JA, Leaf DA, Lee N, et al. A controlled trial of exercise rehabilitation after heart transplantation. N Engl J Med. 1999;340(4):272-277.

40 INDUCTION IMMUNOSUPPRESSION PROTOCOLS FOR HEART TRANSPLANTATION

Leslie W. Miller, MD

Rejection remains one of the leading causes of death, particularly in the first three years following cardiac transplantation. The immunosuppressive therapy used to prevent allorecognition and rejection is one of the determinants of outcome in heart transplantation.

Recognition of foreign antigens begins with initial perfusion of the graft following implantation. Despite copious irrigation of the heart at the time of explantation, thousands of donor-derived antigen-presenting cells (eg, macrophages and dendritic cells) remain in the graft and are released into the recipient's circulation when the graft is reperfused. These cells present donor MHC via the direct pathway of antigen recognition, survive in the recipient circulation for 14 to 21 days, and increase the risk of acute rejection.

The practice of using antibody induction therapy was introduced in the late 1980s. Despite the absence of any prospective randomized trials comparing antibody induction therapy to standard triple-drug therapy, nearly one-half of the heart transplant programs in the country adopted this strategy for all of their patients. A number of polyclonal agents such as antithymocyte globulin (ATG), antilymphocyte globulin (ALG), antithymocyte serum (ATS), and more recently, Thymoglobulin®, have been used as induction therapy in heart transplantation. Prospective comparisons of different antibody preparations have been reported as well as retrospective comparisons using historical controls. The data comparing muromonab-CD3 to these other agents have been mostly retrospective, single-center series, and the few prospective studies of muromonab-CD3 vs ATG were small and open-label. In addition, treatment was for variable durations and involved different preparations of ATG (ie, rabbit vs equine). The results have been inconsistent in demonstrating superiority of one agent.

There is some evidence that would suggest that antibody induction therapy in heart transplant patients may be associated with an increased risk of rejection. Data from the Cardiology Transplant Record Database (CTRD) registry have demonstrated that use of antibody induction therapy is an independent risk factor for

Professor of Medicine; Director, Cardiovascular Division, Department of Medicine, University of Minnesota, Minneapolis, MN

increased total number of rejections at one year. The problem with the interpretation of these data is that variable types, durations, and doses of antibody therapy use were pooled in the analysis of the effect of antibody induction therapy, and may not reflect the individual benefits of a specific regimen.

This trend toward an all-or-none approach to the use of antibody induction therapy persisted for several years until the use of short courses of antibody induction therapy was demonstrated to be a safe way to avoid the early nephrotoxic effects of calcineurin inhibitors. This led to an increased experience with these agents by programs previously reluctant to examine their use. At the same time, the complications associated with their use and the failure to demonstrate an advantage, such as reduced rejection, led many programs that used it for all patients to abandon this strategy.

MURINE MONOCLONAL ANTIBODY

The murine IgG2a monoclonal antibody, known as muromonab-CD3, is directed against the CD3 complex on the surface of the lymphocytes. It has been the agent most used as induction therapy in heart transplantation. The observations made with muromonab-CD3 may not be relevant to the other antibody preparations as well, but is the focus of this review.

Duration of Use

The initial recommended duration of use of muromonab-CD3 was ten days. This was extended to 14 days in an attempt to further prolong the time to first rejection and, theoretically, enhance the effect. The benefits of muromonab-CD3 use, in addition to the hope of reducing rejection, were primarily to delay the time to first rejection from an average of 14 days to more than 30 days with the 14-day course and minimize steroid exposure during wound healing. However, when the duration of antibody therapy was extended to 14 days, it was accompanied by a significant increase in the incidence of severe cellular, as well as antibody-mediated rejection, and an increase in the development of human anti-mouse antibody.

Indication for Use

Initially, programs that used induction therapy applied it to all patients. Currently, the primary indication for use of muromonab-CD3 is to avoid renal insufficiency in the first three to six days posttransplant. It is clear that renal insufficiency is becoming an increasingly common comorbidity in heart transplant recipients. Over 75% of the patients are now in an ICU either on an intravenous inotrope or have a mechanical assist device in place at the time of transplantation. In addition, the average age of transplant recipients is now 50 years, with nearly one-third of the patients aged 55 or older. These risk factors represent a significant incentive to develop and use therapies such as monoclonal antibodies to minimize the nephrotoxicity seen with the use of calcineurin inhibitors during the first three to five days posttransplant.

Barr and Kobashigawa demonstrated equal safety and efficacy of a short course (four to six days) of muromonab-CD3 in small single-center prospective trials. Patients at high risk or with established renal insufficiency were given muromonab-CD3. The control groups received no induction therapy. Both studies showed no difference in outcome with regard to survival, percent of patients free of rejection, or the frequency, severity, or time to rejection for those patients given muromonab-CD3. This confirmed the benefit of short courses of muromonab-CD3 and the apparent safety, as increased rejection did not occur.

Adverse Effects

There are quite a number of adverse effects associated with the use of antibody induction therapy. The pathogenesis of many of these side effects is now known and strategies have been designed to offset their adverse effects.

Thus, the cumulative evidence to date suggests no demonstrable benefit to the empiric use of current induction therapy agents in all heart transplant recipients. Tailored immunosuppression is becoming more of a standard in heart transplantation. There are clearly a number of risk factors that have been demonstrated to be associated with increased risk of rejection including female donor or recipient, younger age, preformed anti-HLA antibodies, and positive donor-specific crossmatch. Patients with these risk factors may greatly benefit from enhanced immunosuppression with antibody induction therapy perioperatively.

In summary, use of antibody induction therapy in heart transplantation is now limited to short courses of four to six days to prevent early nephrotoxicity from cyclosporine or tacrolimus. Development of humanized antibodies may lead to routine use of these agents in place of currently used agents.

RECOMMENDED READING

VanBuskirk AM, Pidwell DJ, Adams PW, Orosz CG. Transplantation immunology. JAMA. 1997;278(22):1993-1999.

Masroor S, Schroeder TJ, Michler RE, Alexander JW, First MR. Monoclonal antibodies in organ transplantation: an overview. Transpl Immunol. 1994;2(3):176-189.

Copeland JG, Icenogle TB, Williams RJ, et al. Rabbit antithymocyte globulin: a 10-year experience in cardiac transplantation. J Thorac Cardiovasc Surg. 1990;99(5):852-860.

Deeb GM, Bolling SF, Steimle CN, Dawe JE, McKay AL, Richardson AM. A randomized prospective comparison of MALG with OKT3 for rescue therapy of acute myocardial rejection. Transplantation. 1991;51(1):180-183.

Laufer G, Laczkovics A, Wollenek G, et al. Impacts of low-dose steroids and prophylactic monoclonal versus polyclonal antibodies on acute rejection in cyclosporine- and azathioprine-immunosuppressed cardiac allografts. J Heart Transplant. 1989;8(3):253-261.

Griffith BP, Kormos RL, Armitage JM, Dummer JS, Hardesty RL. Comparative trial of immunoprophylaxis with RATG versus OKT3. J Heart Transplant. 1990;9 (3 Pt 2):301-305.

Costanzo-Nordin MR, O'Sullivan EJ, Johnson MR, et al. Prospective randomized trial of OKT3 versus horse antithymocyte globulin-based immunosuppressive prophylaxis in heart transplantation. J Heart Transplant. 1990;9(3:Part 2):306-315.

Macdonald PS, Mundy J, Keogh AM, Chang VP, Spratt PM. A prospective randomized study of prophylactic OKT3 versus equine antithymocyte globulin after heart transplantation — increased morbidity with OKT3. Transplantation. 1993;55(1):110-116.

Olivari MT, Kubo SH, Braunlin EA, Bolman RM, Ring WS. Five-year experience with triple-drug immunosuppressive therapy in cardiac transplantation. Circulation. 1990;82(5 Suppl):IV276-IV280.

Kobashigawa JA, Stevenson LW, Brownfield E, et al. Does short-course induction with OKT3 improve outcome after heart transplantation? A randomized trial. J Heart Lung Transplant. 1993;12(2):250-258.

O'Connell JB, Renlund DG, Bristow MR. Murine monoclonal CD3 antibody (OKT3) in cardiac transplantation: three year experience. Transplant Proc. 1989;21(6):31-33.

Norman DJ, Kimball JA, Bennett WM, et al. A prospective, double-blind, randomized study of high- versus low-dose OKT3 induction immunosuppression in cadaveric renal transplantation. Transpl Int. 1994;7(5):356-361.

Alloway R, Kotb M, Hathaway DK, Gaber LW, Vera SR, Gaber AO. Randomized double-blind study of standard versus low-dose OKT3 induction therapy in renal allograft recipients. Am J Kidney Dis. 1993;22(1):36-43.

Hegewald MG, O'Connell JB, Renlund DG, et al. OKT3 monoclonal antibody given for ten versus fourteen days as immunosuppressive prophylaxis in heart transplantation. J Heart Transplant. 1989;8(4):303-310.

Hammond EH, Wittwer CT, Greenwood J, et al. Relationship of OKT3 sensitization and vascular rejection in cardiac transplant patients receiving OKT3 rejection prophylaxis. Transplantation. 1990;50(5): 776-782.

Barr ML, Sanchez JA, Seche LA, Schulman LL, Smith CR, Rose EA. Anti-CD3 monoclonal antibody induction therapy: immunological equivalency with triple-drug therapy in heart transplantation. Circulation. 1990;82 (5 Suppl):IV291-IV294.

41 LEFT VENTRICULAR DYSFUNCTION AFTER CARDIAC TRANSPLANTATION: ETIOLOGIES, DIAGNOSIS AND TREATMENT

Howard J. Eisen, MD

Cardiac Transplantation has become standard therapy for end-stage congestive heart failure. Advances in new immunosuppressive agents in the past fifteen years have resulted in a significant improvement in the survival of cardiac transplant patients. However, left ventricular dysfunction after cardiac transplantation does occur, and its variable etiologies are the subject of this chapter.

ETIOLOGIES OF LEFT VENTRICULAR DYSFUNCTION AFTER CARDIAC TRANSPLANTATION AS A FUNCTION OF TIME AFTER TRANSPLANT

The cardiac allograft is subjected to a series of assaults that are both immunologic and nonimmunologic. The causes of left ventricular dysfunction are related to the time after transplant. Ischemia damage and reperfusion injury are major causes of left ventricular dysfunction in the early posttransplant period. In the immediate posttransplant period, right ventricular dysfunction from severe pulmonary hypertension can also contribute to allograft failure and left ventricular dysfunction. Further, hyperacute rejection, mediated by preformed antibodies directed against HLA or ABO blood group antigens of the donor heart, can also contribute to allograft dysfunction. Beyond the first week after transplantation, the major cause of left ventricular dysfunction is rejection. This is a T cell-mediated assault on the alloantigens of the transplanted heart, and is the process against which immunosuppressive therapy is directed. Although the majority of rejection episodes are asymptomatic and diagnosed by surveillance endomyocardial biopsy, episodes of cellular rejection that result in left ventricular dysfunction can still occur. Further, left ventricular dysfunction can be associated with mild-appearing rejection on biopsy. The pathophysiology in such a case may be different from that of left ventricular dysfunction associated with higher-grade histologic changes. Additionally, infectious etiologies such as cytomegalovirus or Chagas' disease can rarely cause left ventricular dysfunction. Recurrent viral myocarditis also rarely occurs. Further, posttransplant lymphoproliferative disorder (PTLD) can cause left ventricular dysfunction when it involves the allograft. Beyond the first year, the major cause of left ventricular dysfunction is transplant coronary arteriopathy, a disease with both immunologic and nonimmunologic origins that can lead to severe left ventricular dysfunction on the basis of myocardial ischemia and infarction.

Allograft Failure in the Peritransplant Period

The incidence of allograft dysfunction in the peritransplant period is approximately 5%. The etiologies are variable, and often not determined, but include ischemic damage. The Cardiac Transplant Research Database has revealed that ischemia times greater than six hours predispose patients to allograft dysfunction and predict increased 1-year mortality. The role of reperfusion injury is less certain. Reperfusion may induce myocyte apoptosis resulting in left ventricular dysfunction.

Pulmonary hypertension, defined by a pulmonary vascular resistance of 3.0 Wood Units that does not reverse with vasodilators such as Flolan, nitroprusside or nitric oxide, can cause right ventricular dysfunction and subsequent allograft failure. As a result of careful screening during the transplant evaluation and careful management during the waiting period before transplantation, severe pulmonary hypertension can generally be avoided.

Hyperacute rejection is extremely uncommon as a result of the use of ABO-compatible donor organs, pretransplant screening for anti-HLA antibodies and the use of pretransplant crossmatching in patients with detectable antibodies. Patients at risk for developing anti-HLA antibodies are multiparous women, patients who have had prior organ transplants or blood transfusions, as well as those with long-term implantation of left ventricular assist devices. Efforts to reduce antibody levels have included plasmapheresis, cyclophosphamide, intravenous immunoglobulin administration and immunosuppressive agents such as mycophenolate mofetil or tacrolimus. If antibody specificities to particular HLA antigens are identified, donors with those antigens are avoided.

Acute Cellular Rejection

A major cause of left ventricular dysfunction is acute cell-mediated rejection, which is characterized by infiltration of T lymphocytes and macrophages into the myocardium with myocyte necrosis. The severity of rejection is graded using the International Society of Heart and Lung Transplantation (ISHLT) nomenclature system (see Table 41-1). In general, grade 3A rejections or greater are treated with immunosuppressive therapy, usually intravenous or oral corticosteroids. Grade 3A rejections with

Professor of Medicine and Physiology; Medical Director, Advanced Heart Failure and Transplant Center, Temple University School of Medicine, Philadelphia, PA

left ventricular dysfunction and grade 4 rejections are treated with antilymphocyte antibodies. The majority of acute cellular rejection episodes are asymptomatic: only approximately 5% of rejection episodes are associated with some degree of left ventricular dysfunction.

Despite the presence of myocyte necrosis, many episodes of acute cellular rejection associated with hemodynamic compromise can be successfully reversed, and left ventricular function will improve. The pathophysiology of reversible left ventricular dysfunction is thought to be related to cytokines that are elaborated at the time of cardiac allograft rejection. Tumor necrosis factor alpha, interleukin-6 and interleukin-1 beta have negative inotropic effects and are likely contributors to this left ventricular dysfunction. Tumor necrosis factor alpha is elaborated in the myocardium of patients with congestive heart failure and has been shown to play a secondary role in the left ventricular dysfunction that occurs in these patients. Cessation of the production of these cytokines with immunosuppressive therapy may account for the reversibility of left ventricular dysfunction following treatment of acute cellular rejection.

Vascular or Humoral Rejection

The term vascular or humoral rejection generally refers to rejections that are associated with severe hemodynamic compromise in the presence of low-grade (ISHLT Grade 0, 1A, 1B or 2) rejection. Presumably, antidonor antibodies mediate these rejections. In some cases the presence of antibodies on endothelial surfaces has been demonstrated. Patients with preformed anti-HLA antibodies are more likely to develop humoral rejection. The mechanism of left ventricular dysfunction is uncertain but may also be related to cytokines.

Infectious Etiologies of Left Ventricular Dysfunction

On rare occasions, infections can cause left ventricular dysfunction. These are usually infections that can involve the allograft itself. There have been cases reporting cytomegalovirus involvement of the allograft myocardium. Further, there have been reports of recurrence of myocarditis. Chagas' disease has also been observed to recur in cardiac allografts. Posttransplant lymphoproliferative disorders involving the cardiac allograft have been identified as a rare cause of left ventricular dysfunction.

Cardiac Transplant Coronary Arteriopathy

The most common cause of mortality in cardiac transplant recipients after the first year is transplant coronary arteriopathy, also known as cardiac allograft vasculopathy. The etiology of this disease is both immunologic and nonimmunologic. It occurs more commonly in patients with antiendothelial or anti-HLA antibodies, activated T lymphocytes in the coronary arteries, cytokine mRNA in endomyocardial biopsies, and increased endothelial ICAM-1 expression and chronic immune activation expressed as elevated serum interleukin-2 receptors. Nonimmunologic factors that may be associated include hyperlipidemia and diabetes. There is also an epidemiologic association between CMV and transplant arteriopathy, though the relationship is uncertain. Histologically, transplant arteriopathy resembles restenosis after angioplasty and is characterized by diffuse smooth muscle cell proliferation. However, it is far more diffuse than restenosis and can involve both distal and proximal vessels with obliteration of collateral arteries. The mechanism by which transplant arteriopathy can cause left ventricular dysfunction include myocardial infarctions, which are usually silent and not generally characterized by angina because of denervation of the transplanted heart. Further, "hibernating" myocardium, caused by decreased blood flow to the myocardium and a decrease in myocardial energy stores, may also be a cause of left ventricular dysfunction. One of the more common clinical manifestations of transplant arteriopathy is congestive heart failure. Patients with 3-vessel disease have a much poorer prognosis than those with 1- or 2-vessel disease.

Table 41-1. International Society for Heart and Lung Transplantation Nomenclature for Grading of Cellular Rejection

Grade	Histologic Features
0	No rejection
1	1A = focal perivascular lymphocytic infiltrate with no myocyte necrosis 1B = diffuse lymphocytic infiltrate without necrosis
2	One focus of aggressive infiltration and focal necrosis
3	3A = multifocal aggressive infiltrates and myocyte necrosis 3B = diffuse inflammation with necrosis
4	diffuse polymorphous infiltrates with edema, hemorrhage and necrosis

DIAGNOSIS

The diagnosis of left ventricular dysfunction can be made with a variety of tests, most commonly employed when a patient complains of dyspnea, fatigue, orthopnea, or palpitations, or has evidence of congestive heart failure and/or left ventricular dysfunction on physical examination. Left ventricular dysfunction may be asymptomatic and discovered serendipitously on a routine cardiac diagnostic study such as an echocardiogram. Noninvasive tests such as echocardiography and radionuclide ventriculography can provide measurements of left ventricular ejection fraction. The echocardiogram can provide additional information such as ventricular wall thickness, cardiac chamber size and valvular incompetence. Measurement of the pulmonary arterial pressures, pulmonary capillary wedge pressures and cardiac output and index can be performed at the time of right heart catheterization for an endomyocardial biopsy. Echocardiographic and hemodynamic criteria for severe left ventricular rejection are shown in Table 41-2.

For the diagnosis of specific etiologies of left ventricular dysfunction, endomyocardial biopsy should be employed. If acute rejection or infection are not found, vascular rejection should be considered and the presence of anti-HLA antibodies should be determined. It may also be useful to send one biopsy sample to the pathologist for detection of subendothelial antibodies using immunofluorescence or peroxidase technique.

For patients who are (without evidence of allograft rejection) more than nine months out from transplant, coronary angiography should be performed and compared to previous angiograms. Given the concentric nature of transplant arteriopathy, angiography may underestimate the severity of transplant vasculopathy. Intravascular ultrasound may provide additional diagnostic information and may also be useful for prognostic purposes.

Table 41-2. Criteria for Severe Left Ventricular Dysfunction
Echocardiography
Left ventricular ejection fraction ≤30% or 25% decrease from baseline
Fractional shortening ≤20% or 25% decrease from baseline
Hemodynamic Assessment by Pulmonary Artery Catheterization
Cardiac Index ≤2.0 1/min/M2
Need for inotropic therapy

THERAPY

It is crucial to maintain adequate left ventricular function and organ perfusion in patients with left ventricular dysfunction after cardiac transplantation, regardless of the etiology. The therapeutic approaches include: vasodilators and anti-ischemic agents, intravenous inotropic agents, intra-aortic balloon pump counterpulsation and, if needed, left ventricular assist devices and extracorporeal membrane oxygenation.

The early posttransplant graft dysfunction resulting from ischemia can resolve after several days of supportive care, including intra-aortic balloon pump counterpulsation and inotropic and vasodilator therapy. Restoration of function occurs as ischemia resolves and myocardial energy stores and myocyte function are reestablished.

Hyperacute rejection is almost never reversible. When it does not cause immediate death, a combination of antilymphocyte antibodies, plasmapheresis, intravenous immunoglobulin and cyclophosphamide has occasionally proven effective. With severe left ventricular dysfunction and hemodynamic compromise, the only recourse may be support with inotropic agents, left ventricular assist devices, extracorporeal membrane oxygenation or re-transplantation. Acute cellular rejection can usually be treated successfully with corticosteroids and antilymphocyte antibodies. The goal of immunosuppression is to prevent rejection associated with hemodynamic compromise. The one-year analysis of the multicenter mycophenolate mofetil vs azathioprine trial demonstrated a lower incidence of rejection and mortality associated with hemodynamic compromise in patients receiving mycophenolate mofetil compared to azathioprine. Thirty-three of the mycophenolate mofetil-treated patients (11.4%) had rejection with hemodynamic compromise compared to 50 (17.3%) of the azathioprine-treated patients ($P<0.045$). The mortality in the mycophenolate group was also lower (18 [6.2%] vs 33 [11.4%], $P<0.033$). The use of pravastatin has also been shown to reduce the frequency of hemodynamically significant rejection, perhaps because of an inhibition of natural killer cells.

For vascular rejection with hemodynamic compromise, therapy includes maintaining adequate hemodynamic function with intra-aortic balloon counterpulsation or inotropic agents if needed, plasmapheresis to remove potentially offending antibodies, intravenous immunoglobulins to reduce antibody synthesis, cyclophosphamide, antilymphocyte antibodies and corticosteroids. Photopheresis, which has been shown to prevent and treat acute cellular rejection episodes, has also been used in patients with vascular rejection and hemodynamic compromise, but its role is as yet undefined.

Infectious causes of left ventricular dysfunction can be treated with therapies specific for the infectious agents involved. Ganciclovir is used to treat CMV myocarditis. PTLD is treated by reduction of immunosuppressive therapy, especially for the polyclonal form of the disease. The monoclonal form may be refractory to immunosuppression reduction and may require chemotherapy. The role of antiviral therapy in this disease is unknown.

Transplant coronary arteriopathy remains the most difficult challenge to manage after transplant. Therapies that have been successful in reducing the prevalence of this disease include pravastatin and simvastatin, as well as calcium channel blockers. Localized lesions that resemble nontransplant atherosclerosis can sometimes be treated with angioplasty and stenting. The utility of these approaches for treating left ventricular dysfunction is unknown and therapies such as angioplasty or coronary artery bypass grafting have been disappointing in transplant patients with severe 3-vessel disease. For patients with severe 3-vessel disease and left ventricular dysfunction, angiotensin-converting enzyme inhibitors, diuretics, and anti-ischemic agents such as beta-blockers and nitrates may be useful. The utility of these agents for improving survival is unknown. In select patients, especially younger patients without comorbidities, re-transplantation may be considered. However, in general, the survival of re-transplanted patients is shorter than that of first transplants.

RECOMMENDED READING

Barr ML, Meiser BM, Eisen HJ, et al. Photopheresis for the prevention of rejection in cardiac transplantation. N Engl J Med. 1998;339(24):1744-1751.

Billingham ME, Cary NR, Hammond ME, et al. A working formulation for the standardization of nomenclature in the diagnosis of heart and lung rejection: Heart Rejection Study Group. J Heart Transplant. 1990;9(6):587-593.

Day JD, Rayburn BK, Gaudin PB, et al. Cardiac allograft vasculopathy: the central pathogenetic role of ischemia-induced endothelial cell injury. J Heart Lung Transplant. 1995;14(6 Pt 2):S142-S149.

Eisen HJ, Hicks D, Kant JA, et al. Diagnosis of posttransplantation lymphoproliferative disorder by endomyocardial biopsy in a cardiac allograft recipient. J Heart Lung Transplant. 1994;13(2):241-245.

Halle AA, DiSciascio G, Massin EK, et al. Coronary angioplasty, atherectomy and bypass surgery in cardiac transplant recipients. J Am Coll Cardiol. 1995;26(1):120-128.

Hammond EH, Ensley RD, Yowell RL, et al. Vascular rejection of human cardiac allografts and the role of humoral immunity in chronic allograft rejection. Transplant Proc. 1991;23(2 Suppl 2):26-30.

Kirklin JK, Naftel DC, Bourge RC, et al. Rejection after cardiac transplantation: a time-related risk factor analysis. Circulation. 1992;86(5 Suppl):II236-II241.

Kobashigawa JA, Katznelson S, Laks H, et al. Effect of pravastatin on outcomes after cardiac transplantation. N Engl J Med. 1995;333(10):621-627.

Kobashigawa J, Miller L, Renlund D, et al. A randomized active-controlled trial of mycophenolate mofetil in heart transplant recipients. Transplantation. 1998;66(4):507-515.

Kubo SH, Naftel DC, Mills RM, et al. Risk factors for late recurrent rejection after heart transplantation: a multi-institutional, multi-variable analysis. J Heart Lung Transplant. 1995;14(3):409-418.

McNamara D, Di Salvo T, Mathier M, Keck S, Semigran M, Dee GW. Left ventricular dysfunction after heart transplantation: incidence and role of enhanced immunosuppression. J Heart Lung Transplant. 1996;15(5):506-515.

Mills RM, Naftel DC, Kirklin JK, et al. Heart transplant rejection with hemodynamic compromise: a multiinstitutional study of the role of endomyocardial cellular infiltrate. J Heart Lung Transplant. 1997;16(8):813-821.

Ubel PA, Arnold RM, Caplan AL. Rationing failure. The ethical lessons of the retransplantation of scarce vital organs. JAMA. 1993;270(20):2469-2474.

Winters GL, Schoen FJ. Graft arteriosclerosis-induced myocardial pathology in heart transplant recipients: predictive value of endomyocardial biopsy. J Heart Lung Transplant. 1997;16(10):985-993.

42 PATHOLOGIC FINDINGS OF CARDIAC DYSFUNCTION

Michael C. Fishbein, MD

Cardiac dysfunction in the cardiac transplant patient may be cardiac or noncardiac in origin. Patients with fluid and electrolyte imbalance, sepsis, or even rejection, may have abnormal cardiac function, yet morphologically normal myocardium at the time of biopsy or autopsy.

ENDOMYOCARDIAL BIOPSY

The biopsy procedure begins with obtaining an adequate sample, that, according to the International Society of Heart and Lung Transplantation (ISHLT), consists of at least four good fragments of myocardium. Proper fixation is extremely important in preserving morphologic details for pathologic examination. The fixatives used should fix rapidly, allow immunohistochemical studies, and provide adequate cytologic detail of inflammatory cells as well as myocytes. While formalin fixation is used most widely, a Zenker's-based fixative such as Bayley's (half-strength Zenker's) allows much better evaluation of nuclear detail, which is extremely helpful in distinguishing inflammatory cells from other cells present in the biopsy, such as capillary endothelial cells or stromal cells. For the diagnosis of humoral rejection, immunofluorescence studies are often quite helpful. These require the use of fresh-frozen tissue, since use of fixatives (even Zeuss fixative) will interfere with immunofluorescence studies. To freeze tissue, one fragment should be wrapped in saline-soaked gauze (not floating in saline) and sent quickly to the pathology laboratory to be snap-frozen for immunofluorescence staining. It is rote to perform immunofluorescence on the first biopsy after transplantation in every patient. If findings indicate humoral rejection, subsequent studies may be useful to monitor the therapeutic interventions designed specifically to treat this type of rejection episode. A fresh sample collected every time a biopsy is performed is invaluable for research studies.

Proper interpretation of a biopsy also requires that the biopsies be as free as possible from artifact. The most commonly encountered are *drying artifact* from a delay in fixation of the tissue, *crush artifact* related to the biopsy procedure itself, and *contraction band artifact*, which is a spasm of the myocardial fibers that occurs at the time the biopsy is performed. While contraction bands in autopsy material indicate myocyte injury and often necrosis in a biopsy, these are considered artifact and should not be used to attempt to diagnose myocyte injury.

A generally accepted standardized method of reporting rejection has been adopted by the ISHLT. A normal biopsy is composed of myocardium that may be observed in longitudinal, oblique or cross-sections. Normal findings include sparse, sometimes inapparent interstitial connective tissue, vasculature consisting of small arteries and venules, and numerous capillaries, which are present in great volume (one per myocyte). Depending on the orientation of the section, thin, sparsely cellular endocardium may be observed on one or more surfaces of the biopsy. Because the biopsy comes from a very irregular trabeculated surface, it is possible to have endocardium on all sides of the biopsy and even between myocytes. The orientation of the biopsy is important because one's ability to distinguish rejection from a Quilty lesion requires discrimination of endocardial from myocardial tissue. The observation of relatively thick collagen bundles in hematoxylin and eosin or trichrome-stained sections is usually diagnostic for endocardial tissue.

ACUTE CELLULAR REJECTION

Grade 0 is assigned to a normal biopsy with no evidence of rejection. A few perivascular lymphocytes may be present. Because acute cellular rejection may evolve quickly in the early posttransplant period, even a very minimal infiltrate in the first or second biopsy after transplantation should not be ignored. *Grade 1A* rejection, often called focal mild acute rejection (minimal evidence of rejection), consists of focal, primarily perivascular, and perhaps sparse interstitial infiltrates of mononuclear cells, which are mostly T lymphocytes and macrophages (Figure 42-1A). There is no evidence of myocyte injury. *Grade 1B* consists of a more diffuse mononuclear cell infiltration that is multifocal and often involves interstitium to a greater degree, as well as the perivascular spaces (Figure 42-1B). As with grade 1A, there is no myocyte injury. The concept of myocyte injury may not seem to be complex; however, it is quite difficult at times to distinguish real myocyte injury from artifacts in the biopsy. The injured myocytes do not characteristically demonstrate typical coagulation necrosis, but rather "myocytolysis" with loss of cytoplasmic filaments, which can be difficult to assess in the presence of contraction band artifact.

Grade 2 rejection has been called focal moderate acute rejection and consists of one distinct focus of inflammatory cells with injured myocytes present within

Professor of Pathology and Medicine, Department of Pathology and Laboratory Medicine, UCLA Medical School, Los Angeles, CA

this focus (Figure 42-1C). Various studies have indicated that grade 2 cellular rejection is not associated with hemodynamic compromise, and does not progress in the absence of therapeutic intervention. The lesion generally is connected to the endocardium and, therefore, more likely represents a tangential section of a Quilty B-lesion rather than representing true rejection. Thus, one may occasionally make the diagnosis of grade 2 cellular rejection, keeping in mind that it can represent a Quilty lesion. *Grade 3A* rejection, or multifocal moderate acute

rejection consists of multifocal infiltrates of mononuclear cells associated with myocyte injury (Figure 42-1D). *Grade 3B* is a more diffuse inflammatory process, sometimes referred to as diffuse, or borderline severe acute rejection, in which there may be occasional neutrophils present, as well as lymphocytes, macrophages and myocyte injury. Typically, there is no hemorrhage. *Grade 4* rejection, or severe acute rejection, consists of diffuse infiltrates including neutrophils and eosinophils, as well as the other findings noted above. There may also be

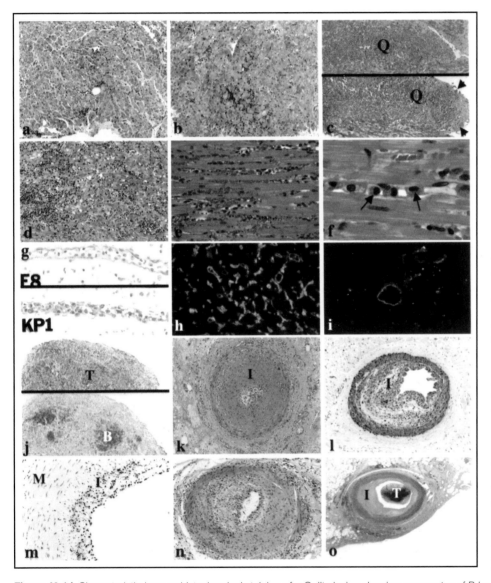

Figure 42-1A. Endomyocardial biopsy showing ISHLT grade 1A rejection (H&E x 16).

Figure 42-1B. Endomyocardial biopsy showing ISHLT grade 1B rejection (H&E x 16).

Figure 42-1C. Endomyocardial biopsy showing lesion that could be considered grade 2 rejection; however, serial sections (lower panel) show that this is actually endocardial (arrowheads), representing a Quilty (Q) lesion (H&E x 16).

Figure 42-1D. Endomyocardial biopsy showing ISHLT grade 3A rejection (H&E x 16).

Figure 42-1E. Section of heart from autopsy of patient who died early after transplantation of humoral rejection. Note congested capillaries (H&E x 40).

Figure 42-1F. Higher magnification of Figure 42-1E showing cells filling capillary lumen (arrows) (H&E x 160).

Figure 42-1G. Immunohistochemical staining for endothelial cells (F8) and macrophages (KP1) showing that intravascular cells are primarily macrophages and not "swollen endothelial cells" (x 80).

Figure 42-1H. Immunofluorescence stain for HLA-DR in case of humoral rejection showing characteristic positive staining of capillaries.

Figure 42-1I. Figure 42-1H showing positive staining in a small artery, a finding that has been associated with accelerated graft vasculopathy.

Figure 42-1J. Characteristic immunohistochemical staining of a Quilty lesion showing aggregates of B lymphocytes and a more diffuse distribution of T cells (x 16).

Figure 42-1K. Graft arteriopathy with small epicardial artery showing marked fibromuscular intimal proliferation (I) (H&E x 16).

Figure 42-1L. Immunohistochemical staining for smooth muscle specific actin showing the smooth muscle cells in the intima (I) (x 16).

Figure 42-1M. "Endothelialitis" in graft arteriopathy, an intimal (I) proliferation of mononuclear cells (M indicates media) (H&E x 80).

Figure 42-1N. Artery demonstrating an actual arteritis, with marked inflammation as well as connective tissue proliferation within the intima (H&E x 16).

Figure 42-1O. Artery from patient who died suddenly, which demonstrates luminal thrombosis (T) occluding as artery with a thickened intima (I) (H&E x 5).

edema, hemorrhage, and small vessel vasculitis. Grade 4 rejection is rarely seen in a biopsy. It has been reported that eosinophils noted in any type of rejection is a worrisome finding that may indicate a more severe rejection episode.

A number of terms have been used to describe the findings on a biopsy obtained following a treated rejection. *Resolved rejection* has been used when a biopsy after treatment shows no cellular infiltration. *Resolving rejection* has been used when there is less cellular infiltration than in the pretreatment biopsy. Caveats to be kept in mind are that rejection is not a uniform process and, whenever small samples are taken from a large organ, a certain degree of sampling error is always present no matter how many fragments of tissue are examined. Also, in the era of cyclosporine immunosuppression, the patient often improves faster than the biopsy, so it is not uncommon to see a biopsy that appears to show no improvement while the patient is clinically better.

HUMORAL REJECTION

Humoral, or vascular, rejection is an antibody-mediated process that usually occurs early, can be a sudden catastrophic event, and is probably more common than appreciated. Patients who develop humoral rejection often have a worse course with poorer survival, and are more likely to develop transplant coronary arteriopathy. There is some controversy regarding the pathogenesis, significance, and even existence of humoral rejection. Some individuals regard these changes as due to ischemia or reperfusion injury, although there are many pathological differences between the findings noted in ischemic injury and humoral rejection. Recent work has demonstrated that ischemia, by itself, and other alloimmunity-independent processes, can initiate an antibody-mediated response in tissue. It is quite likely that insults such as ischemia or induction therapy with muromonab-CD3 may incite an antibody response that manifests itself as humoral rejection. Fewer episodes of humoral rejection have been observed as the use of "induction" therapy has decreased.

The myocardium of the heart that has failed early after transplantation from humoral rejection appears edematous and hyperemic, and often there is hemorrhage in the tissue (Figure 42-1E). Microscopically, there are large cells that appear to be obstructing capillaries (Figure 42-1F). These cells have been referred to as *swollen endothelial cells;* however, most of these cells are intravascular macrophages that may be responding to the endothelial injury (Figure 42-1G). A neutrophilic infiltrate in and around capillaries, referred to as acute capillaritis, is also present. The edema, hemorrhage and capillaritis are generally seen with more severe humoral rejection. Humoral rejection is distinguished from cellular rejection by the absence of significant perivascular and interstitial lymphocyte infiltrates. Immunofluorescence shows deposition of immunoglobulin, usually IgM, in the capillary walls, as well as complement components such as C1Q or C3. HLA-DR (class II MHC antigen) is expressed on the endothelium (Figure 42-1I). HLA-DR, not expressed on normal endothelium, is expressed following endothelial injury. Immunohistochemical studies show numerous macrophages (CD68-positive cells) within the capillaries, which is strong evidence for the diagnosis even if frozen tissue is not available for immunofluorescence studies (Figure 42-1H). It has been noted that the diagnosis of humoral rejection has been made in the presence of a spectrum of symptoms ranging from none to cardiogenic shock. A recent study has demonstrated that if arterial endothelium is positive for HLA-DR in biopsies early after transplantation, the patient is at much greater risk for developing graft arteriopathy at a later date (Figure 42-1I). More work is needed, however, to elucidate the short-term and long-term consequences of humoral rejection.

OTHER BIOPSY FINDINGS

The *Quilty effect* is an endomyocardial infiltrate, composed primarily of B and T lymphocytes and scattered macrophages, that has been shown to be associated with the use of cyclosporine (Figure 42-1J). These lesions, originally described by Margaret Billingham, are quite interesting pathologically. B cells form a cluster resembling a germinal center, and T cells and macrophages organize around these B cells. The deepest parts of these lesions, often consisting of more T cells, sometimes encroach upon the underlying myocardium where there may be focal myocyte injury. These latter lesions, referred to as *Quilty B lesions,* behave in a benign fashion, despite the associated myocyte injury. No therapy is required for Quilty lesions, which may persist for years in endomyocardium. Interestingly, similar lesions are noted in the epicardial fat surrounding the heart, and even in intramyocardial locations where they tend to be present in areas of replacement fibrosis. Numerous theories have been proposed to explain the origin of the Quilty lesion. These include EBV activation of B cells, mild rejection and cyclosporine toxicity. None has been proven, or would completely explain the distribution and morphologic findings associated with Quilty lesions. Immunohistochemical staining may be helpful in distinguishing rejection from a tangential section through the deeper portion of a Quilty lesion. While both demonstrate numerous T lymphocytes, Quilty lesions contain numerous B cells and relatively few macrophages. Lesions of rejection, on the other hand, have few B cells and numerous macrophages, which often exceed the number of T lymphocytes present.

True evidence of ischemic injury can be observed in the myocardium after transplantation. This consists of typical coagulation necrosis of myocytes, which evolves into a granulation tissue response and eventually into nonspecific fibrosis. An early-occurring ischemic injury is important to recognize as it may contribute to early graft dysfunction. Late-occurring ischemic injuries are also important to identify since they are a manifestation of transplant coronary arteriopathy and portend a poor prognosis for the graft and patient.

Rarely, infection can be diagnosed in an endomyocardial biopsy. Cytomegalovirus (CMV) inclusions, or even toxoplasma organisms can be observed, although these are rare events. In situ hybridization studies may be positive for CMV, even in the absence of inclusions. In the presence of infection, it is difficult to diagnose rejection because of the similarity in the type of inflammatory infiltrate.

Posttransplant lymphoproliferative disease (PTLD) is a polyclonal, premalignant or monoclonal malignant proliferation of B cells in transplant patients associated with the presence of Epstein-Barr virus (EBV). EBV can be demonstrated by in situ hybridization techniques. PTLD only rarely has been described in the heart of a transplant patient. This diagnosis should be considered when an intense myocardial infiltrate of plasmacytoid B cells is present.

Because the typical transplantation patient undergoes numerous endomyocardial biopsies, another common finding is a previous biopsy site. Following a distant biopsy, one may only see very well-circumscribed replacement fibrosis in the myocardium. A recent biopsy site will demonstrate a mural thrombus in various stages of organization, with underlying inflammation and granulation tissue in the myocardium.

If the right ventricular free wall is biopsied, one often sees chronic inflammation and fat necrosis of the epicardial tissue related to the transplant procedure. Although perforation of a transplant heart is rare because of the connective tissue response associated with the surgical procedure, it is useful to inform the cardiologist or surgeon that epicardial tissue is present so that they can re-evaluate their methods for monitoring the heart biopsy procedure.

CHRONIC VASCULAR REJECTION (TRANSPLANT CORONARY ARTERIOPATHY)

The greatest obstacle to long-term success remains allograft arteriopathy, which is a proliferation within the coronary arteries that leads to vascular occlusion, graft failure, and often death in the absence of re-transplantation. Angiographic abnormalities, detected by intravascular ultrasound, are present in approximately 50% of patients five years after transplantation. Chronic vascular rejection may cause death less than six months after transplantation and morphologic evidence of this process is present within days of cardiac transplantation.

Transplant arteriopathy is more diffuse and concentric than naturally occurring atherosclerosis (Figure 42-1K). It affects intramyocardial as well as epicardial arteries, but is usually not observed in the arteries that are present within endomyocardial biopsies. Thickened vessels may be observed adjacent to previous biopsy sites and represent *endarteritis obliterans* rather than vascular rejection. While the overwhelming majority of transplant arteriopathy lesions affect epicardial vessels, many more smaller branch vessels are involved than in standard atherosclerosis. The lesions may first consist of proliferating smooth muscle cells and then later become more fibrous. True atheromas with intracellular and extracellular lipid may be present in the large epicardial arteries (Figure 42-1L). The pathognomonic finding of this lesion is called *endothelialitis,* which is an infiltrate of T lymphocytes and macrophages within the vascular intima beneath the endothelium (Figure 42-1M). Many patients have similar infiltrates in the media and adventitia of the vessels, and a small proportion have necrotizing arteritis with intense transmural cellular infiltration, and destruction and necrosis/fibrosis of the vascular wall (Figure 42-1N).

The pathogenesis of these lesions is still uncertain, but contributing factors appear to include risk factors for standard atherosclerosis, as well as cyclosporine, infection, antibody-mediated rejection, and cellular immune responses. It has been suggested that these lesions demonstrate less calcium and less thrombosis than standard atherosclerosis; however, acute thrombosis does occur and may result in sudden death (Figure 42-1O). Calcification may, in fact, be prominent, especially in patients with atheromatous lesions, and in those who have chronic renal disease or other factors that predispose to vascular calcification.

RECOMMENDED READING

Billingham ME, Cary NR, Hammond ME, et al. A working formulation for the standardization of nomenclature in the diagnosis of heart and lung rejection: Heart Rejection Study Group. J Heart Transplant. 1990;9(6):587-593.

Winters GL, Marboe CC, Billingham ME. The International Society for Heart and Lung Transplantation grading system for heart transplant biopsy specimens: clarification and commentary. J Heart Lung Transplant. 1998;17(8):754-760.

Fishbein MC, Bell G, Lones MA, et al. Grade 2 cellular heart rejection: does it exist? J Heart Lung Transplant. 1994;13(6):1051-1057.

Freimark D, Czer LS, Aleksic I, et al. Pathogenesis of Quilty lesion in cardiac allografts: relationship to reduced endocardial cyclosporine A. J Heart Lung Transplant. 1995;14(6 Pt 1):1197-1203.

Hammond EH, Yowell RL, Nunoda S, et al. Vascular (humoral) rejection in heart transplantation: pathologic observations and clinical implications. J Heart Transplant. 1989;8(6):430-443.

Lones MA, Czer LS, Trento A, Harasty D, Miller JM, Fishbein MC. Clinical-pathologic features of humoral rejection in cardiac allografts: a study in 81 consecutive patients. J Heart Lung Transplant. 1995;14(1 Pt 1):151-162.

Billingham ME. Graft coronary disease: old and new dimensions. Cardiovasc Pathol. 1997;6:95-101.

43 LONG-TERM MANAGEMENT ISSUES IN HEART TRANSPLANTATION

Mohamad H. Yamani, MD
Randall C. Starling, MD, MPH

Cardiac transplantation has emerged as a viable therapeutic strategy for selected patients with end-stage heart disease, offering extended survival and improved quality of life. However, it should not be perceived as a curative procedure. Although the patient's primary problem of heart failure is alleviated by a successful transplant, a new set of potential long-term complications may emerge primarily related to the secondary effects of chronic immunosuppression. This chapter focuses on these long-term issues and their management. It also reviews the issue of re-transplantation, and the role of the primary care physician in the long-term management of the heart transplant patient.

CLINICAL ASSESSMENT OF HEART FUNCTION

The function of the newly transplanted cardiac allograft is influenced by an interplay of several important physiologic factors that include allograft denervation, ventricular loading conditions, hormonal milieu, myocardial injury, donor-recipient size relation, pulmonary performance, and atrial function.

Several modalities such as Doppler echocardiography can be used to evaluate the short- and long-term complications following heart transplantation. During the first week after cardiac transplantation, there is generally an increase in the severity of the mitral, tricuspid, and aortic regurgitation. Moderate-to-severe tricuspid regurgitation is the most common (55%), followed by pulmonary regurgitation (42%), moderate mitral regurgitation (32%), and mild aortic regurgitation (23%). These valvular regurgitations are usually asymptomatic at rest, except for tricuspid regurgitation, which is associated with right-sided heart failure in more than half of the patients early postoperatively. Valvular regurgitation, pulmonary hypertension, and right heart failure usually diminish over the initial posttransplant year. Recently, tissue Doppler imaging has emerged as a technique that permits evaluation of myocardial relaxation velocities and, combined with the

Mohamad H. Yamani, MD, Associate Staff, Department of Cardiology, The Cleveland Clinic Foundation, Cleveland, OH

Randall C. Starling, MD, MPH, Director, Heart Transplant Medical Services, Department of Cardiology, The Cleveland Clinic Foundation, Cleveland, OH

transvalvular E-velocity determination, could allow estimation of ventricular filling pressures following heart transplantation. Since allograft rejection results in increased myocardial stiffness and abnormal myocardial relaxation, tissue Doppler imaging can be a useful noninvasive tool for the diagnosis of rejection. Although this technique has not replaced endomyocardial biopsy in diagnosing allograft rejection, it may have a role as a screening technique. However, ongoing research must confirm its sensitivity and specificity in this regard.

Long-term mortality and morbidity of heart transplantation are related to the subsequent development of coronary vasculopathy. Transplant vasculopathy may manifest clinically as proximal obstructive epicardial disease, may be confined to the microcirculation (resistance vessels), but most often is a combination of both. A progressive deterioration of coronary flow reserve, mainly related to dysfunction of the coronary microcirculation, can occur following transplantation. Angiographic evidence of coronary artery disease is very common, occurring in approximately two of five patients by five years. However, up to 80% of patients have lesions detected by intravascular ultrasound (IVUS), which is more sensitive in the detection and quantification of coronary atherosclerosis. Intravascular ultrasound has demonstrated that the severity of transplant coronary vasculopathy progresses after transplantation, most prominently during the first two years. Ultrafast computed tomography can be a useful noninvasive tool for the detection of coronary calcification and appears to be a good predictor of cardiac events in heart transplant recipients. In general, noninvasive techniques (eg, exercise electrocardiography and exercise radionuclide ventriculography) to assess coronary arteriosclerosis are limited by inadequate sensitivity and specificity, and have failed to be significant predictors of cardiac event-free survival following transplantation.

The role of dobutamine stress echocardiography (DSE) in the detection of coronary vasculopathy is currently under evaluation. Regional myocardial dysfunction detected by DSE is associated with moderate-to-severe intimal hyperplasia and predicts a shortened survival following transplant. The use of thallium-201 (^{201}Tl) imaging to diagnose posttransplant coronary vasculopathy remains questionable. While some studies have shown diagnostic usefulness, two other studies did not show significant correlation between the observed pathologic thallium patterns and the extent of coronary vasculopathy identified by IVUS.

SURVEILLANCE ENDOMYOCARDIAL BIOPSIES

Endomyocardial biopsy remains the "gold standard" for the diagnosis of acute rejection after cardiac transplantation. Venous access can be obtained via the internal or external jugular veins, subclavian veins, or the femoral veins. A variety of cardiac bioptomes are available. Fluoroscopic guidance is the standard technique, but two-dimensional echocardiography guidance can also be used. An average endomyocardial biopsy sample has a weight of 3 mg to 5 mg, and a diameter of 1 mm to 2 mm. Multiple samples (usually four to five) are required for histopathologic evaluation. The most commonly used grading scheme for the diagnosis and staging of rejection is that of the International Society of Heart and Lung Transplantation (ISHLT). Rejection is the leading cause of death in the first year after heart transplantation, and accounts for approximately 20% of all deaths. Surveillance endomyocardial biopsies are used to monitor the adequacy of immunosuppressive therapy, especially during the critical initial 6-month period when the incidence of rejection is highest.

Frequency of surveillance biopsy varies from one center to another. In general, routine endomyocardial biopsies are performed weekly for the first month, every two weeks during the second month, every six to eight weeks until the patient is one to three years posttransplant, and every four to six months thereafter. Following a treated episode of rejection, the endomyocardial biopsy is generally repeated within 14 days to assure an adequate treatment. Some centers have reduced the number of surveillance biopsies based on the low frequency of rejection after six months and the excellent medium-term survival results observed. One center conducted a study of 100 consecutive heart transplant recipients for a mean period of 27 months. The mean number of endomyocardial biopsies in the initially evaluated 18 patients was ten. In the next 20 patients, endomyocardial biopsy was performed only three times during the first posttransplant year (at two, four, and eight weeks). In the subsequent 62 patients, endomyocardial biopsy was performed on posttransplant days ten, 20, 30, and 60. The mean number of endomyocardial biopsies in the entire group of 100 patients was 5.9 over the first year. This is a marked reduction from the standard clinical practice of approximately 14 biopsies in the initial posttransplant year. The incidence of acute rejection requiring increased therapy was 24%, and actuarial survivals at 30 days and one year were 98% and 94%, respectively. These findings convinced the authors of a need to reduce the number of surveillance endomyocardial biopsies. In another single-center study, 338 endomyocardial biopsies were performed in 211 patients as part of the routine evaluation at one or more years after transplantation. Only two patients (0.6%) showed histologic evidence suggestive of acute rejection needing treatment. As a result, these investigators believe that routine yearly heart biopsies in asymptomatic patients are not necessary, and recommend that they be performed only if there is clinical suspicion of rejection. These small observational studies provide provocative data, however the necessary frequency of surveillance biopsies remains contentious. A prospective randomized trial will be required to definitively answer this question.

Although endomyocardial biopsy is usually considered very safe, it entails some procedural risk but with few significant long-term sequelae. In a review of 2,454 endomyocardial biopsies performed in 133 cardiac allograft patients, 2.3% of the complications were associated with catheter insertion. Complications during biopsy included arrhythmias (0.25%), and conduction abnormalities (0.2%). Very occasional cases of hepatitis B transmission have been reported, and coronary artery fistula formation has been described in 2.9% of patients, the majority of which close spontaneously without long-term clinical sequelae. Venous thrombosis has also been reported but is very unusual. Iatrogenic tricuspid regurgitation is a known, but fortunately infrequent, complication. Flail tricuspid leaflets following endomyocardial biopsy have been reported to occur in 6% to 14% of the patients necessitating tricuspid valve repair in those with symptomatic right heart failure.

TRICUSPID REGURGITATION

Echocardiographic studies have reported a high prevalence of tricuspid regurgitation following heart transplantation. Moderate-to-severe tricuspid regurgitation is reported in 12% to 32% of patients. Several mechanisms to explain tricuspid regurgitation after cardiac transplantation have been described. The presence of pulmonary hypertension, particularly at the time of transplantation when right ventricular ischemic injury can occur, might initially result in right ventricular and tricuspid annular dilation resulting in tricuspid regurgitation. Tricuspid regurgitation is usually associated with right-sided heart failure in more than 70% of the patients in the early postoperative period and may have a detrimental effect on cardiac performance in those patients with persistent pulmonary hypertension. Tricuspid regurgitation may also account for the subnormal exercise tolerance observed in some patients. Fortunately, perioperative pulmonary hypertension resolves promptly in most recipients.

Another cause of tricuspid regurgitation is related to the surgical technique of atrial anastomosis, which creates a large right atrium and sometimes an abnormality in the geometry of the tricuspid annulus. A significant reduction in posttransplant tricuspid regurgitation has been noted with the bicaval technique. This technique is also associated with significantly lower mean pulmonary arterial pressure and improved overall hemodynamics due to the preservation of the anatomic configuration and physiologic function of the atria. Tricuspid regurgitation may also be due to a size mismatch of the donor heart and recipient pericardial cavity, resulting in distortion of the tricuspid valve ring. Preservation injury and papillary muscle dysfunction may contribute to transient perioperative valvular regurgitation. Tricuspid regurgitation is usually well-tolerated clinically and does not result in significant morbidity. The exception is severe tricuspid regurgitation due to catheter-induced valve damage during endomyocardial biopsy. This form of tricuspid insufficiency, when severe, may ultimately require repair or replacement of the valve.

DIAGNOSIS AND MANAGEMENT OF LONG-TERM COMPLICATIONS
Hypertension

Hypertension developing after cardiac transplantation is nearly universal, occurring in 70% to 90% of cyclosporine-treated, and 30% to 50% of tacrolimus-treated patients. This challenging complication reflects the interplay of several pathogenic mechanisms among which are altered renal vascular reactivity and sympathetic neuro activation. Corticosteroids, which cause sodium retention, play a minor role in the pathogenesis of cardiac transplant hypertension. Abnormal cardiorenal reflexes secondary to cardiac denervation may contribute to salt-sensitive hypertension and fluid retention. Cardiac denervation also explains the lack of normal nocturnal decline in blood pressure.

Careful monitoring of blood pressure is of paramount importance. Generally, blood pressures consistently greater than 140/90 mmHg should be treated. Patients should be encouraged to be discreet with sodium intake, but fluid intake should not be restricted, particularly in patients with renal insufficiency, as this may exacerbate cyclosporine nephrotoxicity. Meticulous blood pressure control is important to provide optimal symptomatic benefits of cardiac transplantation and to preserve graft function. Titrated monotherapy with either angiotensin-converting enzyme (ACE) inhibitors (eg, captopril, enalapril, lisinopril) or calcium channel blockers (eg, diltiazem, verapamil, amlodipine) may be effective in about 50% of the patients. Some patients will be prone to hyperkalemia due to the combined effect of cyclosporine and ACE inhibition on the kidney. Due to decreased metabolism of cyclosporine, the use of diltiazem, verapamil, or amlodipine necessitates the use of lower doses of cyclosporine and initially more frequent cyclosporine level monitoring. Combination therapy with both an ACE inhibitor and a calcium channel blocker is common. Hypertension in some patients is inadequately controlled despite maximally tolerated doses of both calcium channel blockers and ACE inhibitors. Problematic hypertensives requiring multiple agents often require diuretics as part of their regimen. The final tier of man-

agement would be to add an alpha blocker such as clonidine or doxazosin in refractory cases. Beta blockers are usually avoided in the treatment of hypertension due to their known tendency to reduce exercise performance.

RENAL DYSFUNCTION (see also Section IV, Chapter 21)

Immunosuppressive therapy with cyclosporine has improved both graft function and survival in heart transplantation. However, its associated nephrotoxicity still remains a serious clinical challenge. The greatest change in glomerular filtrate rate (GFR) in response to treatment with cyclosporine occurs in the first three to six months. In a retrospective evaluation of renal function in 133 cardiac transplant patients, serial mean serum creatinine levels increased from 1.25 mg/dL at one to two months posttransplant, to 1.48 mg/dL at six months, and to 1.55 mg/dL at nine months, with a subsequent plateau in serum creatinine levels at up to 60 months of follow-up when it had reached 1.66 mg/dL. None of the patients developed end-stage renal disease requiring dialysis. Thus, renal function may remain stable up to five years after transplant if serum cyclosporine levels and cyclosporine doses are monitored and adjusted closely.

In a study of 2,088 Medicare beneficiaries who underwent heart transplantation between 1989 and 1994, the annual risk of end-stage renal disease was reported to be 0.37% in the first year after transplant, and increased to 4.49% by the sixth posttransplant year.

Close monitoring of cyclosporine blood levels is critically important to limit progressive decline in renal function as there is no known treatment that is uniformly effective in preventing or reversing such nephrotoxicity. At the time of transplant, initiation of cyclosporine is delayed postoperatively in patients at high-risk for nephrotoxicity, and antilymphocyte antibody therapy is used for renal sparing purposes.

Osteoporosis (see also Section IV, Chapter 25)

Cardiac transplantation, with its attendant glucocorticoid and calcineurin-inhibitor (ie, cyclosporine and tacrolimus) therapies, is associated with rapid bone loss and high fracture rates. Within two months after heart transplantation, approximately 3% of whole-body bone mineral density is lost, mostly due to decreases in trabecular bone. Glucocorticoids cause dose-related bone loss, particularly in the first six to 12 months of use. In a bone densitometric study of 40 cardiac transplant recipients, osteopenia was noted to be present in 28% of the patients at the lumbar spine, and in 20% of patients at the femoral neck, and vertebral fractures were present in 35%.

The treatment of osteoporosis in heart transplant patients should be directed toward prevention of bone loss. Postmenopausal women should generally receive estrogen replacement. In a recent prospective randomized study of 16 cardiac transplant recipients, exercise training, when initiated early after transplantation, restored bone mineral density toward pretransplantation values. Prophylactic administration of calcium carbonate (1,000 to 1,500 mg/d), alfacalcidol, or bisphosphonate therapy after cardiac transplantation are effective regimens that reduce bone loss and may decrease osteoporotic complications.

Hyperlipidemia (see also Section IV, Chapter 24)

Hyperlipidemia is one of the most frequent metabolic disorders after heart transplantation occurring in 60% to 80% of recipients. It is undoubtedly multifactorial in origin and could be related to preexisting lipid abnormalities, cyclosporine therapy, and corticosteroid administration. Corticosteroid withdrawal has been associated with lower cholesterol levels.

Coronary vasculopathy has emerged as the main determinant of long-term survival in cardiac transplantation. There is controversy as to whether hypercholesterolemia is an important risk factor of allograft vasculopathy. A more consistent observation is that an elevated plasma triglyceride was associated with the development of coronary vasculopathy. Most likely, immune and ischemic mechanisms of endothelial injury in the setting of hyperlipidemia are likely to play a role in the development of coronary vasculopathy.

The complex interactions between lipoprotein metabolism, immunosuppressive drug therapy, and inflammation and the potential benefits of lipid-lowering drug therapy after heart transplantation have been examined recently. Lipid-lowering therapy using gemfibrozil, targeted to the modification of triglyceride levels, appears to confer a survival benefit in cardiac transplant recipients who survive beyond the first year. Moderate-to-severe hypercholesterolemia generally requires the use of an HMG-CoA reductase inhibitor (statin). In a prospective randomized trial, it was observed that the use of pravastatin early after transplantation resulted in a decreased incidence of clinically severe acute rejection episodes, and in a significant improvement in 1-year survival (94% vs 78% in the control group, $P=0.02$). Follow-up at 5-years shows continued survival benefit in patients receiving pravastatin (83% vs 62%). A similar survival benefit result was observed with simvastatin in a randomized prospective trial. This observed survival benefit is probably a "class effect" that is shared among all statins. In vitro studies revealed that pravastatin inhibits natural killer cell cytotoxicity, and acts synergistically with cyclosporine to inhibit cytotoxic lymphocyte activity, thereby implying that the protective effect of pravastatin on survival might be partially immunologically-related.

Gout

Gouty arthritis is the most frequent rheumatological complication among cyclosporine-treated organ transplant recipients. Following heart transplantation, both hyperuricemia and gouty arthritis are observed with increasing frequency in 70% to 80%, and 8% to 17% of patients, respectively. The gout observed is usually polyarticular in nature and often exhibits an accelerated clinical course, with management complicated by the patient's renal insufficiency and interaction with transplant-related medications. The mechanism of hyperuricemia is multifactorial, involving enhanced proximal tubular reabsorption, reduced distal tubular secretion, and alterations in renal blood flow.

Colchicine is generally effective in treating acute gouty episodes and providing prophylaxis against recurrent episodes. However, cardiac transplant recipients treated with cyclosporine may be at increased risk of developing acute colchicine-induced myoneuropathy, especially in the setting of concurrent renal insufficiency. If colchicine is administered, the dose should be reduced, cyclosporine levels should be monitored closely, and patients should be evaluated for signs of neuromuscular toxicity.

Another potential life-threatening drug interaction is the combination of allopurinol and azathioprine resulting in pancytopenia. Since allopurinol blocks the xanthine oxidase pathway by which azathioprine is metabolized, potentially toxic levels of azathioprine may result. This increased risk of myelotoxicity has been reported even after adjustment of the dose of azathioprine to one-third of the usual dose, thus suggesting the need for close hematological monitoring of patients treated with this drug combination. Since mycophenolate mofetil metabolism does not involve the xanthine oxidase pathway, it may be used safely in combination with allopurinol.

Corticosteroids may be the most effective and safest approach to treatment in cyclosporine and azathioprine-treated patients with renal dysfunction. As a rule, nonsteroidal antiinflammatory agents are not used due to their propensity to cause renal dysfunction. Brief courses of indomethacin or sulindac require adequate hydration and close observation of renal function. The potential role of cyclooxygenase-2 inhibitors in heart transplant recipients for the treatment of gout is unknown.

Malignancy (see also Section IV, Chapter 26)

Following heart transplantation, malignancy is identified in 3% to 18% of the recipients with an estimated risk of

1% to 2% per year. It ranks second to coronary vasculopathy as a major cause of mortality, accounting for 10% to 23% of all deaths following heart transplantation. Cutaneous malignancy is the most common type, seen in up to 17% of patients with predominance of squamous cell carcinoma.

Posttransplant lymphoproliferative disorder (PTLD) is a frequently fatal complication occurring in 1.7% to 6% of cardiac transplant recipients. The peak occurrence of PTLD is three to four months after transplantation. A strong association of PTLD with Epstein-Barr virus was observed in several series. The use of muromonab-CD3, which may impact favorably on the rejection rate, has been shown to increase the risk of lymphoma. The total burden of immunosuppression likely impacts the tendency to manifest PTLD, and this principle should always be considered. Initial management of PTLD usually involves reduction in immunosuppression, which may be effective in a proportion of cases. Nonrespondent patients may require aggressive combination chemotherapy, and a mortality rate of 80% is reported for such patients.

Re-Transplantation

Many ethical and fiscal issues have been raised concerning the allocation of a scarce organ to a re-transplant candidate who is 20% less likely to survive one year after transplantation than a primary candidate. Several variables must be considered when examining the issue of re-transplantation: (1) the commitment of the transplant center to the care of the patient; (2) the urgency for re-transplantation; (3) the equity of accessibility to the health care system's benefits; and (4) the efficacy of the allocation process in maximizing the benefits derived from the use of a very limited donor pool. Hence, there is a need for rigorous and consistent criteria to select the "ideal candidate" for re-transplantation.

The ISHLT registry examined factors potentially predictive of outcome after repeat heart transplantation. In their data analysis of 449 recipients of second cardiac allografts, and a matched group of 421 primary transplant recipients, survival was markedly decreased in repeat transplantation patients (1-year actuarial survival rate, 48% vs 79%; $P<0.001$). Four major variables were noted to be predictive of improved survival after repeat transplantation: (1) accelerated coronary artery disease as the cause of allograft failure; (2) an interval longer than six months between transplants; (3) lack of preoperative mechanical assistance; and (4) second transplantation after 1985. An "ideal candidate" defined by these predictive variables had an anticipated 1-year survival rate of 64%, which is still significantly less than that expected for primary transplant recipients. Comparison of causes of death between the primary and re-transplanted groups demonstrated a greater proportion of

deaths from primary graft failure and a lower percentage of deaths from accelerated coronary atherosclerosis in repeat transplant patients. However, the proportion of deaths occurring because of infection and rejection did not differ between the two groups of patients.

Investigators at Stanford University have reported graft survival rates for patients undergoing re-transplantation for severe accelerated coronary artery disease at one and five years of 55% and 10%, respectively. Stanford's published 25-year experience analyzes 66 heart re-transplantations; the actuarial survival estimates for the whole re-transplantation group at one, five, and ten years were 55%, 33%, and 22%, respectively. This survival was significantly lower than that in patients undergoing primary heart transplantation (81%, 62%, 44% at one, five, and ten years, respectively, $P<0.05$). Those patients who underwent re-transplantation for graft atherosclerosis since 1981 had a significantly better 1-year survival than those who underwent re-transplantation for allograft rejection (69% vs 33%, $P<0.05$), but the 5-year survival was similar in both groups (34% vs 33%). Two major determinants of patient survival emerged in their report: (1) intractable rejection as a cause of re-transplantation, and (2) serum creatinine level of greater than 2.0 mg/dL. It is thus recommended to exclude such patients to achieve better survival results.

Very recently, investigators from the Columbia Presbyterian Medical Center reported their 20-year experience in a group of 43 patients who underwent re-transplantation. No significant difference in actuarial patient survival was found at one, two, and five years between patients undergoing primary transplantation and those undergoing re-transplantation (76%, 71%, and 60% vs 66%, 66%, and 51%, respectively). A shorter interval between transplants and an initial diagnosis of ischemic cardiomyopathy were identified as significant risk factors of death after re-transplantation. After revision of the investigators' selection criteria since 1993, by excluding patients with allograft dysfunction as a result of primary graft failure and those with intractable acute rejection occurring less than six months after transplantation, they were able to achieve improved survival in the re-transplant group. The actuarial survivals at one and four years in the re-transplant group were 94% and 94%, respectively, as compared with 81% and 77%, respectively, for the primary transplant group ($P=0.09$).

It is thus apparent that defining the "ideal candidate" poses a challenging dilemma to the transplant team, and may not be easy to accomplish in the face of a worldwide shortage of donated organs. However, based on the aforementioned results of some of the major transplant centers experience, cardiac re-transplantation may be a viable therapeutic strategy for patients with severe coronary artery disease as the cause of allograft dysfunction. Excluding patients with intractable rejection, primary graft failure, and renal dysfunction may improve survival outcome. Additionally, the major contraindications to primary transplantation are also contraindications to re-transplantation.

THE ROLE OF THE PRIMARY CARE PHYSICIAN

Successful long-term care of the transplanted heart is a team effort including the patient, the transplant team, and the primary care physician. A knowledge of cardiac transplantation medicine is fundamental for the health care provider, including the primary care physician who participates in the care of the posttransplant patient.

The primary care physician plays an important role in the management of preexisting and posttransplant medical problems such as diabetes, hypertension, hyperlipidemia, and osteoporosis.

Posttransplant complications such as infection, rejection, coronary vasculopathy, and malignancy pose a major threat to the transplanted organ, and therefore, require a heightened awareness by the primary care physician and an appropriately timed referral to the cardiac transplant team. Symptoms and signs of disease such as fever, dyspnea, fatigue, intractable headache, diarrhea, new appearance of skin lesions, etc., should all be investigated thoroughly in immunosuppressed patients in consultation with the transplant team.

The long-term management of heart transplant patients is continuously evolving with the emergence of new immunosuppressive agents. The key to the safe handling of these agents by the primary care physician requires an in-depth knowledge of the pharmacology including the potential side effects, and the various drug interactions. The alteration of cyclosporine levels with calcium channel blockers is well known and needs to be recognized to avoid unwanted adverse effects such as nephrotoxicity as a result of increased cyclosporine blood level. Combining HMG CoA reductase inhibitors with cyclosporine warrants careful liver function and creatine kinase monitoring. Some drug interactions could be life-threatening, such as the addition of allopurinol to treat gout in a cardiac recipient maintained on an azathioprine immunosuppressive regimen resulting in potentially fatal myelotoxicity. It is thus recommended that newly prescribed medications be given in consultation with the transplant center.

Appropriate antibiotic prophylaxis is recommended for cardiac transplant recipients undergoing dental, genitourinary, or gastrointestinal procedures.

Psychological issues posttransplantation are important and should be addressed by the primary care physician. Appropriate counseling of patients and families is indicated.

Hence, the primary care physician has assumed a growing and vital role in the management of an expanding population of long-term heart transplant recipients.

RECOMMENDED READING

Bhatia SJ, Kirshenbaum JM, Shemin RJ, et al. Time course of resolution of pulmonary hypertension and right ventricular remodeling after orthotopic cardiac transplantation. Circulation. 1987;76(4):819-826.

Puleo JA, Aranda JM, Weston MW, et al. Noninvasive detection of allograft rejection in heart transplant recipients by use of Doppler tissue imaging. J Heart Lung Transplant. 1998;17(2):176-184.

Tuzcu EM, De Franco AC, Goormastic M, et al. Dichotomous pattern of coronary atherosclerosis 1 to 9 years after transplantation: insights from systematic intravascular ultrasound imaging. J Am Coll Cardiol. 1996;27(4):839-846.

Akosah KO, Olsovsky M, Kirchberg D, Salter D, Mohanty PK. Dobutamine stress echocardiography predicts cardiac events in heart transplant patients. Circulation. 1996;94(9 Suppl):II283-II288.

Sethi GK, Kosaraju S, Arabia FA, Rosado LJ, McCarthy MS, Copeland JG. Is it necessary to perform surveillance endomyocardial biopsies in heart transplant recipients? J Heart Lung Transplant. 1995;14(6 Pt 1): 1047-1051.

Williams MJ, Lee MY, DiSalvo TG, et al. Biopsy-induced flail tricuspid leaflet and tricuspid regurgitation following orthotopic cardiac transplantation. Am J Cardiol. 1996;77(15):1339-1344.

Brozena SC, Johnson MR, Ventura H, et al. Effectiveness and safety of diltiazem or lisinopril in treatment of hypertension after heart transplantation. Results of a prospective, randomized multi center trial. J Am Coll Cardiol. 1996;27(7):1707-1712.

Verani MS, Nishimura S, Mahmarian JJ, Hays JT, Young JB. Cardiac function after orthotopic heart transplantation: response to postural changes, exercise, and beta-adrenergic blockade. J Heart and Lung Transplant. 1994;13(2):181-193.

Hornberger J, Best J, Geppert J, McClellan M. Risks and costs of end-stage renal disease after heart transplantation. Transplantation. 1998;66(12):1763-1770.

Kobashigawa JA, Katznelson S, Laks H, et al. Effect of pravastatin on outcomes after cardiac transplantation. N Engl J Med. 1995;333(10):621-627.

Burack DA, Griffith BP, Thompson ME, Kahl LE. Hyperuricemia and gout among heart transplant recipients receiving cyclosporine. Am J Med. 1992;92(2): 141-146.

Armitage JM, Kormos RL, Stuart RS, et al. Posttransplant lymphoproliferative disease in thoracic organ transplant patients: ten years of cyclosporine-based immunosuppression. J Heart Lung Transplant. 1991;10(6):877-886.

John R, Chen JM, Weinberg A, et al. Long-term survival after cardiac retransplantation: a twenty-year single-center experience. J Thorac Cardiovasc Surg. 1999;117(3): 543-555.

**MAINTENANCE IMMUNO-
SUPPRESSION PROTOCOLS FOR
HEART TRANSPLANTATION**

David O. Taylor, MD
Dale G. Renlund, MD
Abdallah G. Kfoury, MD

STANDARD MAINTENANCE IMMUNOSUPPRESSION PROTOCOLS FOR HEART TRANSPLANTATION

Early in the history of clinical heart transplantation, maintenance immunosuppression protocols included only azathioprine and corticosteroids. In the early 1980s, the replacement of azathioprine with cyclosporine led to better survival and allowed a significant reduction in maintenance corticosteroid dosage. The addition of azathioprine back into the cyclosporine and corticosteroid protocols allowed further reductions in both cyclosporine and corticosteroid dosages, and less subsequent toxicities. Today, "standard" maintenance immunosuppression protocols, so-called *triple therapy*, include: (1) a calcineurin inhibitor such as cyclosporine or tacrolimus; (2) an antiproliferative agent such as azathioprine, mycophenolate mofetil (MMF), or rarely, cyclophosphamide; and (3) corticosteroids such as prednisone or prednisolone. Significant controversy remains regarding which agent within each of the first two categories is preferable and whether corticosteroids are required long-term. Currently, national and international surveys suggest that cyclosporine is used more often than tacrolimus, and azathioprine is used more often than MMF. However, these differences appear to be rapidly diminishing as recent data have demonstrated the efficacy of tacrolimus and of MMF in heart transplantation.

David O. Taylor, MD, Associate Professor of Medicine, University of Utah Health Sciences Center, Division of Cardiology, Salt Lake City Veterans Affairs Medical Center, Salt Lake City, UT

Dale G. Renlund, MD, Professor of Medicine, University of Utah Health Sciences Center, Division of Cardiology, Salt Lake City Veterans Affairs Medical Center, Salt Lake City, UT

Abdallah G. Kfoury, MD, Assistant Professor of Medicine, University of Utah Health Sciences Center, Division of Cardiology, Salt Lake City Veterans Affairs Medical Center, Salt Lake City, UT

Cyclosporine vs Tacrolimus Therapy

Two single-center (ie, University of Pittsburgh and University of Munich) and two multicenter (US and European) trials have suggested at least equivalent, and perhaps better, antirejection properties of tacrolimus when compared to cyclosporine, with significantly less hyperlipidemia and hypertension associated with tacrolimus use. The incidence of renal dysfunction is similar between the two agents and the incidence of new or worsening diabetes is only minimally higher with tacrolimus use. The costs and need for blood level monitoring are similar between the two agents. The choice of agents is primarily dictated by the issues outlined below in this chapter.

Azathioprine vs Mycophenolate Mofetil Therapy

In the largest randomized controlled trial in heart transplantation to date, MMF was compared to azathioprine in combination with cyclosporine and corticosteroids. In this study, reported by Kobashigawa et al, 650 primary heart transplant recipients were randomized equally between the two study groups. Intent-to-treat analysis of all 650 randomized patients revealed no significant differences between the two study groups with regard to survival, rejection or safety parameters. Unfortunately, because intravenous MMF was not available during the time of this study, 72 patients unable to take oral medications by the sixth day after surgery were withdrawn without ever receiving the study drug, and three-fourths were placed on open-label azathioprine. In addition, these 72 patients experienced a high mortality or re-transplant rate (56% by one year), and there were more MMF-assigned patients (38 vs 34). These facts, coupled with the 11% early crossover rate (primarily in one direction), significantly affected the discriminatory power of the study. When the data were analyzed in only those 578 patients receiving at least one dose of the study drug (a more clinically relevant group), the MMF group experienced an 11% (2% to 22%, 95% confidence intervals) reduction in treated rejection episodes and a 34% (1% to 56%, 95% confidence intervals) reduction in biopsy-proven rejection episodes associated with severe hemodynamic compromise. In addition, the MMF-treated group experienced less mortality during the first 12 months posttransplant (6.2% vs 11.4%, $P=0.031$). The group of patients with severe hemodynamic compromise deserves further comment. Of particular note is the fact that, during the 12 months posttransplant, there were no deaths in the 19 patients in the MMF group who experienced an episode of severe hemodynamically compromising rejection, as compared to 12 deaths (32%) in the 38 such patients in the azathioprine group. The whole of these data suggest that MMF may be superior to azathioprine in preventing, and successfully treating, the more severe forms of allograft rejection. The adverse events in the two groups were similar except for more diarrhea, esophagitis, and opportunistic infections (primarily herpes virus) in the MMF group and more leukopenia in the azathioprine group. However, at the present time, the pharmaceutical cost of MMF is substantially more than azathioprine (approximately $7,000 per year based on 3.0 g/d of MMF vs $900 per year based on 1.5 mg/kg per day of azathioprine). Thus, when considering the choice between MMF and azathioprine, one must consider not only the efficacy data, but the adverse event profile and cost.

Chronic Corticosteroid Therapy

The role of corticosteroids in chronic immunosuppressive protocols remains unsettled. While there has never been an appropriately-sized, randomized controlled trial addressing this issue, there is much single-center data supporting the use of corticosteroid-free maintenance protocols, at least in a substantial subgroup of patients. Only a few programs still use a true corticosteroid-free protocol (double-therapy with cyclosporine and azathioprine), but most programs attempt to wean off corticosteroids during the first four to 12 months, primarily in patients who experience little or no acute allograft rejection. Most programs using triple-drug protocols without antilymphocyte antibody induction therapy attempt to completely withdraw corticosteroid no sooner that four to six months posttransplant, whereas the programs with the earliest corticosteroid withdrawal (two days to two months) use "quadruple-drug" protocols (standard triple-therapy plus antilymphocyte antibody therapy). While it is arguable whether patients experiencing multiple rejection episodes early after transplant should be weaned completely off corticosteroids late after transplant, it seems clear that the subgroup of patients who experience little or no acute allograft rejection episodes can be safely maintained without corticosteroids. An experience with 374 patients who received antilymphocyte antibody therapy (primarily muromonab-CD3) along with cyclosporine and azathioprine, and tapering doses of corticosteroid until discontinued over a five to six week period postoperatively, was recently reviewed. Early mild or moderate rejection episodes were treated with augmented corticosteroids followed by another weaning attempt. Early corticosteroid weaning was abandoned if a severe cellular rejection, vascular rejection, or more than two treated mild-to-moderate rejection episodes occurred. It was reported that 111 (30%) patients were successfully weaned early from corticosteroids and experienced an excellent long-term survival (82%, 10-year actuarial), which is significantly better than the remaining patients (36%, 10-year actuarial). While these data do not suggest that it was the lack of corticosteroids that led to the excellent survival, it seems unlikely that the resumption of corticosteroids to the regimen of these patients could have improved survival.

Combined Tacrolimus and Mycophenolate Mofetil Therapy

A small, single-center study from the University of Munich suggests that the combination of tacrolimus, MMF and corticosteroids may be more effective than cyclosporine, MMF and corticosteroids, especially when MMF dosing is adjusted to blood levels rather than administered as a fixed dose. The infection risks associated with this combination seemed acceptable. It appears that equivalent doses of MMF are associated with higher mycophenolic acid (MPA) levels when combined with tacrolimus, as compared to cyclosporine. Preliminary evidence suggests that cyclosporine decreases the MPA level slightly by affecting intestinal absorption and enterohepatic recirculation of MPA, whereas tacrolimus has a neutral effect on MPA pharmacokinetics.

DRUG LEVEL MONITORING

Since their application into clinical transplantation, and despite a lack of correlation between drug levels and efficacy or toxicity, cyclosporine and tacrolimus have been carefully dosed according to trough blood (or serum) levels. Currently, whole blood is the sample of choice and there are many different laboratory techniques with which to measure drug levels. Since the major metabolites of both cyclosporine and tacrolimus are far less active than the parent compounds, assays that primarily measure the parent compound are preferred. Tacrolimus is generally measured by an enzyme immunoassay (IMx, Abbott Laboratories), or by HPLC, which is more labor intensive. Cyclosporine is generally measured by a monoclonal fluorescence polarization immunoassay (FPIA) with a TDx analyzer (Abbott Laboratories), by HPLC method, or by a monoclonal radioimmunoassay (RIA). Target ranges for each drug vary widely among programs (and organs transplanted), but in general, cyclosporine whole blood level targets range from 250 to 500 ng/mL for the first few months, 200 to 300 ng/mL for the next few months, and 150 to 250 ng/mL thereafter. Tacrolimus whole blood level targets generally range from 15 to 20 ng/mL for the first few months, 10 to 20 ng/mL for the next few months, and 5 to 10 ng/mL thereafter. These target levels are usually modified upward for ongoing rejection and downward for adverse events.

When MMF was introduced into clinical transplantation it was administered as a fixed dose, adjusted only for adverse events. Clinical and animal data suggest that MMF efficacy and toxicity are somewhat related to blood levels of the active metabolite, MPA. In addition, trough levels of MPA correlate with overall drug exposure (area-under-curve, or AUC) in most patients. However, fixed dosing or even weight-based (mg/kg) dosing is associated with wide variability in trough and AUC levels. This has led some investigators to dose MMF according to trough MPA levels. In a pilot study from the University of Munich, 30 patients maintained on tacrolimus and MMF, which was dosed to keep MPA levels between 2.5 µg/mL and 4.5 µg/mL, experienced a total of only three rejection episodes, all occurring in patients with levels less than the target at the time of rejection. In addition, all patients completing six months of therapy were successfully weaned from corticosteroids. Since toxicity also correlates with blood levels of MPA, one could also simply titrate to the maximum tolerated dose without routine blood level monitoring. Since there are several active, and quite different metabolites of azathioprine, drug level monitoring is not feasible. Like MMF, azathioprine is often administered as either a fixed dose (usually mg/kg), or titrated to a maximum tolerated dose (usually limited by bone marrow suppression). While corticosteroid levels are rarely measured, one must remember that because of cytochrome p450 metabolism, drugs that affect cyclosporine and tacrolimus levels will usually affect corticosteroid levels in a similar fashion.

ADJUSTING MAINTENANCE DRUG PROTOCOLS FOR CLINICAL CIRCUMSTANCES
General Principles of Drug Conversion
Since cyclosporine and tacrolimus share common metabolic pathways and common toxicities, conversion from one to the other should involve minimal "overlap." Usually one can simply hold a single regularly scheduled dose of the current drug and begin the new drug with the next scheduled dose. If one is converting a patient during a rejection episode that is being treated with augmented corticosteroids or antilymphocyte antibody therapy, several doses of the current drug can be omitted prior to beginning the new drug in order to minimize overlap and the chances of additive toxicities. Because of the common metabolic pathways, one can estimate the approximate dose of the new drug needed for target levels based on the dose and levels of the current drug. A milligram-to-milligram dose ratio of approximately 40:1 for cyclosporine-to-tacrolimus will usually result in comparable target level ranges.

Since they lack common metabolism or toxicities, MMF and azathioprine can generally be switched by simply stopping one and starting the other without worrying about overlap. The exception may be patients with severe leukopenia at the time of conversion. Since both agents can cause leukopenia by differing (and perhaps additive) mechanisms, one should stop the current drug and wait for adequate resolution of leukopenia prior to starting the alternative. In addition, patients experiencing severe leukopenia on one agent should be started at a low dose of the alternative. A similar approach should be used for conversions between MMF and cyclophosphamide, or azathioprine and cyclophosphamide. Given the longer half-life of cyclophosphamide and its active metabolites, one should probably hold several doses prior to starting azathioprine or MMF. In general, a milligram-to-milligram dose ratio of 1:3 or 1:4 for cyclophosphamide-to-azathioprine will result in similar bone marrow suppression (usually WBCs).

Long-term cyclophosphamide therapy may not be advisable due to the increased risk of malignancy, particularly urologic and hematopoietic.

Ongoing or Recurrent Rejection
A number of drug adjustments are possible to address the problem of ongoing or recurrent allograft rejection. Increasing the calcineurin inhibitor target levels, increasing the antiproliferative agent to the maximum tolerated dose, or increasing the corticosteroid dose is usually the first approach. If this fails or is associated with excess drug toxicity, the addition of other therapies or conversion to alternative agents must be considered. The addition of weekly methotrexate courses to cyclosporine, azathioprine and corticosteroids has been shown to decrease rejection frequency with acceptable toxicity. Anecdotal experience with methotrexate in combination with cyclosporine and MMF, or tacrolimus and azathioprine suggests similar effects. For recalcitrant or recurrent rejection, total lymphoid tissue irradiation (TLI) has been successfully used with acceptable acute toxicity (primarily leukopenia). However, concern about the late effects of TLI was recently raised when several cases of leukemia were reported in patients previously undergoing TLI for allograft rejection.

There is considerable anecdotal evidence in the literature of resolution of recurrent or ongoing rejection by the conversion from cyclosporine to tacrolimus. With the exception of the US Multicenter FK506 Trial, patient crossover for rejection in the cyclosporine and tacrolimus comparative trials was always from cyclosporine to tacrolimus, rather than the converse. This, coupled with the open-label "rescue" studies, suggests that there exists a subgroup of patients who are cyclosporine-resistant, yet respond favorably to tacrolimus. It has previously been shown that recurrent rejecters can be successfully treated by changing from azathioprine to cyclophosphamide, or by changing from azathioprine to MMF. Given the results of the multicenter MMF trial and its manageable side effect profile, MMF can be used as an initial strategy for recurrent or ongoing rejection.

Infectious Complications
Infection remains a major cause of morbidity and mortality both early and late after transplantation. From the simplest viewpoint, infection represents overimmunosuppression and the natural response to acute infection

is to reduce the level of immunosuppression. The availability of echocardiography and endomyocardial biopsy makes it less risky to markedly reduce immunosuppression in the setting of severe infections. Lower-risk infections, such as urinary tract infections, bacterial bronchitis or sinusitis, and limited herpes infections, can generally be treated with antibiotics without reducing the background immunosuppression. However, severe viral infections generally warrant reduction in both the calcineurin inhibitors and the antiproliferative agents (particularly MMF), whereas severe bacterial or fungal infections may require reduction of all immunosuppressants, especially the corticosteroids.

Malignancy

While malignancy represents only a small overall cause of mortality, its incidence increases with time and represents a major cause of mortality in long-term transplant survivors. Malignancy, like infection, is generally due to a state of overimmunosuppression. However, consideration of the cell type and extent of malignancy is important. Certainly, the early EBV-related, polyclonal B-lymphocyte proliferative disorders should be treated with, and often respond well to, reduction in the calcineurin inhibitors and the antiproliferative drugs, whereas the late monoclonal B cell lymphomas and T cell lymphomas generally do not respond to immunosuppression reduction alone. While it was traditionally taught that azathioprine was primarily responsible for the increased risk of skin malignancies, recent data suggest that it is the overall level of immunosuppression rather than the specific agent. Thus, in response to progressive or recurrent skin malignancies, both azathioprine and cyclosporine/tacrolimus should be reduced to the lowest dose that allows adequate allograft protection. While death from nonmelanoma skin cancer is uncommon, several long-term survivors have died from progressive squamous cell skin cancer. Most other solid tumors are less "immune-related" and the appropriate immunosuppressive management is unclear. Certainly, patients receiving chemotherapy or large-port radiotherapy require reduction in their immunosuppressive drugs to prevent the additive bone marrow suppressive effects and risk for opportunistic infections. A significant reduction (50% or more) in calcineurin inhibitors and elimination of the antiproliferative agents is a reasonable approach to the patient receiving chemotherapy. Corticosteroids appear to offer the lowest risk for malignancy and, in fact, are often a major part of chemotherapy protocols.

Medical Noncompliance

While there are many reasons for medical noncompliance, drug costs and side effects rank high. For patients in whom drug costs threaten compliance, several maneuvers can be attempted. Drugs can be administered that compete with the metabolism of, or augment the gastrointestinal uptake of, tacrolimus or cyclosporine and thus increase blood levels, allowing lower doses. Both diltiazem and ketoconazole have been successfully used to spare cyclosporine dose and cost. Both drugs are well-tolerated and have added ancillary properties. Diltiazem, an effective antihypertensive drug in transplant recipients, may attenuate the development of allograft coronary artery disease and generally allows a 30% to 40% reduction in cyclosporine dosage. Likewise, verapamil has similar antihypertensive effects with a similar effect on cyclosporine metabolism. Ketoconazole is an effective antifungal agent and allows a 60% to 80% reduction in cyclosporine dosage. The other azole antifungals, itraconazole and fluconazole, also increase cyclosporine levels, but to a lesser extent than ketoconazole. As described previously, MMF is substantially more expensive than azathioprine or cyclophosphamide, and conversion from MMF to azathioprine should be considered in this subgroup of patients, particularly if their recent rejection history is benign.

Medication side effects probably represent the major reason for immunosuppressant noncompliance, particularly in the adolescent and young adult. While transplant physicians are often hesitant to alter a successful immunosuppressant protocol simply because of adverse cosmetic side effects, we must realize that these "minor" cosmetic side effects are in fact life-threatening to an adolescent if he or she stops prednisone or cyclosporine. The cosmetic side effects of corticosteroids are well known and can only be minimized by tapering to the lowest effective dose. Using other, perhaps more effective, combinations of immunosuppressive agents to wean corticosteroids could be considered. Changing from cyclosporine to tacrolimus, azathioprine to MMF, and perhaps the addition of low-dose methotrexate, may allow successful corticosteroid weaning. The gingival hyperplasia associated with cyclosporine can be minimized with good gingival hygiene and minimizing the cyclosporine exposure, but may be quite severe and require periodic gingivectomy. The hirsutism associated with cyclosporine can be especially difficult for young women, and the treatment (ie, shaving or depilatory agents) is suboptimal. Since tacrolimus is not associated with gingival hyperplasia or hirsutism, conversion from cyclosporine to tacrolimus could be considered for these patients. However, tacrolimus can be associated with alopecia, an equally concerning side effect for both men and women, and may require conversion to cyclosporine. Given these side effect profiles and the propensity for rejection in young females, many programs now "tailor" the drug protocols by starting young females on tacrolimus and MMF from the beginning and attempt aggressive corticosteroid tapering.

It is well-established that medical compliance is directly related to the complexity of the medical regimen.

Thus, for patients at risk for noncompliance, every effort should be made to keep the drug regimen as simple as possible, avoiding multidose medications and multidrug treatments as able.

Other Clinical Circumstances Affecting Maintenance Drug Protocols

In general, aging is associated with reduced immune responsiveness and an increased risk for malignancy. In addition, the incidence of other chronic diseases is higher in the older transplant recipient. While registry data confirm an increased risk of mortality after heart transplantation for older recipients, their mortality is more often related to infection, malignancy or chronic disease rather than acute or chronic allograft rejection. Accordingly, immunosuppressive protocols for older recipients (particularly men) should be less aggressive with rapid corticosteroid weaning and coupled with aggressive treatment of underlying chronic diseases such as hyperlipidemia, diabetes, diverticulosis, and peripheral vascular disease.

Adjustments of the maintenance immunosuppressive protocols are often required in female transplant recipients who are either pregnant or attempting to become so. Obviously, stopping or changing from drugs known to be a hazard to the fetus is critical and requires the early participation of a high-risk obstetrician. Successful pregnancies have been reported in a number of solid organ transplant recipients taking cyclosporine, tacrolimus, azathioprine and corticosteroids. Despite the lack of clinical data, many transplant physicians lower the doses of azathioprine and cyclosporine during the first trimester hoping to lessen the risk of teratogenicity. However, subsequent allograft rejection may be a greater threat to both the mother and fetus. There is currently little data on MMF and fetal risks, so women who are attempting to become pregnant or become pregnant should be withdrawn from MMF. In a multiinstitutional survey of pregnant heart transplant recipients, it was reported that pregnancy was associated with significantly increased cyclosporine drug requirements in a subgroup of patients. Thus, during pregnancy, cyclosporine (and tacrolimus) levels should be followed closely.

As with any patient on chronic corticosteroid therapy, one must be aware of the risk for acute adrenal crisis during periods of stress. Even after apparently successful corticosteroid withdrawal, the ability of the adrenal glands to react appropriately to stress may remain depressed for months to even years. Patients on chronic corticosteroids undergoing major surgery or a major acute illness should receive supplemental doses of corticosteroids, typically intravenous hydrocortisone (100 mg every six to eight hours), during the acute event. Historically, hydrocortisone was then tapered slowly back to the prior corticosteroid dose; however, current practice is to promptly resume the prior corticosteroid dose once hemodynamically stable. For less major operations, a single dose of hydrocortisone is usually adequate. Patients with no clinical evidence of adrenal insufficiency during a minor illness or minor surgery generally do not require supplementation. Glucocorticoid withdrawal syndrome (distinct from adrenal insufficiency) is characterized by headache, malaise, fatigue, arthralgias, myalgias, low-grade fevers, depression, insomnia, anorexia, nausea, or vomiting. Unlike adrenal insufficiency, these symptoms occur in patients withdrawn from corticosteroid who demonstrate normal hypothalamic-pituitary-adrenal function. The etiology of the symptoms is unclear but may relate to cellular corticosteroid-resistance, prostaglandin rebound, or fluctuations in glucocorticosteroid levels. Like documented adrenal insufficiency, these patients require slower, more physiologic corticosteroid weaning. Early conversion to an alternate-day corticosteroid regimen may reduce the subsequent incidence of adrenal insufficiency and perhaps the corticosteroid withdrawal syndrome as well.

RECOMMENDED READING

Kobashigawa J, Miller L, Renlund D, et al. A randomized active-controlled trial of mycophenolate mofetil in heart transplant recipients. Mycophenolate Mofetil Investigators. Transplantation. 1998;66(4):507-515.

Pham SM, Kormos RL, Hattler BG, et al. A prospective trial of tacrolimus (FK 506) in clinical heart transplantation: intermediate-term results. J Thorac Cardiovasc Surg. 1996;111(4):764-772.

Taylor DO, Bristow MR, O'Connell JB, et al. Improved long-term survival after heart transplantation predicted by successful early withdrawal from maintenance corticosteroid therapy. J Heart Lung Transplant. 1996;15(1): 1039-1046.

Meiser BM, Pfeiffer M, Schmidt D, et al. Combination therapy with tacrolimus and mycophenolate mofetil following cardiac transplantation: importance of mycophenolic acid therapeutic drug monitoring. J Heart Lung Transplant. 1999;18(2):143-149.

Reichart B, Meiser B, Vigano M, et al. European multicenter tacrolimus (FK506) Heart Pilot Study: one-year results—European Tacrolimus Multicenter Heart Study Group. J Heart Lung Transplant. 1998;17(8):775-781.

Taylor DO, Barr ML, Radovancevic B, et al. A randomized, multicenter comparison of tacrolimus and cyclosporine immunosuppressive regimens in cardiac transplantation: decreased hyperlipidemia and hypertension with tacrolimus. J Heart Lung Transplant. 1999;18(4):336-345.

45 EXPECTED CLINICAL OUTCOMES – RISK FACTORS FOR HEART TRANSPLANTATION

Jeffrey D. Hosenpud, MD

Over the past two decades, cardiac transplantation has emerged as definitive care for end-stage cardiac disease. Short-term survival has improved to between 80% and 90% at one year. Long-term survival is still hampered by the development of chronic rejection, manifest by coronary artery disease that occurs in up to 50% of patients by five years. The other major problem is the shortage of donor organs, limiting the total number of transplants performed internationally to around 4,000 per year. It is estimated that the need is at least tenfold this number. The data presented in this chapter was acquired and analyzed by the Joint Thoracic Registry of the International Society for Heart and Lung Transplantation and the United Network for Organ Sharing. The data set used contains information on a total of 45,993 cardiac transplants performed between 1968 and 1998, reported from 301 cardiac transplant programs.

DATA ANALYSIS

Survival was calculated actuarially, and actuarial survival curves were contrasted using the Wilcoxan and log-rank tests. Logistic regression methods were used to determine which variables were associated with survival after transplantation. A multivariate logistic regression analysis was then applied to the entire data set, but limited to those patients who had all of the model variables available in their records, to determine the independent predictors of survival. Furthermore, the odds ratio of each variable was expressed as a comparison of survival between groups, with a value of 1.0 indicating no survival benefit, less than 1.0 indicating increased survival, and greater than 1.0 indicating increased mortality after transplantation.

SURVIVAL

Figure 45-1 presents the actuarial survival following cardiac transplantation over a 14-year period. The overall 1-year survival for cardiac transplantation was 79%. The patient half-life (time to 50% survival) was 8.7 years, and in those surviving the first year, the patient half-life was 11.4 years. The fall-off in survival was almost a straight line from year one through year 14 with a constant mortality rate of 4% per year.

Head, Transplant Cardiology, St. Luke's Cardiac Transplant Program, Milwaukee, WI

The next series of figures represent actuarial survival for year of transplantation, recipient age and re-transplantation. Figure 45-2 demonstrates 5-year actuarial survival over the past 17 years broken down in 3-year time blocks. There was a substantial increase in survival in more recently transplanted patients, compared to those transplanted from 1980 to 1985. There was a marginal, but statistically significant further increase in survival comparing the last five years of the 80s with patients transplanted from 1991 forward. Figure 45-3 demonstrates actuarial survival broken down by recipient age group. There was a statistically significant decrease in survival for each increase in decade of life, with a clinically significant decrease in those patients over the age of 65 years. Figure 45-4 presents 5-year actuarial survival for those re-transplants performed within and beyond nine months after the initial transplantation. Overall, re-transplantation has a significantly worse outcome compared to primary transplantation.

Tables 45-1 and 45-2 show multivariate logistic regression analyses for adult cardiac allograft recipients performed on 17,685 patients at one year and 9,536 patients at five years posttransplantation. The majority of risk factors that affected 1-year mortality persisted at the 5-year time point due to their profound effects on early survival. Recipient factors that had a statistically significant negative impact include prior transplantation, requirement for a ventricular assist device or ventilator support prior to transplantation and increasing age. Recipient factors that had a positive impact include diagnosis of either coronary disease or cardiomyopathy and ABO blood group A. These factors were no longer significant at five years. Center and donor factors that had a negative effect were low volume, increasing ischemia time, donor sex and age. Donor and recipient age, as well as ischemia time, analyzed as continuous variables, were associated with a highly statistically significant increasing risk with increasing values.

Figure 45-5 demonstrates survival following pediatric heart transplantation, both overall and by age groups. The older age pediatric group had survival nearly identical to the adult population while those with the worst outcome were under one year old. Patients one to five years old had intermediate survival rates. Tables 45-3 and 45-4 demonstrate the multivariate logistic regression analysis of risk at one and five years for pediatric heart transplantation. Similar to the adult population, repeat transplantation, use of a ventricular assist device and ventilator mechanical support carried the greatest risks. Other risk factors include very young age, congenital heart disease, low center volume and donor age. Interestingly, recipient age risk in the pediatric population was also linear, but in this case, the risk was inversely correlated to age. At five years, recipient age was no longer a risk factor but recipient sex (female) became one.

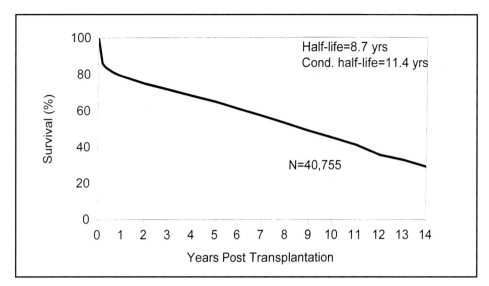

Figure 45-1. Heart transplant actuarial survival for all patients.

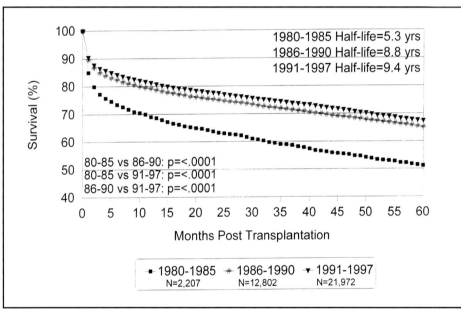

Figure 45-2. Adult heart transplant actuarial survival by era.

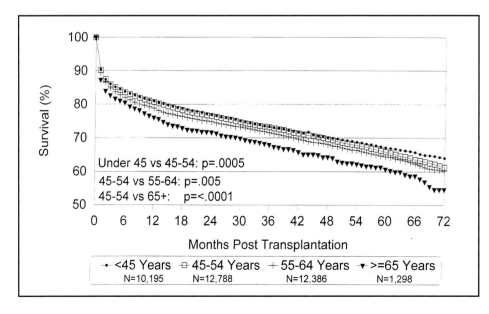

Figure 45-3. Adult heart transplant actuarial survival by age.

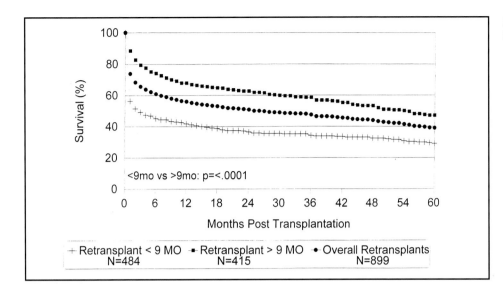

Figure 45-4. Adult heart re-transplant actuarial survival.

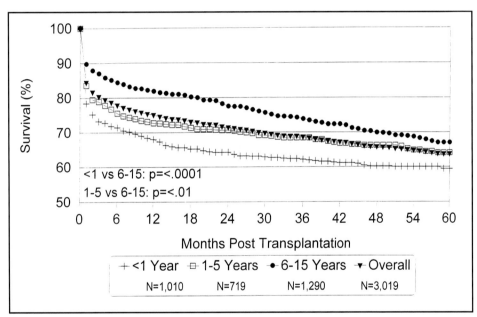

Figure 45-5. Pediatric heart transplant actuarial survival by age.

Figure 45-6 demonstrates the causes of death following cardiac transplantation (both adult and pediatric) at three different time points using the entire data set. Early posttransplantation, nonspecific graft failure accounted for the largest proportion of deaths. In the intermediate period, there was an approximately equal representation by acute rejection and infection. Late after transplantation, the most common causes of death were cardiac allograft vasculopathy (CAV), malignancy and, interestingly, acute rejection. The other category is made up of listed diagnoses not fitting into the more common categories.

MORBIDITY

Morbidity data at one and three years is presented in figures 45-7 through 45-10. Figure 45-7 demonstrates the percent of patients requiring hospital admission

after the initial transplant procedure. Approximately 18% required a hospital admission between the second and third years posttransplantation. Figures 45-8 through 45-10 outline incidences of other morbid conditions in the first three years posttransplantation including drug-treated hypertension, renal dysfunction, drug-treated hyperlipidemia, drug-treated diabetes and malignancy. Hypertension was present in the vast majority of patients, presumably secondary to cyclosporine. The second most common problem was hyperlipidemia seen in approximately half the patients by three years. Both diabetes and renal dysfunction were present in an important minority of patients. Finally, the incidence of malignancy rose over time but the overall incidence of malignancy involving lymphoid tissue (ie, lymphoma, PTLD) remained fairly constant.

CONCLUSIONS

The Registry has allowed for the acquisition of large numbers of patients and has enabled the transplant community to clearly define mortality risks following heart transplantation. With the addition of a substantial amount of morbidity data since 1994, morbidity risk and the impact of various immunosuppressive regimens will begin to be analyzed. It is important to reiterate, however, that only a minority of patients who would benefit from cardiac transplantation are actually being offered this form of therapy.

RECOMMENDED READING

Hosenpud JD, Bennett LE, Keck BM, Fiol B, Boucek MM, Novick RJ. The Registry of the International Society for Heart and Lung Transplantation: fifteenth official report – 1998. J Heart Lung Transplant. 1998;17(7):656-668.

Bourge RC, Naftel DC, Costanzo-Nordin MR, et al. Pretransplantation risk factors for death after cardiac transplantation: a multiinstitutional study. The Transplant Cardiologists Research Database Group. J Heart Lung Transplant. 1993;12(4):549-562.

United Network for Organ Sharing. 1997 Annual Report. Department of Health and Human Services. ISBN 1-886651-25-6.

Table 45-1. Risk Factors for 1-Year Mortality in Adult Heart Transplantation (n=17,685)

Variable	Odds Ratio	95% Confidence Interval	P value
Ventilator	2.66	2.20-3.21	<0.0001
Repeat tx	2.33	1.80-3.01	<0.0001
VAD	1.49	1.23-1.80	<0.0001
Center Vol <9 tx/yr	1.3	1.15-1.47	<0.0001
Female Donor	1.22	1.11-1.33	<0.0001
ABO=A	0.9	0.83-0.98	0.01
DX=CAD	0.79	0.68-0.93	0.005
DX=CM	0.71	0.60-0.83	<0.0001
Ischemia Time*			<0.0001
0 Hours	0.75	0.67-0.83	
2 Hours	0.93	0.90-0.95	
4 Hours	1.15	1.09-1.22	
6 Hours	1.43	1.25-1.64	
8 Hours	1.78	1.43-2.22	
Recipient Age*			< 0.0001
20 Years	0.85	0.69-1.06	
30 Years	0.85	0.76-0.94	
40 Years	0.89	0.85-0.93	
50 Years	1	1.00-1.00	
60 Years	1.19	1.11-1.27	
70 Years	1.5	1.26-1.79	
Donor Age*			< 0.0001
20 Years	0.89	0.84-0.95	
30 Years	0.99	0.99-1.00	
40 Years	1.18	1.14-1.22	
50 Years	1.48	1.34-1.64	
60 Years	1.99	1.59-2.48	

*Linear analysis
VAD indicates ventricular assist device; DX, diagnosis; CAD, coronary artery device; and
CM, cardiomyopathy.
Reprinted with permission from Hosenpud JD, Bennett LE, Keck BM, Fiol B, Boucek MM, Novick RJ. The Registry of the International Society for Heart and Lung Transplantation: fifteenth official report — 1998. J Heart Lung Transplant. 1998;17(7):656-668.

Table 45-2. Risk Factors for 5-Year Mortality in Adult Heart Transplantation (n=9,536)

Variable	Odds Ratio	95% Confidence Interval	P value
Repeat Tx	3.08	2.34-4.05	<0.0001
Ventilator	1.78	1.40-2.27	<0.0001
Center Vol <9 tx/yr	1.29	1.14-1.47	<0.0001
Female Donor	1.15	1.04-1.28	0.006
Ischemia Time*			<0.0001
0 Hours	0.77	0.68-0.88	
2 Hours	0.94	0.91-0.97	
4 Hours	1.13	1.06-1.21	
6 Hours	1.37	1.17-1.60	
8 Hours	1.66	1.29-2.13	
Recipient Age*			<0.0001
20 Years	1.21	0.97-1.51	
30 Years	0.99	0.89-1.10	
40 Years	0.93	0.89-0.97	
50 Years	1	1.00-1.00	
60 Years	1.22	1.10-1.31	
70 Years	1.71	1.40-2.09	
Donor Age*			<0.0001
20 Years	0.89	0.83-0.94	
30 Years	0.99	0.99-1.00	
40 Years	1.19	1.14-1.25	
50 Years	1.53	1.34-1.76	
60 Years	2.21	1.57-2.82	

*Linear analysis
Reprinted with permission from Hosenpud JD, Bennett LE, Keck BM, Fiol B, Boucek MM, Novick RJ. The Registry of the International Society for Heart and Lung Transplantation: fifteenth official report — 1998. J Heart Lung Transplant. 1998;17(7):656-668.

Table 45-3. Risk Factors for 1-Year Mortality in Pediatric Heart Transplantation (n=2,083)

Variable	Odds Ratio	95% Confidence Interval	*P* value
Re-transplant	2.55	1.44-4.51	<0.0001
IABP / VAD	2.54	1.17-5.51	0.02
Ventilator	1.5	1.24-2.06	0.0003
Congenital	1.41	1.10-2.80	0.006
Center Vol <9 tx/yr	1.36	1.08-1.71	0.009
Recipient Age*			<0.0001
0 Years	1.39	1.21-1.61	
3 Years	1.2	1.11-1.29	
6 Years	1.03	1.01-1.04	
12 Years	0.75	0.67-0.85	
17 Years	0.58	0.46-0.73	
Donor Age†			0.003
0 Years	1.08	1.03-1.13	
10 Years	1	1.00-1.00	
20 Years	1.07	1.02-1.12	
30 Years	1.33	1.10-1.60	
40 Years	1.89	1.24-2.87	
50 Years	3.11	0.87-7.86	

*Linear analysis
†Quadratic analysis
IABP indicates intra aortic balloon pump; and VAD, ventricular assist device.
Reprinted with permission from Hosenpud JD, Bennett LE, Keck BM, Fiol B, Boucek MM, Novick RJ. The Registry of the International Society for Heart and Lung Transplantation: fifteenth official report — 1998. J Heart Lung Transplant. 1998;17(7):656-668.

Table 45-4. Risk Factors for 5-Year Mortality in Pediatric Heart Transplantation (n=1,063)

Variable	Odds Ratio	95% Confidence Interval	*P* value
Re-transplant	3.21	1.40-7.35	0.006
Ventilator	1.47	1.08-2.01	0.02
Diagnosis-cong	1.36	1.03-1.79	0.03
Female Recipient	1.31	1.00-1.71	0.05
Donor Age*			0.03
0 Years	1.08	1.01-1.15	
10 Years	1	1.00-1.00	
20 Years	1.08	1.01-1.15	
30 Years	1.34	1.04-1.73	
40 Years	1.95	1.10-3.45	
50 Years	3.28	1.19-9.08	

*Quadratic analysis
Reprinted with permission from Hosenpud JD, Bennett LE, Keck BM, Fiol B, Boucek MM, Novick RJ. The Registry of the International Society for Heart and Lung Transplantation: fifteenth official report — 1998. J Heart Lung Transplant. 1998;17(7):656-668.

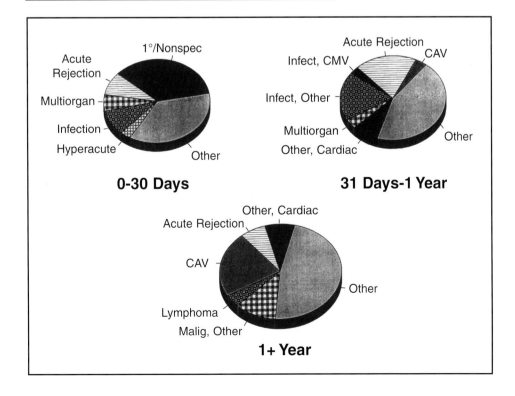

Figure 45-6. Heart transplant cause of death by time post-transplant.

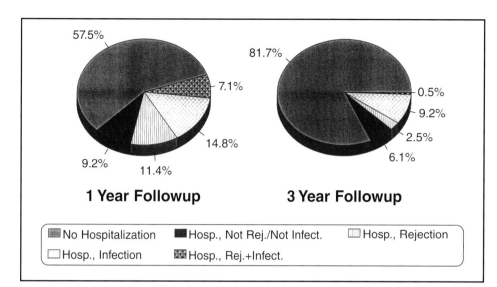

57.5%

7.1%

14.8%

9.2%

11.4%

81.7%

0.5%

9.2%

2.5%

6.1%

1 Year Followup   **3 Year Followup**

No Hospitalization   Hosp., Not Rej./Not Infect.   Hosp., Rejection

Hosp., Infection   Hosp., Rej.+Infect.

Figure 45-7. Readmission to hospital after heart transplantation.

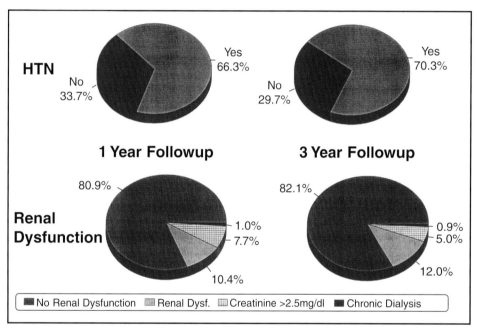

HTN

Yes 66.3%

No 33.7%

Yes 70.3%

No 29.7%

1 Year Followup   **3 Year Followup**

Renal Dysfunction

80.9%

1.0%

7.7%

10.4%

82.1%

0.9%

5.0%

12.0%

No Renal Dysfunction   Renal Dysf.   Creatinine >2.5mg/dl   Chronic Dialysis

Figure 45-8. Hypertension and renal dysfunction after heart transplantation.

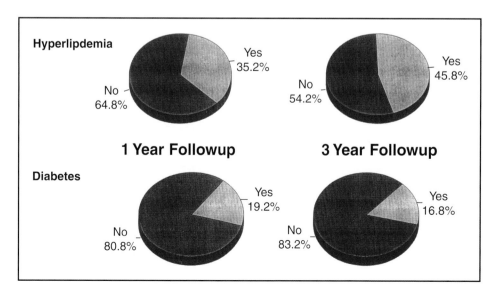

Hyperlipdemia

Yes 35.2%

No 64.8%

Yes 45.8%

No 54.2%

1 Year Followup   **3 Year Followup**

Diabetes

Yes 19.2%

No 80.8%

Yes 16.8%

No 83.2%

Figure 45-9. Hyperlipidemia and diabetes after heart transplantation.

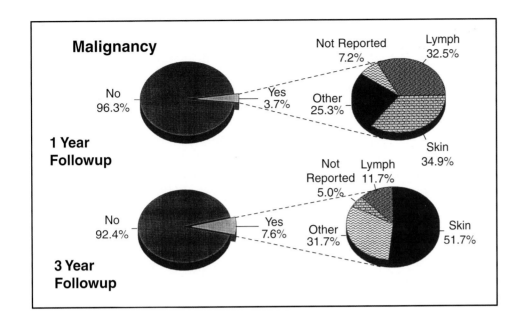

Figure 45-10. Malignancy after heart transplantation.

46 SPECIAL CONSIDERATIONS IN PEDIATRIC HEART TRANSPLANTATION

Linda J. Addonizio, MD

Although cardiac transplantation has been an accepted therapy for end-stage heart disease in the adult patient, it has only been in the last decade that cardiac transplantation has been acknowledged as a standard of care in children. The International Society for Heart and Lung Transplantation (ISHLT) Registry reported 46 pediatric cardiac transplants in 1984, and 25% of the patients were under ten. Early favorable results led to a rapid expansion in the worldwide experience in pediatric cardiac transplantation, with children now comprising about 10% of the total cardiac transplants performed annually. By January 1999, the ISHLT Registry had recorded over 4,100 heart transplants in children between birth and 18 years. Additionally, the mean age of the children receiving transplants decreased remarkably; for the past ten years, over half of the recipients each year have been under five.

Currently, the 5-year actuarial survival is approximately 70% in children, which is equivalent to survival in adults. However, the expectation for pediatric patients is that they will survive for decades. If so, the cumulative side effects of life-long immunosuppression as well as ineffective immunosuppressive protection of the graft will be magnified. The implications of these unique issues in both patient selection and optimal timing of transplantation must be carefully considered against the extensive wait for a donor. Even though results of transplantation continue to improve, the donor pool seems to be relatively fixed, and almost 30% of children die on the waiting list. Further expansion of cardiac transplantation to accommodate the growing number of children surviving palliative repairs of complex congenital heart lesions may prove futile due to the limited supply of donor organs. This chapter will enumerate special considerations that apply to the selection and management of the pediatric cardiac transplant recipient.

INDICATIONS FOR TRANSPLANTATION

Cardiac transplantation is indicated in any child with end-stage heart disease who is refractory to maximal medical therapy, and for whom there is no available sur-

Associate Professor of Pediatrics; Medical Director, Pediatric Cardiac Transplant Program, Columbia University College of Physicians and Surgeons, Babies' and Children's Hospital, New York, NY

gical procedure that could reasonably restore them to an active and productive life. The two main diagnostic indications for heart transplantation in the pediatric age group are myopathic diseases of the heart muscle and complex congenital heart disease. Whereas, in the early 1980s, cardiomyopathy was the most common diagnosis in the young transplant recipient, accounting for 80% of the patients, the proportion of children transplanted with congenital heart disease increased from 16% in 1984 to 46% in 1993, according to the registry of the ISHLT. The predominant diagnostic indications for transplantation varied depending on the age of the child. Seventy-four percent of infants transplanted younger than one year had congenital heart disease and the majority of these had hypoplastic left heart syndrome. Myopathies were the indication in only 17% of infant recipients. Thirty-nine percent of recipients one to ten years old had congenital heart disease and 52% had myopathies. The incidence of re-transplantation was highest (4%) in this pediatric recipient age group compared to 2.6% in adolescents (11 to 17 years) and 1.5% in infants. It is speculated that this represents the "natural history" of eventual graft loss for the large number of infant transplantations that have been performed. Cardiomyopathy and congenital heart disease were the indications for transplantation in 65% and 25% of adolescent patients, respectively.

OPTIMAL TIMING AND EVALUATION OF PROSPECTIVE HEART RECIPIENTS

The evaluation of any child referred for transplantation revolves around two central issues: first, the identification of other treatment options, and second, if none are identified, the optimal timing and management of the child awaiting transplantation. The parameters used in these decisions are variable and dependent on the cardiac diagnosis of the child. (Table 46-1)

CARDIOMYOPATHY

The cardiomyopathies represent a diverse number of diseases affecting the myocardial muscle. In 1993, a multiinstitutional study performed by the Pediatric Heart Lung Transplant Study Group found that idiopathic dilated cardiomyopathy was the diagnosis in 33% of the children who were older than six months at listing; myocarditis occurred in 8%, hypertrophic cardiomyopathy in 8%, and restrictive cardiomyopathy in 3%. The most common type to require cardiac transplantation is dilated cardiomyopathy. The majority of these cases are idiopathic. However, for a number of children thorough evaluation may reveal an etiology resulting in either a potential treatment that would make transplantation unnecessary, or identify other organ system involvement that might preclude transplantation.

Carnitine deficiency, one of the mitochondrial respiratory enzyme deficiencies, is a curable cause of dilated cardiomyopathy. Oral carnitine replacement therapy provides dramatic reversal of cardiac dysfunction. It is also important to determine if cardiomyopathy is secondary to active myocarditis. The treatment of postinfectious myocardial inflammatory disease is controversial in both the adult and pediatric literature. However, it has been shown that pediatric patients may respond to immunosuppressive treatment, which preempts the need for transplant. Gamma-globulin may also improve survival. Additionally, the incidence of spontaneous improvement in myocarditis, using only supportive treatment, has been as high as 30%, a factor that should be considered in the decision for urgent listing in a newly diagnosed case. Other treatable causes of severe myocardial dysfunction in young children include anomalous left coronary artery and chronic arrhythmias. Cardiomyopathy caused by Adriamycin is categorized with the other dilated types, however, it is usually less aggressive in its clinical course. Dilated cardiomyopathies can also be familial, or associated with more global forms of skeletal myopathies. Whereas cardiomyopathy associated with a stable skeletal myopathy is not a contraindication for transplantation, a degenerative

muscular dystrophy would be. Other genetic, biochemical abnormalities of fatty acid, amino acid, glycogen, and mucopolysaccharide metabolism should also be ruled out prior to consideration for transplant.

The natural history of dilated cardiomyopathy has been reported by a number of authors with survival ranging at the best, 84% at ten years, to the worst, 100% mortality in patients presenting over the age of two. Despite the emergence of prognostic factors in heart failure syndromes in adult studies, this wide variability in clinical outcome in the pediatric population has made it difficult to predict impending deterioration. Some children with immeasurable ventricular function are surprisingly free of symptoms, and may do well for years until a viral illness eliminates any cardiac reserve. These are the children who can deteriorate rapidly over a few days, and may be lost before a donor is located. Alternatively, they may have severe pulmonary hypertension from years of left ventricular failure, and be ineligible for transplant except at greatly increased risk. In children it is often too simplistic to stratify their risk for mortality by the severity of their heart failure with the assumption that the greater the severity the poorer the prognosis. The clinical indications for referral to a transplant program include increasing congestive failure despite a maximal regimen including afterload reduction with an angiotensin-converting enzyme inhibitor and beta blockade. A patient with end-stage disease should be evaluated if they are being hospitalized frequently or if their life expectancy is less than 12 months. Malignant arrhythmias that cannot be well-controlled with medications, devices or ablations, are an indication for transplant if the risk of sudden death is considered high. In these patients, an implantable defibrillator may be used as a bridge to transplant. Patients with growth failure, cardiac cachexia or an unacceptably poor quality of life should be referred for transplant evaluation, even when their heart failure appears to be stable, because the wait for a suitable donor can be long and their cardiac reserve is marginal. In dilated cardiomyopathy, a good prognosis was associated with the development of ventricular hypertrophy and a history suggesting a preceding viral illness, thereby implicating inflammation as a cause. Presentation before the age of two was also associated with improved survival. A poor outcome was associated with a left ventricular end diastolic pressure greater than 25 mmHg, decreased left ventricular ejection fraction (LVEF <30%), left ventricular end diastolic dimension (LVEDD) greater than 7 cm in an adolescent, and a family history of cardiomyopathy. These factors correlate with both mortality and clinical symptoms and indicate the need for transplantation. Risk stratification using exercise maximal VO_2 testing, although applicable in adult patients, has never been validated in pediatric series. This technique, which is used as a measure of dis-

Table 46-1. Indications for Heart Transplantation in Children

Cardiomyopathies
Dilated
Idiopathic
Familial
Post-infectious (Myocarditis)
Adriamycin toxicity
Endocardial Fibroelastosis
Restrictive
Idiopathic
Endocardial Fibroelastosis
Hypertrophic
Non-obstructive
Obstructive
Congenital Heart Disease
Complex defects when repair unfeasible
Pulmonary Atresia with Coronary Sinusoids
Single Ventricle Complex with AV valve insufficiency
Ventricular Failure following previous surgery
Failed Physiology (failed Fontan)
Ischemic Disease
Anomalous left Coronary Artery (post-repair)
Kawasaki's Disease

ease progression in some pediatric centers, may become a more valuable tool in the older child and adolescent as more experience is acquired.

Hypertrophic and restrictive cardiomyopathies in pediatric patients have the unique feature of preserved left ventricular systolic function. Hypertrophic cardiomyopathy has a variable natural history and clinical expression. Arrhythmia, the usual etiology of sudden death, is not by itself an indication for transplant because of the availability of implantable defibrillators and newer anti-arrhythmic medications. Although the presence or magnitude of outflow obstruction does not appear to be associated with sudden death, the surgical relief of severe obstruction may help to defer the need for cardiac transplantation. The usual cause for referral is systolic ventricular dysfunction in addition to diastolic dysfunction. This may follow surgical relief of obstruction or other stresses such as a cardiac arrest. Occasionally, the diastolic dysfunction alone is severe enough to warrant transplantation. Other poor prognostic indicators are: (1) young age at diagnosis; (2) history of syncope; (3) a malignant family history; (4) marked left ventricular hypertrophy of greater than 3 cm; or (5) severe chest pains unresponsive to medical management.

Restrictive cardiomyopathy in children is characterized by rapid deterioration and a high mortality rate once patients have significant heart failure. Cardiac transplant appears to be the only viable treatment option. Since there is preservation of left ventricular systolic function, the presentation of these children can be subtle. The progression of pulmonary vascular disease may precede the development of overt heart failure symptoms and thereby preclude successful orthotopic transplantation. Children with idiopathic restrictive cardiomyopathy should undergo serial monitoring of their pulmonary vascular resistance index. A rise in pulmonary vascular resistance index, in association with even subtle symptoms, should prompt a transplant evaluation and early listing.

CONGENITAL HEART DISEASE

It is estimated that perhaps 10% to 20% of children with congenital heart disease might require heart transplantation in their lifetime. Since the outcome from complex surgical repairs has improved dramatically over the years, most children with congenital lesions survive into adulthood with a good quality of life. However, those who eventually need transplantation have usually undergone multiple attempts at palliative or corrective cardiac surgery. Heart transplantation in these patients presents a number of special problems. Their perioperative morbidity and mortality are increased due to poor long-term nutritional status and other end-organ impairment. Children with palliated congenital heart disease also pose the most difficult technical challenges due to their complex anatomy

and anatomic distortion from artificial shunts and baffles that are present from previous surgery. The most common congenital heart lesions that require transplantation are forms of complex single ventricle. In the infant population, this includes both hypoplastic left and right heart lesions. Infants with Hypoplastic Left Heart Syndrome (HLHS) comprise the largest group of infants transplanted. Although the Norwood procedure is available and has been shown to have successful long-term results, it is a palliative operation leading ultimately to a Fontan procedure and its outcome can vary greatly from center to center. However, choosing transplantation as the primary operation incurs an initial significant mortality waiting for a donor organ and a commitment to lifelong immunosuppression. Therefore, selection of the Norwood procedure is driven by center expertise and donor organ availability. Based on current donor availability, less than 10% of all neonates in the USA with HLHS could receive a heart transplant. The use of scarce donor organs for conditions, such as HLHS, that can be palliated by conventional surgery would result in a lack of donor organs for infants with no other option. Pulmonary atresia with intact ventricular septum and right ventricular-dependent coronary circulation has a poor outcome without transplantation. Heart transplantation can be successful in complex heterotaxy syndromes (right and left atrial isomerism) in which traditional palliation with systemic to pulmonary artery shunts, or repair of complex abnormalities would carry an unacceptably high mortality risk. Among older children or adolescents with congenital heart disease, two main diagnostic groups present for transplant. One includes those children with biventricular repairs who subsequently develop ventricular dysfunction and/or severe valvar regurgitation that can not be repaired. The other group includes patients with palliated single ventricles who have developed poor systemic ventricular function or a poor hemodynamics result. The latter are most commonly those patients with failed Fontan physiology. These children and young adults constitute a rapidly expanding group that will need cardiac transplantation in the future.

The majority of patients who require transplantation have severe systemic ventricular dysfunction. However, since there are many children with congenital heart lesions in whom the basis for referral is not left ventricular failure, the clinical indications for transplant evaluation are less easily determined, and the diagnosis of heart failure is dependent on the normal physiology of their specific congenital lesion. A child with severe right ventricular failure and multivalvar insufficiency where the surgical risk for repair is deemed too high, may be a candidate for transplant, even though systemic ventricular dysfunction is only mildly depressed. Ventricular inversion, in which the systemic ventricle is a morphological right ventricle, is an example. A patient with a single ventricle and a Fontan repair has no pulmonary ventricle and therefore the cardiac output from the left ventricle is dependent on passive pulmonary blood flow. Even a mild decrease in left ventricular function or a decrease in diastolic compliance, particularly in combination with an abnormality in lung function or perfusion, can lead to low cardiac output making transplantation the only option for survival. However, occasionally other lesions, such as bronchopulmonary collaterals, may compete with the passive pulmonary flow, and embolization may eliminate the need for a transplant. Additional criteria for transplant referral for congenital heart disease, despite normal ventricular function, include growth failure, severe protein-losing enteropathy, cardiac cachexia and severe cyanosis due to arteriovenous malformations. The complexity of these lesions dictates that all patients with congenital heart disease should first be evaluated at an experienced congenital heart surgery center to ensure that operative and medical alternatives have been exhausted.

RECIPIENT SELECTION

The evaluation and selection process must initially be directed toward determining if other treatment options are appropriate but then subsequently the appropriateness of the candidate for transplantation. Each child referred for transplantation should be evaluated by members of a team including a pediatric cardiologist, cardiothoracic surgeon, transplant nurse specialist, pediatric neurologist, pediatric psychiatrist, social worker, physical therapist, and beyond the infant stage, a pediatric dentist. The patient receives a full physical examination and is assessed for the presence of diseases of the major organs that would affect posttransplant management or make transplantation dangerous or unsuitable. In addition, the psychosocial and financial preparedness of the child and family are evaluated and plans formulated for care and support through the waiting period as well as posttransplant.

Once the evaluation is complete, all data is reviewed by the team, who is responsible, along with the family, for the decision to list a patient for transplantation. Age-appropriate immunizations should be given, but live viral vaccines should be avoided if a patient needs to be listed immediately. Patients on the active waiting list who are not hospitalized need close outpatient follow-up and repeat hemodynamic monitoring every three to six months, depending on their diagnosis, to recheck pulmonary vascular resistance and determine the need and suitability for remaining on the list.

CONTRAINDICATIONS AND EXCLUSION CRITERIA

Contraindications to transplantation have decreased dramatically due to improvements in surgical tech-

niques, perioperative care and selective immunosuppression, which have allowed successful transplantation even in very high-risk patients. Many of the historical absolute contraindications to transplantation now have become relative. Anatomically, since the aorta, pulmonary arteries, and the left atrium are in a relative constant position near the midline, orthotopic cardiac transplantation is feasible in even the most complex of congenital heart lesions if the pulmonary arteries are of reasonable size. The only anatomic contraindication is bilateral "string-like " pulmonary arteries, which would require heart-lung transplant. Orthotopic transplantation has been performed successfully even with only one functional pulmonary artery or lung. Examples are congenital lesions in which one lung is fed by collaterals or if an aortopulmonary shunt is present, there may be systemic pulmonary hypertension in one lung with markedly elevated pulmonary resistance. If there remains a single usable lung with low resistance, an orthotopic transplant can be performed. Pulmonary artery reconstruction can be accomplished successfully at the time of transplantation, and technically creative surgical solutions have been devised to repair systemic and venous anomalies, heterotaxy syndromes, hypoplastic left heart syndrome, dextrocardia and transposition of the great arteries.

High pulmonary vascular resistance has always been an absolute contraindication for orthotopic cardiac transplantation because the new donor right ventricle is unable to pump against this instantaneous workload. However, the physiologic upper limit of resistance has not been determined. Elevated pulmonary resistance is known to be a continuum of risk. An early analysis of pulmonary vascular resistance and transplantation in adult patients showed that no patient developed right heart failure after transplantation if the pulmonary vascular resistance index (PVRI) was less than six indexed units. In the patients with PVRI greater than six, 30% developed right heart failure and 15% died. Some centers rely more on the transpulmonary gradient (TPG) which should be under 15 mmHg to prevent right heart failure. Pediatric patients referred for transplantation often have a higher incidence of elevated pulmonary vascular resistance, whether secondary to unoperated congenital heart lesions or long-term congestive heart failure. Additionally, with some congenital lesions, it is not possible to calculate a true pulmonary resistance. In one pediatric transplant experience of 72 children, 40% had markedly elevated PVRI with a mean of ten indexed units (range from six to 16) and mean TPG of 20 mmHg (80% of patients TPG >15). With maximal vasodilator testing there were 12 patients whose resistance remained greater than six, with eight patients developing right heart failure perioperatively, and two deaths. Two of the eight required temporary right ventricular assist devices and survived. From this extensive experience, the following recommendations for preoperative evaluation of PVRI have been developed. An initial PVRI under six indexed units is acceptable. The medical regimen should be optimized either by the addition of intravenous inotropes and vasodilator therapy when the cardiac index is extremely low, or by alteration of an oral regime if the patient is stable. If the PVRI is over six and the cardiac index is near normal, then the patient should be given a graded nitroprusside infusion to test acute vasoreactivity. If unsuccessful, a one week course of tailored inotropes and vasodilators including dobutamine, milrinone and nitroprusside should be given and a repeat hemodynamic study performed. In select patients, prostacyclin or nitric oxide, if available, can be used for testing and therapy. The purpose of these multiple studies is to determine transplantability and also to find the optimal postoperative regimen. If the resistance remains in the six to nine range despite all these measures, then the patient could still receive an orthotopic transplant, but at greatly increased risk with the knowledge that the severity of the postoperative right heart failure will be unknown and that an assist device may be necessary. If the resistance stays above nine indexed units despite maximal care, then the patient should be evaluated for either a heart-lung, heart-single lung or heterotopic transplantation, unless a longer-term vasodilator and inotrope trial might be deemed useful. Patients with PVRI greater than nine have successfully been transplanted with a higher risk for right ventricular failure (40%), however, only a 10% to 15% mortality.

Another exclusion criterion that has been changing is the history of neoplastic disease. There has been a growing experience with cardiac transplantation in survivors of childhood cancers. Since immune suppression is a risk factor for malignant disease following transplantation, it was speculated that these patients would have an increased risk for recurrence or new tumors. However, in one reported series there was neither a recurrence of the primary tumor following transplant nor an increased incidence of transplant-related neoplasms. Transplantation during active malignancy remains an absolute contraindication to transplantation. Since there is a wide variability in tumor type and behavior, it is unknown what length of time from a patient's oncologic therapy would be considered safe to pursue transplantation.

Hepatitis C virus (HCV) has been considered a relative contraindication to heart transplantation. The controversy concerning heart transplantation of HCV-positive patients or the use of organs from HCV-positive donors is still under discussion. It has been suggested that the risk of acquiring HCV from the donor organ would be better than dying on the waiting list. In the normal host, it can take decades to develop cirrhosis and liver failure from HCV. However, the natural history of HCV can be more variable in the immunosuppressed patient. At the present time, no definitive recommendations exist and most centers continue to list HCV-positive candidates for transplantation and most will use HCV-positive organs. An HCV-positive patient should have a complete pretransplant evaluation, with a liver biopsy, if necessary, by a gastroenterologist, to determine the extent and activity of HCV disease.

Other medical exclusion criteria include irreversible failure of the liver, kidney, lung and brain, degenerative neurological disorders and other systemic diseases that are life-limiting despite treatment, a recent pulmonary embolism, infection with HIV or any significant active infection whether bacterial, fungal or viral. When the infections have resolved, transplantation is again an option. Similarly, with hepatic and renal dysfunction, which are common in shock, stabilization of heart failure or placement of a ventricular assist device may allow the function to improve so that transplantation is feasible.

Psychosocial stability of the child and family has a major effect on the successful outcome of organ transplantation. Noncompliance with medications has been found to occur in at least 20% of pediatric patients with a resultant dismal 30% 5-year actuarial survival compared to 80% in compliant patients. A dependent child must have an actively involved and caring guardian who can ensure that the medical regimen is followed. A stable family support structure or a legal guardian is necessary before transplantation is considered. Lack of an adequate caregiver, active drug or alcohol abuse by the caregiver, or an untreated major psychiatric disorder of the caregiver are absolute exclusions for transplantation. Similarly, a documented history of significant medical noncompliance in the patient and family is a risk factor associated with a poor outcome and should be considered a relative contraindication to transplant. A thorough psychosocial evaluation and plan for psychosocial support and intensive education is as essential for the patient as the proper immunosuppressive regimen. The evaluation must focus not only on the child, but also on the parents, including their parenting skills and ability to understand and follow directions. A financial assessment is also crucial; a lack of insurance to cover the cost of care and medications and/or limited resources can make transplantation untenable. Planned interventions must begin prior to transplant and need not preclude listing if the child is critically ill. In those stable patients who are waiting at home, listing can be contingent on a commitment to a compliance plan. Heightened vigilance and education as well as the development of a support structure for the transplant patient and family can help decrease the incidence of noncompliance.

LABORATORY EVALUATION OF THE RECIPIENT

Prior to transplantation, the child must have a complete echocardiographic examination, a full electrocardiogram and a cardiac catheterization to rule out other operative alternatives and to delineate the extent of the accompanying defects that will affect not only the transplant surgery but also the postoperative care. Angiograms will be necessary to show the size and adequacy of the pulmonary arteries and to provide knowledge of the systemic and pulmonary venous anatomy. For example, a child with a single ventricle complex who was previously cyanotic or post-Fontan procedure should be evaluated for the presence of aortobronchial collateral vessels and pulmonary arteriovenous malformations in addition to the adequacy of the pulmonary arteries. This information is necessary to predict the possibility of high output failure early posttransplant, or continued cyanosis. During the catheterization, the interventional cardiologist could also address and embolize collateral vessels or place stents to stabilize a cyanotic patient for the pretransplant wait. Additionally, it is necessary to know the condition of the femoral arterial and venous systems in children who have had multiple previous sternotomies, as the surgeon might find groin bypass preferable before entering the chest. The catheterization must also include rigorous evaluation of the pulmonary vascular resistance as discussed in the section on contraindications.

Pretransplant testing should also include pulmonary function studies and quantitative ventilation perfusion (VQ) scans, especially for children with congenital heart disease. These studies provide important physiological information that can aid in posttransplant management and add to the understanding of the cardiac dysfunction preoperatively in these patients. In addition, patients with poor ventricular function are at risk for the development of atrial and ventricular thrombi, which can be visualized by echocardiogram. The VQ scans will help determine if there have been any emboli. Preoperative brain imaging should be considered at the request of the neurologist, particularly in those patients with previous neurological events or who are very cyanotic. Head ultrasounds are more routine in the neonatal patient to help rule out congenital abnormalities and intraventricular hemorrhage. In older, stable outpatients with biventricular hearts, a MUGA evaluation of left ventricular function and determination of maximal VO_2 by exercise testing can be helpful in their management.

A general metabolic and end organ functional assessment of the renal, hepatic and endocrine systems is performed in all patients. A hematologic assessment includes a complete blood count, hemoglobin electrophoresis, coagulation profile and iron levels. A serological evaluation for prior infections with: cytomegalovirus (CMV), toxoplasmosis, Ebstein-Barr virus, hepatitis A, B and C, human immunodeficiency virus (HIV) and herpes virus is also performed. Immunoglobulin levels and screening tests for connective tissue diseases are also obtained. Immunity to varicella, measles, mumps, rubella and tuberculosis are measured. The remainder of the immunologic work-up consists of ABO blood and HLA typing, and measurement of anti-HLA antibody levels (panel-reactive antibodies, PRA). If antibodies are present, a pretransplant crossmatch is performed with any potential heart donors. If antibodies to a specific HLA type are demonstrated, donors without HLA specificity will be avoided. Controversy exists over the clinical implications of an elevated PRA in the pediatric patient.

DONOR FACTORS UNIQUE TO PEDIATRICS

ABO blood type compatibility is important, although there has been a report of a series of infants successfully transplanted with ABO-incompatible hearts. Due to the severe organ shortage in the infant weight range, every effort is made to use even marginal donors, and this includes repairing small structural defects (eg, atrial or ventricular septal defects) in the donor heart. In choosing a donor for a pediatric patient, size mismatch of the donor and recipient is very common. In fact, experience has taught that the acceptable weight range for a donor is quite broad, and can be up to triple the body weight of a recipient. Cardiomegaly in the recipient affords a greater potential pericardial space to accommodate the larger donor organ. Surgical expertise is necessary to tailor the disparate great vessel sizes. Care must be taken to more precisely match donor and recipient body size if the recipient has a normal-sized heart, (restrictive cardiomyopathy or certain congenital lesions) to prevent postoperative restriction and tamponade caused by the smaller pericardial space. If there is any question of a mismatch, echocardiographic measurements of cardiac size can be compared to standard nomograms for the recipient body size. Radiographic estimates of heart size taken from plain chest films are not precise.

A unique aspect to donor recovery in pediatrics is the need to procure additional donor tissue to allow for adequate anastomoses and for the creation of conduits. At times, it is important to recover the entire donor aortic arch or the pulmonary artery past the bifurcation to reconstruct the recipient's anatomy. Since the procurement team is usually sent far in advance of the recipient operation, it is paramount to have an operative plan for each complex patient well in advance of the date of surgery. Most hearts can tolerate up to four to five hours of ischemia and still function normally after transplantation. Improved myocardial preservation techniques have diminished the damaging effects of long periods of cold ischemia. Since there are larger glycogen stores in the immature myocardium, it has been suggested that pediatric donor hearts are better able to tolerate longer ischemia times. Successful preservation times of up to ten hours have been associated with good function postimplantation. Long ischemia times may lead to less inotropic reserve requiring maximal exogenous catecholamine support after transplant.

In January 1999, the United Network for Organ Sharing (UNOS) changed its algorithm for the allocation of donor hearts. The new system allows that an adolescent donor will be offered to a pediatric patient in the most urgent status before being given to an adult. Since there are a small number of pediatric recipients, this change could make a tremendous difference in children without adversely affecting adults.

Postoperative Management

The intraoperative and immediate postoperative management of transplant patients is directed at optimizing allograft function in the face of three variables: acute denervation, prolonged ischemia and acclimation to the recipient's hemodynamic environment. Because of denervation, the allograft's stroke volume (assuming adequate preload) is relatively fixed during the first few postoperative days. The cardiac output can be aided by maintaining the heart rate between 100 to 120. Atrial pacing can be used, although using low-dose isoproterenol also adds inotropy and a margin of safety for the allograft which is usually catecholamine depleted. Due to catecholamine depletion and the effects of ischemia, all children should be on a low dose of an inotropic agent even if hemodynamics are excellent coming off bypass. Inotropic support and heart rate control are usually only necessary for one to two days. Since the patient is given a functionally normal heart, the recovery is rapid and the children are extubated and mobilized quickly for rehabilitation.

In children who receive a very large donor heart, care must be taken to maximize pulmonary toilet since there will be compression of the left lower lung early after transplant. Extended intubation or a period of nasal CPAP following extubation to stabilize may be needed. The large stroke volume of an over-sized heart can also cause significant hypertension perioperatively. This should be aggressively managed with nitroprusside or other vasodilators as needed.

In children with high pulmonary vascular resistance, it is crucial to begin specific vasodilators intraoperatively. The preoperative hemodynamic testing helps to tailor the choice of postoperative vasodilators. Right ventricular failure posttransplant can be acute and devastating at the point of separation from cardiopul-monary bypass, or as is more usual, it can be occult and insidious, manifesting itself as low output six to 24 hours later. Myocardial edema as well as mediators released from bypass and transfusions, which affect the microvascular tone in the lungs, prevent the right ventricular myocardium from generating adequate systolic pressure. In this type of right ventricular failure, the central venous pressure is not extraordinarily high and there is simply no flow. The right ventricle becomes increasingly dilated on echocardiography with a relatively empty, snappy left ventricle. Usually the heart tones are soft, but a right ventricular gallop is often heard. Efforts should be directed at minimizing the pulmonary resistance, including continued intubation with deep sedation, arterial pCO2 less-than-or-equal-to 40, and pO2 greater than 100 with no acidosis and maintenance of adequate preload with maximal vasodilation. The right ventricle usually responds in two to three days, first with recovery, and then hypertrophy with resultant adequate systolic function. If the resistance is very high, or the right ventricle is allowed to fail completely before treatment is begun, a right ventricular assist device may be necessary. Recovery of the ventricle can still occur within two to five days.

IMMUNOSUPPRESSION PROTOCOLS UNIQUE TO CHILDREN

Most of the complications that occur following cardiac transplantation are a result of immunosuppressive therapy. Since each recipient must remain on lifelong immunosuppression, it is obvious that the potential years of exposure to these agents will be much greater in the pediatric age group. Additionally, there is substantial data showing heightened immunoresponsiveness in children, out of the neonatal age group, compared to adults.

There are several types of immunosuppressive regimens currently in use and individual transplant programs tailor them to fit their patient's needs. According to the Pediatric Registry of the ISHLT, 90% of pediatric cardiac recipients over the past three years were initially treated with cyclosporine as their main immunosuppressant. By three years postoperative, the use of tacrolimus had risen from an initial 10% to nearly 20%. Azathioprine was part of the initial immunosuppression in 85% of children, but this declined to 60% by three years postoperative. This decrease presumably is attributable to the increased use of mycophenolate mofetil. Prednisone was included in the initial immunosuppressive regimen in 75% of children and 50% remained on prednisone by the third year. From this data it is clear that "triple drug therapy" is still the most common combination therapy in use.

Both cyclosporine and FK506 are metabolized more quickly in children than adults. It is not uncommon to need a thrice daily dosing schedule for cyclosporine to maintain adequate trough levels. Tacrolimus usually can remain at twice daily dosing, but in general, much higher per kilogram doses are needed of both, especially in the young child. By the early teenage years, the metabolism slows and twice daily dosing is feasible. Since their metabolism can change dramatically, and because the nature of young children is to grow, blood levels need to be monitored more frequently than in adults. It is not uncommon to find an unexpected rejection late after transplantation when a child has had a dramatic growth spurt and has not been monitored closely. This ability to "outgrow" their immunosuppression is also partially because of attempts to keep the medications at the lowest safe level to minimize the side effects. Young children have an increased incidence of infections as they grow and gain their natural immunity. Many of the newer antibiotics prescribed by pediatricians can dramatically change the cyclosporine or tacrolimus metabolism and thereby, the blood levels. Families and their physicians should be counseled to review choices of antibiotics with the transplant team to prevent toxicity or inadequate immunosuppression.

INCIDENCE AND DIAGNOSIS OF REJECTION

Rejection of the cardiac allograft is responsible for about 30% of deaths following transplant in children. The incidence of rejection episodes among 332 pediatric cardiac transplant patients in a prospective multiinstitutional study was one per patient by six months and 1.5 per patient at 12 months following transplant. The actuarial freedom from rejection was 61% at one month and only 37% by six months following transplant. The peak hazard for first rejection was at two months after transplant. The rejection detection method in this study was endomyocardial biopsy in 71% of the cases, echocardiography in 23% and clinical criteria in 6% of the cases. Induction therapy made no difference in rejection rates. The incidence of death from rejection in this series was low in infants younger than six months at transplant (6%) and rose to between 23% to 30% in older children.

In the newborn and young child, rejection seems to manifest more symptoms while in the less aggressive stage, which is different than in adolescents and adults. Symptoms of irritability, loss of appetite, fever, tachycardia, and gallop rhythm on physical examination are signs of early rejection in this age group that respond promptly to treatment. In the older child, clinical parameters are usually insensitive indicators of rejection, often until it is so severe that myocardial performance is compromised. Symptoms, when present in the older child, usually center on abdominal complaints and fatigue instead of the classic heart failure signs.

Currently, the most reliable method for detection of acute rejection remains the topic of debate among transplant cardiologists. The "gold standard" has been endomyocardial biopsy, which remains the only direct method of detection of early rejection, as well as an important means for determining adequacy of treatment of rejection episodes. Echocardiographic indices have been investigated for rejection detection. In adult studies with concomitant biopsies, the results have been conflicting and unreliable. The original reports of the efficacy of echocardiography for rejection detection describe an increase in left ventricular mass with rejection in infants after transplantation. A recent study compared the use of echocardiographic indices to biopsy for the detection of acute rejection in infants. Although this study also found that mass increases significantly in acute rejection, the increases were not apparent within the first month. In addition, no threshold value could be determined because of data scatter and the variability ranged from 7% to 80%. One could speculate that this technique may be more applicable to the infant population, in which rejection has more associated edema and clinical signs at an earlier stage, than in older children.

RECOMMENDED READING

Renlund DG, Taylor DO, Kfoury AG, Shaddy RS. New UNOS rules: historical background and implications for transplantation management. J Heart Lung Transplant. 1999;18(11):1065-1070.

Fricker FJ, Addonizio LJ, Bernstein D, et al. Heart transplantation in children. Pediatr Transplant. 1999;3(4):333-342.

Boucek MM, Novick RJ, Bennett LE, Fiol B, Keck BM, Hosenpud JD. The Registry of the International Society for Heart and Lung Transplantation: Second Official Pediatric Report-1998. J Heart Lung Transplant. 1998;17(12);1141-1160.

Morrow WR, Naftel D, Chinook R, et al. Outcome of listing for transplantation in infants younger than six months: predictors of death and interval to transplantation. The Pediatric Heart Transplantation Study Group. J Heart Lung Transplant. 1997;16(12):1255-1266.

Goldstein DJ, Seldomridge JA, Addonizio LJ, Rose EA, Oz MC, Michler RE. Orthotopic heart transplantation in patients with treated malignancies. Am J Cardiol. 1995;75(14):968-971.

Addonizio, LJ, Naftel D, Fricker J, et al. Risk factors for pretransplant outcome in children listed for cardiac transplantation: a multi-institutional study. J Heart Lung Transplant. 1995;14(1 Part 2):S48.

Hsu DT, Addonizio LJ, Smith CR, et al. Cardiac transplantation in children with congenital heart disease. J Am Coll Cardiol. 1995;26(3):743-749.

Addonizio LJ, Gersony WM, Robbins RC, et al. Elevated pulmonary vascular resistance and cardiac transplantation. Circulation. 1987;76 (5 Pt 2):X52-V55.

Rotondo K, Naftel D, Boucek R, et al. Allograft rejection following cardiac transplantation in infants and children: a multi-institutional study. J Heart Lung Transplant. 1996;15(1(2)):S80.

Boucek M, Mathis C, Kanakriyeh M, Hodgkin D, Boucek R, Bailey L. Serial echocardiographic evaluation of cardiac graft rejection after infant heart transplantation. J Heart Lung Transplant. 1993;12:824-831.

Santos-Ocampo S, Sekarski TJ, Saffitz JE, et al. Echocardiographic characteristics of biopsy-proven cellular rejection in infant heart transplant recipients. J Heart Lung Transplant. 1996;15(1 Pt 1):25-34.

Franco KL, ed. Pediatric Cardiopulmonary Transplantation. Armonk, NY: Futura Publishing Company Inc; 1997.

Weller RJ, Addonizio LJ, Kichuk MR, Gersony WM, Hsu DT. Timing of intervention for restrictive cardiomyopathy in children. J Am Coll Cardiol. 1996:27;197A.

Kleinert S, Weintraub RG, Wilkinson JL, Chow CW. Myocarditis in children with dilated cardiomyopathy: incidence and outcome after dual therapy immunosuppression. J Heart Lung Transplant. 1997;16(12):1248-1254.

Shah MB, Schroeder TJ, First MR. Guidelines for immunosuppression management and monitoring after transplantation in children. Transplant Rev. 1999;13(2):83-97.

Webber SA. 15 years of pediatric heart transplantation at the University of Pittsburgh: lessons learned and future prospects. Pediatr Transplant. 1997;1(1):8-21.

47 HEART-LUNG TRANSPLANTATION

James S. Gammie, MD
Robert L. Kormos, MD

HISTORY

Initial clinical experience with transplantation of the heart and both lungs was limited by inadequate immunosuppression. Cooley performed the first human heart-lung transplantation on an infant in 1968. The patient died within 24 hours of operation. Lillehei (1969) and Barnard (1971) performed heart-lung transplants on adults; both recipients succumbed to infection in the perioperative period. In all three cases, immunosuppression was with steroids and azathioprine. The Stanford group continued laboratory work in primates and demonstrated long-term success using a combination of cyclosporine-based immunosuppression, tracheal anastomosis, and avoidance of steroids in the early postoperative period. This work facilitated the first successful transplantation of the heart and both lungs by Reitz in 1981. The first recipient, a 45 year-old woman with primary pulmonary hypertension, demonstrated normal exercise tolerance ten months after operation. Improved results with heart-lung transplantation using cyclosporine-based immunosuppression yielded similar success with single lung transplantation in 1983 and double-lung transplantation in 1985. As a result of the success of isolated lung transplantation and the scarcity of donor organs, heart-lung transplantation is now an uncommon operation. The number of heart-lung transplantations peaked in 1989 and has steadily declined thereafter. In 1997, only 151 heart-lung transplants were performed worldwide (52 in the United States).

EVALUATION AND MANAGEMENT OF THE RECIPIENT

In general, heart-lung transplantation is reserved for patients with end-stage pulmonary parenchymal or vascular disease in combination with irreversible cardiac dysfunction or complex (congenital) cardiac defects not

James S. Gammie, MD, Assistant Professor; Surgical Director, Cardiac Transplantation/Mechanical Circulatory Support, University of Massachusetts Medical Center, Division of Cardiothoracic Surgery, Worcester, MA

Robert L. Kormos, MD, Associate Professor of Surgery; Director, Artificial Heart Program and Adult Heart Transplantation, University of Pittsburgh Medical Center, Division of Cardiothoracic Surgery, Pittsburgh, PA

amenable to repair. Appropriate candidates should have a life expectancy of less than two years and be in NYHA functional class III or IV. Increased application of isolated single- or double-lung transplantation for patients with pulmonary vascular disease arose from the recognition that even substantial right ventricular dysfunction secondary to pulmonary hypertension can improve after lung transplantation alone. Isolated single- or double-lung transplantation is the procedure of choice for patients with normal cardiac function, reversible right-ventricular dysfunction due to pulmonary hypertension, and congenital heart disease that can be repaired. Advantages of a pulmonary-only transplant approach include avoidance of chronic allograft vasculopathy (CAV), a shorter wait for available organs, and an optimal utilization of donor organs. In current practice, most recipients of heart-lung transplants are patients with irreparable congenital heart defects and associated pulmonary vascular disease.

Once a potential recipient has been identified, the presence of comorbid conditions that might compromise outcome after transplantation are identified. Generally accepted contraindications to heart-lung transplantation are detailed in Table 47-1.

Because the waiting time for a heart-lung donor is likely to be protracted, it is desirable to identify potential recipients relatively early in the course of their disease process. Once a patient has been placed on the waiting list, close contact between the transplant team and the potential recipient is essential to identify progression of disease as well as any changes in the status of the patient that would adversely affect outcome after transplantation. Conditions that can be treated are done so aggressively; in some cases recipients will need to be removed from the list.

HEART-LUNG DONOR SELECTION CRITERIA

Proper donor selection is essential for good outcomes after heart-lung transplantation. Generally accepted criteria for donor selection are listed in Table 47-2.

ALLOCATION SCHEME

In 1984, Congress passed the National Organ Transplantation Act, which created the Organ Procurement and Transplantation Network (OPTN). In 1986, the United Network for Organ Sharing (UNOS) was awarded a federal contract to administer the network as a private, nonprofit corporation. The US Department of Health and Human Services has recently renewed this contract for an additional three year period. Solid organs are distributed according to UNOS policies, which are based on medical criteria and intended to yield optimal use of a scarce resource. Allocation schemes are critically

Table 47-1. Contraindications to Heart-Lung Transplantation

Age >55 years
Major chronic disabling illness (eg, lupus, severe arthritis, amyloidosis)

Chronic functional impairment of other vital organs:
 	
  –Renal Insufficiency: serum creatinine >2.5 mg/dL or creatinine clearance <50 mL/min or urine protein excretion >1 gm/24 hours
 	
  –Hepatic Insufficiency: serum total bilirubin >3 mg/dL, serum transaminases >2x normal or elevations in prothrombin time with an INR of >2.0 off anticoagulation
 	
  –Hematologic Disorders: significant coagulation abnormalities, bleeding diathesis

Evidence of end-organ damage from diabetes (eg, retinopathy, nephropathy) and/or brittle diabetes (ie, frequent diabetic ketoacidosis)
Severe peripheral vascular disease or cerebrovascular disease
Active or recent malignancy
Evidence of ongoing or recent substance abuse
History of noncompliance with medical regimens, active mental illness or psychiatric instability
Lack of adequate social support
Morbid obesity – body mass index >50 kg/m2

Table 47-2. Criteria for Donor Selection

General

Age <50 years
    Appropriate size match (donor lung volume ≤ recipient lung volume*, donor weight ± 25% to 30% of recipient weight)
    Blood group compatibility
    Anticipated ischemic time <4 to 5 hours
    Absence of donor malignancy, severe systemic sepsis
    Negative serologies for hepatitis B, C and HIV
    Negative prospective crossmatch for sensitized (PRA >10% to 15%) recipients
    No prior intrapericardial/intrathoracic operation
    Absence of cardiac or pulmonary abnormalities upon inspection by donor surgeon

Cardiac function

Absence of coronary atherosclerosis (mandatory coronary angiography for male donors >40, females >45)
    Absence of underlying cardiac disease
    Acceptable ventricular function on echocardiography
    Acceptable hemodynamics on modest (<15 μg/kg per min dopamine) inotropic support

Pulmonary function

No significant history of pulmonary disease
    No aspiration
    Chest x-ray clear or with minimal infiltrate
    pAO2 >350 mmHg on FiO2 of 100%, 5 PEEP
    Absence of aspiration or significant secretions at bronchoscopy

*Matching donor to recipient height is the most practical way of selecting the appropriate donor size. Transverse thoracic diameter at the aortic knob and at the top of the diaphragm should be within 4 cm.

important for patients in need of a heart-lung transplant, given the high demand for solid organs and the limited supply of donors. Currently, there are 4,114 heart, 3,648 lung, and 219 heart-lung recipients on the UNOS wait list. In 1999, a total of 2,185 heart, 885 lung, and 49 heart-lung transplants were performed. Thus, the ratio of registrants to transplants (R/T) is 1.9 for hearts, 4.1 for lungs and 4.5 for heart-lungs. The allocation of hearts and lungs is based primarily on medical urgency and waiting time. The initial allocation scheme was introduced by UNOS in 1989. An important revision to this system has recently occurred and was introduced into practice in January, 1999. In the original system, heart-lung registrants were considered a separate category and were considered for a heart-lung block after status 1 heart recipients. In the new system, heart-lung recipients are no longer considered a separate category; rather they are listed on both the heart and the lung transplant list. When the patient is eligible to receive a heart, the lungs will be allocated from the same donor. If the patient is eligible to receive a lung in accordance with the allocation policy for lungs, the heart will be offered in combination with the lungs if no suitable status IA isolated heart candidate is eligible to receive the heart. At present, it is unclear if the new algorithm will substantially impact the number of heart-lung transplants performed. In 1998 under the old rules, 47 heart-lung transplants were performed in the United States. In 1999, with the new rules in place, 48 were performed.

SURGICAL PROCEDURE

The surgical techniques for combined heart-lung transplantation are well-described. Key considerations include careful attention to preservation of the phrenic, recurrent laryngeal, and vagus nerves, and meticulous attention to hemostasis with careful control of dilated bronchial and mediastinal collateral vessels.

DONOR OPERATION

Heart-lung procurement usually takes place in the context of a multi-organ donor operation. A median sternotomy provides wide exposure. The donor surgeon provides the final assessment of donor suitability by bronchoscopy, as well as direct inspection of the heart and lungs for evidence of contusion, coronary artery disease, or injury. Following heparinization, PGE1 is administered to counteract reflex pulmonary vasoconstriction secondary to the cold flush solution. The SVC is ligated and the IVC divided at the level of the diaphragm. An aortic cross-clamp is placed high on the ascending aorta and cardioplegia administered into the aortic root. Simultaneously, pulmoplegia is administered via the pulmonary artery. The left atrial appendage is amputated to provide venting of the left heart, and iced

saline is used for topical cooling of the heart and lungs. The heart-lung bloc is then excised by dissecting the plane between the esophagus and pericardium. It is helpful to use electrocautery for this dissection to minimize bleeding after implantation. The trachea is stapled/divided and the graft immersed in cold preservation solution for transport.

RECIPIENT CARDIECTOMY/ PNEUMONECTOMY

While many programs perform heart-lung transplantation via a median sternotomy, others prefer a 4th interspace clamshell incision. Aprotinin is used routinely. The aorta is cannulated at the level of the aortic arch, bicaval cannulae are placed, cardiopulmonary bypass is initiated, and the patient is cooled to 28 degrees Celsius. Cardiectomy is performed at the atrial level. The great vessels are transected 2 cm above the semilunar valves. Following cardiectomy, both phrenic nerves are isolated on generous pericardial flaps. Bilateral pneumonectomies are then performed, dividing both main bronchi with a stapler. A button of the left main pulmonary artery containing the ligamentum arteriosum is left intact to afford protection of the recurrent laryngeal nerve. Traditionally, a tracheal anastomosis has been performed one cartilage ring above the carina. With increasing experience with bilateral sequential lung transplantation, bibronchial anastomoses are now preferred. This has the important advantage of avoiding extensive dissection in the posterior mediastinum.

DONOR IMPLANTATION

Culture swabs of the donor trachea are performed. The right atrium is inspected for the presence of an interatrial communication, which is closed if present. The heart-lung block is then transferred to the recipient, passing both lungs beneath their respective phrenic pedicles. Some surgeons now prefer to place both pulmonary hila anterior to the phrenic nerves. This has the advantage of decreasing the amount of posterior mediastinal dissection, thereby minimizing the chance of phrenic or vagus nerve injury as well as enhancing exposure for control of intraoperative posterior mediastinal bleeding. Bibronchial anastomoses are then performed according to the telescoping technique of Hardesty. The right atrial anastomosis is then performed, followed by the aortic anastomosis. Similar to the trend in cardiac transplantation, many groups have moved to a bicaval technique for heart-lung transplantation.

IMMUNOSUPPRESSION

Current triple-drug immunosuppression protocols are identical to those administered to lung transplant recipients and include tacrolimus or cyclosporine, azathioprine or mycophenolate mofetil, and steroids. Cardiac rejection is rare in the absence of pulmonary rejection. In contrast, acute isolated pulmonary rejection is well-described. Therefore routine right heart catheterizations and biopsies are not performed. Surveillance transbronchial biopsy is performed three to four weeks after operation, and at three, six, nine, and 12 months postoperatively. Thereafter, biopsies are performed at three to four month intervals, or as clinical circumstances dictate. Given the small number of heart-lung transplants performed at many institutions, there is no meaningful clinical data on immunosuppressive protocols for this group of patients. Instead, lessons learned in isolated heart or lung transplantation are applied to the management of the heart-lung recipient.

The introduction of humanized monoclonal antibodies directed against ligands responsible for T cell activation and costimulation are promising for abrogating rejection and appear to have a low incidence of toxicity/global immunosuppression. Beniaminovitz and colleagues recently demonstrated the utility of monoclonal antibody blockade of the high-affinity interleukin-2 receptor in a prospective randomized trial of cardiac transplant recipients. Patients were randomized to induction immunosuppression with daclizumab (a humanized mononucleal antibody directed to the alpha chain of the interleukin-2 receptor) vs placebo, in combination with standard triple-drug immunosuppression. They found an impressive reduction in the frequency and severity of cardiac allograft rejection with no adverse reactions and no increased frequency of infection or malignancy among those treated with daclizumab. Application of this therapy to heart-lung recipients seems justified, and results of the first clinical trials of costimulatory blockade in thoracic organ recipients are anticipated.

DIAGNOSIS AND TREATMENT OF REJECTION

Pulmonary rejection is defined as grade II or higher on transbronchial biopsy, or clinically as dyspnea with a worsening A-a gradient associated with a radiographic infiltrate that resolves with augmented immunosuppression. Additional clinical signs of rejection include fever, tachypnea, a diminished FEV1, and a fall in vital capacity. After the first month, the chest radiograph is frequently normal during an episode of rejection. Empiric treatment of rejection without a histologic diagnosis is discouraged. Once a histologic diagnosis of rejection is secured, patients are treated with intravenous methylprednisolone at 1 gram/day for three days, followed by an augmented prednisone dose that is tapered back to the baseline maintenance dose. Generally a rapid clinical and radiographic improvement occurs after treatment of

an acute rejection episode. Acute rejection that is refractory to methylprednisolone therapy is treated with cytolytic therapy.

Chronic rejection, or obliterative bronchiolitis (OB), is defined either histologically or clinically by a reduction in the FEV1 of greater than 20%. OB is a fibrosing process of the small airways characterized by dense eosinophilic submucosal scar tissue that is partially or completely obstructive. OB remains a common, limiting, and challenging problem after heart-lung transplantation. It is the most common single cause of death late after heart-lung transplantation. The incidence of OB ranges from 55% to 71% five years posttransplantation. Multiple studies have demonstrated that the number of acute pulmonary rejection episodes is the dominant risk factor for subsequent development of OB. At present, therapy is limited to augmented immunosuppression, with equivocal results. OB substantially increases the risk of developing fungal and bacterial pulmonary infections, so caution must be used in exercising this treatment option.

EXPECTED OUTCOMES AND RISK FACTORS

The presence of two pulmonary allografts seems to confer an immunologic advantage to the transplanted heart: the incidence of both acute and chronic cardiac rejection is clearly lower in patients receiving a heart-lung bloc than an isolated heart transplant. In the Stanford experience, 37% of heart-lung recipients were free from (acute) cardiac rejection five years posttransplantation, in comparison with only 7% of isolated heart transplant recipients. Similarly, chronic allograft vasculopathy (CAV) is significantly less common in recipients of heart-lung transplants: freedom from CAV at five years was 89% for heart-lung recipients vs 73% for heart-only recipients. In contrast to chronic cardiac allograft vasculopathy, the lungs do not appear to enjoy an immunologic advantage from being transplanted in the heart-lung configuration. In an early experience at the University of Pittsburgh, Keenan noted a similar incidence of both acute pulmonary rejection and OB among recipients of lung and heart-lung transplants. In the Stanford experience, the freedom from OB was similar in the lung and heart-lung group three years posttransplantation at 50% and 42% respectively.

Results of heart-lung transplantation remain inferior to those of isolated heart or lung transplantation. Current data from the International Society for Heart and Lung Transplantation (ISHLT) show 1-year survival rates of 60% after heart-lung transplantation, with 5-year survival rates of 40%, in contrast to 1-year survival rates of 79% for heart and 71% for lung transplantation. The most common causes of death in the early (0 to 30 days) postoperative period included non-specific graft failure, infection, and bleeding. Mid-term (31 days to one year) deaths were most commonly due to infection, while late deaths were caused by obliterative bronchiolitis and infection. Improvements in early outcomes for patients requiring replacement of both the heart and lungs will require an understanding of the mechanisms of early (lung) allograft dysfunction and the development of techniques to avoid this problem. Similarly, improved long-term outcomes await a solution to the vexing problem of OB.

RECOMMENDED READING

Cooley DA, Bloodwell RD, Hallman GL, Nora JJ, Harrison GM, Leachman RD. Organ transplantation for advanced cardiopulmonary disease. Ann Thorac Surg. 1969;8(1):30-46.

Wildevuur CR, Benfield JR. A review of 23 human lung transplantations by 20 surgeons. Ann Thorac Surg. 1970;9(6):489-515.

Losman JG, Campbell CD, Replogle RL, Barnard CN. Joint transplantation of the heart and lungs. Past experience and present potentials. J Cardiovasc Surg. 1982;23(6):440-452.

Reitz BA, Burton NA, Jamieson SW, et al. Heart and lung transplantation: autotransplantation and allotransplantation in primates with extended survival. J Thorac Cardiovasc Surg. 1980;80(3):360-372.

Reitz BA, Wallwork JL, Hunt SA, et al. Heart-lung transplantation: successful therapy for patients with pulmonary vascular disease. N Engl J Med. 1982;306(10):557-564.

Anonymous. Unilateral lung transplantation for pulmonary fibrosis. Toronto Lung Transplant Group. N Engl J Med. 1986;314(18):1140-1145.

Patterson GA, Cooper JD, Dark JH, Jones MT. Experimental and clinical double lung transplantation. J Thorac Cardiovasc Surg. 1988;95(1):70-74.

Kramer MR, Valantine HA, Marshall SE, Starnes VA, Theodore J. Recovery of the right ventricle after single-lung transplantation in pulmonary hypertension. Am J Cardiol. 1994;73(7):494-500.

Hauptman PJ, O'Connor KJ. Procurement and allocation of solid organs for transplantation. N Engl J Med. 1997;336(6):422-431.

Renlund DG, Taylor DO, Kfoury AG, Shaddy RS. New UNOS rules: historical background and implications for transplantation management. United Network for Organ Sharing. J Heart Lung Transplant. 1999;18(11):-1065-1070.

Griffith BP, Magliato KE. Heart-lung transplantation. Operative techniques in thoracic and cardiovascular surgery. 1999;4:124-141.

Lick SD, Copeland JG, Rosado LJ, Arabia FA, Sethi GK. Simplified technique of heart-lung transplantation. Ann Thorac Surg. 1995;59(6):1592-1593.

Griffith BP, Magee MJ, Gonzalez IF, et al. Anastomotic pitfalls in lung transplantation. J Thorac Cardiovasc Surg. 1994;107(3):743-753.

Griffith BP, Hardesty RL, Trento A, Bahnson HT. Asynchronous rejection of heart and lungs following cardiopulmonary transplantation. Ann Thorac Surg. 1985;40(5):488-493.

Glanville AR, Imoto E, Baldwin JC, Billingham ME, Theodore J, Robin ED. The role of right ventricular endomyocardial biopsy in the long-term management of heart-lung transplant recipients. J Heart Transplant. 1987;6(6):357-361.

Harlan DM, Kirk AD. The future of organ and tissue transplantation: can T-cell costimulatory pathway modifiers revolutionize the prevention of graft rejection? JAMA. 1999;282(11):1076-1082.

Yousem SA, Berry GJ, Cagle PT, et al. Revision of the 1990 working formulation for the classification of pulmonary allograft rejection: Lung Rejection Study Group. J Heart Lung Transplant. 1996;15(1 Pt 1):1-15.

Reitz BA, Poston RS. Heart-Lung Transplantation. In: Franco KL, Verrier ED, eds. Advanced Therapy in Cardiac Surgery. Hamilton, Ontario: BC Decker; 1999:491-501.

Hosenpud JD, Bennett LE, Keck BM, Fiol B, Boucek MM, Novick RJ. The Registry of the International Society for Heart and Lung Transplantation: fifteenth official report – 1998. J Heart Lung Transplant. 1998;7(7):656-668.

Sharples LD, Tamm M, McNeil K, Higenbottam TW, Stewart S, Wallwork J. Development of bronchiolitis obliterans syndrome in recipients of heart-lung transplantation – early risk factors. Transplantation. 1996;61(4):560-566.

Reichenspurner H, Girgis RE, Robbins RC, et al. Stanford experience with obliterative bronchiolitis after lung and heart-lung transplantation. Ann Thorac Surg. 1996;62(5):1467-1472.

Bando K, Paradis IL, Similo S, et al. Obliterative bronchiolitis after lung and heart-lung transplantation. An analysis of risk factors and management. J Thorac Cardiovasc Surg. 1995;110(1):4-13.

McCurry KR, Iacono AT, Dauber JH, et al. Lung and heart-lung transplantation at the University of Pittsburgh. In: Cecka, Terasaki, eds. Clinical Transplants. Los Angeles, CA: UCLA Tissue Typing Laboratory; 1997:209-218.

Sarris GE, Smith JA, Shumway NE, et al. Long-term results of combined heart-lung transplantation: the Stanford experience. J Heart Lung Transplant. 1994; 13(6):940-949.

Keenan RJ, Bruzzone P, Paradis IL, et al. Similarity of pulmonary rejection patterns among heart-lung and double-lung transplant recipients. Transplantation. 1991;51(1):176-180.

Section VI

KIDNEY AND PANCREAS TRANSPLANTATION

48 HISTORY OF KIDNEY AND PANCREAS TRANSPLANTATION

Paul E. Morrissey, MD
Peter N. Madras, MD
Anthony P. Monaco, MD

Many milestones in human achievement were realized in the year preceding December 1954. The USSR launched Sputnik. Roger Banister broke the 4-minute mile barrier. Peter Medawar and colleagues demonstrated acquired neonatal tolerance to skin allografts. Inspired by this development, the first successful treatment of chronic renal failure was administered that December in the form of renal transplantation between identical twins, thereby marking the beginning of an era in transplantation science and medicine. Since the modest and largely unsuccessful beginnings of renal transplantation in the 1950s (identical twin transplants only) and 1960s (first successful cadaver renal transplant), there has been a continuous rise in the annual number of transplants and their success.

At the turn of the 20th century, several investigators hypothesized that organ replacement could be applied as a therapy for organ failure. Emerich Ullmann (1861-1937) performed the first well-recorded studies in organ transplantation in Vienna. He performed several successful allografts in large animal models. Perhaps his most remarkable achievement was the transplantation of a dog kidney to the carotid vessels of a goat with function. Not long afterward, Alexis Carrel began his early experiments in transplantation and the suturing of blood vessels. In 1905, he established the animal model of bilateral nephrectomy followed by renal transplantation, which he published as a single case in *Science* under the title "Successful transplantation of both kidneys from a dog into a bitch with removal of both normal kidneys from the latter." As evidence of the developing surgical confidence of the era, and in desperation to offer some therapy to patients with renal failure, several xeno-

transplants, termed *heterografts*, were carried out from animal donors (ie, pig, goat, lamb, and monkey) to man. Success was nonexistent.

The first attempted renal allograft took place at the Methodist Episcopal Hospital in Philadelphia on November 14, 1911. By report in the *New York Times* (there is no account in the medical literature), a pedestrian was struck dead by a carriage outside the hospital where a patient was dying from renal failure. The cadaver donor organ was quickly procured and transplanted by Doctor LJ Hammond. Although the organ did not function, the brief newspaper article addressed many of the still current issues in solid organ transplantation, including the need for improved methods of organ preservation, the shortage of organs, and the ethics of cadaver organ donation.

Yu Yu Voronoy, in Kiev, described the next human renal allograft from an ABO-incompatible cadaver renal donor to a man with mercury poisoning. The kidney never functioned and the patient died in less than 48 hours. In 1947, a pregnant woman at the Peter Bent Brigham Hospital in Boston developed renal tubulopathy from uterine sepsis. After a prolonged period of anuria it was decided to attempt a renal transplant and the surgical team undertook the task of locating a cadaver donor. Fortunately, one was found and David Hume procured the kidney. The kidney was "transplanted" extracorporeally to the brachial artery and median cubital vein and functioned for a period sufficient to clear the renal waste products, awaken the patient from coma and recover native renal function. Although the functional success of the transplant was limited to a few days, the transplant likely represents the first lifesaving allograft. In 1950, R Lawler performed an orthotopic renal transplant with some limited function. In 1951, eight renal allografts were attempted in France by various groups. Ultimately, it was realized that transplantation without immunosuppression was doomed to failure.

Around the time that enthusiasm for renal transplantation may have been declining, fate brought forth the circumstance of the historic renal transplant between identical twin brothers at the Peter Bent Brigham Hospital. On December 23, 1954, Richard Herrick underwent living-related renal transplant from his twin brother, Ronald, followed a few days later by bilateral nephrectomy for persistent hypertension. He survived 8.5 years and represents the first "successful" renal transplant and, in a broader sense, the first patient "cured" of end-stage renal disease. By 1958, the Peter Bent Brigham Hospital had reported seven living-related renal transplant procedures from twin donors, while the search for adequate immunosuppression continued.

The immune depressant effects of cortisone and x-rays were recognized in the 1950s. The first use of

Paul E. Morrissey, MD, Assistant Professor of Surgery, Brown University; Co-Director, Transplant Services, Rhode Island Hospital

Peter N. Madras, MD, Associate Professor of Surgery, Harvard Medical School; Co-Director, Transplant Services, Rhode Island Hospital

Anthony P. Monaco, MD, Director, Transplant Center, Beth Israel-Deaconess Medical Center; Peter Medawar Professor of Transplant Surgery, Harvard Medical School

clinical immunosuppression was at the Peter Bent Brigham Hospital (1958 to 1960) using total body irradiation with subsequent reconstitution by a bone marrow allograft. In the group's sixth case, the protocol was applied to a living-related renal transplant from a fraternal twin. The allograft was accepted, representing the first successful living-related renal transplant under immunosuppression. Hamburger's group duplicated the feat in Paris and, a year later, Kuss applied the protocol to a sister-to-brother combination with success. In 1959, Schwartz and Dameshek showed that the compound 6-mercaptopurine was capable of blocking antibody production in rabbits injected with human albumin. These findings were applied to transplantation in the animal laboratory the following year by Roy Calne, visiting in the laboratories at the Peter Bent Brigham Hospital, and by Charles Zukoski at the Medical College of Virginia. The group at the Peter Bent Brigham Hospital used 6-mercaptopurine clinically on April 14, 1960, and its imidazole derivative, azathioprine, on March 22, 1961. In 1962, under drug (azathioprine) immunosuppression, the team at the Peter Bent Brigham Hospital succeeded in another first: cadaver renal transplantation. The allograft survived one year and the success quickly produced a flurry of international transplant activity, ushering in the present era of transplantation using drug immunosuppression.

In short course, steroids were introduced to clinical immunosuppression. The subsequent combination of azathioprine and steroids brought kidney transplantation into the mainstream. In the next year, 25 renal transplant programs began in the US. The clinical introduction of antilymphocyte globulin combined with drug therapy resulted in an encouraging 45% 1-year graft survival. Refinements in patient selection, postoperative care and antibiotics eventually resulted in near 80% 1-year graft survival following living-related renal transplantation, although 1-year graft survival for cadaver renal transplantation remained closer to 50%. By the end of the 1970s, living-related renal transplantation was an accepted and effective therapy for end-stage renal disease. However, some of the earlier enthusiasm for cadaver renal transplantation had diminished. Five-year cadaver renal allograft survival was only 35%. Azathioprine and prednisone were routinely used, but antilymphocyte globulin was not readily available. The morbidity of massive infusions of methylprednisolone was prohibitive. Again, advances in pharmacology served as the catalyst for clinical improvement. Calne reported the first use of cyclosporine, used as monotherapy, in human renal transplantation. Protocols were quickly devised to overcome nephrotoxicity, and soon lower doses of cyclosporine were employed in combination with azathioprine and steroids. The results were astounding. Lower doses of all the immunosuppressive agents resulted in a marked decrease in drug-related side effects. Furthermore, the regimens were effective. First-year survival after cadaver renal transplantation surpassed 80% in many centers.

Organ preservation by cooling was first applied in the 1960s. Nonetheless, multiple organ procurement was rare in the early days of transplantation, and it was not until 1978 that two kidneys, the heart and the liver, were procured from a single donor. However, single cadavers provided both kidney and pancreas for simultaneous transplantation beginning in 1966.

PANCREAS

Transplantation of the pancreas, like other solid organs, began in surgical laboratories and was introduced with limited success in the clinical arena shortly thereafter. Prior to undertaking transplantation in humans, investigators had proven endocrine function by documenting serum glucose and circulating insulin levels, and had worked out some of the basic principles of the effect of acute rejection on exocrine function of the gland. Successful canine allotransplantation under azathioprine and steroid immunosuppression established the feasibility of the procedure in humans.

William Kelly and Richard Lillehei pioneered human pancreas transplantation on December 17, 1966. The graft was placed intra-abdominally and vascularized via the iliac blood supply. A long segment of duodenum accompanied the pancreas and was brought out as a cutaneous duodenostomy. The initial allograft, a partial pancreatic allograft, was lost to a pancreatic leak, a complication that did not arise in the nine kidney-pancreas (whole organ) transplants performed over the following two years. Both allografts functioned for greater than a year in only one of ten recipients. As a result, whole organ pancreas transplantation was temporarily abandoned for clinical studies of isolated islet transplantation. These functioned well in the laboratory, but none of the first 24 patients became euglycemic. Islet cell transplantation remains an elusive procedure with less than 2% of grafted islets resulting in long-term survival and insulin independence. New life was breathed into these failed projects with the advent of cyclosporine.

Quantum improvements were noted in pancreas transplantation with the use of better immunosuppression. However, a high rate of morbidity remained with the procedure. In an effort to decrease the perioperative morbidity, a number of technical innovations were developed to improve the procedure. Beyond improved pharmacology, immunologic improvements included better matching, live donor transplantation, a better understanding of the immunogenicity of the pancreas allograft and a variety of clinically applicable methods to detect allograft rejection. Surgical innovations were aimed at treating the metabolic, mucosal and duodenal complications associated with pancreatic exocrine secretion. Pancreatic exocrine secretions were first drained via the recipient ureter. Hans Sollinger modified the technique by directly anastomosing a button of duodenal tissue to the bladder. Robert Corry and Dai Nghiem developed the current practice of duodenocystostomy several years later. Further modifications included the injection of synthetic polymers into the pancreatic duct to obliterate the exocrine secretions as pioneered by Dubernard, and an enthusiastic return at many centers to enteric exocrine drainage combined with portal venous drainage, a technique first attributed to Roy Calne. With these modifications, pancreas transplantation approximates the success of cadaver renal transplantation. Presently, the surgical techniques are well-established, although no consensus is available on the preferred approach. Many clinical studies are underway to evaluate the end-organ benefits of euglycemia achieved by pancreas transplantation and the possible negative vascular effects of hyperinsulinemia resulting from the systemic rather than portal drainage of the pancreas allograft.

RECOMMENDED READING

Ullmann E. Kidney allografts and xenografts in dogs and goats. Experimentielle Nierentransplantation. Wien Klin Wochenschr. 1902;15:281.

Carrel A. Successful transplantation of both kidneys from a dog into a bitch with removal of both normal kidneys from the latter. Science. 1906;23:394-395.

Groth C. Landmarks in clinical renal transplantation. Surg Gynecol Obstet. 1972;134(2):327-328.

New York Times. November 14, 1911, page 2. Editorial Nov. 15, 1911, page 10. This is the first account of human-to-human renal transplantation. An editorial the next day discussed many salient issues including organ preservation by cooling, cadaver organ donation and overcoming the shortage of cadaver organs by xeno-transplantation.

Moore FD, ed. Transplant: The Give and Take of Organ Transplantation. New York, NY: Simon and Schuster; 1972. This book is fascinating reading. The inner workings of the Peter Bent Brigham Hospital are disclosed as the problem of renal replacement is tackled from all aspects. Included are the clinical development of hemodialysis and thirty years of laboratory and clinical work in renal transplantation.

Hamburger J. Memories of old times. In: Terasaki PI, ed. History of Transplantation: Thirty-five Recollections. Los Angeles, Ca: UCLA Tissue Typing Laboratory; 1991.

Brent L, ed. A History of Transplantation Immunology. New York, NY: Academic Press; 1997. This outstanding compilation of transplantation immunology is put together by Leslie Brent, Emeritus Professor of Immunology at Saint Mary's Hospital. Brent, a zoologist by training, performed with Medawar and Billingham the seminal experiments in neonatal tolerance. This work reviews the field from those early days through current times and describes in great detail the cooperation and sharing of information among immunologists, geneticists and transplantation physicians which accounts for the present success of transplantation.

Merrill JP, Murray JE, Takacs F. Successful transplantation of a kidney from a human cadaver. JAMA. 1963;185:347. Although the twin transplant remains the best known, these first successful renal transplantations with immunosuppressive drugs are the basis of modern organ transplantation – the real "landmark" case.

Calne RY, White DJG, Thiru S, et al. Cyclosporin A in patients receiving renal allografts from cadaver donors. Lancet. 1978;2:1323-1327.

Lillehei RC, Simmons RL, Najarian JS, et al. Pancreatico-duodenal allotransplantation: experimental and clinical experience. Ann Surg. 1970;172(3):405-436.

Hering BJ, Ricordi C. Islet transplantation for patients with type I diabetes. Graft. 1999;2(1):12-27.

Di Carlo V, Castoldi R, Cristallo M, et al. Techniques of pancreas transplantation through the world: An IPITA center survey. Transplant Proc. 1998;30(2): 231-241.

49 EVALUATION AND MANAGEMENT OF PROSPECTIVE KIDNEY RECIPIENTS

Bertram L. Kasiske, MD

The pretransplant evaluation should determine whether a patient is an appropriate candidate for transplantation, and adequately prepare the potential recipient to maximize the chances that the transplant will be successful. Not all end-stage renal disease (ERSD) patients are suitable for transplantation, and physicians need to evaluate patients carefully to help them make this important decision. A patient should be denied transplantation if it is felt that the risks outweigh the potential benefits to such a degree that the patient would be better served by remaining on dialysis. However, an equally important goal of the transplant evaluation is to detect and treat reversible medical conditions that increase the risks of transplantation. The major risks of transplantation are attributable to the surgical procedure itself and to the immunosuppressive medications used to prevent rejection. The risk of surgery in a patient with severe renal insufficiency or ESRD is higher than the risk of surgery in healthy individuals. Much of that risk can be attributed to the high prevalence of cardiovascular disease in candidates for renal transplantation. However, if patients survive the immediate postoperative period with a functioning kidney, they must then be subjected to both the immune and the nonimmune risks of the immunosuppressive medications. Those risks can, in part, be assessed in the pretransplant evaluation.

TIMING OF TRANSPLANTATION

The transplant evaluation should begin as soon as it is clear that a patient is destined to develop ESRD. Occasionally, patients with renal disease from malignant hypertension, severe acute tubular necrosis and other causes recover renal function several weeks after initiation of dialysis for presumed ESRD. Transplantation should be delayed in patients who may regain function. On the other hand, some patients who are nearing ESRD can receive a transplant before initiating dialysis. Due to the long waiting times for a cadaver renal transplant, this preemptive transplantation is usually only possible if there is a living donor. Patients without a

Professor of Medicine, Division of Nephrology, Department of Medicine, University of Minnesota, Hennepin County Medical Center, Minneapolis, MN

living donor must be placed on the cadaveric transplantation list. For adults, waiting time can only accrue when transplant evaluation is complete and the measured or estimated creatinine clearance is 20 mL/min or lower. Children (<18 years) can be placed on the list any time the transplant evaluation has been completed.

CARDIOVASCULAR DISEASE

The most common cause of allograft failure after renal transplantation is death with a functioning graft, and the most common cause of death is cardiovascular disease (Figure 49-1).

The risk of surgery is substantially increased by ischemic heart disease, and myocardial infarctions (MIs) are common in the early posttransplant period. Manske et al, conducted a prospective trial in which asymptomatic, diabetic patients with moderately severe coronary artery disease (ie, lesions occluding >70% of the artery on angiography) were randomly allocated to medical management or pretransplant coronary revascularization. Patients who underwent angioplasty or bypass surgery had fewer posttransplant ischemic heart disease events compared to patients who were allocated to medical management. Although this study was very small, it provided the strongest evidence to date that preemptive therapy for ischemic heart disease before transplantation is effective in at least some high-risk patients. This provides a strong rationale for screening and detecting asymptomatic coronary artery disease as part of the pretransplant evaluation. In addition to identifying candidates for coronary revascularization, detecting asymptomatic coronary artery disease may help to identify

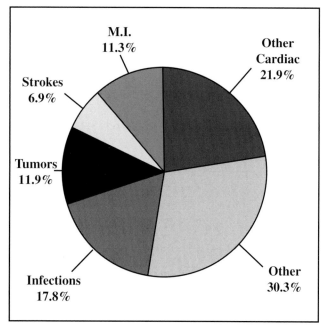

Figure 49-1. Causes of death after renal transplantation. Data are from the United States Renal Data System, 1998.

patients for whom intensive risk factor management will be particularly effective in preventing cardiovascular disease events.

Most transplant centers feel that high-risk individuals should undergo a cardiac evaluation. A history of pretransplant cardiovascular disease is one of the strongest risk factors for posttransplant cardiovascular disease events, and patients with a history of ischemic heart disease should be carefully evaluated as part of the transplant work-up. Patients with a history of peripheral or cerebral vascular disease should also be screened for ischemic heart disease, since the incidence of coronary artery disease is high in this population. Patients with no history of cardiovascular disease, but who have known risk factors, should also be considered for screening. Although there are no fail-safe criteria to predict cardiovascular disease, diabetics, individuals over the age of 45, or younger nondiabetic patients with multiple risk factors can be targeted for screening.

Some centers carry out coronary angiography on all high-risk patients. However, coronary angiography is expensive and is associated with some risk. For example, the radiocontrast used for angiography may accelerate the need for dialysis in patients approaching ESRD. For all of these reasons, most centers first conduct non-invasive stress testing in high-risk transplant candidates. Exercise or pharmacological stress can be used with either radionuclide or echocardiographic imaging. There is no clear advantage of one procedure over another. It is perhaps more important to use the test for which the center has the most expertise.

Patients with severe symptomatic or asymptomatic ischemic heart disease should undergo revascularization prior to transplantation if possible. However, some patients with severe, diffuse coronary artery disease may not be candidates for revascularization. Such patients, especially if myocardial function is markedly reduced, may be candidates for simultaneous heart and kidney transplantation. Some patients with minimal coronary artery disease and decreased myocardial function may do well after renal transplantation, and may have a substantial improvement in myocardial function.

Screening for asymptomatic cerebral vascular disease is controversial. Studies in the general population suggest that patients with asymptomatic carotid bruits and significant narrowing of the carotid arteries on ultrasound examination have better outcomes with prophylactic endarterectomy than with medical management. However, results are dependent on the experience and skill of the local physicians and surgeons. Renal transplant candidates with an asymptomatic carotid bruit should probably undergo carotid ultrasound. Patients with significant, asymptomatic carotid disease, and patients with symptomatic disease should probably be managed like other, nontransplant patients.

MALIGNANCIES

Cancer is a major cause of morbidity and mortality after renal transplantation. The incidence of most tumors is increased when renal transplant recipients are compared to controls matched for age and gender. Most of the increase in cancer is probably due to chronic immunosuppression, and the transplant evaluation should include efforts to reduce the risk of cancer after transplantation. These efforts should include screening for malignancies already present in the potential recipient, and reducing or eliminating risk factors such as cigarette smoking and viral infections known to be associated with cancer after transplantation.

How often subclinical tumors that are present at the time of transplantation lead to disseminated cancer posttransplant is unknown. Nevertheless, it is generally accepted that immunosuppression favors the growth of tumors. Screening for cancer should begin with a thorough physical examination. In addition, screening for colorectal malignancies should include digital rectal examination, stool occult blood test, as well as flexible sigmoidoscopy or colonoscopy in older individuals. Screening for lung cancer should include a chest x-ray. Men should be screened for prostate cancer with a digital rectal examination and possibly prostate-specific antigen, although the latter remains controversial. Women should have a pelvic examination and Pap test. Women over the age of 40 to 50 should have a mammogram, as should younger women with a family history of breast cancer. Screening for renal cell carcinoma usually requires imaging of the native kidneys with ultrasound, computerized tomography or magnetic resonance imaging.

For the transplant candidate who has a history of cancer that is "cured", the most common approach has been to allow an appropriate disease-free interval to elapse before transplantation. Exceptions include non-invasive malignancies such as benign forms of skin cancer, or in situ tumors. Based on registry data that has documented the interval of recurrence for many posttransplant malignancies, it has generally been recommended that a 2-year interval is necessary and sufficient for most invasive tumors (Table 49-1).

Recent evidence has indicated that cigarette smoking at the time of transplantation is associated with an increased incidence of cancer and increased mortality after renal transplantation. Efforts should be made to strongly encourage potential transplant recipients to quit smoking. Organized smoking cessation programs are more successful than cursory advice offered in a busy clinical setting. Transplant candidates who smoke should be encouraged, or perhaps even required, to attend a smoking cessation program. Some have even advocated that a documented, smoke-free interval be required before transplantation.

Table 49-1. Suggested Disease-Free Intervals for Transplantation of Patients with a History of Cancer

Waiting Period	Cancer
None	In situ cancers (bladder, cervical) Duke's A colon cancer Clarke's level I melanoma Basal cell skin cancer Incidental renal tumors
At least two years	Renal tumors Wilm's tumor Invasive bladder cancer Invasive cervical cancer Testicular cancer Thyroid cancer Sarcoma Prostate cancer Lymphoma Squamous cell carcinoma
Greater than two years (about five years)	Breast cancer Colorectal cancer Melanoma

From: Ramos EL, Kasiske BL, Danovitch GM. Pre-Transplant Evaluation of the Recipient. In: Norman DJ, Suki WN, eds. Primer on Transplantation. Primer on Transplantation. 1st ed. Thorofare, NJ: American Society of Transplantation; 1998:183-189.

Emerging evidence indicates that the Epstein-Barr virus (EBV) is responsible for much of the posttransplant lymphoproliferative disorders (PTLDs) that occur after organ transplantation. Most advocate measuring antibodies to EBV pretransplant, since the risk for PTLD is highest for transplant recipients who are EBV antibody-negative at the time of transplantation. Unfortunately, there is as yet no effective vaccine for EBV antibody-negative recipients. Studies are ongoing to determine the effectiveness of intravenous immunoglobulin or antiviral prophylaxis after transplantation.

INFECTIONS

Infections are a major cause of morbidity and mortality after renal transplantation. Pretransplant vaccinations should include influenza, pneumococcus, and hepatitis B. Varicella vaccination may also be appropriate for children and other seronegative individuals. An active, potentially life-threatening infection is usually considered an absolute contraindication to renal transplantation, and screening for infection should be an integral part of the pretransplant evaluation.

Evidence for tuberculosis should be sought with history, physical examination, chest x-ray, and purified protein derivative (PPD) skin testing if there is no history of a positive PPD. Patients who are PPD-positive, who have not already been appropriately treated for tuberculosis, and especially patients from high-risk populations should be considered for isoniazid prophylaxis if there are no contraindications. The duration of isoniazid prophylaxis is usually six months.

Cytomegalovirus (CMV) infection causes more morbidity and mortality after renal transplantation than any other infectious organism. CMV antibody should be measured as part of the pretransplant evaluation, because CMV-negative recipients are at increased risk for infection. High-risk individuals can be targeted for antiviral prophylaxis beginning immediately after transplantation.

All transplant candidates should be tested for human immunodeficiency virus (HIV). HIV has been considered to be an absolute contraindication to renal transplantation. However, the development of effective antiviral therapies has recently led some to reconsider whether all HIV-positive patients should be excluded. Certainly, transplantation of HIV-positive individuals should be considered "experimental" at this time, and should only be done with informed consent.

Patients from areas endemic for *Strongyloides stercoralis* (ie, tropical and subtropical regions) should be screened and treated prior to transplantation. Screening includes stool for ova and parasites and serologic testing. Other, common, occult infections that should be considered include: dental abscesses and periodontal disease; urinary tract infections; and dialysis access sites infections, especially peritoneal dialysis catheters and temporary catheters for hemodialysis.

HEPATOBILIARY DISEASE

Viral hepatitis continues to be a major cause of morbidity after renal transplantation. In some cases, viral hepatitis can cause progressive liver disease and death. However, viral hepatitis is usually not an absolute contraindication to transplantation. Although the risk of transplantation is increased by hepatitis, this risk must be weighed against the risk of remaining on dialysis. Certainly, patients with advanced liver disease and a limited life expectancy should probably not receive a kidney transplant.

The incidence of hepatitis B virus (HBV) infection in ESRD patients has decreased over the last three decades. The reduction in HBV infection resulted from the use of effective isolation techniques in dialysis units, a decrease in the transmission of HBV through blood transfusion, and the introduction of an effective vaccine. Potential transplant candidates with HBV should usually undergo liver biopsy as part of the transplant evaluation. Patients with active disease may sometimes benefit from a course of antiviral therapy prior to transplantation.

Just as HBV has become increasingly rare, hepatitis C virus (HCV) has become relatively common. The consequences of HCV after transplantation have been a source of controversy. In general, most transplant recipients have relatively mild disease and a chronic, indolent course. However, some patients develop progressive disease with cirrhosis. Patients with HCV and clinical evidence of disease activity may need a liver biopsy as part of the pretransplant evaluation. The role of pretransplant, antiviral therapy for HCV is unclear, but some patients may benefit from this approach. Adverse effects of α-interferon, including allograft rejection, make therapy with α-interferon more difficult after transplantation.

With the widespread adoption of erythropoietin, liver disease from iron overload has become unusual in dialysis patients. Drugs and other hepatotoxins should be considered in patients with increased liver enzymes. Although patients with symptomatic cholecystitis generally need a cholecystectomy, most patients with asymptomatic cholelithiasis do not.

GASTROINTESTINAL DISEASES

Routine gastrointestinal x-rays or endoscopy are probably not necessary for all patients. Rather, screening for esophagitis and peptic ulcer disease can be reserved for patients with symptoms. Patients with a history of recent peptic ulcer disease should probably undergo endoscopy to document complete healing.

RENAL DISEASE RECURRENCE

With the exception of Alport's syndrome, polycystic kidney disease, and interstitial nephritis, most kidney diseases can recur in the allograft (Table 49-2).

As graft survival continues to improve, survival with a functioning allograft will also improve and recurrence of renal disease will no doubt become more common. However, renal disease recurrence is rarely a cause of graft failure and, therefore, rarely a contraindication to transplantation. Nevertheless, patients should be fully informed of the likelihood for disease recurrence and its potential consequences during the pretransplant evaluation.

Diabetes is now the most common cause of renal failure leading to transplantation. Diabetes inevitably recurs in the renal allograft, although its clinical onset and rate of progression are usually slow. Nevertheless, in occasional patients diabetes may occur within the first few years after transplant. As graft and patient survival improve, recurrent diabetes will no doubt become a more common cause of graft failure.

One of the most dramatic examples of recurrent renal disease occurs with idiopathic, focal, segmental glomerulosclerosis. The overall chances of recurrence are approximately 10% to 30%, and if the disease recurs, it may lead to graft failure in 40% to 50%. The strongest predictor is a history of recurrence in a previous transplant. Patients with a particularly rapid rate of decline in renal function are also at increased risk for disease recurrence. Reports suggest that there may be an as-yet-unidentified circulating factor that causes disease recurrence, and that aggressive plasmapheresis may induce remission of recurrent disease after transplantation.

Most feel that both systemic and renal manifestations of systemic lupus erythematosus should be clinically quiescent before transplantation. Similarly, serologic evidence of disease activity should be in remission. Interestingly, the risk for clinically significant disease recurrence is quite low, probably under 10%.

Although rare, primary oxalosis was once considered to be a disease that was hopeless. Renal transplantation was felt to be contraindicated due to the rapid deposition of oxalate in the allograft. Current management of primary oxalosis includes preemptive (early) transplantation before ESRD is reached. Patients should be treated aggressively with orthophosphate and pyridoxine, and preemptive liver transplantation should also be considered. Cystinosis in children can be treated with oral analogues of cysteamine to delay the onset of ESRD. Recurrence does not occur because the trans-

Table 49-2. Recurrent Disease in the Kidney Transplant

	Risk (%)	Graft Loss (%)
Primary Disease		
Focal, segmental glomerulosclerosis	10-30	40-50
IgA nephropathy	25-50	10
Membranoproliferative GN type I	20-30	~40
Membranoproliferative GN type II	~80	10-20
Membranous GN	10-20	~30
Secondary Diseases		
Systemic lupus erythematosus	~10	30-40
Hemolytic uremic syndrome	10-25	~50
Henoch-Schönlein purpura	~10	10-20
Diabetes	100	Unusual
Primary oxalosis	100	?
Mixed essential cryoglobulinemia	~50	?
Waldenström's macroglobulinemia	10-25	?
Light chain deposition disease	~50	?
Fibrillary GN	~50	?
Amyloidosis	20-30	?
Scleroderma	~20	?

From: Ramos EL, Kasiske BL, Danovitch GM. Pre-transplant evaluation of the recipient. In: Norman DJ, Suki WN, eds. Primer on Transplantation. 1st ed. Thorofare, NJ: American Society of Transplantation; 1998:183-189.

planted kidney corrects the deficiency in the specific transport system for lysosomal cystine efflux. Survival after transplantation of patients with Fabry's disease is usually acceptable, and histologic disease recurrence does not generally affect allograft function.

Hemolytic uremic syndrome recurs in 10% to 25%. Of those who develop recurrence, approximately 50% will lose their grafts. Anecdotal reports have implicated oral contraceptive use, immunosuppression with calcineurin inhibitors, and other factors as possibly influencing the chances of recurrence. Histologic recurrence of IgA nephropathy is common, but graft failure due to recurrent IgA nephropathy is rare. Similarly, histologic recurrence of Henoch-Schönlein purpura is common, with histologic evidence of recurrence in up to 75%, but in only 10% will recurrence lead to renal dysfunction. In 10% to 20% of patients with membranous glomerulonephritis, the disease will recur in the allograft, and in approximately 30% of these, the recurrence will contribute to allograft failure. However, membranous nephropathy more commonly arises de novo after transplantation. Type I membranoproliferative glomerulonephritis recurs in 20% to 30% and leads to graft loss in about 40% of these. Although type II membranoproliferative glomerulonephritis recurs in 80%, graft loss is seen in only 10% to 20% of cases. Deposition diseases (ie, immunoglobulin light chain deposition disease, Waldenström's macroglobulinemia, fibrillary glomerulonephritis, and amyloidosis) can also recur in the allograft, but outcomes are more often determined by the presence or absence of systemic complications of these diseases than their recurrence in the allograft.

Although graft survival is probably reduced in sickle cell disease (approximately 67% at one year), this is not a contraindication to transplantation. There are some anecdotal reports of recurrence in Wegener's granulomatosus, but most patients appear to do well. It is probably wise to wait until the disease is quiescent before carrying out transplant. Scleroderma recurs in about 20% and can lead to graft failure. However, many patients with scleroderma do very well after renal transplantation.

LUNG DISEASE

The risk from lung disease that is not due to infection is largely the risk of anesthesia and surgery. The risk of surgery in patients with a history of obstructive lung disease can be assessed by measuring the forced, expiratory volume. However, even patients with moderately severe lung disease can usually undergo transplantation successfully. Patients who smoke cigarettes should be strongly encouraged to quit, and should be offered a smoking cessation program.

PSYCHOSOCIAL ISSUES

The psychosocial evaluation should establish that the patient is able to provide informed consent and has the capacity to adhere to posttransplant immunosuppression. Significant impairment in cognitive ability can usually be detected on physical examination. Mild mental retardation is usually not a contraindication to transplantation. Patients with a history of unipolar or bipolar affective disorders can often be transplanted successfully. Patients and caregivers should be aware that high doses of corticosteroids might exacerbate psychiatric symptoms.

Noncompliance with immunosuppressive medications is a major cause of graft failure after renal transplantation. Patients who are noncompliant with therapies prior to transplantation are also more likely to be noncompliant after transplantation. However, predicting whether an individual patient will be noncompliant with immunosuppression is difficult. Great care needs to be taken so as not to unfairly deny transplantation to an individual who has exhibited noncompliant behaviors in the past.

Active drug abuse is a contraindication to transplantation. Most centers insist that patients with a history of drug abuse have a documented, drug-free interval of six to 12 months prior to transplantation. During this time patients should be under the care and supervision of a professional with experience in treating chemical dependencies.

GENITOURINARY TRACT

It is probably not necessary to obtain a voiding cystourethrogram in all patients. Potential problems with bladder emptying and/or infections will usually be evident from the patient's medical history. A urologic evaluation can be reserved for patients with a history of recurrent infection, bladder dysfunction, or other problems. Patients with chronic urinary diversion should be evaluated to see if the bladder could still be used.

A renal ultrasound, computerized tomography, or magnetic resonance imaging study is probably indicated to screen for malignancies and other potential problems. In some cases, a pretransplant bilateral nephrectomy may be indicated. Indications for nephrectomy include reflux nephropathy, a history of recurrent infections, nephrolithiasis, heavy proteinuria, hypertension that is difficult to control, and massively enlarged or symptomatic polycystic kidneys. Patients who are being evaluated for a second transplant need not always have the failed allograft removed.

SYSTEMIC DISEASES

Most patients treated with corticosteroids gain weight after renal transplantation. In some studies obesity has been associated with decreased graft survival. Obesity delays wound healing and increases the risk for wound infections and dehiscence. For all of these reasons, obese patients should be encouraged to lose weight before transplantation. However, the risks associated with obesity are probably not great enough to justify withholding transplantation from most obese patients.

Age is usually only a relative contraindication to transplantation. Most centers offer transplantation to otherwise healthy patients who are in their sixties. Overall health and "physiologic age" are probably more important determinants of outcome than chronological age. However, older individuals are more likely to die and less likely to reject their allografts compared to younger individuals. Some reduction in the amount of immunosuppression is appropriate for older transplant recipients.

Some patients with very difficult to control diabetes may be candidates for pancreas transplantation. Pancreas transplantation can improve quality of life by eliminating the need for insulin injections and reducing the number and severity of severe hypoglycemic episodes. There have been no controlled trials to determine whether other outcomes are better after simultaneous kidney-pancreas transplantation compared to kidney transplantation alone. In general, if a living donor is available, patients should be encouraged to undergo a live-donor transplant. Subsequently, a cadaveric pancreas transplantation may become an option.

BLOOD AND TISSUE TYPING

The immunologic evaluation of the potential transplant recipient is designed to assess the compatibility between the donor and the recipient, and thereby help to predict the likelihood of allograft rejection. The recipient and donor should be ABO blood-group compatible, and should have no preformed antibodies that will cause a rapid (hyperacute) rejection of the donor kidney. Antibodies against a random panel of lymphocytes from the general population are measured periodically. The percent of these random donor lymphocytes that the recipient reacts to is called the *percent panel-reactive antibody* (PRA). Recipients with a high PRA are more likely to have a preformed antibody against a donor kidney, and patients with a high PRA are often said to be "cytotoxic". Over time, the PRA often decreases, particularly if blood transfusions are avoided.

When a potential donor kidney (living or cadaveric) becomes available, the recipient's serum is tested against cells from the potential donor. A recipient whose serum reacts to the donor (indicating the presence of a preformed antibody) is said to have a positive crossmatch and the transplant is generally not possible using that particular donor. Unfortunately, patients who are cytotoxic often have positive crossmatches and must wait for

long periods of time to find a suitable donor kidney. When the potential recipient's current serum reacts to the donor, transplantation is usually contraindicated. Occasionally, the most recent serum fails to react to the donor, but an older serum sample reacts. Transplantation can be carried out safely when the current crossmatch is negative, even if the "historical" crossmatch is positive. Long-term results are probably not as good as for patients with negative current and historical crossmatches.

Major histocompatibility (MHC) antigens are measured on cells from both the recipient and donor. Studies have consistently shown that kidneys with the fewest MHC mismatches survive the longest. Therefore, if more than one potential living donor is available, the number of MHC mismatches may help in choosing which donor is most suitable. If there are no living donors, the number of MHC mismatches may help determine how cadaveric kidneys are allocated. In the United Network for Organ Sharing allocation scheme, first priority is given to kidneys with zero-MHC antigen mismatches. Kidneys without a suitable zero-MHC mismatched recipient are allocated to the recipient with the most waiting list points. Points are awarded for waiting time, fewer MHC mismatches, high PRA, pediatric recipient and having donated for transplantation.

EVALUATION UPDATES

Due to the growing organ shortage, waiting times for cadaveric renal transplantation continue to increase. The median waiting time is now well over two years. Many conditions that can increase the risk of transplantation develop in a relatively short period of time. Therefore, patients should probably be reevaluated at regular intervals. Patients who are at high risk for developing cardiovascular disease complications (eg, diabetics) may need to have a cardiac stress test every one to two years. Similarly, patients with viral hepatitis or a history of cancer should probably be reevaluated periodically.

RECOMMENDED READING

Basgoz N, Rubin RH. Prevention and treatment of infection in the kidney transplant recipient. In: Brady HR, Wilcox CS, eds. Therapy in Nephrology and Hypertension: A Companion to Brenner and Rector's The Kidney. Philadelphia, Pa: WB Saunders Co; 1999:634-640.

Hariharan S, Adams MB, BrennanDC, et al. Recurrent and de novo glomerular disease after renal transplantation: a report from renal allograft disease registry. Transplant Proc. 1999;31(1-2):223-224.

Kasiske BL, Ramos EL, Gaston RS, et al. The evaluation of renal transplant candidates: Clinical practice guidelines. Patient Care and Education Committee of the American Society of Transplant Physicians. J Am Soc Nephrol. 1995;6(1):1-34.

Katznelson S, Terasaki PI. Histocompatibility testing, crossmatching, and allocation of cadaveric kidney transplants. In: Danovitch GM, ed. Handbook of Kidney Transplantation. 2nd Ed. Boston, Ma: Little, Brown and Co., Inc.; 1996:32-54.

Manske CL, Wang Y, Rector T, Wilson RF, White CW. Coronary revascularization in insulin-dependent diabetic patients with chronic renal failure. Lancet. 1992;340(8826):998-1002.

Pereira BJ, Natov SN, Bouthot BA, et al. Effects of hepatitis C infection and renal transplantation on survival in end-stage renal disease. Kidney Int. 1998;53(5):1374-1381.

Penn I. Evaluation of transplant candidates with pre-existing malignancies. Ann Transplant. 1997;2(4):14-17.

Pirsch JD, Armbrust MJ, Knechtle SJ, et al. Obesity as a risk factor following renal transplantation. Transplantation. 1995;59(4):631-633.

Sutherland DE. Pancreas and pancreas-kidney transplantation. Curr Opin Nephrol Hypertens. 1998;7(3):317-325.

50 LIVING KIDNEY DONOR EVALUATION AND SELECTION

Gabriel M. Danovitch, MD

The widening gap between the demand for cadaveric kidneys and the supply, together with new information on the success of transplants from biologically unrelated donors, has led to a critical reevaluation of some long-held tenets regarding the suitability of certain types of live donors. Living donors are used for approximately 33% of all kidney transplants performed in the US, and most transplant centers regard them as the preferred donation modality despite the potential morbidity associated with them. Table 3-1 lists the potential advantages and disadvantages of living vs cadaveric transplantation. The following section reviews the process of selection and evaluation of the living donors. Readers are referred to the clinical practice guidelines for the evaluation of living donors developed by the Patient Care and Education Committee of the American Society of Transplantation.

WHO CAN BE A LIVE DONOR?

For many years, only first-degree relatives (ie, parents, children, and siblings who were at least 1-haplotype-matched) were deemed suitable live kidney donors. This policy was largely based on the premise that the matching of these kidneys compared with all others so improved the prognosis, or "utility," for the recipient that the risk to the donor was justified. The advent of cyclosporine and the widening gap between supply and demand for cadaveric kidneys is changing this attitude. It is now clear that the results of zero-haplotype-matched sibling transplants and transplants from more distant relatives and biologically unrelated donors are similar or even better than those of 6-antigen-matched cadaveric transplants. This suggests that it is not just the matching of the live donor kidney that determines its benefits for the recipient, but the condition of the kidney at the time of its transplantation. There is also a widespread realization that it is unlikely that the cadaveric organ supply will ever keep pace with the need for organs. As a result, there has been a gradual broadening of the definition of who can be a live donor.

Most transplant centers now routinely accept as donors zero haplotype-matched siblings and second-

Professor of Clinical Medicine; Medical Director, Adult Kidney and Pancreas Transplantation, University of California, Division of Nephrology, Los Angeles, CA

degree relatives (ie, cousins, uncles, aunts). Biologically unrelated transplant donors are most frequently spouses or individuals who have an emotional relationship to the recipient (ie, adopted siblings, fiancees, best friends). The term *emotionally related donor* is a good one, since it emphasizes the importance of the relationship between the donor and the recipient. Some transplant centers are more liberal in their definition of an emotionally related donor, and accept a "friend of a friend" or a member of a club, or religious affiliation where the relationship is less personal. Some centers have suggested accepting "altruistic donors" who have no direct relationship with the recipient, but have expressed a strong interest in donating a kidney to a deserving patient. As of 1997, donors who were not first-degree relatives accounted for 21% of all living donations in the US. Paired donor exchange has been proposed as a solution for donor-recipient pairs where there is ABO incompatibility, although experience with the practical and emotional aspects of such practice is limited.

Careful psychosocial examination should be part of the evaluation of all live donors to assess the degree of motivation and volunteerism. This is particularly important when the nature of the motivation is not clear. Live kidney donation, biologically or not biologically related, is an extraordinary act of altruism and love by one individual for another. Follow-up studies of donors show that the great majority are satisfied and gratified by the donation. However, dissatisfaction is more likely if the donor is not biologically related and if the outcome of the transplant is unfavorable. Financial incentives for donation are illegal in the US and in most countries,

Table 50-1. Live vs Cadaveric Kidney Donation

Advantages
Better short-term results (approximately 95% vs 85% 1-year function)
Better long-term results (half-life of 12 to 20 years vs seven to eight years)
More consistent early function and ease of management
Avoidance of long wait for cadaveric transplant
Ability to schedule transplant for medical and personal convenience
Immunosuppressive regime may be less aggressive
Helps relieve stress on national cadaver donor supply
Emotional gain to donor
Thorough medical workup of donor

Disadvantages
Psychological stress to donor and family
Inconvenience and risk of evaluation process

although the ethical underpinnings of this policy have been questioned in the case of countries where the therapeutic options for patients with end-stage renal disease are limited.

A careful family history should be a routine part of the evaluation of all potential transplant recipients, and the advantages and disadvantages of live donation should be discussed when relevant. A brief screening often rules out obviously unsuitable donors. It is reassuring when the donor accompanies the recipient to his or her pretransplant evaluation appointments.

Some patients find it difficult to approach family members, and the nephrologist and transplant team should be prepared to facilitate the discussion of donation. Educational material explaining the donation process often can help to alleviate the fears and anxiety of potential donors, who may also be encouraged by meeting other donors.

DONOR EVALUATION

Evaluation of living donors is a stepwise process that progresses from initial screening through noninvasive to more invasive evaluation and surgery. A practical schema for the process is shown in Table 50-2. Certain basic principles are consistent in the manner that all programs approach and evaluate donors, although details of policy may differ. The pace of the evaluation is often dictated by the donors. The donor can opt to withdraw at any time,

although, clearly, it is wasteful to do so at the more advanced stages of evaluation. Precise definition of renal anatomy with intravenous pyelogram and angiography, or with the spiral computerized tomography (CT), is the final step in the process and should follow psychiatric or social worker evaluation and completion of the recipient workup. The donor who has second thoughts about donation should be provided, if he or she wishes, with a medical alibi to justify his or her hesitation to the family.

EXCLUSION CRITERIA

Potential donors are excluded on medical grounds when it is believed there may be a risk of unrecognized kidney disease or an increased risk of short-term or long-term morbidity and mortality from the operative procedure itself. Table 50-3 reviews some frequent criteria for excluding potentially compatible donors. Many of these criteria are not absolute, and when findings are borderline, it is always wise to err on the side of donor safety. This is because the donor, unlike the recipient, does not need the operation to improve his or her health. Some centers adhere rigidly to an upper age limit, while other centers attempt to judge biological rather than chronological age. A glomerular filtration rate (GFR) of 80 mL/min or more has generally been believed to be adequate to permit donation, although older donors, women with low muscle mass, and vegetarians may

---

Table 50-2. Suggested Evaluation Process for Potential Live Donors

Donor Screening

Educate patient regarding cadaveric and living-related donation

Take family history and screen for potential donors

Review ABO compatibilities of potential donors

Tissue-type and crossmatch ABO-compatible potential donors

Choose primary potential donor with patient and family

Educate donor regarding process of evaluation and donation

Donor Evaluation

Complete history and physical examination

Comprehensive laboratory screening to include complete blood count, chemistry panel, human immunodeficiency virus, HBsAg, anti-hepatitis C virus, cytomegalovirus, glucose tolerance test (for diabetic families)

Urinalysis, urine culture, pregnancy test

24-hour urine collection for protein clearance (twice)

24-hour urine collection for creatinine (twice)

Chest x-ray, cardiogram, exercise treadmill for patients aged 50 years or older

Intravenous pyelogram*

Psychiatric evaluation

Renal angiogram*

Repeat crossmatch prior to transplant

*May be replaced by helical CT urogram in some centers

Table 50-3. Exclusion Criteria Guidelines for Living Donors

Age <18 or >65

Hypertension (>140/90 or necessity for medication)

Diabetes (or abnormal glucose tolerance test)

Proteinuria (>250 mg/24 hr)

Recent or recurrent kidney stones

Abnormal glomerular filtration rate (Ccreat <80 mL/min)*

Microscopic hematuria

Urologic abnormalities in donor kidneys

Significant medical illness (eg, chronic lung disease, recent malignancy)

Obesity (30% above ideal weight)

History of thrombosis or thromboembolism

Psychiatric contraindications including active substance abuse

*Measured by either creatinine clearance or a radio-labeled filtration marker

have a GFR of less than 80 mL/min with no evidence of renal disease. To avoid conflict of interest, it is preferable for a physician other than the one caring for the recipient to determine donor suitability. This physician should be an advocate for the donor, not the recipient or the transplant center. It must be clear to all concerned that donors are not to be "sacrificed" for recipients even in circumstances (particularly parents to children) in which the donor is quite prepared to make the sacrifice.

HEREDITARY KIDNEY DISEASE

The issue of donation in families with hereditary kidney disease occurs most frequently in families with polycystic kidney disease or hereditary nephritis. In families with polycystic kidney disease, a negative ultrasound or CT scan in a potential donor older than age 30 safely rules out the disease and permits donation. Since the polycystic kidney gene is a dominant one, the children of such a donor will not inherit the disease. In hereditary nephritis, the situation may be more complex. A patient in the third decade of life who is free of urinary abnormalities could be deemed free of disease and hence be a donor. It is not inconceivable, however, that the offspring of such a donor could suffer kidney disease; this possibility may be a consideration in the potential donor's decision, particularly when the family history for renal disease is a strong one.

There may also be familial aggregation of renal disease in excess of that predicted by clustering of diabetes and hypertension within families, suggesting that either genetic susceptibility or environmental exposures shared within some families increase the risk of end-stage renal disease. The risk is much higher where two or more first-degree relatives have renal disease and in such families it may be wise to avoid live donation, particularly from young donors. In North America, this situation is most frequently encountered in Hispanic and Native American families with a high incidence of non-insulin-dependent diabetes.

WHICH DONOR TO CHOOSE?

If there is more than one donor in a family, it is logical to commence workup on the relative who is best matched (ie, a 2-haplotype match vs a 1-haplotype match). If the donors are of the same match grade (ie, a 1-haplotype parent and a 1-haplotype sibling), it may be advisable to choose the older donor with the thought that the younger donor would still be available for donation if the first kidney eventually fails.

When more than one 1-haplotype matched sibling is available, it may be worthwhile to check the tissue typing of one parent to determine which sibling shares the non-inherited maternal antigens. Such sharing may improve long-term graft survival. Women of childbearing age are not at increased risk for obstetric problems after donation. Biologically related donors are generally preferred over emotionally related donors.

SURGICAL EVALUATION OF THE DONOR

The two major techniques for donor nephrectomy, the standard open and the newer laparoscopic technique are discussed in Chapter 53 of this section. Spiral CT urography may be sufficiently sensitive to provide accurate anatomic information and has replaced arteriography and intravenous urography in some centers. Usually, the left kidney is selected for donation because the left renal vein is longer than the right vein and thus, easier to transplant. If there are multiple arteries to the left kidney and a single artery to the right kidney, the right kidney can be used. If there are two arteries bilaterally, a kidney may still be used, employing one of several surgical techniques to handle multiple renal arteries. Occasionally, the donor has minor unilateral renal abnormalities, such as renal cysts, or even more severe problems such as uretero-pelvic junction obstruction. Also, one kidney might be smaller than the other. In these situations, the most prudent approach, if such abnormalities are not too severe, is to transplant the abnormal or smaller kidney, leaving the donor with the normal one.

The unexpected finding of unilateral or bilateral fibromuscular dysplasia in a normotensive potential donor presents a difficult dilemma. In the absence of definitive data regarding natural history of this condition, most programs have avoided using such donors.

POSTOPERATIVE COMPLICATIONS

Operative mortality is minimal, but is not nonexistent. In a series of more than 8,000 living donors, there were five deaths due to myocardial infarction, pulmonary embolus, and hepatitis. The rate of major complications was 1.8%, which consisted of pulmonary emboli, myocardial infarctions, sepsis, pneumonia, wound infections, pancreatitis, and injuries to the spleen or the adrenal gland. There are also risks to arteriography, such as femoral artery pseudoaneurysm or thrombosis. Careful and assiduous medical evaluation of the donor, with adherence to strict donation criteria, is the key to minimizing post-nephrectomy complications.

Long-term morbidity has not proved to be a major problem, although postoperative pain and discomfort may continue for several weeks or months in some donors. Follow-up data for up to 45 years (following traumatic wartime uninephrectomy) suggest that having only one kidney does not have a significant health impact. There is a statistically higher risk of low-grade proteinuria. When large numbers of kidney donors have been followed, however, no increase in incidence of hypertension or deterioration of kidney function has been shown. Serum creatinine levels generally remain approximately 20% higher and clearance rates 20% lower than pre-donation values. Long-term mortality is not affected by kidney donation, and most life insurance companies do not penalize donors. The main risk of kidney failure in kidney donors is from trauma to the remaining kidney or unrecognized familial kidney disease.

RECOMMENDED READING

Bia MJ, Ramos EL, Danovitch GM, et al. Evaluation of living renal donors. The current practice of US transplant centers. Transplantation. 1995;60(4):322-327.

Burlingham WJ, Grailer AP, Heisey DM, et al. The effect of tolerance to noninherited maternal HLA antigens on the survival of renal transplants from sibling donors. N Engl J Med. 1998;339(23):1617-1664.

Eberhard OK, Kwem V, Offner G, et al. Assessment of long-term risks for living related kidney donors by 24-h blood pressure monitoring and testing for microalbuminuria. Clin Transplant. 1997;11(5 Pt 1):415-419.

Lei HH, Perneger TV, Klag MJ, Whelton PK, Coresh J. Familial aggregation of renal disease in a population-based case-control study. J Am Soc Nephrol. 1998;9(7):1270-1276.

Kasiske BL, Ravenscraft M, Ramos EL, Gaston RS, Bia MJ, Danovitch GM. The evaluation of living renal transplant donors: clinical practice guidelines. Ad Hoc Clinical Practice Guidelines Subcommittee of the Patient Care and Education Committee of the American Society of Transplant Physicians. J Am Soc Nephrol. 1996;7(11):2288-2313.

Spital A. When a stranger offers a kidney: ethical issues in living organ donation. Am J Kid Dis. 1998;32(4):676-691.

Said MR, Curtis JJ. Living unrelated renal transplantation: progress and potential. J Am Soc Nephrol. 1998;9(11):2148-2152.

Kavoussi LR. Laparoscopic donor nephrectomy. Kidney Int. 2000;57(5):2175-2186.

Gjertson DW, Cecka JM. Living unrelated donor kidney transplantation. Kidney Int. 2000;58(2):491-499.

Matas AJ, Garvey CA, Jacobs CL, Kahn JP. Nondirected donation of kidneys from living donors. N Engl J Med. 2000;343(6):433-436.

51 CADAVER KIDNEY DONOR SELECTION

Carlton J. Young, MD
Robert S. Gaston, MD

Careful selection of appropriate organs from cadaveric donors has always been essential to ensuring a well-functioning allograft. In the early days of renal transplantation, all donors were "non-heart beating" (NHB), a factor that not only limited the number of organs recovered, but also impacted the quality of the allograft and likelihood of early function. After widespread acceptance of the Harvard criteria for brain death in 1968, procurement of kidneys from hemodynamically intact donors resulted in significant improvement in organ quality. More recently, in an attempt to increase the number of kidneys available to meet the overwhelming demand for transplantation, use of "expanded criteria" or "marginal" donors again threatens to compromise quality. Finally, the concept of NHB donors is being revisited at many centers, bringing issues of cadaver organ selection and acceptance full circle. In this changing environment, where the "ideal donor" is becoming a scarce commodity, how do we ensure an adequately functioning, safe allograft for our patients?

The ideal cadaver kidney donor is rather easy to identify: (1) a young adult with no significant medical problems; (2) brain death due to closed head injury; (3) no extracerebral trauma; (4) a brief hospitalization; (5) normal blood pressure and heart rate without pressors; and (6) excellent kidney function. Deviation from these attributes increases the risk of complications in the recipient, and makes the decision to accept or reject a donor kidney more difficult. For example, with aging comes increased risk of vascular disease, glomerular sclerosis, interstitial fibrosis, and cellular senescence. The ability of an older kidney to withstand trauma, brain death, hemodynamic compromise, ischemia, and subsequent immunologic insults is limited. Alternatively, kidneys from very young children (<6 years) pose significant technical challenges for even the most gifted surgeon, and carry increased risk of early vascular and ischemic problems. A donor's history of hypertension or diabetes may not rule out use of a cadaver kidney, but increases the need for close scrutiny of the kidney's condition. Accepting a kidney from an ideal donor is not a difficult decision; assessing the prospects when the kidney comes from a less-than-ideal donor requires greater deliberation.

CADAVER KIDNEYS: CONTRAINDICATIONS TO TRANSPLANTATION

With the current imbalance between the number of transplant candidates and the availability of donor organs, absolute contraindications to using kidneys from a given donor seem to be dwindling (Table 51-1). Those still considered valid exist primarily to minimize risk of transmitting a potentially fatal infectious disease or malignancy. Many variables that were previously considered contraindications (eg, age, preexisting diabetes or hypertension, treatable infections) now require individual assessment to determine whether organs may be used in permissible circumstances, and policies in this regard vary widely from center to center. For example, since hepatitis C virus (HCV) in the recipient may be associated with decreased graft survival, most centers do not offer HCV seropositive kidneys to seronegative recipients. However, some centers transplant HCV seropositive kidneys into seropositive recipients. Clearly, treated or treatable bacterial infections no longer preclude transplantation, and venturesome surgeons are often willing to attempt the technically

Carlton J. Young, MD, Assistant Professor of Surgery, Division of Transplantation, University of Alabama at Birmingham, Division of Nephrology, Birmingham, AL

Robert S. Gaston, MD, Professor of Medicine, Division of Nephrology; Professor of Surgery, Division of Transplantation, University of Alabama at Birmingham, Birmingham, AL

Table 51-1. Contraindications for Using a Cadaver Kidney

Absolute

Unknown cause of death
Extracranial malignancy
Acquired Immunodeficiency Syndrome or HIV +
HBsAg +
Untreated sepsis (especially fungal)
Intravenous substance abuse

Relative (requires individual assessment)

Age <3 or >65
Intracranial malignancy
Hepatitis C antibody +
Hepatitis B core antibody +
Bacteremia or parenchymal bacterial infection
Procurement injury (especially vascular)
Anatomic abnormalities (eg, horseshoe kidney)
Preexisting renal disease, diabetes mellitus, or hypertension

challenging implantation of a kidney with anatomic abnormalities (eg, horseshoe kidney or multiple arteries/veins).

RISK FACTORS FOR DELAYED GRAFT FUNCTION AND ALLOGRAFT FAILURE

Management of cadaver donors has improved in recent years, at least partly as a result of standardization of practices among organ procurement organizations (OPOs). In addition, increasing attention has been focused on the metabolic, hormonal, and hemodynamic consequences of brain death, with development of rational clinical interventions that ultimately have improved the quality of donated organs. In a multi-organ donor, minimal requirements to ensure suitable hearts and livers for transplantation generally guarantee hemodynamic stability of the kidneys. Appropriate management includes: (1) aggressive fluid resuscitation; (2) pressor support to maintain acceptable systemic pressure if necessary; (3) maintenance of adequate oxygenation; (4) vasopressin for diabetes insipidus; and (5) careful attention to body temperature, cardiac rhythm, and other metabolic aberrations. These same principles apply in the kidney-only donor. Hemodynamic stability (systolic blood pressure >100 mmHg), adequacy of urinary output (>100 mL/hour), and terminal serum creatinine levels (<2.0 mg/dL) provide the most common clinical parameters for assessing suitability of kidneys for transplantation.

Prompt onset of renal function after implantation not only makes posttransplant management easier and reduces the financial costs of transplantation, but is a strong predictor of short-term and long-term graft survival. Although it is difficult to discard any potentially transplantable kidney, the factors delineated in Table 51-2, when present, are associated with increased risk of delayed graft function (DGF), or even primary nonfunction. While cold ischemia time (CIT) longer than 24 hours doubles the risk of DGF, there is even greater risk when CIT extends beyond 36 to 48 hours. Kidneys

from very young donors often pose significant technical problems, increasing the risk of DGF. Conversely, DGF is also more common in kidneys from donors over the age of 45. In evaluating cadaver kidneys with one or more of these risk factors, it must be recognized that there is significant interplay among variables; kidneys from a donor between six and 45 years may ultimately function very well despite prolonged CIT, an elevated terminal creatinine level, and/or oliguria.

Apart from the impact of risk factors on the incidence of DGF, a more important question may be the ultimate effect of these variables on graft survival. Kidneys from a donor dying from trauma are associated with better graft survival than are kidneys from a donor dying from medical complications. Donor gender (female) and age (>60 years) both exert adverse impact on long-term graft survival, significantly reducing long-term graft survival. Conversely, kidneys from very young donors (<6 years) increase the risk of DGF and early graft loss, but are not associated with a decrement in long-term graft survival. Likewise, the impact of prolonged CIT on graft survival is typically an early effect; grafts that retain function through the early post-transplant period tend to do well long-term. Preexisting diabetes or hypertension in a donor also reduces long-term graft survival.

As noted earlier, kidneys from NHB donors have been used since the earliest days of transplantation. The use of NHB donors has allowed tolerable time limits for warm ischemia time to be established; kidneys undergoing more than an hour of warm ischemia rarely regained function after adequate circulation was restored. In the current era, the optimal approach to and utility of NHB donors are evolving, with new technologies being developed to prolong permissible warm ischemia time and improve organ quality. For now, a kidney harvested from a young, previously healthy, NHB donor with less than an hour of warm ischemia can be expected to undergo a significant period of DGF, but with a high likelihood of recovering function in an appropriate recipient.

Although CIT is, of itself, a critical variable influencing outcome, data indicate that preservation solution and method are also important. In multiple studies, the University of Wisconsin solution (ViaSpan®) has proved superior to other alternatives in preventing DGF and improving graft survival. Despite a dearth of controlled studies documenting its benefit, there is increasing acceptance that pulsatile perfusion is superior to simple cold storage in improving early allograft function and minimizing DGF. Given the financial costs associated with these complications, the added expense accompanying machine perfusion may be justifiable. At the very least, measurement of resistance to perfusate flow allows some early assessment of how well an allograft will function after engraftment.

Table 51-2. The Cadaver Donor: Risk Factors for Delayed Graft Function

Age <6 or >45 years
Cold ischemia time >24 hours
Warm ischemia time >60 minutes
Non-heart beating donor
Donor hypotension/pressor use
Oliguria
Terminal serum creatinine >1.5 mg/dL
Multiple vessels (arteries/veins)

REDUCING THE RISK OF ADVERSE OUTCOMES IN CADAVER RENAL TRANSPLANTATION

With an increasing percentage of cadaver kidneys originating in less-than-ideal donors, approaches to minimize the adverse impact on outcome are evolving, but remain largely unproved. In a prospective study, the Louisiana Organ Procurement Agency (LOPA) defined "expanded donors" as those aged between 55 and 75, or under five years, those with a history of hypertension/diabetes, and/or those who were seropositive for hepatitis C. Significantly greater expense was associated with procurement and placement of organs from these donors, and graft survival was diminished in recipients relative to those receiving grafts from traditional donors. Other investigators have confirmed these findings.

In the evaluation of kidneys from expanded criteria donors, some have advocated pretransplant or *time-zero* biopsies. In the LOPA study, note is made of biopsies being performed during procurement from many of these donors, but no mention is made of interpretation. In fact, surprisingly little literature exists in this regard. Gaber and coworkers found that pretransplant biopsies from older donors with more than 20% of glomeruli sclerosed were associated with poorer clinical outcomes. The common practice of many organ procurement agencies is that kidneys from donors with preexisting renal disease, hypertension, or diabetes undergo time-zero biopsies, and that significant vascular disease, glomerulosclerosis, or interstitial fibrosis precludes implantation. However, comparative studies regarding the validity of such approaches do not exist.

Several groups have addressed the problems inherent in transplanting kidneys from very young or very old donors by transplanting both kidneys from a marginal donor into a single recipient, either as an "en bloc" procedure (pediatric kidneys) or as a double transplant (expanded criteria kidneys). The technical feasibility of both approaches has been established, with excellent short-term and intermediate-term outcomes. Such approaches may expand the donor pool by using kidneys that would not otherwise be transplanted. However, it has not been established that dual-kidney transplantation offers better outcomes for a single recipient than single-kidney transplantation from the same donors might have done for two recipients.

RECOMMENDED READING

Pratschke J, Wilhelm MJ, Kusaka M, et al. Brain death and its influence on donor organ quality and outcome after transplantation. Transplantation. 1999;67(3): 343-348.

Phillips MG, ed. Organ Procurement, Preservation and Distribution in Transplantation. 2nd Ed. Richmond, Va: United Network for Organ Sharing; 1996.

Jacobbi LM, McBride VA, Etheredge EE, et al. The risks, benefits, and costs of expanding donor criteria: a collaborative prospective three-year study. Transplantation. 1995;60(12):1491-1496.

Gjertson DW. Look-up survival tables for renal transplantation. In: Cecka JM, Terasaki PI, eds. Clinical Transplants 1997. Los Angeles, CA; The Regents of the University of California, UCLA Tissue Typing Laboratory; 1997:337-883.

Koning OH, Ploeg RJ, van Bockel JH, et al. Risk factors for delayed graft function in cadaveric kidney transplantation: a prospective study of renal function and graft survival after preservation with University of Wisconsin solution in multiorgan donors. Transplantation. 1997;63(11):1620-1628.

Ojo AO, Wolfe RA, Held PJ, Port FK, Schmouder RL. Delayed graft function: risk factors and implications for renal allograft survival. Transplantation. 1997;63(7): 968-974.

Gaber LW, Moore LW, Alloway RR, Amiri MH, Vera SR, Gaber AO. Glomerulosclerosis as a determinant of posttransplant function of older donor renal allografts. Transplantation. 1995;60(4):334-339.

Ratner LE, Cigarroa FG, Bender JS, Magnuson T, Kraus ES. Transplantation of single and paired pediatric kidneys into adult recipients. J Am Coll Surg. 1997; 185(5):437-445.

52 SHARING AND ALLOCATION
John F. Neylan, MD

At present, there are 252 kidney transplant programs in the US, and each participates in the national organ procurement and distribution system to obtain cadaveric kidneys for transplantation. The dramatic growth and success of kidney transplantation in the past four decades is, in large measure, due to a combination of developments in immunobiology, organ preservation, surgical technique, medical expertise, and, of equal importance, the development of an integrated system of organ procurement and allocation. As the application of isolated instances of experimental success has undergone the transformation to widely applied and proven clinical therapy, renal transplantation in the US has become dependent upon a supply of organs increasingly insufficient to meet the burgeoning demand. At present, there are over 42,000 patients with end-stage renal disease (ESRD) awaiting a cadaveric kidney. Unfortunately, less than 10,000 cadaveric kidneys are recovered each year for transplantation. Efforts to address this shortfall through allocation schemes have attempted to maintain a balanced approach to both medical utility (ie, the most effective and efficient use of transplantable organs), and medical justice (ie, the fair and equitable distribution to all who are in need). The present system has evolved through compromise and debate and will likely continue in this fashion. The current scheme can only approximate universally accepted solutions, until the day that organ shortage is no longer a problem.

ORGAN PRESERVATION

Early efforts in organ procurement were challenged by the occurrence of irreversible renal damage following the cessation of blood flow for more than 30 minutes. Significant improvement resulted with the acceptance of the diagnosis of brain death in heart beating patients. The concept of brain death, originally taken from the French *coma depasse* in 1959, became codified in the US with the release of the report of the Harvard Ad Hoc Committee on Irreversible Coma in 1968. The report was widely accepted by the medical community because it contained well-defined parameters of diagnosis including the critical apnea test, which were confirmed in subsequent empirical observations. However, legal and societal acceptances were somewhat slower. In fact, it was not

Vice President, Clinical Research & Development, Transplantation/Immunology, Wyeth-Aherst Research, Radnor, PA

until 1989 that the majority of states had brain death laws on the books, and laws that absolved physicians of civil and criminal liability by making such a diagnosis commensurate with a pronouncement of death.

Advances in cold preservation techniques further extended organ viability. The ability to transport organs, to deliberate in the preparation of potential recipients, and to perform histocompatibility testing all enhanced the results of renal transplantation. In addition, these advances also made possible the practicality of other solid organ transplants. Current preservation techniques now predictably lengthen acceptable renal cold ischemic times beyond 48 hours, although most kidneys are transplanted after approximately 24 hours. However, even under the best of conditions, cold ischemia may have an impact upon longer-term graft survival. Cadaveric grafts with under six hours of cold ischemia, as well as grafts from living nonbiologically-related donors, have been shown to have graft survivals comparable to 1-haplotype-matched living-related donor grafts.

ORGAN PROCUREMENT ORGANIZATIONS

Organ Procurement Organizations (OPOs) developed in the 1950s as a consequence of the increasing success in the transplantation of cadaveric kidneys. In the early days, these organizations were offshoots of a small number of transplant programs and were confined to localized operations. After 1972 and the passage of the federal law creating the Medicare entitlement program for patients with ESRD, the proliferation of kidney transplantation as a federally funded therapy for ESRD, and the consequent need for donor organs stimulated a dramatic increase in the number of OPOs nationwide. In the latter half of the 1970s, Medicare funding became available for independent rather than hospital-based OPOs, leading to further refinements of these operations, which facilitated the extension of services to multiple transplant centers. Today, there are 65 active OPOs servicing defined regions throughout the US.

OPOs function with variable effectiveness across the country when assessed according to the traditional, although increasingly contested, measure of organs procured per million population base. Based upon the 1998 record number of 5,788 cadaveric organ donors and an estimate of the US census at 272.6 million population, the national average OPO productivity is 21.23 donors per million population. The wide range for individual OPOs varies from 9.1 to 39.0 donors per million. As a result of the regional differences in medically suitable organ donor candidates, family consent rates and OPO productivity, as well as the variable prevalence of ESRD, there are significant regional variances in patient waiting times. Death audits of hospital records have yielded considerably higher estimates of medically suitable donors, as high as 55 donors per million. In 1998, in an effort to enhance potential donor identification, the Department of Health and Human Services issued a rule for conditions of hospital participation in Medicare, which required hospitals to notify OPOs of all potential deaths. Some have argued that the 5.6% increase in cadaver donors for 1998 may be attributable in part to the implementation of this new rule. However, even with such measures in place, family refusals remain the most significant barrier to organ donation. On average, two of every three requests for organ donations are turned down.

NATIONAL ORGAN TRANSPLANT ACT

In 1984, Congress passed the National Organ Transplant Act (NOTA), which prohibited the sale of human organs, established grants for OPOs, and called for the establishment of a national system of organ sharing. In addition, NOTA created a multidisciplinary task force to conduct an extensive examination of organ donation and transplantation. The task force's extensive list of recommendations included setting performance standards for OPOs and transplant centers, as well as the establishment of protocols within hospitals addressing brain death and organ donation. One important outgrowth of NOTA has been the Uniform Anatomical Gift Act, now established in every state, which maintains the right of every individual aged 18 years or older to donate organs or tissues for purposes including transplantation. The legislation further establishes the right of the individual to designate such direction prior to death, and validates the legality of such methods of declaration as the organ donor card. These declarations are also legally binding even when an attempted contravention by next-of-kin creates conflict.

ORGAN PROCUREMENT AND TRANSPLANTATION NETWORK

The Omnibus Budget Reconciliation Act of 1986 mandated that all OPOs and transplant centers become part of a nationwide Organ Procurement and Transplantation Network (OPTN). The United Network for Organ Sharing (UNOS) successfully bid for that contract and has remained the provider to this day. UNOS was established in 1977 as an outgrowth of the South-Eastern Organ Procurement Foundation (SEOPF), a confederation of transplant programs sharing organs regionally via a computerized matching program. UNOS extended this concept to a national level as a means to optimize matching strategies and improve the efficiency of organ sharing. As the operation grew, UNOS created The Kidney Center in 1982, which was renamed the Organ Center in 1984 to reflect its expanded operations in other transplantable organs. This 24-hour operation coordi-

nated the allocation of available organs to the candidates listed in the computer records.

With the awarding of the national OPTN contract, UNOS changed its structure to that of a nonprofit, private voluntary organization made up of transplant professionals and public members. The organization developed an extensive committee structure and set of bylaws. It has remained dependent upon voluntary efforts, as today, less than one-quarter of its operating expenses are covered by government contracts.

A further outgrowth of UNOS came on the heels of the initial contract for the OPTN. UNOS established a Scientific Registry to track data relating to organs procured and their functional outcomes in transplant recipients. Organ-specific registries were created for each transplanted organ and were maintained by subcontractors. In the case of kidney transplantation, the database is maintained at the University of California at Los Angeles.

According to the 1998 Annual Report of the Scientific Registry and OPTN, 11,990 renal transplants were performed in 1998. Cadaveric kidneys accounted for 66.5%, continuing a trend toward the increased use of living donor organs. A growing number of living unrelated transplants are being performed with results at three years posttransplant comparable to 1-haplotype-matched kidneys.

ORGAN ALLOCATION POLICIES

Organ allocation policies have been developed in an attempt to balance the competing principals of medical utility and justice. The OPTN contractor, with its committee structure, has attempted to find appropriate factors to rank potential recipients of scarce transplantable organs based upon their likelihood of receiving an organ and their likely outcomes after transplantation. For instance, the demonstration of superior longer-term graft survival with 6-antigen matched or 0-antigen mismatched kidneys has led to the mandated sharing of such organs on a national basis. These make up approximately 3% of the cadaveric renal transplants. In the absence of such a match, the donor organ is allocated locally to ABO blood group-identical candidates prioritized on the basis of a computer algorithm that assigns points for recipient age, length of time waiting, present state of alloimmunization, and the quality of human leukocyte antigen (HLA) mismatching. All potential recipients with the same donor ABO blood type are ranked according to these parameters (Table 52-1), and the individual ranked highest is the preferred potential recipient. Factors such as unavailability, intercurrent illness, or a positive final crossmatch may come into play and lead to the designation of alternative candidates.

Alternate Local Units (ALUs) constitute special allocation arrangements that alter this system, some giving greater weight to time on the list, panel reactive

Table 52-1. UNOS Point System for Cadaveric Kidney Allocation

Catagory	Points Assigned
Time of Waiting	1 point assigned to the patient waiting the longest Fractions proportionately assigned to the remainder 1 additional point for each full year waiting
Quality of Antigen Mismatch	7 points for zero B or DR mismatches 5 points for only 1 B or DR mismatch 2 points for only 2 B or DR mismatches
Panel Reactive Antibody	4 points, if the PRA is >80% and a crossmatch is negative
Pediatric	4 points for age <11 years 3 points for age 11 years but <18 years
Prior Kidney Donor	4 points for prior kidney donation

antibody (PRA) or matching strategies. Some incorporate special sharing arrangements between transplant centers within a given region. All ALUs require ratification by the Board of Directors of UNOS, and are periodically reviewed to ensure they are maximizing the efficient use of donor organs and that the allocation scheme is primarily patient-driven rather than transplant center-driven.

PATIENT ACCESS

In 1991, UNOS undertook a feasibility study of a single nationwide list for the sharing of cadaveric kidneys. The study considered the proposal as a means to reduce the inequities associated with the wide regional variations in waiting times. The study concluded that a national single list would create prolonged ischemic times for kidneys transported across broad geographic distances. The consequent preservation injuries would, in turn, have a negative impact upon patient and graft survivals. In addition, the increased transport and laboratory costs of such a system, given present technologies, was deemed to be prohibitive. Moreover, sufficient tissue from recipients and donors would be unavailable to accommodate sensitized patients who would need a crossmatch before transplantation. If the negative impact of such a system upon organ quality, cost and tissue availability for crossmatching could be overcome, it is possible that a single national list might again be considered as a means to more evenly distribute a scarce national resource. In the interim, more widespread regional sharing of kidneys may provide a means to address the present disparities in waiting times for kidneys while still preserving reasonable cost containment and cold ischemia times.

While the number of renal transplants has gradually increased to the present level of nearly 12,000 cadaveric and living donor transplants performed yearly, the supply is vastly insufficient to meet the growing demands. The wait continues to lengthen; in fact, it has more than doubled in the past five years. Presently, the median waiting time for a kidney is more than 1,000 days, with some groups such as African-Americans waiting even longer. Additional considerations that could increase the donation rate include the use of improved public and professional education programs, enforcement of existing required request laws with potential impositions of penalties, financial incentives, presumed consent, the use of marginal donors, as well as expanded use of living donors including nonbiologically related individuals. Ultimately, the solution to these dilemmas of allocation can only be solved by increasing the number of organs available for transplantation.

RECOMMENDED READING

United States Task Force on Organ Transplantation. Organ Transplantation: issues and recommendations: report of the Task Force on Organ Transplantation. In: U.S. Department of Health and Human Services, Public Health Service, Health Resources and Services Administration, Office of Organ Transplantation. Rockville, MD: 1986.

United Network for Organ Sharing. The feasibility of allocating organs on the basis of a single national list. Richmond, VA: UNOS;1991.

United States Public Health Service, Office of the Surgeon General. The Surgeon General's workshop on increasing organ donation: proceedings, Washington, DC, 8-10 Jul 1991. Washington, DC: U.S. Government Printing Office; 1992.

1998 Annual Report of the U.S. Scientific Registry of Transplant Recipients and the Organ Procurement and Transplantation Network: Transplant Data: 1988 - 1997. U.S. Department of Health and Human Services, Health Resources and Services Administration, Office of Special Programs, Division of Transplantation. Rockville, MD: UNOS, Richmond, VA.

53 TECHNICAL ASPECTS OF RENAL TRANSPLANTATION

John M. Barry, MD

This chapter addresses the technical aspects of donor nephrectomy and renal transplantation. The basic techniques for living donor nephrectomy were established in the 1950s, slightly modified during the next two decades, and further modified in the 1990s by the introduction of the laparoscopic-assisted procedure. Cadaver donor nephrectomy was first by removal of the kidneys individually, then by en bloc kidney removal with the inferior vena cava (IVC) and aorta to preserve multiple or anomalous vessels, and then as part of a multiple abdominal and chest organ retrieval process. Evolution of the surgical techniques was complemented by advances in organ preservation. The use of the iliac fossa as the primary site for renal transplantation was established in the 1950s. Subsequently, techniques were developed or modified to transplant kidneys with multiple, anomalous or damaged renal vessels, and to transplant single or double ureters into the bladder or bladder substitute.

DONOR NEPHRECTOMY

The three basic criteria for cadaveric and living renal donors are: (1) absence of renal disease; (2) absence of transmissible infection; and (3) absence of transmissible malignancy. The specific selection criteria are covered in other chapters of this text. The surgical goals for donor nephrectomy are to minimize warm ischemia time, to preserve renal blood vessels, and to preserve ureteral blood supply. In the cadaver donor, it is also necessary to obtain histocompatibility specimens before and at the time of organ retrieval. If there is a choice between kidneys from a living renal donor, the better one should remain with the donor. Because hydronephrosis of pregnancy is more common in the right kidney, and because pyelonephritis of pregnancy is more common with obstruction, many transplant teams prefer to use the right kidney from women with childbearing potential when the kidneys are otherwise equivalent.

CADAVER DONOR

Most cadaver kidney donors are multiple organ donors, and the total midline incision with median sternotomy is the usual approach (Figure 53-1A). An abdominal organ

Professor of Surgery and Chairman, Divisions of Urology and Abdominal Organ Transplantation, Oregon Health Sciences University, Portland, OR

evisceration technique is described below. The chest and abdomen are explored to exclude infection and malignancy, and the kidneys are inspected to be certain there are no gross abnormalities that would preclude their use as transplants. The abdominal organ retrieval team exposes and controls the distal abdominal aorta and IVC, while the thoracic team exposes the heart and lungs and provides control of the proximal IVC. The inferior mesenteric artery is divided between ligatures. The proximal jejunum is divided between staples, the left coronary ligament of the liver is incised, the left lobe of the liver is retracted to the right, the distal esophagus is divided between staples, and the aorta is controlled through the crus of the diaphragm or in the chest. An aberrant left hepatic artery commonly arises from the left gastric artery and this must be preserved. The gall bladder is incised, drained, and flushed with a cold preservation solution to prevent autolysis. Heparin is administered, and the distal aorta and IVC are cannulated (Figure 53-1B). The proximal aorta is occluded and core cooling is initiated by infusion of the distal aortic cannula with ice-cold preservation solution. Although the IVC can be decompressed into the chest, lukewarm effluent will spill into the abdominal cavity; this is prevented by venous drainage through the abdominal IVC cannula. Saline slush is placed in the abdomen to further cool the abdominal organs. After the aortic infusion has washed out the vascular beds of the gastrointestinal tract, spleen, and pancreas, completion of liver preservation is achieved via hepatic artery and portal vein cannulations and infusions. The gastrocolic ligament is divided, the hepatic and splenic flexures of the colon are taken down, the line of Toldt is incised, the transverse mesocolon and small bowel mesentery are opened, and the superior mesenteric artery and vein are divided between ligatures. The right diaphragm is incised, and the en bloc organ specimen that includes the kidneys, adrenals, liver, pancreas, spleen, stomach, duodenum, abdominal aorta, and IVC is retracted anteriorly and to the left. The distal right ureter, the right lumbar veins, and the right lumbar arteries are transected. The en bloc specimen is then retracted to the right, and the distal left ureter, left lumbar arteries and left lumbar veins are transected. The distal abdominal aorta and IVC are transected, the proximal abdominal aorta is transected, the central diaphragm is divided between the aorta and the IVC, and the en bloc specimen is removed from the donor (Figure 53-1C). The organ block is placed face down in a pan of sterile slush to expose the posterior abdominal aorta. When the kidneys are to be transplanted separately, the posterior abdominal aorta is split between the lumbar arteries and then transected between the renal arteries and the superior mesenteric artery (Figure 53-1D). The IVC is transected just cephalad to the entrance of the renal veins, and the kidneys are

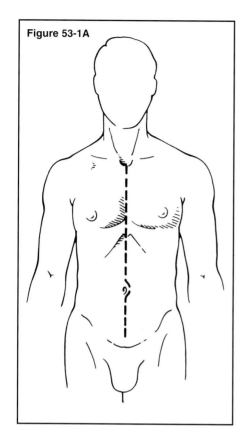

Figure 53-1A

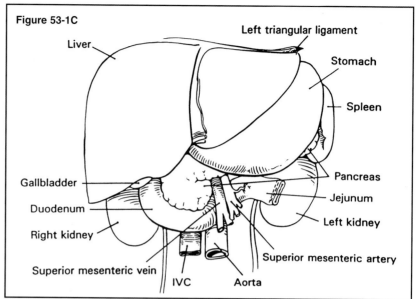

Figure 53-1C

Liver

Left triangular ligament

Stomach

Spleen

Pancreas

Jejunum

Left kidney

Superior mesenteric artery

Aorta

IVC

Superior mesenteric vein

Right kidney

Duodenum

Gallbladder

Figure 53-1A-D. Cadaver kidney retrieval. **A)** Total midline incision exposes all transplantable organs in the chest and abdomen. **B)** Core cooling of the abdominal organs is performed by infusion of the cannulated aorta with ice-cold preservation fluid and drainage through the cannulated inferior vena cava. **C)** Abdominal organ block, anterior view. **D)** After removal, the en bloc specimen is placed "face down" in a pan of slush, and the kidneys are separated from the other abdominal organs as described in the text. Reprinted with permission from Barry JM. Donor nephrectomy. In: Marshall FF, ed. Textbook of Operative Urology. Philadelphia, Pa; WB Saunders; 1996:235-247.

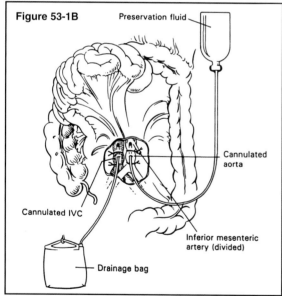

Figure 53-1B

Preservation fluid

Cannulated aorta

Cannulated IVC

Inferior mesenteric artery (divided)

Drainage bag

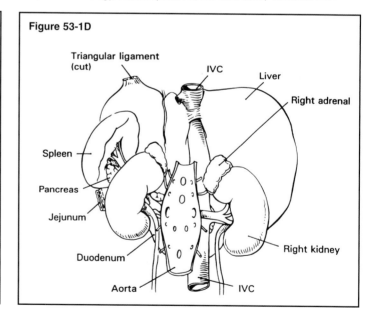

Figure 53-1D

Triangular ligament (cut)

IVC

Liver

Right adrenal

Spleen

Pancreas

Jejunum

Duodenum

Aorta

IVC

Right kidney

dissected from the adrenal glands, liver, duodenum, pancreas and spleen. The kidneys are separated from one another by dividing the anterior aorta between the renal artery ostia and transecting the left renal vein at its entrance into the IVC. The right renal vein is left with the IVC so that it can be extended. If the kidneys are to be transplanted en bloc, the posterior abdominal aorta is not split, and the left renal vein is left attached to the

IVC. The kidney specimen or specimens are then reflushed with ice-cold preservation solution and packaged. Several lymph nodes and the spleen are removed for histocompatibility testing. The external iliac veins and the iliac arteries are usually removed and sent with the liver and pancreas specimens.

The technique is modified for the retrieval of cadaver kidneys from a donor declared dead after heart

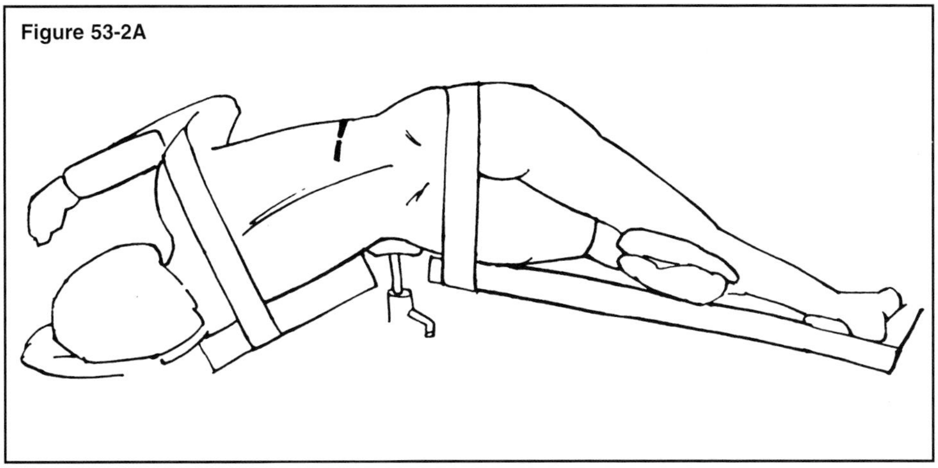

Figure 53-2A

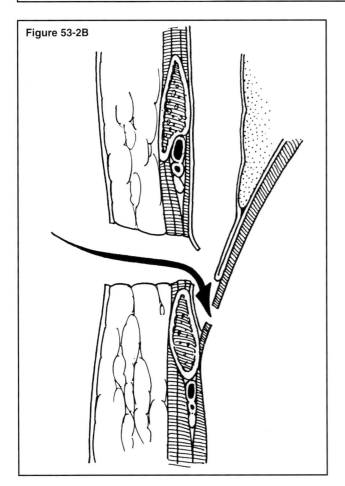

Figure 53-2A-C. Living donor nephrectomy via open flank procedure. **A)** Lateral decubitus position with flexion of the operating table causes rib separation. **B)** Rib-sparing supracostal approach provides excellent exposure of the kidney, regardless of the number of vessels and ureters. Reproduced with permission from Hinman Jr., ed. Atlas of Urologic Surgery. 2nd ed. Philadelphia, Pa: WB Saunders; 1998. **C)** Anterior view of abdomen of patient who underwent left supracostal living donor nephrectomy illustrates minimal extension of scar onto the abdomen.

Figure 53-2B

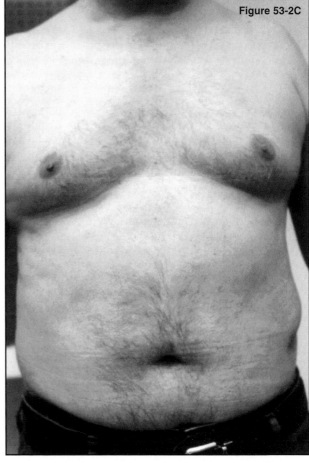

Figure 53-2C

beat cessation. Immediately after cardiac arrest, an intra-aortic double balloon catheter is inserted via a femoral cut-down; the lower balloon is inflated and impacted at the aortic bifurcation; the proximal balloon is inflated above the level of the renal arteries; and core cooling is initiated with an ice-cold preservation solution. The femoral vein is cannulated to allow for drainage of blood and coolant from the IVC. The abdomen is opened through a small incision and filled with saline slush, and the operative procedure for removal of the kidneys is begun as soon as possible.

LIVING RENAL DONOR

Living donor nephrectomy is usually performed by a unilateral flank incision or, less commonly, by a laparoscopic-assisted procedure that includes an abdominal incision to deliver the kidney. Diuresis is promoted by mannitol and intravenous fluid administration. Intravenous fluid administration the night before nephrectomy is unnecessary.

Flank Nephrectomy

The extrapleural, extraperitoneal supracostal approach to living donor nephrectomy is common (Figure 53-2A, 53-2B and 53-2C). Its advantages are excellent exposure of either kidney with or without multiple ureters, arteries or veins; no rib stump to become painful; contribution of the lower rib to the strength of the wound closure; and no risk of bowel adhesions because of the procedure. A corresponding rib-resecting procedure cannot provide the same exposure as a supracostal incision unless the entire rib is removed.

The location of the renal pedicle and the length of the rib determine whether the incision is made over the 11th or 12th rib. As with laparoscopic donor nephrectomy, the upper pole of the kidney is usually mobilized first. The renal vein is exposed. The gonadal vessels are often used to define the medial margin of the ureteral dissection to preserve ureteral blood supply. On the left, the adrenal vein is divided between ligatures. The lumbar vein that commonly drains into the posterior left renal vein is also divided between ligatures. After completion of the upper pole, renal vein, and ureteral dissections, the kidney is retracted anteriorly and the renal artery or arteries are dissected. Renal vasospasm is treated with subadventitial injection of papaverine. The ureter is transected and the presence of a diuresis is confirmed. If there is no urine flow and vasospasm has been corrected, intravenous fluid administration and additional infusions of mannitol and furosemide will correct the problem. On the right, the renal artery or arteries are clamped, and two Satinsky clamps are placed, one within the other, on the side of the IVC. The renal artery or arteries and the renal vein with a patch of IVC are transected. The lateral Satinsky clamp is removed, the opening in the IVC is oversewn, and the remaining Satinsky clamp is removed. On the left, the renal artery or arteries are clamped, the renal vein clamp(s) are placed medial to the previously ligated and divided adrenal vein, and the vessels are transected. The renal vein is oversewn or doubly ligated as the clamps are removed. The stumps of the renal artery or arteries are managed by double ligation, by ligation followed by suture ligation, or by oversewing the renal artery. After nephrectomy, the kidney is immediately placed in a pan of ice-cold slush and flushed with an ice-cold kidney preservation solution. Heparin administration to the patient undergoing open donor nephrectomy is unnecessary. The kidney is taken in an ice bath into the recipient operating room or cold-stored until the time of transplantation. If a pleural entry has

occurred, it is treated by the insertion of a small catheter into the pleural space, suturing the incised edge of the diaphragm to the inferior edge of the seratus posterior inferior and latisimus dorsi muscles, and placing the other end of the catheter under a water seal until the deep wound is closed. Pleural closure is optional with this technique. The catheter is withdrawn after the pleural air has been evacuated. If a pericostal synthetic absorbable suture is to be placed, care is taken to avoid injury to the neurovascular bundles. Drains are usually not used. The muscle layers are closed with far-far, near-near heavy absorbable sutures, and the subcutaneous tissue with an intermediate absorbable suture. A running, fine absorbable suture, subcuticular closure of the skin is more comfortable for the patient than staples or nonabsorbable exposed skin sutures that require later removal. A chest radiograph is taken in the recovery room to check for a pneumothorax.

Laparoscopic Donor Nephrectomy

The reported advantages of laparoscopic-assisted donor nephrectomy when compared with historical cases of open donor nephrectomy are decreased analgesic requirement, earlier return of gastrointestinal continuity, decreased length of hospital stay, and earlier return to work. The disadvantages have been reported to be increased operating time, the increased need for special equipment, and organ damage manifested by delayed graft function and ureteral stricture. An incision large enough to remove the kidney must still be made, donor anticoagulation with heparin is standard practice, warm ischemia time is longer than with the open technique, and the procedure is usually applied only to left kidneys with single renal arteries and veins.

The patient is placed in a lateral decubitus position, similar to that used for standard flank nephrectomy. Oral gastric suction, bladder catheterization, antibiotic prophylaxis and antithrombotic compression devices are used routinely. The positions of the operating surgeon, assistant surgeon, support personnel, and equipment are depicted in Figure 53-3A. A 15 mmHg carbon dioxide pneumoperitoneum is created, and four or five abdominal ports are inserted (Figure 53-3B). The camera port is usually placed in the upper abdomen. The dissection proceeds in a manner similar to that for open donor nephrectomy. The main renal vessels and ureter are controlled with a laparoscopic stapler. The extraction process is through a six to ten centimeter abdominal incision. After extraction, the kidney is immersed in an ice-cold solution and then flushed with an ice-cold kidney preservation solution. The heparin is reversed, the operative site is inspected to assure hemostasis, the instruments are withdrawn, and the abdominal wounds are closed.

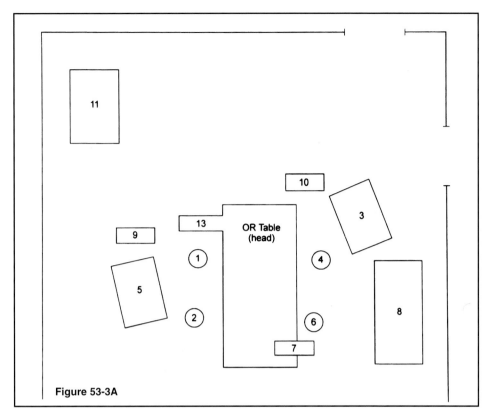

11

10

OR Table
(head)

13

9

3

1

4

5

2

6

8

7

Figure 53-3A

Figure 53-3A-B. Laparoscopic donor nephrectomy. **A)** Locations of patient, personnel, and equipment for left donor nephrectomy. 1 = camera assistant, 2 = surgeon, 3 = primary monitor, 4 = assistant surgeon, 5 = secondary monitor, 6 = scrub nurse, 7 = Mayo stand, 8 = back table, 9 = electrosurgical unit, 10 = irrigation set-up, 11 = covered laparotomy set-up, 12 = anesthesiologist, and 13 = armboard. Modified from Clayman RV, McDougall EM, eds. Laparoscopic Urology. St. Louis, Mo: Quality Medical Publishing; 1993. **B)** Donor position, port locations, and abdominal incision for kidney extraction. Modified from Ratner LE, Kavoussi LR, Siroka M, et al. Laparoscopic-assisted live donor nephrectomy – a comparison with the open approach. Transplantation. 1997;63(2):229-233.

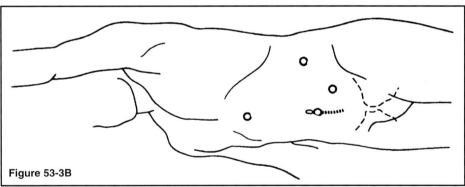

Figure 53-3B

RECIPIENT OPERATION
Preoperative Assessment

The preoperative history and physical examination of the transplant candidate focus on interval problems that will contraindicate transplantation and immunosuppression, and the need for additional crossmatch testing because of recent blood transfusions or an outdated serum sample.

Anesthesiologist's Role

The anesthesiologist is responsible for induction and maintenance of anesthesia, placement of a double or triple lumen central venous catheter, administration of prophylactic antibiotics, intraoperative administration of immunosuppressants, control of bladder volume, administration of heparin, and assurance of the conditions for a diuresis.

Surgical Technique

The genitalia and skin are prepared, and a Foley catheter is placed in the bladder or bladder substitute. Attachment of the catheter to a 3-way drainage system allows intraoperative filling and draining of the bladder. This is especially helpful in the recipient who has a small, defunctionalized bladder or who has had prior pelvic surgery. The bladder or bladder substitute is rinsed with a broad-spectrum antibiotic solution, and gravity-filled to about half capacity. The catheter tubing is clamped until it is time to do the ureteroneocystostomy. It is the practice of some surgeons to prepare the skin over both iliac fossas in case anatomy unsuitable for technical success is unexpectedly detected on the chosen side. The primary surgeon stands on the side opposite the chosen iliac fossa, and the operating table is flexed and rotated towards him. A self-retaining retractor attached to the operating table will allow the operation to be performed by a surgeon and one assistant. Antibiotic irrigation is used liberally during the procedure.

In adults and large children, the kidney graft is usually placed extraperitoneally in the contralateral iliac fossa via a rectus-preserving Gibson incision. This allows the renal pelvis and ureter to be the most medial structures in case subsequent urinary tract surgery is necessary on the kidney graft. If there is doubt about whether a kidney will fit in the left pelvis, placement of the kidney on the right side will allow access to a wider choice of target vessels, including the aorta and IVC, for vascular reconstruction. In women, the round ligament is retracted or divided between ligatures. In men the spermatic cord is preserved to prevent testicular complications such as atrophy, hydrocele, and chronic pain. If the kidney is available, it is placed in the wound to determine which recipient vessels will result in the best fit. The kidney is then replaced in the cold solution until it is time for the vascular anastomoses. The chosen blood vessels are dissected, and the lymphatics are divided between ligatures to prevent the development of posttransplant lymphocele. The genitofemoral nerve should be preserved. It can be mistaken for a lymphatic because it will often cross the distal external iliac artery. In a cadaver kidney transplant, the short right renal vein can be extended with a variety of techniques that use the IVC or the cadaver donor's external iliac vein (Figure 53-4). Techniques for the management of multiple renal arteries are shown in Figure 53-5. Prior to temporary vascular occlusion, heparin is administered intravenously. During the vascular anastomoses, an infusion of mannitol is given to act as a free radical scavenger and as an osmotic diuretic. Infusion of electrolyte solution provides intraoperative volume expansion. An albumin infusion has been found to be helpful in promoting early renal function in cadaver kidney transplantation. The renal artery is usually anastomosed to the end of th children. Prior to 1990, as living transplantation proliferated rapidly in Europe and North America, the dramatic shortage of small cadaveric donors for children led to a waiting list

mortality that approached 50% in many centers. This provided an ethical the splenic artery, or the native renal artery. The atherosclerotic recipient artery can be managed by endarterectomy or arteriotomy with a vascular punch. Many surgeons prefer to do the renal artery anastomosis first because it is the more critical of the two vas-

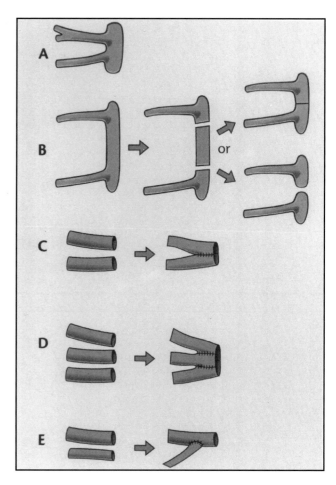

Figure 53-5. Management of multiple renal arteries. A and B, the use of aortic patches when the kidney is from a cadaver donor. C and D, the pair of pants technique when an aortic patch is not available, such as when the kidney is from a living donor. Reproduced with permission from Barry JM. Technical aspects of renal transplantation. In: Schrier RW, ed. Atlas of Diseases of the Kidney; Vol. 5. Philadelphia, Pa: Current Medicine; 1999:14.1-14.12.

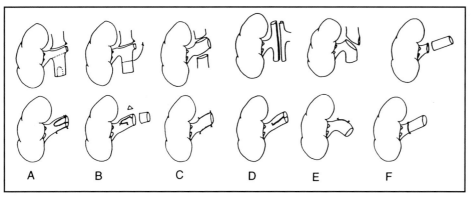

Figure 53-4. Methods of extending the right renal vein in a cadaver kidney graft. A and B are useful when the cephalad portion of the right renal vein has been compromised. F uses a free graft of cadaver donor external iliac vein. Reproduced with permission from Barry JM. Renal transplantation. In: Walsh PC, Retik AB, Vaughan ED Jr., Wein AJ, eds. Campbell's Urology; 7th ed. Philadelphia, Pa: WB Saunders; 1998:505-530.

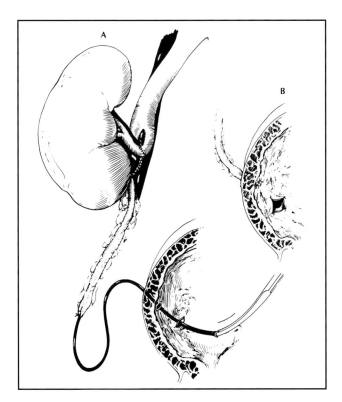

Figure 53-6. Vascular reconstruction and transvesical ureteroneo-cystostomy for left kidney transplant into right iliac fossa. The renal vein is commonly anastomosed to the external iliac vein, and the renal artery is commonly anastomosed to the internal iliac artery. Many prefer to perform renal artery revascularization first because it is the more critical of the two vascular anastomoses, and its exposure is not compromised by limited mobility of the kidney graft when the venous anastomosis has been done first. The spatulated ureter is anastomosed to the bladder with inter-rupted fine absorbable sutures, and the separate cystotomy is closed in one or two layers with intermediate absorbable sutures. Reproduced with permission from Salvatierra O, Jr. Renal trans-plantation. In: Glenn JF, ed. Urologic Surgery; 4th ed. Philadelphia, Pa: Lippincott-Raven Publishers; 1991:243-251.

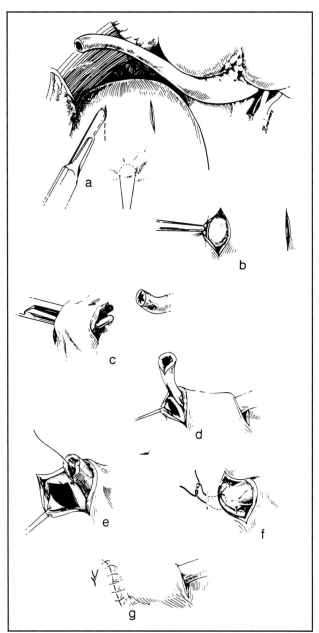

Figure 53-7. Example of extravesical ureteroneocystostomy. The submucosal tunnel is created from outside the urinary bladder which has been filled with antibiotic solution. Prior to the mucosal incision, the bladder is drained. Fine absorbable sutures are used to anastomose and anchor the ureter to the bladder and to close the distal seromuscular bladder incision. Reproduced with per-mission from Barry JM. Unstented extravesical ureteroneocys-tostomy in kidney transplantation. J Urol. 1983;129:918-919.

cular anastomoses, and venous occlusion can be delayed until after the renal artery anastomosis. This results in decreased iliac venous occlusion time and, perhaps, a reduced risk of iliofemoral venous thrombosis. Avoidance of the internal iliac artery in a male candidate for a second kidney graft whose first transplant was anastomosed to the contralateral internal iliac artery will reduce the risk of arteriogenic impotence. The renal vein is usually anasto-mosed end-to-side to the external iliac vein. When the renal vein is short, it is helpful to completely mobilize the external iliac and common iliac veins by dividing the gluteal and internal iliac veins between ligatures. This will allow the recipient vein to be brought up to the venous anastomosis. Blood pressure and central venous pressure criteria and suggestions for diuresis enhancement are described in Table 53-1.

Antireflux ureteroneocystostomy is the most com-mon form of urinary tract reconstruction. An extravesical

(Figure 53-7) rather than a transvesical technique is pre-ferred by many surgeons because the former is more rapid, a separate cystotomy is not required, and less ureteral length is necessary. Regardless of the uretero-neocystostomy technique, it is important to place the ureter posterior to the round ligament or spermatic cord to prevent ureteral obstruction. Ureteroureterostomy and ureteropyelostomy are used when the allograft ureter is short or ischemic, when the recipient has a very limited bladder capacity, when bladder exposure is difficult because of scar from prior pelvic surgery, or when the surgeon prefers it to ureteroneocystostomy. Transplantation into a continent urinary reservoir that has been previously constructed from intestine is by one of the extravesical techniques. When the transplant is done in a patient with an intestinal conduit, the kidney graft is placed in such a way that it does not interfere with the flat surface at the stoma site and thereby contribute to urinary leakage. Double pigtail ureteral stents are used when there is concern about the ureteroneocystostomy technique, when a ureteroureterostomy or ureteropyelostomy has been performed, or when the ureter has been transplanted into an intestinal conduit or reservoir.

Generally accepted indications for the placement of wound drains are anticoagulation, obesity, and complicated urinary tract reconstruction. When used, a closed suction system is preferred in place of the classic Penrose drain. Opinions about the technique of wound closure vary, however, a single layer of far-far, near-near interrupted heavy absorbable sutures will soundly close the deep wound. The rectus muscle is allowed to slide back into its normal position, and the anterior rectus sheath is closed with the same technique. The subcutaneous tissue is approximated with an intermediate absorbable suture, and skin closure with a running fine subcuticular absorbable suture will eliminate the need for subsequent staple or suture removal.

The management of catheters and drains is described in Table 53-2.

CONCLUSIONS

The technical aspects of renal transplantation have gradually evolved over the past five decades to allow the safe retrieval of kidneys from living donors, the retrieval of multiple organs from cadaver donors, the transplantation of kidneys with multiple, damaged or anomalous vessels, and reconstruction of the urinary tract by a variety of techniques.

RECOMMENDED READING

Barry JM. Technical aspects of renal transplantation. In: Schrier RW, ed. Atlas of Diseases of the Kidney. Vol 5. Philadelphia, Pa: Current Medicine; 1999:14.1-14.12.

Illustrated in this chapter are the preparation of a cadaver kidney graft, venoplasties for right renal vein extension, management techniques for multiple renal arteries, 16 plates of a kidney transplant from start to finish, a postoperative clinical pathway, and algorithms for the evaluation of kidney transplant hydronephrosis and perigraft fluid collections.

Table 53-1. Pressure Goals and Methods of Diuresis Enhancement During Renal Transplantation

Goals	Suggestions
Maintain CVP 5-10 cm H_2O	IV crystalloid, albumin 1 g/kg (cadaver kidney recipient), packed RBCs if Hct is ($\leq$) 25
Maintain SBP ($\geq$) 90 mm Hg	Dopamine (less than or equal to 5 mcg/kg per min if CVP ($\geq$) 10 cm H_2O
Diuretic, free radical scavenger	Mannitol 0.20 g/kg (living donor kidney recipient) to 1 g/kg (cadaver kidney recipient) IV over 1 h, start with first vascular anastomosis
Diuretic	Furosemide 0.20 mg/kg (living donor kidney recipient) to 1 mg/kg (cadaver kidney recipient), IV during second half of final vascular anastomosis
Calcium channel blockade	Verapamil 0 to10 mg (cadaver kidney recipient) into renal artery based on BP and weight

IV indicates Intravenous; CVP, central venous pressure; SBP, Systolic blood pressure; RBCs, Red blood cells; Hct, Hematocrit.

Modified from Dawidson IJA, Ar'Rajab A. Perioperative fluid and drug therapy during cadaver kidney transplantation. In: Terasaki PI, Cecka JM, eds. Clinical Transplants 1992. Los Angeles, Ca: UCLA Tissue Typing Laboratory; 1993:267-284.

Table 53-2. Management of Tubes and Drains

Foley catheter	Remove on postoperative day five, administer antibiotic
Ureteral stent, if used	Remove six to 12 weeks postoperatively in clinic
Suction drain(s)	Remove when ($\leq$) 50 mL/24 h or in three weeks if volume is >50 mL/24

Fabrizio MD, Ratner LE, Kavoussi LR. Laparoscopic live donor nephrectomy. Prog Urol. 1999;53(4):665-667.

This article describes the advantages of laparoscopic live donor nephrectomy.

Hinman F Jr., ed. Atlas of Urologic Surgery. 2nd ed. Philadelphia, Pa: WB Saunders; 1998:956-965, 974-977, 993, 1016-1026.

Described within this text are nearly all surgical approaches for renal donation and the basic surgical techniques of renal transplantation in adults and children.

Hume DM. Kidney transplantation. In: Rapaport FT, Dausset J, eds. Human Transplantation. New York, NY: Grune and Stratton; 1958.

This chapter, published more than 40 years ago, describes the principles of kidney transplantation that are still in common use. Among the technical "pearls" is the description of spermatic cord preservation during transplantation in men.

Miller CM, Rappaport FT, Starzl TE. Organ procurement. In: Scientific American Surgery; Vol. 2. New York, NY: Scientific American Medicine; 1998:16.1-16.14.

This chapter presents, in a 1-page algorithm, an approach to the potential multiple solid organ cadaver donor, surgical techniques for removal of the transplantable organs, and current methods of organ preservation.

Novick AC. Laparoscopic live donor nephrectomy. Con Urol. 1999;53(4):667-670.

Read in conjunction with the article by Fabrizio et al, the reader will become aware of the concerns about laparoscopic donor nephrectomy.

Starzl TE. Experience with Renal Transplantation. Philadelphia, PA: W.B. Saunders Company; 1964.

In fewer than 400 pages, one of the pioneers of transplantation describes not only most of the basic surgical techniques of the kidney transplant recipient operation, but also immunology, immunosuppression, candidate selection, donor selection, ABO incompatible transplantation, postoperative complications, renal xenografts into humans, and the "technical triumph and moral muddle" of organ transplantation. For the younger transplant surgeons and physicians, this is a "must read".

54 IMMEDIATE POSTOPERATIVE MANAGEMENT OF THE KIDNEY TRANSPLANT RECIPIENT

Daniel C. Brennan, MD, FACP

The immediate postoperative management of the kidney transplant recipient is made easier by a proper preoperative assessment of the recipient, good communication between the transplant surgeon and nephrologist, and immediate postoperative assessment by the transplant nephrologist in the recovery room. The future of the transplant and recipient is dependent on the early transplant function and characteristics. A team effort is required for long-term success.

PREOPERATIVE EVALUATION

A thorough understanding of recipient and donor characteristics prior to the transplant procedure is essential for postoperative management. It is difficult to predict the future without understanding the past. It is important to know the recipient's cause of end-stage renal disease (ESRD); the particulars of the renal replacement therapy (hemodialysis vs peritoneal dialysis vs transplant vs not-yet-receiving renal replacement therapy); any complications of the renal replacement therapy (eg, thrombosis, hyperkalemia, or hypotension); the amount of residual renal function or daily urine output; medical history — especially cardiovascular risks; prior medications; and the recipient's infection status (eg, the serostatus for cytomegalovirus [CMV], Epstein-Barr virus [EBV], and hepatitis).

DETAILS OF THE TRANSPLANT OPERATION

Immediately postoperatively the nephrologist should be in direct contact with the operating surgeon. It is unlikely that the written operative note will be of sufficient detail to allow for proper postoperative management. Thus, direct communication between the nephrologist and surgeon is essential. Renal transplantation generally takes three to four hours. If the surgeon has not contacted the nephrologist within five hours of the start of the surgery, the nephrologist must contact the surgeon. The initial contact with the surgeon should provide specific information regarding the donor charac-

Associate Professor of Medicine; Director, Transplant Nephrology, Washington University School of Medicine, Barnes-Jewish Hospital, St. Louis, MO

teristics, the operation itself and any intraoperative complications to aid in the immediate postoperative management of the kidney transplant recipient. Accordingly, the transplant nephrologist should confirm the donor age, cause of death, and the details of the period before and after brain death was declared and before the organs were procured. It is important to determine whether pressors were used in the donor, and if so, what and how much. The admitting and final serum creatinine and urine output of the donor and the cold ischemia time may allow one to anticipate the need for postoperative hemodialysis. The anatomy of the donor kidney, the anastomotic connections of the vessels, the quality of the donor and recipient vessels, the rewarm time, and the appearance of the kidney upon anastomosis, provide clues as to the likelihood of the development of vascular complications including stenosis, thrombosis, cholesterol embolization and renovascular hypertension. The integrity of the bladder, whether a urinary stent was required, and whether the kidney made urine in the operating room should be determined. The estimated blood loss, the intraoperative fluid intake and fluid output, whether any drains or intravenous catheters were placed, and the type of analgesia should also be determined.

IN THE RECOVERY ROOM

In the recovery room, the transplant nephrologist should assess the characteristics of the transplant operation as above, and determine whether immediate dialysis is required. The patient should be examined, the urine output noted, and the CBC, electrolytes, and postoperative chest x-ray reviewed. The immediate questions to be answered are: what is the urine output per hour; is the patient acidotic; are the electrolytes, particularly potassium, adequately controlled; and is oxygenation sufficient so that dialysis is not required for ultrafiltration?

Drains

Drains are not commonly placed in kidney transplantation. When they are used, a closed system Jackson-Pratt is preferred to an open system Penrose drain to decrease the risk of infection. The presence of drains may suggest a potential complication of surgery that will require careful scrutiny. Specifically, if a surgeon has placed a drain, one must be concerned about the possibility of either a vascular anastomotic leak or urinary vesicular leak. Alternatively, drains are automatically used by some surgeons if anticoagulation is routinely used postoperatively. If the drainage exceeds 100 cc/d for more than three days, one should analyze the output for creatinine, cell count and Gram stain to differentiate a urine leak from a lymphocele, hematoma, seroma and to rule out infection. A fluid collection with a fluid creatinine greater than the serum creatinine suggests a urine leak, a cell count comprised predominantly of lymphocytes suggests a lymphocele, and a Gram stain primarily of neutrophils and bacteria suggests an infection. When the drainage is less than 50 cc/d, the drain should be removed to prevent superinfection.

Bladder Catheter and Stents

The necessary duration of the bladder catheter is unknown, but staunchly defended. In general, the urinary catheter should be removed by postoperative day five, although many feel that diabetic patients may require an additional day postoperatively to assure sufficient wound healing. Stents are used routinely by some surgeons; more commonly, stents are used when there is concern for the integrity of the anastomosis of the bladder and the ureter. Double-J stents are most commonly used and can be removed cystoscopically, two to six weeks posttransplantation.

The Incision

Sutures or staples should remain for two to three weeks because of slow wound healing associated with the use of steroids, azathioprine, and obesity. A better cosmetic result, however, is achieved with subcuticular sutures compared to external sutures or staples. Steri-Strips® enhance the superficial wound closure and should be inspected daily during the initial hospital stay and weekly thereafter for the first several weeks. They are allowed to fall off "on their own," which usually takes about three to four weeks. Patients are allowed to shower, but should not take prolonged baths until the incision is completely healed. Attention should be paid to the presence of any surrounding erythema that may be the result of usual postoperative inflammation, infection, or impending dehiscence. Wet to dry dressing changes with normal saline twice daily are sufficient for the management of patients with superficial wound dehiscence. Overt wound dehiscence may require placement of retention sutures or surgical debridement and healing by secondary intention.

Pain Control

Immediately posttransplant it is important to establish the current kidney transplant function because the choice of analgesic is dependent on the state of renal function. Nonsteroidal antiinflammatory agents are to be avoided because of their antiprostaglandin effect, which may impair prostaglandin-dependent renal blood flow to the kidney. Meperidine (Demerol®) should be used only with good transplant renal function because the metabolite, normeperidine, accumulates with renal insufficiency and may cause seizures. Morphine sulfate and fentanyl are particularly narcoleptic. Thus, the analgesic of choice is hydromorphone (Dilaudid®) 2 to 4 mg every two to four hours as needed. Patient-controlled analgesia pumps are particularly effective.

Fluid Management

In the early posttransplantation period it is important to maintain the patient's intravascular volume at normal or mildly increased levels. The first principle is that the "tank" must be full to assure a good diureses. With general anesthesia, it is customary to sequester 5% (three to five liters) of fluid in the interstitial space. Diabetic patients are prone to capillary leak syndrome and may require even more fluid resuscitation.

Hourly urine output and nasogastric losses are replaced with half-normal saline on a milliliter-per-milliliter basis because the sodium concentration of the urine from a newly transplanted kidney is 60 to 80 mEq/L. Insensible losses during this period typically are 30 to 60 mL/h of essentially water that can be replaced by a 5% dextrose solution at 30 mL/h. Therefore, during the early posttransplantation period, the patient's maintenance intravenous fluid consists of one-half normal saline at a rate equal to the previous hour's urine and nasogastric output plus 30 mL of a 5% dextrose solution. This necessitates that the patient's volume status be assessed repeatedly.

If the posttransplantation urine output is low (<50 to 100 cc/h) and, if after clinical and hemodynamic evaluation, the patient is felt to be hypovolemic, isotonic saline boluses are given in 250 to 1,000 cc increments. If the patient has normal or increased intravascular volume, furosemide (100 to 200 mg IV for recipients of cadaveric transplant, and 20 to 40 mg IV for those with living donor transplants) should be given. If diuresis follows these maneuvers, the urine output is again replaced milliliter-per-milliliter with half-normal saline.

If the urine output is excessive, the next hour's fluid replacement should be reduced. Thus, if the urine output exceeds 1,000 cc/h, the next hour's rate of fluid replacement may be reduced by 300 cc. If the urine output remains more than 700 cc/h the rate should be again be reduced from the previous rate by 300 cc/h. The goal is to have a urine output rate of approximately 200 to 400 cc/h. This relatively high rate of urine output allows one to feel confident that the urine output is from the transplant kidney. The high urine output may also aid in the clearance of potassium and prevent the need for dialysis for hyperkalemia. Because some newly transplanted kidneys may have impaired concentrating ability, intravenous fluids should not be completely discontinued until the patient is eating and drinking well, unless the kidney has established delayed graft function and remains dialysis-dependent.

An alternative method of replacing fluids in living-donor recipients is to put a patient on a fixed hourly rate of 125 cc to 200 cc D5 NS per hour immediately following transplantation. Hatch et al found this to be a safe protocol that saves valuable nursing time.

Hypertension

Most patients with ESRD have hypertension. Low-dose beta-antagonists are continued perioperatively in patients with a history of coronary artery disease. Patients may be continued on clonidine to avoid rebound hypertension associated with withdrawal. Otherwise, antihypertensive medications are temporarily held in the perioperative period, and the blood pressure is allowed to remain slightly elevated to assure good renal perfusion. However, systolic blood pressures above 200 mm of mercury and diastolic blood pressures above 100 mm of mercury should be treated to prevent vascular anastomotic stress. The first agent of choice is clonidine 0.1 mg orally every twenty minutes until the blood pressure is lower than 180/100 mm of mercury. Short-acting nifedipine (sublingual or oral) is to be avoided. Its use may be associated with a precipitous decline in blood pressure resulting in stroke or graft thrombosis. Intravenous antihypertensive agents may also be used. Common choices of intravenous agents include: hydralazine 10 to 40 mg IV every four to six hours; labetalol 20 mg IV every 20 minutes to a maximum of 300 mg; or esmolol continuous infusion of 50 to 200μL/kg per minute.

Because most patients will require antihypertensive therapy posttransplantation, maintenance antihypertensive therapy is usually initiated during the initial hospital stay. The long-term goal for antihypertensive control should be a blood pressure lower than 130/80 millimeters of mercury. Most patients will require a combination of antihypertensive medications from several classes of agents. After acute control of the blood pressure with clonidine, as above, calcium channel antagonists are usually used first and may confer a survival advantage to the graft. Long-acting nifedipine and amlodipine may be better choices than diltiazem, verapamil, or nicardipine. Nifedipine does not affect cyclosporine or tacrolimus levels and is faster-acting than amlodipine. Amlodipine has a long half-life that allows for convenient dosing in the long-term, but it raises cyclosporine and tacrolimus levels slightly. Diltiazem, verapamil, and nicardipine cause marked elevations in cyclosporine and tacrolimus levels. Use of these agents may significantly reduce the dose needed and the cost of cyclosporine. However, as many physicians may be involved in the care of a renal transplant recipient, many changes in medicines will be made without the transplant nephrologist or center being aware of the changes. Discontinuation of these adjunctive drugs may result in inadequate immunosuppression and rejection. Thus, it may be best to avoid drugs such as diltiazem, verapamil, and nicardipine that have potent interactions with cyclosporine and tacrolimus.

Except as noted above, beta-antagonists are used as the second line agent. They may help control the tremors associated with the sympathetic activation seen with cyclosporine and tacrolimus. Selective beta-antagonists may be used even in patients with diabetes, asthma, and peripheral vascular disease.

Alpha blockers may be particularly useful for men with bladder neck obstruction symptoms. They may cause stress incontinence in women, however. Hydralazine may be useful, especially for afterload reduction, but it requires frequent dosing.

Angiotensin-converting enzyme (ACE) inhibitors and angiotensin II receptor antagonists should probably be avoided in the first several months posttransplant. They may lead to hyperkalemia and acute renal failure, especially when the cyclosporine levels are maintained at relatively high levels during the first several months after transplantation, as is usually done. ACE inhibitors and angiotensin II receptor antagonists also cause anemia and can prevent recovery from anemia. After the first several months, they may decrease the fibrogenic effects of cyclosporine and help prevent chronic rejection. They may also be used to treat posttransplant erythrocytosis.

The chronic maintenance use of diuretics in hypertension of transplantation is controversial. Immediately posttransplant they should probably be avoided unless there is relative oliguria as above, a clear indication of congestive heart failure, or pulmonary edema.

Minoxidil is a potent vasodilator that must be given in combination with a diuretic and a beta-antagonist. It causes hirsutism, which may become uncontrollable with concomitant use of cyclosporine, which also causes hirsutism. Oral labetalol is expensive and ineffective as an antihypertensive agent and other agents are used infrequently.

Ambulation

Early ambulation and good pulmonary toilet are essential after transplant. Most patients should be able to sit in a chair within six to eight hours of the transplant surgery and begin ambulation on postoperative day one. Patients should turn, cough, and practice deep breathing two times an hour. Use of an incentive spirometer prevents atelectasis. Most patients will initially have difficulty achieving a volume above 1,000 cc, but with encouragement, and by describing to the patient that the volume of a soda can is only 360 cc, most patients will rapidly be able to achieve incentive spirometry volumes of 1,500 to 2,000 cc.

Nutrition

INITIAL DIET AND EARLY BOWEL FUNCTION.
One of the benefits of renal transplantation for the patient with ESRD is relaxation of many of the strict

dietary restrictions. Immediately postoperatively most patients experience a mild postoperative ileus and do not pass flatus until postoperative day one or two. Steroids may also cause an adynamic ileus (Ogilvie's syndrome). Thus, patients should begin with clear liquids and rapidly advance, in nondiabetic patients, to a regular diet after flatus is established. The first postoperative bowel movement does not usually occur until postoperative day two or three in nondiabetic patients. In patients with diabetes, the ileus is often prolonged and the diet must be advanced more slowly. All patients should be on stool softeners and most will require mild cathartics such as casanthrol/docusate (Pericolace®) and/or rectal suppositories to stimulate bowel movements. Early intervention with more aggressive cathartics or enemas are appropriate. When allograft function is delayed, lactulose, sorbitol, senna (Senokot®), or non-magnesium-containing laxatives should be the laxatives of choice. If necessary, cottonseed, tap water or soap suds enemas should be used. Magnesium citrate can be used as a laxative, without concern for hypermagnesemia, in a patient with good renal function. Similarly, sodium biphosphate (Fleets®) enemas may be used, without concern for hyperphosphatemia, in patients with good renal function.

ELECTROLYTES AND ACIDOSIS. Electrolyte disturbances and acidosis are common after renal transplantation. Because of the transplanted kidney's inability to concentrate urine maximally, administration of hypotonic fluids commonly results in mild hyponatremia. Pain and narcotics also predispose renal transplant recipients to development of the SIADH (syndrome of inappropriate antidiuretic hormone) which may exacerbate the hyponatremia. Hyponatremia is easily managed by reducing free water intake. Additionally, intravenous fluid replacement should be with isotonic fluids (normal saline) rather than hypotonic fluids (half-normal saline). Hypernatremia is uncommon in the early postoperative period. Hyperkalemia has multiple etiologies after transplantation, but is most commonly seen when there is delayed graft function. Other contributing factors include limb ischemia related to vascular clamping during the transplant operation, hyperglycemia, and various medications including succinyl choline, trimethoprim and beta-antagonists. Hyperkalemia may be treated with dialysis or sodium polystyrene sulfonate (Kayexalate®) 30 to 60 orally in sorbitol. Because use of sodium polystyrene sulfonate retention enemas has been reported to cause bowel necrosis in transplant recipients, they should be avoided. Hypokalemia may occur but is easily corrected with oral potassium supplementation. Mild acidosis also occurs commonly after transplantation and is related to residual renal dysfunction and administration of copious chloride-containing fluids. Renal tubular acidosis associ-

ated with use of cyclosporine is unlikely to occur early after transplantation.

ESRD is associated with hyperparathyroidism, hyperphosphatemia, hypocalcemia, and a propensity to hypermagnesemia. Upon renal transplantation, there is now a functional end-organ (the kidney) on which parathyroid hormone may have its effect. Consequently, hypophosphatemia and hypomagnesemia are almost always seen after renal transplantation — especially when significant hyperparathyroidism is present. Hyperparathyroidism may be considered significant when the intact PTH (parathyroid hormone) is greater than 500 μL equivalents/mL.

PHOSPHOROUS. To avoid hypophosphatemia, all phosphorus binders (eg, calcium carbonate, calcium acetate, Tums®, Basalgel®, and Renagel®) should be held posttransplant unless the patient is still being maintained on dialysis for delayed graft function and has persistent hyperphosphatemia. Likewise, magnesium or aluminum-containing antacids (eg, Mylanta®, Maalox®, Alternagel®, and sucralfate) should not be used after transplant. It is better to use H2 blockers or proton-pump inhibitors to prevent ulcers and treat gastroesophageal reflux. However, if despite these measures, the plasma phosphorus falls below 2.0 mEq/dL, two to three packets of sodium-potassium phosphate (Neutra-Phos®) should be given orally two to three times daily. Rarely, phosphorous needs to be replaced intravenously. If necessary, this should be administered as sodium phosphate to avoid hyperkalemia that may occur with administration of potassium phosphate. Phosphate repletion may only be necessary for the first several weeks after transplantation. Thereafter, liberalization of the diet and ingestion of phosphorous-containing products such as diet colas and milk products is sufficient to prevent hypophosphatemia.

MAGNESIUM. Hypomagnesemia is also almost always seen immediately postoperatively. Cyclosporine causes magnesium wasting. Hypomagnesemia also occurs because of residual hyperparathyroidism and return of renal function. Hypomagnesemia may contribute to poor cardiac function, arrhythmia, muscle cramping, disordered calcium and phosphorus metabolism and metabolic bone disease. Although plasma magnesium levels are unreliable, magnesium should be replaced when the plasma level is below 1.6 mEq/dL to help resolve the postsurgical ileus and other electrolyte disorders. On postoperative day one or two, magnesium sulfate 1 to 2 grams should be administered over four hours. Slow infusion prevents renal wasting of magnesium associated with bolus infusion. On postoperative day two, magnesium oxide 400 to 800 mg can be administered orally at noon. Administration at noon prevents the potential interference of magnesium with absorption of various commonly used medications such as mycophenolate mofetil (CellCept®). Magnesium supplementation may be necessary indefinitely.

CALCIUM. In patients without significant hypophosphatemia, 1,000 mg of elemental calcium should be given away from meals to help prevent progression of metabolic bone disease. Thus, calcium is best taken at night before bed. Several preparations are available and include OsCal®, Tums®, and Viactiv® soft calcium chews. Viactiv may be the most palatable of these preparations. It is a soft, chewable, chocolate flavored calcium supplement that contains 500 mg of elemental calcium, and has only 20 calories and 8 mg of phosphorus. Calcium supplementation should probably be administered indefinitely.

ANEMIA. Anemia is almost always present prior to and immediately following transplantation. With the introduction of erythropoietin, most dialysis patients will have iron deficiency anemia. A significant number will also be deficient in cyanocobalamin (vitamin B12), and folate, particularly if the ESRD patients have not been receiving vitamin supplementation while on dialysis. Rapid correction of anemia may be accomplished through transfusion. To reduce the likelihood of transmission of cytomegalovirus, and to prevent HLA sensitization, it is best to transfuse blood through a leukopoor filter. Oral multivitamin supplements with iron and at least one milligram of folate should probably be given to most patients immediately postoperatively, since most patients will rapidly become iron deficient as anemia corrects posttransplantation. Oral iron supplementation is commonly ineffective, necessitating administration of intravenous iron, such as iron dextran 500 to 1,000 mg.

HOMOCYSTEINE. Hyperhomocystinemia is almost always present in ESRD and common in transplant recipients. It is a major risk factor for arterial and venous thrombosis, atherosclerosis, stroke and myocardial infarction and may contribute to chronic rejection. It is commonly associated with vitamin B12, B6 and folate deficiencies and may be corrected by super-supplementation with these vitamins. The exact amount of supplementation and whether supplementation will reduce these complications is unknown. However, supplementation appears to be innocuous and inexpensive. It appears that at least 500 micrograms of vitamin B12, 50 mg of vitamin B6 and 1 to 5 mg of folate are necessary to lower basal and stimulated levels of homocysteine.

DIABETES AND OBESITY. Approximately one-third of renal transplant recipients have diabetes before transplantation and approximately 10% more become diabetic because of cyclosporine and steroid-based immunosuppressive regimens used posttransplantation. When tacrolimus is used, even more may develop new onset diabetes posttransplantation. In addition, the average transplant patient will regain 10% to 20% of their pretransplant weight posttransplantation, which will further predispose the patient to the development of diabetes. Thus, all transplant patients should be instructed to avoid concentrated sweets and high-fat foods. All patients should be instructed to exercise 20 to 60 minutes, three to five times weekly, to reduce the likelihood of posttransplant diabetes and obesity.

Immediately postoperatively, all patients should receive a low maintenance rate of glucose as D5 normal saline at 30 cc per hour. This will provide almost 150 calories daily of carbohydrate that will help to prevent protein catabolism postoperatively. Patients with diabetes should receive sliding scale insulin or an insulin drip to prevent ketosis during the first two to three days postoperatively.

Thereafter, the maintenance dose of insulin should be re-instituted. Several factors will make the insulin requirements higher and different posttransplant than pretransplant. First, a functioning kidney is gluconeogenic. Second, a functioning renal transplant will excrete insulin, and third, the immunosuppressive medications promote insulin resistance. Typically, patients with diabetes will require at least one unit per kilogram of body weight per day of insulin posttransplantation. A common regimen pretransplant is to administer two-thirds of the daily insulin in the morning and one-third in the evening. Posttransplantation, it is more effective to administer three-quarters of the daily insulin requirement in the morning and one-quarter in the evening to compensate for the late afternoon and early evening hyperglycemia associated with the customary morning steroid administration. Adjunctive use of oral hyperglycemic agents should be used with caution. Troglitazone (Rezulin®) will markedly decrease cyclosporine levels, and metformin may lead to lactic acidosis when renal insufficiency is present.

EARLY POSTOPERATIVE COMPLICATIONS
Urine Leaks
Urine leaks occur in approximately 5% of renal transplant recipients. They usually present as delayed graft function or with a rising serum creatinine that may be easily confused with obstruction. Pain will often be associated with a urine leak and is described as burning in character. The uretero-vesicular junction is the most common site for the leak since this is a watershed area and prone to ischemia. The diagnosis is usually supported by ultrasound, which shows a fluid collection.

Subsequent analysis of the fluid reveals a fluid collection creatinine significantly higher than the serum creatinine and a relative paucity of cells. Alternatively, a nuclear medicine renal scan may also show extravasation of radioisotope supporting the diagnosis of a urine leak. It is important to get delayed images 12 to 24 hours after the first image when poor renal function exists, because initial images may not detect or show a leak if excretion is not great enough. Upon diagnosis, prompt treatment is necessary. The first treatment is placement of a bladder catheter for decompression. Nephrostomy and ureteral stent placement may also be attempted. However, most urine leaks are best treated with prompt surgical revision.

Obstruction

Obstruction of the kidney may occur at any site along the urinary tract. It should be suspected when the serum creatinine rises unexpectedly or fails to fall posttransplantation. Hyperkalemia may be present because of tubular backleak and resorption. A sudden increase in cyclosporine levels on a stable dose may also occur because of failure to excrete cyclosporine and its metabolites. Diminished urine output may or may not be noted. In men, urethral stenosis, particularly if there has been a history of transurethral resection of the prostate, or bladder neck obstruction secondary to prostatism, are common causes of obstruction. In both sexes, the obstruction may be related to ureteral strictures or to fluid collections such as lymphoceles, seromata, hematomata, or urinomata that obstruct the ureter. Fluid collections are commonly associated with ipsilateral lower extremity edema. Occasionally, blood clots or stones may cause obstruction. Diabetic patients may have a functional obstruction from a neurogenic bladder.

Patients in whom a urinary obstruction is expected should have a post-void residual measured and the bladder catheter should remain in place if the post-void residual is greater than 100 to 200 cc. Patients should then have an emergent ultrasound to assess for the presence of hydronephrosis or fluid collections. An aliquot of any fluid collection should be aspirated and analyzed for creatinine, cell count with differential, and sent for Gram stain and culture to determine the character of the fluid collection. A percutaneous antegrade nephrostogram is useful to determine the site of obstruction. Retrograde nephrostograms obtained cystoscopically are difficult to perform because of the difficulty in locating and cannulating the transplant ureteral orifice. The transplant ureteral orifice is typically located in the dome of the bladder. The native ureteral orifices, in contrast, are located in the bladder trigone and are easily accessible cystoscopically.

Drainage of compressing fluid collections may relieve the obstruction. Lymphoceles often recur and may be managed by drainage and sclerosis or through marsupialization performed through an open or laparo-

scopic approach. Short (<2 mm) strictures may sometimes be analyzed endourologically. Longer strictures typically require open revision.

Arterial and Venous Thrombosis

Uremia is associated with platelet dysfunction and poor clotting. Thus, early renal arterial and venous thrombosis are almost always related to surgical technical problems and occur in 1% to 8% of all transplants. Technical factors associated with thrombosis include laparoscopic donor nephrectomy (especially of the right kidney), inadequate flush of the donor kidney, and prolonged cold ischemia and rewarm time. Certain ESRD patient subgroups, however, may be hypercoagulable. These include patients with systemic lupus erythematosus and antiphospholipid (lupus anticoagulant) antibodies; patients with nephrotic syndrome who may be hypercoagulable secondary to urinary loss of antithrombin III and other anti-clotting factors; and patients with hyperhomocystinemia. Rarely, patients will have activated protein C resistance, or protein C or S deficiency.

Renal thrombosis should be expected whenever there is a sudden decrease in the urine output. This is especially true with living-related allografts. Pain, hematuria, and a serum-elevated lactic dehydrogenase (LDH) may or may not be present. After a rapid evaluation to assess volume status, a fluid challenge should be given and then a renal scan or Doppler ultrasound should be obtained immediately. Rarely, immediate thrombolytic therapy or surgical thrombectomy may rescue a thrombosed kidney.

The need for routine antithrombotic prophylaxis is uncertain. Many programs administer heparin 5,000 units during the transplant operation just prior to completion of the venous anastomosis to decrease the incidence of thrombosis. Some programs are now using fractionated heparin and or aspirin. It is important to keep in mind that postoperative mini-dose heparinization has been reported to be associated with an increased incidence of lymphoceles when retroperitoneal surgery is performed.

Deep venous thromboses of the lower extremities were common historically and reported to occur in up to 10% of transplant recipients. Early ambulation and use of sequential pneumatic compression stockings has greatly decreased the incidence in contemporary transplant surgery.

Infections

The infectious risk during the initial hospitalization is primarily nosocomial and related to the surgical procedure, indwelling intravenous catheters, drainage tubes and catheters. Perioperative cefazolin is administered to the recipient during the first 24 hours in most programs. Selective bowel decontamination has been shown to be useful in pediatric liver transplantation, but has no role in kidney transplantation. Reverse isolation or the use of gowns, gloves, and masks for those having contact with the patient is also not warranted, even when the patient is neutropenic. Reverse isolation is also no better at preventing nosocomial spread of vancomycin-resistant enterococci than good hand washing and gloving. Uncooked fruit, vegetables, and fresh flowers and plants harbor many bacteria including *E. coli, Pseudomonas* species, and *Klebsiella* species. Many programs forbid live plants on the transplant floor or do not allow any uncooked food to be served to renal transplant patients. However, simple common sense measures such as food washing and good hand washing are probably all that is necessary.

The classical mnemonic (the five W's) for evaluation of fever in any surgical patient (ie, wind, wound, water, walking, wonder drug) is germane for the kidney transplant recipient. These patients are at risk for conventional bacterial pneumonia from atelectasis; bacterial and candidal wound infection; urinary tract infections associated with indwelling urinary catheters; and infection of hematomata, seromata, urinomata, or lymphoceles. Good pulmonary toilet and early ambulation reduce the risk of pneumonia. The prophylactic use of double dose trimethoprim/sulfamethoxazole (320 mg/1,600 mg) orally, regardless of the serum creatinine while the bladder catheter remains in place, has reduced the risk of urinary tract bacterial infection to less than 10% and the risk of bloodstream infection by tenfold. The optimal duration and dose of continued prophylaxis is unknown. Because of its protection against multiple opportunistic infections, many programs continue trimethoprim/sulfamethoxazole prophylaxis for life in nonallergic patients.

Herpes simplex virus (HSV) 1 and 2 and HHV 6 may be reactivated in the first month. Less commonly, VZV, EBV, and CMV in the recipient may be reactivated in the first month. New or primary viral infection from the donor generally does not become symptomatic until after the first month. Low-dose acyclovir 200 to 400 mg by mouth is effective prophylaxis for reactivation of HSV 1 and 2. Although high-dose acyclovir (800 mg by mouth four to five times per day) was reported to be effective for prevention of CMV, subsequent studies have shown that high-dose acyclovir has little role for prevention of CMV. In contrast, oral ganciclovir 1,000 mg by mouth is highly effective for prevention of most herpes virus infections including HSV 1 and 2, VZV, EBV, CMV, and possibly HHV 6, but not HHV 7.

Use of Imaging Studies

Ultrasonography is most useful to demonstrate hydronephrosis or fluid collections. Doppler ultrasonography may be useful to demonstrate arterial or venous thrombosis. In experienced hands, ultrasonography may demonstrate transplant renal artery stenosis. Threshold arterial velocities of 100 to 200 cm/sec are associated with renal artery stenosis. An elevated "resistive index" above 0.6 to 0.7 and uroepithelial thickening have been felt to be diagnostic of rejection. Unfortunately, both an elevated resistive index and uroepithelial thickening may be seen in any form of renal dysfunction. Thus, ultrasonography is not useful for distinguishing acute rejection from other causes of decreased allograft function.

Radioiodinated contrast angiography remains the "gold standard" for detection of vascular stenosis. The role and availability of carbon dioxide angiography remains to be determined. Magnetic resonance angiography is at present time consuming and expensive.

Nuclear medicine renal scans are useful to show thrombosis, obstruction, leaks, acute tubular necrosis, infarction or to assess renal function. Nuclear medicine scanning may be divided into three phases. The first phase is the angiographic, or first pass, phase and is used to detect blood flow to the kidney. The second phase is the parenchymal phase and is used to assess secretion, filtration and morphology. The third phase is the excretion phase and it is used to assess glomerular filtration rate (GFR) and the presence of leaks. Technetium 99 is the most common isotope used in renal scanning. Several isotope carriers are available that are either primarily excreted by glomerular filtration or tubular secretion and chosen for the clinical situation. Mag 3 (mercaptoacetyltriglycine) is one of the more commonly used isotopes. It is primarily excreted by tubular secretion and is useful for detection of ATN and thrombosis. DTPA (diethylenetriaminepentaacetate), by comparison, is primarily excreted by glomerular filtration and is useful to assess GFR. DMSA (dimercaptosuccinate) binds to renal cortical cells and is useful for imaging areas of infarction in the renal cortex. A mnemonic to keep these isotope carriers clear is: P in DTPA is for performance of the kidney (ie, GFR); M in DMSA is for morphology. Because we are often concerned about ATN, the imaging study of first choice is Mag 3. Nuclear radiology is not useful to diagnose rejection since it is nonspecific.

Computerized tomography and magnetic resonance imaging are not commonly used in the immediate posttransplant period. Computerized tomography is most useful to evaluate for the presence of abscesses. It is not helpful for the diagnosis of rejection or vascular thrombosis. Magnetic resonance imaging is rarely used in the immediate postoperative period, but is particularly useful to diagnose avascular necrosis of the hips either pretransplant or posttransplant.

RECOMMENDED READING

Bigg SW, Catalona WJ. Prophylactic mini-dose heparin in patients undergoing radical retropubic prostatectomy. A prospective trial. Urology. 1992;39(4):309-313.

Bostom AG, Gohh RY, Beaulieu AJ, et al. Treatment of hyperhomocystinemia in renal transplant recipients. A randomized, placebo-controlled trial. Ann Intern Med. 1997;127(12):1089-1092.

Brennan DC, Singer GG. Infectious complications in renal transplant recipients. In: Malluche HH, Sawaya BP, Hakim RM, Sayegh MH, Ismail N, eds. Clinical Nephrology Dialysis and Transplantation. Deisenhofen, Germany: Dustri-Verlag; 1999:1-24.

Brennan DC, Garlock KA, Singer GG, et al. Prophylactic oral ganciclovir compared with deferred therapy for control of cytomegalovirus in renal transplant recipients. Transplantation. 1997;64(12):1843-1846.

Mayforth DR, Lowell JA, Brennan DC, Howard TK. Transplantation. In: Doherty GM, Meko JB, Olson JA, Peplinski FP, Worrall NK, eds. The Washington Manual of Surgery. 2nd ed. Philadelphia, Pa: Lippincott, Williams & Wilkins; 1999:417-440.

Zimmerman P, Ragavendra N, Hoh CK, Barbaric ZL. Radiology of kidney transplantation. In: Danovitch GM, ed. Handbook of Kidney Transplantation. 2nd ed. Philadelphia, Pa: Lippincott Williams & Wilkins Publishers; 1996:417-440.

Bowden RA, Ljungman P, Paya CV, eds. Transplant Infections. Philadelphia, Pa: Lippincott Williams & Wilkins Publishers; 1998.

Hatch DA, Barry JM, Norman DJ. A randomized study of intravenous fluid replacement following living-donor renal transplantation. Transplantation. 1985;40(6): 648-651.

55 PHYSIOLOGY OF THE TRANSPLANTED KIDNEY

Matthew R. Weir, MD

Transplantation has proven to be a successful replacement therapy for end-stage renal disease. However, the recipient of a renal transplant does not usually receive a full complement of nephrons, in part due to the single kidney replacement strategy necessitated by the scarcity of the organs, as well as by the multitude of stresses placed on the organ prior to, during, and after transplantation.

The physiologic function of the transplanted kidney correlates with the adequacy of overall glomerular filtration rate (GFR). This is a composite effect of the adequacy of the donor source, preservation and procurement, and perioperative and postoperative course of the recipient.

EFFECTS OF DIMINISHED NEPHRON MASS

Cadaveric kidneys have a half-life of eight to ten years. This longevity has changed minimally in the last several years (an increase from seven years to 9.4 years) due to more effective immunosuppressive agents, which have been able to substantially reduce acute rejection rates. The fact that the half-life has not improved further suggests that inadequate nephron dosing, or other factors such as noncompliance, may be important for long-term survival.

Since many recipients of cadaveric renal allografts have an impaired creatinine clearance for a variety of different reasons, it is imperative that efforts be made to more carefully control blood pressure, glycemic control, and cholesterol metabolism, as these are known hazards that lead to progressive vascular disease and loss of renal function in nontransplanted patients.

Experimental models of diminished renal mass have demonstrated the importance of reducing systemic and glomerular capillary pressure. This reduces mechanical stretch and shearing forces of the higher pressures on the wall of the blood vessels and glomeruli. Upregulation of angiotensin II production and other mediators of fibrosis, growth and remodeling, such as TGF-beta, are almost always a consequence of vascular injury from stress, turbulence or oxidative damage. Conse-

quently, intensive control of blood pressure is a prerequisite for preventing attrition of renal function. Therapeutic strategies, including angiotensin-converting enzyme (ACE) inhibitors and angiotensin type-1 receptor blockers, that reduce both systemic and glomerular capillary pressure will likely prove to be beneficial in delaying loss of nephrons in transplant recipients. These drugs will need to be combined with other antihypertensive agents in order to ensure adequate reduction in systolic blood pressure, preferably to a level of 150 mmHg or less.

If there is evidence of proteinuria, more intensive blood pressure reduction and the use of antiproteinuric drugs like ACE inhibitors and angiotensin type-1 receptor blockers also assumes more importance. Proteinuria may reflect elevated glomerular capillary pressure and/or damage to the glomerular basement membrane allowing the increased transglomerular passage of proteins. Proteinuria, particularly with glycosylated proteins, as occurs in diabetic patients, can be toxic to the kidney by eliciting an inflammatory response in the phagocytic mesangial apparatus leading to glomerular injury. Thus, more intensive control of blood pressure and glomerular capillary pressure and specific antiproteinuric strategies (ie, dietary salt restriction and pharmacologic blockade of the renin angiotensin system) are critical. In the Modification of Diet in Renal Disease study, which was conducted primarily in nondiabetic patients with chronic renal failure and GFR between 13 mL/min and 55 mL/min, there was a conclusive benefit of more intensive blood pressure reduction (125/75 mmHg) compared to a traditional approach (140/90 mmHg), particularly in proteinuric patients. This level of renal function is comparable to that seen in the transplanted kidney. Thus, the physiology of the transplanted kidney requires careful attention to control many of the factors known to accelerate loss of renal function, most importantly, control of blood pressure and proteinuria.

Chronic deterioration of renal function in transplant recipients more commonly occurs in patients who have received an older or injured kidney, those who have poorly-controlled blood pressure or manifest nephrotoxicity to calcineurin inhibitors, and those who have had acute rejection. All of these situations, alone or together, reduce the amount of nephrons a patient receives with an allograft and places greater stress on the remaining nephron mass (Figure 55-1). The concomitant administration of nephrotoxic immunosuppressive agents, such as the calcineurin inhibitors, can further aggravate intrarenal processes that lead to development of interstitial fibrosis, vascular hyalinosis, and attrition of renal function. Some clinicians have also suggested that older kidneys may be less likely to last longer than younger kidneys because of inherent changes that occur with aging, such as lack of blood vessels to dilate and handle more renal blood flow or an inability of the glomeruli to

Professor and Director, Division of Nephrology and Clinical Research Unit, Department of Medicine, University of Maryland School of Medicine, Baltimore, MD

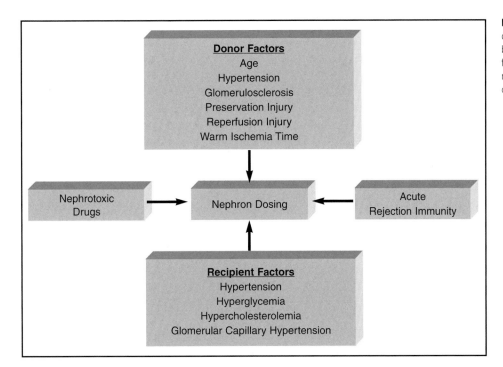

Figure 55-1. This paradigm describes the interrelationship between donor and recipient factors along with immunity and nephrotoxic drugs that lead to chronic allograft nephropathy.

hypertrophy and improve filtration, thus placing more stress on remaining nephrons. Performing double-kidney transplants to establish good initial renal function appears to be the preferred approach to using kidneys from older donors.

Mismatching of donor's and recipient's body size has attracted some interest as a means of impairment of proper nephron dosing, but is not universally accepted as an issue of clinical importance. A more important issue is the use of older donors, as described previously.

Overall, these issues highlight the importance of optimal nephron dosing, but also of protecting transplanted nephrons as best possible by avoiding clinical situations that cause damage or stress.

Recent clinical trials have explored the benefits of reducing the dose of calcineurin inhibitors in patients with chronic allograft nephropathy and deteriorating renal function as these patients have already manifested histologic and functional changes of reduced nephron mass. These drugs may have diminished therapeutic benefit in patients with biopsy-proven interstitial fibrosis and declining kidney function. The early observations from these clinical studies show promise for stabilizing renal function.

Concern about the calcineurin inhibitors stems from their propensity to cause clinical nephrotoxicity but also to promote intrarenal vasoconstriction and to augment matrix protein production leading to interstitial fibrosis, tubular atrophy and vascular hyalinosis. These drugs also have an adverse impact on blood pressure, glucose and cholesterol metabolism. On the other hand, they are essential to prevent acute rejection. Thus, a care-

ful balance has to be achieved between the risk of acute rejection and the risk of toxic effects of these drugs. Interestingly, there is experimental data in rats suggesting that ACE inhibitors and angiotensin type-1 receptor blockers can attenuate cyclosporine-induced interstitial fibrosis independent of changes in blood pressure. This may be another reason to explore the use of these types of drugs in calcineurin inhibitor-treated transplant recipients.

METABOLIC FUNCTION OF THE TRANSPLANTED KIDNEY

The metabolic function of the transplanted kidney parallels its overall GFR. The higher the GFR, the more effective the overall ability to detoxify drugs and to produce necessary hormones that regulate erythropoiesis and calcium and phosphorus homeostasis.

Increased erythropoiesis occurs in most patients within the first few months posttransplantation, provided there is adequate iron storage and no active infection. Recent clinical studies have demonstrated that serum erythropoietin levels increase immediately posttransplantation, usually within the first ten postoperative days. A second, more sustained rise in erythropoietin levels occurs 20 to 50 days posttransplant in patients with good allograft function. Erythrocytosis can occur in 15% to 20% of patients, resulting in a hematocrit greater than 51%. Interestingly, plasma erythropoietin levels are most commonly normal in these patients, suggesting that other humoral factors, perhaps produced by the transplanted kidney, may enhance sensitivity to erythropoietin or directly stimulate erythropoiesis. Drugs that block the renin angiotensin system, such as ACE inhibitors or angiotensin type-1 receptor blockers, are effective in mitigating this effect.

The transplanted kidney is also effective in restoring blood levels of 25-hydroxy vitamin D, and 1, 25-dihydroxy vitamin D. Hypophosphatemia is commonly observed in the first few weeks posttransplantation, primarily related to the phosphaturic effects of elevated concentrations of circulating parathyroid hormone. However, once the intact vitamin D improves calcium homeostasis, parathyroid hormone levels return to normal, resulting in a restoration of serum phosphate levels in the normal range. Early hypophosphatemia associated with normal serum levels of 1, 25-dihydroxy vitamin D indicates that the synthesis of this active form of vitamin D may be transiently impaired since low phosphorus levels should result in elevated 1,25-dihydroxy vitamin D levels. As renal function deteriorates in the transplanted kidney, efforts should be made to provide phosphate binders, replete calcium, and provide the intact form of vitamin D. This is effective in suppressing parathyroid hormone and the risk of osteopenia and metabolic calcification.

Since the transplanted kidney is denervated when procured, there may be an acute inability to increase plasma renin activity in response to a reduction in dietary salt intake. A phenomenon of renal salt wasting could result in volume depletion. However, this is not commonly seen after the immediate polyuric postoperative period, as the concomitant administration of drugs that amplify renal salt and water retention, such as corticosteroids, cyclosporine, or tacrolimus, take hold. Clinical studies have demonstrated that functional regeneration of renal nerves occur within one to three months post-kidney transplantation. This effect and its variable timing no doubt explains some of the contradictory results of early clinical studies trying to evaluate and characterize renal salt and water handling at various times soon after kidney transplantation. However, some well done clinical studies early in the posttransplant period do indicate that sodium and water handling by the kidney can be normal or nearly normal.

THE PHYSIOLOGY OF ELECTROLYTE HANDLING BY THE KIDNEY

Defects in proximal tubule transport have been observed in renal transplant recipients. Glucosuria is most commonly reported and is observed in more than 50% of patients, even in the absence of hyperglycemia. Occasionally, patients may even exhibit the Fanconi syndrome, comprising of phosphaturia, bicarbonaturia, glucosuria, aminoaciduria, and uricosuria. Both proximal and distal renal tubular acidosis may be related to preservation injury, acute proximal tubular necrosis,

acute rejection, or persistent hyperparathroidism. Any of these disorders can resolve over time as the kidney heals; however, these abnormalities, if persistent, may reflect ongoing renal injury or irreparable damage. Reduced ammonia generation resulting from a reduction in renal mass may also contribute to chronic renal tubular acidosis.

Hyperkalemia is not uncommon post-renal transplantation. The mechanism most commonly suspected is a poorly described effect of chronic cyclosporine or tacrolimus therapy. It may be related to impaired renal function, depressed aldosterone levels, or to a primary tubular defect. Cyclosporine may also cause magnesium wasting and subsequent hypomagnesemia. Hyperuricemia may also occur in a substantial number of cyclosporine-treated renal transplant recipients. This abnormality also increases the risk of gouty arthropathy. The presence of hypercalcemia posttransplantation is not indicative of renal dysfunction. It more likely reflects a persistence of hyperparathyroidism. This process may persist over many years, despite the restoration of near-normal renal function.

HEMATURIA AND PROTEINURIA

Hematuria can occur in the early posttransplantation period. Most commonly this is nonglomerular and likely reflects urinary tract infection or structural abnormalities of the urogenital tract. Evaluation with urine culture, renal sonogram, or cystoscopy can be helpful in making the diagnosis. Later in the posttransplantation period, hematuria may reflect urothelial abnormalities, rejection or recurrent glomerular disease. Renal biopsy would be the definitive procedure for this assessment. Renal tissue should be sent for light, immunofluorescence and electron microscopy to make the diagnosis of recurrent glomerular disease.

Proteinuria in the renal transplant recipient indicates glomerular leakage of proteins that overwhelm tubular resorptive mechanisms. In the presence of hematuria it may indicate an acute rejection or recurrent glomerulonephritis. In the setting of deteriorating renal function it most commonly reflects either acute or subacute rejection and/or chronic allograft nephropathy. Renal biopsy should be performed with assessment of light and electron microscopy and immunofluorescence.

Proteinuria should be treated by pharmacologic agents that lower systemic and glomerular capillary pressure as discussed previously. Dietary salt reduction potentiates the antiproteinuric properties of ACE inhibitors. Reducing proteinuria (along with blood pressure) will likely prove to be beneficial in delaying deterioration of allograft function, much as it has been shown to be beneficial in other forms of renal disease.

RECOMMENDED READING

Halloran PF. Nonimmunologic tissue injury and stress in chronic allograft dysfunction. Graft. 1998;1:25-29.

Ojo AO, Wolfe RA, Held PJ, Port FK, Schmouder RL. Delayed graft function: risk factors and implications for renal allograft survival. Transplantation. 1997;63(7): 968-974.

Cosio FG, Pelletier RP, Falkenhain ME, et al. Impact of acute rejection and early allograft function on renal allograft survival. Transplantation. 1997;63(11):1611-1615.

Cosio FG, Qiu W, Henry ML, et al. Factors related to the donor organ are major determinants of renal allograft function and survival. Transplantation. 1996;62(11): 1571-1576.

Klahr S, Levey AS, Beck GJ, et al. The effect of dietary protein restriction and blood-pressure control on the progression of chronic renal disease: Modification of Diet in Renal Disease Study Group. N Engl J Med. 1994;330(13):877-884.

Weir MR, Dworkin LD. Antihypertensive drugs, dietary salt, and renal protection: how low should you go, and with which therapy? Am J Kid Dis. 1998;32(1):1-22.

Weir MR, Anderson L, Fink JC, et al. A novel approach to the treatment of chronic allograft nephropathy. Transplantation. 1997;64(12):1706-1710.

DiBona GF. Renal innervation and denervation: lessons from renal transplantation reconsidered. Artif Organs. 1987;11(6):457-462.

Kamel KS, Ethier JH, Quaggin S, et al. Studies to determine the basis for hyperkalemia in recipients of a renal transplant who are treated with cyclosporine. J Am Soc Neph. 1991;2(8):1279-1284.

Sun CH, Ward HJ, Paul WL, Koyle MA, Yanagawa N, Lee DB. Serum erythropoietin levels after renal transplantation. N Engl J Med. 1989;321(3):151-157.

Wilson DR, Siddiqui AA. Renal tubular acidosis after kidney transplantation. Natural history and significance. Ann Int Med. 1973;79(3):352-361.

Hatch DA, Barry JM, Norman DJ. A randomized study of intravenous fluid replacement following living-donor renal transplantation. Transplantation. 1985;40(6): 648-651.

56 INDUCTION IMMUNOSUPPRESSION PROTOCOLS FOR KIDNEY TRANSPLANTATION

Flavio Vincenti, MD

Induction immunosuppression therapy was introduced in the late 1960s by Monaco and Starzl with the use of polyclonal antilymphocyte sera derived from horses or rabbits. The concepts for the use, the mechanisms of action and the benefit of induction therapy have evolved appreciably over the past 30 years. In addition, there has been an evolution in the use of these biological agents, from a full course for induction, to an abbreviated course for delaying the introduction of calcineurin inhibitors, referred to as sequential immunosuppression. The initial purpose of induction therapy with biological agents was to produce selective depletion of circulating and tissue lymphocytes to change the host immune response to the graft from activation to tolerance. Induction therapy with biological agents has been proposed to result in a number of effects that facilitate successful engraftment. Biological agents may have a modulatory effect on T cells when administered at the time of antigen presentation (ie, transplant surgery). In addition, induction therapy may induce a quiescent inflammatory state in an organ that could be replete with inflammatory cells associated with the reperfusion injury. Immunosuppression has been shown to occur during the period of T cell depletion and persists following peripheral recovery of the T cells.

In recent years, specific analysis of some of the polyclonal antilymphocyte preparations showed that they contained antibodies against numerous functional leukocyte surface molecules including CD3, CD45, CD11A/18, CD2, CD4, CD8, HLA-DR and CD25. In addition, in some preparations, high titer antibodies were also found to CD28 and CD40. In 1986, muromonab-CD3, a murine monoclonal antibody directed to the epsilon chain of the CD3 complex, was shown to be more effective than corticosteroids in reversing acute rejection episodes. Soon thereafter, muromonab-CD3 was used in induction protocols. The most recent biological agents to be introduced have been the anti-interleukin-2 receptor antibodies, daclizumab, a humanized monoclonal antibody, and basiliximab, a chimeric monoclonal antibody. These last two agents were the first biological agents to undergo vigorous clinical trials as induction agents in randomized, prospective and double-blind trials. Induction therapy may evolve in yet another direction with biological agents that block the co-stimulatory pathways such as CD40, CD28 and B71 and B72. Other potential targets for humanized monoclonal antibodies include adhesion molecules such as LFA1 and ICAM.

POLYCLONAL ANTIBODIES

There is currently over 30 years of experience with the use of polyclonal antibodies as induction agents in organ transplantation. The most commonly used preparations have been MALG (Minnesota Antilymphocyte Globulin®) which is no longer available, antilymphocyte globulin (ATGAM®), Fresenius ATG (available in Europe but not to the US) and rabbit antithymocyte globulin (Thymoglobulin®), which was approved for use in renal transplantation in 1999. None of these agents underwent the rigors of placebo-controlled, blinded, randomized trials for safety and efficacy as induction agents. In fact, the phase III trial of Thymoglobulin® was performed for reversal of acute rejection, although it will likely be used more frequently for induction of immunosuppression.

Antilymphocyte preparations are produced by immunization of laboratory animals with human lymphoid cells such as cultured lymphoblasts and thymocytes. The animal species used most often are the horse and the rabbit. Unwanted antibodies are largely removed by adsorption with erythrocytes, platelets and serum proteins. The desired antibodies reside exclusively in the IgG fraction, and thus this fraction is often isolated to yield the antilymphocyte or antithymocyte globulin. Disadvantages of polyclonal antilymphocyte agents include the batch-to-batch variation in immunopotency, as well as the unavoidable presence of cross-reacting antibodies that may cause thrombocytopenia, leukopenia or anemia. Two polyclonal agents are currently available for use in the US.

ATGAM®

ATGAM® is a horse polyclonal antilymphocyte globulin prepared by immunizing horses with human thymocytes. The immunoglobulin fraction isolated from the sera of the immunized horses is purified by adsorption with erythrocytes, platelets and serum proteins to remove the unwanted antibodies and to yield a preparation with relatively high-specificity for lymphocytes. The usual daily dose of ATGAM® is 10 mg/kg to 20 mg/kg administered through a 0.22 to 1.9 micron filter as an intravenous infusion in normal saline (250 cc to 500 cc) over four to six hours. The infusion is given via a central line because of the frequent occurrence of chemical phlebitis when the drug is given in a peripheral vein. In

Professor of Clinical Medicine, Kidney Transplant Service, University of California, San Francisco, CA

view of the possibility of anaphylactic reactions, intradermal skin testing with horse IgG is sometimes advised, but rarely done. A safer approach is to infuse the first 15 mL over 30 minutes before proceeding with the full infusion. When using all polyclonal agents, premedication with acetaminophen and diphenhydramine is advisable.

THYMOGLOBULIN®

Thymoglobulin® is a purified, pasteurized, gamma immune globulin obtained by immunization of rabbits with human thymocyte. Thymoglobulin® should be administered by slow, continuous infusion through a high flow vein, preferably a central vein. The first dose should be infused over six hours through an in-line 0.22 μm filter. Subsequent doses may be infused over a period of at least four hours. Skin testing is not recommended in patients who receive Thymoglobulin®. The recommended dose of Thymoglobulin® is 1.5 mg/kg administered for seven to 14 days.

Adverse Effects

The first dose of these agents is often associated with the development of fever and chills, which may be mediated by cytokines produced by activated cells and perhaps released during lymphocytolysis. Other side effects that have been reported include nausea, vomiting, diarrhea, myalgia, arthralgia, rash and pruritus. Thrombocytopenia and leukopenia are the most frequent hematologic abnormalities, and usually respond readily to dose reduction or discontinuation of the polyclonal agents. Rarely, the adult respiratory distress syndrome may occur with the use of polyclonal antibodies. In a minority of patients, signs or symptoms of serum sickness may develop in response to the administration of a large volume of xenoantibodies.

Clinical Use

In clinical trials in the pre-cyclosporine era, polyclonal agents were used to improve the dismal graft outcome with immunoprophylaxis with prednisone and azathioprine. However, the results of these studies were conflicting. A major problem was the increased incidence of infectious complications, especially cytomegalovirus, at a time when antiviral therapy did not exist. Although a definite increase in graft survival with the use of polyclonal antilymphocyte agents could not be demonstrated in all studies, prophylactic use of these agents was often associated with delayed onset of rejection and a steroid sparing effect. In contrast to the conflicting results from studies of antilymphocyte agents used for induction therapy, more convincing results were achieved with the use of these agents in the treatment of primary rejection or in steroid-resistant rejection.

Following the introduction of cyclosporine in 1983, the use of polyclonal agents was advocated as part of a sequential immunoprophylaxis therapy. This approach used antilymphocyte agents immediately after transplantation until the renal function improved sufficiently to initiate cyclosporine. The advantage of this sequential therapy approach was to minimize the potential nephrotoxicity of cyclosporine when renal function was still compromised and prevent the occurrence of early rejection due to subtherapeutic levels of cyclosporine. These low levels may result from under-dosing or poor bioavailability of cyclosporine. In 1999, Thymoglobulin®, a rabbit antihuman thymocyte globulin was approved for use by the Food and Drug Administration (FDA) for reversal of acute rejection. In a phase III multicenter, double-blind, randomized trial, patients with acute rejections received seven to14 days of Thymoglobulin® (1.5 mg/kg per day) or ATGAM® (15 mg/kg per day). The primary endpoint was reversal of rejection. Thymoglobulin® had a higher rate of reversal than ATGAM® (88% vs 76%, $P=0.027$), although there was no difference in the two treatment groups in day 30 graft survival, serum creatinine levels as a percentage of baseline, or in improvement of posttransplant biopsy results. T cell depletion was maintained more effectively with Thymoglobulin® than ATGAM®. Recurrent rejection occurred significantly less at day 90 after therapy with Thymoglobulin® (17%) vs ATGAM® (36%), $P=0.011$. There was a similar incidence of adverse events with the use of both agents. The conclusion was that Thymoglobulin® was more potent than ATGAM® in reversing acute rejection, which is consistent with a long-held belief that rabbit antibody preparations are more potent than horse-derived antibody preparations. Additional studies are required to assess the effectiveness of Thymoglobulin® in induction therapy.

MUROMONAB-CD3

Hybridoma technology has made it feasible to prepare large quantities of monoclonal antibodies (mAb) with a defined antigen specificity. This technology has had a major impact in many fields of basic research as well as in clinical medicine. The synthesis of second generation antilymphocyte preparations has used this new technology, and a series of mAbs directed against T lymphocyte surface antigens, the OKT series, was described in the late 1970s. One of these mAbs, muromonab-CD3 was evaluated for reversal of acute rejection in the early 1980s, and was approved by the FDA in 1986. Muromonab-CD3 is a murine IgG_{2A} antibody specifically directed against the epsilon sub-chain of the CD3 complex, which is positioned adjacent to the T cell receptor on mature T lymphocytes. Monitoring of CD3 levels during muromonab-CD3 therapy is recommended. The number of circulating CD3-positive cells during muromonab-CD3 therapy is usually below 25 cells/mm^3. A gradual or rapid rise in circulating CD3-positive cells during muromonab-CD3 therapy almost invariably is a result of the formation of human anti-mouse antibodies (HAMA) resulting in clearance of muromonab-CD3 from the circulation. Completion of successful therapy can be attempted by increasing the dose of muromonab-CD3 from 5 mg to 10 mg. However, titers of HAMA greater than 1:1000 contraindicate the further use or reuse of muromonab-CD3.

Muromonab-CD3 is administered rapidly in an intravenous dose of 5 mg. The usual course for induction therapy, or for reversal of rejection is seven to 14 days. On repeated dosing of muromonab-CD3, the mean trough level is approximately 800 mcg/mL to 900 mcg/mL, a steady state trough serum muromonab-CD3 concentration that is required for in vitro inhibition of cytotoxic T cell function. Patients who develop HAMA have a precipitous fall in muromonab-CD3 serum concentrations.

ADVERSE EFFECTS (see Section II, Chapter 14g)

The administration of the first dose of muromonab-CD3 is frequently associated with a clinical syndrome referred to as the *cytokine release syndrome*. This syndrome is caused by the transient activation of CD3 cells and the release of IL-2, TNF, γ interferon and IL6.

Clinical Use

Muromonab-CD3 was initially approved for treatment of first acute rejections. It soon became apparent that it was also effective in treating rejections that did not respond to steroids, and in recent years muromonab-CD3 has been used more frequently for induction therapy than for reversal of acute rejection. The initial experience of the use of muromonab-CD3 for induction therapy was reviewed in a consensus conference. Most of these trials involved small numbers of patients, few were randomized, and none were double-blind, controlled studies. Despite these limitations, prophylactic muromonab-CD3 regimens resulted in a reduction of acute rejection rate, especially during the first month posttransplant, and delayed the onset of acute rejection when compared to conventional immunosuppression (usually cyclosporine, azathioprine, prednisone). There is no consistently beneficial effect of muromonab-CD3 on 1-year graft survival, on the reduction of the incidence of delayed graft function, or on the duration of dialysis posttransplant.

In 1995, Dr. Opelz published, on behalf of the collaborative transplant study, data collected by the registry on the effect of immunoprophylaxis with muromonab-CD3. Patients treated with muromonab-CD3 prophylaxis and sequential (ie, delayed) addition of cyclosporine were compared to patients treated with a similar maintenance immunosuppression regimen, but without muromonab-CD3. The muromonab-CD3 – CsA sequential regimen was associated with a significantly higher overall 3-year graft survival rate in recipients of first transplants (75 ± 1% vs. 71 ± 1%, respectively; $P<0.0001$) and in recipients of retransplants (68% ± 2% vs. 62% ± 1%, respectively; $P < 0.001$). In contrast the simultaneous administration of muromonab-CD3 and cyclosporine from the first post-transplant day was not associated with improved graft survival when compared to patients treated without muromonab-CD3. Significantly improved 3-year graft survival rates with muromonab-CD3 and sequential cyclosporine were likewise obtained in highly sensitized patients (PRA>50%), African-American and pediatric recipients. However, results of analysis from registry data should be interpreted with caution, because other differences between patients and centers could make therapy appear to be better or worse than it actually is.

In 1996, Abramowicz et al published the pooled data from two randomized prospective studies with similar maintenance immunosuppressive regimens (cyclosporine, azathioprine, steroids) to evaluate the long-term effects of muromonab-CD3 on renal grafts with prolonged cold ischemia time. Patients were randomly allocated to receive either muromonab-CD3 (5 mg for 14 days) plus maintenance immunosuppression or maintenance immunosuppression alone. The patients in the muromonab-CD3 arm had delayed initiation of cyclosporine until postoperative day 11. The mean number of rejection episodes per patient was significantly lower in the muromonab-CD3 group compared to the non-muromonab-CD3 group, both at one and five years. Overall graft survival rates during the first five years following muromonab-CD3 induction were numerically higher in the muromonab-CD3 group, but did not reach statistical significance. However, in recipients of kidneys with long cold ischemia time (≥24 hours), the muromonab-CD3 group had a significantly higher graft survival than the control group ($P=0.045$). The conclusion from these studies is that muromonab-CD3 induction with delayed cyclosporine introduction was superior to non-induction therapy, especially in high-risk patients as well as in patients with prolonged cold ischemia time. While there are several studies comparing polyclonal antilymphocyte agents to muromonab-CD3 for induction, there is no convincing evidence that one agent is superior to another.

ANTI-INTERLEUKIN-2 ANTIBODIES

In the late 1980s, several rodent anti-interleukin-2 receptor (IL-2R) α mAbs were introduced in clinical renal transplantation to test the hypothesis of whether blockade of the interleukin-2 (IL-2) activation pathway with mAb therapy can provide effective and safe immunosuppression. These mAbs were effective while they were administered, but the overall outcome of the patients treated was reduced because of their immunogenicity. In these clinical trials, almost all patients developed a rapid immune response against the xenoantibodies. Human anti-mouse or anti-rat antibodies accelerated the clearance of the anti-IL-2R mAbs and further reduced an already short half-life below the level necessary for clinical efficacy. These limitations were overcome by the introduction of the fully-humanized anti-IL2-R α mAb daclizumab and the chimeric mAb basiliximab. These agents were approved by the FDA for immunoprophylaxis in 1997 (daclizumab) and 1998 (basiliximab).

Daclizumab is a humanized monoclonal IgG_1 antibody. It retains from its murine antiTac parent antibody almost exclusively the complimentary determining regions. It binds with high-affinity to the α chain of the IL-2R and blocks IL-2-mediated responses. Pharmacokinetic and pharmacodynamic analysis showed that patients who received 1 mg/kg every two weeks for a total of five doses had complete saturation of the IL-2R α chain on circulating lymphocytes for 120 days posttransplant. Two international multicenter phase III trials were conducted using this regimen of daclizumab to test its efficacy (the primary end point was biopsy-proven rejection at six months) and safety (patients' survival, opportunistic infections, malignancies and serious adverse events at 12 months). The maintenance therapy in one phase III trial (predominantly in Europe) was double therapy consisting of cyclosporine and prednisone, while in the second phase III trial (predominantly in North America) the maintenance therapy consisted of cyclosporine, azathioprine and prednisone. In the intent-to-treat analysis, daclizumab prophylaxis resulted in a significant reduction in the incidence of biopsy-proven acute rejection during the first six months following transplantation (40% in the double therapy, 36% in the triple therapy). The number of rejection episodes per patient and the number of patients receiving antilymphocyte preparations for severe rejection were also reduced in daclizumab-treated patients. The median time to rejection was delayed in daclizumab-treated patients in both studies. There was a trend towards improved graft survival in both the double and the triple therapy studies. In the double therapy trial at six months, daclizumab-treated patients received a significantly lower cumulative dose of corticosteroids. Administration of daclizumab was not associated with any increase in serious adverse events, opportunistic infections or malignancies.

In a subsequent phase I/II blinded, randomized trial, 75 patients treated with maintenance immunosuppression, consisting of cyclosporine, mycophenolate mofetil and steroids, were administered daclizumab or placebo. Patients receiving their first renal transplant from either a cadaver or a non-HLA identical living donor were enrolled in the study. The combination of daclizumab and mycophenolate mofetil was safe and well-tolerated. There were no pharmacokinetic interactions between the two drugs, and, at six months, biopsy-proven rejection episodes occurred in 12% vs 20% of the daclizumab and placebo groups, respectively. An open-label trial of daclizumab is currently being conducted in pediatric patients treated with triple therapy maintenance immunosuppression consisting of either cyclosporine (74%) or tacrolimus (26%), mycophenolate mofetil (87%), or azathioprine (11%) and corticosteroids. With a mean follow-up of 263 days, three out of 47 patients (6%) had biopsy-proven acute rejection episode. Thus, the combination of daclizumab and maintenance triple therapy with mycophenolate mofetil appears to result in a very low acute rejection rate.

Basiliximab is a chimeric anti-CD25 antibody derived from the murine RFT5 IL-2R αmAb. The half-life of basiliximab is seven days. The regimen of basiliximab used in the phase III studies consisted of two doses of 20 mg administered at day zero (preoperatively) and at day four posttransplant, with maintenance dual therapy consisting of cyclosporine and prednisone. The two-dose basiliximab regimen was designed to be simple and practical. It was found to result in drug concentrations that provide saturation of the IL-2 α chain on circulating lymphocytes for a period of 30 to 45 days posttransplant. To test the efficacy and safety of basiliximab, two phase III randomized double-blind, placebo-controlled trials were conducted in Europe and the US. In both trials, the maintenance immunosuppression consisted of cyclosporine and steroids. The European trial enrolled only primary cadaver renal transplants, while both primary cadaveric and living-related transplants were enrolled in the US trial. Basiliximab was associated with a significant reduction in biopsy-proven rejection at six months in the European and US trials. In both trials, patients treated with basiliximab had significantly less steroid-resistant rejections. In the US trial, basiliximab-treated patients had significantly higher mean calculated creatinine clearances than placebo-treated patients in the first year after transplantation. Patient and graft survival were comparable in basiliximab-treated and placebo-treated patients in both phase III trials. Anti-idiotypic antibodies to basiliximab were not developed by the patients. Basiliximab was found to have an excellent safety profile with no increase in infections or malignancies.

Since being approved for use in clinical transplantation, daclizumab and basiliximab have been used in regimens somewhat different than those used in the pivotal phase III trials. Daclizumab is being increasingly used in one to two dose regimens similar to basiliximab, with the first dose administered preoperatively and the second dose at seven to 14 days following transplantation. Basiliximab is being used with triple immunosuppression regimens that include mycophenolate mofetil. Preliminary results have indicated that these regimens are safe and efficacious. Increasingly, daclizumab and basiliximab have replaced the polyclonal agents and muromonab-CD3 in induction regimens, primarily because of their safety profiles. However, additional studies are needed to assess their effectiveness in delayed graft function and highly sensitized recipients.

CORTICOSTEROIDS

Corticosteroids are still used at the time of transplantation as part of the immunosuppressive regimen. The initial use of high doses of corticosteroids may be beneficial in inducing a quiescent state in the renal allograft, especially in patients with delayed graft function and reperfusion injury. Both the immunosuppressive and antiinflammatory properties of corticosteroids play an important role in altering the immune response to the graft early after transplantation. The importance of corticosteroids in the early phase of immunosuppression was demonstrated by the high rates of acute rejection in patients treated with cyclosporine monotherapy. Whether the introduction of newer immunosuppressive agents can eliminate the need for corticosteroids altogether remains to be determined.

ANTIBODY FREE INDUCTION PROTOCOLS

The most frequently used immunosuppression regimens in the US consist of triple therapy with a calcineurin inhibitor (either cyclosporine or tacrolimus), mycophenolate mofetil and corticosteroids started at the time of transplantation or soon thereafter. These regimens have been reported to result in rejection rates of 20% or lower in the first year after transplantation. However, while these regimens are cost-effective and easy to administer in patients receiving kidneys from living donors, or from cadaver donors with immediately functioning grafts, they are more difficult to implement in patients with delayed graft function. The use of full doses of calcineurin inhibitors in patients with appreciable delayed graft function may delay the recovery of function of the allograft and may initiate the process of chronic nephropathy from nephrotoxicity.

IMMUNOSUPPRESSION FOR PATIENTS RESTRICTED TO INTRAVENOUS THERAPY

Patients following renal transplantation are "NPO" (nothing per mouth) for only a few hours and immunosuppression drugs can be administered by mouth within 24 hours of transplantation. However, all the current immunosuppression agents can be administered intravenously if the patient is required to be NPO for over 24 hours. Both calcineurin inhibitors cyclosporine and tacrolimus can be administered intravenously, although their toxicities are enhanced with intravenous administration. Acute renal failure, as well as acute neurotoxicity (especially with tacrolimus) may occur. The intravenous dose of cyclosporine should be approximately 25% of the oral dose, and should be infused over 24 hours. Since tacrolimus is more toxic when it is administered intravenously, the usual dose is 1 mg per 24 hours by continuous infusion. Therapeutic levels can be easily attained with these regimens. Azathioprine has been administered intravenously for a number of years, but the intravenous dose need only be 50% of the oral dose. However, in practice, the intravenous dose has been the same as the oral dose. Recently an intravenous preparation of mycophenolate mofetil has become available and can be administered over four hours at the same dose and interval as the oral dose.

USE OF CALCIUM CHANNEL BLOCKERS TO PREVENT EXACERBATION OF DELAYED GRAFT FUNCTION OF DGF

Calcium channel blockers have been proposed to be clinically useful in patients immunosuppressed with cyclosporine. Calcium channel blockers are frequently used for the therapy of cyclosporine-induced posttransplant hypertension. Calcium channel blockers have been noted to reduce cyclosporine-induced intrarenal vasoconstriction. In several studies, calcium channel blockers, when administered immediately after transplantation, were shown to reduce the incidence of delayed graft function as well as reduce cyclosporine-induced chronic renal dysfunction. Furthermore, calcium channel blockers may potentiate the immunosuppressive effect of cyclosporine, although it is not clear whether this is an independent effect or is related to the decreased metabolism of cyclosporine by calcium channel blockers. In fact the dose of calcineurin inhibitors needs to be adjusted with the use of nondihydropyridine calcium channel blockers. While the therapeutic effectiveness of calcium channel blockers in posttransplant hypertension is well-established, the renal hemodynamic and immune effects of calcium channel blockers are still controversial.

TIMING OF INITIATION OF IMMUNOSUPPRESSION

Recipients of living donor kidneys are usually admitted several hours (and up to one day) before the transplant surgery. This allows better assessment of their immuno-suppression requirements and allows administration of the immunosuppression drugs prior to transplantation. Azathioprine or mycophenolate mofetil should be started before transplantation and preferably a few days before the transplant. There are no specific guidelines for the timing of the initiation of the calcineurin inhibitors, but both cyclosporine and tacrolimus can be started before the transplant surgery. A potential concern is that at the time of engraftment the patient may already have thera-peutic or elevated concentrations of calcineurin inhibitors which may produce vasoconstriction. Usually calcineurin inhibitors are started within the first 24 hours after trans-plantation. Anti-IL-2R mAbs can be administered within 24 hours prior to transplantation. The polyclonal antilym-phocyte agents and muromonab-CD3 are preferably administered following intubation in surgery. Many of the same guidelines apply to recipients of cadaveric kidneys.

SELECTION OF INDUCTION PROTOCOL BY PATIENT TYPE

Transplant physicians at different transplant centers use a variety of immunosuppression regimens for immuno-prophylaxis. At one extreme are centers that do not use any biological induction therapy and may rely on intra-venous calcineurin inhibitors in the first few days post-transplant to achieve immediate immunosuppression. On the other extreme are centers that use routine induc-tion therapy for all their patients. However, at most transplant centers, an attempt is made to base the selec-tion of patients for induction therapy with biological agents on multiple factors including immunologic risk, age, race, cold ischemia time, and the quality of function immediately after transplantation. The categories of patients that can be regarded at immunologic high risk are variable, but consist of re-transplants (especially if the graft loss was due to rejection in the first year), patients with high panel-reactive antibodies, patients with a channel shift by fluorescence-activated cell sort-ing in the crossmatch, patients with systemic lupus erythematosus, and African-Americans. Children have an immunologically active immune system and tradi-tionally have had high rejection rates. Therefore, children are frequently considered to be high-risk. Adult patients who receive pediatric kidneys en bloc may be at risk for renal artery thrombosis with an episode of acute rejec-tion, and therefore are also candidates for induction therapy. Patients who are transplanted with a kidney with prolonged cold ischemia time (>24 hours) or who develop posttransplant delayed graft function are at

higher risk of rejection and are frequently considered candidates for induction therapy.

The introduction of the new anti-IL2 receptor anti-bodies, daclizumab and basiliximab, has widened the choice of agents for use in induction therapy. The safety, ease of administration, and proven effectiveness of these agents in phase III trials have catapulted them as agents of choice for biological induction. However, the phase III trials were performed in primary transplant patients, and therefore additional data needs to be accumulated on the effectiveness of these agents in higher immunologic risk groups and in patients with delayed graft function. Polyclonal antilymphocyte agents and muromonab-CD3 should still be used in patients where T cell depletion is desirable, such as second transplant patients who are highly sensitized.

In summary, induction therapy with biological agents offers transplant physicians a greater degree of flexibility in individualizing immunosuppression regi-mens to different groups of transplant recipients.

RECOMMENDED READING

Gruber SA, Chan GLC, Canafax DM, Matas AJ. Immunosuppression in renal transplantation II. Corticosteroids, antilymphocyte globulin, and OKT3. Clin Transplant. 1991;5:219-232.

Sommer BG, Henry M, Ferguson RM. Sequential anti-lymphoblast globulin and cyclosporine for renal trans-plantation. Transplantation. 1987;43(1):85-90.

Cosimi AB. The clinical usefulness of antilymphocyte antibodies. Transplant Proc. 1983;15:617-621.

Abouna GM, Al-Abdullah IH, Kelly-Sullivan D, et al. Randomized clinical trial of antithymocyte globulin induction in renal transplantation comparing a fixed daily dose with dose adjustment according to T cell monitoring. Transplantation. 1995;59(11):1564-1568.

Gaber OA, First MR, Tesi RJ, et al. Results of the double-blind, randomized, multicenter, phase III clinical trial of Thymoglobulin vs ATGAM in the treatment of acute graft rejection episodes after renal transplantation. Transplantation. 1998;66(1):29-37.

Goldstein G. Overview of the development of Orthoclone OKT3: monoclonal antibody for therapeutic use in transplantation. Transplant Proc. 1987;19 (2 Suppl 1):1-6.

Goldstein G, Fuccello AJ, Normal DJ, Shield CF 3d, Colvin RB, Cosimi AB. OKT3 monoclonal antibody plasma levels during therapy and the subsequent devel-opment of host antibodies to OKT3. Transplantation. 1986;42(5):507-511.

Abramowicz D, Schandene L, Goldman M, et al. Release of tumor necrosis factor, interleukin-2, and gamma-interferon in serum after injection of OKT3 monoclonal antibody in kidney transplant recipients. Transplantation. 1989;47(4):606-608.

Opelz G. Efficacy of rejection prophylaxis with OKT3 in renal transplantation. Transplantation. 1995;60(11): 1220-1224

Abramowicz D, Norman DJ, Vereerstraeten P, et al. OKT3 prophylaxis in renal grafts with prolonged cold ischemia times: Association with improvement in long-term survival. Kidney Int. 1996;49(3):768-772.

Vincenti F, Kirkman R, Light S, et al. Interleukin-2-receptor blockade with daclizumab to prevent acute rejection in renal transplantation. New Engl J Med. 1998;338(3):161-165.

Nashan B, Light S, Hardie IR, Lin A, Johnson JR. Reduction of acute renal allograft rejection by daclizumab. Daclizumab Double Therapy Study Group. Transplantation. 1999;67(1):110-115.

Nashan B, Moore R, Amiot P, Schmidt AG, Abeywickrama K, Soulillou JP. Randomised trial of basiliximab versus placebo for control of acute cellular rejection in renal allograft recipients. CHIB 201 International Study Group. Lancet. 1997;350(9086):1193-1198.

Kahan BD, Rajagopalan PR, Hall M. Reduction of the occurrence of acute cellular rejection among renal allograft recipients treated with basiliximab a chimeric anti-interleukin-2-receptor monoclonal antibody. United States Simulect Renal Study Group. Transplantation. 1999;67(2):276-284.

Ahmed K, Michael B, Burke JF Jr. Effects of isradipine on renal hemodynamics in renal transplant patients treated with cyclosporine. Clin Nephrol. 1997;48(5):307-310.

Epstein M. Calcium antagonists and renal protection. Current status and future perspectives. Arch Intern Med. 1992;152(8):1573-1584.

Bantle JP, Paller MS, Boudreau RJ, Olivari MT, Ferris TF. Long-term effects of cyclosporine on renal function in organ transplant recipients. J Lab-Clin Med. 1990;115(2):233-240.

57 DIAGNOSIS AND TREATMENT OF RENAL DYSFUNCTION EPISODES

V. Ram Peddi, MD
M. Roy First, MD

Allograft dysfunction frequently complicates the post-transplant course. The differential diagnosis is extensive and is best understood in the context of the timing of its occurrence. Allograft dysfunction can therefore be divided into (1) early, occurring less than 90 days posttransplant and (2) late, occurring greater than 90 days after transplantation. It can be further differentiated into medical and mechanical problems. These are outlined in Table 57-1.

DELAYED GRAFT FUNCTION

Delayed graft function (DGF) or renal dysfunction in the immediate posttransplant period is a serious and frequent problem in cadaver renal transplantation. The risk factors associated with an increased incidence of DGF include: donor hypovolemia or hypotension, particularly in the presence of nephrotoxic drugs or vasopressors; prolonged cold or warm ischemia times; older donors and donors with hypertension or vascular occlusive disease; injury incurred during procurement, preservation, or implantation; and a high (>50%) panel-reactive antibody level in the recipient. The pathophysiology leading to DGF is complex and incompletely understood, and appears to be due to ischemia-reperfusion injury. The presence of DGF is associated with acute rejection in the short-term and chronic rejection in the long-term. Because of the increased incidence of rejection and the possible adverse effects of calcineurin inhibitors when DGF is present, some centers use antilymphocyte antibodies initially and hold calcineurin inhibitors until renal function is restored. Others do not use antibodies but avoid high doses of the calcineurin inhibitors initially.

The optimal initial dose of cyclosporine (CsA) or tacrolimus has not been established. One approach is to use low doses together with prednisone and azathioprine or mycophenolate mofetil (MMF) immediately posttransplantation, until recovery of renal function has

V. Ram Peddi, MD, Associate Professor of Medicine, Division of Nephrology and Hypertension, Department of Internal Medicine, University of Cincinnati College of Medicine, Cincinnati, OH

M. Roy First, MD, Professor of Medicine, Division of Nephrology and Hypertension, Department of Internal Medicine, University of Cincinnati College of Medicine, Cincinnati, OH

occurred, at which time full doses are administered. An alternative approach is to use full doses of CsA or tacrolimus with concomitant administration of nephroprotective agents such as calcium channel blockers, and misoprostol, a prostaglandin E1 analogue. At the present time, no clear consensus exists as to the ideal induction therapy for patients with DGF. Furthermore, there is no treatment available for the prevention of DGF. Monoclonal antibodies against adhesion molecules, which target the interaction between host leukocytes and allograft endothelium, may have a protective effect against ischemia-reperfusion injury. These antibodies are still in experimental stages and may hold promise for the future.

HYPERACUTE REJECTION

Hyperacute rejection is a rare and largely preventable cause of immediate graft failure. It is caused by preformed antibodies against donor antigens present in the recipient's serum at the time of transplantation. These antibodies are the consequence of previous exposure to donor antigens due to blood transfusions, prior transplantation, or pregnancy. Hyperacute rejection may occur when transplantation is attempted across ABO-incompatible barriers. The events that lead to hyperacute rejection occur with such rapidity that the kidney becomes visibly ischemic while the patient is still on the operating table. It always occurs within 24 hours of transplantation. Renal histology shows fibrin thrombi occluding the glomerular capillaries and small vessels with extensive tissue necrosis. Although plasmapheresis and anticoagulation have been advocated, there is no effective treatment. A kidney with hyperacute rejection should always be removed promptly. The current cross-match techniques, because of their increased sensitivity, have greatly diminished the incidence of hyperacute rejection.

ACUTE REJECTION

Although acute allograft rejection is the most common cause of graft dysfunction both in the early and late periods, it most commonly occurs during the first 90 days after transplantation. Based upon the analysis of over 40,000 kidney transplants reported to the United Network for Organ Sharing (UNOS) Scientific Renal Transplant Registry between October 1987 and August 1992, 24% of the recipients of first cadaver renal transplants developed one or more rejection episodes during the initial transplant hospitalization, and 52% during the first six months following transplantation. Recipients of transplants from living donors had a significantly lower incidence of rejection episodes. Factors significantly associated with the development of acute rejection were HLA mismatch, anti-HLA antibodies reactive to greater than 50% of a lymphocyte panel, re-transplantation,

Table 57-1. Differential Diagnosis of Renal Allograft Dysfunction

Early (0 to 90 days posttransplantation)	Late (>90 days posttransplantation)

Medical
   Hyperacute rejection
   Delayed graft function
   Acute rejection
   Acute CsA/tacrolimus nephrotoxicity
   Dehydration
   Other drug toxicities
   Infection
   De novo/recurrent disease
	Medical
	   Acute rejection
	   CsA/tacrolimus nephrotoxicity
	   Chronic rejection
	   Dehydration
	   Other drug toxicities
	   Infection
	   De novo/recurrent disease

Mechanical
   Lymphocele
   Ureteric obstruction
   Urine leak
   Vascular thrombosis
	Mechanical
	   Renal artery stenosis
	   Ureteric obstruction
	   Urine leak
	   Vascular thrombosis

African-American race, and recipient age under 16. These data were derived from the period before Neoral®, MMF and tacrolimus were in routine use. The classic clinical features associated with acute rejection are fever, oliguria, weight gain, edema, hypertension and the presence of an enlarged tender graft. However, with the current immunosuppression, these features are frequently absent, and the most common presentation may be an asymptomatic rise in serum creatinine. An increase in serum creatinine greater than 20% is often the cardinal feature of rejection. A variety of tests have been devised in an attempt to increase the diagnostic accuracy of acute rejection, but percutaneous needle biopsy of the allograft remains by far the most reliable method for the diagnosis of acute rejection. A biopsy can also differentiate among nonrejection causes of renal dysfunction. Sonographically-guided biopsies using an automated biopsy gun have provided diagnostic information in approximately 99% of cases, are safe, and can be performed as an outpatient procedure. The approach to the management of a patient with a rise in serum creatinine is illustrated in Figure 57-1.

Histologic Classification and Treatment of Acute Rejection

Based on histological severity, the recently published Banff 97 classification of renal allograft pathology has three distinct diagnostic categories for acute rejection. These are grades I (interstitial infiltration and tubulitis), II (intimal arteritis), and III (transmural arteritis). Depending upon the severity of interstitial infiltration and intimal arteritis, grades I and II are further differentiated into types A and B. There is also a category referred to as *borderline changes* that is suspicious for acute rejection. This category is indicated by foci of mild tubulitis

(one to four mononuclear cells/tubular cross-section) and no intimal arteritis. The introduction of the Banff classification has resulted in the standardized schema for transplant pathology and classification of renal rejection severity.

The principles and the management of acute rejection include rapid diagnosis, accurate classification, and prompt administration of antirejection therapy. Currently, corticosteroids and antilymphocyte antibodies represent the main components of antirejection treatment protocols. The decision on treatment of acute rejection is based on histological severity. One approach is to treat mild acute cellular rejection (Banff 97 Grade IA) with a 4-day course of 250 mg of intravenous methylprednisolone administered dialy, and moderate and severe acute cellular rejection and acute vascular rejection (Banff 97 Grades IB, IIA, IIB and III) are treated with a 7- to 10-day course of an antilymphocyte antibody, currently either Thymoglobulin® or muromonab-CD3.

In a double-blind, randomized, multicenter, phase III clinical trial, Thymoglobulin® was compared with ATGAM®, for the treatment of acute rejection episodes after renal transplantation. Patients were stratified based on the severity of rejection according to the Banff classification of the kidney biopsy specimen, to receive a 7- to 14-day course of either Thymoglobulin® (1.5 mg/kg per day) or ATGAM® (15 mg/kg per day). The primary endpoint of the study was a successful response defined as a return of the serum creatinine level to or below baseline (day 0 value). Successful response was seen in 88% of Thymoglobulin®-treated patients vs 76% of the ATGAM®-treated patients ($P=0.027$). In each Banff rejection severity category there was a tendency towards improved response in the Thymoglobulin®-treated group when compared with the ATGAM®-treated group. In

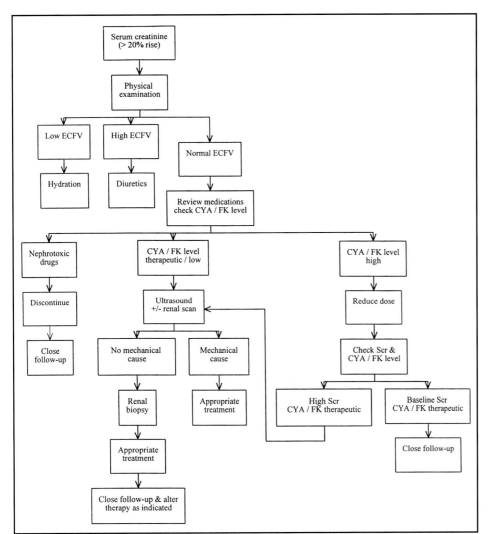

Figure 57-1. Approach to the management of the renal transplant recipient with an increase in the serum creatinine level. (abbreviations: ECFV indicates extracellular fluid volume; CYA, cyclosporine; FK, tacrolimus; Scr, serum creatinine)

addition, recurrent rejection occurred less frequently in Thymoglobulin®-treated patients when compared with ATGAM®-treated patients. Thymoglobulin® use was associated with a significantly greater depletion of CD2+, CD3+, CD4+, and CD8+ cells, indicating that the superior T cell depletion may be responsible for the lower rate of recurrent rejection. Although polyclonal antibodies are effective for the treatment of acute rejection, in most instances, the monoclonal antibody, muromonab-CD3 has tended to supersede the use of polyclonal antibodies. The initial multicenter randomized prospective study using muromonab-CD3 for the treatment of acute rejection reported a rejection reversal rate of 94%, which was significantly better than the 75% reversal rate obtained with steroid treatment. The 1-year graft survival rate for the muromonab-CD3-treated group was 62%, as compared with 45% for the steroid-treated group. This study was performed in the pre-cyclosporine era. Following this initial study, there have been numerous similar experiences reported with muromonab-CD3 in reversing primary and steroid-

resistant acute renal allograft rejection, as well as acute vascular rejection. Given the observation that acute rejection is associated with poor long-term graft survival, several centers have employed muromonab-CD3 as first-line treatment for Banff 93 grades IIA, IIB, and III acute rejection episodes. Rejection reversal rates of up to 98%, with 1-year post-muromonab-CD3 graft and patient survival rates of 87.5% and 95.5% respectively, have been reported when muromonab-CD3 was used as first-line therapy for the treatment of acute rejection episodes. The determination of anti-muromonab-CD3 antibody titer is useful in patients in whom re-treatment with muromonab-CD3 may be necessary. Previous muromonab-CD3 treatment does not preclude its reuse. However, it is important to know the patient's antibody status before and during reuse. Muromonab-CD3 therapy can be reinstituted successfully in patients who are antibody negative or have a low titer (≤1:100) anti-muromonab-CD3 antibody following their first course of muromonab-CD3. These patients have rejection reversal rates that are equivalent to those obtained with primary therapy. In patients with low-titer antibodies it may be necessary to increase the dose of muromonab-CD3 during reuse to overcome the antibody response and achieve depletion of all CD3+ cells. Reappearance of CD3+ cells and fall in serum muromonab-CD3 levels during muromonab-CD3 therapy are associated with increasing antibody formation. Patients who have a high-titer antibody response (≥1:1000) should be treated with antirejection therapy other than muromonab-CD3.

CHRONIC REJECTION

With the advent of newer immunosuppressive agents, dramatic improvements in the 1-year allograft survival rates have occurred over the last decade. Despite these impressive short-term results, the rate of long-term graft failure has remained relatively unchanged until recently. More recent analysis of the UNOS Scientific Registry Data indicate improved graft half-lives in the modern era of immunosuppression. Chronic rejection (CR) is considered to be the single most important cause of late allograft failure. The course of CR is slow and insidious. It is characterized clinically by a progressive decline in renal function, persistent proteinuria, and hypertension. CR often occurs in conjunction with other histologic causes of allograft dysfunction, namely, acute rejection, CsA and tacrolimus nephrotoxicity, and recurrent or de novo glomerular diseases. The diagnosis of CR should therefore be based on morphological characteristics of allograft histology and the clinical observation of a gradual decline in renal allograft function. CR that includes chronic vascular rejection and transplant glomerulopathy is diagnosed histologically in the presence of obliterative arteriopathy, tubular atrophy and interstitial fibrosis, glomeruli with wrinkled basement membranes, glomerular sclerosis or enlarged glomeruli with prominent swollen endothelial cells, spongy mesangial matrix and reduplication of the basement membrane. The pathophysiology of CR is not completely understood, but most likely involves both immune and nonimmune factors. Risk factors for the development of CR in renal allograft recipients include delayed graft function/ischemia-reperfusion injury, degree of HLA mismatching/histoincompatibility, acute rejection episodes, inadequate renal mass, hypertension, hyperlipidemia, and cytomegalovirus infection. Histologically proven CR has been shown to have a very poor outcome, with a graft half-life of 5.2 years, which is significantly lower than the 17 years in patients without chronic graft dysfunction. There is no treatment for CR at the present time. It is speculated that immunosuppressive agents such as MMF and Sirolimus® (rapamycin), which have an effect on the B lymphocytes and endothelial cell proliferation, may slow the progression of CR. Supportive treatment should include aggressive control of hyperlipidemia with an HMG-CoA-reductase-inhibitor, and adequate control of blood pressure. An angiotensin-converting enzyme inhibitor or angiotensin II receptor blocker should be used for the control of hypertension and proteinuria, whenever feasible.

RECURRENT DISEASE IN THE ALLOGRAFT

With the introduction of the newer immunosuppressive agents, and the resultant improvement in allograft survival, recurrent disease in the kidney has become an increasingly more important problem. A recent report from the European Renal Association-European Dialysis and Transplant Association Registry evaluated recurrence of glomerulonephritis and resultant graft loss following transplantation. Recurrence of the original disease resulted in graft loss in 24% of 723 patients with childhood focal segmental glomerulosclerosis (FSGS), 19% of 397 with mesangiocapillary glomerulonephritis (MCGN) Type II, 6% of 564 with MCGN Type I, and 6% of 1,810 with IgA nephropathy. Graft loss within the first two years was due to recurrent disease in 65% of patients with FSGS, 57% with MCGN Type II, 33% with Henoch-Schönlein nephritis, 14% with MCGN Type I, and 9% with IgA nephropathy. Overall graft failure rate due to recurrent disease was 3% in first grafts (n=14,565), but rose to 48% in second grafts when the first graft had failed because of recurrent disease. In the US Renal Allograft Disease Registry, recurrent disease in the allograft was also shown to result in significantly reduced long-term graft survival and half-life in those patients with recurrent diseases vs those who did not develop recurrence. In patients with recurrent disease, graft half-life was 2,038 days, compared to 3,135 days in those allografts without recurrence (P=0.002).

NEPHROTOXICITY
Nephrotoxicity of Calcineurin-Inhibitors

CsA and tacrolimus are associated with both acute and chronic nephrotoxicity. The nephrotoxicity caused by these drugs both clinically and histologically is identical. The acute toxicity is due in part to hemodynamic changes secondary to their vasoconstrictor effects on the afferent arteriole of the glomerulus. This results in a reduction in the glomerular filtration rate, manifested by an increase in the serum creatinine concentration. This acute change is dose-related and reversible. Chronic nephrotoxicity is caused by the chronic exposure of a patient to either drug and has been well-demonstrated in patients with autoimmune diseases treated with CsA, as well as in the various organ transplant recipients: heart, liver, kidney, lung, heart-lung and bone marrow. The pathologic lesions in the kidney are characterized by a focal or striped form of tubulointerstitial fibrosis, afferent arteriolopathy with nodular hyaline deposits, and global or focal glomerular sclerosis or collapse. Although the exact pathophysiology and mechanism by which these lesions are produced is unclear, it has been shown to be associated with cytokines such as transforming growth factor-beta (TGF-β). Nephrotoxicity may occur with therapeutic CsA or tacrolimus doses and target trough concentrations. It often occurs together with other causes of graft dysfunction such as acute rejection, chronic rejection, and recurrent or de novo glomerular disease. Hence, it may be difficult to differentiate the effects of CsA or tacrolimus on the renal structure and the relative role of other causes of renal allograft dysfunction. Studies in heart transplant recipients elucidated the structural and functional changes in the native kidneys of heart transplant recipients. CsA-treated patients, compared to azathioprine-treated controls, showed a decrease in the glomerular filtration rate with a concomitant rise in serum creatinine level and fall in renal plasma flow, and an increase in the renal vascular resistance during the first year posttransplantation, which stabilized thereafter. Additional evidence of glomerular injury was an elevation in the urinary albumin excretion rate. There was an increased incidence of hypertension in the CsA-treated group. Renal biopsies in a subset of CsA-treated patients showed global or segmental glomerular sclerosis, afferent arteriolopathy and striped interstitial fibrosis. A subsequent tissue sample obtained six to 24 months after the initial biopsy in some of these patients revealed progressive renal damage with a significant increase in the percentage of glomeruli exhibiting either sclerosis or ischemic collapse of the glomerular tuft. There was a cumulative incidence of end-stage renal failure of 10%, after eight years of CsA therapy. Sequential renal biopsies, before and after stopping CsA in renal transplant recipients with a histological diagnosis of CsA-associated nephrotoxicity, showed that the arteriolar hyalinosis and interstitial fibrosis of the striped form progressed after discontinuation of CsA in about half of the twenty patients studied. CsA-associated arteriolopathy decreased significantly after discontinuation of CsA therapy only in patients with less severe arteriolar lesions in the initial biopsy. This finding suggests that the severity of the preexisting lesions of CsA-associated arteriolopathy are responsible for the final outcome, and that early diagnosis and intervention are essential to prevent persistence or progression of the CsA-associated arteriolopathy. The progression of interstitial fibrosis could be attributed to the development of chronic vascular rejection after stopping CsA. Although the histologic distinction of chronic rejection from CsA toxicity may be difficult and sometimes impossible, as both disorders affect vessels, glomeruli and the tubulointerstitial compartment, these disorders can be differentiated from each other in most instances, when early allograft biopsies for graft dysfunction are obtained.

No clear consensus exists as to the management of patients with CsA or tacrolimus nephrotoxicity. Calcium-channel antagonists, misoprostol, and fish oil have been shown to have an ability to mitigate CsA-induced nephrotoxicity. Data on CsA withdrawal protocols have produced conflicting results. While some studies have reported an increased incidence of acute rejection following CsA withdrawal, others have reported either no difference, or a beneficial effect in long-term graft survival after withdrawal of CsA. In patients who are on azathioprine, most centers replace this agent with MMF. Thereafter, patients are maintained on low-dose CsA or tacrolimus. Substitution of calcineurin-inhibitors with sirolimus as an option is currently being evaluated in several prospective studies. There have been no well-controlled studies which examine the issue of CsA or tacrolimus nephrotoxicity and its management in renal transplant recipients.

Other Nephrotoxic Agents

The same agents that cause nephrotoxicity in the native kidneys can also be nephrotoxic to the allograft. The transplant recipient who is already on CsA or tacrolimus, and has some degree of renal vasoconstriction induced by these agents, may in fact be more sensitive to the nephrotoxic effects of other agents. This needs to be kept in mind in any allograft recipient who is to receive radio-contrast agents, aminoglycoside antibiotics, nonsteroidal antiinflammatory drugs, amphotericin B, and other potentially nephrotoxic antibiotics. Judicious use of such agents, dosage modification, and the possible use of alternative drugs should be considered in such situations. Synergistic toxicity of calcineurin-inhibitors has been reported with acyclovir, ganciclovir, trimethoprim-sulfamethoxazole, vancomycin, furosemide, H2-antagonists, and melphalan in addition to those drugs mentioned above. CsA or tacrolimus toxicity can also result from the co-administration of drugs that inhibit metabolism of these two immunosuppressive agents resulting in elevated blood concentrations. Important in this area are diltiazem, verapamil, nicardipine, fluconazole, itraconazole, ketoconazole, and erythromycin. On the other hand, sub-therapeutic drug levels, and resultant risk of acute rejection, can occur with co-administration of agents that stimulate more rapid metabolism of the calcineurin-inhibitors; important drugs in this category include isoniazid, rifampin, phenobarbital, phenytoin, and carbamazepine. Therefore, caution needs to be applied when co-administering drugs that interact with the calcineurin inhibitors, along with careful monitoring of renal function and drug levels.

PROTEINURIA

Persistent proteinuria following renal transplantation occurs in up to 30% of renal allograft recipients. Proteinuria in the immediate posttransplant period occurs frequently and has little prognostic significance. However a poor prognosis has been described in patients with persistent heavy proteinuria in later stages of the posttransplant course. The causes that have been attributed to posttransplant proteinuria are: CR, recurrent or de novo glomerulonephritis, renal vein thrombosis, reflux nephropathy, and CsA or tacrolimus nephrotoxicity. CR is the most common cause of persistent posttransplant proteinuria and close to 50% of patients with persistent proteinuria have CR. Proteinuria due to allograft glomerulonephritis is responsible for approximately 30% of cases, and is the second most common cause. Persistent proteinuria is associated with a poor outcome. The allograft half-life in patients with proteinuria of greater than 2g/d is 5.6 years compared to 16.5 years for those with proteinuria less than 2g/d. Among patients with proteinuria there was no difference in the graft half-life if the proteinuria was due to chronic rejection (5.2 years) or due to other causes (5.7 years).

INFECTION
Urinary Tract Infection

Urinary tract infections are a frequent complication of renal transplantation. Although they are frequently asymptomatic, they constitute the major source of bacteremia in this patient population. Therefore, all urinary tract infections, even asymptomatic ones, should be treated appropriately. Fortunately, renal dysfunction is an uncommon complication of urinary tract infections in the transplant recipient. It usually occurs with severe pyelonephritis involving the allograft, usually in the setting of ureteric obstruction or vesicoureteral reflux.

Cytomegalovirus Infection

Cytomegalovirus (CMV) is the most important viral infection affecting transplant recipients. Renal allograft dysfunction during active CMV infection has been noted by some investigators, but not by others. An association between CMV viremia and glomerulopathy causing a transient rise in serum creatinine level has been reported, and was felt to be due to immune complex-mediated damage to the glomerular capillaries. Subsequently, doubt has been cast on the entity of CMV glomerulopathy. Currently, it is not clear whether the renal impairment is due to graft rejection, which may occur in the context of the decreased immunosuppression dictated by a virus-associated leukopenia, or because of an adverse effect of the virus directly on the kidney.

POSTTRANSPLANT SURGICAL COMPLICATION

The incidence and severity of surgical complications have gradually decreased in the past 30 years as a result of improved surgical techniques and better diagnostic tools. Nevertheless, these complications may cause graft dysfunction and account for a small percentage of graft losses.

Vascular Complications

RENAL ARTERY THROMBOSIS. Renal artery thrombosis occurs in less than 1% of transplant recipients. Thrombosis may occur due to a technical complication such as dissection under the distal intimal flap, torsion or kinking of the renal artery, atherosclerotic disease in the donor or the recipient, disparate donor/recipient arterial segment as in transplantation of pediatric kidneys into adult recipients, or the presence of multiple renal arteries. Thrombosis may also occur due to hyperacute rejection, CsA-related or tacrolimus-related arteriolopathy, or a hypercoagulable state such as the presence of antiphospholipid antibody in a patient with lupus nephritis. It may present as a sudden cessation of urine output in the setting of a previously functioning graft. In the early posttransplant period, after the possibility of an occluded Foley catheter and hypovolemia are excluded, the diagnosis is established by nonvisualization of the transplant kidney with a radionuclide renal scan or renal angiography. Immediate surgical exploration is mandatory. Treatment consists of thrombectomy and identification and correction of the underlying cause. Graft loss is not unusual.

RENAL ARTERY STENOSIS. Renal artery stenosis is diagnosed in approximately 2% of renal transplant recipients and can occur early or several years after transplantation. It may be caused by atheromatous occlusive vascular disease either in the donor or the recipient vessels, intimal hyperplasia in response to intraoperative trauma, or by immunologic factors. Renal artery stenosis is suspected in the presence of severe hypertension with worsening renal function in the absence of rejection and CsA or FK nephrotoxicity. A bruit may be heard over the allograft. A sudden decline in renal function following treatment with an ACE inhibitor is highly suggestive of renal artery stenosis. The diagnosis is confirmed by renal angiography. Percutaneous transluminal angioplasty is the preferred initial intervention whenever feasible. It is successful in up to 85% of cases, but there is a high restenosis rate. Surgical correction is more difficult than in nontransplant recipients because of dense scar tissue surrounding the allograft.

RENAL VEIN THROMBOSIS. Allograft renal vein thrombosis is a relatively rare complication and occurs in less than 1% of transplant recipients. The symptoms of renal vein thrombosis include pain and tenderness over the allograft with hematuria, proteinuria and oliguria. The allograft is swollen on examination with accompanying swelling of the ipsilateral lower extremity. The causes of renal vein thrombosis include: mechanical causes such as angulation and kinking of the renal vein, compression by hematoma or lymphocele, stenotic lesion at the anastomosis, or a hypercoagulable state. Although Doppler sonography or radionuclide scan usually establish the diagnosis, a renal venogram may be necessary to confirm the diagnosis in a few cases. Thrombosis of the main renal vein generally causes permanent allograft injury, as the transplanted kidney has a single venous drainage system without capsular collaterals. Although graft salvage is rare, prompt exploration and thrombectomy are mandatory.

ATHEROEMBOLIC DISEASE. Atheroembolic renal disease, also referred to as cholesterol emboli, can also involve the transplanted kidney. This condition usually occurs in patients with generalized atheromatous disease following angiography or aortic surgery. Now that more elderly patients are receiving renal allografts, it is important to keep this complication in mind following angiography in the transplant recipient. It manifests as either acute oliguric renal failure or an insidious, gradual decline in renal function. Unlike radiocontrast-associated nephropathy, atheroembolic disease is usually irreversible and may result in failure of the transplanted organ.

Lymphocele

Following transplantation, lymphatic fluid collection between the bladder and the transplant kidney occurs in up to 15% of recipients. The development of lymphocele has been ascribed to disruption of normal lymphatic channels along the recipient iliac vessels, or from the hilum of the allograft. The majority of lymphoceles are asymptomatic and are discovered during routine transplant ultrasonography. Some however, become manifest clinically by causing pressure on the adjacent structures including the bladder, ureter, iliac vein or lower extremity lymphatics, and thereby cause impaired renal function and ipsilateral lower extremity, abdominal wall, scrotal or labial edema. Symptomatic lymphoceles require therapy. Percutaneous aspiration under ultrasound or computed tomography guidance is associated with a high recurrence rate with a potential for persistent lymph leak and exogenous infection. The procedure of choice is either an open surgical marsupialization or a laparoscopically-created peritoneal window. These procedures connect the lymphocele with the peritoneal cavity, whereby the lymphatic fluid drains freely into the abdominal cavity and is absorbed by the peritoneum. Both procedures have excellent long-term results.

Urologic Complications

URINE LEAK. Urine leak is an infrequent but serious problem that occurs in 1% to 2% of renal transplant recipients. Leaks occurring at the ureterovesical junction are usually due to technical failures, whereas those occurring in the upper urinary tract are due to ischemia and necrosis resulting from vascular compromise during organ procurement. Urine leaks present with pain, swelling, and discharge from the wound or through the drain, when present. These symptoms occur together with increasing serum creatinine levels and decreased urine output. Transplant ultrasonography and radionuclide scan demonstrate perinephric fluid collection and extravasation of radioisotope outside of the collecting system. Fluid may be aspirated and comparison of the fluid urea, creatinine, and potassium concentration to serum concentrations may confirm or exclude urine leak. Management of the urine leak depends upon the site and the degree of disruption. Placement of a percutaneous antegrade nephrostomy and a ureteric stent may control the urine leak and allow the surrounding tissue to heal and seal the perforation. This procedure, however, is associated with the risk of infection and fistula formation. If stenting fails, and with urine leaks near the renal pelvis or with significant ureteral necrosis, surgical revision or reconstruction to restore urinary tract continuity provides definitive treatment. The stent is removed four to six weeks after placement, provided that contrast administration fails to detect extravasation.

URINARY TRACT OBSTRUCTION. This is the most common urologic complication following transplantation and may occur as an early or late complication. The majority of the lesions occur at the distal ureter and are due to ureteral ischemia leading to fibrosis and stricture formation. It is usually asymptomatic and is suspected when the transplant recipient has an elevated serum creatinine level. Ultrasonography demonstrates hydronephrosis. A percutaneous antegrade pyelography confirms the diagnosis and also determines the site of obstruction. Ureteric obstruction is initially managed by placement of a percutaneous nephrostomy that relieves obstruction and allows the renal function to improve. Treatment options include balloon dilation or surgical reconstruction.

STONES. Urinary calculi are a relatively uncommon complication of renal transplantation. Calculi may have been present in the donor kidney or may develop after transplantation. Predisposing factors include obstruction, recurrent urinary tract infection, hypercalciuria, hyperoxaluria, internal stents and nonabsorbable suture material. Open removal of a calculus from the transplanted kidney is rarely necessary. Complete stone removal is usually possible by standard urological techniques.

RECOMMENDED READING

Amante AJ, Kahan BD. Technical complications of renal transplantation. Surg Clin North Am. 1994;74(5):1117-1131.

Bennett WM, DeMattos A, Meyer MM, Andoh T, Barry JM. Chronic cyclosporine nephropathy: the Achilles' heel of immunosuppressive therapy. Kidney Int. 1996;50(4): 1089-1100.

Kamath S, Dean D, Peddi VR, et al. Efficacy of OKT3 as primary therapy for histologically confirmed acute renal allograft rejection. Transplantation. 1997;64(10): 1428-1432.

Mihatsch MJ, Ryffel B, Gudat F. The differential diagnosis between rejection and cyclosporine toxicity. Kidney Int. 1995;48(Suppl 52):S63-S69.

Paul LC. Chronic renal transplant loss. Kidney Int. 1995;47(6):1491-1499.

Peddi VR, Dean DE, Hariharan S, Cavallo T, Schroeder TJ, First MR. Proteinuria following renal transplantation: correlation with histopathology and outcome. Transplant Proc. 1997;29(12):101-103.

Racusen LC, Solez K, Colvin RB, et al, The Banff 97 working classification of renal allograft pathology. Kidney Int. 1999;55(2):713-723.

Ramos EL, Tisher CC. Recurrent diseases in the kidney transplant. Am J Kidney Dis. 1994;24(1):142-154.

Troppmann C, Gillingham KJ, Benedetti E, et al. Delayed graft function, acute rejection and outcome after cadaveric renal transplantation. Transplantation. 1995;59(7):962-968.

58   PATHOLOGIC FINDINGS OF RENAL ALLOGRAFT DYSFUNCTION

Kim Solez, MD

Lorraine C. Racusen, MD

The diagnosis of causes of renal transplant dysfunction based on pathological findings on biopsy studied by traditional methods is one of the most important subjects in renal transplantation today. An internationally agreed upon standard for interpretation of such biopsies now exists – the Banff '97 classification – and repeated clinical validation studies have shown that the biopsy has a very important influence on proper treatment and prognosis. This chapter serves to further disseminate the specifics of the Banff '97 classification as well as bringing further information and recommendations from the June 7 to 12, 1999 Fifth Banff Conference on Allograft Pathology. Further information and images related to this chapter are available on the World Wide Web at: http://cnserver0.nkf.med.ualberta.ca/banff.

There is an analogy between large-scale political change and scientific advancement. With the dawning of the new millennium we are entering a time of great possibilities in transplantation, when events analogous to, and as momentous as, the fall of the Berlin wall or the end of apartheid in South Africa may occur. As was true of these political events, the scientific events we are waiting for are probably inevitable, but no one knows whether they will take one, five, ten, or 20 years to occur. The reader may predict a longer time course and yet surprises abound in both science and politics. So the systems and observations described in the rest of this chapter need to be balanced against the possibility of one or more of the following seminal changes occurring:

- Development of a new immunosuppressive agent or protocol that results in a completely different histologic pattern of toxicity and/or rejection.
- Development of a molecular biology assessment of the transplant biopsy that completely supplants traditional microscopic examination of paraffin sections.

Kim Solez, MD, Professor of Pathology, University of Alberta; Director of NKF cyberNephrology, President of Transpath, Edmonton, Alberta, Canada

Lorraine C. Racusen, MD, The Johns Hopkins University School of Medicine, Department of Pathology, Baltimore, MD

- Development of a robust noninvasive test for acute rejection that is both more specific and sensitive than the percutaneous biopsy.
- Development of means for making a specific diagnosis of chronic rejection prior to renal functional decline on protocol biopsies, perhaps using Sirius Red quantification of interstitial fibrosis and immunostaining for C4D.
- Universal acceptance by AST/ASTS/Eurotransplant of the Banff clinical practice guidelines which recommend:
  - Implantation biopsies in every renal transplant.
  - Rapid paraffin (microwave) processing for rapid reading of biopsies rather than frozen sections.
  - Routine ("protocol") biopsies performed at set time intervals in the absence of clinical signs of rejection to detect "subclinical" rejection and/or incipient chronic rejection.
  - Uniform employment of H&E, PAS (+/o silver), and trichrome or Sirius red stains in all renal transplant biopsies.

Despite the timeliness of this chapter, the authors are in the unusual position of hoping that parts of the chapter become outdated rapidly, as that would signal important and much-anticipated breakthroughs in the field of transplantation. Breakthroughs in the areas of noninvasive rejection diagnosis, new pathology techniques, molecular biology, tolerance-induction, cell and organ senescence, and chronic rejection are among those anticipated. We do not know that these positive events will unfold in the near future, but need to be prepared for that possibility, which could radically change the role of the transplant biopsy in patient management.

THE IMPORTANCE OF PROTOCOL BIOPSIES/HISTORY OF THE KIDNEY TRANSPLANT BIOPSY

Needle biopsies of the kidney transplants were first attempted in 1954, but it was not until the late 1970s and 1980s that the practice of performing percutaneous needle biopsies of renal allografts became popular in transplant centers in Europe and North America. The introduction of the semiautomated, small caliber biopsy needle replacing the traditional Tru-Cut needle, combined with the application of real-time ultrasound to visualize the renal cortex and the needle pathway encouraged increased use of renal transplant biopsies. The safety of the procedure has been repeatedly investigated, with most reports showing a low complication rate.

The introduction of cyclosporine in 1980 and subsequent newer therapies for the treatment of acute rejection resulted in great improvements in the 1-year graft survival. However, these agents also complicated the care of the transplant recipients through their nephrotoxic effects. Percutaneous biopsies are the most reliable current test that distinguishes rejection from drug-nephrotoxicity and other causes of acute allo-graft dysfunction. Most current clinical trials of new anti-rejection agents require confirmation of the renal pathology by biopsy prior to treatment of rejection.

Indications for renal allograft biopsies have been widening to accommodate new concepts in patient management. For example, a major current focus in clinical transplantation is expansion of the donor pool. Broadening of the donation criteria and improved donor management permit accepting kidneys from marginal donors that would not have been considered 15 years ago. A biopsy of the kidneys of such donors is now widely used to assess the suitability of the kidney for transplantation. Donor biopsies also provide important information about the baseline status of the transplanted kidney and serve as a reference for later investigation of chronic allograft injury. A new, but rapidly-evolving concept in transplantation medicine is to use sequential protocol or "routine" biopsies of clinically stable grafts to study the development of chronic rejection and potentially intervene in its progression.

The ultimate goal of transplantation medicine for the 21st century, if attainable, is to achieve graft tolerance. For now, improving the long-term results of renal transplantation remains the primary challenge. The poor rates of 5-year and 10-year survival of kidney allografts continue to overshadow the marvelous accomplishments in the field of transplantation, and point to our current inability to prevent or to arrest progression of chronic allograft nephropathy/chronic rejection.

There is probably no area of nephrology and transplantation today in greater need of sharper more precise definitions than the area of chronic transplant changes. In the Banff classification, the severity of chronic transplant nephropathy is based on extent of interstitial fibrosis and tubular atrophy, with new onset of fibrous intimal thickening in the arteries and the relatively rare light microscopic lesion of transplant glomerulopathy noted as suggesting the specific diagnosis of chronic rejection.

The recently described use of Sirius Red staining for quantitation of allograft fibrosis and chronic allograft nephropathy is of great interest, and may refine morphologic assessment of these parameters because of it's specificity in staining interstitial collagen. Sirius Red (which eliminates false-positive staining of structures other than the interstitium) is an affordable and easy-to-perform stain that can be readily implemented in histology laboratories. Another important property of Sirius Red is autofluorescence, making it ideal for stereologic

systems that depend on fluorescence such as confocal microscopy.

The great excitement in this area is derived in part from the potential for improved clinical management based on the application of sequential protocol biopsies in kidney transplantation. Biopsies done in normally functioning grafts without clinical signs of rejection have been found to quite frequently reveal smoldering subclinical rejection. Although there is preliminary evidence that treatment of these subclinical rejections improves functional performance of the allograft, there is no proof to date that such treatment prevents long term renal scarring. Importantly, fibrosing changes seen on protocol biopsy appear to precede chronic progressive renal functional impairment by several years and thus act as an "early surrogate marker" for chronic rejection by providing an opportune window for intervention. Overall, this area of inquiry into using histology to guide pharmacologic prevention of chronic allograft nephropathy is exciting and should yield interesting and beneficial new management strategies for renal allograft recipients.

RETURNING TO THE BEGINNING: THE DONOR/IMPLANTATION BIOPSY

Although the major emphasis of this chapter has been on biopsies obtained at times of transplant dysfunction and protocol (routine) posttransplant biopsies, the donor or implantation biopsy is of great importance as well. Many donor kidneys have vascular or parenchymal scarring/glomerulosclerosis changes that might be interpreted as chronic rejection or cyclosporine/FK506 toxicity if they were not already known to be preexisting. Thus, the presence of an implantation biopsy considerably improves the interpretation of later biopsies in the same kidney and should be mandatory in every renal transplant program. Changes in later biopsies such as hyaline arteriolar change to diagnose cyclosporine toxicity, and fibrous intimal thickening interstitial fibrosis and tubular atrophy need to be evaluated for degree of change from the implantation biopsy baseline, rather than as absolutes.

In addition, changes present in the implantation biopsy have important long-term and short-term prognostic value. The degree of apoptosis in implantation biopsies may predict severity of posttransplant ATN, though is not predictive of function at six months. Late graft function can be predicted from glomerular size in implantation biopsies; enlarged glomeruli may reflect underlying glomerular hyperfiltration. Hyaline arteriolar change and (when the sample has >25 glomeruli) the degree of glomerulosclerosis likewise predict long-term outcome.

ADDENDUM
The Banff 97 Working Classification of Renal Allograft Pathology

Owing to its importance, the abstract and tables from the recent publication describing the Banff'97 classification are reproduced here by permission. These are modified in format from the original but the basic information remains the same.

Abstract – The Banff 97 Working Classification of Renal Allograft Pathology. Used with permission from Kidney Int. 55;1999:713-723.

Background – Standardization of renal allograft biopsy interpretation is necessary to guide therapy and to establish an objective end point for clinical trials. This manuscript describes a classification, Banff 97, developed by investigators using the Banff Schema and the Collaborative Clinical Trials in Transplantation (CCTT) modification for diagnosis of renal allograft pathology.

Methods – Banff 97 grew from an international consensus discussion begun at Banff and continued via the World Wide Web. This schema developed from: (1) analysis of data using the Banff classification; (2) publication of and experience with the CCTT modification; (3) international conferences; and (4) data from recent studies on impact of vasculitis on transplant outcome.

Results – Semiquantitative lesion scoring continues to focus on tubulitis and arteritis, but including a minimum threshold for interstitial inflammation. Banff 97 defines "types" of acute/active rejection. Type I is tubulointerstitial rejection without arteritis, Type II is vascular rejection with intimal arteritis, and Type III is severe rejection with transmural arterial changes. Biopsies with only mild inflammation are graded as "borderline/suspicious for rejection". The schema grades chronic/sclerosing allograft changes based on severity of tubular atrophy and interstitial fibrosis. Antibody-mediated rejection, hyperacute or accelerated acute in presentation, is also categorized, as are other significant allograft findings.

Conclusions – Banff 97 Working Classification refines earlier schemas and represents input from two classifications most widely used in clinical rejection trials and in clinical practice world-wide. Major changes include: rejection with vasculitis is now separated from tubulointerstitial rejection; severe rejection now requires transmural changes in arteries; "borderline" rejection can only be adequately interpreted in clinical context; antibody-mediated rejection is now better defined, and lesion scoring focuses on most severely involved structures. Criteria for specimen adequacy have also been modified. Banff 97 represents a significant refinement of this important pathologic schema, developed via international consensus discussions.

Table 58-1. Specimen Adequacy (a necessary prerequisite for numeric coding)

Unsatisfactory	No glomeruli or arteries
Marginal	Seven glomeruli with an artery
Adequate	Ten or more glomeruli with at least two arteries
Minimum Sampling	Seven slides: three H&E; three PAS or silver strains, and one trichome

Table 58-2. Quantitative Criteria for Tubulitis ("t") Score*

t0	No mononuclear cells in tubules
t1	Foci with 1 to 4 cells/tubular cross-section or 10 tubular cells
t2	Foci with 5 to 10 cells/tubular cross-section
t3	Foci with >10 cells/tubular cross-section, or the presence of at least two areas of tubular basement membrane destruction accompanied by i2/i3 inflammation and t2 tubulitis elsewhere in the biopsy.
*Applies to tubules no more than mildly atrophic	

Table 58-3. Quantitative Criteria for Intimal Arteritis ("v")

v0	No arteritis
v1	Mild-to-moderate intimal arteritis in at least one arterial cross section
v2	Severe intimal arteritis with at least 25% luminal area lost in at least one arterial cross-section
v3	Arteritis with arterial fibrinoid change and/or transmural arteritis with medial smooth muscle necrosis

Note number of arteries present and number affected. Indicate infarction and/or interstitial hemorrhage by an asterisk (with any level v score).

Table 58-4. Quantitative Criteria for Mononuclear Cell Interstitial Inflammation ("i") Scores

i0	No or trivial interstitial inflammation (<10% of unscarred parenchyma)
i1	10% to 25% of parenchyma inflamed
i2	26% to 50% of parenchyma inflamed
i3	% >50 of parenchyma inflamed

Indicate presence of remarkable numbers of eosinophils, polys, or plasma cells (specify which) with an asterisk*.

Table 58-5. Quantitative Criteria for Early Allograft Glomerulitis ("g") Score

g0	No glomerulitis
g1	Glomerulitis in a minority of glomeruli
g2	Segmental or global glomerulitis in 25% to 75% of glomeruli
g3	Glomerulitis (mostly global) in all or almost all glomeruli

Table 58-6. Acute Rejection – Overview: Banff 97 Banff 93 CCTT

Suspicious for acute rejection, borderline Type I	
Type IA	(tubulointerstitial with t2) Grade I
Type IB	(tubulointerstitial with t3) Grade IIA
Type IIA	(vascular with v1) Grade IIB Type II
Type IIB	(vascular with v2) Grade III
Type III v3	fibrinoid change/transmural arteritis) Grade III Type II

Table 58-7. Quantitative Criteria for Interstitial Fibrosis ("ci")

ci0	Interstitial fibrosis in up to 5% of cortical area
ci1	Mild interstitial fibrosis in 6% to 25% of cortical area
ci2	Moderate-interstitial fibrosis of 26% to 50% of cortical area
ci3	Severe-interstitial fibrosis of 50% of cortical area

Table 58-8. Quantitative Criteria for Tubular Atrophy ("ct")

ct0	No tubular atrophy
ct1	Tubular atrophy in up to 25% of the area of cortical tubules
ct2	Tubular atrophy involving 26% to 50% of the area of cortical tubules
ct3	Tubular atrophy of >50% of the area of cortical tubules

Table 58-9. Quantitative Criteria for Allograft Glomerulopathy ("cg")

cg0	No glomerulopathy-double contours in (less than)10% of peripheral capillary loops in most severely affected glomerulus
cg1	Capillary loop thickening with double contours affecting up to 25% of peripheral capillary loops in the most affected of nonsclerotic glomeruli
cg2	Double contours affecting 26% to 50% of peripheral capillary loops in the most affected of nonsclerotic glomeruli
cg3	Double contours affecting more than 50% of peripheral capillary loops in the most affected of nonsclerotic glomeruli

Note number of glomeruli and percentage sclerotic.

Table 58-10. Quantitative Criteria for Mesangial Matrix Increase ("mm")*

mm0	No mesangial matrix increase
mm1	Up to 25% of nonsclerotic glomeruli affected (at least moderate matrix increase)
mm2	26% to 50% of nonsclerotic glomeruli affected (at least moderate matrix increase)
mm3	>50% of nonsclerotic glomeruli affected (at least moderate matrix increase)

*The threshold criterion for the moderately increased "mm" is the expanded mesangial interspace between adjacent capillaries. If the width of the interspace exceeds two mesangial cells on the average in at least two glomerular lobules the "mm" is moderately increased.

Table 58-11. Quantitative Criteria for Vascular Fibrous Intimal Thickening ("cv")

cv0	No chronic vascular changes
cv1	Vascular narrowing of up to 25% luminal area by fibrointimal thickening of arteries ± breach of internal elastic lamina or presence of foam cells or occasional mononuclear cells*
cv2	Increased severity of changes described above with 26% to 50% narrowing of vascular luminal area*
cv3	Severe vascular changes with >50% narrowing of vascular luminal area*

*in most severely affected vessel. Note if lesions characteristic of chronic rejection (breaks in the elastica, inflammatory cells in fibrosis, formation of neo-intima) are seen.

Table 58-12. Quantitative Criteria for Anteriolar Hyaline Thickening ("ah")

ah0	No PAS-positive hyaline thickening
ah1	Mild-to-moderate PAS-positive hyaline thickening in at least one arteriole
ah2	Moderate-to-severe PAS-positive hyaline thickening in more than one arteriole
ah3	Severe PAS-positive hyaline thickening in many arterioles.

Indicate arteriolitis (significance unknown) by an asterisk on ah.

Table 58-13. Diagnostic Categories for Renal Allograft Biopsies – Banff '97*

1.	Normal, see Definitions	
2.	Antibody-mediated rejection demonstrated to be due, at least in part, to anti-donor antibody	
	A. Immediate (Hyperacute) B. Delayed (Accelerated Acute)	
3.	Borderline Changes – "Suspicious" for acute rejection. This category is used when no intimal arteritis is present, but there are foci of mild tubulitis (1 to 4 mononuclear cells/tubular cross-section)	
4.	Acute/Active Rejection Type (Grade) Histopathological Findings	
	IA	Cases with significant interstitial infiltration (>25% of parenchyma affected) and foci of moderate tubulitis (>4 mononuclear cells/tubular cross-section or group of 10 tubular cells)
	IB	Cases with significant interstitial infiltration (>25% of parenchyma affected) and foci of severe tubulitis (>10 mononuclear cells/tubular cross-section or group of 10 tubular cells)
	IIA	Cases with mild to moderate intimal arteritis (v1)
	IIB	Cases with severe intimal arteritis comprising >25% of the luminal area (v2)
	III	Cases with "transmural" arteritis or fibrinoid change and necrosis of medial smooth muscle cells (v3)
5.	Chronic/Sclerosing Allograft Nephropathy†	
	Grade Histopathological Findings	
	Grade I (mild) Mild interstitial fibrosis and tubular atrophy without (a) or with (b) specific changes suggesting chronic rejection	
	Grade II Moderate interstitial fibrosis and tubular atrophy (moderate) (a) or (b)	
	Grade III Severe interstitial fibrosis and tubular atrophy and tubular loss (severe) (a) or (b)	
6.	Other Changes not considered to be due to rejection, see Table 14	

*The recommended format of report is a descriptive narrative sign out followed by numerical codes in parentheses. Categorization should in the first instance be based solely on pathologic changes, then integrated with clinical data as a second step. More than one diagnostic category may be used if appropriate.
†Glomerular and vascular lesions help define type of chronic nephropathy; chronic/recurrent rejection can be diagnosed if typical vascular lesions are seen.

RECOMMENDED READING

Hume DM, Merrill JP, Miller BF, Thorn GW. Experiences with renal homotransplantation in the human: report of nine cases. J Clin Invest. 1955;34:327-382.

Kark RM. The development of percutaneous renal biopsy in man. Am J Kidney Dis. 1990;16(6):585-589.

Hanas E, Larsson E, Fellström B, et al. Safety aspects and diagnostic findings of serial renal allograft biopsies, obtained by an automatic technique with a midsize needle. Scand J Urol Nephrol. 1992;26(4):413-420.

Beckingham IJ, Nicholson ML, Kirk G, Veitch PS, Bell PR. Comparison of three methods to obtain percutaneous needle core biopsies of a renal allograft. Brit J Surg. 1994;81(6):898-899.

Wilczek HE. Percutaneous needle biopsy of the renal allograft. Transplantation. 1990;50(5):790-797.

Al-Awwa IA, Hariharan S, First MR. Importance of allograft biopsy in renal transplant recipients: Correlation between clinical and histological diagnosis. Am J Kidney Dis. 1998;31(6 Suppl 1):S15-S18.

Colvin RB, Cohen AH, Saiontz C, et al. Evaluation of pathologic criteria for acute renal allograft rejection: reproducibility, sensitivity, and clinical correlation. J Am Soc Nephrol. 1997;8(12):1930-1941.

Gaber LW, Gaber AO, Tolley EA, Hathaway DK. Prediction by postrevascularization biopsies of cadaveric kidney allografts of rejection, graft loss, and preservation nephropathy. Transplantation. 1992;53(6):1219-1225.

Gaber LW, Moore LW, Alloway RR, Amiri MH, Vera SR, Gaber AO. Glomerulosclerosis as a determinant of post-transplant function of older donor renal allografts. Transplantation. 1995;60(4):334-339.

Table 58-14. Other Non-Rejection Diagnoses in Renal Allograft Biopsies Posttransplant
Lymphoproliferative disorder
Nonspecific changes focal intersitial inflammation without tubulitis reactive vascular changes venulitis
Acute tubular necrosis
Acute interstitial nephritis
Cyclosporine or FK506-associated changes, acute or chronic
Subcapsular injury "healing in"
Pretransplant acute endothelial injury
Papillary necrosis
de novo glomerulonephritis
Recurrent disease
Immune complex glomerulonephritis
Focal segmental glomerulosclerosis
Diabetes
Hemolytic-uremic syndrome
Other
Preexisting disease
Viral infection
Obstruction/reflux, urine leak

Nickerson P, Jeffery J, Gough J, et al. Identification of clinical and histopathologic risk factors for diminished renal function 2 years posttransplant. J Am Soc Nephrol. 1998;9(3):482-487.

Grimm PC, Nickerson P, Gough J, et al. Quantification of allograft fibrosis and chronic allograft nephropathy. Ped Transplantation. 1999;3(4)249-251.

Racusen LC, Solez K, Colvin RB, et al. The Banff 97 working classification of renal allograft pathology. Kidney Int. 1999;55(2):713-723.

Nickerson P, Jeffery J, Gough J, et al. Effect of increasing baseline immunosuppression on the prevalence of clinical and subclinical rejection: a pilot study. J Am Soc Nephrol. 1999;10(8):1801-1805.

Grimm PC, McKenna R, Nickerson P, et al. Clinical rejection is distinguished from subclinical rejection by increased infiltration by a population of activated macrophages. J Am Soc Nephrol. 1999;10(7):1582-1589.

Gaber L, Solez K. Renal allograft pathology: crossing over to the new millennium. Pediatr Transplantation. 1999;3(4):249-251.

Oberbauer R, Rohrmoser M, Regele H, Muhlbacher F, Mayer G. Apoptosis of tubular epithelial cells in donor kidney biopsies predicts early renal allograft function. J Am Soc Nephrol. 1999;10(9):2006-2013.

Abdi R, Slakey D, Kittur D, Burdick J, Racusen L Baseline glomerular size as a predictor of function in human renal transplantation. Transplantation. 1998;66(3):329-333.

Wang HJ, Kjellstrand CM, Cockfield SM, Solez K. On the influence of sample size on the prognostic accuracy and reproducibility of renal transplant biopsy. Nephrol Dial Transplant. 1998;13(1):165-172.

59 LONG-TERM MANAGEMENT ISSUES IN KIDNEY TRANSPLANTATION

Donald E. Hricik, MD

Steady improvements in short-term renal allograft survival rates during the past two decades have mandated increased attention to the long-term management of kidney transplant recipients. Initial posttransplant management focuses on the recognition and treatment of delayed allograft function, surgical complications, and acute rejection episodes. Beyond the first few posttransplant months, the risk of acute rejection in compliant patients declines substantially, and attention turns to the recognition and treatment of various causes of chronic allograft dysfunction and of the metabolic complications of immunosuppressive therapy. This chapter focuses on the causes and management of chronic renal allograft dysfunction. Metabolic disturbances and related issues are reviewed in Section IV, Chapter 24.

CLINICAL ASSESSMENT OF RENAL FUNCTION

Periodic assessment of renal function is an important component of the long-term care of kidney transplant recipients. Renal allografts have the capacity to function for decades. However, the average half-life of a cadaver transplant is approximately 11 years, implying that many transplanted kidneys fail over relatively short periods of time. The major causes of chronic renal dysfunction in kidney transplant recipients are listed in Table 59-1. Even "stable" kidney transplant recipients often have mild renal insufficiency and therefore are also more vulnerable than normal subjects to common forms of acute renal failure resulting from sepsis, hypotension, or administration of radiocontrast dye, nonsteroidal antiinflammatory drugs, and other nephrotoxins.

As is true in the general population, estimates of glomerular filtration rate (GFR) provide the best assessment of overall renal integrity in transplant recipients. Isolated abnormalities of tubular function (eg, defective potassium or hydrogen ion secretion) or synthetic capacity (eg, vitamin D deficiency) are sometimes clinically significant, but most of the adverse consequences of renal failure can be attributed directly or indirectly to a decreased GFR. Measurement of the serum creatinine concentration is a simple, inexpensive, and universally

available method for estimating GFR and is a reliable means of detecting acute changes in renal function. However, a number of studies have shown that the serum creatinine concentration is relatively unreliable for detecting chronic changes in renal function. Over long periods of time, alterations in tubular secretion of creatinine and changes in muscle mass, particularly relevant in patients receiving corticosteroid therapy, make the serum creatinine level a less sensitive marker for detecting subtle, chronic fluctuations in GFR.

Measurement of creatinine clearance using timed urine specimens theoretically eliminates the confounding influence of muscle mass in estimating GFR. However, the usefulness of such clearance determinations is limited by practical difficulties in obtaining complete and well-timed collections. Furthermore, as renal function worsens, tubular secretion of creatinine may increase, resulting in progressive overestimation of GFR. Conventional formulas used to estimate GFR based on clinical parameters that correlate with muscle mass (eg, age, gender, and weight) are also subject to substantial variability. Urinary or plasma clearance of isotopic (eg, iothalamate) or non-isotopic (eg, iohexol) substances that mimic the properties of inulin (ie, freely filtered by the glomerulus, neither reabsorbed nor secreted by renal tubules) provides accurate, albeit expensive and cumbersome, estimates of GFR. Although some transplant physicians recommend the routine use of such clearance techniques to monitor long-term renal function, further studies are needed to determine whether this approach improves patient outcomes when compared to standard serial measurements of serum creatinine concentration or creatinine clearance.

Kidney transplant recipients should be screened periodically for the presence of urinary protein. Persistent proteinuria (exceeding 1 gm) is common in patients with chronic allograft nephropathy or recurrent glomerular disease, may be detected prior to any measurable reduction in GFR, and portends a poor long-term prognosis for the renal allograft. Diseased native

---

Professor of Medicine; Chief, Division of Nephrology, Case Western Reserve University; Medical Director of Transplantation Services, University Hospital of Cleveland, Cleveland, OH

Table 59-1. Major Causes of Chronic Renal Allograft Dysfunction
Chronic allograft nephropathy (ie, "chronic rejection")
Drug toxicity (including the effects of cyclosporine and tacrolimus)
Recurrence of original renal disease
Ischemic nephropathy (renal artery stenosis)
Obstructive uropathy
De novo glomerulopathies

kidneys may contribute to urinary protein excretion. In addition, transient proteinuria is common during episodes of acute rejection and other forms of acute renal failure. Thus, in assessing prognosis, trends in urine protein excretion over long periods of time are more meaningful than measurements obtained at any single point in time. The standard dipstick is a convenient, inexpensive method for measuring urinary protein excretion but is only semiquantitative and best used for screening. Despite the limitations of timed urine collections noted above, measurement of total protein excretion in a 24-hour collection is the definitive method for assessing proteinuria quantitatively. Protein/creatinine ratios measured in spot-urine specimens correlate reasonably well with 24-hour protein excretion rates, although some studies suggest that the correlation decreases with progressively increasing amounts of urinary protein.

The frequency with which renal functional parameters are monitored after kidney transplantation varies widely. The Clinical Practice Guidelines Committee of the American Society of Transplantation currently recommends measurement of serum creatinine concentration at least twice weekly in the first posttransplant month, weekly in the second month, biweekly until the fourth month, monthly until the end of the first transplant year, every two months during the second posttransplant year, and every four to six months thereafter for the lifespan of the allograft, in uncomplicated patients. Patients with acute or chronic allograft dysfunction require more frequent monitoring. Some transplant centers obtain a urinalysis during each office appointment. For the purposes of monitoring patients for proteinuria, it is probably sufficient to screen for proteinuria with a dipstick every three to six months for the first year, and every six to 12 months thereafter. In patients with a positive dipstick test of 2+ (corresponding to 40 gm to 100 gm of protein/dL) or greater, a 24-hour urine should be obtained to quantify daily protein excretion. Thereafter, serial 24-hour urine collections or protein/creatinine ratios in spot specimens should be employed for continued monitoring.

PREVENTION, DIAGNOSIS AND MANAGEMENT OF RECURRENT DISEASE

Kidney diseases that can recur in renal allografts and the risks of their recurrence are summarized in Chapter 57 of this section. Clinical manifestations of recurrence vary with the underlying disease process. Recurrences of glomerular diseases such as focal glomerulosclerosis or membranoproliferative glomerulonephritis frequently present with new onset proteinuria, sometimes associated with the nephrotic syndrome. Hematuria may be the primary clinical manifestation of recurrent IgA nephropathy or Henoch Schoenlein purpura. Microangiopathic hemolysis and thrombocytopenia usually herald recurrent hemolytic uremic syndrome. Renal biopsy is essential in confirming clinically suspected recurrence of renal disease. In many cases, recurrent disease is discovered unexpectedly when biopsy is performed in patients with otherwise unexplained renal insufficiency. Both immunofluorescence and electron microscopy may be required to supplement information obtained on light microscopy when renal biopsy is performed to determine the presence of recurrent disease.

Specific therapies are lacking for many of the diseases that recur in transplanted kidneys. In fact, recurrent diseases do not predictably cause renal dysfunction, perhaps because of the mollifying effects of immunosuppressive drug therapy, and specific therapy may not be required. Plasmapheresis is sometimes beneficial in patients with rapidly recurrent focal glomerulosclerosis, although the benefit may be limited to a subset of patients with detectable plasma levels of a glomerular permeability factor that is not measured routinely in most laboratories. In patients with recurrent hemolytic uremic syndrome, plasmapheresis, plasma replacement, antiplatelet agents, and reduction or discontinuation of calcineurin inhibitors have been used with reported success, but controlled clinical trials are lacking to confirm the efficacy of such measures. Recurrence of primary oxalosis can sometimes be averted with intensive hemodialysis and treatment with pyridoxine, phosphorus and magnesium.

MANAGEMENT OF CHRONIC ALLOGRAFT DYSFUNCTION AND PROTEINURIA

Chronic allograft nephropathy and death are currently the two most common causes of renal allograft loss beyond the first posttransplant year. Also referred to as chronic rejection, chronic allograft nephropathy usually occurs more than six months after transplantation and is clinically characterized by a slow, relentless decline in GFR, and by proteinuria; it is the most common cause of nephrotic syndrome in kidney transplant recipients. The pathologic hallmarks include an occlusive vasculopathy, glomerulosclerosis, and interstitial fibrosis. Renal biopsy is required for definitive diagnosis, and should be considered in all patients with slowly deteriorating renal allograft function to exclude a component of acute rejection and recurrent or de novo renal diseases. A simultaneous imaging study, most often ultrasound, serves the dual purpose of excluding obstructive uropathy.

The pathophysiology of chronic allograft nephropathy is poorly understood. It is widely acknowledged that both immunologic and nonimmunologic factors play a role in pathogenesis (Figure 59-1). However, there is little evidence that intensification of immunosuppressive therapy is beneficial. Indeed, the interstitial fibrosis and vascular changes induced by the calcineurin inhibitors can be difficult to differentiate from the lesions of chronic allograft nephropathy and may play an additive role. Recent reports suggest that addition of mycophenolate mofetil, or conversion from azathioprine to mycophenolate mofetil, may stabilize or improve renal function in patients with chronic allograft nephropathy; however, the benefit may be limited to patients in whom cyclosporine dosage is simultaneously reduced. Sirolimus blocks the development of chronic allograft vasculopathy in a number of animal models, but clinical trials are needed to determine whether this agent is capable of preventing or treating vasculopathy in humans.

Currently, the management of patients with chronic allograft nephropathy focuses on nonimmunologic factors (eg, systemic hypertension, hyperlipidemia) that are amenable to therapy. There is no evidence that dietary protein restriction is beneficial in this form of chronic progressive renal failure. In fact, severe dietary protein restriction may lead to malnutrition in patients under the catabolic influence of chronic corticosteroid therapy. A number of cytokines and growth factors have been implicated as pathophysiologic links between early ischemic and immunologic injuries and the later expression of chronic allograft nephropathy. Pharmacologic inhibition of the mitogenic and pro-inflammatory effects of these mediators may prove to be useful in the preven-

tion and treatment of this disorder. Angiotensin plays a pivotal role in mediating chronic renal injury by promoting intraglomerular hypertension, and by stimulating the expression of profibrotic cytokines such as transforming growth factor beta (TGFβ). Ongoing clinical trials may help to determine whether pharmacologic inhibition of angiotensin can halt the progression of chronic allograft nephropathy. In the absence of definitive data, a trial of either an angiotensin-converting enzyme (ACE) inhibitor or an angiotensin receptor blocker is probably reasonable in kidney transplant recipients with heavy proteinuria, based on evidence that these agents can reduce urinary protein excretion and slow the rate of deterioration of other kidney diseases.

DIAGNOSIS AND MANAGEMENT OF HYPERTENSION

Hypertension occurs in 50% to 80% of kidney transplant recipients and has been attributed to a number of etiologic factors including the effects of diseased native kidneys, acute and chronic allograft rejection, recurrent disease in the allograft, transplant renal artery stenosis, and the effects of immunosuppressive drugs. More than one of these factors is involved in many cases. In diabetic patients, the incidence of hypertension is lower after kidney-pancreas transplantation than it is after kidney transplantation alone; however, the "protective" effect of the dual transplant may be limited to recipients of bladder-drained pancreatic allografts. Although there have been no large randomized trials demonstrating a

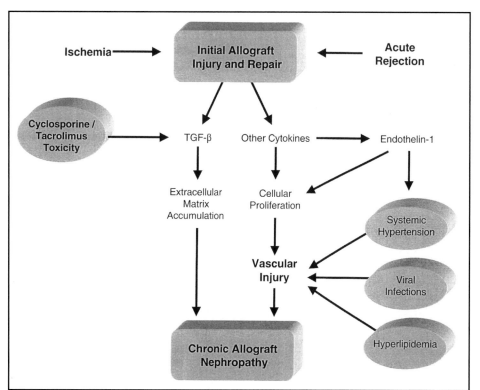

Figure 59-1. Schema of possible mechanisms involved in the pathogenesis of chronic allograft nephropathy. Early immunologic and ischemic injuries in combination with the effects of cyclosporine or tacrolimus lead to the generation of transforming growth factor (TGFβ) and other cytokines resulting in extracellular matrix accumulation and cellular proliferation, including smooth muscle proliferation that contributes to progressive vascular occlusion. Nonimmunologic factors such as systemic hypertension, viral infections, and hyperlipidemia may contribute to the vascular injury. Endothelin-1 may play a key role by directly promoting vascular injury and by increasing systemic blood pressure.

beneficial effect of blood pressure reduction in kidney transplant recipients, it seems likely that hypertension contributes to the risk of posttransplant cardiovascular disease based on abundant data suggesting this relationship in the general population. In addition, results from a number of studies indicate that elevated blood pressure adversely effects renal allograft survival, especially in black patients. Thus, posttransplant hypertension should be treated aggressively. Management depends on the underlying etiology.

Corticosteroids induce hypertension, in part, by promoting sodium retention and weight gain. Cyclosporine, and to a lesser extent, tacrolimus, exacerbate hypertension via renal or peripheral vasoconstriction, sodium retention, and activation of the sympathetic nervous system. Complete withdrawal of corticosteroids or cyclosporine from patients receiving multi-drug immunosuppressive regimens generally has been accompanied by reductions in blood pressure. However, the benefits of eliminating or reducing the dose of these agents must be weighed against a risk of precipitating allograft rejection.

Diseased native kidneys may continue to produce renin and other vasoactive substances that probably contribute to posttransplant hypertension in many cases. Unfortunately, measurements of peripheral or renal vein renin levels have not proved to be reliable as indicators for bilateral nephrectomy. Ablation of the native kidneys using embolization techniques is an alternative to nephrectomy, but large studies have not been performed to judge the effectiveness of these radiologic procedures. With the availability of potent antihypertensive drugs and drug combinations, most transplant nephrologists consider native kidney ablation or nephrectomy only in rare cases of intractably severe posttransplant hypertension.

Functionally significant renal artery stenoses have been observed in 5% to 10% of kidney transplant recipients. Stenoses may occur at the site of the arterial anastomosis (most commonly with end-to-end anastomoses), in the recipient artery, or in the donor artery, and may result from either surgical or immunologic injury or de novo atherosclerosis. Transplant renal artery stenosis should be suspected in patients with new onset hypertension or severe hypertension that is resistant to medical therapy, particularly in patients with otherwise unexplained renal dysfunction. Recalling that posttransplant erythrocytosis typically occurs in patients with normal renal allograft function, polycythemia in the presence of impaired renal function suggests renal artery occlusion and associated renal ischemia. Administration of ACE inhibitors to transplant recipients with renal artery stenosis affecting a functionally solitary kidney may cause acute renal failure based on the well-known dissociation in the autoregulation of renal blood flow and GFR that occurs under these circumstances. However, the commonly used calcineurin inhibitors

(eg, cyclosporine, tacrolimus) tend to suppress the renin-angiotensin system and thus reduce the predictive value of using ACE inhibition as a provocative test for renal artery stenosis. The presence of a bruit over the allograft is not specific; however, new or loud bruits detected in the appropriate setting may increase suspicion for renal artery occlusion. Conventional or digital subtraction angiography remains the "gold standard" for confirmation of the diagnosis, although noninvasive techniques such as color Doppler ultrasound and magnetic resonance arteriography are reasonably sensitive and warrant further study. Percutaneous transluminal angioplasty is the treatment of choice, but is technically infeasible in many cases and is associated with recurrence of the stenosis in up to 20% of cases. Graft loss has been reported in up to 30% of patients requiring surgical repair for transplant renal artery stenosis.

Most patients with posttransplant hypertension require pharmacologic antihypertensive treatment, but there is no consensus regarding optimal drug therapy. Calcium channel blockers generally are effective and well-tolerated, and may ameliorate the vasoconstrictive effects of the calcineurin inhibitors. Some (eg, diltiazem, verapamil), but not all (eg, nifedipine, isradipine) calcium channel blockers impair hepatic metabolism of cyclosporine, tacrolimus and sirolimus, leading to increased blood levels. The dihydropyridine compounds (eg, nifedipine, isradipine, amlodipine) are synergistic with cyclosporine in causing gingival hyperplasia. Diuretics are appealing agents in transplant patients with hypertension and edema, however, even mild drug-induced volume depletion may exacerbate the prerenal azotemia caused by calcineurin inhibitors. The ACE inhibitors are relatively ineffective in patients receiving calcineurin inhibitors. Furthermore, hyperkalemia, anemia, or acute renal failure may complicate the use of these drugs. However, ACE inhibitors or the newer angiotensin receptor blockers ultimately may prove to be useful in retarding the development or progression of chronic allograft nephropathy (see above). The indications and contraindications for beta-blockers, alpha-blockers, central-acting sympatholytics, and vasodilators in the management of posttransplant hypertension generally are similar to those relevant to the management of essential hypertension in the general population.

MANAGEMENT OF HYPERLIPIDEMIA

Hyperlipidemia occurs in approximately 70% of renal transplant recipients and may contribute not only to the development of cardiovascular disease, but also to chronic allograft dysfunction. Posttransplant hypercholesterolemia and hypertriglyceridemia have been linked to a number of factors including genetic predisposition, proteinuria, advancing age, and diuretic therapy.

However, most authorities agree that immunosuppressive drugs, especially corticosteroids, cyclosporine, and sirolimus, play a preeminent role (see Section IV, Chapter 24). In patients receiving cyclosporine and steroids, the most commonly observed lipoprotein profile consists of elevations of both LDL and HDL cholesterol. Hypertriglyceridemia is more common in patients receiving sirolimus. Although it is not clear whether the risks of hyperlipidemia in organ transplant recipients are similar to those in the general population, many transplant physicians adhere to the management guidelines established for the general population by the National Cholesterol Education Program. Single studies and a meta-analysis suggest at least a short-term benefit of dietary management in hyperlipidemic renal transplant recipients. Thus, a low cholesterol diet with a relatively high content of polyunsaturated fats should be recommended for hypercholesterolemic patients. Those with hypertriglyceridemia may benefit from total caloric restriction, weight loss, and restriction of alcohol intake. The HMG-CoA reductase inhibitors have emerged as the pharmacologic agents of choice in the treatment of posttransplant hypercholesterolemia, despite concerns about an increased incidence of myositis in patients taking these agents in combination with cyclosporine. By inhibiting bile acid synthesis, cyclosporine decreases the biliary excretion of the HMG-CoA reductase inhibitors, resulting in blood levels threefold to tenfold higher than those observed in patients not receiving cyclosporine. This phenomenon mandates the use of relatively low doses of HMG-CoA reductase inhibitors. Treatment with fibrates such as gemfibrozil may be necessary for management of patients with severe hypertriglyceridemia.

RESUMPTION OF DIALYSIS AND EVALUATION FOR RE-TRANSPLANTATION

In patients with failing renal allografts, neither the indications for initiation of dialysis nor the selection criteria for re-transplantation differ from those in the general population of patients with kidney disease. Renal replacement options should be discussed with the patient when it becomes clear that allograft failure is inevitable. However, the timing of this discussion varies substantially depending on the rate of decline in renal function, local waiting times for cadaver organs, and the availability of living donors for a second transplant. Management of immunosuppression following resumption of dialysis is a subject of great controversy. Most transplant physicians gradually withdraw immunosuppression. However, recognizing that withdrawal of immunosuppressive drugs may precipitate acute rejection manifested by local or systemic symptoms, there is no consensus about the timing or pace

of withdrawing immunosuppressive drug therapy. Some centers advocate continuation of immunosuppressive drugs in patients who are candidates for expeditious re-transplantation, based on the premise that withdrawal of immunosuppression may be associated with a rise in the titer of anti-HLA antibodies, especially in patients in whom the failed allograft has not been removed surgically.

INDICATIONS FOR REMOVAL OF A RENAL ALLOGRAFT

Although allograft nephrectomy rates vary widely from center to center, as many as 50% of grafts that fail beyond the first posttransplant year are surgically removed. Indications for allograft nephrectomy include otherwise unexplained fever, graft swelling or tenderness, hematuria, and/or general malaise. Because these signs and symptoms generally reflect acute rejection of the allograft, some transplant physicians recommend a short course of corticosteroids to treat the symptoms and possibly to avoid nephrectomy. The effect of allograft nephrectomy on anti-HLA antibody titers and on the outcome of subsequent transplants is another subject of controversy. Some studies suggest that allograft nephrectomy has an unfavorable impact on the outcome of subsequent transplants. However, it is likely that nephrectomies are performed more commonly in patients who are "high immunologic responders," and it is difficult to separate the effects of nephrectomy per se from the tendency of such patients to reject multiple allografts.

ROLE OF THE PRIMARY PHYSICIAN IN LONG-TERM MANAGEMENT

As the population of kidney transplant recipients grows, long-term management increasingly requires cooperation between transplant nephrologists and primary care physicians. However, the exact role of the primary physician is in a state of evolution and varies greatly based on local medical practices and the regionally disparate influences of managed care. Most physicians would agree that the transplant center should remain intimately involved in all decisions related to immunosuppressive drug therapy or the diagnosis and management of renal allograft dysfunction. The primary physician that follows a kidney transplant recipient must possess at least a minimal understanding of the principles of immunosuppression, including the basic pharmacology and side effects of commonly-used immunosuppressive drugs. Most importantly, the physician responsible for prescribing other medications to the organ transplant recipient must make an effort to understand drug-to-drug interactions that could ultimately result in under-immunosuppression or over-immunosuppression or serious drug toxicity.

RECOMMENDED READING

Abouljoud MS, Deierhoi MH, Hudson SL, Diethelm AG. Risk factors affecting second renal transplant outcome with special reference to primary allograft nephrectomy. Transplantation. 1995;60(2):138-144.

Bia MJ. Nonimmunologic causes of late renal graft loss. Kidney Int. 1995;47(5):1470-1480.

Cosio FG, Dillon JJ, Falkenhain ME, et al. Racial differences in renal allograft survival: the role of systemic hypertension. Kidney Int. 1995;47(4):1136-1141.

Kobashigawa JA, Kasiske BL. Hyperlipidemia in solid organ transplantation. Transplantation. 1997;63(3): 331-338.

Massy ZA, Guijarro C, Wiederkehr MR, Ma JZ, Kasiske BL. Chronic renal allograft rejection: immunologic and nonimmunologic risk factors. Kidney Int. 1996;49(2): 518-524.

Nankivell BJ, Gruenewald SM, Allen RD, Chapman JR. Predicting glomerular filtration rate after kidney transplantation. Transplantation. 1995;59(12):1683-1689.

Opelz G, Wujciak T, Ritz E for the Collaborative Transplant Study. Association of chronic kidney graft failure with recipient blood pressure. Kidney Int. 1998;53(1):217-222.

Ramos EL, Tisher CC. Recurrent diseases in the kidney transplant. Am J Kidney Dis. 1994;24(1):142-154.

Savin VJ, Sharma R, Sharma M, et al. Circulating factor associated with increased glomerular permeability to albumin in recurrent focal segmental glomerulosclerosis. N Engl J Med. 1996;334(14):878-883.

Vathsala A, Verani R, Schoenberg L, et al. Proteinuria in cyclosporine-treated renal transplant recipients. Transplantation. 1990;49(1):35-41.

Weir MR, Anderson L, Fink JC, et al. A novel approach to the treatment of chronic allograft nephropathy. Transplantation. 1997;64(12):1706-1710.

60 MAINTENANCE IMMUNOSUPPRESSION PROTOCOLS FOR KIDNEY TRANSPLANTATION

Barbara T. Murphy, MD, FRCPI

Until recently, maintenance immunosuppression consisted of corticosteroids, azathioprine and the original formulation of cyclosporine (CsA) – Sandimmune®. Data from the United Network for Organ Sharing (UNOS) registry in 1997 show that 78% of first cadaveric renal transplants received a cyclosporine-based triple therapy regimen. With the introduction of new drugs, in particular mycophenolate mofetil (MMF), tacrolimus and the microemulsion version of CsA, and the promise of many newer agents on the horizon, the number of options available has increased dramatically. The optimal combination, however, has yet to be established. Several important issues need to be considered when deciding on an appropriate immunosuppressive protocol for a particular patient. As a rule, the risk of acute rejection is highest in the first three months posttransplant, therefore, the number and dosages of immunosuppressive drugs should be highest during this period. However, the particular immunological history of an individual must also be considered. Factors such as the HLA matching or mismatching; the degree of sensitization of the patient; living-related vs cadaveric transplant; a history of a previously rejected graft; and the race of the patient all help stratify the immunological risk. Based on these broad criteria, the immunosuppressive protocol can be tailored to the needs of the individual patient. The side effect profile of a certain medication may also play a role in whether it is chosen. Thus, when planning a protocol, one must consider all aspects of immunosuppression: the immunosuppressive, immunodeficiency and nonimmune toxic effects.

CORTICOSTEROIDS

There is no consensus on the optimal dose or maintenance schedule for steroids. Suggested guidelines are shown in Table 60-1. A concerted effort has been made, particularly since the introduction of CsA, to reduce or withdraw steroids so as to minimize many of their associated side effects. Early withdrawal, within three to six

Assistant Professor of Clinical Medicine; Director of Transplant Nephrology, Renal Division, Mount Sinai School of Medicine, New York, NY

months posttransplant, and rapid tapering are associated with an increased frequency of acute rejection and decreased long-term graft survival, requiring recommencement of steroid therapy in more than 50% of patients. Acute rejection has been reported in 26% to 74% of recipients after steroid withdrawal in various studies. This wide variability most likely reflects differences in the patient population studied, and the timing of the withdrawal. Data from uncontrolled studies of stable patients who have had no rejection episodes for more than six months, or an uneventful course in the first year with good renal function, have noted successful outcomes in approximately 80% of patients maintained on CsA and azathioprine alone. It has also been suggested that racial mismatching of renal allografts and African-American race are predictors of acute rejection upon withdrawal of steroids. The Canadian multicenter transplant study found that, despite initially good results, withdrawal of steroids was associated with a deterioration in allograft survival that was only appreciated five years posttransplant. These results are tempered by the fact that patients in this study were rapidly tapered over a period of 90 days. The ability to withdraw steroids with patients remaining on newer immunosuppressants, and the long-term effects on chronic rejection remain to be seen. Maintenance therapy with alternate-day dosing has been used as a means to reduce the overall dose of steroids. In two large randomized controlled trials, alternate-day steroids were as effective in maintaining graft function, and were as well-tolerated as daily dosing.

Stress dose steroids are routinely given to renal transplant patients undergoing major surgery or suffering from a major illness (Table 60-1). Only two prospective, nonrandomized studies have been conducted looking at the need for stress dose steroids in renal transplant patients in particular. Both of these studies concluded that stress dose steroids were not required in patients on a stable low dose of prednisone (5 to 10 mg/day). Further studies will be required before this is broadly accepted.

ANTIPROLIFERATIVE AGENTS
Azathioprine

Azathioprine (AZA) has been the mainstay of immunosuppression since the 1960s. Triple drug protocols using prednisone, CsA and AZA were the standard regimen until the emergence of several newer agents in the past few years. Several studies have reported the successful withdrawal of AZA in an initial drug regimen without deleterious effects on graft survival (see below). Indeed, many centers in Europe use prednisone and CsA alone immediately posttransplant. AZA should be temporarily withheld if the white cell count falls. Centers vary in their threshold for withholding AZA, with values ranging between 2,000 to 4,000/mm^3. Recovery usually occurs after one to two weeks, at which point AZA can be restarted at a lower dose and increased gradually while monitoring the white cell count. Due to the inhibition of breakdown of active metabolites of AZA by allopurinol, if allopurinol needs to be given in conjunction with AZA, the dose of AZA should be reduced by at least one-half, and the white cell and platelet count closely monitored so as to avoid bone marrow suppression.

Mycophenolate Mofetil

AZA has been replaced in many programs by MMF. Three large prospective, randomized, double-blind trials have been conducted in the US, Canada, Europe and Australia comparing MMF with AZA or placebo as adjunctive therapy to CsA and steroids. Two MMF treat-ment groups, 2g/d and 3g/d, were included to compare dosing. All three studies had similar results. The com-bined data showed that treatment with MMF resulted in a reduction in the incidence of acute rejection by almost 50% at one year, with an associated reduction in severity. Renal function was consistently better for both MMF groups; however, there was no effect on graft or patient survival. While both doses of MMF had similar effects on the incidence of acute rejection, MMF 3g was considered to be less tolerated with a greater number of reported gastrointestinal side effects and an increased incidence of invasive CMV. Hence, MMF 2g/d in two divided doses is recommended. MMF may cause a leukopenia, though at 2g/d this is less frequent than with AZA. The dose of MMF should be reduced to 500/mg twice daily in the event of leukopenia and the white cell count closely monitored. If no response is seen MMF should be

Table 60-1. Maintenance Immunosuppression: Dosing and Therapeutic Levels

1. Prednisone	
Oral Dosing	Month 1 = 0.5 mg/kg per day Month 2 = 0.4 mg/kg per day Month 3 = 0.3 mg/kg per day Month 4 = 0.2 mg/kg per day Month 5 = 0.15 mg/kg per day Thereafter = 0.1 mg/kg per day
Intravenous Dosing	Equivalent dose of Methylprednisolone (4 : 5, MP : P)
Stress Dose Steroids	Major illness: 100 mg hydrocortisone q8o for 24 hours taper by half per day to maintenance levels. Major surgery: As above plus additional 100 mg preoperatively.
2. Calcineurin Inhibitors (one drug chosen)	
CsA	Oral dose: 8 to 10 mg/kg per day initially taper to a maintenance dose of 3 to 5 mg/kg per day
	Intravenous dose: one-third the PO dose

	Target whole blood trough levels:
	    Zero to six months: 300-250 ng/mL
	    Six to 12 months: 200-250 ng/mL
	    >2 months: 150-200 ng/mL

Tacrolimus	Oral dose: 0.1 to .15 mg/kg per day b.i.d.
	Intravenous dose: one-third the PO dose

	Target whole blood trough levels:
	    Zero to one month posttransplant: 15-20 ng/mL
	    One to three month posttransplant: 10-15 ng/mL
	    >3 month posttransplant: 5-12 ng/mL

3. Antiproliferative agents (one drug chosen)	
AZA MMF	Oral dose: 1.5 - 2 mg/kg per day Oral dose: 1g b.i.d. Both have a 1:1 ratio for intravenous administration.

held. The gastrointestinal side effects may be similarly managed. A trial of MMF at the higher dose may be attempted two weeks or so after the resolution of symptoms. The long-term effects of MMF on graft survival have not been established.

CALCINEURIN INHIBITORS
Cyclosporine

The introduction of CsA in the 1980s was associated with a 10% to 15 % improvement in graft survival. The majority of renal transplant patients are maintained on CsA and prednisone with or without a purine synthesis inhibitor. There are also a few centers in Europe in which selected patients are maintained on CsA monotherapy with reportedly good results. Despite the definite advantage offered by CsA with regard to 1-year graft survival, a therapeutic dilemma arises due to the nephrotoxic effects of this drug, an issue that now also applies to tacrolimus. Optimal dosing of CsA is key to avoiding nephrotoxicity. Several groups have shown that a low mean daily dose leads to an increase in the number of late acute rejections. Many studies have also examined the withdrawal of CsA at various times posttransplant in an attempt to see if, once the initial immunologically high-risk period is over, withdrawal of CsA would prevent the progressive decline in renal function. A meta-analysis examining the effect of elective CsA withdrawal demonstrated that there is a highly significant risk of acute rejection in those patients that had CsA withdrawn, however, no difference was seen in graft or patient survival over the short-term. African-Americans and patients with a higher number of HLA-DR mismatched appear to be at particularly high risk of rejection. A newer microemulsion formulation of CsA (Neoral®) has been developed to overcome the problems associated with poor and variable absorption of the traditional formulation, an issue that is particularly true in diabetic and African-American patients. This preparation exhibits less inter-patient and intra-patient variability and its absorption is not bile-dependent. In comparative studies with Sandimmune® and Neoral®, the latter has had fewer rejection episodes with the same safety and tolerability profile. Patients are now routinely commenced on the Neoral® preparation. For conversion, Neoral® is commenced at the same dose as Sandimmune®, trough levels are closely monitored and dosing adjusted appropriately.

The success of CsA has been accompanied by increased expense, a factor particularly troublesome for those without adequate insurance coverage. The inhibition of the metabolism of CsA by the P450 system through the coadministration of drugs such as ketoconazole and calcium channel blockers has been used as a potential mechanism for reducing the requirement for CsA, while still maintaining therapeutic drug levels. Several reports have demonstrated up to a 70% reduction in the dose of CsA when given in conjunction with ketoconazole, with similar outcomes in graft and patient survival. It is important to note that ketoconazole requires an acid medium for absorption, therefore it should not be given at the same time as antacids or drugs which inhibit gastric acid production. Non-dihydropyridine calcium channel blockers have been associated with a reduction in CsA dose in the order of 30%. In addition, several uncontrolled studies have found that the early administration of calcium channel blockers in the perioperative period is associated with a reduced incidence of delayed graft function and improved graft survival.

Tacrolimus

Tacrolimus, which had been used successfully in liver transplantation, was first approved by the Federal Drug Administration (FDA) for use in the prevention of graft rejection in kidney transplantation in 1997. Two large multicenter, randomized trials were conducted in the US and Europe comparing tacrolimus with CsA in recipients of cadaveric kidney transplants. The US trial demonstrated that patient and graft survival were similar at one and two years in both groups, however there was a significant reduction in the incidence of acute rejection episodes in the tacrolimus group at 30.7% compared to 46.4%, with significantly fewer number of steroid resistant rejections. These findings were corroborated by the European trial, which differed only in that induction therapy was not used. Subgroup analysis in the US trial showed that for African-Americans, considered to be a higher immunological risk group, these findings also held true with lower incidence and lower severity of rejection episodes. No significant difference in the incidence of nephrotoxicity was seen between groups; however, those treated with tacrolimus were more likely to suffer from neurotoxicity and 19.9% developed new onset insulin-dependent diabetes mellitus compared with 4% on CsA. African-Americans were at increased risk overall of posttransplant diabetes mellitus, particularly those treated with tacrolimus. Half of these cases were reversible at two years. It is important to note that African-American patients required, on average, a 37% mean higher dose of tacrolimus than Caucasians to achieve comparable blood concentrations.

Conversion from CsA to tacrolimus has been undertaken for the management of side effects, such as hypertension and hyperlipidemia, and failure to prevent rejection at therapeutic CsA levels. Alternatively, conversion from tacrolimus to CsA would predominantly occur for neuropathy and posttransplant diabetes mellitus. Both agents have been associated with hemolytic uremic syndrome with case reports of resolution upon conversion to the other drug. If it is necessary to convert a patient from one drug to the other, this is best accomplished by discontinuing one and starting the other at the next dose. They should not be overlapped. There is no absolute indication for choosing either calcineurin inhibitor over the other. The use of tacrolimus in children and women offers the advantage of avoidance of the cosmetic side effects of CsA, such as gum hypertrophy and hirsutism, thus potentially influencing the issue of noncompliance.

RAPAMYCIN

Multicenter, randomized controlled trials have been conducted in the US and Europe to examine the efficacy of rapamycin. Results from the phase II European study investigating the efficacy of Rapamycin vs CsA in a triple therapy regimen with AZA and prednisone showed no difference in acute rejection rate, or graft or patient survival at 12 months. Preliminary results from the US phase III trial were presented at the World Congress of Transplantation in Montreal. In this study patients received Rapamycin or AZA in conjunction with CsA and prednisone. At six months Rapamycin significantly reduced the incidence of acute rejection episodes. Hyperlipidemia was found to be a significant side effect, however, this responded to dose reduction. Interestingly, in the European trial a significant number of patients treated with Rapamycin complained of arthralgias. Rapamycin was approved for use in the US during the fourth quarter of 1999. Its ultimate role in kidney transplantation will be determined by phase IV and single-center studies.

DOUBLE VS TRIPLE THERAPY

This issue classically refers to the regimen containing CsA and one additional agent, usually prednisone, compared to CsA, prednisone and AZA. No single study has demonstrated an advantage of triple therapy over double therapy as defined in this sense, with respect to patient or graft survival, the number of rejection episodes, or to infection. It remains to be seen whether triple therapy with a combination of some of the newer agents and CsA will be more efficacious than currently used immunosuppression regimens. Indeed, it may be possible to eliminate or greatly reduce the use of CsA after transplantation. The rapamycin study (discussed above) examined a regimen that could prove to be a useful alternative to CsA-based immunosuppression. Similarly, other studies have explored the potential role of tacrolimus in replacing CsA. For example, prospective and retrospective studies have shown the feasibility of eliminating CsA from prophylactic immunosuppression regimens. A randomized prospective and a retrospective study comparing tacrolimus and prednisone with tacrolimus, MMF and prednisone have been conducted,

further highlighting the need for clarification when using the terms double and triple therapy. Both studies failed to demonstrate a difference in 1-year patient or graft survival; however, there was a statistically significant reduction in the number of rejection episodes in those patients who received the triple drug protocol. The results differed between the studies on the impact of increased immunosuppression on infection, with the latter demonstrating a significant increase in both CMV viremia and invasive CMV in the tacrolimus-MMF group, while the prospective study demonstrated no such increase.

THE ELDERLY

The elderly transplant patient (>60 years) is regarded as having decreased immune responsiveness with a lower incidence of rejection episodes, and an increased likelihood of death with a functioning graft. Immunosuppressive protocols are not well-established in this group and often are not specifically modified for the decreased immunological risk. Several small studies have been conducted looking at various regimens, including studies with either induction therapy or tacrolimus, with no overall difference in patient or graft survival demonstrated. The elderly deserve special consideration when developing new protocols, since greater degrees of immunosuppression in this group may put them at increased risk of opportunistic infections and neoplasms.

PREGNANCY

There are few data on the management of the pregnant transplant recipient. It is generally advised that the patient wait 18 months to two years posttransplantation before considering pregnancy. At this point they should be on a stable maintenance regimen, and once pregnant should remain at prepregnancy doses unless side effects occur. There are several reports that show that alterations in the level of CsA may occur during pregnancy due to physiological or metabolic changes. In addition, a significant percentage of recipients with reported graft dysfunction during pregnancy had either decreased or discontinued CsA. Thus, close monitoring and appropriate adjustment of CsA dosage is required during pregnancy. Neoral® that has less inter-patient and intra-patient variability and may prove to be easier to manage during pregnancy. However, if a patient is switched to Neoral®, she should be well established and on a stable dose before becoming pregnant. Switching preparations is not recommended during pregnancy or within three months postpartum. The epidemiological data available to date on AZA-based regimens is favorable, despite the fact that there is evidence of risk to the human fetus. Relatively little information is available regarding the safety of some of the newer immunosuppressive agents.

Several centers have reported successful pregnancies in both liver and renal recipients on tacrolimus-based therapy.

INFECTION AND NEOPLASMS

When a neoplasm or severe infection develops in a renal transplant patient, consideration should be given to reducing the dose of immunosuppressive drugs. There are no universally agreed upon protocols for the adjustment of immunosuppression in these patients. Fortunately, in renal transplantation the decision to withdraw immunosuppressive drugs is an option, since an alternative replacement therapy in the form of dialysis is available. For example, in the case of Kaposi's sarcoma or lymphoma, both of which are caused by viruses, the first line treatment is the reduction or cessation of immunosuppression, with or without the use of adjunct therapy, depending on the severity at presentation. Usually if the patient is on CsA and an antiproliferative agent, one agent will be stopped while the other is reduced initially. Further adjustment will be determined by the response. There have been many case reports of total regression of these neoplasms upon reduction or withdrawal of immunosuppressive therapy. For severe infections and bowel perforation a similar approach is adopted. Immunosuppression should be reduced or eliminated since the risk of rejection appears low in most patients in whom severe infection is present, and the mortality rate is extremely high. In the case of CMV or other viral illnesses with an associated leukopenia, the discontinuation of MMF or AZA is an obvious first option, since these agents may further aggravate the decreasing white cell count.

SUMMARY

Larger multicenter prospective trials are required to fully evaluate the pros and cons of the different potential regimens, in particular, the ability of a particular regimen to effect the incidence of acute or chronic rejection, its impact on patient and graft survival, while also considering the effect on the rate of infections, neoplasms, cardiovascular risk factors and other side effects. With 1-year graft survivals at an all time high it is going to be increasingly difficult to demonstrate benefits between different immunosuppressive regimens. The protocols that will be used in the future will be determined by alternative endpoints such as long-term graft survival, and will have to take into consideration the morbidity associated with increased immunosuppression. The development of new immunosuppressive agents afford us the opportunity to consider what can be withdrawn rather than simply increasing the cumulative dose of immunosuppression. Studies are currently being conducted to better understand which immunosuppressive agents can safely be withdrawn, and what combination of agents have the highest long-term, benefit-to-risk ratio.

RECOMMENDED READING

Hricik DE, Almawi WY, Strom TB. Trends in the use of glucocorticoids in renal transplantation. Transplantation. 1994;57(7):979-989.

Helderman JH, Van Buren DH, Amend WJ, Pirsch JD. Chronic immunosuppression of the renal transplant recipient. J Am Soc Nephrol. 1994;4(8 Suppl):S2-S9

Halloran P, Mathew T, Tomlanovich S, Groth C, Hooftman L, Baker C. Mycophenolate mofetil in renal allograft recipient: a pooled efficacy analysis of three randomized, double-blind, clinical studies in prevention of rejection. Transplantation. 1997;63(1):39-47.

Mathew TH. A blinded, long-term, randomized multicenter study of mycophenolate in cadaveric renal transplantation: results at three years. Transplantation. 1998;65(11):1450-1454.

Sanders CE, Curtis JJ, Julian BA, et al. Tapering or discontinuing cyclosporine for financial reasons — a single-center experience. Am J Kidney Dis. 1993;21(1):9-15.

First MR, Schroeder TJ, Michael A, Hariharan S, Weiskittel P, Alexander JW. Cyclosporine-Ketoconazole interaction. Long-term follow-up and preliminary results of a randomized trial. Transplantation. 1993;55(5):1000-1004.

Laskow DA, Neylan JF 3rd, Shapiro RS, Pirsch JD, Vergne-Marini PJ, Tomlanovich SJ. The role of tacrolimus in adult kidney transplantation: a review. Clin Transplant. 1998;12(6):489-503.

61 EXPECTED CLINICAL OUTCOMES – RISK FACTORS IN KIDNEY TRANSPLANTATION

Arthur J. Matas, MD

Many approaches are possible when analyzing transplant outcome. Each gives a different perspective. When studying patient survival, one can compare the survival of transplant recipients vs the expected survival in the age-matched general population; within the group of transplant recipients, one can also compare outcome for those with vs without different risk factors. From a patient perspective, the most important comparison is to a matched group of individuals with end-stage renal disease who are not undergoing a transplant. Not surprisingly, many risk factors for decreased posttransplant survival rates (eg, older age) are also risk factors for decreased survival rates in the general population or in the matched group with renal failure not undergoing a transplant.

Early nonrandomized studies suggested that patients undergoing transplantation survive longer than those maintained on dialysis. However, a major criticism of those studies was that patient selection for transplantation may explain the results (ie, the sicker patients would have been left on dialysis). More recently, Port et al compared survival for patients accepted for transplantation and transplanted vs those accepted for transplantation but still on the waiting list vs those never accepted for transplantation (most never having been referred) and remaining on dialysis. Overall, those accepted for transplantation had better survival than those staying on dialysis (suggesting that the transplant population truly is a selected population). But, those who had undergone transplantation have significantly better survival than those accepted but still on the waiting list, suggesting transplantation does provide an advantage.

When studying graft survival, one can compare survival between groups of recipients (eg, diabetic vs nondiabetic) or study variables affecting individual subgroups (eg, donor source, immunosuppressive protocol). Not adequately emphasized is that some factors affecting survival can be changed (eg, allocation algorithm, immunosuppressive protocol) whereas others are fixed for any given recipient (eg, age).

Finally, what should be the "gold standard" for measuring of outcome? Most transplant and dialysis studies measure patient and graft survival. Yet, mere survival without adequate quality of life should not be considered an acceptable outcome. Numerous studies have now demonstrated improved quality of life with successful transplantation (vs dialysis).

EXPECTED CLINICAL OUTCOMES

With improvement in immunosuppressive protocols and in overall care of transplant recipients, both short-term and long-term graft survival rates have steadily improved. Figure 61-1 shows actuarial graft survival, by decade, for living and cadaver donor transplants at the University of Minnesota. Each decade brought a stepwise improvement in survival. National data is shown in Figure 61-2. Between January 1, 1991 and December 31, 1997, a total of 70,549 kidney transplants were reported to the UNOS Scientific Renal Transplant Registry. Living donor kidney recipients had significantly higher patient and graft survival rates than cadaver kidney recipients ($P<.001$). After five years, a 14% difference in graft survival rates was seen between these two groups. Importantly, about half of the difference could be explained by better patient survival rates.

In both Figure 61-1 and 61-2, as in many transplant studies, graft survival was calculated with death with a functioning graft considered a transplant failure. This approach made sense when a significant proportion of deaths was related to immunosuppressive complications. More recently, older patients are increasingly having transplants, and death often occurs from causes completely unrelated to the transplant. If death with function is considered a graft loss in survival analyses, both deaths related to the transplant and deaths due to other causes in the aging patient population will be included. Using current data, Gjertson has calculated that most deaths in the first three posttransplant years are not transplant-related and that after five years, only 25%, 15%, 10%, and 6% of deaths among patients who were 30, 42, 54, and 66 years old, respectively, should be regarded as treatment failures. Calculating graft survival while censoring for death with a functioning graft provides a better estimate of immunologic graft loss.

FACTORS AFFECTING OUTCOME

One can conceptualize a graph of renal function in transplant recipients plotting serum creatinine (Cr) (or 1/Cr) vs time. Long-term outcome can be affected by the initial Cr (axis) or the slope of the curve. There are two major theories as to factors affecting slope. The first holds that immunologic factors predominate, that chronic deterioration of graft function is only seen in those recipients with previous acute rejection episodes. The second theory holds that limited nephron mass, that may be present at the time of the transplant

Professor of Surgery, Department of Surgery, University of Minnesota Medical School, Minneapolis, MN

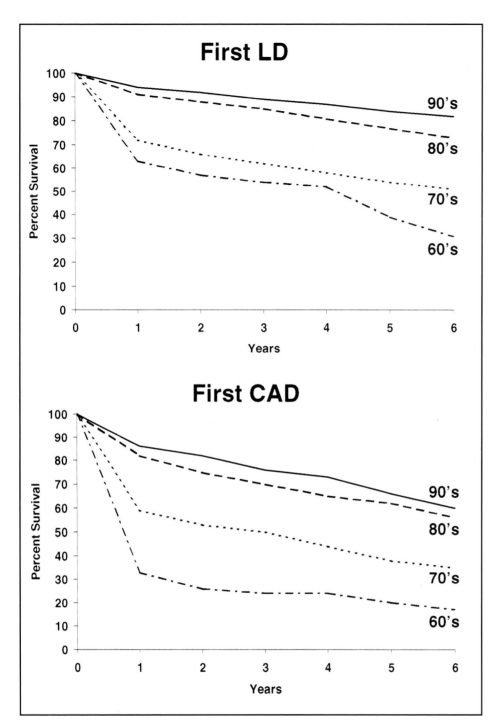

Figure 61-1 Actuarial graft survival by decade at the University of Minnesota for living (a) and cadaver (b) donor transplants. There is an incremental improvement in each decade.

(eg, with older donors), or that may occur after the transplant (immunologic destruction), leads to hyperfiltration of the remaining nephrons; this hyperfiltration then results in further damage to the kidney.

Numerous variables have been noted, in univariate or multivariate analyses, to have an impact on short-term and long-term outcome. Most multivariate analyses consider these variables together and discuss their relative importance. Yet for any one recipient, some variables are fixed (eg, sex, age, race, original disease) whereas others can be changed (eg, donor source, immunosuppressive protocol).

Fixed Variables

Recipient age and donor age have each been shown to affect graft survival. Both young and old recipients have worse survival (vs those 18 to 50 years old); pathogenesis differs. For pediatric recipients, decreased graft survival is due to an increased immune responsiveness, the resultant increased rejection rate, and, in part, to the relatively high rate of noncompliance seen in children and adoles-

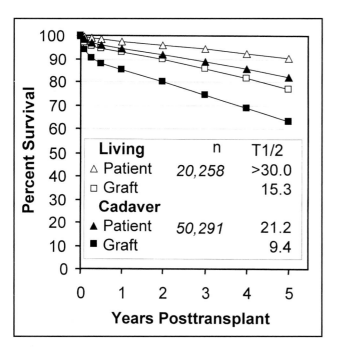

Figure 61-2 Patient and graft survival for 70,549 kidney transplants reported to the UNOS Scientific Renal Transplant Registry. Reprinted with permission from Cecka JM. The UNOS Scientific Renal Transplant Registry. In: Cecka JM, Terasaki PI, eds. Clinical Transplants, 1998. Los Angeles, CA: The Regents of the University of California, UCLA Tissue Typing Laboratory; 1999; 1-16.

cents. Decreased graft survival in older recipients is due to patient death. Older recipients have less rejection; calculation of death-censored graft survival reveals no difference in graft survival rates between recipients older than 60 vs those 18 to 60.

Increased donor age has a marked impact in cadaver transplantation. In the UNOS registry, 5-year graft survival for recipients with donors 19 to 30 years old was 68%; with donors age 46 to 50, 55%; and with donors over 60, 44% (*P*<.001). Avoiding older cadaver donors would alleviate this problem, but is impractical given the tremendous organ shortage. For living-donor recipients, donor age has less of an impact, perhaps due to better opportunities to evaluate donors and to minimize preservation time.

The interaction of preservation time and donor age is important in cadaver transplantation. Recipients of kidneys from older donors are more likely to have delayed graft function (DGF) posttransplant. And, as preservation time increases, so does the likelihood of developing DGF, especially for recipients with older (vs younger) donors.

Both donor and recipient race affect outcome. Recipients of donor kidneys from whites (vs African-American or Asian donors) have better outcome. This difference may be due to greater nephron mass in white donors or to a higher incidence of underlying disease (eg, hypertension) in other donors. African-American

(vs white) recipient race has been associated with worse outcome. Asian recipient race has been associated with better outcome.

Primary renal disease has an important impact. Some diseases recur posttransplant (FSGS, HUS); others are associated with significant comorbidity that affects patient survival (Type I and Type II diabetes). It has been found that for patients with diabetes, extensive pretransplant evaluation and intervention, when indicated, improves posttransplant survival.

Mutable Variables

The variable most amenable to change is donor source. As shown in Figures 61-1 and 61-2, short-term and long-term patient and graft survival rates are better for recipients with living (vs cadaver) donors. A major change in recent years is the increased acceptance of living unrelated donors. Accumulated data clearly shows that survival for recipients with unrelated donors is similar to that for recipients with non-HLA-identical living donors (Figure 61-3). Only HLA-identical recipients do better. The excellent survival seen with living unrelated donors is not due to HLA matching (most are a poor HLA match), but it is likely due to the combination of donor selection, optimal timing (elective surgery when donor and recipient are in the best shape), and a minimal ischemia time, all of which lead to immediate graft function in most cases. In fact, outcome for the subset of cadaver kidney recipients with young donors, minimal ischemia time, and immediate graft function, is

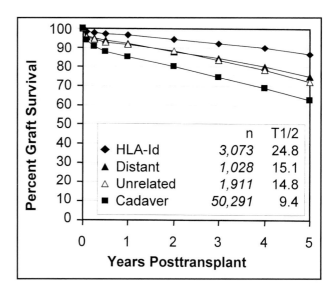

Figure 61-3 Graft survival by donor source for transplants reported to the UNOS Scientific Renal Transplant Registry. Living unrelated transplant recipients have survival equal to non-HLA-identical related recipients. Reprinted with permission from Cecka JM. The UNOS Scientific Renal Transplant Registry. Cecka JM, Terasaki PI, eds. Clinical Transplants, 1998. Los Angeles, Ca: The Regents of the University of California, UCLA Tissue Typing Laboratory; 1999;1-16.

similar to outcome for non-HLA-identical living donor recipients.

One of the most important variables is the transplant center. For recipients transplanted between January 1, 1991, and December 31, 1995, center-specific 1-year graft survival varied by 20%. Part of the difference may be recipient demographics and patient selection. However, when the data is stratified for other risk factors, center effect remains significant.

In the University of Minnesota series, the major risk factor for decreased graft survival is an acute rejection episode. Recipients who have a late rejection episode (>6 months posttransplant) and recipients who have multiple acute rejection episodes are at markedly increased risk. Of note, their grafts are not ultimately lost to the acute rejection episode itself but rather to the subsequent development of chronic rejection. In the absence of acute rejection, chronic rejection is rare. Acute rejection may be a common underlying risk factor for many previously identified variables shown to be risks for decreased graft survival in both univariate and multivariate analyses. Importantly, many of these analyses study variables present at the time of transplant or during the transplant admission and do not control for subsequent development of at least one or more acute rejection episodes. For example, DGF has been shown to be a risk factor for poorer long-term outcome. There may be an increased risk of acute rejection for recipients with DGF; however, for recipients with DGF and without acute rejection, graft survival is not decreased. Similarly, African-American recipients have worse outcomes, but when controlled for rejection there is no difference between African-Americans and non-African-Americans.

For both living and cadaver donors, HLA match has an effect on outcome. Recipients with HLA-identical living donors have better long-term outcome than do recipients with mismatched living donors. However, there is little difference in outcome between other subgroups (or between living unrelated vs related but mismatched recipients). Similarly, zero-mismatch cadaver recipients have excellent long-term survival (comparable to those with living donors). But there are only small differences in outcome between grades of mismatch. In theory, transplant outcome would improve by decreasing the average HLA mismatch. But doing so would require more transportation of kidneys from one area of the country to another and a resultant increase in preservation time. The penalty would be increased DGF, which must be balanced against the potential benefit of better matching.

One factor that is difficult to quantitate is noncompliance. Numerous studies have demonstrated a correlation between noncompliance and an increased rate of acute rejection, chronic rejection, and graft loss. Commonly, only complete cessation of drugs by a patient is recognized and reported in studies. Incomplete cessation of drugs most probably also plays an important role in chronic graft loss.

As described above, the preservation time of cadaver kidneys has an impact on outcome via an association with DGF. Shortening preservation time (especially when using older donor kidneys) will decrease DGF and improve outcome.

The immunosuppressive protocol plays a major role, especially in the first year posttransplant. Patient and graft survival rates have improved dramatically since the introduction of calcineurin inhibitors. Other new agents for induction (monoclonal and polyclonal antibodies) and maintenance immunosuppression will likely result in further improvements in long-term outcome. Currently, numerous combinations of immunosuppressive agents are possible. Randomized, prospective studies are needed to determine which combination is best for each recipient subgroup.

More recently, posttransplant blood pressure has been described as a significant risk indicator for death-censored graft survival. When controlled for rejection episodes and graft function, elevated blood pressure posttransplant was associated with worse outcome. In addition, active smoking has been shown to be detrimental to outcome; whether this is just an effect on mortality or whether other factors are also involved is controversial.

Multivariate Analysis

Gjertson, using the UNOS database, analyzed the percent of variability in outcome between groups that could be attributed to specific risk indicators excluding rejection episodes and noncompliance. More than 50% of the variability in short-term (1-year) survival was due to factors that can be controlled. Fixed variables affecting long-term outcome cannot be altered (Table 61-1). It would be important to repeat these analyses looking at the relative impact of rejection and noncompliance.

CONCLUSION

Incremental improvements have occurred in outcome (patient and graft survival) for kidney transplant recipients. Numerous risk factors have been identified that significantly affect outcome. Although some are fixed for any one recipient, others can be optimized. Future studies need to address transplant-related morbidity and quality of life, along with further efforts to improve patient and graft survival.

ACKNOWLEDGMENTS

I would like to thank Mary Knatterud for editorial assistance and Stephanie Daily for preparation of the manuscript.

Table 61-1. Total Assignable Variation (%) in Graft Survival, by Variable		
	Variables Affecting 1-Year Survival	Variables affecting long-term graft survival (for those with 1-year survival)
Transplant center	21%	16%
Drug regimen	20%	–
Donor relationship	15%	3%
Donor age	7%	31%
Donor cause of death	6%	5%
Recipient race	5%	20%
Transplant year	4%	—
Recipient age	3%	4%
Dialysis time	3%	—
CMV status	2%	1%
Donor race	2%	1%
Recipient sex	2%	7%
PRA	1%	—
HLA – A, B, DR	1%	3%
Donor sex	1%	—
Medical status	—	2%
Original disease	—	2%

RECOMMENDED READING

Port FK, Wolfe RA, Mauger EA, Berling DP, Jiang K. Comparison of survival probabilities for dialysis patients vs cadaveric renal transplant recipients. JAMA. 1993;270(11):1339-1343.

Cecka JM. The UNOS Scientific Renal Transplant Registry. Cecka JM, Terasaki PI, eds. Clinical Transplants, 1998. Los Angeles, Ca: UCLA Tissue Typing Laboratory; 1999: 1-16.

Gjertson DW. The role of death in kidney graft failure. In Cecka JM, Terasaki PI, eds. Clinical Transplants, 1998. Los Angeles, Ca: UCLA Tissue Typing Laboratory; 1999: 399-412.

Kasiske BL. Clinical correlates to chronic renal allograft rejection. Kidney Int. 1997;63:S71-S74.

Matas AJ. Risk factors for chronic rejection – a clinical perspective. Transpl Immunol. 1998;6(1):1-11.

Kerr SR, Gillingham KJ, Johnson EM, Matas AJ. Living donors >55 years: to use or not to use? Transplantation. 1999;67(7):999-1004.

Matas AJ. Noncompliance and late graft loss: implications for long-term clinical studies. Transplant Rev. 1999;13:78-82.

Opelz G, Wujciak T, Ritz E. Association of chronic kidney graft failure with recipients' blood pressure. Collaborative Transplant Study. Kidney Int. 1998;53(1):217-222.

62 SPECIAL CONSIDERATIONS IN PEDIATRIC KIDNEY TRANSPLANTATION

Amir H. Tejani, MD

All modalities of dialytic replacement therapy are inadequate for the needs of the growing child. Both peritoneal dialysis, delivered either as continuous ambulatory peritoneal dialysis or continuous cycling peritoneal dialysis, and hemodialysis lead to a deceleration of growth. Data from the dialysis component of the North American Pediatric Renal Transplant Cooperative Study (NAPRTCS) registry show that during dialysis the overall height deficit (-1.8 standard deviation [SD]) becomes more negative (-2.16 SD) at 24 months. Additionally, dialysis dependency induces loss of self-esteem and emotional maladjustment in children. Transplantation permits the child to attend regular school, and studies have demonstrated that, following transplantation, cognitive functioning measured by standardized tests such as the Wide Range Achievement Test and the Test of Nonverbal Intelligence show marked improvement. A functioning transplant is, therefore, the optimal replacement therapy for end-stage renal disease in children.

INCIDENCE AND FREQUENCY OF TRANSPLANTATION

Donor Source

The NAPRTCS has recorded about 500 pediatric transplants each year since 1987. This accounts for 80% of all pediatric transplants performed in North America. Whereas living donors (LD) accounted for only 28% of all transplants done in the US in 1997, the rate of living-related transplants in the pediatric population is much higher. In 1987, only 40% of all transplants performed in children were from a LD source; by 1991, LD source kidneys accounted for 53% of all transplants and for the last seven years LDs account for at least 50% of all pediatric renal transplants. Parents comprise 85% of donors, and the parental contribution is 56% maternal to 44% paternal. There is no outcome advantage between the parental donation in our registry, though it has been suggested that maternal donation may have a slight decreased number of rejections in very young infants. 1- or 2-haploidentical sibling transplants are rare in children because the siblings of children requiring a trans-

Professor of Pediatrics and Surgery, New York Medical College, Valhalla, NY

plant are frequently minors and unable to donate. We have recorded only 182 sibling donors and 42 unrelated donors. Only 10 LDs were under 18; of these, nine were transplants between siblings, and one was between a parent and a child. Young donors are rarely used for cadaveric donor (CD) transplants in pediatrics, with only 56 recovered from a child under two and 12% being from donors ages two to five. NAPRTCS' studies have shown that the outcome of CD kidneys recovered from donors under ten years is inferior to that of older donors. It is noteworthy that only 26% of all CDs are under the age of ten and that the use of young donors has progressively declined. From 1987 to 1990, 59% to 68% of CD kidneys were recovered from donors over ten, whereas for the years 1991 to 1995, this figure rose to 78% to 88%. Coincidentally, infants (<2 years) represented 3.5% of all CDs for 1987 to 1990, however the use of infant CD kidneys ceased by 1996. These changes in practice patterns have occurred as a result of widespread dissemination of data showing that the preferential placement of infantile CD kidneys into infant recipients is extremely deleterious to patient and graft survival. Given the nonhomogeneous US population, 30% of CD transplant recipients are mismatched with their donor at both the B and DR loci, and 36% have either a B or a DR mismatch. Similarly, a 6-antigen match among pediatric kidney recipients is rarely seen (76/2457). This is unfortunate since recent analysis has shown that the long-term outcome of 6-antigen-matched CD transplants is better than an LD 1-haplotype parental transplant.

Recipient Characteristics

Overall, Caucasian children account for 64% of all recipients in the pediatric age range, however there is a significant variation in the racial make-up of transplanted children when reviewed by diagnostic category. Sixty transplants were performed in children under the age of 12 months, and 222 were performed in patients between the ages of 12 to 24 months. Approximately 200 total transplants have been recorded in the NAPRTCS registry for the three, four and five year-olds. Children under the age of six, whose graft outcome continues to remain poor, constitute about 21% of all transplants in the pediatric age group. Similar figures for total transplants for children in the age range ten to 13 are about 300 for each age year, and 400 for children 15 to 17. Table 62-1 depicts the frequency of transplantation, the donor source and the age groupings over the ten years from 1987 through 1996.

Diagnosis

A major focus of effort in pediatric transplantation has been to identify the disease processes that lead to end-stage status in the anticipation of intervention. Three major disorders, renal aplasia/hypoplasia, obstructive uropathy, and focal segmental glomerulosclerosis (FSGS), account for over 2,000 patients who have received a renal allograft in the pediatric age range. Whereas developmental defects of the kidney are currently not amenable to therapy, the nephrotic syndrome caused by FSGS has in recent years been treated effectively; however, the number of children undergoing a renal transplantation for FSGS has remained constant at between 40 and 50 each year since 1987. The causes of end-stage renal disease vary according to the racial background. For developmental disorders, Caucasian children constitute 68% of all transplants, however for FSGS they form only 50% of the patients. For certain rare disorders, such as hemolytic uremic syndrome, oxalosis, and cystinosis, Caucasian children account for 80% to 90% of all transplants, and for diseases such as lupus nephritis almost 50% of the recipients of a kidney are African-American. Renal disorders that account for large numbers of transplants among adult patients, such as diabetes, are a rare cause for pediatric transplantation (five of almost 5,000 patients); similarly, membranous nephropathy and IgA nephropathy are rare. A detailed description of diseases that lead to transplantation in the pediatric age range is shown in Table 62-2.

INDICATIONS FOR TRANSPLANTATION AND PREEMPTIVE TRANSPLANTATION

Good patient care has resulted in evaluation guidelines for prospective recipients in adult transplant programs; similar guidelines for donation to children are in the process of being formulated. In pediatrics, almost all children reaching ESRD are considered candidates for transplantation. Initiation of dialysis is generally carried out in children at creatinine clearances of 10 to 15 mL/min per

1.73 meters^2. A crucial management difference between adults and children is the institution of preemptive CD transplantation in pediatric centers. In a review of 4,329 children transplanted from 1987 through 1996, the NAPRTCS noted that 1,064 (25%) had never received maintenance dialysis. The primary reason for preemptive transplantation is parental desire to avoid dialysis (35%); a secondary reason is attributed to the recommendation by the nephrologist (20%). When outcome is reviewed, patients transplanted preemptively have similar graft survival at one and four years, compared to patients who undergo dialysis, and the incidence of noncompliance is no higher among children who have never received dialysis. Since the publication of data showing that preemptive transplantation does not confer a disadvantage, the use of this modality has increased and currently there are over 1,400 pediatric transplant recipients who have never undergone maintenance dialysis. Thirty-four percent of LD pediatric recipients have a preemptive transplant, and because the UNOS guidelines for allocation favor children, 14% of CD recipients are also transplanted prior to the need for dialysis. Transplantation without dialysis is observed more often among Caucasian patients (30%), vs 15% for other races, however the rates of preemptive transplantation are 20%, 26%, 29%, 22%, and 19% for recipients zero to one, two to five, six to 12, 13 to 17, and 18 to 20 years, respectively.

There are almost no absolute contraindications for transplantation in children, except in situations where a child is harboring active infection or undergoing chemotherapy. The concern of further immunosuppressing an already compromised host makes human immunodeficiency virus (HIV) a relative contraindication, however there is a considerable debate regarding this issue, now that a significant number of HIV-infected patients survive for prolonged periods. Another relative

Table 62-1. Patient Registrations, Transplants, and Selected Characteristics, by Year of Registration

	1987	1988	1989	1990	1991	1992	1993	1994	1995	1996	Total
Patients Registered	530	495	459	490	495	537	557	505	545	285	4898
% Male	60.9	61.6	59.7	60	59.2	57.4	56.6	60.2	62.2	63.5	59.9
% White	72.5	66.3	62.3	65.5	66.3	63.7	61	58	60.7	60	63.8
Number of Transplants	541	523	499	542	559	592	602	578	596	330	5362
% Living Donors	43.4	40.3	46.1	41.3	53.3	49.5	52	44.8	51.5	53.6	47.5
% Age Distribution (at index transplant)											
0 - 1	6.2	6.5	7.4	4.3	5.5	6.3	7.5	4.4	3.7	3.9	5.7
2 - 5	18.7	14.9	15.9	16.7	17.2	14.9	16.3	11.1	12.8	18.9	15.6
6 - 12	35.3	37.4	38.1	38	38	33.5	31.6	30.9	29	31.9	34.3
13 - 17	39.8	41.2	38.6	41	39.4	36.1	35.2	41	42.9	37.5	39.3
18 - 20	0	0	0	0	0	9.1	9.3	12.7	11.6	7.7	5.1

contraindication is a preexisting malignancy, though the pediatric registry records 26 children with Wilm's tumor who have received a kidney transplant without recurrence. Patients with preexisting metastatic disease and those with neurological dysfunction are also unsuitable transplant candidates. In recent years there has been significant improvement in the management of infants (<2 years) on dialysis, and a CD transplant before the end of the second year may not be advisable since the graft survival in these infants is uniformly poor. Experience in over 600 patients with FSGS who have received a transplant has resulted in data that is beginning to indicate that LD transplantation in this disease has a higher rate of recurrence compared to CD transplantation. Oxalosis, which once was considered an absolute contraindication because of its high rate of recurrence, can be treated successfully with combined liver and kidney transplants.

PRETRANSPLANT PREPARATION
Recipient Preparation

Two areas are of major concern – eradication of the uremic milieu, which is common to all patients with chronic renal insufficiency, and additional preparation for patients with urologic abnormalities. Uremia leads to the development of anemia, protein/calorie malnutrition, and growth retardation. Correction of the anemia is carried out by early initiation of erythropoietin therapy. The use of recombinant human growth hormone prior to transplantation has significantly improved the height standard deviation deficit of these children. In patients with congenital nephrotic syndrome, additional prophylactic native nephrectomy may be required to control the urinary protein losses. A suggested standard preparation of pediatric transplant candidates is shown in Table 62-3.

It has been shown that almost 30% of children undergoing a renal transplant have urologic abnormalities, ie, posterior urethral valves, neurogenic bladder, prune belly syndrome, vesicoureteral reflux, outflow obstruction, or bladder extrophy. Prior to transplantation, measurement of urinary flow and ultrasound estimation of post-micturition urine volume are essential. For successful transplantation, urine flow should be at least 15 mL/second and the residual volume should not exceed 30 mL. To adequately evaluate the urinary bladder in patients suspected of urethral stricture, a voiding

Table 62-2. Sex and Race by Primary Renal Diagnosis

Diagnosis	N (4898)	% Male (60)	% White (64)
Obstructive uropathy	804	87	69
Aplastic/hypoplastic/dysplastic kidneys	783	61	67
Focal segmental glomerulosclerosis	582	59	51
Reflux nephropathy	274	45	73
Systemic immunologic disease	232	31	53
Chronic glomerulonephritis	206	38	46
Syndrome of agenesis of abdominal musculature	138	97	64
Congenital nephrotic syndrome	132	51	67
Polycystic kidney disease	131	50	76
Medullary cystic disease/juvenile nephronophthisis	131	51	83
Familial nephritis	116	79	61
Pyelo/interstitial nephritis	112	48	73
Cystinosis	111	50	88
Membranoproliferative glomerulonephritis Type I	111	47	56
Renal infarct	87	53	80
Idiopathic crescentic glomerulonephritis	84	36	62
Membranoproliferative glomerulonephritis Type II	47	47	74
Oxalosis	33	61	85
Wilms tumor	30	50	83
Membranous nephropathy	27	70	59
Drash syndrome	27	52	67
Sickle Cell nephropathy	9	56	0
Diabetic glomerulonephritis	5	40	20
Other	326	56	61
Unknown	235	52	37

Table 62-3. Pretransplant Work-Up Pediatric Candidates	
History & Physical Exam	

Blood Tests
   Hematology
   Coagulation
   Chemistry
	CBC w/Platelets & Differential
	PT, PTT, TT
	Electrolytes
	BUN, Creatinine
	Liver Function Tests
	Lipid Profile

Virology	Titers for CMV, EBV, VZV, MMR
Blood Bank/Immunology	ABO & HLA Typing Antileukocyte Antibody Screening Hepatitis Profile HIV
Urine Tests	Urinalysis C & S 24-hour Protein
X-Ray	Voiding Cystourethrogram Chest X-ray Bone Age
Vaccines, etc.	Hepatitis B Pneumococcus Varivax PPD
Consults	Social Worker Nutritionist

cystometrogram and a urethrocystoscopy are essential. When additional information regarding bladder capacity, pressure rise and the efficiency of voiding are necessary, urodynamic studies with radioisotope imaging should be done.

Most pediatric patients with urologic anomalies will have a urinary bladder that will adapt to the new kidney, particularly if the bladder wall is compliant and the bladder is distensible.

Criteria for a usable bladder are an end-filling pressure of less than 30 cm of water and a good flow rate. In those rare patients with low bladder capacity or high pressures, bladder augmentation prior to transplantation may be necessary. Augmentation cystoplasty, which is adding bowel or gastric wall to the bladder, is preferred to substitution cystoplasty, which consists of excision of most of the bladder and replacement with bowel. Gastric remnants have been popular for augmentation, however the loss of excessive amounts of gastric acid in the urine will lead to repeated episodes of metabolic alkalosis.

Presensitization

In children, the major cause of high sensitization (>50%) is a previous failed graft, particularly when the graft failure occurred in the first three months posttransplant. Additional factors include blood transfusions, viral infections and autoimmune disorders such as lupus nephritis. Since 10% of all transplants in children are secondary, presensitization is emerging as a barrier in this subset of patients who not only have difficulty obtaining an allograft because of a positive crossmatch against the donor, but also have a high incidence of acute irreversible rejection. Currently, a study is underway to determine if administration of intravenous gamma globulin can effectively decrease the level of the panel reactive antibody in children with levels higher than 50%, and thus enable them to undergo a successful transplant.

Donor Evaluation

LIVING DONORS. From 1987 through 1990, 42% of pediatric transplants were from a living donor. In this decade there has been a steady increase in the percentage of LD transplants, so that in 1996 and 1997, 54% were from an LD source. Hence, careful evaluation of the donor is essential. Candidates with systemic disease, such as diabetes and established hypertension requiring substantial therapy, are not potential donors. Prospective donors are tested for ABO compatibility and for a negative lymphocytotoxic crossmatch with recipient sera. Transplantation across the ABO barrier is rare in children, however it has been shown that such transplants involving recipients whose anti-A titer is low do have excellent graft survival. The work-up of a potential LD for a pediatric transplant is similar to that done in adults, however because of the emotional attachment of the care giving physician to the child it is imperative that the evaluation of the donor be done by an independent physician not involved in the transplant process

CADAVER DONORS. Donor age and organ ischemia are critical issues in pediatric transplantation. Strong input from the nephrologist involved in the care of the potential recipient is necessary regarding acceptance of a given kidney. For a number of years it was standard practice to transplant kidneys recovered from young donors into young recipients with disastrous consequences for graft survival. Studies from the NAPRTCS forced a change in this allocation system with dramatic improvement in graft survival. Kidneys recovered from donors up to two years old must not be used for pediatric transplantation; the ideal donor for a pediatric recipient is an adult 20 to 40 years old. Cold ischemia times greater than 24 hours lead to delayed graft function (DGF) which increases the risk of graft failure threefold.

TECHNICAL PROBLEMS IN PEDIATRIC TRANSPLANTATION

Whereas the surgical techniques used in children with body weight of 15 kg or more is identical to that in adult patients, the operative technique for young infants requires a midline incision and the use of the recipient aorta and inferior vena cava for anastomosis with the donor kidney vessels. After reflection of the cecum and the right colon, the anterior wall of the aorta and the inferior vena cava are exposed and dissected. The aorta is mobilized from above the inferior mesenteric artery to the external iliac artery on the right side. The cava is mobilized from the left renal vein to the iliac veins. An end-to-side anastomosis of the donor renal vein to the cava is carried out, followed by an end-to-side anastomosis of the donor renal artery to the recipient aorta. Careful monitoring of the recipient's hemodynamics is necessary and a central venous pressure of 15 to 18 cm of water must be maintained prior to unclamping of the major vessels. A large adult (parental) kidney placed in an infant will take up a significant portion of the infant's normal blood volume. To preclude vascular compromise upon unclamping the vessels, volume replacement is critical and will also protect against vascular thrombosis.

The ureteral anastomosis is done by implanting the donor ureter into the recipient's bladder. The technique is generally a modified Leadbetter-Politano procedure. Upon completion of the ureteric anastomosis and release of vascular clamps, immediate function of the transplanted kidney is manifested by the production of urine.

DIAGNOSIS AND TREATMENT OF RENAL DYSFUNCTION

Failure of immediate urine production may be due to a variety of factors and the differential diagnosis of immediate nonfunction is a critical component of the transplant physician's role.

Acute Tubular Necrosis

Delayed graft function due to acute tubular necrosis (ATN) is observed in 5% of LD and 19% of CD transplants in children. Risk factors for DGF in LD kidneys are repeat transplant and the use of frequent (>5) random transfusions. For CD kidneys, additional risk factors are prolonged cold ischemia (>24 hours), and the absence of T cell induction therapy. Diagnosis is confirmed in most cases by radionuclide scan, however, in cases where the DGF is prolonged, an allograft biopsy may be necessary to distinguish acute rejection. Early acute rejection can mimic ATN or coexist with it. Data from the NAPRTCS show that ATN increases the risk of graft failure sixfold for a LD kidney and that the 4-year graft survival for CD grafts without ATN is 71%, compared to 51% for those with ATN in the immediate posttransplant period.

Graft Thrombosis

Graft vessel thrombosis is the third most common cause of graft failure for primary renal transplants in children (12%) and the second most common cause of graft failure for repeat transplants (20%). Although a major cause of immediate nonfunction, it can also manifest later in the course, and has been documented as late as 15 days posttransplant. Graft thrombosis should be suspected in cases where immediate function is followed by oligo-anuria. The diagnosis is established by radionuclide scan using diethylenetriamine pentacetic acid (DTPA), which reveals a defect with no uptake by the transplant kidney. Currently there are no established remedies to reverse a fixed thrombosis, although numerous procedures have been tried. A careful analysis of risk factors for graft thrombosis has been prepared by the NAPRTCS, and attention to this should reduce the risk in an individual case. Repeat transplants and young recipient age are risk factors, and the use of prophylactic T cell antibody reduces the risk for LD kidneys. Risk factors for CD kidneys are young recipient, prolonged cold ischemia, and donor age under five, whereas T cell antibody is protective.

Obstruction and Urinary Leak

Decreasing urinary output and a developing hydronephrosis should alert the clinician to this rare but correctable technical problem. A radionuclide scan with furosemide wash-out is necessary to confirm the diagnosis, which can be suspected by ultrasound. Obstruction can be due to kinking of the ureter, to edema or blockage at the implantation site of the ureter, or to the development of a large lymphocele. A more sudden and ominous cause of immediate nonfunction is the very rare case of urinary leak caused by the disintegration of the distal ureter or rupture of the bladder. Extravasation of the urine into the peritoneal cavity is extremely painful and needs immediate exploration. Diagnosis is established by radionuclide scan which reveals the tracer either in the peritoneal cavity or in the scrotal or vulval regions.

IMMUNOSUPPRESSION PROTOCOLS FOR CHILDREN
Induction Therapy

The role of T cell antibody induction therapy has been well-demonstrated in pediatric transplantation. In a review of LD transplants, 5-year graft survival for 1,143 patients who received T cell antibody prophylaxis was 82% compared to 76% for 1,636 patients who did not.

Similarly, for CD transplants the 5-year graft survival for 1,157 patients who did not receive T cell antibody prophylaxis was 58% compared to 68% for 1,578 patients who did receive the prophylactic therapy. As can be seen from these figures, 57% of CD and 41% of LD transplants are treated with induction therapy. The efficacy of T cell antibody induction therapy in decreasing the incidence of acute rejections and improving long-term graft survival has been shown only in these retrospective data, however a major National Institutes of Health-funded, randomized clinical trial testing muromonab-CD3 induction is currently in progress in 21 centers of the NAPRTCS, and when completed the trial should provide definitive guidelines regarding the need for induction therapy. Information on the efficacy of the two newer anti-CD 25 antibodies (basiliximab and daclizumab) in children is not available, although the safety of both has been demonstrated.

Maintenance Therapy

Cyclosporine remains the primary calcineurin inhibitor used for maintenance immunosuppression. In a review of 5,362 patients 91% were receiving cyclosporine at six months posttransplant and 89% of those with a functioning graft were continuing to receive the drug at five years posttransplant. The recommended dose of cyclosporine for children under the age of six is 500 mg/m^2 daily, administered in three divided doses; for children over six the dose is 15 mg/kg daily, administered in two divided doses. A calcium channel blocker is frequently given with cyclosporine to reduce renal toxicity. Recommended cyclosporine blood levels are 200 to 300 ng/mL HPLC whole blood trough levels for the first three months and 100 to 200 ng/mL after that. Equivalent TDX whole blood levels should be 300 to 500 ng/mL in the first three months and 200 to 450 ng/mL thereafter. Constant dosage adjustment is necessary with the older (Sandimmune®) preparation, however, 81% of the children transplanted in 1997 were initiated with the newer (Neoral®) preparation of cyclosporine. Maintenance cyclosporine dose at six months should be 8 mg/kg. Rejection is more frequent (24%) in children maintained on lower cyclosporine doses (5 to 7 mg/kg) compared to those maintained on 8 mg/kg (16 %).

Tacrolimus, another calcineurin inhibitor, has very limited usage in pediatric renal transplantation due to the high rate of posttransplant lymphoproliferative disorder (PTLD). Eight cases were noted in 48 tacrolimus-initiated patients (16%) compared to 46 cases in 4,084 (1.1%) cyclosporine-initiated patients. The incidence of insulin-dependent diabetes in pediatric patients treated with tacrolimus also appears to be high. The most recent publication from the NAPRTCS notes that of 520 patients transplanted in 1996, only 13 (2.5%) were being maintained on tacrolimus. The recommended oral dose is 0.10-0.15 mg/kg twice daily and should be reduced to 0.1 mg/kg as maintenance dose. Target whole blood trough level should be 10 to 20 ng/L.

Azathioprine and mycophenolate mofetil (MMF): The use of azathioprine, a purine analogue, as an adjuvant drug has dropped significantly since the introduction of mycophenolate mofetil. Azathioprine is used in a dose of 1 to 2 mg/kg daily, whereas MMF should be given at 1,200 mg/meter^2 divided into two, three, or four doses. Gastrointestinal disturbances are a major difficulty with the use of MMF in children, leaving approximately 10% to 15 % of the patients unable to accept the drug due to intractable diarrhea.

Prednisone, starting at a dose of 2 mg/kg per day, is rapidly tapered so that most children receive 0.2-0.3 mg/kg daily by the end of the first year posttransplant. The median dose in children at six months posttransplant is 0.27 mg/kg, tapering to 0.16 mg/kg at three years posttransplant. At four years posttransplant, 30% of LD and 23% of CD patients are receiving alternate-day steroid therapy.

ACUTE REJECTION: INCIDENCE DIAGNOSIS AND MANAGEMENT

The incidence of acute rejection in the pediatric age range is higher than that observed in adult patients. In a review of rejection, the NAPRTCS observed a rejection ratio of 1.1 in 2,520 LD transplants (2,540 rejection episodes), and a ratio of 1.32 in 2,520 CD patients (3,653 rejection episodes). At days 15, 30 and 45 posttransplant, 21%, 29% and 35% of LD patients and 21%, 39%, and 48% of CD patients have had one rejection episode, respectively. By the end of the first year posttransplant, 49% of LD and 63% of CD patients have had an acute rejection. The NAPRTCS has also demonstrated that the initial rejection episode in recipients younger than six is more likely to be irreversible, leading to graft loss. For LD recipients, irreversible graft failure is noted in 11% of zero to one year-old, 7% of two to five year-old, and 4% of six to 17 year-old patients. For CD patients, irreversible graft failure occurs in 21% of zero to one year-old, 15% of two to five year-old and 7% of six to 17 year-old patients. For both donor groups, recipients younger than six have a significantly (P=0.001) poorer outcome.

Because of the poor outcome of the initial rejection episode in younger children, an early diagnosis is imperative. Decreasing urine outflow and a rising serum creatinine should alert the clinician. Although obstruction, renal stenosis, infection and urinary leakage may all produce the same picture, after ultrasound examination to rule out obstruction, a renal biopsy is mandatory. Attempts to diagnose the rejection by radionuclide scan are frequently done, but definitive diagnosis can rarely be obtained by this technique. The safety of percutaneous renal biopsy in children done as early as days five and 12 posttransplantation for surveillance and at any time post-transplantation for suspected rejection has been clearly demonstrated by recent data from the Cooperative Clinical Trials in Pediatric Transplantation. This study from 21 pediatric centers evaluated 182 biopsies done per protocol and noted an exceptionally low rate of complications and no graft loss. Initial treatment of acute rejection is bolus methylprednisolone given in the dose of 20 to 25 mg/kg daily for three consecutive days. Most grade 1 and 2 lesions, as scored by the Banff criteria, respond to the 3-day course. Steroid-resistant rejection episodes are treated with anti-T cell antibody, either muromonab-CD3 or antithymocyte globulin (ATGAM®). Muromonab-CD3 is administered in the dose of 2.5 mg for children under 30 kg, and 5 mg for children over 30 kg, for ten days. ATGAM® is administered in the dose of 15 mg/kg daily through a central vein for ten to 14 days.

OUTCOMES AND RISK FACTORS

Graft survival data presented here are from the 1997 NAPRTCS Annual Report, which is pooled data from 71 pediatric renal transplant centers in North America. Four thousand, eight hundred ninety-eight patients received 5,362 grafts. Of these, 1,333 (25%) grafts have failed. Of 4,898 index transplants, 1,183 (24%) have failed. Table 62-4 displays causes of graft failure. Figure 62-1 displays 5-year graft survival rates for LD and CD source index transplants. Actuarial 1-, 2-, and 5-year survival rates for LD transplants are 91%, 87%, and 77%, and for CD transplants the rates are 81%, 75%, and 61%, respectively.

Graft survival for LD transplants is significantly better at all time periods. Other factors impact on graft survival. Figure 62-2 displays LD graft survival by recipient age, race, induction therapy, transfusion history and annual cohorts. At five years, graft survival for all age groupings is similar (76%), however it is significantly better in Caucasian children (79%) than in African-American children (62%). Both induction therapy and fewer than five random transfusions improve graft survival.

Figure 62-3 displays graft survival for CD transplants by recipient age, race, induction therapy, transfusion history and prior transplant, donor age, cold ischemia time, and by annual cohorts. Young infants and children of African-American ethnicity have a poorer outcome. Kidneys with a prolonged cold ischemia time are at a disadvantage, whereas kidneys recovered from an individual over ten have a better outcome. Absence of induction therapy, more than five transfusions and a repeat transplant also produce a poorer graft survival,

Table 62-4. Causes of Graft Failure

Cause	Index Graft Failures (n=1183)	(%)	Subsequent* Graft Failures (n=150)	(%)	Total Graft Failures (n=1333)	(%)
Primary nonfunction	35	(3.0)	3	(2.0)	38	(2.9)
Vascular thrombosis	137	(12.4)	28	(18.7)	175	(13.1)
Miscellaneous technical	20	(1.7)	4	(2.7)	24	(1.8)
Hyperacute rejection, <24 hours	9	(0.8)	3	(2.0)	12	(0.9)
Accelerated acute rejection, 2 to 7 days	29	(2.5)	6	(4.0)	35	(2.6)
Acute rejection	216	(18.3)	23	(15.3)	239	(17.9)
Chronic rejection	352	(29.8)	41	(27.3)	393	(29.5)
Rental Artery Stenosis	12	(1.0)	0	(0.0)	12	(0.9)
Infection/Discontinue Meds	26	(2.2)	2	(1.3)	28	(2.1)
Cyclosporine Toxicity	9	(0.8)	0	(0.0)	9	(0.7)
(De Novo) Kidney Disease	4	(0.3)	2	(1.3)	6	(0.5)
Patient discontnued medication	31	(2.6)	2	(1.3)	33	(2.5)
Malignancy	13	(1.1)	1	(0.7)	14	(1.1)
Recurrence of original disease	67	(5.7)	15	(10.0)	82	(6.2)
Death	136	(11.5)	12	(8.0)	148	(11.1)
Other	77	(6.5)	8	(5.3)	85	(6.4)

*Eleven patients have had three graft failures, one patient has had four failures.

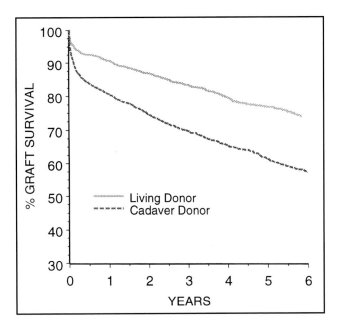

Figure 62-1. Five-year graft survival rates for index transplants by donor source.

whereas graft survival shows improvement for transplants done in more recent years.

Using proportional hazards, modeling relative risk (RR) factors for index LD transplant graft survival are: African-American race, RR=2.1, indicating a twofold increase in the risk for graft failure (*P*<0.001); more than five random transfusions, RR=1.6 (*P*<0.001); absence of HLA-B locus match, RR=2.1 (*P*<0.006); infant recipient, RR=1.4 (*P*<0.04). Induction therapy was protective (RR=0.76, (*P*<0.009). Risk factors for CD transplants are more numerous and are displayed in Table 62-5. It should be noted that cadaver graft survival shows a steady improvement when reviewed by biannual cohorts and that the 1992 cohort has a 5-year graft survival which is almost 20% better than that observed for the 1987 cohort.

POSTTRANSPLANT GROWTH

With a steady improvement in graft survival, attention has turned to the quality of life of children posttransplantation. A functioning graft not only relieves the child from dialysis dependency, but also improves self-esteem. Studies have shown that both reading and writing skills also improve. Instead of attending special classes, which may be necessary during dialysis, children posttransplant are able to attend regular school. Children with a functioning transplant should be able to interact normally with other children, except for their height disadvantage.

Chronic renal insufficiency beginning in infancy invariably leads to reduction in growth potential. Growth retardation continues in children on a dialysis regimen whether the mode of dialysis is continuous peritoneal or hemodialysis. Thus, most children whose renal insufficiency begins in early infancy will, at the time of transplantation, have a significant degree of growth retardation. Since individual heights vary tremendously, for uniformity, all growth measurements are indicated as Z score or height standard deviation (SD), which is defined as height at the 50th centile minus height of the patient, divided by the SD for the age of the patient. In reviewing over 4,000 transplants, the NAPRTCS has noted that, at transplantation, the mean height Z score for all patients was -2.08, over two SDs below the appropriate age and sex-matched mean heights. The natural history of growth posttransplantation has been studied by NAPRTCS in special serial studies.

In the first study, patients with a functioning graft at two years posttransplant were analyzed (n=300). The mean baseline deficit at transplant was a Z score of -2.41, and at two years posttransplant the mean improvement in the Z score was only 0.18. The second study reviewed height SD score at three years posttransplant. For these 412 patients the baseline deficit was -2.46, and the improvement was only 0.16. The third study had 587 patients and reviewed the height improvement at 4.5 years posttransplant. The baseline deficit was -2.29 and the improvement was only 0.11. Additionally, the improvement in the height deficit posttransplant was not distributed uniformly across all ages. Improvement in the Z score was observed in zero to one year-old (0.94) and in two to five year-old (0.77) children, whereas for those over six, who constituted 74% of the patients in the study, there was an actual deceleration. Catch-up growth (gain of 1 SD) was noted in only 47% of zero to one year-old, 43% of two to five year-old, 16% of six to 12 year-old, and 9% of 13 to 17 year-old children.

The studies also noted that improvement in growth posttransplantation was only observed in the Caucasian

Table 62-5. Risk Factors for Cadaver Donor Transplantation

	Relative Risk Increase	*p*-value
Recipient Age (<2)	2.00	<.001
Donor Age (<6)	1.30	.005
Prior Transplant	1.41	.001
No ATG/ALG/muromonab-CD3 Early Administration	1.31	<.001
>5 Lifetime Transfusions	1.32	.001
No HLA-B Match	1.27	.001
No HLA-DR Matches	1.30	.001
Annual Cohort (1987 vs 1992)	1.36	<.001
African-American Race	1.29	.005
Prior Dialysis	1.31	.04
Cold Storage Time >24 Hours	1.16	.06

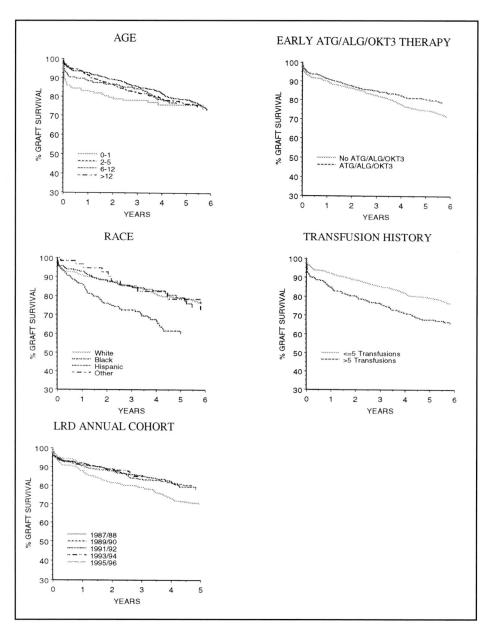

Figure 62-2. Five-year living donor graft survival rates by notable risk factors.

children (0.19), with African-American and Hispanic children showing an actual deceleration of growth of -0.05 and -0.018 SD, respectively. In a more recent evaluation the NAPRTCS looked at the effect of a transplant on the final adult height achieved by children. For 589 patients who received a transplant in childhood and who are now over 22, the Z score was -1.79 SD; 25% of these children had a Z score more negative than -2.8 and 10% had a score more negative than -4.0 SD.

Growth failure prior to transplantation is multifactorial involving caloric malnutrition due to uremia, bone demineralization due to hyperparathyroidism, renal acidosis and hypocalcemia. A functioning transplant, which corrects the uremic milieu and restores the renal function to near normal, ought to enable the child to achieve catch-up growth. As we have demonstrated,

catch-up growth, however, is not seen in the great majority of children posttransplantation. Current maintenance immunosuppressive therapy consists of calcineurin inhibitors and adjunct therapy with corticosteroids. Steroids inhibit growth by reducing growth hormone output, by reducing growth hormone receptor expression, and by uncoupling the receptors from their signal transduction mechanisms. The growth-inhibiting effects of corticosteroid therapy are universal and are seen in children who receive liver or heart transplants as well.

Attempts to overcome the steroid inhibition of growth have consisted of reduction in steroid maintenance dose, however, doses as low as 5 mg daily will still inhibit growth. An alternative method has been the use of alternate-day steroid therapy, which has shown improvement in growth but has found only a limited use

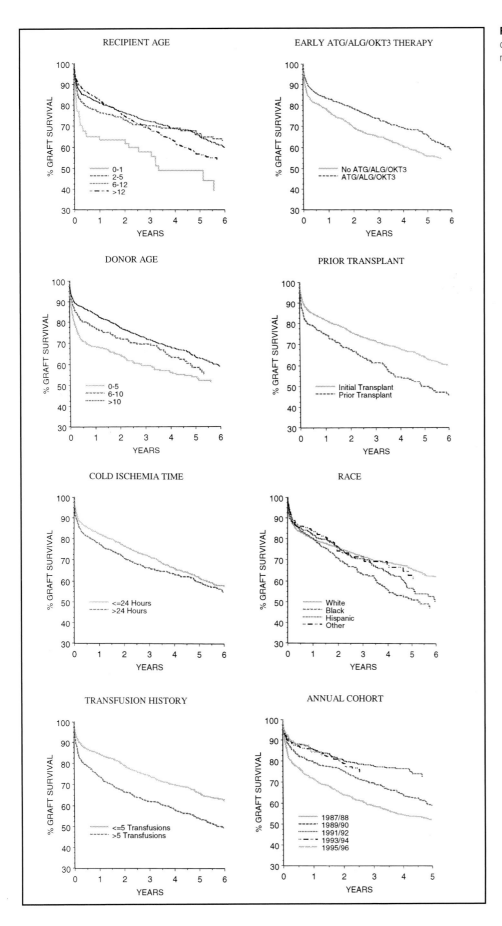

Figure 62-3. Five-year cadaver donor graft survival rates by notable risk factors.

in pediatric centers due to concerns for noncompliance. Attempts to improve growth posttransplantation by the use of recombinant human growth hormone (RhGh) are handicapped by the facts that RhGh is currently not approved for posttransplantation use and that its efficacy in the presence of corticosteroids is suboptimal. Additionally there has been a concern that the use of RhGh may trigger an episode of acute rejection. Anecdotal studies have documented an increased risk of acute rejection with the use of RhGh, however confirmation awaits the results of a controlled trial of the NAPRTCS which is currently ongoing. Since growth retardation posttransplant continues to remain the major area of concern, total steroid withdrawal is the ideal goal in pediatric renal transplantation. Successful steroid withdrawal will permit catch-up growth. Unfortunately, acute rejection episodes are common in children maintained on steroid-free protocols under current immunosuppressive therapies. The rejection rate in uncontrolled studies in the first year postwithdrawal is about 20%, but rises to 40% at three years postwithdrawal. Such high rates will obviously lead to graft attrition, and novel immunosuppressives, other than the current calcineurin inhibitors, are essential for steroid-free protocols which will enable the pediatric patient to achieve catch-up growth.

RECOMMENDED READING

Warady BA, Hebert D, Sullivan EK, Alexander SR, Tejani A. Renal transplantation, chronic dialysis, and chronic renal insufficiency in children and adolescents. The 1995 Annual Report of the North American Pediatric Renal Transplant Cooperative Study. Pediatr Nephrol. 1997;11(1):49-64.

United States Renal Data System (USRDS) The 1997 Annual Report. Bethesda, Md: National Institutes of Health, National Institute of Diabetes and Digestive and Kidney Diseases, 1997.

Kohaut EC, Tejani A. The 1994 Annual Report of the North American Pediatric Renal Transplant Cooperative Study (NAPRTCS). Pediatr Nephrol. 1996;10(4):422-434.

Cecka JM, Gjertson DW, Terasaki PI. Pediatric renal transplantation: A review of the UNOS data. Pediatr Transplant. 1997;1(1):55-64.

Feld LG, Stablein DM, Fivush BA, Harmon WE, Tejani A. Renal transplantation in children from 1987-1996: the 1996 Annual Report of the North American Pediatric Renal Transplant Cooperative Study (NAPRTCS). Pediatr Transplant. 1997;1(2):146-162.

McEnery P, Stablein DM, Arbus G, Tejani A. Renal transplantation in children: a report of the North American Pediatric Renal Transplant Cooperative Study (NAPRTCS). N Engl J Med. 1992;326(26):1727-1732.

Tejani A, Sullivan EK, Alexander S, Fine R, Harmon W, Lilienfeld D. Posttransplant deaths and factors that influence the mortality rate in North American children. Transplantation. 1994;57(4):547-553.

Harmon WE, Alexander SR, Tejani A, Stablein D. The effect of donor age on graft survival in pediatric cadaver renal transplant recipients. A report of the North American Pediatric Renal Transplant Cooperative Study (NAPRTCS). Transplantation. 1992;54(2):232-237.

Balachandra S, Tejani A. Recurrent vascular thrombosis in an adolescent transplant recipient. J Am Soc Nephrol. 1997;8(9):1477-1481.

Singh A, Stablein D, Tejani A. Risk factors for vascular thrombosis in pediatric renal transplantation: a special report of the North American Pediatric Renal Transplant Cooperative Study. Transplantation. 1997;63(9):1263-1267.

Morris PJ. Cyclosporine. In: Morris PJ, ed. Kidney Transplantation: Principles and Practice, 4th Ed. Philadelphia, Pa: WB Saunders; 1994:179-201.

Tejani A, Sullivan EK, Fine RN, Harmon WE, Alexander S. Steady improvement in renal allograft survival among North American children: a five year appraisal by the North American Pediatric Renal Transplant Cooperative Study. Kidney Int. 1995;48(2):551-553.

Jabs K, Sullivan EK, Avner ED, Harmon WE. Alternate-day steroid dosing improves growth without adversely affecting graft survival or long-term graft function. A report of the North American Pediatric Renal Transplant Cooperative Study (NAPRTCS). Transplantation. 1996;61(1):31-36.

Tejani A, Cortes L, Stablein D. Clinical correlates of chronic rejection in pediatric renal transplantation: a report of the North American Pediatric Renal Transplant Cooperative Study (NAPRTCS). Transplantation. 1996;61(7):1054-1058.

Tejani A, Cortes L, Sullivan EK. A longitudinal study of the natural history of growth post-transplantation. Kidney Int. 1996;53:S103-S108.

Broyer M. Results and side-effects of treating children with growth hormone after kidney transplantation – a preliminary report. Pharmacia & Upjohn Study Group. Acta Paediatr Suppl. 1996;417:76-79.

Harmon WE. Opportunistic infections in children following renal transplantation. Pediatr Nephrol. 1991;5(1):118-125.

63 PANCREAS AND SIMULTANEOUS KIDNEY-PANCREAS TRANSPLANTATION

John D. Pirsch, MD
Robert J. Stratta, MD

Insulin-dependent diabetes mellitus is the leading cause of end-stage renal disease (ESRD), accounting for one-third of new ESRD patients each year. In 1997, diabetes (both insulin- and non-insulin-dependent) accounted for 25% of transplants performed in the US. The poor five year survival of diabetic patients on dialysis makes kidney transplantation the treatment of choice for end-stage diabetic nephropathy. Increasingly, pancreas transplantation (PTX) is also being offered to patients who require a kidney transplant (simultaneous pancreas-kidney [SPK]) or had a previously successful transplant (sequential pancreas after kidney [PAK]). A few centers are also performing PTX alone (PTA) in diabetic patients with hyperlability and severe hypoglycemic unawareness in the absence of advanced nephropathy. The appropriateness of PTX has been questioned because of the increased morbidity associated with the procedure and the lack of controlled trials that demonstrate a significant benefit on secondary complications of diabetes. Despite these concerns, PTX has continued to grow in popularity as an option for diabetic patients with complications, since it can enhance quality of life and is the single most effective method of achieving tight glucose control.

Vascularized PTX was first developed as a means to reestablish endogenous insulin secretion responsive to normal feedback controls. PTX is currently the only known therapy that establishes an insulin-independent euglycemic state with complete normalization of glycosylated hemoglobin levels. The penalties for normal glucose homeostasis are the operative risks of the transplant procedure and the need for chronic immunosuppression. With improvements in organ retrieval technology, refinements in surgical techniques, and advances in clinical immunosuppression, success rates for vascularized PTX have improved dramatically. As a

John D. Pirsch, MD, Professor of Medicine and Surgery; Director of Medical Transplantation Service, University of Wisconsin Medical School, Madison, WI

Robert J. Stratta, MD, Professor of Surgery, Division of Transplantation Surgery, University of Tennessee at Memphis, Memphis, TN

result, PTX (particularly SPK) has become an accepted treatment option in appropriately selected diabetic patients.

REGISTRY RESULTS

From 1996 through 1998, 11,442 pancreas transplants were performed worldwide and reported to the International Pancreas Transplant Registry (IPTR). Since October 1, 1987, all US cases have also been reported to the United Network for Organ Sharing (UNOS) Registry through a subcontract with the IPTR. At present, about 85% of pancreas transplants reported to the IPTR are performed in the US. The vast majority (87%) of pancreas transplants in the US have been performed in conjunction with a simultaneous kidney transplant (SPKT) in diabetic patients who have imminent or projected renal failure (preemptive) or are already on dialysis. The remaining pancreas transplants have been performed as a sequential PAK transplant (9%), as a PTA (3.9%), or in conjunction with a single organ other than the kidney or with multiple organs (<1%).

Most of the current UNOS Registry analysis is restricted to US cadaveric pancreas transplants performed from January 1994 to October 1998. The group analyzed included 3,409 SPKT, 375 PAK, and 181 PTA cases. The number of pancreas transplants performed with enteric drainage has steadily increased, accounting for one-third of cases from 1994 to 1998 and more than 50% of cases in 1998. The 1-year patient survival rate for all three categories is 94% to 95%. The 1-year pancreas graft survival rates are 83% after SPKT, 71% after PAK, and 64% after PTA. The 1-year kidney graft survival rate after SPKT is 90%. Compared to kidney transplantation alone (KTA) in diabetic patients, the kidney graft survival rate for SPKT recipients is higher. This may be due in part to patient selection and better donors in SPKT recipients. Therefore, patients are not disadvantaged in terms of kidney graft survival if they are selected for SPKT. At present, about 40% of diabetic patients below age 50 undergoing kidney transplantation in the US actually receive SPKT.

The results of pancreas transplantation are similar for US and non-US cases. Of the three types of pancreas transplants performed, SPKT has a significantly better pancreas graft survival rate compared to PAK and PTA. With the emergence of new immunosuppressive agents, the 1-year rates of immunologic graft loss have decreased to 2% after SPKT, 9% after PAK, and 16% after PTA. In patients receiving both tacrolimus (FK) and mycophenolate mofetil (MMF), the 1-year rates of pancreas graft survival are 86% after SPKT, 83% after PAK, and 75% after PTA.

The latest Registry results are notable for an expanded analysis of pancreas transplants performed with bladder vs enteric drainage as well as a new analysis relative to maintenance immunosuppression. In the last few years, the results of SPKT with enteric drainage have steadily improved and are now comparable to bladder drainage. In patients with bladder drainage, a finite incidence of enteric conversion remains (7% at one year, 11% at two years). With regard to PAK and PTA, enteric drainage is associated with an inferior graft survival rate, predominantly due to a higher technical failure rate. In all three categories, the rate of thrombosis is significantly higher after enteric drainage vs bladder drainage. However, the rates of graft loss due to either technical failure or rejection are much lower than previous Registry reports.

The results of SPKT without anti-T cell induction are now comparable to treatment regimens employing polyclonal or monoclonal induction (1-year graft survival rates of 84% with ATG, 83% with muromonab-CD3, and 81% with no induction). However, anti-T cell induction therapy is still associated with superior pancreas graft survival in the PAK and PTA categories. In all three categories, immunosuppression with MMF is associated with improved graft survival vs azathioprine. In the SPKT category, patients receiving either cyclosporine and MMF or FK and MMF fare equally well, particularly in combination with anti-T cell induction therapy. In the PAK category, FK-MMF is associated with improved graft survival, particularly in patients receiving bladder drainage and ATG induction. In the PTA category, improved graft survival occurs in patients receiving FK-MMF, without a significant co-variate effect of either bladder vs enteric drainage or anti-T cell induction therapy.

The Registry report also includes logistic and multivariate regression analyses of outcomes according to

transplant category. In general, older donor or recipient age (>45 years) is associated with either reduced patient or graft survival rates. Re-transplantation is also a risk factor for graft loss after SPKT and PAK. The use of MMF after SPKT and FK after PAK or PTA are both associated with a decreased risk of graft loss. In each successive Registry report over the last decade, the volume and outcomes of pancreas transplantation in the US have steadily improved.

PRETRANSPLANT EVALUATION

Because of the increased morbidity of PTX compared with KTA, recipients selected for PTX should be free of significant comorbid illness. At most centers, the major contraindication to PTX is significant uncorrectable cardiovascular disease. Other relative contraindications include severe vascular disease, psychiatric illness, the lack of well-defined diabetic complications and obesity. The primary determinants for recipient selection are degree of nephropathy, cardiovascular risk, and presence of diabetic complications. Selection criteria for solitary PTX are based on the presence of early diabetic complications or exogenous insulin failure with hyperlabile diabetes.

Patients with IDDM and impending or established ESRD who have minimal or limited secondary complications of diabetes (usually between the ages of 20 and 40 years) are considered optimal candidates for SPKT. However, not all patients with IDDM and renal failure are acceptable candidates. Some centers regard a history of blindness, major amputation, or heart disease as relative contraindications to transplantation. Age over 60, active smoking, an ejection fraction below 30%, and severe obesity (>150% over ideal body weight) are usually viewed as absolute contraindications to PTX. Other contraindications that are applicable to all solid organ transplant recipients include the presence of active infection or recent malignancy, active substance abuse or dependence, recent history of noncompliance, or psychiatric illness.

In patients with established diabetic nephropathy, the choice between SPKT or PAK transplantation can be problematic, particularly if there is a living donor willing to donate a kidney. Historically, living-related KTA in diabetic recipients is associated with a survival advantage compared with cadaver KTA. The increased morbidity of PTX has led to a reluctance of some centers to recommend SPKT to appropriate candidates with living donors. On the other hand, the results of PAK transplantation are worse than receiving an SPKT. Some patients with a suitable living donor may elect to receive a cadaver SPKT despite the increased risks associated with the procedure. In general, diabetic patients with an HLA-identical donor should receive an HLA-identical kidney since the long-term patient and graft survival rates far exceed those of

Table 63-1. Overall Survival Rates Between 1994 and 1998 in the UNOS Registry

	Years Posttransplant		
Patient Survival	**1 Year (%)**	**2 Year (%)**	**3 Year (%)**
SPK (n=3409)	94	92	91
PAK (n=375)	95	92	88
PTA (n=181)	95	95	95
Graft Survival			
SPK (n=3409)			
Kidney	90	88	85
Pancreas	83	80	77
PAK (n=375)			
Pancreas	71	61	55
PTA (n=181)			
Pancreas	64	58	50

any cadaver transplant. The results of haplo-identical or living nonrelated transplantation are comparable to SPKT and the decision should be based on patient preference and projected waiting time. Finally, if the patient is an acceptable candidate for a PTX and has no living donor available, then SPKT should be considered as primary treatment to establish insulin-independence and provide renal replacement therapy.

DONOR SELECTION AND MANAGEMENT

Donor selection and organ procurement are of paramount importance to the success of PTX. Most heart-beating donors who have been declared brain dead and are appropriate for kidney, heart, lung, and liver donation are also suitable for pancreas donation. Although there is some evidence that donor hyperglycemia may have a deleterious effect on allograft function, the presence of hyperglycemia or hyperamylasemia as such are not usual contraindications for pancreas donation.

In general, the ideal pancreas donor is between ten and 40 years old and weighs between 30 and 80 kg. Expanded criteria pancreas donors range in age from six to 60 and range in weight from 20 to 100 kg, depending on height and gender. A basic principle of pancreas donation is that the quality of the donor is more important than the quality of the HLA-match.

Management of the multiple organ donor includes aggressive resuscitation to maintain hemodynamic stability, organ perfusion, and oxygenation. Resuscitative efforts usually result in significant hyperglycemia, and intensive control with insulin may have a favorable effect on initial allograft function and survival. Liberal use of intravenous colloid fluids and Mannitol is recommended to minimize pancreatic edema. Judicious administration of vasopressors such as Dopamine are indicated to maintain a systolic blood pressure above 90 mmHg and promote diuresis. High doses of vasopressors and other agents that impair the splanchnic circulation and pancreatic perfusion should be avoided, if possible, to avoid ischemic hypoperfusion and the possibility of reperfusion pancreatitis.

Contraindications for pancreas organ donation include a history of diabetes mellitus (type 1, type 2, or gestational), previous pancreatic surgery, severe pancreatic trauma, active acute or chronic pancreatitis, or the presence of significant intraabdominal contamination or active infection. With increasing experience in pancreas donation, previous absolute contraindications have become relative contraindications, and relative contraindications have become risk factors for organ utilization. Donor age above 45 years and cardiovascular or cerebrovascular causes of brain death have been identified as risk factors for thrombosis after PTX. Relative contraindications for pancreas organ donation include significant fatty infiltration, moderate to severe atherosclerosis, severe irreversible pancreatic edema, and donor instability. Risk factors for pancreas organ donation include massive transfusions, prior splenectomy, aberrant hepatic artery anatomy, and prolonged length of hospital stay. The importance of an experienced retrieval team must be emphasized for the in situ assessment of pancreatic anatomy. Living-related pancreas donation is reserved for patients in whom cytotoxic antibody titers have developed, rendering it difficult, if not impossible, to finding a crossmatch-negative cadaver donor. A portion of the body and tail of the pancreas can be removed from a living donor based on a vascular pedicle of the splenic vessels. In highly selected cases, this procedure may be performed simultaneous with or sequential to kidney donation, with the left kidney usually removed. Although the results of living-related segmental PTX have been acceptable, the potential short-term and long-term risks to the donor are such that this procedure is reserved for exceptional situations.

ORGAN PROCUREMENT, PRESERVATION, AND PREPARATION

Advances in organ retrieval and preservation technology have played an important role in the improving results of PTX. Combined liver, kidney, and whole organ pancreaticoduodenal retrieval can be safely performed in virtually all donors, irrespective of vascular anatomy. At present, whole organ pancreas retrieval is not compatible with small bowel procurement. Although a number of techniques have been described, many authors advocate combined en bloc hepaticopancreaticoduodenosplenectomy. Bilateral en bloc nephroureterectomy is next performed by standard techniques. Back table ex vivo separation of the liver and pancreas is then performed. The liver, pancreas, and kidneys are packaged separately in sterile cold UW (University of Wisconsin) solution. Rapid removal of both the liver and pancreas is possible with a minimal dissection technique in an otherwise unstable donor. In highly selected cases, the liver, pancreas, and kidneys can all be removed as an en bloc specimen with subsequent separation ex vivo.

The introduction of UW solution into clinical transplantation has permitted safe and extended cold storage preservation of the pancreas up to 30 hours without compromise of graft function. The enhanced margin of safety afforded by extended preservation in UW solution has increased the capability for distant organ procurement and sharing, minimized organ wastage, improved the efficiency of organ retrieval, allowed time for crossmatching and adequate preparation of the recipient, and has enabled semi-elective performance of the recipient operation. Moreover, the quality of preservation has improved, resulting in better initial graft function with fewer complications such as pancreatitis or vascular thrombosis. However, even with an ideal donor, most centers are reluctant to extend preservation times beyond 20 hours. With an expanded criteria donor, preservation times are kept to a minimum, usually 12 hours or less. Before the recipient operation, the pancreas is prepared for transplantation under cold storage conditions in UW solution. Bench reconstruction of the pancreas comprises several steps that require careful attention to detail to avoid organ injury and facilitate the transplant procedure. The spleen is left attached to provide a "handle" during the transplant procedure as the vessels are reconstructed and the duodenal segment is prepared.

SURGICAL TECHNIQUE AND MANAGEMENT

Over the past five years there has been a major change in the type of drainage procedure employed for pancreas transplants. While bladder drainage (Figure 63-1) remains the most common technique for management of the pancreas exocrine secretions, the number of enteric drained pancreas transplants (Figure 63-2) is increasing. In 1994, only 6% of SPK transplants were enteric drained. In 1997, enteric drained pancreas transplants increased to 48%. The increase in enteric drainage is likely due to a number of factors that include improvement in immunosuppression with less rejection and improved surgical techniques. Bladder-drained pancreas transplants have a high frequency of metabolic and infectious complications and up to 20% of patients eventually require enteric conversion. A successful enteric drained pancreas transplant obviates the need for another surgical procedure and results in a lower overall infection rate, particularly UTIs. The major problem with

enteric drainage is a higher rate of technical failures: 11% vs 8% for bladder drained pancreas transplants in the most recent Registry analysis.

The operation usually lasts three to five hours, depending on whether the patient is receiving a PTA, PAK, or SPKT. During the transplant procedure, no recipient organs are removed, and the patient receives a "second" pancreas, a "third" kidney, or both. In highly selected cases in which donor renal function may be marginal, a double-kidney transplant can be performed in conjunction with the PTX. The major nonphysiologic aspects of the procedure include transplantation of a completely denervated organ into an ectopic location with systemic venous drainage of insulin. A few centers have reported limited success transplanting the pancreas to a mesenteric vein of the recipient to establish portal venous drainage of insulin. This technique can be performed with enteric drainage to further improve the physiology of the transplant procedure.

In the initial postoperative period, serum glucose levels are followed closely and an intravenous insulin infusion is continued to maintain the serum glucose below 200 mg/dL. Persistent elevation or acute rises in the serum glucose to more than 200 mg/dL require immediate evaluation with duplex ultrasonography or radionuclide scanning to assess graft perfusion and function. Rejection parameters that are prospectively monitored may include urine cytology, serum glucose and amylase, serum lipase, 12 hour timed and spot-urine amylase, serum anodal trypsinogen, and pancreas specific protein. Immune monitoring may consist of serum muromonab-CD3 levels, flow cytometry for determination of T-lymphocyte subsets, or cytokine levels. Metabolic monitoring may include fasting serum insulin, C-peptide, lipid profiles, glucagon levels, proinsulin levels, or glycohemoglobin levels.

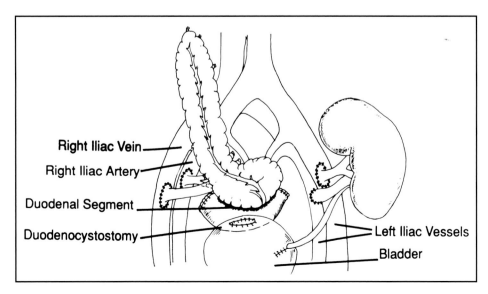

Right Iliac Vein

Right Iliac Artery

Duodenal Segment

Duodenocystostomy

Left Iliac Vessels

Bladder

Figure 63-1. Surgical technique of combined pancreas-kidney transplant through a midline intraperitoneal approach showing whole organ PTX with the duodenal segment method of bladder drainage. Reprinted by permission of the publisher from Ozaki CF, Stratta RJ, Taylor RJ, Langnas AN, Bynon JS, Shaw BW Jr. Surgical complications in solitary pancreas and combined pancreas-kidney transplantations. Am J Surg. 1992;164(5):546-551. Copyright 1992 by Excerpta Medica Inc.

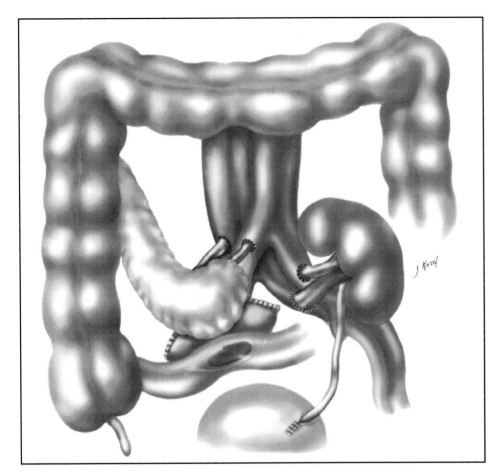

Figure 63-2. Enteric drainage technique. Enteric drainage is most often performed with the donor duodenal segment anastomosed side-to-side to the ileum or distal jejunum. It is less commonly performed with a Roux-en-Y anastomosis. Enteric drainage is more physiologic than bladder drainage, allowing pancreatic secretions to drain into the bowel. Reprinted with permission from Pirsch JD, Odorico JS, Sollinger HW. Kidney-pancreas transplantation. In: Schrier RW, Henrich WL, Bennett WM. Atlas of Diseases of the Kidney, Volume 5. Philadelphia, PA; Current Medicine; 1999: 15.1-15.17.

PTX with bladder drainage may result in the obligatory loss of at least 1 to 2 L/d of pancreatic exocrine and duodenal mucosal secretions rich in bicarbonate and electrolytes into the urine. The early postoperative period of most PTX recipients is characterized by an increased need for supplemental fluids and bicarbonate. To minimize problems with fluctuating drug levels due to gastroparesis or malabsorption, patients may be given metoclopramide, erythromycin, vitamin E, or oral pancreatic enzyme supplements.

IMMUNOSUPPRESSION

Most pancreas transplant centers initially use quadruple drug immunosuppression to control early rejection. In the past, antilymphocyte therapies such as muromonab-CD3 or antilymphocyte globulin were used for induction. The recent introduction of daclizumab and basiliximab offers another less toxic, choice for induction immunosuppression. The use of mycophenolate mofetil has dramatically reduced the incidence of rejection for pancreas recipients. Many centers are also employing tacrolimus for chronic immunosuppression, despite the diabetogenic effect of tacrolimus on pancreatic islet cells. In the Pancreas Registry, the role of various immunosuppressive regimens has been analyzed. For SPK, myco-

phenolate mofetil significantly reduced the incidence of acute rejection, but the use of antilymphocyte therapy or tacrolimus had less impact. In solitary pancreas groups (PAK and PTA), maintenance immunosuppression with tacrolimus and mycophenolate was associated with the highest pancreas graft survival rates.

REJECTION

Pancreas transplant rejection remains a significant clinical problem, despite the use of more potent immunosuppressive agents to prevent rejection. The overall incidence of rejection for all pancreas transplants has declined from nearly 80% in the late 1980s to 10% to 40% in the most recent era. However, graft loss from pancreas rejection has decreased in the most recent transplant era. In the most recent registry data, pancreas graft loss from rejection in the first year was 2% for SPK, 9% for PAK, and 16% for PTA recipients. The decrease in rejection frequency is largely attributed to the use of mycophenolate mofetil and tacrolimus for prevention of rejection.

Despite a decrease in pancreas graft loss from rejection, the diagnosis of pancreas rejection remains problematic. Clinical criteria consistent with rejection include fever, allograft swelling and tenderness, ileus, abdominal pain, or hematuria (in bladder drained pancreas transplants). Laboratory findings can include an increase in serum creatinine (after SPK), serum amylase, lipase or anodal trypsinogen, a reduction in urine amylase or pH, or positive urine cytology. An elevated blood sugar is a late manifestation of acute rejection and portends a poor prognosis, but can be elevated with chronic rejection, high dose steroids or tacrolimus toxicity. Most centers monitor serum amylase, lipase and creatinine (for SPK) because of their universal availability. In SPK recipients with both grafts from a single donor, an elevated serum creatinine usually precedes any manifestation of pancreas graft dysfunction and the diagnosis of rejection is made easily with a kidney biopsy. For PAK and PTA recipients, a definitive diagnosis of rejection can only be made with a pancreas biopsy.

A number of techniques of pancreas allograft biopsy have been described. Percutaneous biopsy with ultrasound or CT guidance is most often performed with a very low rate of complication. In patients with bladder drainage, cystoscopic transduodenal needle biopsy with ultrasound guidance has also been performed successfully. Both techniques utilize a semiautomated instrument such as the Biopty® gun, which sets a predetermined length of needle penetration to obtain an adequate tissue sample for diagnosis.

A classification system for the histologic diagnosis of pancreas rejection has been proposed and has helped standardize interpretation of pancreas transplant biopsies (Table 63-2). The degree of septal and acinar inflammation, eosinophils, and the presence of endotheliitis or vasculitis determine the severity of rejection. The grade of rejection has prognostic implications and therapeutic considerations. Very mild forms of rejection may respond to an increase of corticosteroids alone, but for more severe forms of rejection (grade II and higher), antilymphocyte therapy is necessary to reverse rejection.

Table 63-2. Grading Scheme for Pancreas Transplant Biopsies	
Grade 0	Normal
Grade I	Inflammation of undetermined significance
Grade II	Minimal rejection Septal inflammation with venous endotheliitis
Grade III	Mild rejection Septal inflammatory infiltrates with lymphocytes and acinar inflammation
Grade IV	Moderate rejection Arterial endotheliitis and/or necrotizing arthritis (vasculitis)
Grade V	Severe rejection Extensive acinar inflammation with cell necrosis

PHYSIOLOGY OF THE TRANSPLANTED PANCREAS

Successful PTX restores euglycemia within minutes to hours after the procedure. In addition, long-term metabolic control, as measured by glycosylated hemoglobin levels, remains normal as long as the pancreas is functioning. Another potential benefit is reestablishment of glucagon responses to hypoglycemia. The exocrine functions of the pancreas are potentially problematic, particularly when the PTX is bladder-drained. Pancreatic enzyme activation in the bladder can cause dysuria, hematuria, urine leaks, and severe urethritis with urethral stricture or disruption. The loss of bicarbonate in bladder-drained PTXs can lead to metabolic acidosis and dehydration. If the pancreas is drained into the bowel, these exocrine side effects are minimized.

COMPLICATIONS

SPKT is associated with a higher morbidity than KTA. Because most pancreas donors are young, and cold ischemia times are short, delayed graft function of the pancreas and kidney grafts is unusual. Since SPKT is usually performed by an intraabdominal approach, prolonged ileus and delayed return of bowel function are common. Early surgical problems resulting in graft loss include vascular thrombosis, pancreatitis and infection. In contrast to other solid organs transplanted, the pancreas is susceptible to a unique set of complications because of its exocrine elements and low microcirculatory blood flow. Furthermore, intraperitoneal placement of a denervated pancreas allograft in a paratopic location, with systemic venous drainage of insulin and exocrine drainage into the urinary bladder, is associated with a number of unusual problems. Because of the potential for surgical complications, the rate of early reoperation is higher, and the length of hospital stay is longer, for SPKT as compared to KTA. Early graft loss usually results in allograft pancreatectomy.

Exocrine

The management of exocrine complications continues to be an area of controversy after PTX. For patients with bladder drainage, enteric conversion is recommended for refractory problems, such as dehydration with intractable metabolic acidosis, chronic urethritis with urethral disruption or stricture, recurrent urine leaks with severe duodenal pathology, persistent hematuria, chronic urinary tract infections with foreign body formation or urosepsis, transitional cell dysplasia, and recurrent reflux pancreatitis. The most common technique of enteric conversion involves a side-to-side anastomosis between the allograft duodenal segment and recipient small bowel (Figure 63-3). Collected series have reported enteric conversion rates ranging from 10% to 20%. The operative complication rate after enteric conversion is 10% to 20%, with an enteric leak rate of 6% to 10%. However, the rate of death or graft loss after enteric conversion is very low and the procedure is indisputably therapeutic and yields excellent results in the setting of refractory problems related to the duodenal segment, metabolic alterations, or urologic complications. In general, conversion should be delayed as long as possible because many of the previously mentioned problems are self-limited and healing may be compromised by the higher doses of immunosuppressants in the early postoperative period.

Metabolic

PTX recipients with bladder drainage are susceptible to metabolic acidosis and volume depletion due to the loss of sodium, bicarbonate and alkaline enzyme-rich pancreatic fluid into the urinary tract. Dehydration in the setting of diabetic autonomic neuropathy can result in significant problems with orthostatic hypotension. Although usually self-limited and easily managed with oral or intravenous supplementation of fluids and bicarbonate, severe volume depletion and refractory metabolic acidosis may develop in a small subset of patients. In extreme cases, this metabolic derangement can lead to malnutrition, chronic abdominal pain, hemoconcentra-

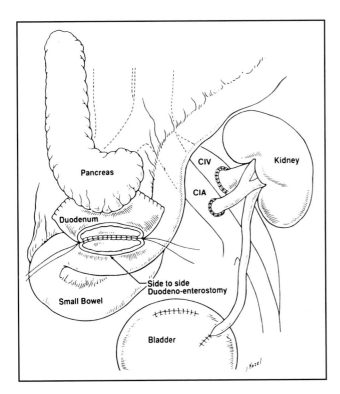

Figure 63-3. Technique of exocrine drainage conversion from bladder to enteric drainage with side-to-side duodenoenterostomy. Reprinted from Sollinger HW, Sasaki TM, D'Alessandro AM, et al. Indications for enteric conversion after pancreas transplantation with bladder drainage. Surgery. 1992;112(4):842-845.

tion, and syncope. In addition to oral fluid and bicarbonate supplementation, medical management can include long-term vascular access with periodic intravenous fluid and bicarbonate supplementation, oral sodium chloride tablets, fludrocortisone to promote salt and water retention, and acetazolamide therapy to reduce bicarbonate secretion from the pancreas and duodenum. A potential benefit of this condition is that hypertension appears to be less of a problem in PTX recipients. If patients have continued problems with fluid and electrolyte imbalance, they may be considered candidates for enteric conversion, which is performed for this complication in 5% to 7% of patients.

Enzyme Activation

Another complication of urinary drainage of the exocrine pancreas is enzyme (trypsinogen) activation, leading to "chemical" cystitis, urethritis, or balanitis. The enzyme activation can be aggravated both by volume depletion and bladder dysfunction and may result in or exacerbate catheter-induced urethral mucosal injury. This condition can result in persistent urethritis manifesting as dysuria, hematuria, or recurrent urinary tract infections and may intensify leading to urethral disruption or stricture. These problems are much more frequent in men than in women. Although the reported overall incidence is low (3% to 9%), refractory cases may be encountered. Management includes oral or intravenous fluid hydration, urethral catheter drainage, alkalinization of the urine, urinary tract analgesics, and antibiotics to treat any associated urinary tract infection. Refractory cases may require suprapubic cystostomy or enteric conversion to divert enzymes and allow for the healing of the urethral mucosa. For the most part, however, this problem is self-limited and can be managed non-operatively.

Hyperamylasemia

An elevation in serum amylase is common following PTX due to donor factors, procurement and preservation injury, and surgical implantation. Pancreatic ascites may occur as a result of a leak from the duodenal segment or from the distal pancreatic duct secondary to necrosis or injury during the surgical procedure. Hyperamylasemia may or may not signify allograft pancreatitis. Patients with pancreatitis may be asymptomatic or present with fever, lower abdominal pain, allograft swelling or tenderness, ileus, distension or constipation. The diagnosis of allograft pancreatitis is usually based on clinical presentation; hyperamylasemia; ultrasonographic evidence of pancreatic edema; hyperperfusion with loss of border resolution on radionuclide scanning; CT findings of pancreatic enlargement with edema, peripancreatic fluid, or inflammation; or direct evidence of pancreatitis at laparotomy with edema and saponification. Initial management consists of urethral catheter drainage, urine culture, intravenous fluid hydration, radiologic studies, and blood and urine studies to rule out rejection or infection. Since many patients may have a neurogenic bladder from diabetes, reflux pancreatitis from inadequate bladder emptying is a frequent cause of hyperamylasemia that usually responds to urethral catheter drainage and may necessitate short-term intermittent self-catheterization. In selected cases, the administration of Sandostatin may help reduce the exocrine output of the denervated pancreas allograft. Allograft pancreatitis may be due to surgical complications, such as leak, fistula, or infection, with the development of fluid collections, pseudocysts, or abscesses surrounding the pancreatic graft. The combination of pancreatitis with local tissue breakdown and bacterial contamination may lead to peripancreatic abscess formation that can be difficult to treat. Initial therapy of a peripancreatic fluid collection usually consists of percutaneous drainage. When an infection develops or persists, operative exploration is often required. The reported incidence of abscess formation requiring operative drainage ranges from 5% to 22%. The presence of peripancreatic infection portends a poor prognosis, resulting in multiple procedures and eventual allograft pancreatectomy in 30% to 50% of cases.

Urologic Complications (Bladder Drainage)

Urologic complications are common with bladder drainage of the pancreas. Urinary tract infections in bladder-drained recipients are common and multifactorial in nature. The incidence of urosepsis (4%), however, is relatively low. Many of these urinary tract infections are caused by normally nonvirulent organisms that are not commonly associated with infection. Among these organisms are *Staphylococcus epidermidis, citrobacter species,* and *enterococcus.* The combination of pancreatic enzyme activation, an alkaline environment, and immunosuppression seems to predispose the bladder to infection by these atypical organisms, and makes the eradication of these organisms difficult. Urinary tract infections may actually change the pH of the bladder environment and therefore initiate or exacerbate enzyme activation.

With enzyme activation, patients are predisposed to developing urethritis, cystitis, or actual ulceration, which may manifest as hematuria. Gross hematuria is the most frequent major urologic complication, occurring in about 10% of patients with bladder-drained PTXs. Urethral catheter drainage is the mainstay of therapy, with most episodes being self-limited. In severe cases, cystoscopy and clot evacuation with or without cauterization may be required. At times, an ulcer in the duodenal segment or granulation tissue at the suture line may be implicated as a source of bleeding. In cases

of chronic life-threatening hematuria, conversion to enteric drainage may be necessary.

Perforation of the duodenal segment and urinary extravasation occurs nearly as frequently as gross hematuria (4% to 14%) and, if unrecognized, may result in significant morbidity. Most patients present with the sudden onset of lower abdominal pain and hyperamylasemia. A high degree of clinical suspicion is sometimes required because patients may present with only vague abdominal symptoms and fever in the setting of immunosuppression. If a standard cystogram does not demonstrate the leak, a CT scan-cystogram or radionuclide voiding cystourethrogram can be helpful in confirming the presence of a perforation. Duodenal segment leaks may occur early or late, with early cases usually due to technical causes or ischemia and late cases due to rejection or infection. Treatment is usually by direct open repair, although some small leaks can be managed nonoperatively with prolonged urethral catheter drainage. In some cases, an enteric conversion can be performed for duodenal or anastomotic leaks, particularly if recurrent or if associated with significant duodenal segment pathology.

Vascular Complications

In addition to urologic and exocrine complications, PTX is associated with other operative complications inherent to the procedure. Pancreas allografts are prone to vascular problems because the arterial blood supply is based on collateral flow. Vascular complications include hemorrhage, thrombosis, stenosis, pseudoaneurysm formation, and arteriovenous fistulas. Complications may involve the reconstructed vascular supply to the pancreas, the intrinsic blood supply, or the recipient's native vessels. Clinical presentation is variable, but usually includes allograft dysfunction. Diagnosis is usually confirmed by duplex ultrasonography and/or angiography. Arterial or venous thrombosis is a dreaded complication after PTX because it almost always results in allograft pancreatectomy. Patients usually present with the new onset of abdominal pain, acute hyperglycemia, hematuria, and a dramatic reduction in urine amylase levels. The incidence of thrombosis is about three times higher after solitary PTX.

Mycotic pseudoaneurysm is another dreaded complication that usually results in allograft pancreatectomy. Infection of the vascular supply to the pancreas allograft may occur during the donor operation, preservation, bench reconstruction, or result from an endogenous source of contamination in the recipient. Patients usually present with fever and positive blood cultures in association with other signs or symptoms such as a pulse deficit, tender or pulsatile mass, ipsilateral venous thrombosis, hematuria, or rupture with intraabdominal hemorrhage and shock. In addition to allograft pancreatectomy, vascular reconstruction is usually required because the infectious process involves the native circulation. Vascular complications are an important source of morbidity in PTX recipients, ranging in incidence from 10% to 20%. Early diagnosis is critical to graft survival, but prompt surgical intervention may still result in a high (50%) rate of graft loss. Although vascular complications are associated with reduced pancreas allograft survival, they are rarely a cause of mortality.

Infection

Infection following pancreas transplantation is common. Most early infectious complications relate to the transplant procedure itself and the type of drainage employed for pancreatic exocrine secretions. Intra-abdominal infection is the most feared complication and most frequently is associated with postoperative transplant pancreatitis or leak from the duodenal-vesical or enteric anastomosis. Abdominal pain, fever, leukocytosis or prolonged ileus following pancreas transplantation should be evaluated with a CT scan to look for intraabdominal or peripancreatic fluid collections. When present, percutaneous drainage or surgical drainage is indicated to ascertain the etiology of the infection. Infection associated with posttransplant pancreatitis is usually associated with a single organism and high serum amylase in the infected fluid. A leak from the duodenal-vesical anastomosis can be diagnosed with a cystogram using standard radiographic contrast or DTPA (diethylenetriaminepentaacetic acid) and nuclear scanning. Infections following an enteric anastomosis are often polymicrobial with a high serum amylase in the fluid. The character of the fluid suggests an enteric leak when it has the appearance of small-bowel contents. Recent data suggests that the overall incidence of a leak from enteric drainage is less frequent than leak from a bladder-drained pancreas transplant, but is more often associated with loss of the pancreas transplants.

Pancreas transplantation is associated with a higher rate of rejection and more use of antilymphocyte therapies for induction and the treatment of rejection. For this reason, the incidence of opportunistic infection, especially CMV, is higher in pancreas transplant recipients. Aggressive prophylaxis strategies with ganciclovir have been employed to decrease the incidence and severity of CMV infection. Interestingly, the overall incidence of posttransplant lymphoproliferative disease is not higher in pancreas transplant recipients.

The most common long-term infectious complication in pancreas transplant recipients is urinary tract infection, particularly for bladder-drained pancreas transplants. The drainage of pancreatic exocrine secretions into the bladder can predispose patients to recurrent urinary tract infections that can lead to resistant organisms. Chronic or recurrent urinary tract infections

may require enteric conversion to eradicate the infection. One of the major advantages of primary enteric drainage is a dramatic reduction in the overall incidence of infection, particularly urinary tract infection.

Other Complications

The benefits of PTX must be weighed against the morbidity associated with the operative procedure and long-term immunosuppression. Most centers report an operative complication rate of 20% to 30% after PTX related to vascular problems, urologic problems, problems related to exocrine pancreatic drainage and allograft pancreatitis, wound or infectious problems, and miscellaneous problems. Placement of an intraperitoneal PTX can be associated with general surgical complications, such as small bowel obstruction, cholecystitis, and superficial or deep wound infections. With longer follow-up, the incidence of cholelithiasis after PTX may exceed 30%. In the setting of symptoms or biliary complications, laparoscopic or open cholecystectomy can be performed in these patients with minimal morbidity. Similar to other immunosuppressed transplant recipients, PTX patients are at risk not only for bacterial but also opportunistic infections due to viruses (particularly cytomegalovirus), fungi (especially *Candida* species) and *Pneumocystis* species. Postoperative management should include prophylactic regimens specifically directed against these otherwise unusual infections.

BENEFITS OF PANCREAS TRANSPLANTATION

In addition to correcting dysmetabolism and freeing the patient from exogenous insulin therapy, data on the course of secondary complications after PTX is emerging. Because of the lack of randomized controlled trials, the effects of PTX on secondary diabetic complications has been somewhat difficult to ascertain. However, several comparative trials have examined the effects of SPKT over KTA and have shown improvement in some of the secondary complications. The major benefit of PTX is an enhanced quality of life. Freedom from daily insulin injections and blood glucose monitoring is a major benefit for patients with a successful PTX. Although the long-term commitment to immunosuppression is the major trade-off, most diabetic patients find the transition to transplantation easier because of the freedom from continued insulin therapy, and an improved sense of well-being with fewer dietary and activity restrictions.

PTX does not appear to alter established severe retinopathy, but in some studies of longer duration (four years or more), successful PTX is associated with stabilization of retinopathy, more than that observed in other patient groups. Both prospective and cross-sectional studies have suggested that PTX prevents the recurrence of diabetic nephropathy in a newly transplanted kidney. Whether early intervention with solitary PTX can prevent progression of native diabetic nephropathy to complete renal failure is unknown at this time. A number of studies have reported improvements in both motor and sensory nerve function as assessed by nerve conduction velocity in SPKT recipients compared both to diabetic patients receiving a KTA or after pancreas graft failure. Studies of autonomic function following PTX are less clear. However, in some studies, PTX was associated with greater improvements in autonomic symptoms, even if they were accompanied by little objective evidence of change. A report of decreased mortality following PTX in patients with autonomic neuropathy is intriguing, and other studies have reported improvements both in gastric and cardiac function with successful PTX.

Events associated with atherosclerotic vascular disease are among the most common cause of morbidity and mortality following solid organ transplantation, particularly in IDDM patients. Several groups have studied the effects of PTX on lipids and have shown that SPKT recipients have an increased HDL-cholesterol and decreased triglyceride and cholesterol-HDL ratio. Resolution of renal failure and possibly improved sex steroid secretion in women both contribute to these changes, but improved insulin delivery is also important, since PTX appears to ablate the hyperlipidemic effects of immunosuppression. Changes in weight, exercise, hypertension, and diet following PTX have been incompletely studied. An important area currently being examined is the effect of PTX on microvascular disease. Although there is some evidence for increased blood flow to the microvasculature, whether successful PTX alters cardiovascular events or mortality requires further study and longer follow-up.

SURVIVAL

Recipients of SPK transplants have significantly better graft survival than diabetics receiving a kidney alone. Selection criteria and the quality of the organs likely account for some of the difference. Studies of the contralateral kidney of SPK donors also have had better long-term graft survival. Recent studies have also suggested an improved patient survival of SPK recipients over diabetic kidney transplant recipients. According to life-table analysis, diabetic recipients attain more of their projected life-expectancy when transplanted with both a kidney and pancreas transplant.

SUMMARY

Vascularized PTX has assumed an increasingly important role in the treatment of insulin-dependent diabetes mellitus (IDDM). SPKT is gaining acceptance as a viable alternative to KTA in diabetic transplant recipients because of its ability to provide superior glycemic control and an improved quality of life. Although morbidity is still higher after SPKT compared to KTA, most complications are easily managed and the addition of the PTX does not appear to jeopardize either the patient or the kidney transplant, since many centers report comparable survival rates. The most common complication, rejection, does not appear to adversely influence long-term kidney graft survival compared to KTA in diabetic recipients. The greater morbidity of SPKT can be justified by the evidence that a pancreas graft will prevent recurrent diabetic nephropathy, result in greater improvements in motor and sensory neuropathy, and in some but not all studies, provide greater stabilization of eye disease. Improvements in lipid profiles observed after SPKT may predict better cardiovascular outcomes as well.

Indications for solitary PTX are less clearly defined and are based on the presence of early diabetic complications or hyperlability with poor quality of life. Success rates are lower compared with SPKT. At present, the type of transplant being considered has a strong influence on patient and physician acceptance. Although PTX results in euglycemia and complete insulin independence, this occurs at the expense of hyperinsulinemia and chronic immunosuppression. The net result of these changes on diabetic complications in the long-term remains to be determined. In the short-term, improvement in the quality of life and possible prevention of further morbidity associated with diabetes makes PTX an important therapeutic option for selected diabetic patients.

In the future, advances in immunosuppressive strategies and diagnostic technology will only enhance the already good results achieved with PTX. Further documentation of the long-term benefits and effects of PTX may lead to wider availability and acceptance, particularly from a reimbursement standpoint. Effective control of rejection with earlier diagnosis or better prevention may soon permit solitary PTX to become an accepted treatment option in diabetic patients without advanced complications. Although there is significant associated morbidity unique to the PTX, this is usually manageable without influencing the outcome. PTX will remain an important option in the treatment of IDDM until other strategies are developed that can provide equal glycemic control with less or no immunosuppression or less overall morbidity.

RECOMMENDED READING

Drachenberg CB, Papadimitriou JC, Klassen DK, et al. Evaluation of pancreas transplant needle biopsy: reproducibility and revision of histologic grading system. Transplantation. 1997;63(11):1579-1586.

This series examines a number of histologic features found in a large number of pancreas transplant needle biopsies and proposes a grading system for pancreas transplant histology.

Gruessner AC, Sutherland DER. Analysis of United States (US) and non-US pancreas transplants as reported to the International Pancreas Transplant Registry (IPTR) and to the United Network for Organ Sharing (UNOS). In: JM Cecka JM, PI Terasaki, eds. Clinical Transplants 1998. Los Angeles, Ca: UCLA Tissue Typing Laboratory; 1999: 53-71.

Latest update of UNOS data from the International Pancreas Transplant Registry.

Pirsch JD, Odorico JS, D'Alessandro AM, Knechtle SJ, Becker BN, Sollinger HW. Posttransplant infection in enteric versus bladder-drained simultaneous pancreas-kidney transplant recipients. Transplantation. 1998;66(12):1746-1750.

A single-center analysis of infectious complications in enteric- versus bladder-drained simultaneous pancreas-kidney transplant recipients demonstrating a significantly lower incidence of overall infection with enteric drainage.

Sollinger HW, Odorico JS, Knechtle SJ, D'Alessandro AM, Kalayoglu M, Pirsch JD. Experience with 500 simultaneous pancreas-kidney transplants. Ann Surg. 1998;228(3):284-296.

This series represents the world's largest experience with SPK and bladder drainage and is a comprehensive review of both surgical and medical complications following simultaneous kidney-pancreas transplantation.

Sollinger HW, Messing EM, Eckhoff DE, et al. Urological complications in 210 consecutive simultaneous pancreas-kidney transplants with bladder drainage. Ann Surg. 1993;218(4):561-568.

A large experience with urologic complications in SPKT recipients with bladder drainage.

Stratta RJ, Taylor RJ, Larsen JL, Cushing K. Pancreas transplantation. Int J Pancreatol. 1995;17(1):1-13.

A recent "state of the art" review on the benefits, risks, and consequences of pancreas transplantation.

Stratta RJ, Taylor RJ, Wahl TO, et al. Recipient selection and evaluation for vascularized pancreas transplantation. Transplantation. 1993;55(5):1090-1096.

A single center report discussing indications, patient selection, and evaluation for the different types of pancreas transplants.

Smets YF, Westendorp RG, van der Pijl JW, et al. Effect of simultaneous pancreas-kidney transplantation on mortality of patients with type-1 diabetes mellitus and end-stage renal failure. Lancet. 1999;353(9168):1915-1919.

Tydén G, Bolinder J, Solders G, Brattström C, Tibell A, Groth CG. Improved survival in patients with insulin-dependent diabetes mellitus and end-stage diabetic nephropathy ten years after combined pancreas and kidney transplantation. Transplantation. 1999;67(5): 645-648.

These two studies show the striking benefit in both patient and graft survival for simultaneous pancreas-kidney transplant recipients.

64 PANCREATIC ISLET CELL TRANSPLANTATION

Bernhard J. Hering, MD
Camillo Ricordi, MD
David Sutherland, MD, PhD
Jeffrey A. Bluestone, PhD

Diabetes mellitus affects 16 million people in the US, including one million patients with type 1 diabetes, and continues to be a therapeutic challenge. More than 14% of US health care dollars are spent on diabetes, a total of $122 billion in 1994 alone. Yet, diabetes remains the fourth leading cause of death by disease and the leading cause of blindness, kidney failure, and nontraumatic amputations.

The principal risk-factor for the devastating complications of diabetes is the total lifetime exposure to elevated blood glucose. Therefore, establishing safe and effective methods of achieving and maintaining normoglycemia will have substantial implications for the health and quality of life of individuals with diabetes. Intensive insulin treatment does not achieve normal levels of blood glucose, is labor intensive, difficult to implement for many patients, and is limited by the accompanying increased frequency of severe hypoglycemia. Pancreas transplantation is currently the only treatment of type 1 diabetes that routinely achieves both sustained normoglycemia and insulin-independence.

Despite the tremendous impact pancreas transplantation has on the life of recipients, much of current research efforts are focused on islet cell transplantation. This alternative procedure has even greater potential: First, islet transplantation is a minimally invasive procedure; second, unique options exist for tolerance induction because islet cells can be pretreated in culture (eg, gene transfer), transplanted to immunoprivileged sites, and transplanted days to weeks after recipient pretreatment with donor antigen; third, donor tissue avail-

Bernhard J. Hering, MD, Assistant Professor of Surgery and Medicine, University of Minnesota, Minneapolis, MN

Camillo Ricordi, MD, Professor of Surgery and Medicine, University of Miami, Miami, FL

David Sutherland, MD, PhD, Professor of Surgery, University of Minnesota, Minneapolis, MN

Jeffrey A. Bluestone, PhD, A.W. and Mary Margaret Claussen Distinguished Professor; Director, UCSF Diabetes Center, University of California at San Francisco, San Francisco, CA

ability could become unlimited with in vitro islet cell expansion, genetically-engineered cell lines, and xenogeneic islets. Finally, avoiding surgical complications and circumventing the need for chronic immunosuppressive therapy would greatly lower costs and increase the applicability of transplantation therapy.

Taken together, the potential for wide-spread application of islet cell transplantation for the treatment of diabetes is significant. The challenge is to capitalize on the extraordinary opportunities now available in the areas of cell biology and transplantation immunology and to translate unparalleled research achievements into practical benefits for people afflicted with diabetes.

PAST OBSTACLES TO SUCCESS

Clinical data indicate that insulin-independence can be achieved and maintained in approximately 80% of totally pancreatectomized autograft and single-donor allograft recipients and in up to 100% of immunosuppressed type 1 diabetic islet multi-donor allograft recipients. The inferior outcome in the single-donor islet allotransplantation has been attributed to three obstacles unique to the setting of islet allotransplantation in type 1 diabetic recipients.

First, during preparation, islets encounter serious cellular stresses including hypoxia, shear forces, growth factor deprivation, and disruption of cell matrix interactions which lead to imbalances in MAP kinase signaling and activation of proapoptotic effectors. As a cellular, primarily avascular graft, islets are exquisitely susceptible to proinflammatory mediators. They also have a finite potential to repair injury, and are directly exposed to beta cell-toxic proinflammatory cytokines, nitric oxide, and reactive oxygen intermediates generated as part of a nonspecific inflammatory response. While a critical mass of autologous islets required to maintain an insulin-independent state survives this early innate immune response, clinical observations strongly suggest that a smaller and insufficient proportion of allogeneic islets function and engraft in an environment of destructive, islet-directed autoimmunity. It is hypothesized that the magnitude of alloantigen-independent inflammatory responses and the associated generation of inflammatory mediators and expression of cellular adhesion molecules are greatly augmented in recipients with persistent autoimmunity.

Second, several lines of evidence now suggest that destructive anti-islet autoimmunity constitutes a major barrier to success in clinical islet transplantation. Syngeneic islet beta cells transplanted to spontaneously diabetic BB rats or NOD mice are rapidly destroyed by a persistent autoimmune response which has been found to be resistant to immunosuppressive drugs. Along these lines, cyclosporine (CsA) failed to protect intraportal islet transplants from recurrent autoimmunity. Notably, whole pancreas isografts are protected from recurrent autoimmunity in CsA-treated spontaneously diabetic BB recipients. It is now becoming appreciated that this protection is functionally related to the inclusion of a significant quantity of lymphoid tissue (possibly containing an immunoregulatory T cell subset) as part of the pancreas graft and not to immunosuppression alone. Clinical evidence also indicates that destructive anti-islet autoimmunity persists for decades after manifestation of type 1 diabetes and that type 1 diabetic individuals with long disease duration do not spontaneously anergize their autoreactive effector Th1 cells and/or restore Th2 or other regulatory T cell function. Accordingly, reprogramming the recipient's immune system seems to be of paramount importance if autoimmune recurrence in transplanted islets is to be prevented.

Third, although the immunosuppressive regimens currently used to ensure allograft acceptance are effective, their diabetogenic effects are particularly deleterious in the situation of reduced beta cell mass, contributing to the historically poor success rate of graft function. The combination of calcineurin-inhibitors and prednisone is associated with the development of an insulin-dependent diabetic state in up to 25% of non-diabetic kidney transplant recipients. To maintain normoglycemia, immunosuppressed nondiabetic kidney transplant recipients must increase insulin secretion 2.5 times. Even when systemic drug levels are carefully controlled, intraportally-transplanted islets bathed in portal blood are exposed to higher and potentially toxic local concentrations of orally administered immunosuppressive drugs. This may not matter when there is a normal beta cell mass, as with a whole pancreas transplant. The limited mass of engrafted islet beta cells, however, is inadequate to restore insulin independence in the presence of impaired insulin secretion, calcineurin inhibitors, and corticosteroids.

FUTURE DIRECTIONS

Islet transplant protocols that mitigate early inflammation, restore self-tolerance, and induce donor-specific allotolerance will be most likely to succeed. Clinical evaluation of selective immunomodulatory therapies is justifiable in the setting of solitary islet transplantation because: (1) islet autografts are consistently successful; (2) the procedural risk of islet transplantation is minimal; (3) graft failure is not life-threatening; (4) islet grafts in conjunction with diabetogenic immunosuppressive therapy have been largely unsuccessful; and (5) perhaps most importantly, tolerogenic protocols have shown promise in preclinical NOD mice and nonhuman primate (NHP) islet transplant models. Taken together, in contrast to kidney transplantation, islet transplantation provides a unique opportunity to test tolerogenic proto-

cols in the absence of standard immunosuppressive drugs, which are known to interfere with the induction of tolerance.

Unparalleled progress made over the past few years in understanding the mechanisms operative in the induction of allotolerance and restoration of self-tolerance has led to the development of unique and selective immunomodulatory strategies. Prime examples of progress include: (1) the demonstration of long-term islet allograft survival in NHPs receiving anti-CD154 antibody monotherapy; (2) the induction of robust tolerance to murine islet allografts by allo-antigen pretreatment under the cover of short-term anti-CD154 therapy; and (3) the restoration of self-tolerance to beta cell autoantigens in overtly diabetic NOD mice by partial TCR-signaling mediated cytokine deviation and selective inhibition of the inflammatory subset of primed autoreactive effector T cells. Moreover, selective costimulatory blockade and partial TCR signaling may counteract innate immunity and established autoimmunity. This may, in turn, diminish alloantigen-independent cell loss, maximize engraftment and functional survival of transplanted islets, lessen the incidence and severity of acute cellular rejection, and foster the environment necessary for the induction of tolerance. These accomplishments signal a quantum leap in our approaches to circumvent islet graft failure due to nonspecific inflammation, autoimmune destruction, and rejection; they now provide realistic opportunities for major advances in clinical islet transplantation.

TOLERANCE INDUCTION STRATEGIES

Proposed areas of emphasis need to include strategies both for the induction of donor-specific allotolerance and restoration of self-tolerance. Particular attention should be paid to non-diabetogenic protocols targeting signal 1, signal 2, and clonal inactivation/deletion.

Targeting Signal 1

NONDEPLETING ANTI-CD4 ANTIBODIES. Treatment with monoclonal anti-CD4 antibodies can generate a tolerogenic environment for the development of specific unresponsiveness to alloantigens in murine transplant models and reprogram the immune system towards restoration of operational self-tolerance in murine models of autoimmune diabetes. Combined pretreatment with donor alloantigen in the form of donor-specific transfusion (DST) and a single dose of nondepleting anti-CD4 antibody, induced donor-specific tolerance to mouse heart allografts and to rat heart and kidney allografts, provided that a critical period of time was allowed between pretreatment and transplantation. Results of experiments in rodents indicate that the specific type of antibody used is of critical importance, and a short course of treatment with a non-depleting anti-CD4 antibody obviates the need for alloantigen pretreatment in rat islet, skin, and kidney allograft models. The potential applicability of a short peritransplant course of nondepleting anti-CD4 immunotherapy in type 1 diabetic islet allograft recipients is highlighted by the induction of robust tolerance to MHC-incompatible allografts in nondepleting CD4 monoclonal antibody-treated sensitized recipients (ie, in the presence of an ongoing immune response) of rat heart allografts. Interestingly, the same antibody (RIB/5-2) prevented autoimmune but not allogeneic islet

destruction in spontaneously diabetic BB/OK rats. Translation of selective immunotherapy based on non-depleting anti-CD4 antibodies to the clinical setting of islet transplantation seems possible, provided a suitable antibody can be developed and results of rodent studies can be confirmed in a NHP islet allotransplant model. Pending the definition of the precise regimen (ie, type, timing and dosing of antibody and alloantigen) in a NHP model, clinical evaluation of the elaborated protocol could be initiated in totally pancreatectomized islet allograft recipients, ie in immunologically naive recipients in the absence of autoimmunity. Pending demon-

Table 64-1. Candidate Tolerance Induction Strategies in Islet Transplantation

Approach	Elements
Peripheral Nondeletional Approach	1. Donor antigen infusion under cover of either nondepleting anti-CD4 or anti-CD154 antibodies. 2. Short-term course of FcR-nonbinding anti-CD3 antibodies or rapamycin.
Central Deletional Approach	1. High-dose donor bone marrow under cover of anti-CD154 antibodies. 2. Costimulatory blockade with CTLA4-Ig.
Local Inflammatory Approach	Generation of an immunoprivileged environment by transplantation of anti-transfected islets or co-transplantation of testicular cell aggregates or bystander cells engineered to express/secrete immunoregulatory p molecules.

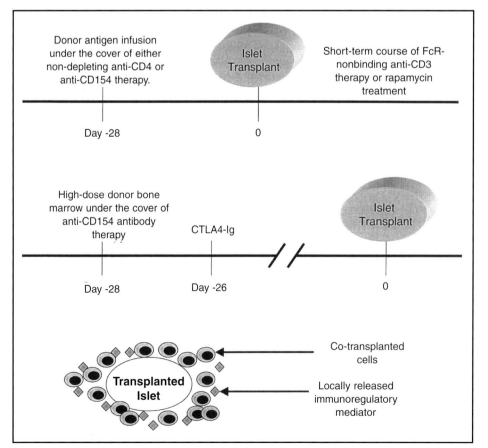

Figure 64-1. Candidate tolerance induction strategies in islet transplantation. Peripheral nondeletional approach (upper panel) based on donor antigen pretreatment under the cover of short-term coreceptor or costimulatory blockade and partial TCR-signaling or rapamycin immunotherapy at the time of islet implantation. Central deletional approach (middle panel) based on the pretransplant establishment of hematopoietic mixed chimerism via high-dose donor bone marrow/hematopoietic stem cell infusion under the cover of combined costimulatory blockade. Local immunotherapy approach (lower panel) based on the generation of an immunoprivileged environment by transfection of transplanted islets or co-transplantation of testicular cell aggregates or bystander cells engineered to express/secrete immunoregulatory molecules.

stration of safety and operational tolerance in non-autoimmune recipients, clinical evaluation could be extended to type 1 diabetic recipients.

FcR NONBINDING ANTI-CD3 ANTIBODIES. Immunotherapy strategies that tolerize autoreactive effector T cells and/or restore immunoregulatory T cell function in recipients with persistent anti-islet autoimmunity are critical to success in type 1 diabetic islet transplant recipients. The autoimmune process in NOD mice can be prevented by a number of immunomodulatory interventions early in the ontogeny of the immune system, before or shortly after the appearance of extensive islet infiltration. Conversely, it has proven much more difficult to arrest established autoimmune disease and restore self-tolerance. A genetically engineered FcR nonbinding form of antimurine and antihuman CD3 mAbs can induce selective immunomodulation without the toxicity associated with conventional anti-CD3 mAb therapy. FcR nonbinding anti-CD3 Abs have short-lived effects on naive T cells, but deliver a partial signal in activated T cells resulting in clonal inactivation of Th1 cells and proliferation/cytokine production by Th2 cells. These selective effects make these new agents particularly useful for targeting the imbalance of autoreactive Th1 cells and immunoregulatory T cells that mediate autoimmune diabetes. Remarkably, short-term treatment with low doses of the anti-CD3 mAb, 145-2C11, restored self-tolerance to beta cell-associated antigens in overtly diabetic NOD mice and protected subsequent islet isografts from autoimmune destruction. The ability to induce tolerance in the face of an ongoing immune response is unparalleled. The humanized FcR non-binding anti-CD3 mAb hOKT3$_\gamma$1 (Ala-Ala), a genetically engineered derivative of the parental murine OKT3 mAb, has proven safe and effective in the clinical setting, as demonstrated by prompt reversal of vigorous rejection episodes in kidney and kidney-pancreas recipients and clinical improvement in patients with psoriatic arthritis, each in the absence of first dose reaction. Clinical evaluation has now been expanded to Phase I trials into patients with new onset type 1 diabetes. Collectively, these results highlight the accumulated evidence that the FcR nonbinding hOKT3$_\gamma$1 (Ala-Ala)-mAb provides an unprecedented opportunity for restoring self-tolerance (and possibly inducing allotolerance) in the setting of islet transplantation for patients with type 1 diabetes. To prevent allorejection, hOKT3$_\gamma$1 (Ala-Ala) must be combined with a suitable complementary agent with therapeutic compatibility and efficacy in preventing allorejection. Promising agents for nondiabetogenic combination therapy with the FcR nonbinding anti-CD3 mAb are the cell cycle progression inhibitor rapamycin, anti-CD154-specific mAbs, and CD28 antagonists (anti-CD80/anti-CD86 mAbs).

ANTI-CD45RB ANTIBODIES. CD45 is a potent immunotherapeutic target that may act through distinct mechanisms that include alteration of CD45 isoform expression, modulation of regulatory T cell subsets and upregulation of CTLA-4. CD45RB$^{Hi)}$ CD4 cells have been shown to preferentially secrete IL-2. Transient recipient treatment with anti-CD45RB results in a low molecular weight isoform, with a prevalence of CD45RB$^{(Lo)}$ CD4 cells that preferentially secrete IL-4. Recent studies demonstrated that the low molecular weight isoform switch that follows anti-CD45RB treatment, is also associated with up-regulation of CTLA-4. The induction of CTLA-4 was recently shown to be potentially important in donor-specific tolerance induction. CTLA-4 signaling could be required for down regulation of already activated T cells, and may also be a critical regulator of resting memory CD4 T cells.

Targeting Signal 2
ANTI-CD154 ANTIBODIES. Blockade of the CD154:CD40 costimulatory pathway represents a powerful treatment option for prevention of islet allograft failures in patients with type 1 diabetes. Anti-CD154 monoclonal antibody therapy has been shown to be effective for prevention of rejection, autoimmunity (timing of treatment is critical), and inflammatory events, all of which are thought to contribute to the poor outcome of clinical islet cell transplants. Studies in NHPs support this notion. Blockade of the CD40-CD154 T lymphocyte costimulatory pathway in NHP recipients of allogeneic islets allowed for (1) successful engraftment, (2) long-term maintenance of function, and (3) preservation of islet mass at levels comparable to prepancreatectomy. Of note, monkeys treated with anti-CD154 are maintaining renal allograft function for months after discontinuation of therapy, with no evidence of rejection. However, donor-specific tolerance has not yet been demonstrated. The mechanism(s) responsible for the encouraging results obtained in both the renal and islet allograft models have not been clearly delineated. However, a loss of donor-specific MLC reactivity, with maintenance of anti-third party responsiveness, has been demonstrated in both models. There are strong preliminary results indicating that anti-CD154 treatment of NOD mice receiving an islet allograft after the onset of diabetes, significantly prolonged islet allograft survival with a mean survival time of 58 days in the treatment group vs nine days in the control group (*P* <0.001). Interestingly, these results were obtained only with a 20 mg/kg dose, identical to what was successfully used in the NHP studies and to the dose proposed for clinical trials. Lower doses had marginal effect on diabetes recurrence. Carefully designed clinical trials will have to clarify whether anti-CD154 therapy also protects allogeneic human islets from autoimmune

destruction. The addition of anti-CD80/anti-CD86 could further enhance islet allograft survival and induction of donor-specific unresponsiveness. The combination of anti-CD80/anti-CD86 and anti-CD154 consistently prevented anti-donor antibody production in NHP recipients of kidney allografts. Although antibodies blocking costimulation are attractive clinical immunotherapeutic agents, additional therapies to control aggressive CD8[+] T cell responses may be required to induce tolerance. Alternatively, a short course of anti-CD45RB antibody therapy may represent another option for combination therapy with costimulatory blockade strategies.

CD28 ANTAGONISTS. Short-term anti-CD86 and CTLA4Ig therapy induced prolonged C3H islet allograft survival in B6 mice. Trials with humanized anti-CD80/anti-CD86 therapy have been initiated in a primate model of islet allotransplantation. These primate studies will be extended and CD80/CD86 mAbs will be administered in combination with rapamycin to support the clinical trials. Issues such as an appropriate initial dosing strategy (both level and duration), the probable need for and nature of ancillary treatment are currently addressed in the primate model.

COMBINATION OF COSTIMULATORY BLOCKADE AND DONOR HEMATOPOIETIC CELL INFUSION. Early studies of CTLA4-Ig fusion protein in experimental transplantation indicated that CTLA4-Ig promoted graft survival more efficiently if combined with exposure to alloantigen by DST. Administration of CTLA4-Ig by itself was insufficient to prevent heart allograft rejection, but when combined with DST, all animals had long-term graft survival and accepted donor-matched second cardiac allografts. In addition, donor antigen was found to be necessary for the prevention of chronic rejection in CTLA4-Ig treated murine cardiac allograft recipients. The synergistic effect of DST was subsequently confirmed in anti-CD154-treated recipients. A single dose of anti-CD154 at the time of transplantation was able to induce long-term survival of vascularized cardiac allografts in 70% of murine recipients. The addition of DST led to indefinite survival in all animals. Anti-CD154 antibody therapy administered for two to seven weeks combined with DST blocked the rejection of murine islet allografts, although tolerance was not demonstrated. Using this approach, long-term skin allograft survival in NHPs (>225 days and still ongoing) has been achieved. However, anti-CD154 mAb plus DST treatment failed to prolong islet and skin allograft survival in spontaneously diabetic female and non-diabetic male NOD mice, respectively, suggesting the existence of a general defect in tolerance mechanisms in NOD mice. Rapamycin synergizes with DST plus anti-CD154 to block autoimmune and alloimmune responses to transplanted islets, thus permitting prolonged islet allograft survival in spontaneously diabetic NOD recipients. The type, dose, route and timing of donor hematopoietic cell infusion and the precise regimen of costimulatory blockade and concomitant rapamycin therapy most appropriate for induction of allotolerance, as well as the underlying mechanism, remain to be identified in NHP studies. Whether or not the ultimate protocol also confers protection from autoimmune destruction of transplanted islets will need to be addressed in carefully designed clinical trials.

Targeting Clonal Inactivation or Deletion
MIXED CHIMERISM WITHOUT MYELOABLATION. Treatment of mice with single injections of an anti-CD154 mAb and CTLA4Ig, a low dose of whole body irradiation, plus fully major mismatched allogeneic bone marrow transplantation reliably induced extrathymic donor-reactive host T cell deletion, high levels of stable multilineage chimerism, followed by central T cell tolerance. Recent findings indicate that high-dose bone marrow infusion completely eliminated the need for low-dose total body irradiation. It is therefore conceivable that an appropriate combination therapy of donor hematopoietic cell infusion and costimulatory blockade may substantially reduce or completely eliminate the need for recipient radiation conditioning. This non-myeloablative, clinically applicable approach would not only provide thymo-deletional tolerance, it should also abrogate defective negative intrathymic selection and thereby help correct the imbalance of autoreactive and immunoregulatory T cells in recipients with type 1 diabetes. Experimental studies in NOD mice support this notion. Mixed allogeneic reconstitution protected transplanted islet tissue from recurrent autoimmunity and rejection in previously diabetic NOD recipient mice are effective in preventing islet isograft destruction in diabetic NOD mice. Protection against autoimmune diabetes in mixed bone marrow chimeras may, however, require high levels of chimerism (eg, >25%).

Other/Concomitant Immunotherapeutic Approaches
TRANSIENT T CELL DEPLETION. The majority of successful islet allografts in patients with type 1 diabetes have required an induction course with antithymocyte globulin (ATG)/antilymphocyte globulin (ALG) at the time of, or before islet transplantation. One of the possible mechanisms for the facilitatory effect of ATG on islet graft survival is that it possesses numerous specificities for cell lineages including macrophages, B lymphocytes and memory T lymphocytes. Targeting these cells might be required to prevent inflammatory events and recurrence of both cellular and humoral autoimmunity.

In addition, the use of ATG in combination with costimulatory blockade could enhance engraftment of donor marrow cells at levels that will drive the immune system towards a state of donor-specific tolerance. The use of a depleting agent may also bias the immune system towards tolerance by reducing the number of mature T cells and allowing for reeducation and/or deletion of newly emerging donor-specific T cells. This could be important also in view of recent experimental evidence suggesting that the level of chimerism necessary to prevent recurrence of autoimmunity may be higher than what may be sufficient to induce tolerance in a non-autoimmune allograft setting.

Alternatively, the use of a short course of the anti-CD3-specific immunotoxin (IT) could be potentially administered in place of ATG. A short course of anti-CD3-IT was very effective in allowing long-term survival of intrahepatic islet grafts in three of three monkeys, suggesting that this agent could be of assistance to induce operational tolerance following islet transplantation. It has been postulated that the encouraging results may be related to the transient but intense CD3- depleting effect of the treatment, not only on circulating CD3-positive cells, but also on tissue CD3-positive cells (unlike ATG). If these results are confirmed in additional NHP studies, this strategy could be tested as a potential alternative to ATG.

INTRATHYMIC INJECTION OF ANTIGEN. This central deletional tolerance induction approach, based on intrathymic injection of cellular alloantigen combined with depletion of preexisting alloreactive peripheral T cells was first applied to experimental models of islet transplantation in chemically diabetic rodents, and subsequently extended to spontaneously diabetic rodents and experimental models of skin, heart, liver, and kidney transplantation.

ANTI-INTERLEUKIN-2 RECEPTOR ANTIBODIES. Recipient treatment with anti-interleukin-2 receptor (anti-IL-2R) antibodies (Ab) could represent an alternative strategy to ATG. Also, in this case, the anti-IL-2R Ab could complement costimulatory blockade, since a percentage of T lymphocytes may escape or bypass efficient costimulatory blockade and progress to an activated state. Although high levels of activation would not be expected in the presence of costimulatory blockade, cells which escape blockade, memory cells, and preexisting anti-islet or anti-donor-specific T cells could lead to graft failure. Administration of anti-IL-2R Ab post-antigen administration could specifically target these cells.

ADJUVANT, CYTOKINE AND AUTOANTIGEN-BASED IMMUNOTHERAPIES. Stimulating the host's own immunoregulatory mechanisms may represent an appealing approach to prevent autoimmune mediated islet destruction in recipients with type 1 diabetes. Among the few as yet unmentioned strategies that protected islet isografts from autoimmune destruction in overtly diabetic NOD mice (possibly through the regeneration of immunoregulatory T cells) are adjuvant immunotherapy with complete Freund's adjuvant (CFA), bacillus Calmette-Guerin (BCG), or Q-fever antigen (QFA), combined therapy with IL-4 and IL-10, and GAD65-based immunotherapy.

IMMUNOPRIVILEGED SITES. The fact that islets can be transplanted to immunoprivileged sites provides a unique opportunity for tolerance induction. Immunoprivileged sites may not be limited to classical sites such as the thymus or intraabdominal testes, but may include immunoprivileged environments generated by co-transplantation of testicular cell aggregates or bystander cells engineered to express/secrete immunoregulatory molecules, direct transfection of transplanted islets, or by semipermeable immunobarrier devices, to name a few.

CONCLUSIONS

The next few years will see pilot clinical islet transplant trials evaluating immunotherapeutic strategies designed to induce robust and permanent donor-specific allotolerance as well as restore self-tolerance in recipients of human islet allografts. Combination strategies of multiple agents may prove particularly useful. The field of tolerance induction is rapidly progressing and it is fair to assume that with refined understanding of the mechanisms operative in the induction and maintenance of allotolerance, more sophisticated combination strategies will emerge. The NHP model will continue to be critical in providing crucial information for the rational design of clinical trials. In view of the efficacy of novel immunotherapeutic agents noted in NHP models, it seems possible, if not likely, that recent promising preclinical findings in allotransplant models will translate into the clinic. The challenge will be to induce tolerance to alloantigens in the presence of a diverse, islet-directed, autoreactive T cell repertoire. It will be critical to determine the therapeutic compatibility of approaches chosen to target alloimmunity and autoimmunity and to incorporate, as an integral part of the clinical trials, mechanistic studies designed to advance the understanding of the mechanisms underlying induction/restoration and maintenance of tolerance. Mechanistic studies performed in close collaboration with the clinical trials will add considerably to the strength of the clinical trials, as valuable new information will also be generated in the event of graft failure. The information provided would assist in identifying how to correctly use tolerogenic agents available. It is hypothesized that correct use of currently available immunotherapeutic agents will mitigate early inflammatory responses, restore peripheral self-tolerance, and induce donor-specific allotolerance, thereby leading to sustained insulin independence in islet allograft recipients without associated procedural risks and drug toxicity.

RECOMMENDED READING

Shapiro AM, Lakey JR, Ryan EA, et al. Islet transplantation in seven patients with type 1 diabetes mellitus using a glucocorticoid-free immunosuppressive regimen. N Engl J Med. 2000;343(4):230-238.

Kenyon NS, Chatzipetrou M, Masetti M, et al. Long-term survival and function of intrahepatic islet allografts in rhesus monkeys treated with humanized anti-CD154. Proc Natl Acad Sci USA. 1999;96(14):8132-8137.

Rossini AA, Greiner DL, Mordes JP. Induction of immunologic tolerance for transplantation. Physiol Rev. 1999;79(1):99-141.

Smith JA, Bluestone JA. T cell inactivation and cytokine deviation promoted by anti-CD3 mAbs. Curr Opin Immunol. 1997;9(5):648-654.

Thomas FT, Ricordi C, Contreras JL, et al. Reversal of naturally occurring diabetes in primates by unmodified islet xenografts without chronic immunosuppression. Transplantation. 1999;67(6):846-854.

Waldmann H, Cobbold S. How do monoclonal antibodies induce tolerance? A role for infectious tolerance? Ann Rev Immunol. 1998;16:619-644.

Wekerle T, Sykes M. Mixed chimerism as an approach for the induction of transplantation tolerance. Transplantation. 1999;68(4):459-467.

Zheng XX, Markees TG, Hancock WW, et al. CTLA4 signals are required to optimally induce allograft tolerance with combined donor-specific transfusion and anti-CD154 monoclonal antibody treatment. J Immunol. 1999;162(8):4983-4990.

Section VII

LIVER AND INTESTINAL TRANSPLANTATION

65 HISTORICAL OVERVIEW OF LIVER TRANSPLANTATION

Sue V. McDiarmid, MD
Michael R. Lucey, MD, FRCPI

"Orthotopic homotransplantation of the human liver," published in 1968 in the Annals of Surgery by Starzl et al, reported the first case of liver transplantation with extended survival and opened the era of modern liver transplantation. Despite the historic success achieved, the author himself foresaw the struggle ahead. Starzl was later to write:

> "The appalling early mortality after liver transplantation has prompted exhaustive clinical-pathologic analyses…Mortality figures included the use of grafts damaged by ischemia, massive operative hemorrhage, thrombosis of the reconstituted homograft blood supply, intra-operative cerebral embolism, unsuspected recipient abnormalities, hopeless anatomical situations created by multiple previous operations, irreversible pre-existing debilitation and (above all) defective biliary tract regarding reconstruction… [however] the conclusion was reached that even after a perfect operation, the unacceptable acute mortality would remain until improved immunosuppression became available."

Until the first clinical use of cyclosporine in 1979, the intervening years were marked more by the unflagging determination of surgeons to persevere than by impressive survival figures. Adult patient 1-year survivals of only 23% to 27% invited professional censure and recommendations that the procedure should be abandoned. The motivation to persist must surely have come from an all-too-intimate familiarity with the helplessness felt at the bedsides of patients dying inexorably of liver disease.

The advent of cyclosporine vindicated the vision of the early surgical pioneers and proved that rejection had been one of the major barriers to successful liver transplantation. In 1983, the National Institutes of Health

Sue V. McDiarmid, MD, Associate Professor of Pediatrics and Surgery; Director, Pediatric Liver Transplantation, Departments of Pediatrics and Surgery, University of California, Los Angeles Medical Center, Los Angeles, CA

Michael R. Lucey, MD, FRCPI, Professor of Medicine; Associate Chief, Division of Gastroenterology; Director of Hepatology; Medical Director, Liver Transplant Program, University of Pennsylvania, Philadelphia, PA

convened a consensus conference to review the efficacy of liver transplantation. This conference proved to be a watershed for the procedure, and for patients with life-threatening liver failure. The consensus panel concluded that liver transplantation was no longer an experimental procedure, but rather was an appropriate therapy for many patients with serious liver disease. They included patients with previously contentious indications such as alcoholic liver disease, non-A and non-B hepatitis, and hepatic malignancy. As a consequence, the number of centers offering liver transplantation increased throughout North America. At the same time, waiting lists for liver transplantation have grown exponentially, whereas the procurement of donors showed a modest increase only.

Recently in the US, there has been an intense national controversy regarding the distribution and allocation of donor livers. It has proven to be a difficult task to devise a system that strikes a balance between the demands of providing livers to the sickest patients first (who may have a poorer outcome) and the utility of allocating livers to stable patients (who are more likely to survive). To complicate the controversy further, there are geographic differences in donor availability and length of waiting lists. Although a sense of fairness would require that all patients waiting should have equal access and similar waiting times, the practicalities of achieving this goal remain formidable. At the time of writing, the allocation system in the US continues to prioritize donor livers to more urgent patients, at the expense of greater utility of outcome. The cost of favoring the 'sickest first' is unknown, in part because overall survival data have improved despite the 'sickest first' policy.

The allocation of donor livers has relied on two predominant recipient characteristics: severity of liver disease and duration on the waiting list. The determination of severity is confounded by the heterogeneity of liver diseases being treated with liver transplantation. For example, fulminant hepatic failure, liver failure in cirrhosis due to chronic hepatitis or alcoholic liver disease, chronic cholestatic liver disease, and primary hepatocellular carcinoma are four diagnostic categories that require separate instruments to estimate prognosis. This heterogeneity has led to a complicated system of allocation rules with special provisions for specific cases, such as fulminant hepatic failure and hepatocellular carcinoma.

On the other hand, greater consensus has been achieved about rules governing entry to the waiting list: so-called *minimal listing criteria*. While the allocation rules focus on identifying the sickest patients and giving those patients priority, the need for minimal listing criteria stems from the use of waiting time as a factor in allocation donor livers. The minimal criteria focus on distinguishing patients whose liver failure is likely to progress to death from those who can wait safely without risk. The Childs-Turcotte-Pugh classification is the basis of the minimal listing criteria rules for chronic liver disease.

The current success of liver transplantation is reflected in 1-year and 5-year actuarial patient survivals of 87% and 72.3%, respectively, as recorded by the United Network for Organ Sharing (UNOS) database. Short-term causes of graft loss are mostly nonimmunologic; for example, primary nonfunction, hepatic artery thrombosis and multi-organ failure. Chronic rejection, an important cause of long-term graft loss in heart and kidney grafts, is relatively uncommon in liver grafts, with an incidence of less than 10%. The most important cause of long-term liver graft dysfunction is recurrent disease. Although malignancy, autoimmune disease, and primary biliary cirrhosis may all recur in the graft, by far the most important problem is the recurrence of hepatitis C. In many programs, chronic hepatitis C is the indication for transplant in about 50% of adults. With such large numbers of patients transplanted for this indication, the long-term impact of recurrent hepatitis C on both patient and graft survival is yet to be realized. Antiviral treatment for hepatitis C and strategies to prevent histological reoccurrence in the graft have yet to be met with any clear success.

About 50% of recipients will experience at least one episode of acute cellular rejection after liver transplantation. In the past 25 years many immunosuppressive agents have been developed, including cyclosporine, tacrolimus, sirolimus, rapamycin, mycophenolate mofetil, and monoclonal antibodies against lymphocytes or lymphocyte subsets. There remains little consensus on the best immediate or extended immunosuppressive regimens, and each transplant program tends to develop its own local preferred protocols. Calcineurin inhibitors such as cyclosporine or tacrolimus remain the mainstay of immunosuppressive protocols after liver transplantation. At the same time, it has become clear that the toll of acute cellular rejection on the liver allograft is less than that for other solid organ allografts. There appears to be a qualitative distinction between severe acute cellular rejection that is resistant to treatment, and that may progress to chronic ductopenia and graft loss, and mild acute cellular rejection that responds readily to modest adjustments in immunosuppressive management. One of the most striking developments in posttransplant management in the past five years has been the recog-

nition that many patients thrive at lower doses of immunosuppressives than previously used. This has lead to the widespread practice of withdrawing or greatly reducing corticosteroids in many patients in the first year after liver transplantation.

Long-term complications of liver transplantation require further study. The incidence and severity of nephrotoxicity after years of cyclosporine or tacrolimus exposure are not yet fully realized. Of particular importance in pediatric patients will be the effects on long-term growth and development. Other issues will be the ongoing risk of de novo malignancy, cardiovascular and diabetic risk, and the cause of graft loss.

The biggest challenge to the immediate future of liver transplantation is the donor shortage. Xenotransplantation offers exciting new frontiers. Most progress has been made in pediatric liver transplantation with the increased use of living-related donors, reduced-size grafts, and most especially split liver transplantation. Recently, the use of adult to adult living donation has been widely reported, although it poses special ethical questions regarding the risks to the donor. In addition, the societal questions of who will pay for liver transplantation for what diseases and for what expected outcome become increasingly more pertinent as health care costs are scrutinized. The current generation of transplant physicians and surgeons may find their biggest obstacles to providing this life-saving advance to all who require it are no longer surgical and immunologic challenges, but crises in supply of both donors and dollars.

RECOMMENDED READING

Starzl TE, Iwatsuki S, Van Thiel DH, et al. Evolution of liver transplantation. Hepatology. 1982;2(5):614–636.

Anonymous. National Institutes of Health Consensus Development Conference Statement: liver transplantation – June 20-23, 1983. Hepatology. 1984;4(1 Suppl): 107S-110S.

Lucey MR, Brown KA, Everson GT, et al. Minimal criteria for placement of adults on the liver transplant waiting list: a report of a national conference organized by the American Society of Transplant Physicians and the American Association for the Study of Liver Diseases. Liver Transpl Surg. 1997;3(6):628-637.

66 EVALUATION AND MANAGEMENT OF PROSPECTIVE LIVER TRANSPLANT CANDIDATES

John R. Lake, MD

ESTABLISHING THAT A LIVER TRANSPLANT IS NECESSARY
Indications for Orthotopic Liver Transplantation

Most patients undergoing liver transplantation have cirrhosis and are experiencing complications of portal hypertension. The most common etiologies for which orthotopic liver transplantation (OLT) is performed in adults include chronic hepatitis C, alcoholic liver disease (or a combination of the two), chronic hepatitis B, primary biliary cirrhosis (PBC), primary sclerosing cholangitis (PSC) and autoimmune hepatitis. The most common disease indications for liver transplantation in pediatric patients are extrahepatic biliary atresia and α-1-antitrypsin deficiency, accounting for 55% and 6.6% of the pediatric recipients, respectively.

In the past, the most common disease indications for OLT were the cholestatic forms of liver disease. The major change that has occurred in the last decade is the increased number of patients with hepatitis C and alcoholic liver disease now being offered liver transplantation. This largely reflects a maturation of the hepatitis C epidemic that occurred in the late 1960s and the 1970s. In addition, fewer patients receive transplants for malignant disease, although this number is also likely to increase for several reasons. First, cirrhosis caused by chronic hepatitis C is the most important risk factor for hepatocellular carcinoma (HCC). Second, studies that have shown patients with relatively small HCCs do well after liver transplantation. This has been recognized formally by the transplant community by allowing patients with early stage HCC to be listed at a higher priority status.

However, diseases by themselves are generally not the indications for OLT. Rather, it is the complications of these diseases that create the indications for OLT. The complications of chronic liver disease fall in two broad categories. The first are those complications that reflect the presence of portal hypertension. These complications include gastrointestinal bleeding caused either by gastro-esophageal varices or portal hypertensive gas-

tropathy. Fluid retention resulting in either ascites or hepato-hydrothorax is also included. Finally, porto-systemic encephalopathy may either reflect a reduced liver cell mass or shunting of blood flow around the liver related to the presence of portal hypertension. The second class of complications are those that reflect a reduced liver cell mass. These include coagulopathy, jaundice, impaired drug metabolism and as mentioned above, hepatic encephalopathy.

The evaluation of patients for liver transplantation represents team efforts including hepatologists, transplantation surgeons, social workers, and consultants. The initial evaluation involves assessing whether indications for OLT are present. In the past, indications for liver transplantation were discussed in the context of quality of life and severity of disease indications. However, because of the increase in the number of patients referred for OLT and the relative shortage of donor organs, distrust increased among transplant programs, and as a result, standardized listing criteria have been developed. A recent development in this area is the adoption of minimal listing criteria. These minimal listing criteria have largely endorsed the use of the Childs-Turcotte-Pugh score as a reflection of the severity of chronic liver disease (Table 66-1). In order to be placed on the waiting list, one must have sufficient liver dysfunction to rate a Childs-Turcotte-Pugh score of at least seven, which indicates a Childs Class B. Certain complications including refractory variceal bleeding, encephalopathy, ascites, and spontaneous bacterial peritonitis are given appropriate consideration in both listing criteria as well as in the criteria for establishing priority on the

Professor of Medicine and Surgery; Director, Division of Gastroenterology, Hepatology and Nutrition; Director, Liver Transplantation Program, University of Minnesota

Table 66-1. Childs-Turcotte-Pugh Classification

Variable	Points		
	1	2	3
Encephalopathy	None	Moderate	Severe
Ascites	None	Slight	Moderate
Albumin	>3.5	2.8-3.5	<2.8
Prothrombin time (sec. prolonged)	<4	4-6	>6
(INR)	<1.7	1.7-2.3	>2.3
Bilirubin Primary Biliary Cirrhosis/Primary Sclerosing Cholangitis	1-4	4-10	>10
All other diseases	<2	2-3	>3

Scores are summed to determine Childs class: A indicates 5-6; B,7-9; C,10-15.

waiting list. Patients with unusual indications including pruritus, metabolic bone disease, and xanthomatous neuropathy (seen in cholestatic diseases), representing impaired quality of life must be approved by regional review boards to be listed for OLT. Examples are listed below.

Fatigue is likely one of the more troublesome quality-of-life indications due to the difficulty in differentiating it from depression, which is common in people with chronic disease.

Several quality-of-life indications are unique to patients with cholestatic liver disease (ie, primary biliary cirrhosis, primary sclerosing cholangitis, and extrahepatic biliary atresia). The most common of these is intractable pruritus. Many patients with cholestatic liver disease develop pruritus that fails to respond to medical therapy, including ursodeoxycholic acid and rifampicin. These patients are also at risk for metabolic bone disease, which can lead to fractures prior to development of advanced liver disease. Liver transplantation is the only therapy that has been shown to increase bone mineralization in such patients. OLT is also effective therapy for xanthomatous neuropathy, a rare but disabling complication that can occur in patients with cholestatic liver disease.

With the marked improvement in patient survival, it is now reasonable to consider OLT for correction of non-hepatic manifestations of certain metabolic disease in which the genetic defect is expressed in the liver; for example Crigler-Najjar syndrome, severe familial hypercholesterolemia, and hereditary oxalosis.

The minimal listing criteria for patients with fulminant hepatic failure (FHF) are the acute onset of liver dysfunction leading to hepatic encephalopathy within eight weeks of the onset of jaundice, with at least some other indicator of severe liver dysfunction (eg, coagulopathy). These patients are critically ill and generally require transplantation within 48 hours if they are to have a good chance for survival. As will be discussed later in this section, only patients with FHF, primary nonfunction, acute Wilson's disease and hepatic artery thrombosis can be listed as status 1, the highest priority for potential liver recipients. In order to increase the probability of transplanting patients with FHF, and thus decrease waiting list mortality for patients with FHF, UNOS recently adopted a policy of regional sharing of livers for these most desperate patients. As mentioned, patients with acute Wilson's disease are also considered to have poor short-term prognosis and can be listed as status 1. These patients are typically children or young adults and present with severe liver dysfunction a Coomb's (-) hemolytic anemia. In addition to the hemolysis, other clinical findings that may suggest acute Wilson's include only modest elevation of serum AST activity and an AST/ALT ratio much greater than one, a very low serum alkaline phosphatase activity and a low serum uric acid level.

While chelation therapy may be tried, most of these patients will require liver transplantation.

CONTRAINDICATIONS TO LIVER TRANSPLANTATION

Contraindications to liver transplantation (Tables 66-2 and 66-3) can be divided into two categories. Absolute contraindications are clinical conditions in which the results of liver transplantation are so poor that it should not be offered. Relative contraindications are clinical conditions that negatively affect survival, but not to the degree that transplantation should never be considered.

Patients with failure of three or more organ systems should not be regarded as candidates for OLT. In the early 1990s, there were a number of reports of patients with MSOF being rescued with OLT. The issue is no longer whether someone might be saved, but rather what is the likelihood that they will be saved; and, perhaps it should be added, at what cost. Several studies have suggested that patients with three or more organ systems failing have a 1-year survival of less than 20%. This is really too low to justify the use of a donor organ. Moreover, patients with renal failure have poorer outcomes and their transplants cost substantially more as well. It is important to point out that these patients currently can be listed as high priority for OLT.

It goes without saying that extrahepatic malignancy represents an absolute contraindication to OLT. The only potential exception is recipients with hemangioendothelioma, where survival, even with metastatic disease, can be for extended periods of time. At this time, OLT should never be used as palliative therapy for malignant disease.

Some patients with neuroendocrine tumors metastatic to liver may be candidates for OLT, if there is no evidence of disease outside the hepato-biliary tract

---

Table 66-2. Absolute Contraindications

Multisystem organ failure (MSOF)
Extrahepatic malignancy
Advanced cardiac or pulmonary disease
Severe and uncontrolled extrahepatic infection
Active substance abuse

Table 66-3. Relative Contraindications

Renal insufficiency
HIV infection
Primary hepatobiliary malignancy
Hemochromatosis
Inability to comply with an immunosuppression protocol

and if there is an expected 5-year patient survival with OLT of greater than 50%.

Advanced cardiopulmonary disease is generally regarded as an absolute contraindication to OLT. However, it is important that patients with hypoxemia undergo an evaluation to determine the exact cause of the hypoxemia. Patients with the hepatopulmonary syndrome, defined as severe hypoxemia caused by noncardiac, right-to-left shunting, improve substantially after liver transplantation and are often transformed from completely disabled patients to active people with few physical limitations. However, there is probably a limit to this statement. Patients who fail to markedly increase their PO2 (ie, >80 mmHg) on 100% FIO2 are relatively unlikely to survive the transplant procedure and should not be offered OLT. Approximately 1% of patients with portal hypertension develop pulmonary hypertension. In patients with cirrhosis, pulmonary hypertension (like portal hypertension) is driven by both increases in resistance and an increase in flow as a result of increased cardiac output. Given that the hyperdynamic state at least in part reverses following transplantation, those candidates with a normal pulmonary vascular resistance and no evidence of right heart dysfunction may be candidates for OLT. However, if either the PVR is elevated or there is evidence of right heart dysfunction, the likelihood of a favorable outcome precludes OLT. Similarly, if the ejection fraction is less than 40%, the likelihood for a favorable outcome precludes OLT.

Extrahepatic infection not controlled by appropriate antibiotic therapy (ie, CNS infection, septicemia, or pneumonia) also remains an absolute contraindication to transplantation. Many patients experience spontaneous bacterial peritonitis prior to liver transplantation. It has been shown that the peritoneal fluid is sterile after only 48 hours of antibiotic therapy and transplantation need not be delayed much beyond this 48-hour period.

Renal insufficiency has been associated with decreased patient survival after OLT. This is independent of the cause of renal insufficiency or whether combined liver and kidney transplantation is performed. Similarly, the survival of patients undergoing OLT for end-stage hemochromatosis has been relatively poor. This appears to be the result of increased early mortality due to occult cardiac disease.

Heretofore, HIV infection was regarded as an absolute contraindication to OLT. This was because of the almost inevitability of developing post-OLT AIDS. Moreover, the early reports of the outcome of HIV (+) recipients suggested early mortality related to opportunistic infections. Fortunately, times have changed. HIV infection can be controlled using highly effective antiretroviral therapy (HAART) and the survival of HIV-infected patients has improved dramatically. We now are

beginning to see patients with HIV infection, but never a diagnosis of AIDS, who are dying of liver disease.

HIV should be viewed like any other comorbid condition. It should be determined to what degree it is going to impact patient survival and/or can a subgroup of potential candidates be identified where the expected outcome is satisfactory. Several programs, after consultation with HIV treatment experts, have agreed to transplant patients who meet the following criteria: no diagnosis of AIDS, HIV RNA (-) on antiviral therapy and CD4 count greater than 300/mL.

The assessment of the likelihood of compliance with medical therapy is important, as one of the most important causes of late allograft rejection is noncompliance with medical therapy. The results of OLT for hepatobiliary malignancy and acute liver failure will be discussed below.

THE LIVER TRANSPLANT EVALUATION

The evaluation process is designed to address several key issues: (1) Confirm the etiology of liver disease; (2) Determine if any of the indications listed above, are present; (3) Identify any contraindications to liver transplantation; (4) Clarify conditions that need to be addressed prior to transplantation that may alter the posttransplant protocol. In order to address these issues, the following testing is performed.

Patients being considered for OLT should be evaluated by a hepatologist, surgeon, social worker and financial counselor. Laboratory testing should include: complete blood count, prothrombin time, PTT, electrolytes (including calcium and phosphorous levels), BUN, creatinine, liver enzymes, liver function tests, hepatitis B and C serologies, CMV and EBV serology, ANA, AMA, ferritin, α-fetoprotein, thyroid function testing, fasting blood sugar, urinalysis, total protein, cholesterol and triglycerides levels, and drug and alcohol testing.

All patients should undergo ultrasonography with Doppler, chest x-ray, EKG and PaO_2 testing. All patients with an abnormal cardiac exam and anyone over 40 should undergo echocardiography and anyone with risk factors for coronary artery disease should undergo a dobutamine echocardiogram. Potential recipients with a PaO_2 less than 70 mmHg require formal pulmonary function testing and "bubble-contrast" echocardiography to look for intrapulmonary right to left shunting.

Most programs do not routinely perform upper or lower endoscopy. All patients with PSC and ulcerative colitis, however, should undergo colonoscopy with biopsy of suspicious lesions. Similarly, most programs also do not perform routine MRI or CT scanning of the abdomen. However, if the ultrasound exam is suspicious for malignancy, additional imaging studies are indicated. One should avoid biopsies of suspicious lesions and, rather, diagnose HCC by imaging studies and α-fetoprotein because of a fear of spreading tumor cells outside the liver. Healthcare maintenance should be updated. This includes a gynecologic exam including Pap smear and mammography, if appropriate, in women and PSA testing in appropriate men. We also perform colo-rectal cancer screening in appropriate patients.

All patients with a history of alcohol or drug abuse within the past five years should see a substance abuse specialist who makes recommendations regarding pretransplant substance abuse treatment. The specialist also should help assess the likelihood of long-term sobriety.

Other consultations are obtained only if dictated by a specific medical problem.

Most programs have a patient care conference where candidates are discussed by the entire team. Recommendations are made regarding any additional evaluation that is required (eg, angiography to rule out portal vein thrombosis). Indications and contraindications for transplantation are also assessed. This is also the opportunity to alert the members of the team regarding any special considerations that would impact posttransplant care.

COMORBID CONDITIONS

It is not uncommon that the pretransplant evaluation reveals an unexpected comorbid condition. Several of these have been discussed above. It then becomes important to consider how these comorbid conditions will impact post-OLT outcome. Given that the recent UNOS statistics show a mean 5-year survival after OLT of ~70%, most programs feel that OLT is contraindicated if the expected 5-year survival after OLT in a particular candidate with significant comorbid illness is less than 50%. This means that any comorbid condition that decreases 5-year survival by more than 30% probably represents a contraindication to OLT. This reasoning should apply to all comorbid conditions including end-organ disease such as cardiomyopathy, or significant clinical history such as a recent cancer.

Perhaps the best example of this is the coincidentally discovered HCC. While some of these lesions represent the reason why the patient with stable cirrhosis has developed decompensated liver disease, in some, it is truly a coincidental finding in someone with advanced liver disease. If these are small lesions, they have a minimal effect on post-OLT survival. However, most would agree that this increases the urgency for OLT. This has been recognized by the liver transplantation community who have allowed patients with small HCC, representing single lesions less than 5 cm in diameter, or fewer than three lesions, the largest of which is greater than

3 cm, and, of course, without evidence of disease outside the liver, to be listed as status 2B.

Other comorbid conditions may require treatment prior to OLT. One of the best examples here is the patient with a (+) PPD, who has not been previously treated. Many programs would recommend the patient receive isoniazid for some period of time before OLT, given the risk of post-OLT tuberculosis.

TIMING OF TRANSPLANTATION AND PRIORITIZING ON THE WAITING LIST

Currently, about 4,500 liver transplants are performed each year in the US. The number of available donors limits the number of transplants that are performed such that the waiting list continues to increase each year. Thus, the challenge is to maximize the use of every potential donor. This means not only increasing organ donation rates but also carefully examining the outcome of recipients undergoing liver transplantation. It also has become increasingly important to lower the costs of liver transplantation. Unfortunately, the most important predictor of the cost of transplantation is the severity of illness at the time of transplantation. Thus, with the current system of organ allocation that gives priority to those with the most advanced liver disease, it is difficult to appropriately time transplantation in order to minimize costs.

The challenge for transplantation physicians and surgeons is how to allocate organs equitably, in an era where demand is exceeding supply, and costs are mounting. The development of cirrhosis is, by itself, not an indication for OLT. For example, the 5-year survival for patients with well-compensated cirrhosis caused by chronic hepatitis C is 91%. This is better than can currently be achieved with liver transplantation. By contrast, the survival of those who have experienced a complication of their chronic liver disease is far less.

The most common decompensating event is the development of ascites. Intractable ascites, generally defined as ascites resistant to diuretic therapy, can be an indication for more urgent listing. Several recent reports have demonstrated the efficacy of TIPS in such patients. While for some patients TIPS provides long-term relief from intractable ascites, it may simply function as a bridge to OLT in many of these patients.

Encephalopathy is the second most common decompensating event. Patients who experience repeated bouts of encephalopathy despite therapy with lactulose and/or neomycin should be referred for liver transplantation. The differentiation between chronic encephalopathy and irreversible organic brain syndromes can sometimes be difficult. Formal psychomotor testing may be helpful in this regard.

Bleeding from gastroesophageal varices is a common decompensating event but has become a less common indication for urgent liver transplantation, largely reflecting improved methods for managing patients with recurrent variceal hemorrhage, including use of β-blockers, variceal banding, and TIPS. TIPS has been shown to be effective for patients with bleeding refractory to other forms of therapy. However, the long-term results of TIPS remain to be defined. The major advantages of TIPS are that they do not alter extrahepatic anatomy, avoid surgery in the right upper quadrant, and are entirely removed with the explant at the time of transplantation.

Ideally, one would like to identify patients who have less than a 50% chance of surviving one year, in order to adequately prioritize patients on the waiting list. Unfortunately, the natural history of most common forms of liver disease, such as postviral cirrhosis and alcoholic liver disease, is not well-defined, making accurate predictions of the risk of death difficult. Hepato-renal syndrome represents a very poor prognostic factor and, generally, these patients require urgent transplantation. Similarly, patients with two or more episodes of recurrent spontaneous bacterial peritonitis have limited life expectancy as well. The use of daily oral antibiotics has been shown effective in decreasing recurrent episodes of spontaneous bacterial peritonitis.

On the other hand, there is good natural history data for the cholestatic forms of liver disease, in particular, PBC and PSC. Prognostic models have been developed and allow prediction of survival. The Mayo model for PBC uses five independent clinical variables: serum bilirubin and albumin concentrations, age, prothrombin time, and the presence or absence of peripheral edema. Serum bilirubin concentration is the most predictive of these variables. Generally, the chance of surviving two years is less than 50% when it reaches 10 mg/dL in patients with primary biliary cirrhosis. Similar scoring systems also have been developed for primary sclerosing cholangitis (PSC). As with primary biliary cirrhosis, the most predictive variable is in PSC serum bilirubin. Thus, once patients with these diseases develop clinical jaundice, they should be evaluated for liver transplantation.

For patients to be listed at a higher status (ie, status 2B, for transplantation) they either must have a Childs-Pugh score of ten (ie, Childs' Class C) or meet minimal listing criteria and be experiencing a decompensating event. For patients with chronic liver disease to be listed at the highest status (ie, 2A) they must have Childs-Pugh score of ten, be in the ICU with a decompensating event, and be judged to have a life expectancy of more than seven days (see below).

PRETRANSPLANT MANAGEMENT

In terms of the management of patients awaiting transplantation, two main principles apply. First, the complications of chronic liver disease are predictable and many can be prevented. Examples of this include spontaneous bacterial peritonitis (SBP) in patients with ascites and GI bleeding in patients with large esophageal varices. Certainly, anyone with a previous bout of SBP or who experiences variceal bleeding should receive one of the antibiotic regimens shown to be effective for the prevention of SBP. These include daily norfloxacin or trimethoprim-sulfamethoxazole, or weekly ciprofloxacin. Generally prophylactic antibiotics may be given to all patients with ascites awaiting OLT, even if they have not previously experienced SBP.

β-blockers can be given prophylactically to patients with large esophageal varices, even if they have not previously bled. If they have bled a variceal band ligation can be performed as mentioned earlier. In addition, TIPS is used for patients with refractory variceal bleeding. It is clear that the outcomes of patients who were managed with TIPS are superior to those treated with surgical shunts. TIPS has also been shown to be effective for diuretic-refractory ascites. In fact, at many medical centers, refractory ascites has become the most common indication for TIPS. In addition, TIPS has emerged as the treatment of choice for diuretic-refractory hepatohydrothorax. Unfortunately, 25% of patients develop post-TIPS encephalopathy and up to 60% of patients will require TIPS revision because of a stenosis or occlusion leading to recurrence of portal hypertension. Moreover, the hope had been that not only would TIPS stabilize these patients with complications such as variceal bleeding and ascites but that they would also decrease intraoperative blood loss, decrease operating time and improve patient and graft survival. Unfortunately, TIPS has not been shown to alter the outcome of patients undergoing transplant.

Many patients with advanced liver disease are malnourished pretransplant. Pretransplant malnutrition has been associated with a worse outcome after liver transplantation. The best method for nutritional support has not been established. Moreover, whether nutritional support with enteral or parenteral hyperalimentation improves outcomes has not been proven. It is also unclear whether one can positively impact metabolic bone disease prior to transplant, particularly in those who are at or below the fracture threshold.

Prior to transplant, patients should receive both the hepatitis A and B and pneumococcal vaccines.

Finally, recurrence of hepatitis B virus (HBV) infection and posttransplant hepatitis occurs in the vast majority of untreated patients transplanted for chronic HBV. Passive immunization with high-dose hepatitis B immune globulin (HBIg) clearly reduces the risk of reinfection. However, HBIg likely needs to be given for life and is expensive. It also is less effective in patients with chronic disease who exhibit serologic evidence of active viral replication (ie, HBeAg [+] or HBV DNA [+]).

Lamivudine is a nucleoside analogue that blocks HBV replication. It is given orally with few side effects. Lamivudine has now been shown to be an effective treatment for post-OLT hepatitis B. In HBV DNA (+) patients, lamivudine markedly decreases the level of HBV DNA, and also lowers serum transaminase but generally doesn't lead to clearance of HBsAg from serum. This agent has also been used to decrease rates of recurrent HBV infection peritransplant and appears to be quite effective even when given alone pre- and post-OLT. The main limitation to this agent is acquired drug resistance through the development of mutations at the YMDD locus of the reverse transcriptase molecule. This occurs at a rate of 20% to 30% per year. To even further lessen the risk of HBV reinfection, several programs are now using lamivudine in combination with HBIg, particularly in patients who are HBV DNA (+) in serum pre-OLT.

RECOMMENDED READING

Charlton M, Seaberg E, Wiesner R, et al. Predictors of patient and graft survival following liver transplantation for hepatitis C. Hepatology. 1998;28(3):823-830.

Wiesner RH, Porayko MK, Dickson ER, et al. Selection and timing of liver transplantation in primary biliary cirrhosis and primary sclerosing cholangitis. Hepatology. 1992;16(5):1290-1299.

Lucey MR, Brown KA, Everson GT, et al. Minimal criteria for placement of adults on the liver transplant waiting list: a report of a national conference organized by the American Society of Transplant Physicians and the American Association for the Study of Liver Diseases. Transplantation. 1998;66(7):956-962.

Hoofnagle JH, Kresina T, Fuller R, et al. Liver transplantation for alcoholic liver disease: executive statement and recommendations. Summary of a National Institutes of Health workshop held December 6-7, 1996, Bethesda, Maryland. Liver Transpl & Surg. 1997;3(3):347-350.

Seaberg E, Belle S, Beringer K, Schivens J, Detre K. Long-term patient and retransplantation –free survival by selected recipient and donor characteristics: An update from the Pitt-UNOS Liver Transplant Registry. In: JM Cecka, PT Terasaki, eds. Clinical Transplants. Los Angeles, Ca: UCLA Press; 1997:15-29.

Showstack J, Katz PP, Lake JR, et al. Resource utilization in liver transplantation: effects of patient characteristics and clinical practice. NIDDK Liver Transplantation Database Group. The association of patient and clinical characteristics with resource use for liver transplantation. JAMA. 1999;281(15):1381-1386.

Everhart JE, Lombardero M, Detre KM, et al. Increased waiting time for liver transplantation results in higher mortality. Transplantation. 1997;64(9):1300-1306.

Samuel D, Muller R, Alexander G, et al. Liver transplantation in European patients with the hepatitis B surface antigen. N Engl J Med. 1993;329(25):1842-1847.

Everhart JE, Wei Y, Eng H, et al. Recurrent and new hepatitic C virus infection after liver transplantation. Hepatology. 1999;29(4):1220-1226.

Rossle M, Haag K, Ochs A, et al. The transjugular intrahepatic portosystemic stent-shunt procedure for variceal bleeding. N Engl J Med. 1994;330(3):165-171.

O'Grady JG, Alexander GJ, Hayllar KM, Williams R. Early indicators of prognosis in fulminant hepatic failure. Gastroenterology. 1989;97(2):439-445.

Lake, JR. Changing indications for liver transplantation. Gastroenterol Clin North Am. 1993;22(2):213-229.

Osorio RW, Ascher NL, Avery M, Bacchetti P, Roberts JP, Lake JR. Predicting recidivism after orthotopic liver transplantation for alcoholic liver disease. Hepatology. 1994;20(1 Pt 1):105-110.

67 LIVING-RELATED LIVER TRANSPLANTATION: SELECTION OF RECIPIENT AND DONORS

Jean Emond, MD

Living-related liver transplantation (LRT) was introduced as an alternative to cadaveric transplantation one decade ago. Its initial use was in pediatrics, both for technical reasons and in the response to an apparently greater scarcity of donor organs for children. Prior to 1990, as living transplantation proliferated rapidly in Europe and North America, the dramatic shortage of small cadaveric donors for children led to a waiting list mortality that approached 50% in many centers. This provided an ethical imperative for the development of alternative techniques for pediatric liver transplantation, such as reduced-size liver transplantation (RLT). While RLT decreased the mortality for children on the waiting list, it did not increase the overall supply of organs and its use has diminished as the overall demand for organs has continued to increase. Split livers were introduced in 1988 as an attempt to increase the number of organs.

Although LRT was initially performed in individual cases in South America and Australia, Broelsch was the first to systematically apply left lateral segment living donation in a pediatric program, reporting these results in 1990. This initial experience was greeted with great concern by the transplant community, focused on questions about the safety of the donor. Nonetheless, opponents of LRT could no longer deny the enormous need for increasing access to liver transplantation. Expansion of the use of LRT was limited by the technical difficulty of the procedure, requiring familiarity with intrahepatic surgical anatomy and the use of microvascular techniques for optimal results. While the use of LRT in children increased gradually in North America, rapid expansion occurred in Asia, led by Tanaka in Kyoto whose team has now performed over 500 cases.

As alluded to earlier, the rapid growth of demand for liver transplantation since 1990 led to sporadic efforts to extend the benefits of LRT from the pediatric population to adults. Initial efforts were extremely disappointing, due to a high rate of technical complications and functional graft failure. In 1996, a syndrome of cholestatic hepatic insufficiency that seemed to be a direct conse-

quence of small graft size was described. It became clear that extension of LRT to adults would require an increase of the extent of hepatectomy in the donor, resulting in an uncertain modification in the extent of risk for the donor.

In 1999, there was a rapid proliferation of LRT for adults, subjecting the donor to right hepatectomy with promising preliminary results. The added risk of right lobe donation is likely to be substantial, and a mortality has already occurred in a US center, leading to an estimated mortality risk of 1% (a fivefold increase over estimates for left lateral segment donation). In the coming decade, the challenge will be to make the benefits of LRT available to an ever-increasing population of patients, without compromising the safety of the donor.

ETHICAL CONSIDERATIONS

While there are clearly issues of magnitude in considering liver donation by a healthy adult, the underlying ethical arguments have long been debated in the literature of renal transplantation. A comprehensive clinical/ethical analysis preceded the initial trial of LRT in Chicago. The introduction of this therapy needed to meet three critical standards: the need for the innovation, the expectation of acceptable risk and benefit to the participants, and a secure process to ensure informed consent of the donor.

Need for the Innovation

Initial studies of access to pediatric liver transplantation established a convincing argument to justify the introduction of LRT. Estimates of mortality on the pediatric waiting list in North America have been readily accepted and, today parents rarely hesitate to consider living donation for a child who needs liver transplantation. The great majority of the 500 children who receive liver transplants each year are young, under five years old. According to United Network for Organ Sharing (UNOS) data, fewer than 300 organs from small children are available for these patients. The arguments are even more dramatic for adults (Figure 67-1). Currently, over 13,000 patients are listed for transplantation on the UNOS waiting list, with an annual supply of under 4,000 cadaveric livers. Because of limited regional sharing of livers, the acuity of the shortage of livers varies between centers, creating disparate pressure to consider living donation from region to region.

In other countries, varying scenarios are observed. LRT has been attempted in several third world nations, where limited capabilities of the health care system coexist with an inability to organize cadaveric liver procurement. In general, results in these situations have been dismal, and the risk to the donor is hard to justify since the probability that the recipients will benefit is low. In many developed societies such as Japan, the

Professor of Surgery, Columbia College of Physicians and Surgeons; Surgical Director, Center for Liver Disease and Transplantation, The New York Presbyterian Hospital, New York, NY

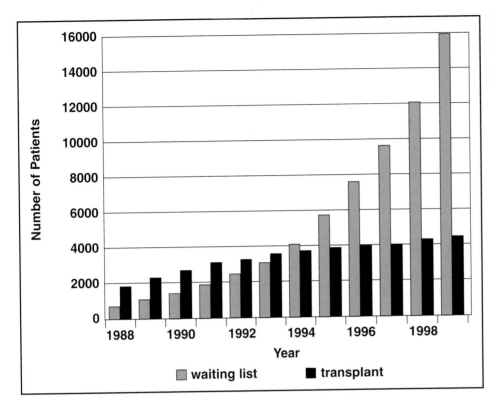

Figure 67-1. The growth in demand of liver transplantation in the last decade (UNOS data). The size of the waiting list at year's end is plotted against the number of transplants.

political and cultural barriers to brain death legislation have created a unique imperative to expand LRT. In fact, the largest series of LRT for adults have been reported from centers in Hong Kong, Kyoto, and Tokyo.

Acceptable Risk and Benefit

The second ethical mandate is that the participants in the trial of innovative therapy face an acceptable risk and the probability of benefit. When we designed the original trial of LRT for pediatric recipients, we extrapolated from the known risks of hepatic resection surgery in noncirrhotics to predict a risk of mortality for donors of less than 1%. In fact, the choice of an "acceptable" risk is somewhat arbitrary, but most transplant surgeons accept the notion that renal donation, which has an estimated risk between 0.1% and 0.2%, is an appropriate standard. The notion of the probability of success with the recipient was based on experience with both RLT and SLT, which had rates of graft survival comparable to cadaveric liver transplants. Today, results of LRT in children appear superior to standard OLT, approaching 95% in some centers. Several reasons contribute to these results. LRT is generally performed when both donor and recipient are in optimal medical condition. Second, LRT in pediatrics has largely been confined to centers with specific expertise in the transplantation of small recipients, familiar with partial transplants and the precise microvascular techniques required for optimal results.

The limited results of LRT for adults to date do not yet permit us to precisely predict risk for these recipients.

As noted earlier, approximately 600 cases of adult LRT have been reported with three donor deaths. With respect to recipients, the right lobe seems to provide an adequate-size graft for satisfactory function in the recipient. In initial series, biliary fistulas seem to be much more common in recipients of right lobe donation (40% to 50%) than has been observed in recipients of left lobes (10%) or standard cadaveric grafts (2%). While these results are concerning, it can be assumed that experience will progressively decrease the risks faced by both donors and recipients. While most of the initial published reports of right lobe donation have come from centers with vast experience in hepatobiliary surgery, this has not always been the case. Therefore, centers contemplating the initiation of such a program should conduct a critical review of their capabilities prior to subjecting the donor to this significant intervention.

Informed Consent

The greatest ethical challenge to the initiation of LRT is the establishment of a process to optimize informed consent. Coercion of the potential donor, either overt or concealed, is the greatest difficulty in this process, and has led some extremists to argue that LRT is always coercive and, therefore, inherently unethical. A legitimate point can be made that, in a society that values altruism, living donation is always coercive. Just as legitimately, based on a doctrine of self-interest, restoration of health to a loved one can be justified as conferring substantial benefit to the donor. Finally, the enhanced self-esteem brought on by the heroic act of the donor should not be underestimated as a benefit. Ultimately, we accept the premise that the harm of coercion can be balanced and mitigated by a strict process of psychosocial evaluation and a clear recognition of the benefits both donor and recipient reap in the process.

Initial protocols for LRT went to great lengths to mitigate coercion. Emergencies were excluded, the consent process required two separate steps, and the donor evaluation was conducted by a physician who was not a member of the transplant team, to decrease the conflict of interest inherent when the recipient's physician makes medical decisions regarding the suitability of the donor. These rigorous criteria have gradually been modified in recent years with the routine acceptance of LRT in pediatrics for both elective and urgent transplantation. The initiation of new programs for LRT in adults should include rigorous protocols to ensure donor safety and optimize informed consent.

TECHNICAL AND PHYSIOLOGIC CONSIDERATIONS
Functional Reserve and Regeneration

The success of LRT is predicated on the ability of the liver to regenerate, providing a functional graft for the recipient and restoration of full health for the donor. For infant recipients of LRT, the graft is often larger than the recipient requires and has been observed to rapidly decrease in size in the days following transplantation. When the liver is smaller than the needs of the host, the regenerative response, which has been well-studied in the clinic and the laboratory, appears to regulate mass restoration in both donors and recipients. When the limits of graft size are exceeded (ie, when the liver is too small), progressive damage to the graft may occur, leading to acute graft failure and death of the recipient. The lower limit of safe grafting has been studied empirically in a variety of centers. The first important contribution was to develop a formula for accurately predicting the size of the "normal" liver needed for the recipient. CT imaging has been shown to be reliable in predicting the size of a grafted liver and, therefore, useful in planning the operation. A liver graft as small as 25% of the expected liver size of the recipient has been successfully transplanted, though this is clearly at the limits of safe transplantation. Our studies suggest that grafts smaller than 50% of the recipient's needs will be associated with poor function and an increased risk of complications.

Anatomic Considerations (Figures 67-2a and 67-2b)

Extensive studies of reduced size and split liver transplantation preceded the introduction of LRT. These clarified the anatomic foundation needed to obtain functional grafts of appropriate size for the recipients. The smallest liver that can be practically created is the left lateral segment graft (Segments II and III of Couinaud) and can be used for a recipient approximately 1/10th the size of the donor. Smaller disparities can be overcome using the full left lobe (Segments II, III, and IV) in which the donor is larger than the recipient. Finally the right lobe, which typically comprises 60% of

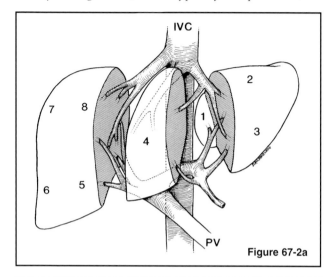

Figure 67-2a

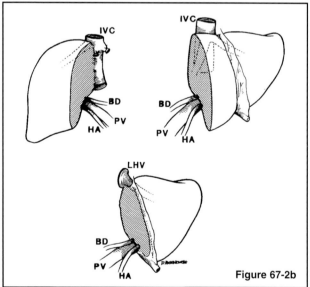

Figure 67-2b

Figure 67-2a & 67-2b. A) Segmental anatomy as modified from Couinaud. Hepatic segments are numbered 1 through 8. Segments 2 and 3 comprise a functional unit that is optimal for an infant. The addition of segment 4 forms the full left lobe, which is used for a large child or small adult. Segments 5 to 8 comprise the right lobe and are needed for an adult recipient. PV indicates portal vein; IVC, inferior vena cava. **B)** The use of partial grafts is schematically depicted. The left upper sketch is the full right lobe, the right upper sketch is the full left lobe, the left lateral lobe is depicted below. Reprinted with permission from: Emond JC, Whitington PF, Thistlethwaite JR, Alonso EM, Broelsch CE. Reduced-size orthotopic liver transplantation: use in the management of children with chronic liver disease. Hepatology. 1989;10(5):867-872.

the mass of the liver, is used to transplant a recipient of comparable, or even larger size than the donor.

Technical Considerations

Transplantation of a segmental liver graft always requires hepatico-jejunostomy for reconstruction of the biliary system. This requires detailed understanding of the intrahepatic biliary anatomy and careful preparation of the bile ducts during donor hepatectomy. Reconstruction requires meticulous technique and the creation of very fine anastomoses, ideally under high magnification to minimize technical flaws.

Tanaka and the Kyoto group introduced the most important technical advance in liver transplantation in the recent era: the routine use of the microscope for arterial reconstruction in LRT. The demonstration that vessels as small as 2 mm could be reconstructed with a 99% patency rate dispelled the notion that arterial thrombosis is anything other than a technical failure. Competence with microvascular technique has become an essential technical skill for LRT.

The careful positioning of the liver in all types of partial transplantation is important. The liver is exquisitely sensitive to obstruction of the hepatic vein outflow, thus the anastomosis must be designed to accommodate the final resting position of the liver as the abdomen is closed. Failure to adhere to this principle led to lethal complications initially. As use of the right lobe becomes more common, similar care must be applied for these transplants.

CURRENT RESULTS OF LRT
(Table 67-1)
Pediatrics

LRT is routine in pediatrics and accounts for 75% of children transplanted at Columbia College. This is obviously an extreme example, and the proportion of LRT varies from region to region based on the supply of livers and the preferences of the team. Nationally, fewer than 20% of children have received LRT. As noted above, recipient outcomes are comparable to those receiving standard liver transplants: patient and graft survival should exceed 90%. Technical complications differ somewhat, and in general, biliary problems are more common after LRT, while nonfunction of a graft from a living donor is exceedingly rare.

The left lateral lobe donor operation has been refined substantially over the last decade and is accomplished with minimal blood loss in approximately three hours. The gall bladder is spared and there is a minimum of dissection of the structures supplying the right lobe (the donor's liver). The effect on hepatic function is minimal and patients generally leave the hospital in three to five days. The need for reoperation is approximately 1%, although percutaneous treatment of biliary complications is slightly more frequent. One reported death has been published (from a pulmonary embolus), and one other has been described, for a total donor mortality of two in 1,000, a risk comparable to renal donation. Because the liver is able to regenerate, no long-term risk to the donor is anticipated, however, since the longest follow-up is ten years, this expectation has not yet been verified.

Adults

In our earliest attempts to use LRT for adults, left lateral segment grafts were found to be uniformly inadequate, leading to a recipient mortality exceeding 50%. Recent reports suggest that recipients of right lobe grafts have an outcome comparable to recipients of standard transplants. This observation must be tempered to take into account the inevitable patient selection that must influence results. In addition to reports from Hong Kong and Japan, a recent series of more than 30 patients was

Table 67-1. Results of LRT in Children and Adults
(frequencies estimated from personal experience and reported series)

Donors

Type	Mortality	OR time	Hospital stay	Reoperations	Peak bilirubin
Left lat	0.2%	3-4.5h	3-6 days	<1%	2.5 mg/dL
Left	0.2%	4-6h	4-7 days	<1%	2.5 mg/dL
Right	1%	4.5-10hrs	5-10 days	1-5%	8 mg/dL

Recipients:

Type	Patient Survival	Biliary Leaks	Peak Bilirubin		
Left lat	95%	5-10%	<5 mg/dL		
Left	90%	5-10%	5-15 mg/dL		
Right	80-90%	30-50%	5-15 mg/dL		

reported by Marcos from Virginia. Recipients of right lobes have a clearly increased incidence of biliary leakage (60% in the early experience in the Marcos series) that seems to improve with experience.

Donors of the right lobe undergo a very significant reduction in hepatic parenchyma. The operation takes much longer (eight to 12 hours in the Marcos series). Postoperatively, the patients are extremely fatigued, and are at risk for narcotic overdose in the early postoperative period. Transient elevations of prothrombin time and bilirubin attest to the clear impact of the donation on hepatic function. Although little data are available, it is likely that complications will be more frequent. The single reported mortality in a donor was apparently the consequence of a biliary fistula complicated by pancreatitis following postoperative ERCP.

SELECTION OF RECIPIENTS FOR LRT

The first step in the evaluation of a potential transplant patient is the comprehensive assessment of the recipient. The indications for liver transplantation are well-outlined elsewhere in this textbook and are not modified in patients receiving LRT. The assessment permits the transplant team to confirm the diagnosis of the liver disease and determine the timing of transplantation. In fact, LRT permits elective planning of transplantation, an enormous advantage that has been lost in cadaveric transplantation in the face of the scarcity of donor livers. Rather than specifically transplanting the sickest patients, it is possible to plan the transplant based on the condition of the patient, and to respond to social constraints the family may face, such as coordination of the transplant with school holidays, or vacations from work. In children with biliary atresia, it has long been accepted that the optimal time for transplantation is when growth failure occurs, but prior to frank hepatic decompensation or the development of complications of portal hypertension. This optimal practice is only possible with LRT.

LRT in patients with fulminant hepatic failure is now frequently recommended. The rapidly progressive nature of this disease, leading to brain edema within hours to days of admission, makes it uncertain whether a cadaver donor will be located in time. In patients who are admitted in stage 3 or 4 hepatic coma, the donor evaluation has been compressed to an overnight process, and the transplant proceeds within 24 to 36 hours of admission. The inherently coercive nature of the situation is recognized by offering the family the option of waiting for a cadaver donor, ultimately making a collaborative decision with the family to proceed with LRT if it seems unsafe to wait.

The underlying principle in patients for LRT is that the source of the donor organ should not modify the choice of the recipient. This concept is most often tested in patients in whom the indication for transplantation is hopeless, such as in a recurrent hepatoblastoma. Somehow, the use of a living donor is seen to allow an extreme choice in the selection of the recipient. While it is true that the heroic transplant does not deprive another patient on the cadaveric list the chance to receive a liver, the donor's gift is an equally precious resource and should not be squandered if the recipient has no chance of survival.

There is one note of technical caution that might affect the use of a living donor in primary hepatic malignancy. In LRT, the donor is able to provide few extra vessels as is standard with cadaver donors. This may limit the scope of the cancer operation in the recipient since, ideally, the cancer hepatectomy should include all the vessels and nodes of the portal hepatis. Prosthetic vascular grafts have been liberally used to replace the vena cava, and saphenous vein to replace the portal vein and hepatic artery in a patient undergoing total hepatectomy for hepatoblastoma. This technical constraint of LRT in cancer patients is unfortunate, since the group most affected by the current organ shortage is the population with small hepatomas who have been shown to be curable if transplanted early. These patients are an obvious group in which living donation is crucial in restoring the appropriate timing of transplantation.

Because of the greater complexity of LRT in adults, and the fact that the graft will always be smaller than the ideal liver for the recipient, it recommended that LRT not be used in patients with advanced decompensation of chronic liver disease (currently listed as 2A in the UNOS scheme). In these recipients, the operation is often prolonged with increased blood loss, impaired renal and pulmonary function, and a decreased overall probability of a good outcome. With the exception of patients with fulminant hepatic failure who clearly benefit from LRT even in emergencies, LRT should be done electively in ideal recipients to ensure optimal outcomes for both donors and recipients.

SELECTION OF DONORS (Table 67-2)

A donor evaluation process that proceeds in phases has been described, one that is coordinated with the evaluation of the recipient. The process is summarized in Table 67-2 and this approach has changed little in the past five years. The three principal changes in strategy include the acceptance of unrelated donors, early completion of serologic testing and blood type to save time and stress for the family, and modification in the morphologic imaging of the donor. In the initial phase, as the family is educated about the nature of the liver disease and the need for liver transplantation, the possibility of living donation is introduced systematically as part of the informational materials about transplantation. It is true

Table 67-2. Living Donor Evaluation Criteria

Phase: I	I	II	II	II	III
Age	Relation	Psychosocial Support	Medical Evaluation	Laboratory Evaluation	Graft Assessment
18-60	Emotionally related to recipient. ABO compatible Negative serology for hepatitis and HIV viruses.	Psychosocial support systems adequate as determined by independent psychosocial assessment.	Comprehensive history and physical examination negative for acute or chronic illness affecting operative risk.	Hematologic, serum chemistry, liver, and kidney function normal. Normal EKG and CXR.	MR assessment of liver, vessels and bile ducts. Graft represents > 50% of expected recipient liver mass. Selective liver biopsy and angiography.

that presentation of this information could be regarded as inherently coercive, but it is done in the context of the alternative of cadaveric transplantation. Families are educated about the listing and selection process and the function of UNOS and the allocation of livers. All patients are put on the cadaveric list even if a potential donor is available, so that the patient does not lose waiting time if subsequent events preclude use of the living donor.

Many donors do not meet obvious criteria and are excluded without any invasive investigation in phase I. The donor and recipient do not need to be genetically related. There is widespread acceptance of the appropriateness of emotionally-related donors, most typically donation between spouses. If the donor is obviously healthy and desires to proceed, blood typing and serologic testing for HIV and hepatitis viruses is carried out. This initial phase identifies the majority of potential contraindications to donation. In phase II, the donor undergoes a comprehensive psychosocial assessment by the transplant social worker and psychiatrist. This process serves both an educational and diagnostic function, familiarizing the family with the steps involved in the procedure, and once again, helping the family decide whether living donation is appropriate. Significant constraints may include a limited ability of the family to care for two patients, or significant financial hardship if the primary breadwinner is the donor. It is the responsibility of the transplant team to help the potential donor recognize and accept contraindications to donation. This phase also includes a comprehensive medical assessment by a physician whose primary responsibility is the safety of the donor. In selecting the physician who will conduct the donor evaluation, the need for objectivity in this assessment must be balanced by adequate experience with the medical issues surrounding transplantation that will affect both donor and recipient.

The investigations of phase III have undergone some evolution since earlier descriptions of the process.

For pediatrics, reliance on volumetric scanning for determination of appropriate graft size has decreased. Because most infants with liver disease have enlarged livers, there is always room to accommodate the graft, even from very large donors. Enlargement of the recipient abdominal cavity with a prosthetic closure can overcome even very great disparities. MR with vascular and biliary enhancement is the principal study for the evaluation of the donor liver. This gives an ideal combination of arterial and venous anatomy for planning the procedure. If further information about the arteries is required, arteriography may be necessary. The benefits of preoperative cholangiography do not outweigh the risks of the procedure to the healthy living donor.

The evolution of techniques for LRT have made a number of choices available in planning the transplant. Naturally, if the recipient is a small child, the graft is limited to the left lateral lobe. If the recipient is an adult, the right lobe will probably be necessary for an optimal procedure. An intermediate choice is the use of the left lobe graft for adult recipients, as championed by Miller. This is an appealing alternative, since the operation seems safer than the right lobe donation, and has been used in larger children since the earliest days of LRT. The primary constraint is that in most patients, the full left lobe is only about 40% of the total liver parenchyma. This option is ideal for donation when the donor is larger than the recipient, such as in most husband-to-wife pairs. Ultimately, the choice of the technique of donation is made to optimize the balance between the safety of the donation and the expectation of an optimum outcome for the recipient.

ROLE OF LRT IN THE OVERALL STRATEGY OF LIVER TRANSPLANTATION TODAY

The sequential strategy for the use of LRT is presented schematically in Figure 67-3. LRT should be considered for all potential adult recipients of liver transplantation. While it is clear that LRT can pose great hardship to the family, the worsening of the organ shortage forces this option. Elective LRT as an alternative to the progressive deterioration of the patient on the waiting list has sufficient merit to justify its expansion for use on a scale comparable to that of renal donation. This statement is predicated on the assumption that the transplant team has adequate experience to perform LRT with acceptable risk and benefit.

In conclusion, LRT must meet three major ethical requirements: a convincing need for the innovation, an acceptable risk and benefit, and a satisfactory process for ensuring optimal informed consent of the participants. While the need is clear, the ability of centers to offer adequate expertise in LRT requires a major commitment and preparation on the part of the transplant centers. The proliferation of right lobe donation in the next several years may run the risk of creating great harm if transplant surgeons do not approach LRT with the appropriate balance of humility and expertise needed to truly do no harm.

RECOMMENDED READING

Emond JC, Whitington PF, Thistlethwaite JR, Alonso EM, Broelsch CE. Reduced-size orthotopic liver transplantation: use in the management of children with chronic liver disease. Hepatology. 1989;10(5):867-872.

Broelsch CE, Whitington PF, Emond JC, et al. Liver transplantation in children from living related donors. Surgical techniques and results. Ann Surg. 1991;214(4): 428-437.

Singer PA, Siegler M, Whitington PF, et al. Ethics of liver transplantation with living donors. N Engl J Med. 1989;321(9):620-622.

Lo CM, Fan ST, Liu CL, et al. Adult-to-adult living donor liver transplantation using extended right lobe grafts. Ann Surg. 1997;226(3):261-269.

Marcos A, Fisher RA, Ham JM, et al. Selection and outcome of living donors for adult to adult right lobe transplantation. Transplantation. 2000;69(11):2410-2415.

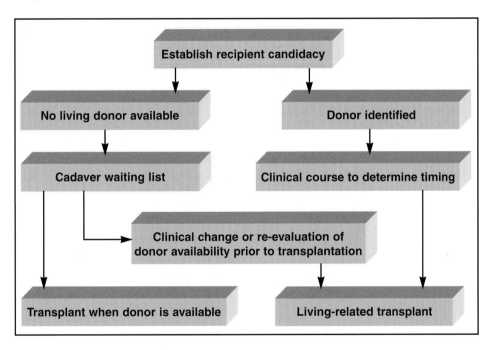

Figure 67-3. The algorithm of routine use of LRT is depicted. Establishing the candidacy of the recipient is the first step in the process.

68 CADAVER LIVER DONOR SELECTION CRITERIA

Kim M. Olthoff, MD

Not all donor livers should be used in every recipient. Each donor needs to be assessed with the specific recipient in mind, and an appropriate donor for one patient may be contraindicated in another. As the gap between the number of patients waiting and the number of available donors enlarges, there is a need to try to expand the use of donors, but also to be more aware of outcome and cost-effectiveness.

DONOR TESTING AND MANAGEMENT

To determine if an individual is suitable for organ donation, a detailed evaluation is performed by the local organ procurement organization staff regarding donor demographics, medical and surgical history, hospital course, cause of death, hemodynamics, social history, laboratory data and serologies (Table 68-1). This information is then relayed to the transplant surgeon who must decide whether to recover the liver. The surgeon may ask for more detailed information or that additional studies be done to further evaluate the donor and the liver. Pathology reports or consultations may need to be obtained if there is a history of malignancy or other significant medical conditions. If there is a history of significant alcohol use, ultrasound has been shown to be beneficial in evaluating livers for fat content.

Management of the potential donor is extremely important in maximizing the quality of the organs that can be used. Profound hypotension, acidosis, hypoxia, hypernatremia and renal insufficiency due to the effects of brain death and ineffective donor management can cause a potential liver donor to be eliminated. It is critical to have an on-site coordinator experienced in donor management for minute-to-minute critical care decisions. The intensivists at the donor hospital are a valuable resource. Since thyroxine replacement may enhance the hemodynamic and metabolic stability of the organ donor, thyroid hormone (Levothyroxine/T-4) replacement therapy protocols are now in place in many organ procurement organizations. Although elevated serum liver chemistries are common after a period of hypotension and resuscitation and minor elevations are not a contraindication for liver donation, massively elevated or

rising serum enzymes indicate a severely damaged and untransplantable liver.

FACTORS PREDICTING OUTCOME AND THE "MARGINAL" DONOR

Many variables have been found to predict poor outcome due to primary nonfunction or early graft dysfunction following transplantation. The studies identifying these factors were usually retrospective, univariate or multivariate in design, while lacking uniformity of definition of primary nonfunction or early allograft dysfunction. Each study focused on different characteristics, set different guidelines (such as age or cold ischemia cutoffs), and evaluated different end-points. Therefore, it is difficult to determine which variables truly lead to a significant change in long-term survival. Characteristics that have been associated with worse clinical outcome from all these studies are listed in Table 68-2.

A recently completed UNOS Expanded Donor Study analyzed data from 27,671 transplants from 9,283 donors in an attempt to determine which donor characteristics, alone or in combination, might provide a detrimental or beneficial effect on transplant outcome in all organs. Results from liver transplants identified the following donor factors associated with poorer graft outcome: donor race (ie, African-American vs non-African-American), increasing cold ischemia time, cause of death due to stroke, elevated serum creatinine and history of alcohol dependency. One or two detrimental character-

Table 68-1. Donor Evaluation by Local Organ Procurement Organization

Donor History	Laboratory Tests	Studies
Age	ABO	CXR
Sex	Arterial blood gas	EKG
Race	Chemistries	Echocardiogram
Physical Exam*	Liver enzymes and bilirubin	Cardiac catheterization†
Cause of death	PT/PTT	Ultrasound‡
Medical history	Blood/urine/sputum cultures	
Surgical history	HIV 1/HIV 2/HTLV RPR/VDRL	
Social history	Hepatitis B/C serologies	

*including height and weight
†older donors, coronary risk factors
‡if requested

Assistant Professor of Medicine, University of Pennsylvania Liver Transplantation Program, Philadelphia, PA

Table 68-2. Potential Donor Risk Factors Associated with a Worse Clinical Outcome

Donor Characteristics

Prolonged cold ischemic time
Older donor
Long ICU/hospital stay
Preprocurement acidosis
Death due to stroke
Severe steatosis
ABO mismatch
Female gender
Race other than Caucasian
Elevated serum creatinine/BUN
High pressors
History of alcohol dependency

istics should not eliminate a potential donor, but a combination of several factors, or a high-risk recipient, may be reason enough to pass on a liver.

There are few tests performed preprocurement that can determine if a liver will function adequately after transplantation, and nothing may be more accurate than an experienced surgeon's visual evaluation at the time of organ recovery. Characteristics regarding fat content, color, texture, sharpness of the edges, quality of flush, and just "how it looks", are all subjective reasons for a surgeon to decline the use of a liver. In support of this, the large NIDDK Liver Transplantation Database has identified the surgeon's assessment of liver quality and texture as one significant factor predictive of early allograft dysfunction.

The concept of the "marginal donor" has changed with increasing experience and improved outcomes, as well as more aggressive surgical teams. Traditionally, "marginal" has included fatty livers, older age, positive serologies for hepatitis B and C, and history of malignancy in the donor. Many of these livers are used routinely at large centers and are no longer considered "marginal", but are very acceptable donors in the face of the great need that exists. Perhaps the terminology should change to "expanded donor criteria" in order to reflect this wider acceptance.

THE FATTY LIVER

Fatty livers have long been associated with increased incidence of primary nonfunction. Many livers with severe steatosis (lipid content greater than 50%) are discarded, and those with moderate fatty infiltration are often only used in high-urgency patients. The growing waiting list, and increased death on the list, has renewed

an interest in the use of these "marginal" livers in a broader recipient population. Unfortunately, liver biopsies at the time of procurement are unreliable and imprecise, particularly if done in the middle of the night by a pathologist at a donor hospital with little experience in the reading of frozen liver biopsies for total fat content. Procuring surgeons should have experience in reviewing these biopsies, and may need to bring the biopsy back to their liver center for more experienced interpretation. There are several reports that moderate hepatic steatosis (30% to 60%), in and of itself, may not be a significant risk factor for primary nonfunction. However, the presence of significant steatosis does contribute to initial poor function, and in combination with other risk factors, can have a higher rate of primary nonfunction. Many of these livers will recover and the steatosis frequently resolves, but the stress of early marginal liver function in a recipient who is high-risk may lead to increased postoperative complications and poor patient survival. Careful clinical judgement is required in the decision to use a fatty liver, including the presence of other donor risk factors, and the status of the recipient. Controllable risk factors, such as cold ischemic time, should be kept to an absolute minimum.

THE OLDER DONOR

Older donor age is frequently cited as a significant independent predictor of worse outcome, particularly in high-risk recipients, such as candidates in the ICU or requiring re-transplantation. However, in ideal circumstances, donors older than 60 have similar results to younger donors. Donor age is one of the few donor factors that increases resource utilization, resulting in higher hospital costs. It is therefore imperative that the liver should look acceptable at the time of procurement, cold ischemic time must be kept as short as possible, and the recipient brought to the operating room once the liver is visualized.

DONORS WITH POSITIVE SEROLOGIES

Most transplant centers will use hepatitis C-positive donors in recipients with chronic hepatitis C. Under these circumstances, there is no difference in patient and graft survival at five years in grafts infected with hepatitis C. However, a baseline liver biopsy at the time of recovery demonstrating active hepatitis and/or cirrhosis is a contraindication to donation.

Other "marginal" donors are those that test positive for hepatitis B core antibody (anti-HBc). These donors have been found to have a high transmission rate into naive recipients regardless of the donor hepatitis B surface antibody status. The presence of antibody to hepatitis B surface antigen (anti-HBs) in the recipient can protect from infection, but the recipient with only anti-HBc can still become infected. Although treatment with antivirals or hyper immune globulin may prevent infection, there is always risk of drug resistance and mutant infections. Therefore, these livers should be used in a select group of hepatitis B surface antigen-positive recipients. If they are to be used in patients with anti-HBs or anti-HBc, than HBV prophylaxis should be instituted, and the recipient should be informed of the possible risk.

CONTRAINDICATIONS TO LIVER DONATION

There are few contraindications to selection of a donor. A positive HIV test, cirrhosis, hepatitis B surface antigen positivity, and the presence of extracerebral malignancies eliminate these potential donors. The use of donors with intracerebral malignancies confined to the central nervous system is controversial, due to a few reported instances of spread outside the central nervous system. Profound, irreversible hypotension is considered a contraindication. Severe trauma to the liver may be a contraindication, but CT scans frequently overestimate the degree of injury, and examination of the liver at the time of recovery should still be performed on stable, othewise acceptable donors. Sometimes, the damaged portion of a liver may be resected and the remaining segment transplanted. Certain high-risk social activities by the potential donor are relative contraindications. These include recent multiple sexual partners, active intravenous drug use characterized by fresh track marks, and recent sexual contact with an HIV-positive person.

THE NON-HEART BEATING DONOR

Before the advent of brain death guidelines, livers from donors whose hearts had stopped were the only source of allografts. Several organ procurement organizations and transplant programs across the country have instituted programs to use non-heart beating donors. The use of these livers should be extremely selective, taking into account the age of the donor, hemodynamic stability prior to withdrawal of life support, total warm ischemic time, and visualization of the liver. If the liver is recovered by an experienced surgeon with "super-rapid" technique, the above parameters optimized, and cold ischemia kept to a minimum, successful transplantation can be accomplished with these donors. In general, ideal non-heart beating liver donors should be under 50 years old, with controlled withdrawal of life support and cold in situ perfusion occurring within 30 minutes of extubation.

THE MULTIPLE ORGAN DONOR

When a patient is waiting for multiple organs, particularly thoracic organs such as liver-heart or liver-lung, the requirement for "ideal" donor organs is much greater. Marginal donors are acceptable for isolated liver transplants only. An exception is liver-kidney transplantation, in that older donors, and even non-heart beating donors, may be used as long as the renal function is adequate in the donor prior to recovery.

THE SPLIT-LIVER DONOR

Only young, hemodynamically stable multiorgan donors are considered for in situ splitting. These donors should not have experienced any significant compromise prior to procurement, such as a long period of resuscitation, prolonged hypotension, or irreversible acidosis. Donor hospitals and the other organ teams should be made aware that the liver is being split, as this adds approximately 1.5 hours to the procedure. Livers can be split into a left lateral segment/right tri-segment combination or a right lobe/left lobe split. The size of the segment should be at least 1% to 1.5% of recipient body weight to provide adequate hepatic function. With this technique, a whole adult cadaveric liver can be divided into two functioning allografts, effectively increasing the donor pool.

RECOMMENDED READING

Gilbert JR, Pascual M, Schoenfeld DA, Rubin RH, Delmonico FL, Cosimi AB. Evolving trends in liver transplantation: an outcome and charge analysis. Transplantation. 1999;67(2):246-253.

Marino IR, Doria C, Doyle HR, Gayowski TJ. Matching donors and recipients. Liver Transpl Surg. 1998;4(5 Suppl 1):S115-S119.

Seu P, Imagawa DK, Olthoff, et al. A prospective study on the reliability and cost effectiveness of preoperative ultrasound screening of the 'marginal' liver donor. Transplantation. 1996;62(1):129-130.

Pratschke J, Wilhelm MJ, Kusaka M, et al. Brain death and its influence on donor organ quality and outcome after transplantation. Transplantation. 1999;67(3):343-348.

Ploeg RJ, D'Alessandro AM, Knechtle SJ, et al. Risk factors for primary dysfunction after liver transplantation – a multivariate analysis. Transplantation. 1993;55(4):807-813.

Strasberg SM, Howard TK, Molmenti EP, Hertl M. Selecting the donor liver: risk factors for poor function after orthotopic liver transplantation. Hepatology. 1994;20(4 pt 1);829-838.

Deschenes M, Belle SH, Krom RA, Zetterman, RK, Lake JR. Early allograft dysfunction after liver transplantation: a definition and predictors of outcome. National

Institute of Diabetes and Digestive and Kidney Diseases Liver Transplantation Database. Transplantation. 1998;66(3):302-310.

Alexander JW, Vaughn WK. The use of "marginal" donors for organ transplantation. The influence of donor age on outcome. Transplantation. 1991;51(1):135-141.

Trevisani F, Colantoni A. Caraceni P, Van Thiel DH. The use of donor fatty liver for liver transplantation: a challenge or a quagmire? J Hepatol. 1996;24(1):114-121

D'Alessandro AM, Kalayoglu M, Sollinger HW, et al. The predictive value of donor liver biopsies for the development of primary nonfunction after orthotopic liver transplantation. Transplantation. 1991;51(1):157-163.

Markin RS, Wisecarver JL, Radio SJ, et al. Frozen section evaluation of donor livers before transplantation. Transplantation. 1993;56(6):1403-1409.

Detre KM, Lombardero M, Belle S, et al. Influence of donor age on graft survival after liver transplantation – United Network for Organ Sharing Registry. Liver Transpl Surg. 1995;1(5):341-343.

Marino IR, Doyle HR, Aldrighetti L, et al. Effect of donor age and sex on the outcome of liver transplantation. Hepatology. 1995;22(6):1754-1762.

Washburn WK, Johnson LB, Lewis WD, Jenkins RL. Graft function and outcome of older(> or = 60 years) donor livers. Transplantation. 1996;61(7):1062-1066.

Grande L, Matus D, Rimola A, et al. Expanded liver donor age over 60 years for hepatic transplantation. Clin Transplant. 1998;14:297-301.

Seaberg EC, Belle SH, Beringer KC, Schivins JL, Detre KM. Liver transplantation in the United States from 1987-1998: updated results from the Pitt-UNOS Liver Transplant Registry. Clin Transplant. 1998;14:17-37.

Markmann JF, Markowitz JS, Yersiz H, et al. Long-term survival after retransplantation of the liver. Ann Surg. 1997;226(4) 408-420.

Gayowski T, Marino IR, Singh N, et al. Orthotopic liver transplantation in high-risk patients: risk factors associated with mortality and infectious morbidity. Transplantation. 1998;65(4):499-504.

Showstack J, Katz PP, Lake JR, et al. Resource utilization in liver transplantation: effects of patient characteristics and clinical practice. NIDDK Liver Transplantation Database Group. JAMA. 1999;281(15):1381-1386.

Testa G, Goldstein RM, Netto G, et al. Long-term outcome of patients transplanted with livers from hepatitis C-positive donors. Transplantation. 1998;65(7):925-929.

Laskus T, Wang LF, Rakela J, et al. Dynamic behavior of hepatitis C virus in chronically infected patients receiving liver graft from infected donors. Virology. 1996; 220(1):171-176.

Dodson SF, Issa S, Araya V, et al. Infectivity of hepatic allografts with antibodies to hepatitis B virus. Transplantation. 1997;64(11):1582-1584.

Ascher NL. Expanded donor pool. Liver Transpl Surg. 1998;4(3):249-250.

Hauptman PJ, O'Connor KJ. Procurement and allocation of solid organs for transplantation. N Engl J Med. 1997;336(6):422-431.

Casavilla A, Ramirez C, Shapiro R, et al. Experience with liver and kidney allografts from non-heart-beating donors. Transplantation. 1995;59(2):197-203.

Edwards JM, Olthoff KM, Zamir G, et al. The changing pattern of referral and utilization of intra-abdominal organs from non-heart beating donors. Transplantation. 1999;67(9):S582.

Busuttil RW, Goss JA. Split liver transplantation. Ann Surg. 1999;229(3):313-321.

69   LIVER DONOR ALLOCATION SCHEME

Abraham Shaked, MD, PhD
Michael R. Lucey, MD, FRCPI

THE DONOR-RECIPIENT IMBALANCE

Although it is clear there are not enough donor livers to meet the potential pool of recipients, the disjunction between donor supply and candidate number is more complex than it first might appear. Evans has defined six overlapping categories of potential patients for liver transplantation: unrecognized need (people never listed); unmet need (people never listed and those listed but untransplanted); unmet demand (people on the waiting list and those who die waiting); met demand (transplants done); total demand (those placed on the waiting list and those transplanted); and finally total need (all these groups). This nomenclature is valuable because it accounts for the changing populations applicable to liver transplantation that have made it difficult to project the future societal requirements for liver transplantation. There is a great difficulty in estimating the true denominator of unrecognized and unmet need. It is clear that biases exist in referral practices. The best data come from Great Britain, where retrospective chart review of referral practice in a community hospital showed that a substantial proportion of potential candidates for transplantation were not referred to a regional liver transplant center, and that the bias against referral was greatest toward patients with alcoholic liver disease. The same researchers have shown that family practitioners tend to discriminate against patients with alcoholic liver disease when asked in an opinion survey to allocate scarce donor livers to hypothetical candidates. However, these are malleable opinions, and one reason for the unexpected expansion of the candidate pool (ie, unrecognized need becoming unmet demand) is a change in referral practices as the transplant community educates referring physicians that previously unsuitable patients (eg, alcoholics, IV drug users, patients with malignancies or previously untreatable conditions such as HIV infection,

Abraham Shaked, MD, PhD, Professor of Surgery; Chief, Liver Transplant Program, Hospital of the University of Pennsylvania, Philadelphia, PA

Michael R. Lucey, MD, FRCPI, Professor of Medicine; Associate Chief, Division of Gastroenterology; Director of Hepatology; Medical Director, Liver Transplant Program, University of Pennsylvania, Philadelphia, PA

patients at the extremes of age), are potential liver transplant candidates.

Most of the data from the US has concentrated on patients who have already been evaluated and placed on the waiting list (ie, unmet and met demand). Even using these limited perspectives, it is seen that numbers of patients on the waiting list are growing faster than numbers receiving transplants. Consequently, numbers dying on the list are also increasing. At the same time, the number of centers performing liver transplants in the US grew to 125 in 1998, resulting in competition between individual centers for transplant candidates and donor organs. These competing service and economic factors have led to a contentious debate that has pitched smaller center against larger center, the United Network of Organ Sharing (UNOS) against the Department of Health and Human Services, and State against Federal governments.

In 1998, the Secretary of State for Health and Human Services, Dr. Shalala, issued an injunction to the transplant community to make liver transplantation more fair. She urged continuation of the "sickest first policy," while avoiding futile transplantation. The department held public meetings and commissioned a review of solid organ procurement and transplantation policy by the Institute of Medicine (IOM). Among the recommendations of the IOM was that accumulated time by candidate on the waiting list should have diminished value as a criterion for allocation of donor livers. In 1999, the Department issued an amended Final Rule under the National Organ Transplant Act that called for the establishment of policies that reflected, "the following core principles:

- Organs must be allocated according to uniform medical criteria, which are developed by the transplantation community. Likewise, the transplantation community should design fair and effective criteria by which the performance of the system can be measured.
- Organ sharing must take place over broad enough areas to ensure that organs can reach the patients who need them most, and for whom transplantation is most medically appropriate."

To date, UNOS has moved to change the allocation rules to meet these challenges (see below).

PREDICTING THE OUTCOME OF LIVER TRANSPLANTATION

The cause of the underlying liver disease in the recipient influences outcome after liver transplantation. The best outcomes are observed in patients with chronic cholestatic disorders, and in chronic liver failure from cirrhosis of many causes. In contrast, the outcome is somewhat worse in patients transplanted for fulminant liver failure, and significantly worse in patients with malignant disease of the liver. The outcome of liver transplantation is little affected by a history of alcoholism, while recognizing that only a select population of alcoholic persons receive liver transplantation. Re-transplantation carries a poorer outcome than primary grafting, especially in patients undergoing re-transplantation soon after the initial graft. The outcome of liver transplantation is influenced by the severity of illness of the recipient prior to surgery. Patient and graft survival is significantly impaired in recipients who require intensive care unit management, or in patients with multisystem failure prior to transplant. In summary, the outcome is worst in patients with greatest urgency.

EXPANDING THE DONOR POOL

The increasing imbalance between the available donors and the number of candidates with life-threatening liver disease has led to strategies to expand the pool of donor organs. Such strategies have included requiring by law that families of brain dead persons are asked to consent for organ donation *(mandatory request)*, or even presuming that the brain dead person has consented to organ donation, rather than requiring consent by the donor family *(presumed consent)*. An alternative approach is to supplement altruism with payments to donor families, usually characterized as small sums to assist in funeral expenses. Innovative responses to the donor shortage, including the division of a cadaveric organ between two recipients (often referred to as a split-liver transplant), or the harvesting of liver segments from living donors, are dealt with elsewhere in this textbook. Finally, the donor organ shortage has led to the more frequent use of donor organs that hitherto would have been discarded: so-called *marginal donor organs*. Marginal organs include those from older donors, or from patients infected with present or past viral hepatitis B or C. The latter are matched to a recipient already infected by the same virus. Other marginal grafts include steatotic livers with a certain percentage (>25% to 30%) of micro vesicular or macro vesicular fat seen on frozen biopsy, although these grafts are associated with a higher incidence of primary nonfunction. At present, allocation priority schemes have not provided for a separate allocation system for less-than-ideal donor organs. All organs are allocated on the presumption that they have an equal chance of success.

Donation of a partial graft by a living donor is a novel response to the inadequate supply of cadaveric donor organs. Live liver donation began with removal of left lateral segments from adults (usually parents or grandparents) for transplantation into children. More recently, removal of right lobe partial grafts has allowed donation by adults to adult candidates. Live liver dona-tion is conducted within the same constraints of ABO compatibility as cadaveric donation. Concern for the health of the donor is the major impediment to live donation. Donor deaths have been recorded. Live liver donation affords the donor and the recipient the opportunity to avoid the uncertainties of waiting for a cadaveric allograft. This consideration becomes particularly pressing when the potential recipient is deteriorating either from worsening liver failure, or because of discovery of carcinoma. Whether the advent of live liver donation will result in an expansion in the recipient pool by expanding accepted indications for liver transplantation remains to be seen.

ORGAN ALLOCATION, URGENCY AND UTILITY

It is necessary to define organ allocation, urgency and utility and contrast this with organ distribution. *Organ allocation* refers to the system of prioritizing candidates on the waiting list. It is often characterized as the choice between urgency and utility. *Urgency* refers to the practice of giving priority to the most sick patient (ie, the patient at *greatest* risk of dying *before* a transplant). *Utility* refers to the practice of giving priority to the recipient who maximizes the chances of a successful outcome (ie, the patient at *least* risk of dying *after* a transplant). The rules on liver allocation must resolve the conflict between urgency and utility when determining the appropriateness of a particular candidate, relative to others on the waiting list.

Up to November 2000, donor livers in the US have been allocated through a points system that mixes prioritization according to urgency of the potential recipient and utility of outcome. In this system, which is administered by UNOS, points are awarded up to a capped maximum on the basis of three clinical attributes of the potential *recipient*. These are: severity of liver failure (urgency), ABO type matching with the donor (utility), and length of time on the waiting list (a notion of justice independent of either urgency and utility). Points for severity of liver failure are awarded according to the presence of fulminant hepatic failure, Childs-Turcotte-Pugh class among patients with chronic liver failure (Chapter 66) and requirement for intensive care unit management. Since points are also awarded for accumulated time on the waiting list, there are standardized criteria for placement of patients on the waiting list.

Further complicating the development of allocation rules are the arguments in favor (or against) "special cases". The present (circa 1999) rules for UNOS give additional priority to categories such as pediatric cases, patients with small malignancies confined to the liver or patients with fulminant hepatic failure. Similarly, there have been proposals to assign lower priority to "special cases": multiple organ failure, overweight, old, or alcoholic candidates or patients requiring re-transplantation. The present UNOS system does not incorporate penalty points for these or other circumstances.

In response to the directives of the Department of Health and Human Services, and the report of the IOM alluded in the foregoing, UNOS has proposed to change the rules that govern the allocation of donor organs to patients with chronic liver disease. These rules do not alter the special priority given to patients with fulminant hepatic failure. In particular, the new rules propose to replace the Childs-Turcotte-Pugh class as the basis for determining urgency for liver transplantation with a recently described prognostic instrument called the Mayo End-Stage Liver Disease (MELD) score. Like the Childs classification, the MELD score was designed to predict the outcome of decompressive therapy for portal hypertension. In contradistinction to the Childs classification, MELD was derived from prospectively gathered data, rather than empirically constructed. Calculation of the MELD score is based on serum bilirubin, prothrombin time as presented as INR, and serum creatinine, and is easily done through software displayed on the Mayo Clinic website. The MELD score has advantages when compared to the Childs score, including that it uses less subjective parameters, that its objective parameters are less prone to center-to-center variability than the Childs class, and that the MELD score increases as the three constituent parameters deteriorate, whereas the individual scoring elements in the Childs score remain fixed once a defined threshold has been reached.

The MELD score has been verified in four independent pretransplant populations: (1) a cohort of patients hospitalized for decompensated liver disease; (2) ambulatory patients with noncholestatic liver cirrhosis; (3) patients with primary biliary cirrhosis; and (4) unselected patients from the 1980s with cirrhosis, and found to have a clinically useful ability to classify patients according to their risk of death at three time intervals relevant to determination of urgency for liver transplantation (ie, one week, three months and one year). Furthermore, the addition to the scoring system of clinical phenomena often associated with decompensation and worse outcome, such as ascites, encephalopathy, variceal bleeding or spontaneous bacterial peritonitis does not substantially improve the degree of fit between the MELD score and the actual outcome. Finally, the inclusion of a broad diagnostic category (ie, cholestatic or alcoholic vs the rest), which was included in the original score, has been found to be unnecessary. The latter point was a potential area of contention whenever MELD was to be applied to populations awaiting liver transplantation. It remains to be determined how UNOS will allocate livers to special cases that fall outside the MELD criteria, such as patients with hepatocellular carcinoma.

DISTRIBUTION

Distribution refers to the system of prioritization of transplant centers according to their geographic location (local, regional, super-regional or national) in relation to a specific donor. In the US, these geographical distinctions are based on the boundaries of organ procurement organizations (OPOs). The present UNOS rules mandate distribution to centers within the OPO first, then to regional centers and, finally, an organ not claimed already will be offered nationally. Since OPOs differ both in size and in number of transplant programs they contain, this scheme has resulted in marked differences between OPOs in waiting times for liver transplantation of patients with similar degrees of liver failure. These disparities in distribution led the Secretary of State to issue a Final Rule that mandated, "Organ sharing…over broad enough areas to ensure that organs can reach the patients who need them most, and for whom transplantation is most medically appropriate." As yet, UNOS has not determined how to achieve this goal throughout the US.

THE PAYORS' PERSPECTIVE

Throughout the debate on allocation and distribution, little attention has been paid to the influence of the payers. Both Medicare and many insurance carriers have developed networks of preferred transplant centers (ie, "centers of excellence") to which they direct their covered lives. Participation in a center of excellence program is dependent on external review that usually includes survival statistics and other quality measures. The consequence of the center of excellence concept is to exert pressure on transplant centers to select more utilitarian and less urgent cases, since tilting the balance in favor of urgency will likely lower that transplant center's survival statistics, jeopardizing the continued access of the transplant center to patients with that insurance carrier, while simultaneously increasing center costs, thereby lowering the margin on the fixed payment.

RECOMMENDED READING

Evans RW. Need for liver transplantation. Lancet. 1995;346(8983):1169.

Davies MH, Langman MJ, Elias E, Neuberger JM. Liver disease in a district hospital remote from a transplant centre: a study of admissions and deaths. Gut. 1992;33(10):1397-1399.

Neuberger J, Adams D, MacMaster P, Maidment A, Speed M. Assessing priorities for allocation of donor liver grafts: survey of public and clinicians. BMJ. 1998;317(7152):172-175.

Annual Report of the US Scientific Registry for Transplant Recipients and the Organ Procurement and

Transplantation Network – Transplant Data: 1988-1996. United Network for Organ Sharing, Richmond, VA, and the Division of Transplantation, Office of Special Programs, Health Resources and Human Services Administration, US Department of Health and Human Services, Rockville, MD.

Lucey MR, Brown KA, Everson GT, et al. Minimal criteria for placement of adults on the liver transplant waiting list: a report of a national conference organized by the American Society of Transplant Physicians and the American Association for the Study of Liver Diseases. Liver Transpl Surg. 1997;3(6):628-637.

Statement by Donna E. Shalala, Secretary of Health and Human Services Regarding Issuance of OPTN Final Rule Amendments:
http://www.hhs.gov/news/press/1999pres/991018.html

Institute of Medicine. Analysis of waiting times. In: Committee on Organ Procurement and Transplantation Policy, ed. Organ Procurement and Transplantation: Assessing current policies and the potential impact of the DHHS final rule. Washington, DC: National Academy Press; 1999:57-78.

Malinchoc M, Kamath PS, Gordon FD, Peine CJ, Rank J, ter Borg PC. A model to predict poor survival in patients undergoing transjugular intrahepatic portosystemic shunts. Hepatology. 2000;31(4):864-871.

Forman LM, Lucey MR. Predicting the prognosis of chronic liver disease: an evolution from Childs to MELD. Hepatology. 2001;33:473-475.

70 SURGICAL TECHNIQUES IN LIVER TRANSPLANTATION

Hasan Yersiz, MD
Ronald W. Busuttil, MD, PhD

Liver Transplant Surgical Procedure

Multiple advances in surgical techniques have been developed throughout the past 40 years. A successful outcome is heavily influenced by the employment of highly refined technical skills during organ recovery, recipient hepatectomy, and organ allografting. Many liver transplant centers have tailored the procedure to meet the needs of their own center and patient population. In assessing the experience derived in over 3,000 cases, the Dumont-UCLA Transplant Center believes the following techniques to be most beneficial to a broad patient population. Application of such techniques provides maximum safety to the organ at the time of procurement and ensures the least morbidity to recipients at the time of transplantation.

THE LIVER PROCUREMENT TECHNIQUE. A midline incision from the suprasternal notch to the pubis is made with electrocautery. After the sternum is split and self-retaining retractors are placed, the dissection commences with electrocautery.

The round ligament, falciform ligament and left triangular ligaments are cut (Figure 70-1). The left lateral segment of the liver is elevated and retracted to the donor's right and the gastro-hepatic omentum is divided with care not to injure a replaced left hepatic artery (prevalence of this anomaly is 15%).

The right colon and the small bowel are mobilized cephalad and moved out of the incision to the donor's left and a Kocher maneuver is performed. The peritoneal reflection between the duodenum and the retroperitoneal area is cut, which allows full exposure of the entire retroperitoneal structures, including the infrahepatic vena cava, both renal veins, the superior mesenteric artery, the abdominal aorta and the inferior mesenteric vein (IMV). The inferior mesenteric vein is isolated close

Hasan Yersiz, MD, Assistant Professor of Surgery, Division of Liver and Pancreas Transplantation, The Dumont-UCLA Transplant Center, Los Angeles, CA

Ronald W. Busuttil, MD, PhD, Professor and Chief, Division of Liver and Pancreas Transplantation; Dumont Chair in Transplantation Surgery; Director, The Dumont-UCLA Transplant Center, Los Angeles, CA

to the root of the transverse mesocolon and cannulated for infusion with cold Plasmalyte solution for precooling. The peritoneum and lymphatic-rich tissue overlying the distal aorta are divided; the aorta is exposed and encircled with two umbilical tapes to cannulate the aorta later for flushing.

After the right colon and the small bowel are moved back to the abdominal cavity, the common bile duct is visualized just above the duodenum and, by palpation behind the hilum, a replaced right hepatic artery (prevalence is 10%) pulse is sought. The common bile duct is turned around with a right angle, paying special attention to not go beyond the bile duct. This precaution will prevent injuring the possible replaced right hepatic artery or the low take-off right hepatic artery. The distal common bile duct is tied with a 2-0 silk and the bile duct is cut sharply (Figure 70-2). The gallbladder is flushed with saline solution until the effluent from the cut common duct is clear. After mobilizing the left colon to make a space for ice around the left kidney, the supraceliac aorta is prepared for cross-clamping. In this maneuver the left lateral segment of the liver is elevated and retracted medially and a vertical incision is made to the diaphragmatic crura at the midline while retracting the esophagus to the left. The aorta is then dissected anteriorly and laterally and is encircled with an umbilical tape to identify it easily before cross-clamping.

At this point 30,000 U of heparin (500 U/kg for pediatric donors) is given via central line and distal abdominal aorta is cannulated (Figure 70-3). A long straight vascular clamp is placed around the supraceliac aorta and is held by the first assistant unclamped. The

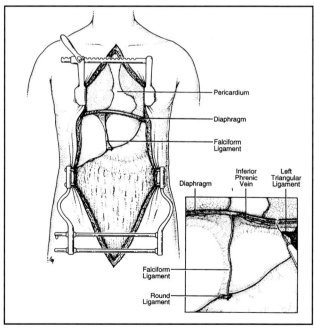

Figure 70-1. The round ligament, falciform ligament and left triangular ligaments are cut.

surgeon transects the vena cava at the caval-atrial junction to allow exsanguination of the abdominal organs. Simultaneously the first assistant cross-clamps the supraceliac aorta. When there is a heart team, the vena cava is cut by the heart surgeon. Cold University of Wisconsin (UW) solution is run through the aortic and portal cannulas without pressure. The suprahepatic inferior vena cava is vented into the pericardium and right pleural space. If there is lung procurement, the distal inferior vena cava can be vented. Ice slush is poured into the abdominal cavity to facilitate rapid cooling of the viscera. Usually, two liters of cold preservation solution through

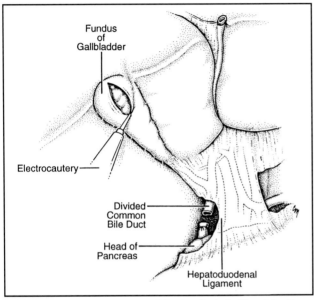

Figure 70-2. The distal common bile duct is tied with a 2-0 silk and the bile duct is cut sharply.

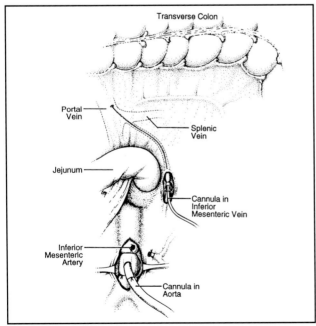

Figure 70-3. The distal abdominal aorta is cannulated.

the aortic cannula and one liter through the portal cannula are enough to flush and to cool the liver (50 mL/kg UW solution is enough for pediatric and small donors).

After flushing is completed, the pericardium and the posterior wall of the suprahepatic inferior vena cava are divided. The first assistant pulls the esophagus to the left and the surgeon divides the diaphragm in an anterior-to-posterior direction down to the aorta in the midline. The right diaphragm is cut along the right lobe towards the left kidney and the liver is left to fall back into the right chest. The liver is covered with slush and pool suction is placed behind the hilum to provide a dry field. The duodenum is retracted from the liver and the gastroduodenal artery is identified at the level of the superior edge of the duodenum where it is dissected towards the liver until the common hepatic artery is reached. After seeing the common hepatic artery going both directions proximally and distally, the gastroduodenal artery is tied at a distance from the hepatic artery and cut. While dissecting the gastroduodenal artery toward the common hepatic artery, if the portal vein traverses at the right side of the common hepatic artery, it is most likely that the totally replaced hepatic artery originating from the superior mesenteric artery (prevalence is 1%) is supplying arterial circulation to the liver. The hepatic artery is dissected back to the aorta. As the splenic artery is encountered it is ligated, divided and gently pulled to the right. Dissection of the celiac trunk to the aorta is continued until the aorta is reached. All the fibrous tissue, the celiac plexus nerves and the diaphragmatic crura located to the left of the celiac trunk and the aorta are divided. The dissection should be carried out at the inferior edge of the celiac trunk so that the left gastric artery is not encountered. If there is a replaced left hepatic artery, the left gastric artery must be preserved. In this case, the lesser omentum is mobilized off the stomach before dissecting the celiac trunk. Then the supraceliac aorta is transected below the cross-clamp.

Dividing the avascular fibrous tissue along the superior margin of the pancreas then identifies the portal vein. If the pancreas is not procured, the head of the pancreas is divided and the superior mesenteric vein is identified, tied, cut and held up and mobilized toward the liver. The dissection is continued with the portal vein. As the splenic, the inferior mesenteric and the coronary veins are encountered, they are cut at a distance from the portal vein. If the pancreas is to be procured, then the portal vein is divided distal to the coronary vein. The portal vein dissection is stopped at the level of the bile duct tie. While mobilizing the portal vein, the presence of a replaced right hepatic artery originating from the superior mesenteric artery or a low take-off right hepatic artery may be noted. The rest of the fibrous tissue of the liver hilum and the dense nerve tissue of the celiac plexus between celiac trunk and the superior mesenteric artery are cut towards the aorta. A hole is made to the aorta anteriorly, between the celiac trunk and the superior mesenteric artery, it is extended obliquely to the left and the aorta is opened on the left side, taking special care not to cut a left renal artery. The right side of the aorta now can be observed from the inside and is then cut toward the transection line. Together with the surrounding tissues the aortic patch and the celiac trunk are mobilized and held up to the liver side. If a replaced right hepatic artery exists, it is followed to the superior mesenteric artery and the superior mesenteric artery is mobilized toward the aorta. The aortic patch now includes both the celiac and the superior mesenteric artery openings. Occasionally, a renal artery arises above the origin of the superior mesenteric artery, and this must be recognized.

The infrahepatic inferior vena cava is transected above the renal veins. The remaining diaphragmatic and peritoneal attachments are divided and the liver is removed and placed in a sterile plastic bag with a liter of cold UW solution and the bile duct is flushed with 20 mL of cold UW solution. Two more plastic bags are used for storage and the liver is placed in the ice-filled cooler.

After the kidneys are removed, the iliac arteries and veins are excised and placed in cold preservation solution. These vessels may be needed as vessel grafts during the recipient procedure. In elderly donors, if the iliac arteries are atherosclerotic and cannot be used, other medium-sized arteries, such as the carotid artery or the superior mesenteric artery, may be removed. In small pediatric donors, the iliac arteries are not suitable as a graft because of the small size. The neck vessels may be used for this purpose.

This technique allows rapid flushing and safe procurement of the abdominal organs. Even if the donor is unstable, it can be used without damaging any organ. In case of a non-heart beating donor, the abdominal aorta is rapidly cannulated and UW flushing is started. The suprahepatic inferior vena cava is transected below the right atrium, the pericardium is opened and the thoracic aorta is cross-clamped in the lower mediastinum. Iced slush is applied around the organs. Then the superior mesenteric vein is identified and cannulated for portal flushing. All dissection is made cold after the flushing.

SEGMENTAL LIVER TRANSPLANTATION
The Surgical Technique of In Situ Splitting of the Cadaveric Liver
This technique for liver splitting results in two liver grafts, in the conventional technique a left lateral segment graft (segments 2 and 3) and a right trisegmental graft (segments 1 and 4-8). The liver can be split to left (segments 1-4) and the right lobes (segments 5-8) or

vena cava and the segment 1 may be left with right lobe, resulting in a left graft with segments 2-4 and a right graft with segments 1 and 5-8.

In order to permit rapid perfusion, in the event of donor instability, the initial steps of the standard multi-organ procurement procedure are completed before further dissection.

In the conventional in situ splitting, the first vascular structure isolated in the liver hilum is the left hepatic artery along its entire length. Special attention is paid to the arterial branch to segment 4. The segment 4 branch is preserved whenever possible. The right hepatic artery is identified at the level of the common hepatic artery but not dissected free. Next the entire left portal vein is isolated, which requires ligation and division of all the branches entering the caudate lobe of the liver. Portal vein branches to segment 4 of the liver are ligated and divided to the right of the umbilical fissure. This maneuver is followed by extrahepatic mobilization of the left hepatic vein.

After total vascular control of the left lateral segment, the parenchymal cut line is marked using electrocautery. The line is 1 cm above the left bile duct in the umbilical fissure and traverses between the segment 3 hepatic vein and the middle hepatic vein. The superior part of the liver parenchyma is divided by electrocautery along the right of the falciform ligament. The left hilar plate and bile duct are cut sharply. The rest of the liver parenchyma is divided, using electrocautery and suture ligation as required. When this dissection is completed, the left lateral segment (segments 2 and 3), and the rest of the liver parenchyma (segments 1 and 4-8) are separated, each with its own vascular pedicles and venous drainage.

Perfusion is the next step. Three (3) L of UW solution is used for perfusion: 2 L in the aorta and 1 L in the portal vein. After perfusion, the left hepatic artery, the left portal vein and the left hepatic vein are divided. The left bile duct is flushed with UW solution and the left lateral segment is stored in cold UW solution. The right graft is then removed in the usual fashion and stored at 4° C in UW solution.

THE BACK TABLE SPLITTING OF THE LIVER. This technique is used for both reduction and splitting of the liver. After dissecting the vessels, parenchyma is cut with a knife and the cut surfaces are prepared by oversewing the vessel and bile duct openings. To avoid rewarming of the liver graft, finger fracture should not be use.

THE BACK TABLE PREPARATION OF THE LIVER GRAFT. The liver graft is prepared for the implantation on the slush machine to avoid excessive rewarming. The purpose of this preparation is to trim off the diaphragm and connective tissue around the liver and its vessels and to provide a single arterial inlet if there is an arterial variation requiring reconstruction. Injured vessels can also be reconstructed on the back table. The phrenic veins and the adrenal vein are tied to avoid bleeding from the vena cava after reperfusion in the recipient. The portal vein is cannulated and checked for its integrity. This cannula is later used to flush out the preservation solution and the air. The celiac trunk is dissected from its origin to the gastroduodenal artery. Dissecting the hepatic artery distal to the gastroduodenal juncture should be avoided, since it may compromise extra hepatic bile duct circulation.

An arterial reconstruction is required if the donor artery does not have a single inlet. The replaced left hepatic artery does not require a reconstruction unless it originates from the aorta. In this latter case it is either anastomosed to the splenic artery or to the gastroduodenal artery. The totally replaced hepatic artery, originating from the superior mesenteric artery, also does not require any reconstruction. The most common arterial variant that requires reconstruction is the replaced right hepatic artery, originating from the superior mesenteric artery. In this case, either proximal end of the superior mesenteric artery is anastomosed to the Carrel patch and the distal superior mesenteric artery is used for anastomosis in the recipient or the replaced right hepatic artery is anastomosed to the splenic or the gastroduodenal stump.

The left lateral segment of the in situ split liver does not need any back table preparation. The right trisegment of the liver is trimmed as the usual whole liver graft and then the vessel and the bile duct openings are oversewn. The left hepatic vein opening on the suprahepatic vena cava and left portal vein opening on the portal vein are oversewn using running 7-0 Prolene. The left hepatic artery stump is also oversewn with a running 7-0 prolene. The left bile duct opening is oversewn on the cut surface with 6-0 Prolene. The bile duct is flushed with UW solution and the cut surface is observed for any biliary leakage. If there is any leaking point, they are closed with 6-0 Prolene stitch.

ORTHOTOPIC LIVER TRANSPLANTATION

The abdomen is opened via a bilateral subcostal incision with midline extension. Except for the superficial skin incision, the skin, subcutaneous tissue, and muscle layers are opened with the electrocautery unit. The right-sided incision is brought so far lateral as to allow horizontal view into the vena cava. The left-sided incision is shorter and extends beyond the lateral border of the rectus. If splenomegaly is present, care should be taken to avoid making this incision very long because the spleen may be injured. The midline incision is extended to the point at which the surgeon has a direct perpendicular view of the suprahepatic vena cava. This may necessitate a complete or partial xiphoidectomy. After placement of a mechanical retractor, the falciform ligament is divided to the suprahepatic vena cava and the tissue with all the collaterals along the falciform ligament and the midline fascia are removed up to the xiphoid, thus totally preventing further collateral bleeding and obstruction of the field from the tissue mass itself. The left triangular ligament is then opened with cautery up to its tip, which often requires ligature for hemostasis. The left lateral segment is now retracted up out of the wound and to the right. The gastrohepatic ligament is now visualized and requires either cautery division or suture ligation depending on the extent of the collateral vessels.

The anteroinferior edge of the liver is now lifted up by an assistant, allowing an unobstructed view of the porta hepatis. The dissection is carried down to the hepatic artery, which is then divided above its bifurcation. Next proceed to the right side of the porta hepatis and divide the common duct. Complete the dissection around the portal vein. In most cases, the dorsal pancreatic vein drains into the anterior portion of the portal vein and must be divided. If adhesions are present after previous operations or from spontaneous bacterial peritonitis, they are taken down with electrocautery. The tip of the electrocautery is kept and run parallel to the liver surface at all times, never venturing more than 1 mm from the liver surface but never violating the liver capsule.

In an uncomplicated case, proceed to dissect the right triangular ligament. This is done completely with cautery, beginning lateral and inferior and dividing the ligament carefully all the way into the vena cava. If there are technical problems with an unusual amount of collaterals, scarring, and inflammation, this part of the procedure is deferred until after the patient is on total venovenous bypass. With the portal vein transected, the anterior aspect of the infrahepatic inferior vena cava (IVC) is exposed, allowing easy circumferential mobilization for placement of a vascular clamp (ie, Blalock clamp). If the portal vein is not transected at this point, the vena cava is dissected inferior to superior, using cautery. The right adrenal vein is ligated and divided. At this time, allow the right lobe to fall back into the hepatic fossa and expose the left side of the vena cava by retracting the left lateral segment and the caudate lobe to the right. The peritoneal reflection is opened longitudinally along the vena cava with cautery. In most cases, the retrohepatic caval tissue can be taken down with finger dissection. Any resistance to this dissection usually signifies retrohepatic collaterals entering the vena cava, which require ligation. With this dual-sided approach, the posterior aspect of the retrohepatic cava can be quickly and safely liberated from the retroperitoneum.

At this juncture the patient is prepared for venovenous bypass by cannulation of the left saphenous and left axillary veins. Wire-reinforced cannulas are preferred to prevent kinking and to allow safe securing to the drained vessel. The portal vein cannula size is usually 24 to 28 French, and the axillary and saphenous vein cannulas, 18 to 22 French (Research Medical, Midvale, UT). Forced cannulation is contraindicated; if the cannula does not go in easily, it should be downsized. The axillary cannula is often the more difficult one to introduce because of inadvertent kinking of the axillary vein and the presence of valves. By pulling the axillary vein out and distally as straight as possible, the cannula usually goes in without difficulty.

Once the axillary and saphenous vein cannulas have been introduced and secured, the portal vein is cannulated and secured by snugging down a Romel tourniquet. Total venovenous bypass is now started.

In cases in which the portal vein is injured or, even more important, when dense adhesions with large collateral veins are surrounding the liver, the inferior mesenteric vein can be used for bypass purposes.

In patients with organized portal vein thrombus, a formal thromboendovenectomy can be performed in the majority of situations, removing thrombus all the way down to the superior mesenteric and splenic vein confluence. In patients with portal vein thrombosis, partial or complete, utmost care should be taken to avoid any further traumatization of the portal vein. In cases in which this is impossible, iliac vein graft from the superior mesenteric vein is used to establish portal venous inflow to the liver.

Vascular clamps are now placed on the suprahepatic vena cava and the lower infrahepatic vena cava (Figure 70-4). Care should be taken to place these clamps horizontally and with the liver in its normal anatomical position to prevent rotation of the vessels. The suprahepatic vena cava clamp should be placed on the very edge of the diaphragmatic reflection to avoid phrenic nerve injuries.

Now divide the vena cava, taking care to retain as much of the right and left hepatic veins as possible, pulling up the veins by almost cutting into the liver substance. The lower cava is then divided as far distal as possible. The previously ligated retrocaval tissue is divided and the liver is removed.

To achieve hemostasis, the bare area can be reperitonealized using a 2-0 Prolene (monofilament polypropylene suture, Ethicon, Somerville, NJ) (Figure 70-5). Care should be taken to ensure that the needle passes superficially under the bottom of the entire wound to obtain hemostatic control.

In patients with difficult dissections, the vena cava can be clamped above and below the liver before all the right-sided and retrohepatic dissection is done. In such cases, it is often expedient to retain the dorsal side of the vena cava to eliminate the need for elaborate hemostatic control of the retrocaval tissue.

The suprahepatic vena cava is now prepared by opening the right and left hepatic veins into a common cloaca of the IVC. All phrenic vein ostia are oversewn with 4-0 Prolene with knots placed outside of the suprahepatic vena cava cuff. The liver is now brought into the wound. By placing a lap in the hepatic fossa, the liver receives support from below to prevent it from sinking down too far into the wound.

Corner stitches are placed on the two opposing ends. With a 3-0 Prolene, the suprahepatic vena cava anastomosis is run; care is taken to ensure perfect intimal adaptation. The dorsal suture is run to the right-

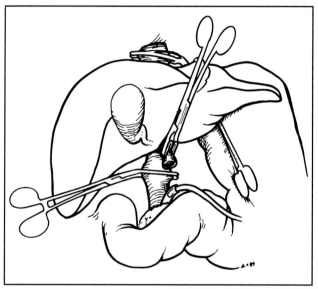

Figure 70-4. Vascular clamps are placed on the suprahepatic vena cava and the lower infrahepatic vena cava.

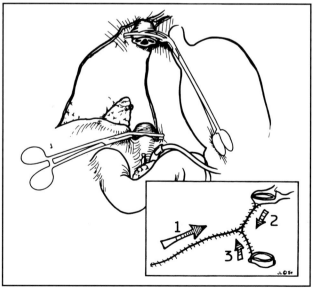

Figure 70-5. To achieve hemostasis, the bare area can be reperitonealized using a 2-0 Prolene.

sided stay suture and the front wall closure is completed in a simple running suture fashion.

A portal flush with normal saline or lactated Ringer's solution and 25 g of albumin per liter is run through the portal vein during the completion of the infrahepatic vena cava. This is to empty the graft of air to prevent air emboli as well as to remove the excessively high concentrations of intravascular potassium, resulting from the preservation solution. The infrahepatic vena cava is sewn in exactly the same manner as that of the suprahepatic vena cava, including a 1½-cm growth factor. Care must be taken to prevent too long a vena cava. Excessive length of vena cava is the main cause of folding, and kinking can cause formidable postoperative problems that require extraordinarily difficult reconstructions in a later stage.

The portal bypass cannula is now clamped, continuing only the systemic venovenous bypass. The cannula is removed from the portal vein, and an atraumatic clamp is carefully placed proximal on the portal vein. The donor portal vein is now shortened to the appropriate length. One should not cut the recipient portal vein shorter than 1 cm because length should be conserved in the event that re-transplantation is needed. As with the vena cava, it is crucially important to prevent portal vein kinking, folding, and flow obstruction. The portal vein is run with a 6-0 running Prolene suture, also with the everting stitch in the back wall using a growth factor that is ½ of the portal vein diameter. If size must be adjusted, to either the donor or the recipient portal vein, a fish-mouth reconstruction is recommended. There are several methods to reperfuse the liver after portal venous reconstruction: (1) reperfusion through portal vein with or without vena cava venting; (2) opening IVC followed by portal reperfusion; and (3) reperfusion with portal and hepatic artery simultaneously. To date, no randomized trial has conferred superiority to any of these methods. It is our preference to release the portal vein clamp slowly with an eye on the electrocardiogram. We usually open the portal vein in stages after any T-wave segment elevations have reversed. Once these are normalized, the portal vein is completely opened. It usually takes three or four partial decompressions before the vein is completely open.

After making sure that there is no significant bleeding from the vena cava, portal vein, or its anastomoses, the systemic bypass is now discontinued and the cannula removed from the groin, allowing the blood in the bypass system to be reinfused into the patient. The saphenous vein is later ligated, and the axillary vein is either reconstructed or ligated. If the axillary vein becomes thrombosed postoperatively, it usually recanalizes and can be used later if necessary. No difference has been found in arm swelling or venous hypertension between patients whose axillary veins are reconstructed or ligated. When the portal vein is unusable, a portal venous conduit is

used. In these cases, the arterial reconstruction with reperfusion of the liver is done before the portal conduit is sewn in. For portal venous conduit, the donor iliac vein is perfect material. The superior mesenteric vein (SMV) is most commonly used for inflow and accessed at the base of the colon mesenterium. After the SMV has been identified and is side-occluded, the venous conduit is anastomosed using running 6-0 Prolene. It should be pointed out that when the side-occluding clamp on the SMV is released, there must be an outflow already established from the venous conduit. Otherwise, the anastomosis line may completely rupture, causing an immediate catastrophe.

Successful hepatic artery reconstruction is crucial for graft function. A variety of methods can be used. In principle, the type of reconstruction with regard to specific recipient and donor arteries is secondary to achieving excellent inflow and outflow at the first anastomosis. In the routine case, the celiac trunk of the donor is anastomosed end to end to the recipient common hepatic artery or to a branch patch of the bifurcation between the gastroduodenal and the hepatic artery proper. The arterial anastomosis is sewn with 6-0 or 7-0 Prolene and a ¼-diameter growth factor is tied in place to provide the full expansion of the arterial anastomosis without any constriction.

In some patients, despite a perfect technical result, inflow is inadequate as a result of arcuate ligament compression of the celiac axis. This is demonstrated by marked respiratory variation and can be documented by flow measurement. In this situation, the celiac artery must be dissected proximal to the aorta and the arcuate ligament is cut.

Arterial reconstruction varies greatly depending on the particular circumstances of each patient. Occasionally, in the case of dual blood supply to the liver from an accessory right hepatic artery and from a hepatic artery proper, the accessory right hepatic stemming from the SMA is dominant and serves a source of inflow. When the recipient hepatic artery is insufficient, the donor celiac artery can then be anastomosed directly to the supraceliac recipient aorta. This approach to the aorta is more commonly done in pediatric transplants than in adult transplants. When there is no acceptable common hepatic artery or right hepatic artery to which to anastomose the donor celiac artery, a donor iliac artery conduit is used. This is done by exposing the infrarenal aorta just above the inferior mesenteric artery. After the aorta is side-occluded, the iliac arterial conduit is sewn end-to-side using 5-0 Prolene. The conduit is then tunneled through the transverse mesocolon, pulled behind the stomach in front of the pancreas and up toward the liver hilum, where it is anastomosed end-to-end to the donor celiac artery using 6-0 Prolene. By sewing the arterial conduit to the aorta before it is attached to the donor celiac artery, the conduit is completely mobile and access to the completion of the anastomosis is made easier. When extensive scarring is found around the stomach or the pancreas, it is sometimes advantageous to curve the arterial conduit lateral to the pancreas after first having mobilized the duodenum. The attachment to the aorta is the same as in the shorter conduit, but after the aortal anastomosis is completed the arterial conduit is pulled lateral – care is taken not to traumatize the pancreas – and up toward the hepatic hilum behind the duodenum.

After the gallbladder is removed, the common duct is shortened proximal to the cystic duct. Usually a lap is placed superior to the liver, pushing the liver down to approximate donor and recipient ducts better. It is important to prevent redundancy of the bile duct because this is an important cause of biliary obstruction in the postoperative period. The donor cystic duct, if allowed to remain in order to preserve common duct length, has to empty freely into the remaining common duct to prevent the development of cystoceles, which can compress the duct, causing biliary obstruction and serious long-term consequences. If the cystic duct does not empty into the common duct, it has to be excised. The biliary anastomosis is sewn with interrupted 6-0 monofilament absorbable suture, PDS (polyglyconate, Davis & Geck, American Cyanamid Company, Wayne, NJ), and a T-tube that exits through the recipient common duct wall is secured with a purse-string or similar suture. Doing the choledochocholedochostomy without T-tube is preferred, unless the liver is marginal and there is a large size discrepancy between the donor and the recipient bile ducts.

If there is any size discrepancy in the bile duct size, or if both donor and recipient ducts are of normal or small size, it is best to spatulate the small one; if equal size, we spatulate both. In the equally-sized normal or small ducts, the spatulation is done to compensate for the tissue that is effectively lost in the suture line to prevent the stricturing effect of the suture line. If one of the ducts – usually in the recipient - is excessively large, as is frequently seen in patients with previous cholecystectomies, a part of the large duct is closed with a running or interrupted 6-0 Prolene suture. This leaves a duct opening large enough to accommodate the donor duct, which is then sewn in the usual fashion with an interrupted 6-0 PDS suture.

In patients with very small donor common ducts or with extraordinarily large biliary collateral veins, a Roux-N-Y choledochojejunostomy can be performed. In patients with a thrombosed portal vein or Budd-Chiari syndrome, the huge venous collaterals that parallel the bile duct can cause excessive blood loss and make the choledochocholedochostomy difficult because collateral veins can completely encase the common duct. Placement of the Roux-N-Y is usually retrocolic. The choledochojejunostomy is done with interrupted 5-0

PDS. A silastic catheter is placed in the anastomosis and secured with one of the bacula stitches. Three drains are now introduced (Figure 70-6). These drains are always placed in the same sequence, allowing secure identification of the location of any postoperative hemorrhage. The drains are numbered from right to left, with no. 1 draining behind the liver and up above the dome toward the right side of the vena cava, no. 2 draining the subhepatic space, and no. 3 draining the left quadrant and the medial side of the vena cava. The wound is closed with interrupted sutures; each layer is carefully identified. The inguinal and axillary wounds for the venovenous bypass are closed with two layers of subcutaneous running suture to prevent the collection of wound seroma. The skin is finally closed with staples.

The procedure as explained provides only the initial guidelines for the recipient hepatectomy and implantation of the graft. The secret of this operation, as for all surgery, is to have complete mastery of the anatomy to avoid wandering into places or structure where you are not supposed to be. Even the most minute, careless move can have a devastating impact on the outcome of a liver transplantation.

RECOMMENDED READING

Busuttil RW, Klintmalm GB, eds. Transplantation of the Liver. Philadelphia, Pa. WB Saunders Company; 1996.

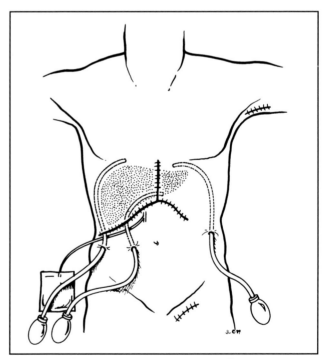

Figure 70-6. Three drains are now introduced. The drains are always placed in the same sequence, numbered from right to left. No. 1 drains behind the liver and up above the dome toward the right side of the vena cava. No. 2 drains the subhepatic space. No. 3 drains the left quadrant and the medial side of the vena cava.

71 IMMEDIATE POSTOPERATIVE MANAGEMENT OF THE LIVER TRANSPLANT PATIENT

Timothy McCashland, MD
Michael F. Sorrell, MD

The immediate care of the patient after transplantation is best handled by a multidisciplinary team effort. The complexity of care demands the attention of a diverse and experienced team of individuals. The experienced transplant team anticipates potential complications that include graft dysfunction, sepsis, pulmonary and renal failure as well as technical problems arising from the transplant itself.

GENERAL PRINCIPLES OF ICU CARE

Daily rounds by a multidisciplinary team of physicians, nurses, transplant coordinators, dieticians and pharmacists are essential in the care of the new recipient. Data pertinent to the patient's condition must be carefully organized and available.

Cardiopulmonary Management

All patients require a period of ventilatory management in the immediate postoperative period. The length of time on the ventilator and the degree of difficulty in achieving adequate gas exchange depends in large measure on the preoperative condition of the recipient. A patient with a relatively normal nutritional status as exemplified by the absence of hypoalbuminemia and muscle wasting often has a short period of mechanical ventilation. Marked ascites and/or pleural effusion can prolong intubation. A tidal volume of 10 mL/kg is usually adequate. The respiratory rate and FiO2 are adjusted to maintain satisfactory pH and arterial blood gases. Daily chest x-rays should be ordered to monitor tube placement and look for early evidence of fluid overload, pneumothorax, pleural effusions and pulmonary consolidation. Pulmonary hypertension can produce severe hemodynamic consequences. A fall in PaO2 usually signifies a problem in oxygen delivery and all possible explanations must be examined. Intrapulmonary shunt-

ing and ventilation/perfusion mismatch are the two usual culprits. The team must distinguish between hypoxia secondary to alveolar hypoventilation vs intrinsic pulmonary disease. As pulmonary function improves, extubation can be attempted, using generally accepted weaning parameters as a guideline (Table 71-1).

Patients with chronic liver disease present a special challenge because they exhibit a markedly hyperdynamic circulation. The not-so-ill patient will come to the ICU in a euvolemic or somewhat hypervolemic state. The use of a pulmonary artery pressure catheter (Swan Ganz®) should be used to maintain a euvolemic state. Pulmonary artery wedge pressures of 12 to 15 mmHg are usually satisfactory. Low filling pressures, a rising systemic vascular resistance and fall in cardiac output all signal the need for colloid or red blood cell infusions. Patients with more advanced liver disease present a more difficult challenge. These patients may have severe hypoalbuminemia, hyponatremia, striking ascites and some degree of renal failure. These advanced cases usually have an extremely hyperdynamic state and may have chronic myocardial dysfunction as well. Cautious use of fluid and colloid challenges is in order. Since renal failure is often present, it is prudent to avoid overhydration and rapid shifts in sodium balance. It is important to keep in mind that many of the problems of fluid shifts, electrolyte balance and the hyperdynamic state will not resolve without restoration of normal donor liver function.

Hypertension and Pain Control

Hypertension is common after transplantation and should be aggressively treated to prevent intracerebral bleeding in patients who already have coagulation defects. Early on, intravenous sodium nitroprusside may be necessary to adequately control hypertension. Later, control can be maintained on combination therapy with diuretics, beta blockers and calcium channel blockers, the current favored antihypertensive agents. Satisfactory blood pressure control equals pressures below 140 to 150 mmHg systolic and below 90 mmHg diastolic. The common practice of using sublingual nifedipine with sudden elevations of blood pressure is to be deplored since precipitous drops in blood pressure can initiate CNS

Timothy McCashland, MD, Associate Professor of Medicine, Liver Transplant Program, University of Nebraska Medical Center, Omaha, NE

Michael F. Sorrell, MD, Robert L. Grissom Professor of Medicine, Liver Transplant Program, University of Nebraska Medical Center, Omaha, NE

Table 71-1. Acceptable Weaning Parameters

PaO2 >70 torr
FiO2 40% or less
Vital Capacity >10 to 15 mL/kg
Minute Volume <10 L/min
Peak Inspiratory Pressure >25 cm H2O
Adequate cough reflex and satisfactory chest x-ray

strokes. Adequate pain control is important in the treatment of hypertension. Satisfactory pain control is mandatory, but one should not oversedate in a misguided attempt to relieve all vestige of pain. Oversedation can lead to late mobilization, diminished respiratory function and often sepsis due to lack of satisfactory pulmonary toilet.

Ulcer Prophylaxis

Administration of high-dose corticosteroids, surgical stress and intubation combine to increase the risk of upper gastrointestinal bleeding. Although major hemorrhage in the immediate posttransplant period is rare, it is advisable to use ulcer prophylaxis with either H2 blockers or proton pump inhibitors.

Nutrition

With the exception of the fulminant liver failure patient, almost all patients with chronic liver disease are malnourished. Muscle wasting, hypoalbuminemia, low serum transferrin and prealbumin are characteristic of the patient with advanced liver disease. Fat soluble vitamins and electrolytes are variably deranged depending upon the severity of the liver disease and the degree of renal failure. The transplant recipient is invariably catabolic and protein deficient as the result of surgery and prior liver disease and often coupled with preoperative dietary protein restriction. The patient with early return of allograft function to normal allows for the prompt use of enteral nutrition and the quick resolution of their hypermetabolic state. The early use of enteral nutrition via nasoduodenal feeding tube maintains enterocyte integrity and aids in the prevention of bacterial translocation. Most often parenteral nutrition is required for a period after transplantation. The use of parenteral nutrition is complicated by shifts in electrolyte composition, hypervolemia and the presence of renal failure and cardiac dysfunction. The availability of concentrated parenteral solutions allowing adequate delivery of nutrients and caloric needs with less volume has been an important aid in managing these problems. Intravenous lipids are an important high calorie/lower volume source since lipids deliver 9 kcal/gm, as compared to glucose which contains 4 kcal/gm. It is important not to give excess calories since overfeeding can generate excess carbon dioxide production with precipitation of respiratory failure in the patient with borderline respiratory reserve.

Renal

Oliguria is common in the postoperative patient and results from a combination of ascites production from fluids weeping from raw surgical surfaces, preexisting renal dysfunction, inadequate volume replacement and the administration of nephrotoxic drugs, including tacrolimus or cyclosporine. Clinical signs of fluid overload such as pulmonary congestion and rapid weight gain should be carefully monitored. Pulmonary artery wedge pressure should be kept in the range of 12 to 15 mmHg to ensure adequate filling pressures and to avoid overhydration. Renal dose dopamine (2 to 3 µg/kg per minute) is routinely administered to improve renal perfusion, although the efficacy of the routine use of dopamine has not been proven in rigorous trials. Renal failure can persist and worsen despite adequate fluid administration and attention to renal perfusion. At that point, other explanations for renal dysfunction should be sought (Table 71-2).

Electrolyte and acid-base abnormalities are common in the postoperative period. Metabolic alkalosis results from a combination of factors including volume contraction, administration of sodium bicarbonate during surgery, administration of citrated blood, corticosteroid use and hydrogen ion loss via nasogastric suction. Patients with end-stage liver disease are usually volume and sodium overloaded. Postoperatively, hyponatremia and hypokalemia are common. Hyponatremia responds to diuresis and avoidance of excessive sodium replacement. Wide shifts in serum sodium concentrations should be avoided since central pontine myelinolysis can be the consequence. Hyperkalemia can result from poor allograft dysfunction, excessive potassium administration, renal tubular acidosis and worsening renal function. Persistent and worsening hyperkalemia may require the use of potassium-binding resins or dialysis. Blood calcium, magnesium and phosphate levels must be monitored on a daily basis. Deficiencies of each of these electrolytes have serious clinical consequences. Total serum calcium levels are usually low because of hypoalbuminemia, therefore, ionized calcium levels should be monitored daily. Hypomagnesemia is common, particularly in the alcoholic, and often results from type 4 renal tubule acidosis induced by cyclosporine or tacrolimus. The development of hypophosphatemia can result in myocardial depression and respiratory muscle weakness, making weaning from the ventilator difficult.

Table 71-2. Causes of Renal Failure After Transplantation

Acute tubular necrosis
Hepatorenal syndrome prior to transplantation
Antibiotic and immunosuppressive medications
Antiviral agents
Worsening allograft function
Sepsis
Inadequate volume replacement

73 INDUCTION IMMUNOSUPPRESSION PROTOCOLS FOR LIVER TRANSPLANTATION

Frederick Nunes, MD

The optimal immunosuppressive regimen for initial, maintenance and rejection therapy after liver transplantation has not yet been identified. The term induction therapy is sometimes equated with initial therapy (ie, antirejection therapy) at the initiation of the recipients' immunologic response to the newly-engrafted liver. Initial therapy to prevent liver allograft rejection generally consists of higher doses of the same medications used in maintenance therapy. Others more narrowly define induction therapy as potent immunosuppression effected by an antibody compound directed against a component or components of the T cell (Table 73-1). This definition will be used for this chapter. Acute cellular rejection prophylaxis made possible through induction therapy must be balanced against the potential increased risk of infection and malignancy. Induction therapy has not gained widespread use in liver transplant centers, except in the setting of renal insufficiency.

OBJECTIVES OF INDUCTION THERAPY

The highest incidence of acute rejection is soon after transplantation. The primary objective of induction therapy is to decrease the incidence of acute cellular rejection (Table 73-2). However, the hypothesis that a decreased incidence of acute cellular rejection will lead to better graft and patient survival has not been conclusively demonstrated in randomized controlled studies.

In addition to decreasing the incidence of acute rejection, delaying the onset of the first rejection episode is an objective of induction therapy. A delayed acute rejection episode may often be treated on an outpatient basis and often occurs past the first month posttransplantation, when the risk of infection is highest.

A third objective of induction therapy is delaying the introduction of calcineurin inhibitors, primarily to ameliorate calcineurin inhibitor-associated renal toxicity. The aim to decrease the use of intravenous cyclosporine and its associated toxicities has largely been achieved by the use of newer formulations of cyclosporine or tacrolimus, rather than the routine use of induction therapy.

Assistant Professor of Medicine, Division of Gastroenterology, University of Pennsylvania, Philadelphia, PA

ANTILYMPHOCYTE AGENTS
Antilymphocyte Globulin and Antithymocyte Globulin

Antilymphocyte globulins (ALG) (ATGAM®) and antithymocyte globulin (ATG) (Thymoglobulin®) are polyclonal antibodies derived by immunizing horses against human lymphocytes, or rabbits against human thymocytes, respectively. These polyclonal antilymphocyte preparations bind multiple antigens on both T and B lymphocytes. They are administered for seven to 14 days at a fixed dose, depending on the preparation. ATG and ALG are associated with significant adverse reactions. Systemic signs such as fever and chills occur in up to a third of treated individuals. Arthralgias, nausea and vomiting may occur in up to 20% of treated patients. Leukopenia and thrombocytopenia may necessitate dose adjustment.

The long-term efficacy of ATG in liver transplantation has not been conclusively demonstrated. Retrospective reviews of ATG induction therapy, in combination with conventional cyclosporine-based immunosuppression in liver transplant recipients, suggest that there is lower incidence of rejection during the first 30 days and a delay to the first rejection episode. Nonrandomized studies of data collected in a prospective fashion do not conclusively demonstrate the utility of ATG or ALG. The liver transplant database is a prospective study of patients undergoing liver transplantation at three US centers. A cohort of 762 consecutive liver transplantation recipients was studied to determine the incidence, timing and risk factors for acute rejection. Eight days is the median time to the first rejection episode. Overall, 65% of liver transplant recipients develop an episode of acute cellular rejection during the first year posttransplantation. Induction therapy with antilymphocyte globulin significantly decreased the six week incidence of acute rejection by univariate analysis. However, in multivariate analysis, antilymphocyte globulin was not significantly associated with a decrease in the incidence of acute rejection. Randomized controlled trials are needed to determine whether there exists a long-term benefit of ATG.

Muromonab-CD3

Muromonab-CD3 (Orthoclone OKT®3) is a murine monoclonal antibody that binds to the CD3 complex of the T cell receptor. Within minutes of muromonab-CD3 infusion, CD3+ lymphocytes are cleared from the circulation. During therapy, CD3+ cells remain undetectable unless neutralizing antibodies develop. A cytokine release syndrome characterized by fever, chills, chest pain, shortness of breath, nausea, vomiting, diarrhea, hypertension and headache generally occurs within one hour of muromonab-CD3 administration. The severity and presentation of the syndrome is variable, but is ame-

Table 73-1. Induction Therapy Agents

Compound	Brand Name	Antibody Source	Target	Major Side Effects	Comment
Antilymphocyte globulin (ALG)	MALG®	Horse	multiple antigens on lymphoid cells	Serum sickness Leukopenia Thrombocytopenia	Not available at the present time
Antithymocyte globulin (ATG)	ATGAM®	Horse	Multiple antigens on lymphoid cells	Serum sickness Leukopenia Thrombocytopenia	Immunosuppressive potency variability by lot
Antithymocyte globulin (ATG)	Thymoglobulin®	Rabbit polyclonal	Multiple antigens on lymphoid cells	Serum sickness Leukopenia Thrombocytopenia	
Monoclonal anti-CD3 antibodies	Orthoclone OKT®3	Mouse monoclonal	CD3 complex of the T cell receptor	Cytokine release syndrome (fever, chills, pulmonary edema, headache) Neuropsychiatric (seizures, aseptic meningitis, encephalopathy)	Increased risk of infection and malignancy
Basiliximab	Simulect®	Human/mouse chimeric monoclonal antibody	Interleukin-2 receptor (CD25)	potential hypersensitivity reaction	two dose regimen
Daclizumab	Zenapax®	Humanized antibody	Interleukin-2 receptor (CD25)	potential hypersensitivity reaction	five dose regimen

Table 73-2. Induction Therapy

Objectives	Limitations	Concerns
Prophylaxis against first rejection Delay onset of first rejection	No improved survival	Impact on recurrent disease (ie, HCV)
Delay calcineurin inhibitor to decrease renal toxicity	Antibody development (muromonab-CD3)	
Therapy in patients not suitable for conventional immunosuppression	Cost	

liorated somewhat with acetaminophen, antihistamines and steroid pretreatment. Neuropsychiatric toxicity including headache, seizures, confusion and aseptic meningitis may complicate therapy. Muromonab-CD3-induction therapy with delayed introduction of cyclosporin A significantly decreases the incidence of acute rejection. Reported graft and patient survival rates, however, are similar with muromonab-CD3-, tacrolimus- or cyclosporin A-based protocols. The major side effects of muromonab-CD3 therapy, such as cytokine release syndrome and neuropsychiatric toxicity described above

have limited the use of muromonab-CD3 induction therapy. Infectious complications precipitated by muromonab-CD3 therapy, such as CMV disease, can be ameliorated with antiviral prophylactic therapy. The increased risk for posttransplant lymphoproliferative disease (PTLD) is another consequence of muromonab-CD3 therapy that has limited its adoption for induction therapy. A randomized controlled trial demonstrated the efficacy of low-dose muromonab-CD3 induction therapy in renal transplantation; however only pilot data exist in liver transplantation.

Anti-Interleukin-2 Receptor

A number of antibody compounds have been developed against the interleukin-2 (IL-2) receptor complex present on the surface of activated T lymphocytes. Basiliximab (Simulect®) is a human/mouse chimeric monoclonal antibody that binds to the alpha chain of the IL-2 receptor complex. Placebo-controlled trials in renal transplant recipients demonstrate that the recommended two dose regime of basiliximab decreases the frequency of acute rejection during the first six months posttransplantation. Basiliximab is administered in conjunction with cyclosporine and corticosteroids. The adverse event profile of basiliximab is comparable to placebo. Placebo-controlled trials of basiliximab combined with cyclosporine and corticosteroids have not been reported in liver transplant recipients.

Daclizumab (Zenapax®) is a humanized (10% mouse) monoclonal antibody that binds to the alpha chain of the IL-2 receptor complex. Randomized controlled trials of recommended five dose regimen of daclizumab reduces the frequency of acute rejection during the first six months postrenal transplantation when combined with cyclosporine, azathioprine and prednisone. Randomized controlled trials of daclizumab have not been reported in liver transplant recipients.

A randomized trial of 40 liver transplant recipients, comparing a monoclonal anti-IL-2 receptor antibody (BT563) and placebo, found a lower incidence of acute cellular rejection, but no difference in patient survival. Both groups received an immunosuppression regimen consisting of cyclosporin A, prednisone and azathioprine. No difference in infectious complications was found. The same group compared BT563 anti-IL-2 receptor antibody and ATG as part of a quadruple immunosuppressive induction regimen following liver transplantation. The prospective randomized trial included 80 consecutive patients. Patients treated with BT563 had a lower incidence of steroid-sensitive rejection episodes and fewer adverse medication effects. No difference in infectious complications were noted.

CONCLUSION

The hypothesis that a decreased incidence of acute cellular rejection post-liver transplantation will lead to better graft and patient survival has not been conclusively demonstrated in randomized controlled studies. Acute cellular rejection prophylaxis made possible through induction therapy must be balanced against the potential increased risk of infection and malignancy. Induction therapy has not gained widespread use in liver transplant centers, except in the setting of renal insufficiency. Further studies are needed to determine the utility of the newer monoclonal antibodies directed against a component of the IL-2 receptor. Newer strategies that attempt to restrict inhibition to only those T cells that respond to donor antigen may successfully decrease the incidence of rejection and improve survival.

RECOMMENDED READING

Tchervenkov J, Flemming C, Guttmann RD, des Gachons G. Use of Thymoglobulin® induction therapy in the prevention of acute graft rejection episodes following liver transplantation. Transplant Proc. 1997;29(7A): 13S-15S.

Wiesner RH, Demetris AJ, Belle SH, et al. Acute hepatic allograft rejection: incidence, risk factors, and impact on outcome. Hepatology. 1998;28(3):638-645.

McDiarmid S, Millis M, Terasaki P, Ament ME, Busuttil R. OKT3 prophylaxis in liver transplantation. Dig Dis Sci. 1991;36(10):1418-1426.

Wall WJ, Ghent CN, Roy A, McAlister VC, Grant DR, Adams PC. Use of OKT3 monoclonal antibody as induction therapy for control of rejection in liver transplantation. Dig Dis Sci. 1995;40(1):52-57.

Fung J, Starzl T. Prophylacic use of OKT3® in liver transplantation: a review. Dig Dis Sci. 1991;36(10):1427-1430.

Bailey TC, Powderly WG, Storch GA, et al. Symptomatic cytomegalovirus infection in renal transplant recipients given either Minnesota antilymphoblast globulin (MALG®) or OKT3® for rejection prophylaxis. Am J Kid Dis. 1993;21(2):196-201.

Turgeon N, Fishman JA, Basgoz N, et al. Effect of oral acyclovir or ganciclovir therapy after preemptive intravenous ganciclovir therapy to prevent cytomegalovirus disease in cytomegalovirus seropositive renal and liver transplant recipients receiving antilymphocyte antibody therapy. Transplantation. 1998;66(12):1780-1786.

Whiting JF, Rossi SJ, Hanto DW. Infectious complications after OKT3® induction in liver transplantation. Liver Transpl Surg. 1997;3(6):563-570.

Swinnen L, Constanzo-Nordin M, Fisher S. Increased incidence of lymphoproliferative disorder after immunosuppression with monoclonal antibody OKT3® in cardiac transplant recipients. N Engl J Med. 1990; 323(25):1767-1769.

Whiting JF, Fecteau A, Martin J, Bejarano PA, Hanto DW. Use of low-dose OKT3® as induction therapy in liver transplantation. Transplantation. 1998;65(4):577-580.

Nashan B, Moore R, Amlot P, Schmidt A, Abeywickrama K, Soulillou J. Randomized trial of basiliximab versus placebo for control of acute cellular rejection in renal allograft recipients. CHIB 201 International Study Group. Lancet. 1997;350(9086):1193-1198.

Kahan B, Rajagopalan P, Hall M. Reduction of the occurrence of acute cellular rejection among renal allograft recipients treated with basiliximab, a chimeric anti-interleukin-2-receptor monoclonal antibody. United States Simulect® Renal Study Group. Transplantation. 1999;67(2): 276-284.

Vincenti F, Kirkman R, Light S, et al. Interleukin-2-receptor blockade with daclizumab to prevent acute rejection in renal transplantation. Daclizumab Triple Therapy Study Group [see comments]. New Engl J Med. 1998;338(23): 1700-1701.

Langrehr JM, Glanemann M, Guckelberger O, et al. A randomized, placebo-controlled trial with anti-interleukin-2 receptor antibody for immunosuppressive induction therapy after liver transplantation. Clin Transplant. 1998;12(4): 303-312.

Langrehr JM, Nussler NC, Neumann U, et al. A prospective randomized trial comparing interleukin-2 receptor antibody vs antithymocyte globulin as part of a quadruple immunosuppressive induction therapy following orthotopic liver transplantation. Transplantation. 1997;63(12):1772-1781.

74 DIAGNOSIS AND TREATMENT OF HEPATIC ALLOGRAFT DYSFUNCTION

Fatima A.F. Figueiredo, MD, PhD
K.V. Narayanan Menon, MD, MRCP
Russell H. Wiesner, MD

Orthotopic liver transplantation (OLT) is now the therapy of choice for end-stage liver disease, with 1-year patient survival rates of 80% to 85% being achieved at most major centers. However, there is a growing disparity between the supply and demand of organs that has generated the need for alternate donor sources, such as marginal donors, split-livers and living-related donors. With this widening gap between the need and availability of donor organs, and with the use of marginal donors, preventing or minimizing posttransplant allograft dysfunction has become increasingly important.

Hepatic allograft dysfunction may occur any time after OLT and for purposes of classification and discussion, this period can be arbitrarily divided into early (<2 months) and late (>2 months) intervals. This arbitrary division provides a useful framework to develop a differential diagnosis in patients with hepatic allograft dysfunction and to initiate appropriate therapy promptly (Table 74-1).

PRESERVATION INJURY

Preservation injury (PI) is a universal phenomenon that occurs in every transplanted liver and is characterized by elevated aminotransferase levels in the posttransplant period. Although these levels may reflect the severity of the underlying injury, most of the patients do not develop significant clinical manifestations and the serum aminotransferase levels progressively decrease and reach normal values by the end of the first week. However, approximately 40% of patients with aspartate aminotransferase (AST) levels greater than 5,000 IU/L in the first 72 hours after OLT develop primary nonfunction. Some patients may also present with prolonged cholestasis related to PI.

The likely cause of preservation injury is multifactorial, however, donor factors and events occurring during

Fatima A.F. Figueiredo, MD, PhD, Fulbright Scholar, Division of Gastroenterology and Hepatology, Mayo Clinic, Rochester, MN

K.V. Narayanan Menon, MD, MRCP, Fellow, Division of Gastroenterology and Hepatology, Mayo Clinic, Rochester, MN

Russell H. Wiesner, MD, Professor of Medicine; Medical Director, Liver Transplantation, Mayo Clinic, Rochester, MN

cold/warm ischemia and reperfusion are thought to play a major role (Table 74-2). Excess fat in the donor liver seems to be detrimental and, even in patients who receive donor livers with up to 30% fat, short-term graft and patient survival rates have been found to be significantly worse, with primary nonfunction being a major cause of graft failure. Problems during organ procurement related to intraoperative hypotension or to technical misadventures may also contribute to preservation injury. Preservation injury may also be caused by cold ischemia and a cold ischemic time longer than 12 hours

Table 74-1. Causes of Hepatic Allograft Dysfunction

Early (0 to 2 months)

Preservation injury
Primary allograft dysfunction
Acute cellular rejection
Infections
Vascular stenosis / thrombosis
Biliary complications
Drug reactions

Late* (>2 months)

Chronic rejection
Recurrence of the original liver disease

*Includes all causes of early allograft dysfunction except preservation injury and primary allograft dysfunction.

Table 74-2. Causes of Preservation Injury and Primary Allograft Dysfunction

Donor factors

Age >65 years
Race other than Caucasian
Hepatic steatosis >30%
Preexisting liver diseases
Donor hospital stay >3 days
Preprocurement acidosis
Small graft size

Procurement complications

Cold ischemic injury

Warm ischemia / reperfusion injury

Recipient factors

Elevated pretransplant bilirubin or prothrombin time
Awaiting transplant in hospital or intensive care unit
Renal insufficiency
Re-transplantation

has been shown to increase the incidence of primary nonfunction and ischemic-type biliary complications. Preservation injury may further result from warm ischemia and a warm ischemic time longer than 180 minutes has been associated with allograft dysfunction and diminished graft survival.

Reperfusion injury appears to be related to the degree of injury sustained during cold and warm ischemic times. Neutrophil and monocyte activation coupled with generation of reactive oxygen species (ROS) and apoptosis are thought to be major pathogenic mechanisms of reperfusion injury with Kupffer cells and sinusoidal endothelial cells playing a central role.

Improved operative and preservation techniques may help prevent the development of PI. Prostaglandin E_1 (PGE$_1$) has been shown to reduce PI in rats and canine livers and may be beneficial in reducing the incidence of PI in humans. Neutralizing the effects of ROS generation using antioxidant therapy and the inhibition of apoptosis by caspase inhibitors are therapeutic options that may prove useful in the future.

PRIMARY ALLOGRAFT DYSFUNCTION

Primary allograft dysfunction comprises primary nonfunction (PNF) and initial poor function (IPF). In general, there is a lack of agreement on the definitions of both these terms. PNF can be defined by the irreversible absence of hepatic allograft function in the first one week after OLT and the diagnosis is made primarily by exclusion of other causes of allograft failure. Clinical features include hypoglycemia, acidosis, coagulopathy, absent or poor bile flow, high serum aminotransferase levels, coma, renal failure and shock that culminates in death unless the patient is re-transplanted. The prevalence of PNF ranges widely among centers, and is reported to occur in 1.4% to 9.5% of orthotopic liver transplants.

Initial poor function is even less well-defined, but is much more common, and is defined as a hepatic allograft with marginal function during the first week after OLT. IPF affects 5% to 23% of liver grafts and results in a significantly lower patient and graft survival. IPF may be defined by the presence of at least one of the following: serum bilirubin greater than 10 mg/dL, prothrombin time more than 17 seconds or hepatic encephalopathy occurring between day two and seven after OLT. Additionally, AST levels greater than 2,000 IU/L observed on any occasion from the second to the seventh postoperative day is another criterion by which IPF may be defined.

The cause of primary allograft dysfunction is usually multifactorial and the presence of multiple risk factors may increase its incidence (Table 74-2). There are no tests available that can predict the occurrence of primary allograft dysfunction. The only effective treatment for PNF is re-transplantation as soon as possible. Prophylactic strategies using PGE$_1$ reveal that PGE$_1$-treated patients have better renal function and reduced use of healthcare resources, although there does not seem to be a difference in the overall prevalence of PNF or in patient or graft survival. The treatment of IPF depends on its clinical course. Avoiding the combination of multiple risk factors may also help decrease the incidence of primary allograft dysfunction.

VASCULAR COMPLICATIONS

Vascular problems occurring after OLT are a major cause of graft failure and loss and include arterial and venous complications.

Arterial Complications

The incidence of hepatic arterial complications ranges from 5% to 15% and includes thrombosis, stenosis, pseudoaneurysm formation and rupture. Hepatic artery thrombosis remains the most common arterial complication with an incidence ranging from 1.6% to 8%. There is a significantly increased incidence in the pediatric population. Factors predisposing to hepatic arterial thrombosis include anatomical factors (eg, arteriosclerosis, small arterial size, complex anatomy, use of extension grafts for the arterial anastomosis), hypercoagulable states, rejection, prolonged ischemia time and transplantation for primary sclerosing cholangitis. In the majority of cases, however, the etiology remains unknown. The clinical spectrum of hepatic artery thrombosis includes fulminant hepatic failure and sepsis, hepatic abscesses, biliary complications and asymptomatic liver test abnormalities. The most dramatic presentation of hepatic artery thrombosis is fulminant hepatic failure due to necrosis of the graft and is characterized by markedly elevated aminotransferase levels, refractory metabolic acidosis, hypoglycemia, coagulopathy, encephalopathy and renal failure. Other patients may present with multiple hepatic abscesses and bacteremia. Biliary complications occur four to six weeks after OLT and are common in patients with hepatic artery thrombosis as the intrahepatic biliary epithelium is perfused solely by the hepatic artery and decreased arterial perfusion results in biliary ischemia and necrosis. These patients may present with biliary strictures and cholangitis or with bile leaks due to necrosis of the biliary anastomosis. Hepatic artery thrombosis can sometimes present with asymptomatic liver test abnormalities or may occasionally be detected during routine Doppler ultrasound examination.

Doppler ultrasonography is the initial modality of choice in screening patients with suspected hepatic artery thrombosis. It is noninvasive and has a high sensitivity and specificity enabling early diagnosis. Doppler spectral wave analysis may provide additional information compared to conventional Doppler ultrasonography. Arteriography should be performed to confirm the diagnosis and should also be performed in patients with a high degree of clinical suspicion even if a Doppler ultrasound is normal. Treatment modalities available for the treatment of hepatic artery thrombosis include percutaneous transluminal angioplasty, thrombectomy and surgical revision. Re-transplantation may ultimately be required for 50% to 75% of patients with hepatic artery thrombosis. Anticoagulation and antiplatelet therapy may be necessary in patients with hepatic artery thrombosis in whom there is no evidence of technical problems.

Hepatic artery stenosis, pseudoaneurysms and rupture are rare complications seen after OLT. Stenosis of the hepatic artery predisposes to subsequent hepatic artery thrombosis. Angioplasty may be effective for relatively short stenosis involving the hepatic artery but patients may ultimately need to be re-transplanted. Pseudoaneurysm formation and rupture of the hepatic artery are rare complications that can be related to infections, particularly fungal. These patients can present with massive gastrointestinal bleeding. Treatment is problematic and options include primary repair in the absence of infection, or excision and ligation.

Portal Vein Thrombosis or Stenosis

Portal vein thrombosis is a relatively infrequent finding in adult liver transplantation with an incidence of about 2%. Risk factors include pretransplant portal vein thrombosis or shunt surgery in the recipient, trauma, or hypercoagulable states. Stenosis or thrombosis at the anastomotic site can cause clinical symptoms of portal hypertension, such as esophageal varices, gastrointestinal bleeding and ascites. Diagnosis is based on Doppler ultrasonography, late-phase arteriography or magnetic resonance imaging (MRI). If diagnosed in the immediate postoperative period, surgical thrombectomy is advised. The use of interventional radiological procedures such as balloon dilatation/stenting and thrombectomy may help avoid surgical intervention.

Hepatic Vein and Inferior Vena Caval Problems

Stenosis or thrombosis of the inferior vena cava (IVC) and/or hepatic veins is quite rare and is usually the result of recurrence of Budd-Chiari syndrome or to technical problems related to the vascular anastomoses. Hepatic vein stenosis occurs with piggy-back technique of hepatic vein-IVC anastomosis while inferior vena caval problems occur more commonly with the conventional anastomosis. Patients usually present with abdominal pain, ascites, hepatomegaly and edema. The diagnosis can be made by Doppler ultrasonography and confirmed by hepatic and inferior vena cavography with simultaneous measurement of the transanastomotic pressure gradients. Treatment options range from percutaneous balloon dilatation to surgical revision. For patients with recurrent Budd-Chiari Syndrome, thrombolysis followed by anticoagulation may be attempted. Re-transplantation may be necessary for patients with persistent and progressive liver dysfunction.

ACUTE CELLULAR REJECTION

The cumulative incidence of acute cellular rejection (ACR) varies from 50% to 90% depending on the criteria by which rejection is defined and whether protocol biopsies are performed. Acute cellular rejection can cause bile duct damage by directly affecting the interlobular bile ducts. Additionally, the bile ducts may also be affected by ischemia resulting from damage to the vascular endothelium by acute rejection.

Risk factors for acute cellular rejection (ACR) include the type of immunosuppressive regimen used, nature of the underlying liver disease and cytomegalovirus (CMV) infection. Immunosuppressive regimes with low dose cyclosporine, or cyclosporine mono or dual therapy have been associated with higher rates of acute cellular rejection compared to regimens containing tacrolimus. Both acute and steroid-resistant rejection appear to occur more frequently in patients transplanted for autoimmune disease, fulminant hepatic failure and primary sclerosing cholangitis (PSC). Patients transplanted for autoimmune liver disease have the highest rates of ACR (70% to 80%) while patients transplanted for alcoholic and cryptogenic cirrhosis have the lowest rates. CMV infection may also constitute a risk factor for ACR as it has multiple effects on the immune response. However, a direct cause and effect relationship between CMV and ACR has been difficult to demonstrate because ACR frequently precedes CMV infection and the increased risk of ACR after CMV infection may be related to the decrease in immunosuppression required to treat CMV infection.

ACR is typically seen between day five and day 30 after OLT (median time of ten days), but can occur at any time. Patients are usually asymptomatic although severe rejection can cause fever, changes in bile color (pale), jaundice and occasionally ascites. Laboratory testing reveals elevated aminotransferase levels although leukocytosis and eosinophilia may also be frequently present.

The differential diagnosis for moderate to severe ACR includes hepatic artery thrombosis, CMV hepatitis, bile duct obstruction, viral hepatitis or systemic sepsis. These conditions should be excluded by Doppler ultrasound, appropriate cultures, cholangiography and liver biopsy.

The diagnosis of ACR is made exclusively by liver biopsy. Characteristic features include: (1) mixed portal inflammation, but a predominantly mononuclear infiltrate containing activated lymphocytes, neutrophils and eosinophils; (2) bile duct inflammation/damage; and (3) subendothelial inflammation of portal veins or terminal hepatic venules. An international panel of experts proposed the Banff schema for grading ACR, which provides a measure of the severity of the necro-inflammatory process. However, the global assessment of histology by an experienced pathologist yields similar results in terms of diagnosis.

The differential diagnosis of the histological changes of ACR includes preservation injury, chronic viral hepatitis, biliary tract disease and recurrence of autoimmune disorders. Differentiating these conditions from ACR histologically is dealt with in a separate chapter.

The histological diagnosis of rejection does not necessarily render it clinically significant, especially in mild cases. Currently there is no consensus on treatment of mild ACR and if the patient remains asymptomatic and the liver enzymes are stable, some centers routinely obtain a follow-up biopsy after one week before recommending specific treatment.

Treatment is, however, recommended for moderate and severe ACR and usually consists of bolus intravenous methylprednisolone therapy. More than 90% of patients with ACR will usually respond to this regimen. If ACR persists in a follow-up liver biopsy, it suggests the presence of steroid-resistant rejection and an antilymphocyte globulin or muromonab-CD3 is recommended. In patients on a cyclosporine-based regimen, rescue therapy with tacrolimus appears to result in successful treatment of rejection in almost 80% of the grafts. Treatment of acute cellular rejection is dealt with in greater detail in Chapter 73 of this section.

Graft loss directly as a result of ACR is extremely rare and, unlike other solid organ transplants like the kidney and the heart, there appears to be no significant impact of ACR per se on either patient or graft survival. In fact, patients experiencing a single episode of early mild ACR showed a trend toward better survival when compared to grafts without ACR. However, recurrent episodes of ACR may result in poor graft function in the long term and can lead to chronic rejection. Additionally, in patients undergoing liver transplantation for hepatitis C, treatment of ACR is thought to contribute to early recurrence of hepatitis C in the allograft.

CHRONIC REJECTION

Chronic rejection, also called ductopenic rejection or vanishing bile duct syndrome, is a complex process characterized by an obliterative vasculopathy and progressive loss of bile ducts. Today this entity is relatively uncommon, with an incidence of less than 5%, and typically occurs several months or more following OLT.

Factors that predispose to the development of chronic rejection in liver allografts include age, steroid-resistant ACR, recurrent and late ACR, previous chronic rejection, and etiology of liver disease. Recipients younger than one year old are particularly at risk for developing chronic rejection. Most cases of chronic rejection are preceded by one or more episodes of moderate or severe ACR and patients who develop ACR more than six months after OLT are at a significantly higher risk of developing chronic rejection. There is also a trend toward a higher incidence of chronic rejection in patients with autoimmune liver disease and PSC, compared to patients with alcoholic liver disease. The role of other factors such as HLA mismatch, interferon therapy, and CMV infection in the development of chronic rejection is controversial.

Chronic rejection usually presents with a cholestatic biochemical profile presumably related to a progressive loss of small bile ducts. Radiological investigations such as ultrasound, CT, and MRI are useful in excluding other causes of allograft dysfunction, but are not helpful in diagnosing chronic rejection. Hepatic arteriography may reveal narrowing or pruning of the vessels in some patients, while others with chronic rejection may have a completely normal study.

The diagnosis of chronic rejection is made by liver biopsy and is defined by the absence of interlobular septal bile ducts in 50% or more of portal tracts. Additionally, it should be strongly suspected when there is atrophy and pyknosis of the biliary epithelium, in the absence of other causes of injury to the biliary tree. Chronic rejection is often accompanied by an obliterative or foam cell arteritis of the hilar and septal branches of the hepatic artery. The resultant arterial stenosis is thought to cause an ischemic-type injury and contributes to graft dysfunction. These arteries are generally only assessed at the time of re-transplantation, as they are rarely sampled in a percutaneous needle liver biopsy.

New immunosuppressive agents are currently available that may be effective for patients with early chronic rejection. Corticosteroids in general have little effect on chronic rejection, while mycophenolate mofetil, tacrolimus or rapamycin rescue therapy can reverse ductopenic chronic rejection in some patients. Patients with early chronic rejection (<90 days after OLT), serum bilirubin levels greater than 10 mg/dL, and absent interlobular bile ducts in over 90% of portal tracts have a poor long-term prognosis. If hepatic synthetic function deteriorates irreversibly, re-transplantation must be considered.

BILIARY TRACT COMPLICATIONS

In spite of the success of orthotopic liver transplantation, biliary complications continue to occur in up to 30% of patients after OLT and are a significant source of morbidity. The biliary tree, which relies heavily on the hepatic artery for its blood supply, has a poor collateral blood supply and hepatic arterial problems usually result in biliary complications as well. Biliary tract complications after OLT include bile leaks, biliary strictures and choledocholithiasis.

Bile leaks typically present early after OLT and mandate immediate intervention to avoid sepsis. Bile leaks may occur at the site of the biliary anastomosis, the cut surface of a reduced-sized graft, a T-tube exit site or following removal of a T-tube. The use of a ureteral catheter through the donor cystic duct and held in place by a hemorrhoidal rubber band may result in a lower incidence of bile leaks at removal, when compared with the conventional T-tube.

Biliary strictures are generally divided into anastomotic and nonanastomotic types. Strictures confined to the site of anastomosis are thought to be related to surgical technique. Nonanastomotic bile duct strictures, either single or multiple, involving only the donor biliary tree are usually seen between one and three months after OLT and are thought to be ischemic in origin. Other, less well-established causes of nonanastomotic biliary strictures are ABO incompatibility, chronic rejection, prolonged ischemia time, CMV infection and recurrent primary diseases such as primary sclerosing cholangitis.

Less common causes of biliary obstruction in post-OLT patients are choledocholithiasis and compressions secondary to a fluid collection. Following OLT, a number of factors such as increased lithogenicity of bile, biliary dyskinesia, strictures, and bacterial invasion of the bile ducts in patients with a choledochojejunostomy predispose patients to the development of pigment stones in the biliary system. Collections of blood or bile around the biliary tree may also result in secondary obstruction to bile flow.

Manifestations of biliary tract complications include cholangitis, a cholestatic biochemical profile, biliary dilatation on ultrasound or evidence of biliary obstruction on liver biopsy. Although the diagnosis of biliary obstruction can be made noninvasively using computed tomography, ultrasound or MRI, endoscopic or percutaneous cholangiography better localize the level of obstruction and also define what therapeutic options may be used. Bilomas, abscesses, hematomas and loculated ascites are best diagnosed by ultrasound or computed tomography and percutaneous drainage is the treatment of choice. All patients with bilary strictures should have patency of hepatic artery assessed with Doppler ultrasound and/or hepatic arteriography if necessary.

Anastomotic strictures can be treated by either endoscopic or percutaneous dilatation I stenting or by

surgery, while nonanastomotic strictures are usually treated by percutaneous or endoscopic dilatation and stenting. Intrahepatic strictures are usually dilated when symptomatic. Biliary stents are commonly changed at eight to 12 week intervals to avoid bacterial cholangitis caused by stent occlusion. Patients with biliary strictures treated successfully have comparable mortality and re-transplantation rates to those who do not experience these complications. Patients with progressive allograft dysfunction or repeated episodes of cholangitis in spite of adequate biliary drainage should be considered for re-transplantation.

INFECTIONS

Infections seen after liver transplantation are largely related to the patient's immunosuppression status and can cause considerable allograft dysfunction. The most common infections causing hepatic allograft dysfunction are bacterial, fungal and viral (eg, CMV, herpes simplex and Epstein-Barr virus). In the first month after OLT, the most common infections are nosocomial Gram-negative bacterial and candidal infections. Between one and six months after OLT, infections with CMV, Epstein-Barr virus (EBV), *Pneumocystis carinii* and *Aspergillus* are commonly seen. Infections beyond six months after liver transplantation are similar to that seen in the normal population. However, patients on high-dose immunosuppressive regimens or those undergoing treatment for rejection may have an increased incidence of infection. Surveillance cultures of blood and urine, prophylactic intravenous antibiotics and selective bowel decontamination are some of the strategies used in the prevention and early recognition of infection.

Bacterial Infections

Bacterial infections occur in over 50% of liver transplant recipients and are usually seen in the first three months after transplant. Frequent sites of bacterial infection include intravascular lines, wounds, biliary tract, urinary tract, respiratory tract and the blood stream. Infections are commonly caused by Gram-positive and Gram-negative organisms. Although patients with infection and sepsis commonly present with fever, jaundice and cholestasis may also be seen. Proinflammatory cytokines released in sepsis are thought to be responsible for this phenomenon and seem particularly effective in causing cholestasis in the hepatic allograft. Histologically these changes are characterized by bile ductular proliferation with prominent bile plugging and usually resolve with treatment of the underlying infection. These changes differ from those seen in extrahepatic obstruction where the proliferating bile ductules are located within the portal connective tissue and bile plugs are uncommon.

Fungal Infections

Fungal infections usually occur between one and six months after OLT and are associated with a high mortality. Risk factors for fungal infection include pretransplant renal failure and dialysis, re-transplantation, prolonged operative time, increased transfusion requirements, high levels of immunosuppression, antibiotic usage and CMV infection. Fungal infections also have a high propensity to infect vascular grafts resulting in mycotic aneurysms and rupture. About 75% of all fungal infections are caused by *Candida* species, followed by *Aspergillus* in about 20%. Invasive fungal disease should be considered in all patients with unexplained allograft dysfunction or fever of unknown origin in the setting of OLT. In general, candidial infections occur earlier than other fungal infections and colonization at mucocutaneous sites represents the primary risk factor. The incidence of invasive fungal infections may be lowered by better operative techniques, judicious use of antibiotics and better control of immunosuppression. It is yet to be proven if high-risk patients will benefit from routine prophylactic administration of antifungal agents such as amphotericin.

Cytomegalovirus Infection

The majority of CMV infections occur within eight weeks of OLT and CMV hepatitis accounts for more than 50% of CMV disease. Seronegative recipients of seropositive donors have the highest risk of developing symptomatic disease (>50%). However, a latent CMV infection can be activated by therapy with antilymphocyte antibodies or cytotoxic drugs, systemic infection or rejection. In addition to hepatitis, CMV can also cause fever, leukopenia, thrombocytopenia, atypical lymphocytosis, pneumonitis, and retinitis. CMV hepatitis may clinically, biochemically and histologically mimic rejection. Serologic tests have little value in the diagnosis of CMV hepatitis and the diagnosis is made by demonstrating the typical nuclear inclusions or microabscesses on liver biopsy or by detection of viral DNA by polymerase chain reaction. "Mini" microabscesses may also be part of a syndrome unrelated to CMV and is characterized by a female preponderance, hepatocellular pattern of liver injury, absence of CMV DNA in liver biopsy tissue and lack of impact on long-term graft or patient survival. Treatment of CMV requires administration of intravenous ganciclovir for two to four weeks, until clearance of viremia. Resistant cases may be treated with foscarnet. Administration of low-dose ganciclovir to high-risk patients (eg, CMV-seropositive patients receiving antilymphocyte antibody therapy, patients undergoing re-transplantation or those with fulminant hepatic failure) reduces the risk of clinical disease from 65% to below 20%. Oral ganciclovir has been shown to be safe and effective for CMV prophylaxis.

Other Herpes Virus

Other herpes viruses causing hepatic allograft dysfunction include herpes simplex and EBV. Herpes simplex infections are commonly seen in the first three weeks after transplant and can involve oral and genital mucosa, eye, esophagus or liver. Herpes hepatitis can lead to serious allograft dysfunction and may be fatal. The drug of choice for treating herpes simplex is acyclovir. Herpes simplex can be virtually eliminated by the prophylactic use of low-dose acyclovir (400 mg orally twice a day) for the first six weeks posttransplant.

The most common manifestations of EBV infection in the posttransplant patient are hepatitis and posttransplant lymphoproliferative disorder (PTLD). EBV hepatitis usually occurs four to six months after OLT and may be associated with increased immunosuppression, particularly the use of muromonab-CD3. EBV may also be associated with PTLD, a B cell lymphoproliferative disorder. PTLD not uncommonly involves the liver and may present as hepatic dysfunction. Both EBV hepatitis and PTLD can occasionally cause massive hepatic necrosis. EBV infection is diagnosed by the presence of the EBV genome, usually detected by PCR. In PTLD, the presence of the EBV genome usually signifies active EBV infection. Histologic features of PTLD are similar to that seen in rejection, but a monomorphic mononuclear B lymphocytic portal infiltrate without bile duct damage may suggest PTLD. In situ immunohistologic staining for EBV can be useful in confirming the diagnosis. Unfortunately, effective antiviral agents are not available for the treatment of EBV. In patients with documented PTLD withdrawal or a marked decrease in immunosuppression may be helpful if conventional chemotherapy is not planned. The mortality from polymorphic PTLD ranges from 0% to 20% while that from monomorphic PTLD ranges from 67% to 87%.

DRUG HEPATOTOXICITY

Hepatic allograft dysfunction can occur secondary to drug therapy and a detailed drug or toxin history is therefore essential in all patients. Although the temporal relationship between the onset of symptoms and commencement of the drug may provide a clue to the presence of drug-related hepatotoxicity, it can sometimes be difficult, if not impossible, to completely exclude drug hepatotoxicity as a cause of hepatic allograft dysfunction. The most important aspect of investigating a possible drug-induced injury is to rule out other possible causes of liver injury by appropriate testing.

Drug-related hepatic injury is conventionally divided into cytotoxic (hepatocellular), cholestatic or mixed patterns. Occasionally, acute steatosis may occur. Hepatic injury may or may not be accompanied by systemic manifestations of hypersensitivity, such as fever, rash, and eosinophilia. Biochemical parameters show hyperbilirubinemia associated with elevated amino-transferase and/or alkaline phosphatase levels. The histologic picture caused by drugs may resemble those of any known type of liver dysfunction in liver transplantation setting. In addition to the usual agents causing hepatic dysfunction in the nontransplant population, drugs such as azathioprine, trimethoprim-sulfamethoxazole, antifungal agents such as amphotericin B and ketoconazole, cyclosporine and tacrolimus are especially important to keep in mind while dealing with posttransplant patients.

Azathioprine-induced hepatotoxicity can present with a mixed hepatocellular-cholestatic picture but additionally has also been associated with venooclusive type disease, peliosis hepatis, sinusoidal dilatation and nodular regenerative hyperplasia. Cyclosporine-induced hepatotoxicity is predominantly cholestatic in nature but is now relatively rare at the lower doses currently in use. Cyclosporine has also been associated with the increased formation of biliary sludge and calculi. Toxic doses of tacrolimus can result in elevated liver enzymes, and a histologic picture characterized by centrizonal hepatocellular dropout, sinusoidal dilatation and congestion has been attributed to tacrolimus by some investigators. However, recent studies indicate that these changes may be components of ACR and, in fact, tacrolimus has been safely used in the setting of severe liver dysfunction associated with refractory allograft rejection. Corticosteroids produce macrovesicular steatosis, with hepatomegaly being the most important clinical finding.

The offending drug must be immediately discontinued if suspected of causing hepatic dysfunction. Fortunately, most of the drug-induced abnormalities reverse upon dose reduction or discontinuation of the drug. However, hepatocellular injury may occasionally result in fulminant hepatic failure and this must be borne in mind when treating these patients.

RECURRENT DISEASE

Recurrence of the original liver disease after OLT is one of the most frequent causes of late hepatic allograft dysfunction and graft loss. Recurrent diseases commonly seen after OLT include viral hepatitis (hepatitis B and C), primary biliary cirrhosis (PBC), PSC, autoimmune liver disease, nonalcoholic steatohepatitis (NASH), alcoholic liver disease, and malignancy.

Hepatitis B

Hepatitis B infection of the hepatic allograft can result from transmission of the virus from the donor, or from recurrence of the disease in the recipient. All donors with active viral replication, and 30% to 50% of donors with isolated antibodies to hepatitis B core antibody, will transmit hepatitis B to the recipient. Recipients with active viral replication, as evidenced by the presence of the hepatitis B antigen or hepatitis B virus DNA (HBV DNA), have a higher recurrence rate compared to recipients with hepatitis B who have neither marker of active viral replication. Recurrent hepatitis B is diagnosed by the presence of hepatitis B surface antigen or HBV DNA in the recipient's serum and hepatitis B surface and core antigen in liver tissue.

Patients with recurrent hepatitis B frequently progress to liver dysfunction and cirrhosis. Additionally, a particularly virulent form of recurrent hepatitis B called *fibrosing cholestatic hepatitis* results in marked cholestasis without a significant elevation of aminotransferase levels and a paucity of inflammatory cells on liver biopsy. Rapid deterioration of liver function and death is common and usually occurs in under six months in these patients. Strategies to prevent HBV reinfection include passive immunoprophylaxis with hepatitis B immunoglobulin (HBIG) alone or in combination with antiviral therapy. Recurrent hepatitis B is almost universal in the absence of HBIG therapy. Our patients receive HBIG at a dose of 10,000 IU during the anhepatic phase, followed by 10,000 IU daily for a week. Subsequently, the dose of HBIG is titrated to maintain an anti-HBs level greater than 500 IU/L and therapy is maintained indefinitely. The risk of developing mutants during long-term HBIG therapy is unknown. After an allograft is infected clinically with HBV, passive immunization has no known role and should be discontinued.

Antiviral therapy with lamivudine, either alone or in combination with HBIG, is also being tried at many transplant centers. Lamivudine, at a dose of 100 to 150 mg/day, is associated with prompt disappearance of HBV DNA from the serum and improvement in liver biochemistries and histology. Long-term use of lamivudine, however, is associated with the appearance of YMDD mutants in about 1/3 of patients at the end of two years of treatment. The significance of this mutant remains unclear at this point in time. The best time to institute lamivudine pre-OLT is uncertain. It should ideally be given with a view to rendering patients HBV DNA negative at the time of transplantation. The use of famciclovir as a rescue therapy is an option in patients with the pre-core mutant virus. Additionally, the use of combination therapy with lamivudine and famciclovir may delay or prevent the emergence of resistant strains of HBV. Another antiviral agent with activity against HBV, adefovir dipivoxil, is currently undergoing phase I/II studies. Preliminary results suggest that it is effective against the YMDD mutant associated with the long-term use of lamivudine.

Hepatitis C

Recurrence of hepatitis C in the allograft from HCV present in the mononuclear cells of the recipient is almost universal. Although published reports show no difference in survival after OLT between patients with and without hepatitis C, longer periods of observation are needed to detect true differences in outcome. The development of cirrhosis in these patients, however, is associated with decreased survival.

Multiple factors play a role in the development of aggressive recurrent hepatitis C and these include viral genotype, viral load, degree of immunosuppression and ACR. In some studies, genotypes 1b and 1a have been associated with a more severe degree of recurrence. Genotype 1b-infected recipients have a high incidence of developing cirrhosis, particularly after treatment for rejection. Pretransplantation HCV-RNA titers greater-than-or-equal-to 1×10^6 vEq/mL and the use of high-dose immunosuppression (corticosteroid boluses and muromonab-CD3) are also strongly associated with a poorer outcome. Patients with recurrent hepatitis C usually present with elevated transaminase levels. Occasionally, a cholestatic hepatitis similar to that seen in recurrent hepatitis B, can also be seen. The diagnosis is made by demonstrating viremia in the blood and coexisting histologic hepatitis. Histologically, hepatitis C should be differentiated from acute cellular rejection, ischemia and recurrent autoimmune disease. Serial biopsies are helpful in demonstrating progression of recurrent hepatitis C.

The optimal treatment of recurrent hepatitis C in the hepatic allograft remains unclear. Reducing immunosuppression by rapid tapering of steroids or by using mycophenolate mofetil may help retard the progression of recurrent hepatitis C. Results of monotherapy with interferon are poor. However, combination therapy with interferon and ribavirin has resulted in sustained response rates of about 10% to 15%. The potential for interferon to precipitate allograft rejection is still the subject of continuing debate. Re-transplantation for severe recurrent hepatitis C is controversial, but should be considered an option for patients who develop end-stage liver disease.

Other Causes

Other causes of hepatic allograft dysfunction include recurrence of PBC, PSC, autoimmune hepatitis, NASH, alcoholic liver disease and malignancies. All these conditions are dealt with in greater detail in a separate chapter.

RECOMMENDED READING

Strasberg SM. Preservation injury and donor selection: it all starts here. Liver Transpl Surg. 1997;3(5 Suppl 1): S1-S7.

Marsman WA, Wiesner RH, Rodriguez L, et al. Use of fatty donor liver is associated with diminished early patient and graft survival. Transplantation. 1996;62(9): 1246-1251.

Piratvisuth T, Tredger JM, Hayllar KA, Williams R. Contribution of true cold and rewarming ischemia times to factors determining outcome after orthotopic liver transplantation. Liver Transpl Surg. 1995;1(5):296-301.

Clavien PA, Harvey PR, Strasberg SM. Preservation and reperfusion injuries in liver allografts. An overview and synthesis of current studies. Transplantation. 1992;53(5): 957-978.

Pesonen EJ, Hockerstedt K, Makisalo H, et al. Transhepatic neutrophil and monocyte activation during clinical liver transplantation. Transplantation. 2000;69(7): 1458-1464.

Sanchez-Urdazpal L, Gores GJ, Ward EM et al. Ischemic-type biliary complications after orthotopic liver transplantation. Hepatology. 1992;16(1):49-53.

Ploeg RJ, D'Alessandro AM, Knechtle SJ, et al. Risk factors for primary dysfunction after liver transplantation – a multivariate analysis. Transplantation. 1993;55(4): 807-813.

Deschenes M, Belle SH, Krom RA, Zetterman RK, Lake JR. Early allograft dysfunction after liver transplantation: a definition and predictors of outcome. National Institute of Diabetes and Digestive and Kidney Diseases Liver Transplantation Database. Transplantation. 1998;66(3):302-310.

Henley KS, Lucey MR, Normolle DP, et al. A double-blind, randomized, placebo-controlled trial of prostaglandin E1 in liver transplantation. Hepatology. 1995;21(2):366-372.

Abbasoglu O, Levy MF, Vodapally MS, et al. Hepatic artery stenosis after liver transplantation – incidence, presentation, treatment, and long term outcome. Transplantation. 1997;63(2):250-255.

Wiesner RH, Goldstein RM, Donovan JP, Miller CM, Lake JR, Lucey MR. The impact of cyclosporine dose and level on acute rejection and patient and graft survival in liver transplant recipients. Liver Transpl Surg. 1998;4(1):34-41.

Berlakovich GA, Imhof M, Karner-Hanusch J, et al. The importance of the effect of underlying disease on rejection outcomes following orthotopic liver transplantation. Transplantation. 1996;61(4):554-560.

Berlakovich GA, Rockenschaub S, Taucher S, Kaserer K, Muhlbacher F, Steiniger R. Underlying disease as a predictor for rejection after liver transplantation. Arch Surg. 1998;133(2):167-172.

Hayashi M, Keeffe EB, Krams SM, et al. Allograft rejection after liver transplantation for autoimmune liver diseases. Liver Transpl Surg. 1998;4(3):208-214.

Prieto M, Berenguer M, Rayon JM, et al. High incidence of allograft cirrhosis in hepatitis C virus genotype 1b infection following transplantation: relationship with rejection episodes. Hepatology. 1999;29(1):250-256.

Anonymous. Banff schema for grading liver allograft rejection: an international consensus document. Hepatology. 1997;25(3):658-663.

Wiesner RH. A long-term comparison of tacrolimus (FK506) versus cyclosporine in liver transplantation: a report of the United States FK506 Study Group. Transplantation. 1998;66(4):493-499.

Charco R, Murio E, Edo A, et al. Early use of tacrolimus as rescue therapy for refractory liver allograft rejection. Transpl Int. 1998;11 Suppl 1:S313-S317.

Wiesner RH, Demetris AJ, Belle SH, et al. Acute hepatic allograft rejection: incidence, risk factors, and impact on outcome. Hepatology. 1998;28(3):638-645.

Feller RB, Waugh RC, Selby WS, Dolan PM, Sheil AG, McCaughan GW. Biliary strictures after liver transplantation: clinical picture, correlates and outcomes. J Gastroenterol Hepatol. 1996;11(1):21-25.

Patel R, Portela D, Badley AD, et al. Risk factors of invasive Candida and non-Candida fungal infections after liver transplantation. Transplantation. 1996;62(7):926-934.

Falagas ME, Paya C, Ruthazer R, et al. Significance of cytomegalovirus for long-term survival after orthotopic liver transplantation: a prospective derivation and validation cohort analysis. Transplantation. 1998;66(8):1020-1028.

Paya CV, Wiesner RH, Hermans PE, et al. Risk factors for cytomegalovirus and severe bacterial infections following liver transplantation: a prospective multivariate time-dependent analysis. J Hepatol. 1993;18(2):185-195.

Gane E, Saliba F, Valdecasas GJ, et al. Randomised trial of efficacy and safety of oral ganciclovir in the prevention of cytomegalovirus disease in liver-transplant recipients. The Oral Ganciclovir International Transplantation Study Group. Lancet. 1997;350(9093):1729-1733.

Van Hoek B, Wiesner RH, Krom RA, Ludwig J, Moore SB. Severe ductopenic rejection following liver transplantation: incidence, time of onset, risk factors, treatment, and outcome. Semin Liver Dis. 1992;12(1):41-50.

Demetris AJ, Seaberg EC, Batts KP, et al. Chronic liver allograft rejection: a National Institute of Diabetes and Digestive and Kidney Diseases interinstitutional study analyzing the reliability of current criteria and proposal of an expanded definition. National Institute of Diabetes and Digestive and Kidney Diseases Liver Transplantation Database. Am J Surg Pathol. 1998;22(1):28-39.

Douglas DD, Rakela J, Wright TL, Krom RA, Wiesner RH. The clinical course of transplantation-associated de novo hepatitis B infection in the liver transplant recipient. Liver Transplant Surg. 1997;3(2):105-111.

Samuel D, Muller R, Alexander G, et al. Liver transplantation in European patients with the hepatitis B surface antigen. N Engl J of Med. 1993;329(25):1842-1847.

Lau GK, Tsiang M, Hou J, et al. Combination therapy with lamivudine and famciclovir for chronic hepatitis B-infected Chinese patients: a viral dynamics study. Hepatology. 2000;32(2):394-399.

Wright TL, Donegan E, Hsu HH, et al. Recurrent and acquired hepatitis C viral infection in liver transplant recipients. Gastroenterology. 1992;103(1):317-322.

Boker KH, Dalley G, Bahr MJ, et al. Long-term outcome of hepatitis C virus infection after liver transplantation. Hepatology. 1997;25(1):203-210.

Charlton M, Seaberg E, Wiesner R, et al. Predictors of patient and graft survival following liver transplantation for hepatitis C. Hepatology. 1998;28(3):823-830.

75 THE HISTOPATHOLOGY OF LIVER ALLOGRAFT DYSFUNCTION

A.J. Demetris, MD
Randall G. Lee, MD

INTRODUCTION AND OPTIMAL UTILIZATION OF PATHOLOGY SERVICES

Optimal care of the liver transplant recipient requires an integrated team of healthcare professionals, including a pathologist with an interest in liver and transplantation pathology. The pathologist's services can be used most effectively when there is direct and open communication and an understanding of the pathophysiology of allograft dysfunction, the techniques available to study tissue samples, and the limitations on diagnostic interpretation. For proper histopathologic evaluation, certain clinical information is required with the biopsy specimen: a brief clinical history, the original liver disease, and the time since transplantation. Specimens should be reviewed and discussed with the pathologist regularly (ideally, on a daily basis) to correlate the histopathologic findings with other diagnostic tests and therapeutic interventions. This provides essential feedback to both the clinician and pathologist to assure that they share a common understanding of each case and to avoid "diagnostic drift."

An important point to remember is that the various causes of allograft dysfunction occur during relatively well-defined periods following transplantation (Table 75-1), so that even without biopsy results, the diagnostic possibilities can be narrowed. A biopsy diagnosis not corresponding to the characteristic time period should be made and interpreted with caution. Also keep in mind that more than one insult can often contribute to allograft injury (eg, preservation injury and acute rejection).

ISCHEMIA/PRESERVATION INJURY

Ischemia/preservation injury is a generic term for the multiple potential insults suffered by the allograft before and during implantation. Clinically, this injury usually manifests with poor bile production and variable elevations of serum aminotransferases during the first few

A.J. Demetris, MD, Professor of Pathology, Director, Transplant Pathology, University of Pittsburgh Medical Center, University of Pittsburgh, Pittsburgh, PA

Randall G. Lee, MD, Medical Director, Pathology Services, Providence St. Vincent Medical Center, Portland, OR

days following transplantation. The more severe the insult, the higher the aminotransferase values, and a subsequent increase in serum bilirubin is also typical of moderate or severe injury.

The histopathologic changes entail varying degrees of hepatocellular injury and consequent regeneration with mitosis, thickened hepatic plates and cholangiolar proliferation. In general, the magnitude and duration of the dysfunction and regenerative response is proportional to the severity of the initial insult. Mild injury is characterized by mild hepatocellular swelling, spotty acidophilic necrosis, and cholestasis, which usually resolves within a week or so. More severe injury is distinguished by greater hepatocyte injury and necrosis with cholangiolar proliferation, and hepatocellular swelling and cholestasis can persist for up to several months. Persistent damage should prompt a search for additional insults.

BILIARY/VASCULAR COMPLICATIONS

Although the hepatic parenchyma is protected from ischemia by its dual blood supply, the biliary tract is supplied only by the hepatic artery and its branches. This renders the bile ducts especially vulnerable to ischemic injury, and consequently, hepatic artery complications (such as thrombosis or strictures) frequently present as biliary tract pathology.

Most posttransplant biliary/vascular complications can be traced to technical operative complications, pre-existing donor atherosclerosis, and difficulties with donor/recipient anatomic compatibility. These problems are most frequently encountered during the first several months after transplantation, but a second peak occurs between 16 and 36 months. The clinical manifestations very widely, as the patient may be entirely asymptomatic or may present with fever and intermittent bacteremia or fulminant hepatic failure.

Routine percutaneous needle biopsies are not reliable for diagnosing vascular thrombosis. Because ischemic injury predominantly affects the hilar and perihilar tissues, usual liver biopsies can be normal or show varying degrees of hepatocellular swelling, ischemic necrosis, and cholangiolar proliferation. Consequently, radiographic methods represent the diagnostic "gold standard".

The biliary tract complications (ie, obstruction, strictures, or acute cholangitis) yield the same histopathologic changes seen in non-allograft livers. Key features include portal and periductal edema, neutrophilic or eosinophilic portal inflammation, and bile ductular proliferation; cholestasis and intra-lobular neutrophil clusters are variably present. Incomplete or intermittent obstruction (especially late after transplantation) can give rise to predominantly mononuclear or mixed portal inflammation, which may be indistinguishable from that seen in acute rejection.

Table 75-1. Causes of Allograft Dysfunction and Their Characteristic Time of Onset

Cause of Allograft Dysfunction	Time of Onset	Comments
Ischemia/preservation injury	Immediately	Graft dysfunction may persists for several months
Humoral rejection	Immediately	Graft dysfunction may not become apparent for several days
Acute rejection	3-30 days	Late onset unusual, unless immunosuppression inadequate or complicating viral infection.
Biliary/vascular complications	Biphasic: first month; 16-36 months	Occurs as a result of immediate (1st peak, most common) or delayed (2nd peak, less common) technical complications.
Opportunistic Viral Infections		More common and severe in seronegative recipients.
CMV hepatitis	3-8 weeks	Very unusual out of time frame unless patient is seriously over-immunosuppressed.
EBV hepatitis/PTLD	Anytime	Hepatitis more common early (<6 months), PTLD later (>6 months).
Herpes simplex/varicella zoster	First 6 weeks Anytime	Seronegative recipients more likely to develop disease shortly after transplantation, but can occur anytime.
Adenovirus	First 6 weeks Anytime	Seronegative recipients more likely to develop shortly after transplantation, but can occur anytime.
Recurrent Original Disease		
HBV/HCV	Usually 3-6 weeks	Earlier onset (1-2 weeks) can be seen and often associated with aggressive clinical course
Primary biliary cirrhosis/ Primary sclerosing cholangitis	>1 year	Earlier onset can occasionally occur; perhaps more common under tacrolimus
Autoimmune hepatitis	>1 year	More common without steroids
Alcoholic liver disease	>6 months	More common in severe alcoholics

REJECTION
Humoral Rejection

Humoral rejection is an uncommon cause of allograft injury that occurs immediately (hyperacute) or during the first week (acute) after transplantation. It develops most predictably in ABO-incompatible allografts, is very uncommon with ABO compatibility, and can also occur in the 1% to 3% of recipients (especially females and presensitized patients) who harbor preformed lymphocytotoxic antibodies with high titer IgG.

Most commonly, the clinical presentation involves a persistent rise in serum bilirubin during the first post-transplant week, accompanied by refractory thrombocytopenia, low serum complement activity, and a biopsy showing ischemia/preservation injury. In severe cases, graft swelling, cyanosis, and mottling together with slowing of bile flow can develop soon after transplantation. Hepatic angiography may demonstrate changes indicative of vasospasm.

Histopathologic findings in severe cases include sinusoidal sludging of platelets and neutrophils (with lymphocytotoxic antibodies) and red blood cells (with isoagglutinins) in post-reperfusion biopsies, progressing to small infarcts in subsequent specimens. Endothelial cell hypertrophy may be evident, and arteries occasionally show neutrophilic and/or necrotizing arteritis. Late manifestations include ischemic biliary necrosis as manifest by biliary sludge, obstructive cholangiopathy and loss of small bile ducts. Immunofluorescent and immunoperoxidase stains in early biopsy samples can help establish the diagnosis by demonstrating clearcut, selective deposition of IgG, IgM and complement components in the arterial and venous tree.

Acute (Cellular) Rejection

Acute (cellular) rejection most commonly occurs between five and 30 days after transplantation, with at least 60% of all episodes occurring within the first six weeks. Between 30% to 70% of recipients are affected, and it is more common in inadequately immunosuppressed recipients, pediatric recipients, and patients with a positive crossmatch or donor/recipient DR mismatch. Unless the patient is inadequately immunosuppressed, acute rejection becomes less common as the time after transplantation lengthens; it thereby accounts for less than 30% of allograft dysfunction episodes occurring after one year posttransplant.

Clinical findings are often absent in early or mild examples. In late or severe cases, fever and graft enlargement, cyanosis, and tenderness can occur. Nonselective elevations of some or all of the standard liver injury tests are typical.

The histopathologic diagnosis is based on allograft inflammation together with damage of the small bile ducts, portal and/or hepatic venules, or occasionally the hepatic artery branches. The inflammatory component, located in the portal tracts and/or around the terminal hepatic venules, consists predominantly of blastic or activated lymphocytes, neutrophils and eosinophils. The mononuclear cells infiltrate the bile ducts and often tunnel beneath the subendothelial space of portal or terminal hepatic veins (so-called "endotheliitis"). The diagnosis is strengthened when more than 50% of the ducts are damaged or if unequivocal endotheliitis can be identified.

Once the diagnosis of acute rejection has been established, its severity can be graded based on the Banff Schema (Table 75-2), which is based on the overall severity of inflammation and evidence of rejection-related ischemia. A descriptive grade of indeterminate, mild, moderate, or severe can be designated, and, if desired, a semi-quantitative score, the Rejection Activity Index, provided as outlined in Table 75-3.

Chronic Rejection

Chronic rejection, which affects less than 10% of recipients, usually evolves from severe or persistent acute rejection. Risk factors include the number and severity of acute rejection episodes, late onset acute rejection episodes, younger recipient age, male-to-female sex mismatch, a primary diagnosis of autoimmune liver disease, non-Caucasian recipient race, donor age over 40 years, and the type of immunosuppression regimen.

It is usually first recognized within several months after transplantation, and later onsets are typically associated with inadequate immunosuppression. The diagnosis may become evident only because of a persistent, progressive cholestatic pattern of liver injury tests. Biliary strictures, hepatic infarcts, and finally loss of hepatic synthetic function occur in the later stages. Because similar laboratory and histopathologic changes can be seen with biliary and hepatic arterial complications, cholangiography or angiography may be required for diagnosis.

In biopsy specimens, the minimal histopathologic criteria of chronic rejection involve the presence of bile duct atrophy/pyknosis involving a majority of the ducts (with or without bile duct loss); convincing foam cell obliterative arteriopathy; bile duct loss affecting more than 50% of the portal tracts. Unfortunately, arteries with obliterative arteriopathy are rare in needle biopsy specimens, and bile duct injury and loss thereby become the major diagnostic focus. However, because a similar clinical and histopathologic picture is seen with non-rejection-related complications (eg, obstructive cholangiopathy, hepatic artery stricturing or thrombosis, and adverse drug reactions), these should be appropriately excluded before a final diagnosis is rendered.

As summarized in Table 75-4, chronic rejection can be staged according to the extent and severity of potentially irreversible damage to the three target structures – bile ducts, hepatic arteries and hepatic venules. Early-stage disease is present if only one or no late histologic changes are found, with such changes in two or more structures required in the late stage. In general, the changes progress from early to late, although this is not well-established for the perivenular alterations. Some patients appear to persist in the early stage for months or

Table 75-2. Banff Schema for the Grading of Acute (Cellular) Rejection

Global Assessment	Criteria
Indeterminate	Portal inflammatory infiltrate that fails to meet the criteria for the diagnosis of acute rejection
Mild	Rejection infiltrate in a minority of the triads, that is generally mild, and confined within the portal spaces
Moderate	Rejection infiltrate expanding most or all of the triads
Severe	As above for moderate, with spillover into periportal areas and moderate to severe perivenular inflammation that extends into the hepatic parenchyma and is associated with perivenular hepatocyte necrosis
Verbal description of mild, moderate or severe acute rejection could also be labeled as Grade I, II and III, respectively.	

Table 75-3. Rejection Activity Index (RAI) for Acute (Cellular) Rejection

Category	Criteria	Score
Portal Inflammation	Mostly lymphocytic inflammation involving, but not noticeably expanding, a minority of the triads	1
	Expansion of most or all of the triads, by a mixed infiltrate containing lymphocytes with occasional blasts, neutrophils and eosinophils	2
	Marked expansion of most or all of the triads by a mixed infiltrate containing numerous blasts and eosinophils with inflammatory spillover into the periportal parenchyma	3
Bile Duct Inflammation Damage	A minority of the ducts are cuffed and infiltrated by inflammatory cells and show only mild reactive changes such as increased nuclear:cytoplasmic ratio of the epithelial cells	1
	Most or all of the ducts infiltrated by inflammatory cells. More than an occasional duct shows degenerative changes such as nuclear pleomorphism, disordered polarity and cytoplasmic vacuolization of the epithelium	2
	As above for 2, with most or all of the ducts showing degenerative changes or focal luminal disruption	3
Venous Endothelial Inflammation	Subendothelial lymphocytic infiltration involving some, but not a majority of the portal and/or hepatic venules	1
	Subendothelial infiltration involving most or all of the portal and/or hepatic venules	2
	As above for 2, with moderate or severe perivenular inflammation that extends into the perivenular parenchyma and is associated with perivenular hepatocyte necrosis	3

Total RAI score = sum of scores for the three components (range 0-9)

Table 75-4. Features of Early and Late Chronic Liver Allograft Rejection

Structure	Early Chronic Rejection	Late Chronic Rejection
Small bile ducts (< 60 m)	Degenerative change involving a majority of ducts: eosinophilic transformation of the cytoplasm; increased N:C ratio; nuclear hyperchromasia; uneven nuclear spacing; ducts only partially lined by biliary epithelial cells.	Degenerative changes in remaining bile ducts
	Bile duct loss in < 50% of portal tracts.	Loss in > 50% of portal tracts.
Terminal hepatic venules and zone 3 hepatocytes	Intimal/luminal inflammation	Focal obliteration
	Lytic zone 3 necrosis and inflammation	Variable inflammation
	Mild perivenular fibrosis	Severe fibrosis
Portal tract hepatic arterioles	Occasional loss involving < 25% of portal tracts.	Loss involving > 25 % of portal tracts.
Other	So-called "transition" hepatitis with spotty necrosis of hepatocytes	Sinusoidal foam cell accumulation; marked cholestasis
Large perihilar hepatic artery branches	Intimal inflammation, focal foam cell deposition without luminal compromise	Luminal narrowing by subintimal foam cells
		Fibrointimal proliferation
Large perihilar bile ducts	Inflammation damage and focal foam cell deposition	Mural fibrosis

years, while others rapidly develop severe fibrosis and late-stage disease.

OPPORTUNISTIC VIRAL HEPATITIS

The opportunistic viruses, primarily adenoviruses and the herpesviruses, seldom result in hepatic injury in the general population, but can give rise to significant allograft hepatitis. Usually these agents are acquired in childhood and lie dormant in the immunocompetent adult, but they can be reactivated in the transplant recipient. In addition, some patients may develop a primary infection, which is more common in children and is associated with a greater frequency and severity of allograft injury.

Adenovirus

Allograft hepatitis due to adenoviral subtypes 1, 2 and 5 occurs predominantly in the pediatric population, usually one to ten weeks after transplantation. Histopathologic findings include randomly scattered, "pox-like" granulomas, consisting almost entirely of macrophages and encompassing small groups of necrotic hepatocytes. The characteristic infected cells found near the edge of the necrotic zones or granulomas contain smudged nuclei with marginated chromatin that imparts a "muffin-shaped" appearance. Because such cells are difficult to identify with certainty, immunohistochemical and in situ hybridization studies are needed for confirmation.

Cytomegalovirus

Despite effective prophylaxis and treatment, CMV remains the most common opportunistic viral hepatitis. Symptomatic infection is usually encountered between three and eight weeks posttransplantation, during or shortly after increased immunosuppressive therapy used to treat rejection. The clinical presentation entails fever, leukopenia and low-grade elevations of liver injury tests, sometimes with diarrhea, gastrointestinal ulcers and respiratory insufficiency and retinitis in severe disease.

The histopathologic manifestations depend, in part, on the patient's immune status and prior antiviral treatment. In seronegative recipients, the changes include variable portal inflammation, mild lobular disarray with spotty hepatocyte necrosis, Kupffer cell hypertrophy, and microabscesses or microgranulomas scattered randomly throughout the lobules. The portal infiltrate may include conspicuous plasma cells, and focal bile duct inflammation and damage can also be seen. The diagnostic CMV-infected cells, which are generally located in or near the microabscesses or microgranulomas, are enlarged and display characteristic large eosinophilic intranuclear inclusions, and/or multiple small, basophilic to amphophilic cytoplasmic inclusions. In some patients, particularly in those treated with antiviral drugs, CMV inclusions may be absent, fragmented, or smudged, and difficult to recognize without immunohistochemical confirmation.

Epstein-Barr Virus

Epstein-Barr virus (EBV) can give rise to both allograft hepatitis and posttransplant lymphoproliferative disorder (PTLD), an oligoclonal and/or monoclonal B cell proliferation that may act like an aggressive lymphoma. The systemic viral syndrome seen with EBV can resemble that of classical infectious mononucleosis, but atypical features (ie, jaw pain, arthralgia, joint space effusions, diarrhea, encephalitis, pneumonitis, mediastinal lymphadenopathy and ascites) can also be seen. Laboratory findings usually include elevated liver injury tests and circulating atypical lymphocytes.

The histopathological picture of EBV hepatitis is typically a low-grade lobular hepatitis with focal hepatocellular swelling, mild acidophilic necrosis, and mild lobular disarray with occasional granulomatoid aggregates of Kupffer cells. Mononuclear infiltrates accumulate in the portal and periportal regions and form linear arrays and small aggregates within the sinusoids; these cells comprise small and blastic lymphocytes, some of which are atypical, admixed with plasmacytoid lymphocytes and plasma cells. In PTLD, sheets of monomorphic atypical immunoblastic cells (cytologically resembling those found in immunoblastic lymphoma) expand the portal tracts and obscure normal architectural landmarks; smaller aggregates of these cells collect in the sinusoids, occasionally with focal areas of necrosis.

Both EBV hepatitis and PTLD can mimic acute rejection histopathologically, but as the treatments are diametrically opposed, distinguishing the two is essential. Features favoring acute rejection include a mixed portal inflammatory infiltrate, numerous eosinophils, prevalent bile duct damage and venulitis (especially involving the terminal hepatic venules), whereas a monomorphic portal infiltrate of cytologically atypical cells with only rare eosinophils is more suggestive of an EBV-related disorder. In situ hybridization with the EBER probe for EBV RNA is often required to make the final distinction.

HERPES SIMPLEX AND VARICELLA-ZOSTER VIRUSES.

Both HSV subtypes I and II and varicella-zoster (VZ) can give rise to allograft hepatitis. This has been seen as early as three days posttransplant, but may occur anytime thereafter; the clinical presentation includes fever, vesicular skin rashes, fatigue, body pain, and elevated liver injury tests. Unrecognized HSV hepatitis can rapidly lead to submassive or massive hepatic necrosis with hypotension, disseminated intravascular coagulation, and metabolic acidosis.

Early biopsy detection of these agents is crucial for prompt intervention. They characteristically produce circumscribed, randomly scattered foci of coagulative-type necrosis with central hepatocyte "ghosts" intermixed with neutrophils and nuclear debris. The hepatocytes along the periphery contain the typical intranuclear inclusions, which can appear as smudgy, ground glass, or eosinophilic (Cowdry type A) bodies. Multinucleate cells are occasionally present. Not infrequently, diagnostic changes will be not identified on routine sections, and immunohistochemical confirmation is required.

RECURRENT AND DE NOVO VIRAL HEPATITIS

Hepatitis A Virus

Liver transplantation may be necessary for the rare case example of fulminant, prolonged, or relapsing hepatitis A. Recurrence of the disease has not been a problem, although the virus can be detected for a short time after transplantation in some patients.

Viral Hepatitis Types B and C

Virtually all hepatitis B patients with pretransplant evidence of viral replication (ie, HBeAg +; HBV-DNA +) reinfect their allograft and develop recurrent hepatitis. This complication is less predictable in those patients with HBV-induced fulminant liver failure or with chronic HBV in the low replicative state (anti-HBe +; HbeAg -; HBV-DNA-), and, despite screening, occasional HBV-negative patients will unfortunately acquire the infection during or after transplantation. In hepatitis C recipients, reinfection and disease recurrence is nearly universal.

In general, the manifestations of recurrent HBV and HCV are similar, although untreated HCV tends to be a less aggressive disease. Recurrence is usually first detected three to six weeks after transplant because of elevated aminotransferases found during routine monitoring. More dramatic initial presentations (especially with HBV) include nausea, vomiting, jaundice and hepatic failure.

The histopathologic changes mimic those seen in non-allograft livers. The earliest finding is an acute lobular hepatitis characterized by lobular necro-inflammatory activity, lobular disarray, and Kupffer cell hypertrophy with variable portal inflammation. A small percentage of HBV recipients will quickly progress to submassive necrosis, particularly if immunosuppression is withdrawn, but this is not seen with HCV. In most patients, this acute phase partially resolves with evolution toward a typical chronic hepatitis with a predominantly mononuclear portal and periportal inflammatory process. Cirrhosis can sometimes develop with striking rapidity.

Unusual histopathologic patterns of HBV and HCV can also be seen, and are likely related to the potent immunosuppression and MHC non-identity between the liver and recipient. One such pattern is fibrosing cholestatic hepatitis characterized by marked hepatocyte swelling (attributed to massive viral replication), lobular disarray, and cholestasis together with minimal or no inflammation and variable cholangiolar proliferation. Follow-up biopsies often show progressive portal expansion because of cholangiolar proliferation, periportal sinusoidal fibrosis and lobular collapse, often without a significant inflammatory component.

OTHER CAUSES OF ALLOGRAFT DYSFUNCTION

Unfortunately, many of the leading diseases leading to liver transplantation can recur in the allograft (Table 75-5). In addition, the transplanted liver can fall victim to any of the causes of hepatic dysfunction seen in native livers

Table 75-5. Recurrent Disease after Liver Transplantation

Disease	Approximate Prevalence at Five Years	Methods of Diagnosis
Viral Hepatitis		
HBV	60-90%	Viral serology, viral DNA levels and histopathology
HCV	Nearly universal	Viral serology, viral RNA levels and histopathology
Autoimmune Disorders		
PBC*	10-30%	Histopathology, auto-antibody serology and clinical symptoms
PSC†	10-30%	Cholangiography and histopathology
Autoimmune hepatitis	20-30%	Histopathology, auto-antibody serology and absence of other causes of hepatitis
Other		
Alcoholic Liver Disease	20%	Histopathology, clinical history and serologic studies and absence of other causes of steatohepatitis

*PBC indicates Primary Biliary Cirrhosis; †PSC, Primary Sclerosing Cholangitis

including adverse drug reactions and systemic disorders such as sepsis. The histopathologic changes produced by these insults are identical to those used in biopsies from non-allograft livers, and will not be reviewed here.

RECOMMENDED READING

Banff schema for grading acute liver allograft rejection: An international consensus document. Hepatology. 1997;25(3):658-663.

Blakolmer K, Seaberg EC, Batts K, et al. Analysis of the reversibility of chronic liver allograft rejection. Implications for a staging schema. Am J Surg Pathol. 1999;23(11):1328-1339.

Demetris A, Adams D, Bellamy C, et al. Update of the International Banff Schema for Liver Allograft Rejection: working recommendations for the histopathologic staging and reporting of chronic rejection. An International Panel. Hepatology. 2000;31(3):792-799.

Pappo O, Ramos H, Starzl T, Fung JJ, Demetris AJ. Structural integrity and identification of causes of liver allograft dysfunction occurring more than 5 years after transplantation. Am J Surg Pathol. 1995;19(2):192-206.

Shuhart MC, Bronner MP, Gretch DR, et al. Histological and clinical outcome after liver transplantation for hepatitis C. Hepatology. 1997;26(6):1646-1652.

76 LONG-TERM ISSUES IN LIVER TRANSPLANTATION

Rafik M. Ghobrial, MD, PhD
Hugo R. Rosen, MD
Paul Martin, MD

The past decade has witnessed a dramatic growth of orthotopic liver transplantation (OLT) with more than 20,000 patients transplanted worldwide. In the United States, more than 4,000 OLTs are performed yearly with expected patient survival of greater than 85% at one year and greater than 70% at five years. Thus much attention is currently focused towards long-term management of liver transplant recipients.

LATE MORTALITY AND GRAFT LOSS

Common late causes of hepatic allograft dysfunction after orthotopic liver transplantation include recurrence of original disease, hepatic allograft rejection, biliary tract complications and drug-induced hepatotoxicity. Clinical differentiation of such causes is often difficult. The patterns of enzyme elevation might be identical in various entities and histological pictures are often overlapping. Inappropriate management of such problems may lead to graft loss and patient death. For example, in hepatic allograft rejection, immunosuppression must be promptly increased, while infectious causes of liver dysfunction demand lower immunosuppressive therapy. Therefore, such frequently encountered clinical dilemmas demand meticulous assessment of hepatic allograft dysfunction (Table 76-1) to ensure successful outcomes.

Recurrence of Original Disease

Undoubtedly, recurrence of underlying liver diseases poses the greatest threat to long-term graft survival. The largest series to date of liver transplant recipients surviving for at least five years (n=116) demonstrated an unexpectedly high prevalence of histological abnormalities, even in the presence of normal biochemical liver tests in long-term survivors. In nearly half of the patients with histological changes consistent with chronic allograft hepatitis, the cause could not be identified. No evidence of HBV, HCV, or recurrent disease was demonstrated. Thus, other causes such as poorly-treated acute rejection episodes and initial graft injury may influence long-term graft survival in addition to disease recurrence.

CHOLESTATIC LIVER DISEASE. Primary biliary cirrhosis (PBC) may recur following liver transplantation. In one study, of 60 patients transplanted for PBC, antimitochondrial antibodies persisted in 43 (72%) of the patients, and although the median titer dropped from 1:640 dilution pretransplant to 1:40 posttransplant, five patients exhibited florid duct lesions and portal granulomas. However, these five patients were asymptomatic and had normal liver tests and only two had detectable antimitochondrial antibodies. Although considerable overlap exists between histologic features of PBC and other entities such as chronic rejection, most authors agree that PBC can recur, but that the clinical impact of recurrence remains unclear.

Speculation that primary sclerosing cholangitis (PSC) may recur is based on the high frequency of posttransplant nonanastomotic biliary strictures. One study suggested that biliary complications were six times more likely after OLT for PSC. However, another group demonstrated that patients transplanted for conditions other than PSC, who had a Roux-en-Y hepaticojejunostomy that is commonly employed in PSC patients, developed features of biliary obstruction and periductal fibrosis. Such studies suggest that the type of anastomosis, not the original disease, may lead to such complications. Further PSC-like lesions are seen with hepatic artery thrombosis, preservation-related ischemic injury, ABO-

Rafik M. Ghobrial, MD, PhD, Assistant Professor of Surgery, Division of Liver and Pancreas Transplantation, Dumont-UCLA Transplant Center, University of California Los Angeles, Los Angeles, CA

Hugo R. Rosen, MD, Associate Professor of Medicine, Molecular Microbiology, and Immunology, Division of Gastroenterology/ Hepatology; Medical Director, Liver Transplantation Program, Oregon Health Sciences University Portland Veterans Affairs Medical Center, Portland, OR

Paul Martin, MD, Associate Professor of Medicine Director, Hepatology, Division of Digestive Diseases and Dumont-UCLA Transplant Program, University of California at Los Angeles; Los Angeles, CA

Table 76-1. Evaluation of Liver Allograft Dysfunction
Review of original liver disease
Pattern of biochemical abnormalities
Medication history
Review of previous posttransplant complications
Review of immunosuppressive medications
Ultrasonography and Doppler studies
Hepatitis serologies and cultures
Liver biopsy
Cholangiography and angiography

incompatible grafts, and chronic rejection. Large series of patients are required in which PSC patients are carefully matched with appropriate controls to prove recurrent disease.

CHRONIC VIRAL HEPATITIS. The significance of chronic viral hepatitis as a cause of end-stage liver disease is reflected in the large number of patients referred for OLT. Identification of prognostic markers, for hepatitis B virus (HBV) recurrence post-OLT, enabled the development of effective immunoprophylaxis that contained and prevented HBV recurrence and dramatically improved patient and graft survival in HBV-infected recipients. A seminal European multicenter study evaluating 372 consecutive HBV-infected patients undergoing OLT demonstrated that long-term treatment (>6 months) with hepatitis B immune globulin (HBIg) was effective in preventing or delaying graft reinfection. However, a protective effect of HBIg was not observed in patients with active viral replication as indicated by HBV DNA or hepatitis B e antigen (HBeAg) positivity pretransplant. Such patients exhibited recurrence rates that were similar to patients who received short-term or no prophylactic therapy. Nevertheless, high-dose HBIg prophylaxis (fixed dose of 10,000 IU monthly) has recently been shown to reduce HBV recurrence, even in patients with pre-OLT indices of active viral replication. The excellent patient and graft survival now possible with long-term HBIg and with the more recently reported lamivudine prophylaxis suggest that HBV recurrence post-OLT has been contained. Transplantation for HBeAg-positive patients, which until recently was a controversial issue, is now a commonplace practice with lamivudine therapy. However, the significance of lamivudine-induced HBV mutations in this setting remains to be determined. Furthermore, lamivudine and HBIg therapy have also been successful in preventing further graft loss after re-transplantation for recurrent HBV. Although early reports of re-transplantation in patients with HBV recurrence suggested a more accelerated natural history and a shorter window to graft failure, recent analysis demonstrated that HBV recurrence was preventable in six of seven re-transplanted patients treated with aggressive immunoprophylaxis that maintained an anti-HBs antibody level over 500 IU/L.

Although recurrence of for hepatitis C virus (HCV) as detected by PCR is almost universal after liver transplantation, OLT is performed with excellent results. To date the largest series that included 374 patients transplanted for HCV over an 8-year period, demonstrated an overall patient survival of 86% and 76% at one and five years, respectively. Comparison to a contemporary cohort of 701 patients who underwent transplantation for causes other than viral infections did not reveal any difference in patient survival. Overall graft survival in this series was 70% and 60% at one and five years,

respectively. Two other series that included a cohort of 183 and 149 transplant recipients, patient and graft survival was not significantly different from HCV-negative patients at one and five years posttransplantation.

The spectrum of allograft injury related to HCV recurrence ranges from minimal evidence of biochemical or histologic injury to mild abnormalities or frank graft failure in a small minority of recipients. A major difficulty in managing OLT recipients with HCV is that histological differentiation between recurrent hepatitis C and rejection is difficult, and may be only evident following evaluation of serial allograft biopsies. The mechanisms by which HCV causes liver damage following OLT are poorly understood. However, the recent findings that higher serum HCV RNA levels just prior to, and in the first two weeks following OLT were associated with a higher rate of chronic active allograft hepatitis and increased mortality suggest that early events are critical and that antiviral therapy should be started early. Interferon treatment of recurrent HCV post-OLT has lacked convincing efficacy, with concern about an increased incidence of rejection associated with its use. However, recent studies using the combination of interferon-α and ribavirin have been encouraging. Whether preemptive antiviral treatment prior to the development of histological recurrence alters the natural course of HCV post-OLT is currently under investigation. Moreover, it is likely that in the near future, HCV-positive donors will be routinely used for HCV-positive recipients, given the preliminary data suggesting that donor HCV serostatus does not adversely impact outcome.

Much attention is currently directed towards factors that influence the rate and severity of recurrent hepatitis C. Although, graft re-infection with HCV is universal, graft loss and death due to hepatitis C appears to be much less common. In one study that included 149 patients who were transplanted for HCV, graft loss occurred in 27 of 149 patients, but only eight patients suffered graft loss secondary to HCV. In another series of 166 HCV-infected transplant recipients, recurrent HCV with ensuing graft failure was the cause of death in only 11 of 39 patients.

Effects of immunosuppression on viral replication may accelerate the natural history of HCV recurrence after transplantation. Muromonab-CD3 treatment for steroid-resistant rejection has been convincingly shown by several groups to be associated with early and severe HCV recurrence in allografts. In a study from UCLA, allograft cirrhosis was documented in 26.3% of recipients who received muromonab-CD3 during their posttransplant course, compared with 6% of patients who had steroid-responsive rejection. Similarly, severe or multiple rejection episodes were associated with early recurrence. Higher levels of viral replication was documented with excessive steroid use for treatment of rejection episodes. Tacrolimus was implicated to increase recurrence rates in one study and was associated with a poor clinical outcome in another. However, in the first study, patients received excessive doses of steroids for treatment of rejection, and in the second, excessively high doses of tacrolimus were used. More recently, the same group demonstrated that the use of lower doses of tacrolimus resulted in patient and graft survivals that were similar to non-HCV transplant recipients. In a more recent study that included 374 patients transplanted for HCV, tacrolimus demonstrated excellent patient and graft survival rates that were not significantly different from cyclosporine (CsA). Further, tacrolimus immunosuppression may be particularly useful in patients with hepatitis C due to the lower incidence of acute rejection when compared to CsA. Thus, tacrolimus may prevent rejection episodes that demand the use of steroids and/or muromonab-CD3, which have been associated with progressive allograft injury.

Initial reports of poor outcomes associated with re-transplantation for recurrent hepatitis C and the suggestion that viral reinfection may negatively influence the prognosis of re-transplanted livers questioned the wisdom of the procedure. However, re-transplantation carries a worse prognosis than primary OLTs, for all indications. Evaluation of 250 patients that underwent re-transplantation at UCLA for a variety of indications, revealed 55%, 47% and 44% survival rates from the date of the second transplant, at one, five, and ten years, respectively. Patient survival from the date of the second transplant for all causes of re-transplantation, was 63% and 58%, and for recurrent hepatitis C was 59% at one and two years. Thus, there appears to be no difference in survival in re-transplantation for recurrent hepatitis C when compared with other causes of re-transplantation. A number of independent variables were found to predict a poor outcome for re-transplantation. Such factors included the UNOS status and the poor preoperative condition of the patients but not the recipient primary diagnosis. Another study demonstrated a patient survival of 64% at one and two years following re-transplantation for hepatitis C and that poor outcomes were associated with critically ill recipients. Thus, re-transplantation early in the course of recurrent disease, prior to deterioration of the patient, exhibits a better outcome and remains a viable option in treatment of allograft failure due to recurrent HCV.

Transplantation for hepatitis C is performed with excellent results. Despite the risk of recurrence, the clinical outcome of transplantation for HCV is equivalent to that performed for other causes of ESLD. To date, HCV recurrence has not resulted in decreased patient and graft survivals. However, longer periods of follow-up may demonstrate different results. There appears to be no distinct advantages for the use of tacrolimus or CsA when patient and graft survivals are considered. Re-transplantation for recurrent HCV achieves good results in healthy patients, and should be considered an important option for the treatment of recurrent disease.

ALCOHOLIC LIVER DISEASE. The rate of recidivism and the effect of alcohol on hepatic allografts raise controversial issues regarding selection and exclusion criteria for patients with alcoholic liver disease (ALD). Although six months' abstinence prior to OLT remains a widely accepted prognostic model, other measurements based on social functioning and stability, hope and self-esteem can stratify patients into low-, moderate-, and high-risk for recidivism and noncompliance following OLT. However, the effect of alcohol on graft function is not well characterized, and the consequences of recidivism, occurring in 10% to 15% of patients, is difficult to assess. Further, evolving data suggest that alcohol does not impact the recurrence of HCV following transplantation, and may even have immunosuppressive properties that protect the recidivist from allograft rejection. Some reports suggested that even alcoholics who return to abusive drinking comply with their regular medications, and that death posttransplant is rarely attributable to alcohol abuse alone. Others demonstrate that drinking after OLT is associated with considerable morbidity, requiring hospital admissions and occasionally leading to graft loss and death. A recent National Institutes of Health-sponsored conference summarized the experience to-date with liver transplantation for alcohol-related liver failure and identified a major need for clinical research for prediction and treatment of relapse in patients with long-term follow-up.

HEPATIC MALIGNANCY. Hepatocellular carcinoma (HCC) is the most common of the primary liver malignancies, with a worldwide incidence of one million cases per year. Surgical resection remains the mainstay of therapy for HCC, but less than 30% of patients presenting with HCC have resectable tumors. OLT for unresectable HCC offers the advantage of removal of the entire liver, eliminating the problem of multifocality or bilobar involvement, and replacement with a functional liver, allowing patients with advanced cirrhosis to be treated. *Incidental* carcinomas are typically lesions less than 2 cm and discovered by the pathologist at the time of sectioning the explant and are associated with a good prognosis. Penn's recent analysis of compiled worldwide data demonstrated that patients with "usual hepatomas" (ie, diagnosed pre-OLT) excluding incidental and fibrolamellar tumors, had a post-OLT recurrence rate of 39% and a five year overall survival of 18%. Moreover, of the 365 patients transplanted for HCC, only 34 (9%) survived tumor free for more than two years, and another 21 had recurrences after two years. Numerous studies have reported similarly disappointing results. Iwatsuki et al identified tumor size (greater than 5 cm), multiple nodules, vascular invasion, and tumor shape (noncircumscribed) as poor prognostic indicators for recurrence in nonfibrolamellar HCC. Recent mathematical models that predict HCC recurrence have been developed using five risk factors: gender, tumor number, lobar tumor distribution, tumor size, and grade of vascular invasion. Using specific criteria for selection of unresectable patients with HCC, a recent Italian study demonstrated an overall actuarial survival of 75% post-OLT if the tumor size was less than 5 cm diameter, if single or if multiple less than 3 cm, and three or less in number. The fibrolamellar variant of HCC, which is characterized by unique histologic features and is not typically associated with cirrhosis, generally grows more slowly and has a higher resectability rate. Although recurrence post-OLT appears to be similar to usual HCC, the one, two, and three year survival rates (70%, 60%, and 55%, respectively) are considerably better for the fibrolamellar variant.

Because micrometastatic disease may account for the high rate of recurrence of HCC, several programs have explored the role of adjuvant chemotherapeutic protocols in patients transplanted for HCC with improved survivals reported in patients with poor prognosis. In summary, there definitely appears to be a role for OLT in the management of HCC, and further long-term evaluation of adjuvant therapy including preoperative hepatic artery chemoembolization and postoperative adjuvant chemotherapy will help define the optimal approach in these patients.

Biliary Complications

Biliary complications, once considered the "Achilles heel" of liver transplantation, are less common today and often can be managed either radiologically or endoscopically without the need for surgical intervention or re-transplantation. Biliary tract complications, which can occur in up to 20% of liver transplant recipients, represent a heterogeneous group of complications consisting of bile leaks, strictures, and obstruction due to stones and/or biliary sludge formation. A study from the University of Pittsburgh of 1,792 consecutive OLT recipients found that just over one-third of biliary complications were diagnosed within one month of surgery and 80% were diagnosed within six months, with leaks and strictures being the most common findings. After the first postoperative year, the incidence of biliary complications drops significantly. The most common cause of late biliary leaks is the T-tube site, following its removal in 10% to 15% of patients. Such leaks are managed endoscopically and rarely require laparotomy. Moreover, it is important to point out that any biliary tract complication may be due to hepatic artery thrombosis (HAT), which should be excluded by a Doppler ultrasound study.

However, the etiology of biliary strictures post-OLT is multifactorial and numerous studies have suggested an association between the development of multiple and/or late intrahepatic nonanastomotic strictures in the absence of HAT with preservation injury (specifically prolonged donor cold ischemia time), ABO-incompatibility, and CMV infection (Table 76-2). Often, such problems progress, and re-transplantation may be eventually indicated because of graft failure. Moreover, biliary stricturing in PSC patients may represent recurrent disease or may be caused by the Roux-en-Y choledochojejunostomy. Nonanastomotic strictures generally appear one to four months after transplantation and are often treated with balloon dilatation or stenting either using a transhepatic or endoscopic approaches. Although long-term patency of the biliary tree can be established in 80% of patients, approximately 20% will eventually develop secondary graft failure and require re-transplantation. The fact that recurrence of intrahepatic biliary strictures occurs following re-transplantation further suggests that an autoimmune mechanism is important.

Vascular Complications

Hepatic artery thrombosis (HAT) is the most common vascular complication after liver transplantation and generally occurs early after OLT. If HAT occurs late (>2 months posttransplant), the patient generally develops stricturing and obstruction of the biliary tree with bacteremia, recurrent bacterial cholangitis, and on occasion the development of hepatic abscesses. Several studies have suggested an association with cytomegalovirus infection and/or viral hepatitis and the development of late HAT. Frequently, HAT leads to graft failure and requires re-transplantation.

The second most common vascular complication is portal vein thrombosis. The diagnosis can be difficult, and the presentation is often insidious. Patients can present with increasing ascites or recurrent variceal bleeding. Patients at risk include those with a preexisting recanalized portal vein thrombosis or previous portocaval shunt and patients in whom an interposition graft was required for the portal vein anastomosis. Compli-

---

Table 76-2. Risk Factors of Nonanastomotic Biliary Strictures

Prolonged cold ischemic time (>12 hours)
Hepatic artery thrombosis (HAT)
ABO-incompatible graft
Chronic rejection
Biliary infection
Recurrent primary sclerosing cholangitis

cations of portal hypertension including bleeding from varices and ascites formation may demand re-transplantation. Hepatic vein thrombosis is an unusual complication post-liver transplantation, except in transplantation for Budd-Chiari syndrome. Such patients should be systemically anticoagulated indefinitely and myeoloproliferative disorders should be excluded.

Acute and Chronic Rejection

Although the frequency of acute cellular rejection is highest in the first 30 days, it can occur any time. Late rejection episodes (>6 weeks posttransplantation) occur infrequently and are often related to reduction in immunosuppression therapy, altered absorption of immunosuppressive drugs caused by gastrointestinal problems or other medications, and/or poor compliance. Typically, late rejection episodes are often associated with a delay in diagnosis and are often more difficult to treat.

Chronic rejection, often referred to as ductopenic rejection, affects approximately 5% of patients and is usually diagnosed six weeks or more after transplantation. The incidence of chronic rejection appears to be decreasing with the advent of more effective immunotherapy such as tacrolimus and mycophenolate mofeteil. Chronic rejection is usually preceded by multiple bouts of acute cellular rejection that are resistant to corticosteroid and/or muromonab-CD3 therapy. With greater than 90% reduction of the bile ducts in portal tracts, the process is often irreversible and unresponsive to additional immunosuppressive therapy and often requires re-transplantation. Unfortunately a high incidence of chronic rejection occurs in patients undergoing re-transplantation for chronic rejection.

Drug-Induced Hepatotoxicity

Drugs commonly associated with hepatotoxicity in the liver transplant recipient include sulfa medications such as Bactrim™ and antibiotics such as erythromycin. Azathioprine (AZA) has also been associated with hepatotoxicity and can present with a mixed hepatocellular-cholestatic picture and has also been associated with a venoocclusive-type disease (see Chapter 22). Frequently, withdrawal of a potentially hepatotoxic drug is indicated with close follow-up of liver function tests. However, in all instances of potential hepatotoxicity, it is important that hepatic allograft rejection be excluded on the basis of hepatic histology.

LATE NONALLOGRAFT COMPLICATIONS
Infectious Complications

The most common opportunistic infections following OLT are viral, which include cytomegalovirus (CMV), Epstein-Barr virus (EBV), and herpesvirus infections.

Despite recent advances in diagnosis and treatment, CMV continues to be a common cause of infection and disease in solid organ transplant recipients. Risk factor analyses have provided important clues to identify those patients at high risk for symptomatic CMV infection. The major risk factors for the development of CMV infection and disease are seronegativity for CMV, treatment with muromonab-CD3 or other antilymphocyte preparations, hepatic artery thrombosis, and re-transplantation. In addition to producing protean clinical manifestations including fever, hepatitis, malaise, arthralgias, and pneumonitis in the first six months after transplantation, CMV infection appears to have an immunosuppressive effect and is a risk factor for superinfection with opportunistic pathogens. Indeed, two recent studies have demonstrated that CMV infection is associated with increased severity of HCV recurrence and graft failure.

EBV infection has been strongly implicated as a cause of a lymphoproliferative syndrome. On the basis of serological testing before and after transplantation, primary reactivated EBV infection occurs in 25% to 50% of liver transplant patients. The incidence is higher in pediatric patients, especially in those who are under two years old. The majority of patients present within the first six months after transplantation. EBV is a B cell lymphotrophic virus capable of inducing proliferative changes that lead to frank lymphomas in 1% to 2% of all patients undergoing liver transplantation. Use of muromonab-CD3, EBV and CMV seronegativity were all demonstrated as important risk factors for the development of posttransplant lymphoproliferative disorders related to Epstein-Barr infection.

Candida is most common post-OLT fungal infection. However, *aspergillosis* and *cryptococcus* are the most severe, and often fatal, fungal infections. Risk factors for the development of fungal infections include antilymphocyte preparations, re-transplantation, previous bacterial infection, long-term antibiotic use, and vascular complications, massive blood transfusions, and prolonged pretransplant hospitalization. Some centers have advocated prophylactic antifungal therapy for such high-risk patients. Regimens using low-dose intravenous amphotericin or intravenous immune globulin have been administered as a means of preventing fungal infection. However, the efficacy of such measures remains to be determined.

TMP/SMX prophylaxis for *Pneumocystis carini*, has been extremely successful. However, allergic reactions and hepatic toxicity have been associated with long-term use of sulfa medications. In such patients, pentamidine inhalation administered monthly for at least one year posttransplantation has been shown to provide adequate prophylaxis. Other prophylactic therapy include vaccination with Pneumovax® and also for hepatitis B, although antibody responses are typically low in cirrhotic patients. While many programs recommend flu vaccination, its efficacy in the liver transplantation recipient has not been established.

De Novo Malignancy

A recent report from the Cincinnati Transplant Tumor Registry demonstrated a disproportionately high incidence of de novo lymphomas in hepatic vs renal transplant recipients. Lymphomas comprise by far the largest group of tumors (57%) following liver transplantation. The shorter interval to the development of these tumors may be a reflection of more intense immunosuppression, including the more frequent use of triple therapy and antilymphocyte preparations as compared with renal allograft recipients. In contrast, a decreased incidence of skin cancers, carcinomas of the cervix, and carcinomas of the vulva and perineum, which typically occur late following organ transplantation, is noted in liver transplant recipients and may reflect the relatively shorter follow-up of liver patients in this study. Patients with inflammatory bowel disease should be advised to have surveillance for colonic dysplasia as carcinoma is not an infrequent development following liver transplantation for PSC.

Renal Complications

Long-term therapy with either cyclosporine (CsA) or tacrolimus is plagued with a significant number of side effects, the most important of which is renal dysfunction. Initial studies, in patients receiving high doses of CsA, suggested that a substantial number of transplant recipients develop progressive renal insufficiency. However, more recent long-term studies have clearly shown that when CsA is administered at doses that maintain whole blood trough levels within low therapeutic ranges, renal function tends to stabilize after the initial deterioration observed in the first few months. Most patients demonstrate stable long-term renal function, even after years of therapy. However, deterioration of renal function, although rare, does occur, and therefore, close monitoring of both CsA and tacrolimus levels, as well as renal function is warranted. The managing physician must also be aware of drugs that may worsen renal impairment by altering CsA or tacrolimus metabolism. Both immunosuppressive agents are metabolized by the cytochrome P450 system. Thus, drugs such as erythromycin and ketoconazole, that can affect the P450 function produce significant renal toxicity. In addition, nephrotoxicity can be potentiated by nephrotoxic agents such as aminoglycosides, aspirin and nonsteroidal antiinflammatory agents.

Hypertension

Hypertension developing after liver transplantation is nearly universal and likely reflects multiple pathogenic mechanisms that include altered vascular reactivity and vasoconstriction related to CsA, and to a lesser extent tacrolimus immunosuppression. Contributing mechanisms are impaired glomerular filtration rate and sodium retention by corticosteroids. Hypertension poses considerable long-term cardiovascular risks for the liver transplant recipients. One series from Mayo Clinic, reported that 75% of patients undergoing liver transplantation developed hypertension within the first two months posttransplant. In the US Multicenter tacrolimus randomized trial, the incidence of documented hypertension in the CsA group was 56% vs 47% in the tacrolimus group. However, relatively few data address optimal treatment of tacrolimus-induced or CsA-induced hypertension.

Selection of antihypertensive therapy must recognize the impairment of glomerular infiltration rate, the vasoconstricted state of the kidney, and the elevated uric acid levels. Further, CsA and tacrolimus impair renal potassium, and hydrogen ion excretion and may induce hyperkalemic metabolic acidosis. Therefore, diuretics are to be used with caution to prevent worsening azotemia and uric acid elevation. Potassium-sparing agents are generally avoided. Angiotensin-converting enzyme inhibitors when used alone have limited efficacy and may aggravate both hyperkalemia and acidosis. Several calcium channel blockers, particularly verapamil, nicardipine, and diltiazem, interfere with CsA removal and, therefore, may lead to significant elevations in CsA levels and worsening of renal function. In some circumstances, this feature of these drugs is used to reduce CsA dosage. However, calcium channel blocking agents are currently a preferred class of drugs for hypertension in the transplant patient. This is related partly to their effect on smooth muscles. It appears that dihydropyridine agents in particular can overcome even intense vasoconstriction produced by endothelin in vitro. Thus, the agents of choice have included nifedipine, isradipine, and felodipine, all of which have virtually no effects on CsA disposition and are potent vasodilators that may allow renal vasodilatation. Labetolol is an equally effective antihypertensive agent. However, approximately 30% of patients on labetolol can develop intolerable levels of edema, headache, and postural intolerance.

Endocrine and Metabolic Complications

DIABETES MELLITUS. Approximately 15% to 18% of patients develop diabetes mellitus that may be related to corticosteroid therapy and the use of CsA or tacrolimus. While neither the European nor US tacrolimus trials showed a marked increase in the frequency of diabetes associated with tacrolimus, the need for less long-term steroid treatment did not translate into an advantage with regard to the incidence of diabetes mellitus. Thus, it is suspected that tacrolimus may be more diabetogenic as compared to CsA. Further studies are needed to confirm such findings in liver recipients.

HYPERLIPIDEMIA. Nearly 40% of liver transplant recipients develop sustained hypercholesterolemia and/or hypertrigyceridemia. after transplantation. The pathophysiology of post-OLT hyperlipidemia is complex, and recent analyses have identified female sex, cholestatic liver disease, greater than three steroid bolus treatments for rejection, and a pre-OLT cholesterol level greater than 141 mg/dL as predictive of posttransplant hyperlipidemia. Whether CsA-based or tacrolimus-based immunosuppressive regimens are linked to different risk levels of hyperlipidemia and therefore atherosclerotic disease post-OLT is not currently known. A preliminary analysis demonstrated that the prevalence of hypertension, hypercholesterolemia, and obesity was less at one year post-OLT in patients treated with tacrolimus, and this difference was unrelated to cumulative steroid dose.

HYPERURICEMIA. Hyperuricemia is also a frequent complication in patients on CsA, particularly in those who are treated with concurrent diuretic therapy for hypertension. One report quoted a 90% increase in uric acid levels in renal transplant recipients who were treated with CsA and diuretic therapy. In this series, 7% of patients developed attacks of gouty arthritis in the posttransplant period. Detailed studies of uric acid metabolism in six patients indicated that CsA caused hyperuricemia by decreasing renal urate clearance. Acute attacks of gouty arthritis should be treated with colchicine. Treatment with allopurinol, particularly in patients on AZA, should be avoided as allopurinol inhibits xanthine oxidase, a major enzyme in AZA metabolism. The combination of these two agents can lead to severe bone marrow suppression.

METABOLIC BONE DISEASE. Osteopenia, with associated bone fractures, is a common source of morbidity in patients with chronic cholestatic liver disease, and is initially augmented by liver transplantation. Risk factors for bone fractures include a history of osteoporosis documented by a bone mineral density level of the lumbar spine that is below the fracture threshold. Other important factors include high-dose corticosteroid therapy in the early posttransplant course and prolonged immobilization after surgery. Most of the bone loss occurs in the first three to four months after surgery. Thereafter, bone mineral density increases and fractures become infrequent. Approximately 80% of PBC patients with bone mineral densities below the fracture threshold experience one or more fractures in the first six months posttransplant.

Currently, totally effective therapy to prevent osteoporotic fractures in the posttransplant course is not available. However, early mobilization, calcium and vitamin D supplementation to maintain 25-hydroxy vitamin D serum levels in the normal range are important in reducing bone loss after liver transplantation.

Neurological Complications

Neurological complications have been reported in between 30% to 50% of all patients undergoing OLT and include mild disorders in levels of alertness to seizures, stroke, and even death. The majority of neurological complications occur within the first two months posttransplantation. Both focal and generalized seizures can be seen and are often related to intravenous administration of either CsA or tacrolimus. Vascular events such as ischemic infarction or hemorrhage can occur after liver transplantation and are most often related to coagulopathy frequently associated with the liver patient. Disorders of white matter are also frequently seen including those related to CsA or tacrolimus and, in the extreme case, central pontine myelinolysis that frequently leads to death.

The most prevalent cause of neurological disorders is related to the neurotoxic effects of medications such as CsA and tacrolimus. In addition to tremor, headache, and seizures, focal and diffuse leukoencephalopathy have been described as a sequelae of the use of both of these calcineurin inhibitors. Other less common side effects described in the literature include complex visual hallucinations, cortical blindness, cerebellar syndrome, and akinetic mutism. Finally, peripheral neuropathy is also commonly seen in the liver transplant patient. The etiology is usually multifactorial but often is related to CsA and tacrolimus administration. In addition, periviral processes including chronic post-infectious demyelinating polyradiculoneuropathy and mononeuropathy multiplex have been reported to be associated with chronic viral syndromes including CMV infection. Central nervous system infections with *Aspergillosis, Candida, Cryptococcus*, and other viral infections (eg, HHV-6) are not rare.

HEALTH MAINTENANCE
Management of Patients by Primary Care Physician

Long-term management of the OLT recipient, as outlined in Table 76-3, requires continuing cooperation and communication between the primary care physician (PCP) and the transplant center. As in nontransplanted individuals, OLT recipients require immunization updates and boosters, screening for malignancy, and management of coronary artery disease risk factors. In addition, frequent monitoring of liver function tests and levels of immunosuppressive medications are required.

Table 76-3. Long-Term Care of OLT Recipient by the PCP
Routine Laboratory Monitoring
Complete blood count, electrolytes, BUN and creatinine, liver function tests, cyclosporine or tacrolimus level
Immunization
If not given prior to OLT, hepatitis B virus and pneumococcal vaccines should be given after OLT.
Patients should receive the current influenza vaccine each Fall.
Dental Prophylaxis
Increased risk of periodontal disease in patients on long-term immunosuppression
Need for dental prophylaxis even for basic cleaning.
Health Maintenance
Common management issues include diabetes mellitus, hypertension, hyperlipidemia (see text).
Flexible sigmoidoscopy recommended every three years, more frequent surveillance with colonoscopy in patients with ulcerative colitis.
Discourage any ethanol use, especially in alcoholic patient. Recidivism should be reported to OLT center and patient encouraged to obtain rehabilitation.
Bone Disease
Accelerated osteoporosis not an infrequent problem post-OLT; bone pain and avascular necrosis also occur. Calcium intake of 1,250 mg daily should be prescribed for all patients.
Contraception
Restoration of normal sexual function usually occurs within few months after OLT.
Post-OLT pregnancies are complicated by high rate of prematurity and low birth weight, and therefore, should be followed as high-risk pregnancies.
Immunosuppressive agents should be continued throughout pregnancies; drug levels often vary because of changes in volume of distribution.
Neurologic/Psychiatric Problems
Chronic headaches and peripheral neurotoxicity (ie, intention tremor) are frequently associated with immunosuppressive drugs. PCP should contact OLT center to discuss lowering dosing of drug or conversion to another immunosuppressive agent.
Seizures usually associated with CNS structural abnormality.
Frequent psychological symptoms include depression, mood swings, nervousness, and difficulty in concentrating.

Table 76-4 outlines common signs, symptoms, and problems that warrant a call to the transplant center. When an unexplained abnormality of liver tests occurs, it is imperative to do a complete workup for causes. Percutaneous liver biopsy can be performed by either the local physician or the transplant center. As the local pathologist may be inexperienced in allograft pathology, the pathological specimen should be reviewed at the transplant center to make appropriate decisions regarding management (eg, recurrent HCV vs rejection). Additionally, many programs prefer to perform interventional biliary tract studies, as therapeutic intervention is often required and immediate access to the transplant team permits more rapid decisions. Any sign of graft failure needs to be attended to immediately by referral to the transplant center.

Parenting After Liver Transplantation

With an increase in long-term survival and restoration of hormonal derangements associated with liver failure, has come the possibility of parenthood after liver transplantation. Issues of concern revolve around the potential teratogenic effects of immunosuppressive drugs during pregnancy. The outcomes of pregnancy have been monitored in the National Transplantation Pregnancy Registry database. To date, outcomes from 48 pregnancies in 34 female liver transplant recipients have been reported. All but two of these recipients were on immunosuppressive medications before, during, and after pregnancy. All recipients were on CsA-based regimens except for two that were on tacrolimus therapy. The mean age of conception was 26.1 years and the mean time interval from transplantation to conception was 2.9 years. Female liver recipients with hypertension before pregnancy had a higher proportion of premature infants than normotensive patients. In the female liver transplant population, acute rejection was diagnosed during six pregnancies, two of which were ended by therapeutic abortion. Four recipients treated with methylprednisolone for rejection continued with their pregnancies and delivered live born infants. Mean birth weights (2,176 grams) and gestational age (35 weeks) were lower in the offspring of the rejection-treated group when compared with the group without rejection. No birth defects or neonatal deaths were reported in the offspring of female liver transplant recipients, although six newborns had complicated courses, including one with a hypoglycemic episode, two with prolonged neonatal jaundice, and three who required ventilatory support.

The outcome of 22 pregnancies fathered by 17 recipients revealed that the incidence of prematurity and low birth weight of newborns is significantly lower than the female liver recipient population and is similar to the general population. Of the four complications reported in male recipient offsprings, one newborn had multiple malformations including a tracheoesophageal fistula, tetralogy of flow, and a cleft palate; one infant had a ventricular septal defect; and one developed pyloric stenosis. A neonatal death was reported in a newborn with respiratory failure without reported associated gross malformations.

In summary, the data from the National Transplantation Pregnancy Registry support the concept that female liver transplant recipients can safely undergo pregnancy and male recipients are able to father pregnancies. The true incidence of malformations in both populations needs further study. It is recognized that female liver transplant recipients have a high rate of premature and low birth weight infants. Therefore, pregnancies in the female population must be considered high-risk and require close monitoring of liver function. Data also suggest that graft dysfunction during pregnancy may represent rejection and must be thoroughly investigated, including the performance of a liver biopsy.

RECOMMENDED READING

Recurrent liver disease after liver transplantation: Diagnosis and management. Liver Transpl Surg. 1997;3(5 Suppl 1):S1-S67.

Summary of National Institute of Health Workshop on Liver Transplantation for Alcoholic Liver Disease. Liver Transpl Surg. 1997;3:197-347.

Gane EJ, Portmann BC, Naoumov NV, et al. Long-term outcome of hepatitis C infection after liver transplantation. N Engl J Med. 1996;334(13):815-820.

Mazzaferro V, Regalia E, Doci R, et al. Liver transplantation for the treatment of small hepatocellular carcinomas in patients with cirrhosis. N Engl J Med. 1996;334(11): 693-699.

Wiesner RH, Therneau TM, Porayko MK, et al. Prognostic models to assist in the timing of liver transplantation. In: Maddrey WC, Sorrell MF, eds. Transplantation of the Liver, 2nd ed. Norwalk, Ct: Appleton & Lange; 1995:123-144.

Zetterman RK, McCashland TM. Long-term follow-up of the orthotopic liver transplantation patient. Sem Liver Dis. 1995;15(2):173-180.

Table 76-4. When to Contact Transplant Center

Fever	Sustained more than 38.5°C for more than 24 hours
	Any fever associated with abdominal pain, severe headache, or other neurologic symptoms
Medications	Recommendations for changes in immunosuppressive regimens, whenever discontinuing or starting new medications
Neurologic	Persistent headaches, visual disturbances, new onset seizures
Metabolic	New onset endocrine disorders
Graft Function	Any acute increase in LFTs or signs of graft failure (increased bilirubin)
Surgery	Before any elective or emergent surgery
Other	Any time questions arise

Ghobrial RM, Colquhoun S, Rosen H, et al. Retransplantation for recurrent hepatitis C following tacrolimus or cyclosporine immunosuppression. Transplant Proc. 1998;30(4):1470-1471.

Rosen HR, Martin P. Hepatitis C infection in patients undergoing liver retransplantation. Transplantation. 1998;66(12):1612-1616.

Rosen HR, Corless CL, Rabkin, J, Chou S. Association of cytomegalovirus genotype and graft rejection after liver transplantation. Transplantation. 1998;66(12):1627-1631.

Rosen HR, Martin P. Liver Transplantation. In: Schiff ER, Maddrey WC, Sorrell MF, eds. Schiff's Disorders of Liver Disease (8th edition); Philadelphia, Pa: Lippincott-Raven Publishers; 1999:1589-1615.

Rosen HR, Madden JP, Martin P. A model to predict survival following liver retransplantation. Hepatology. 1999;29(2):365-369.

77 MAINTENANCE IMMUNOSUPPRESSION FOR LIVER TRANSPLANTATION

Gregory T. Everson, MD

Maintenance immunosuppression is defined as a regimen of stable long-term immunosuppressive medications that successfully prevents allograft rejection. Currently approved drugs used for maintenance immunosuppression induce nonspecific suppression of cellular immunity and are classified into three groups: calcineurin inhibitors (cyclosporine or tacrolimus), corticosteroids, and inhibitors of purine biosynthesis (azathioprine, mycophenolate mofetil). Maintenance immunosuppression is associated with risk of acquisition of certain metabolic disorders, such as hypertension, hypercholesterolemia, obesity, hyperuricemia and diabetes mellitus, and renal failure. Excessive immunosuppression increases the risk of malignancy, particularly lymphoproliferative disease, and opportunistic infections and is associated with more severe manifestations of the metabolic complications mentioned above.

Acute cellular rejection occurs in 30% to 80% of liver allografts and if untreated may lead to graft destruction and loss. Fortunately, current therapy to control cellular rejection is highly effective and immunologic graft loss is an extremely rare event. The degree of immunosuppression varies greatly during the first three posttransplant weeks due to variations in plasma concentrations of immunosuppressive drugs. The occurrence of breakthrough rejection indicates that the patient is not yet on effective maintenance therapy. Acute cellular rejection occurs rarely after the first three months, indicating that maintenance immunosuppressive therapy is effective for most patients. Acute cellular rejection occurring after three months is usually due to inadequate or fluctuating levels of immunosuppression medications or intercurrent illness.

FIRST LINE IMMUNOSUPPRESSIVE THERAPY: CYCLOSPORINE VS TACROLIMUS

Cyclosporine is available in two forms: original (Sandimmune®), and modified (Neoral®, Gengraf®).

Professor of Medicine; Director, Section of Hepatology; Medical Director of Liver Transplantation, University of Colorado School of Medicine, Denver, CO

The absorption of the original cyclosporine from the gut is highly dependent upon micellar solubilization by bile acids. Interruption of the enterohepatic circulation by biliary diversion (T-tubes) necessitates administration of cyclosporine intravenously to ensure adequate levels of immunosuppression. In contrast, use of indwelling internal common duct stents maintains the enterohepatic circulation, facilitating absorption of orally administered cyclosporine. Although absorption is more efficient and reproducible, the modified form of cyclosporine still requires adequate luminal concentrations of bile acids. Maintenance doses of cyclosporine usually range from 50 to 200 mg po bid; dose is adjusted by adherence to target concentrations in plasma (maintenance trough concentrations after three months posttransplant usually range from 150 to 250 ng/mL.

Tacrolimus is a more potent immunosuppressive agent than cyclosporine. Maintenance doses of tacrolimus usually range from 0.5 to 5 mg po bid and trough blood concentrations usually range from 3 to 10 ng/mL. Tacrolimus absorption is not dependent upon bile but the variations in dose requirements are similar to or greater than that observed with cyclosporine.

Two large trials comparing cyclosporine to tacrolimus demonstrated similar patient and graft survivals (Table 77-1). Although steroid-resistant rejection and use of monoclonal antibodies (muromonab-CD3) were significantly higher in cyclosporine-treated groups, the clinical significance of this difference is questionable since patient survival, graft survival, and re-transplantation rate were unaffected. Cyclosporine-treated patients, who also received higher maintenance doses of steroids, had more hirsutism and slightly greater risk of developing hypertension. Tacrolimus-treated patients had more nephrotoxicity, neurotoxicity, hyperglycemia and a greater incidence of diabetes mellitus (Table 77-2). Infection rates were similar. Crossovers from cyclosporine to tacrolimus were usually for treatment of rejection. Crossovers from tacrolimus to cyclosporine were usually for untoward adverse effects of tacrolimus.

Toxicity and metabolic consequences of cyclosporine and tacrolimus are, at least in part, related to the dose used. Attempts to lower immunosuppression to prevent or reduce complications must be balanced by the potential risk of precipitating rejection. Changes in immunosuppressive regimens, new and emerging therapies, practice patterns, pharmaceutical costs, and even definitions of rejection (vs HCV) have complicated the ability to perform adequate, comprehensive, and generally applicable cost-effectiveness comparisons between cyclosporine and tacrolimus.

Table 77-1. Multicenter Trials Comparing the Efficacy of Cyclosporine (CsA) and Tacrolimus (FK) in Hepatic Transplantation

	USA (N=529)				Europe (N=545)		
	CsA	FK	p		CsA	FK	p
Primary Endpoints				%			
Patient Survival	88	88	NS		78	83	NS
Graft Survival	79	82	NS		73	78	NS
Secondary Endpoints*							
Acute Rejection	76	68	<.002		50	41	<.04
Steroid Resistant Rejection†	36	19	<.001		—	—	—
Refractory Rejection‡	15	3	<.001		5	1	<.005
Withdrawal for Drug Toxicity§	5	14	<.001		NA	NA	—
Re-transplantation Rate	8	7	NS		11	8	NS

Abbreviations: p indicates probability value; NS, not significant; NA, not available for analysis.

*Secondary endpoints included rejection, withdrawal for drug toxicity, and rate of re-transplantation.

†The diagnosis of acute rejection required histologic confirmation. Steroid-resistant rejection was histologically-confirmed rejection after a course of pulse/recycle steroids and was treated with muromonab-CD3.

‡Refractory rejection was persistence of rejection despite the above therapy.

§Nephrotoxicity and neurotoxicity accounted for this difference. These toxicities are observed with both cyclosporine and tacrolimus but more frequently with tacrolimus.

Table 77-2. Incidence of Side Effects of Cyclosporine (CsA) and Tacrolimus (FK) from US and European Multicenter Trials

	USA (N=529)				Europe (N=545)		
	CsA	FK	P		CsA	FK	P
Constitutional Symptoms				%			
Fever	56	48	NS		NA	NA	—
Anorexia	24	34	<.01		NA	NA	—
Nausea	37	46	<.05		NA	NA	—
Nephrotoxicity / Hypertension							
Hyperkalemia	26	45	<.001		NA	NA	—
Hypertension	56	47	NS		42	35	<.01
Renal Dysfunction	NA	NA	—		21	31	<.05
Neurotoxicity							—
Headache	60	64	NS		NA	NA	—
Paresthesia	30	40	<.04		15	14	NS
Tremor	46	56	<.04		35	45	<.05
Gastrointestinal							
Diarrhea	47	72	<.001		NA	NA	—
Vomiting	15	27	<.001		NA	NA	—
Hyperglycemia	38	47	NS		20	31	<.05
Diabetes Mellitus	—	—	—		9	15	<.05
Dermatologic							
Alopecia	6	20	<.001		NA	NA	—
Hirsutism	31	7	<.001		9	0	<.05
Rash	19	24	NS		NA	NA	—

Abbreviations: P indicates probability value; NS, not significant; NA, not available.

WITHDRAWAL OF CORTICOSTEROIDS FROM MAINTENANCE IMMUNOSUPPRESSION IN LIVER RECIPIENTS

Corticosteroids are potent medications with global antiinflammatory and immunosuppressive actions (greater inhibition of cellular than humoral immunity). The immune system, however, is not their only target. Nearly every cell in the body expresses receptors for glucocorticoids and is regulated by these potent hormones, accounting for the wide array of side effects and toxicities observed clinically (Table 77-3). Many of these adverse effects are dose-dependent and ultimately limit the use of glucocorticoids as immunosuppressive agents. The discovery of additional, effective immunosuppressants immediately stimulated the development of steroid-sparing or steroid-free protocols. Withdrawal of corticosteroids from immunosuppressive regimens after liver transplantation is desirable to reduce drug toxicity, so long as the new regimen does not precipitate rejection. Concern that patients will experience breakthrough acute cellular rejection has limited the widespread application of steroid withdrawal by the transplant community.

Since 1989 there have been 16 reports of steroid withdrawal in liver transplantation involving 901 patients, 749 adults and 152 children. The average rates of success in withdrawing steroids, without their reinstitution as maintenance immunosuppression, are 93% in adults (N = 749), and 76% in children (N=162). The most common reason for reinstitution of maintenance steroids was exacerbation of underlying autoimmune conditions (ie, autoimmune hepatitis, inflammatory bowel disease). Failure of steroid withdrawal in patients with autoimmune hepatitis correlated with underlying inflammatory bowel disease and HLA-DR52.

ACUTE OR CHRONIC REJECTION AFTER STEROID WITHDRAWAL

Uncontrolled trials have indicated that 5% to 14% of patients on stable chronic immunosuppression experienced acute rejection when steroids were withdrawn. Episodes of rejection were easily controlled by high-dose, pulse steroids or reinstitution of maintenance steroids.

Controlled trials have demonstrated that steroid withdrawal is not associated with an increased risk for rejection. McDiarmid et al, compared acute rejection rates in 17 adults and 13 children undergoing steroid withdrawal, to 17 adults and ten children maintained on steroids. All patients in the trial received cyclosporine and azathioprine and were greater than one year post-OLTx. Seven percent of patients in the withdrawal arm and 7% in the control group experienced acute rejection. The authors concluded that steroid withdrawal did not cause acute rejection. Belli et al, compared acute rejection in 54 adult patients undergoing steroid withdrawal three months posttransplant to 51 patients maintained on steroids in the absence of azathioprine. Acute rejection occurred in 4% of the steroid withdrawal group and 8% of controls. These authors also concluded that steroid withdrawal was not associated with an increased risk of acute rejection.

We withdrew steroids 14 days after transplantation in 71 patients who were treated with mycophenolate mofetil plus either cyclosporine or tacrolimus. The incidence of acute rejection was 46% for cyclosporine+ mycophenolate and 42% for tacrolimus+mycophenolate. There were no cases of refractory rejection and no episodes of immunologic graft loss. We concluded that early withdrawal of steroids, even as soon as 14 days post-OLTx, is not associated with an increased risk of acute rejection.

Two studies examined the risk of chronic ductopenic rejection after steroid withdrawal. Chronic rejec-

Table 77-3. Changes in Metabolic Complications after Liver Transplantation in Response to Steroid Withdrawal

	Prednisone Taper			
	Study 1		Study 2	
	10 → 5 mg/d	*P*	5 → 0 mg/d	*P*
Number of Patients	61		28	
Cholesterol (mg/dL)*	-22	<.005	-19	<.05
Hypertension (%)	-13	<.01	-22	NS
Diabetes (%)	-7	<.01	-8	NS
Obesity (%)	8	NS	11	NS

Abbreviations: P indicates probability value; NS, not significant.
*Prior to steroid withdrawal, hypercholesterolemia was more prevalent in women vs men: 39% vs 23%, p<.06.

tion was observed in 3.9% of patients in Padbury's uncontrolled trial, in which three patients experienced graft loss related to rejection, that resulted in death or need for re-transplantation. In Belli's controlled trial, chronic ductopenic rejection was not observed during a followup of five years in any patient who underwent steroid withdrawal and in only one patient (3%) on maintenance steroids. Given the small sample sizes of these studies and the relatively short duration of followup, it is not possible to be certain that steroid withdrawal is free of risk of chronic rejection.

METABOLIC BENEFITS REAPED BY STEROID WITHDRAWAL

The effect of steroid withdrawal on the incidence of posttransplant metabolic complications was first examined by Padbury. The prevalence of hypertension requiring antihypertensive therapy was only 26%, nearly half that of the approximately 50% prevalence (at two years posttransplant) reported with steroid-containing protocols. There were no new cases of posttransplant diabetes mellitus (compared to 11% to 17% reported from steroid-containing protocols). Six additional studies examined the effects of steroid withdrawal on the posttransplant hypertension, hypercholesterolemia, diabetes mellitus and obesity .

HYPERTENSION

Steroid withdrawal improves management of hypertension as indicated both by a reduction in the mean number of antihypertensive medications per patient and a decrease in systemic blood pressure related to the dose reduction in prednisone. We observed a prevalence of treated hypertension of 30% under cyclosporine and only 12% under tacrolimus in our study of 14 day steroid withdrawal. In Belli's prospective controlled trial, 58% of the group treated with steroids had treated hypertension, after one year of follow-up, compared to only 17% of patients in the group that underwent steroid withdrawal (*P*<.001).

HYPERCHOLESTEROLEMIA

Steroid withdrawal improves cholesterol homeostasis. For example, Stegall et al, demonstrated lowering a decline in serum cholesterol levels as patients were weaned from 10 mg (224 ± 65 mg/dL) to 5 mg (203 ± 66 mg/dL) to 0 mg (188 ± 33 mg/dL) of prednisone. Belli's controlled trial demonstrated mean serum cholesterol levels of 253 + 76 mg/dL and 183 + 81 mg/dL for control and withdrawal groups, respectively, 1.25 yr posttransplant (*P*< .001).

DIABETES MELLITUS

The incidence of posttransplant diabetes mellitus on maintenance steroids was defined in the European trial

comparing tacrolimus to cyclosporine. Hyperglycemia occurred in 31% vs 20% and diabetes in 15% vs 9%, respectively.

Six studies have demonstrated that steroid withdrawal improves posttransplant diabetes mellitus. We examined the effects of steroid withdrawal in nine patients who were diabetic prior to transplantation and another 13 who acquired diabetes posttransplantation (total N = 22). Six of the 22 died within the first year posttransplant. Of the 16 remaining diabetics, nine had hypercholesterolemia and all nine were hypertensive. Seven of these 16 died in subsequent followup. Of the remaining nine, four were removed from insulin but five continued to be insulin-dependent when prednisone was decreased from 10 to 5 mg/day. Three of the remaining five diabetics were able to eliminate insulin when prednisone was decreased from 5 to 0 mg/day. Tchervenkov observed significant reductions in fasting blood glucose with steroid withdrawal and he observed that seven of ten diabetics (70%) were able to discontinue insulin or oral hypoglycemic agents. In one study of early steroid withdrawal it was found that four of eight pretransplant diabetics randomized to cyclosporine treatment were able to discontinue insulin or oral hypoglycemics. There were no new cases of posttransplant diabetes. In contrast, the only diabetic randomized to tacrolimus was unable to discontinue insulin and one additional patient developed posttransplant diabetes in this group. The latter patient was ultimately able to be weaned from insulin on steroid-free maintenance with tacrolimus monotherapy. In Belli's study the prevalence of patients requiring antidiabetic therapy 1.25 year posttransplant was 25% in controls and only 6% in the steroid-withdrawal arm (*P*<.007). Although there are some inconsistencies, the majority of the data supports the notion that steroid withdrawal is associated with reduction in posttransplant diabetes and improvement in diabetic control.

OBESITY

Many patients experience a dramatic improvement in sense of well-being and appetite after successful liver transplantation and become obese. Studies have yielded conflicting results regarding the benefit of steroid withdrawal on weight gain.

MODIFICATION OF MAINTENANCE IMMUNOSUPPRESSION IN PATIENTS WITH CHRONIC RENAL FAILURE

Chronic renal failure occurs in at least 10% of liver transplant recipients within two years of transplantation. In most cases the renal failure is due to either cyclosporine or tacrolimus, although one must exclude urate nephropathy and obstructive uropathy. Renal failure is not systematically improved or worsened by steroid withdrawal per se, but may benefit from regimens that allow reduction in dosing of either cyclosporine or tacrolimus. Ideal regimens remain to be defined but cyclosporine-sparing or tacrolimus-sparing can be achieved by reinstitution of steroids in those previously withdrawn, addition of azathioprine, or use of mycophenolate mofetil or rapamycin. Partial improvement or reversal of the decline in renal function is often observed when cyclosporine or tacrolimus doses are reduced. In some cases, despite further reduction or even elimination of cyclosporine or tacrolimus, renal dysfunction may persist or worsen.

Nonsteroidal antiinflammatory drugs should be avoided. Management consists of: aggressive treatment of hypertension, urologic evaluation to rule out obstructive uropathy, and treatment of hyperuricemia, if present, with allopurinol. Allopurinol is contraindicated in patients on azathioprine, since inhibition of xanthine oxidase impairs the metabolism of azathioprine, raising its serum level, and leading to severe bone marrow suppression.

AZATHIOPRINE FOR MAINTENANCE IMMUNOSUPPRESSION?

Azathioprine has been used in immunosuppressive regimens for liver transplantation for over 30 years. However, there is little or no evidence that it provides any additional benefit over maintenance immunosuppression with cyclosporine or tacrolimus as monotherapy or in combination with prednisone. The current major use for azathioprine posttransplantation is as a prednisone-sparing agent or in the treatment of underlying or associated autoimmune conditions. Side effects of azathioprine include dose-related bone marrow suppression (mainly neutropenia) and idiosyncratic pancreatitis (rare).

MYCOPHENOLATE FOR MAINTENANCE IMMUNOSUPPRESSION?

Recent controlled trials have established the superiority of mycophenolate mofetil over azathioprine in liver transplantation. Use of mycophenolate was associated with a reduction in the rate of allograft rejection, and use of muromonab-CD3. There was no significant difference in side effects between mycophenolate and azathioprine, although renal trials demonstrated dose-related neutropenia, anemia and gastrointestinal distress (eg, nausea, abdominal pain, cramps, diarrhea) with mycophenolate. Mycophenolate may also be useful as either a steroid-sparing, cyclosporine-sparing or tacrolimus-sparing agent. Several centers are exploring the possible use of mycophenolate to reduce or elimi-

nate use of cyclosporine and tacrolimus in patients with neurotoxicity or nephrotoxicity due to calcineurin inhibitors.

RAPAMYCIN FOR MAINTENANCE IMMUNOSUPPRESSION

The role of rapamycin in maintenance immunosuppression after liver transplantation is not yet defined. Limited data from a few centers suggests that rapamycin may be useful for sparing either steroids, cyclosporine, or tacrolimus. Rapamycin exhibits little or no nephrotoxicity but is associated with neutropenia and hyperlipidemia.

COMPLETE WITHDRAWAL OF IMMUNOSUPPRESSION

One series of 95 patients from the University of Pittsburgh suggested that as many as 19% of liver recipients on maintenance therapy may be completely withdrawn from immunosuppressives. However, the period of followup was highly variable, ten months to 4.8 yrs, and the potential long-term consequences of this strategy, such as chronic rejection and immunologic graft loss, were not defined. A recent study examined lymphocyte subpopulations in liver biopsies from patients selected for withdrawal of immunosuppression. Six of 27 patients (22%) were tolerant of withdrawal but there was no long-term followup. Interestingly, the tolerant group was characterized by reduced amounts of CD8+ and CD3+ lymphocytes, suggesting that lymphocyte markers in prewithdrawal liver biopsies may be useful is selecting patients for withdrawal of immunosuppression. Nonetheless, the existing data is inadequate regarding the role of total withdrawal of immunosuppression in liver recipients.

RECOMMENDED READING

Padbury RTA, Gunson BK, Dousset B, et al. Steroid withdrawal from long-term immunosuppression in liver allograft recipients. Transplantation. 1993;55(4):789-794.

Anonymous. A comparison of tacrolimus (FK506) and cyclosporine for immunosuppression in liver transplantation. US Multicenter FK506 Liver Study Group. N Engl J Med. 1994;331(17):1110-1115.

Anonymous. Randomized trial comparing tacrolimus (FK506) and cyclosporin in prevention of liver allograft rejection. European FK506 Multicentre Liver Study Group. The Lancet. 1994;344(8920):423-428.

Sollinger HW. Mycophenolate mofetil for the prevention of acute rejection in primary cadaveric renal allograft recipients. US Renal Transplant Mycophenolate Mofetil Study Group. Transplantation. 1995;60(3):225-232.

Anand AC, Hubscher SG, Gunson BK, McMaster P, Neuberger JM. Timing, significance, and prognosis of late acute liver allograft rejection. Transplantation. 1995;60(10):1098-1103.

Stegall MD, Wachs M, Everson GT, et al. Prednisone withdrawal 14 days after liver transplantation with mycophenolate: a prospective trial of cyclosporine and tacrolimus. Transplantation. 1997;64(12):1755-1760.

Mazariegos GV, Reyes J, Marino IR, et al. Weaning of immunosuppression in liver transplant recipients. Transplantation. 1997;63(2):243-249.

Belli LS, de Carlis L, Rondinara G, et al. Early cyclosporine monotherapy in liver transplantation: a 5-year follow-up of a prospective randomized trial. Hepatology. 1998;27(6):1524-1529.

Wong T, Nouri-Aria KT, Devlin J, Portmann B, Williams R. Tolerance and latent cellular rejection in long-term liver transplant recipients. Hepatology. 1998;28(2):443-449.

Everson GT, Trouillot T, Wachs M, et al. Early steroid withdrawal in liver transplantation is safe and beneficial. Liver Transpl Surg. 1999;5(4 Suppl 1):548-557.

78 EXPECTED CLINICAL OUTCOMES/ RISK FACTORS FOR LIVER TRANSPLANTATION

Kimberly Ann Brown, MD
Dilip Moonka, MD

UNITED NETWORK FOR ORGAN SHARING SURVIVAL DATA

The 1998 Annual Report of the US Scientific Registry of the Transplant Recipients and the Organ Procurement and Transplantation Network documents several demographic factors that influence long-term survival following liver transplantation. Both graft and patient survival have increased steadily from 1988 (Table 78-1). Nevertheless, several recipient and donor factors continue to have an adverse affect on outcome. These include age of donor and recipient at transplantation, and the following recipient factors: race, history of a previous transplant, degree of illness at transplantation, and etiology of liver disease.

RECIPIENT AGE

One-year and 5-year survivals for patients over 65 years are 80% and 58.7%, respectively, which are significantly worse than the results (89.4% and 76.7%) in their 35 to 49 year-old counterparts. The factors that control these differences are unclear. United Network for Organ Sharing (UNOS) data also suggest that survival of very young recipients is lower than for older children, or young adults. One-year and 5-year patient survivals were 81.4% and 74.6%, respectively. Contrary to these

Table 78-1. Percent Graft and Patient Survival Rates

Survival	1 Year	3 Year	5 Year
Graft	79.2%	67.4%	62.0%
Patient	86.9%	78.1%	73.2%

1998 Annual report of the US Scientific Registry of Transplant Recipients and the Organ Procurement and Transplantation Network – Transplant Data: 1988-1997. UNOS, Richmond, VA and the Division of Organ Transplantation, Bureau of Health Resources Development, Health Resources and Services Administration, US Department of Health and Human Services, Bethesda, MD.

Kimberly Ann Brown, MD, Liver Transplantation, Henry Ford Hospital, Detroit, MI

Dilip Monka, MD, Liver Transplantation, Henry Ford Hospital, Detroit, MI

data, Van der Werf reported excellent results in 99 children, with no effect of age shown in recipients younger than six months, compared to children in the six to 12 month, 12 to 24 month, or over two years strata.

DONOR AGE

Livers from older donors (>65 years) have significantly worse 5-year graft (44.6%) and patient (57.9%) survivals when compared to the outcomes in recipients of younger organs. It is likely that older organs are less able to tolerate ischemia.

RECIPIENT RACE

Five-year patient survival among recipients of livers from African-American (69.3%) or Asian (62.2%) donors is less than for Caucasian (73.7%) or Hispanic (76.3%) donors.

Donor and recipient sex affects outcome, with worse outcome being observed in male recipients of female organs.

Patient and graft survival declines with worsening clinical status of the recipient at the time of transplantation. For example, 1-year patient survival varies from 94.4% in recipients not requiring hospitalization, to 76.8% in recipients on life support prior to transplant.

RECIPIENT DIAGNOSIS

The etiology of disease in the recipient influences graft and patient survival. As shown in Table 78-2, chronic cholestatic diseases have the best patient and graft outcome. Graft and patient survival is worst in patients undergoing transplantation on account of intrahepatic malignancy. Recurrence of malignant disease is the main reason for this difference. These data do not reflect the current trend to limit liver transplantation to persons with single or small multiple tumors. Whether protocols designed to limit the spread of malignancy in the perioperative period will alter these statistics remains uncertain.

Hepatitis C virus (HCV) persists in almost all persons who are viremic at the time of transplantation. Five-year survival in liver transplant recipients infected with HCV is similar to unaffected recipients. Nevertheless, the occasional occurrence of a severe cholestatic disorder resulting in graft loss, and the increased fibrosis seen in follow-up biopsies at five years suggests that when adequate numbers are followed for sufficient time, HCV will have a negative impact on patient and graft survival.

The early experience with liver transplantation in persons infected with hepatitis B virus (HBV) was marked by a recurrent aggressive form of HBV and associated graft and patient loss. Chronic administration of hyperimmune gammaglobulin (HBIg) as an immunoprophylactic agent has resulted in markedly improved survival in HBV-infected individuals. However, HBIg does not eliminate HBV, and antivirals such as lamivudine may provide further protection to the graft, albeit at the risk of developing escape mutant forms of HBV.

QUALITY OF LIFE AFTER LIVER TRANSPLANTATION

Belle et al evaluated 346 patients enrolled in the NIH liver transplant database prior to and one year after liver transplantation, using a variety of instruments to assess general well-being, symptom-related distress, and ability to perform physical and social functions. The overall assessment of well-being after transplantation was similar to that in the normal population. The percentage of patients who described themselves as unhappy declined from 50% before transplantation, to 10% after transplantation. Fifteen out of 21 symptoms were improved. The three symptoms that worsened significantly after transplantation were excess appetite, headaches, and poor vision. Sixty-nine percent felt that their medical state did not prevent them from working. Similar data were reported by Gross in a survey of transplant recipients with prior cholestatic liver disease.

Despite these overall encouraging results, specific patient groups may experience less salutary outcomes. Patients with recurrent HCV infection report lower quality of life, greater depression, and less physical functioning than other liver transplant recipients. These data indicate that while liver transplantation provides a clear benefit to patients, there remain significant problems with fatigue, symptoms related to immunosuppressive medications and obstacles to employment.

RECOMMENDED READING

1998 Annual Report of the US Scientific Registry of Transplant Recipients and the Organ Procurement and Transplantation Network – Transplant Data: 1988-1997. UNOS, Richmond, VA and the Division of Organ Transplantation, Bureau of Health Resources Development, Health Resources and Services Administration, US Department of Health and Human Services, Bethesda, MD.

Brooks BK, Levy MF, Jennings LW, et al. Influence of donor and recipient gender on the outcome of liver transplantation. Transplantation. 1996;62(12):1784-1787.

Van der Werf WJ, D'Alessandro AM, Knechtle SJ, et al. Infant pediatric liver transplantation results equal those for older pediatric patients. J Pediatr Surg. 1998;33(1):20-23.

Markmann JF, Gornbein J, Markowitz JS, et al. A simple model to estimate survival after retransplantation of the liver. Transplantation. 1999;67(3):422-430.

Rosen HR, Madden JP, Martin P. A model to predict survival following liver retransplantation. Hepatology. 1999;29(2):365-370.

Table 78-2. One-Year Graft and Patient Survival Rates by Year of Liver Transplantation

	1988	1989	1990	1991	1992	1993	1994	1995	1996
% Graft Survival	68	66.7	71.1	72.2	74.6	76.9	79.1	79.9	78.4
% Patient Survival	81.2	80.0	82.8	81.5	83.6	84.9	87.2	86.8	87.1

1998 Annual report of the US Scientific Registry of Transplant Recipients and the Organ Procurement and Transplantation Network - Transplant Data: 1988-1997. UNOS, Richmond, VA and the Division of Organ Transplantation, Bureau of Health Resources Development, Health Resources and Services Administration, US Department of Health and Human Services, Bethesda, MD.

Table 78-3. Patient Survival Rates after Liver Transplantation According to Primary Diagnosis

Diagnosis	N	One-year Survival	Three-year Survival	Five-year Survival
Noncholestatic Cirrhosis	13293	86.6%	77.5%	71.4%
Cholestatic Cirrhosis	4112	90.8%	84.9%	81.2%
Biliary Atresia	1726	93.8%	85.1%	82.9%
Acute Hepatic Necrosis	1594	79.7%	71.5%	68.9%
Metabolic Disease	1148	90.0%	82.4%	79.5%
Malignant Neoplasms	872	85.6%	48.5%	38.9%

1998 Annual report of the US Scientific Registry of Transplant Recipients and the Organ Procurement and Transplantation Network – Transplant Data: 1988-1997. UNOS, Richmond, VA and the Division of Organ Transplantation, Bureau of Health Resources Development, Health Resources and Services Administration, US Department of Health and Human Services, Bethesda, MD.

Nery JR, Weppler D, Rodriguez M, Ruiz P, Schiff ER, Tzakis AG. Efficacy of lamivudine in controlling hepatitis B virus recurrence after liver transplantation. Transplantation. 1998;65(12):1615-1621.

Charlton M, Seaberg E, Wiesner R, et al. Predictors of patient and graft survival following liver transplantation for hepatitis C. Hepatology. 1998;28(3):823-830.

Penn I. Hepatic transplantation for primary and metastatic cancers of the liver. Surgery. 1991;110(4):726-735.

Mazzaferro V, Regalia E, Doci R, et al. Liver transplantation for the treatment of small hepatocellular carcinomas in patients with cirrhosis. N Engl J Med. 1996;334(11): 693-699.

Belle SH, Porayko MK, Hoofnagle JH, Lake JR, Zetterman RK. Changes in quality of life after liver transplantation among adults. National Institutes of Diabetes and Digestive and Kidney Diseases (NIDDK) Liver Transplantation Database (LTD). Liver Transpl Surg. 1997;3(2):93-104.

Gross CR, Malinchoc M, Kim WR, et al. Quality of life before and after liver transplantation for cholestatic liver disease. Hepatology. 1999;29(2):356-364.

Singh N, Gayowski T, Wagener MM, Marino IR. Quality of life, functional status, and depression in male liver transplant recipients with recurrent viral hepatitis C. Transplantation. 1999;67(1):69-72.

INDICATIONS FOR TRANSPLANTATION

Unlike adults, in whom postnecrotic cirrhosis is the most common indication for orthotopic liver transplantation (OLT), children are transplanted predominantly for cholestatic diseases (eg, biliary atresia) and metabolic disorders. A complete list is provided in Table 79-1.

Biliary Atresia

Occurring approximately in one in 10,000 births, biliary atresia is the most common indication for OLT in children. However, early diagnosis and timely surgical attempts to provide biliary drainage may delay transplantation for several years. Any infant with conjugated hyperbilirubinemia must be aggressively investigated until biliary atresia is unequivocally ruled out. If a biliary drainage procedure is performed after 90 days, the chance of establishing biliary flow is less than 25%; whereas if performed before 60 days, successful biliary drainage may be obtained in up to 90%. However, even with optimal timing of the drainage procedure, about 75% of children will eventually require transplantation. Despite this, it is still recommended to perform the Kasai before OLT if the child is younger than 90 days, as this will afford many children the chance to grow before OLT is indicated. After 90 days, many surgeons do not advocate biliary drainage as the chances of success are very low and the difficulty of the impending transplant surgery will be increased by what is very likely a futile, previous laparotomy. If further surgical attempts to obtain biliary drainage are considered after the Kasai, the transplant center should be advised. Attempts to redo the Kasai are generally ill-advised, unsuccessful, and increase the morbidity of the transplant procedure itself. The risk of perforation posttransplantation increases, which in turn increases both morbidity and mortality.

Metabolic Diseases

Table 79-2 is a comprehensive list of metabolic diseases for which OLT has been considered. The most common

Associate Professor of Pediatrics and Surgery; Director, Pediatric Liver Transplantation, Departments of Pediatrics and Surgery, University of California Los Angeles Medical Center, Los Angeles, CA

are α-1 antitrypsin deficiency, hereditary tyrosinemia, and Wilson's disease.

α-1 antitrypsin deficiency is the indication for OLT in up to 10% of children transplanted and is the most common metabolic disease for which OLT is performed. Cirrhosis with portal hypertension may develop by midchildhood. Following OLT, α-1 antitrypsin levels normalize in the serum, and a phenotypic cure is affected. No cases of emphysema occurring after OLT have been described. Hereditary tyrosinemia may present in infancy as fulminant liver failure, or later in childhood as cirrhosis. This disease is of particular importance because of the early onset of hepatocellular carcinoma: a 37% incidence by age three years. Many centers advocate preemptive transplantation before age two, even if other criteria for end-stage liver disease have not yet been met. Wilson's disease typically presents in the teenage years

Table 79-1. Indications for Liver Transplantation

Cholestatic Liver Disease	Chronic Active Hepatitis/Cirrhosis
Biliary Atresia Paucity Intrahepatic Bile Ducts • syndromic (Alagille's) • nonsyndromic Familial Cholestasis Syndromes Sclerosing Cholangitis	Autoimmune Neonatal hepatitis Chronic hepatitis C, B Cryptogenic cirrhosis
Fulminant Liver Failure	**Malignancy**
Viruses Drugs (eg, acetaminophen, isoniazid) Toxins Metabolic (eg, Wilson's)	Hepatoblastoma Hepatocellular CA Sarcomas Hemangioendothelioma
Metabolic Liver Disease	**Miscellaneous**
α_1-antitrypsin deficiency Wilson's Tyrosinemia Urea cycle defects Glycogen storage disease (I and IV) Crigler Najjar syndrome Neonatal iron storage disease Disorders of Bile Acid Metabolism Hyperoxaluria Type 1 Selected lipid storage diseases, eg, Hematologic disorders • Hemophilia A, B • Protein C deficiency, porphyria • Familial Hypercholesterolemia	Budd-Chiari Trauma Cystic fibrosis Cirrhosis 2° to parental nutrition Caroli's disease

as either fulminant liver failure mandating urgent OLT or chronic liver disease. If cirrhosis with portal hypertension is already established, chelating therapy will not be useful, and OLT should be planned.

In assessing whether OLT is indicated for treatment of metabolic disease, it is essential that it is clearly understood where the defect lies, whether extra-hepatic systems are involved, and what the impact of liver replacement will have on extra-hepatic disease. For example, in the mucopolysaccharidoses, the enzyme deficiency is not confined to the liver. OLT will provide temporary relief of symptoms related to liver dysfunction, but ongoing accumulation of storage material in the central nervous system leads to continued neurologic deterioration. In contrast, the threat of life-threatening kernicterus is completely obviated by successful liver transplantation for Crigler Najjar syndrome.

Ornithine transcarbamylase deficiency, a rare X-linked inherited disorder, deserves special mention as this urea cycle defect, which is almost exclusively con-

Table 79-2. Summary of Metabolic Disease for which Liver Transplantation may be Indicated

Disease	Defect	Inheritance	Comments
α_1-antitrypsin deficiency	↑α_1-antitrypsin serum levels	Codominant	OLT restores -AT serum levels to normal, prevents lung disease
Wilson's Disease	↓biliary copper excretion	Autosomal recessive	OLT improves or reverses neurologic manifestations
Tyrosinemia	Fumarylacetoacetate hydrolase deficiency	Autosomal recessive	OLT for fulminant neonatal form or OLT at about 2 yrs to avoid hepatocellular carcinoma
Urea Cycle Defects	Ornithine transcarbamylase deficiency	X-linked dominant	OLT may be needed in neonatal period to prevent irreversible CNS damage
	Carbamoyl phosphate synthetase deficiency	Autosomal recessive	Variants may present in later childhood
	Arginosuccinate synthetase deficiency	Autosomal recessive	
Galactosemia	Galactose 1 - phosphate uridyl transferase deficiency	Autosomal recessive	May develop cirrhosis and risk of hepatocellular carcinoma
Glycogen Storage Diseases •Type 1A	Glucose 6 phosphatase deficiency	Autosomal recessive	Dietary management alone sometimes successful. Risk of hepatic adenoma
•Type IV	Brancher enzyme deficiency	Autosomal recessive	Cirrhosis often early Amylopectin accumulation liver, heart, muscle may not be completely reversed by OLT.
Familial Hypercholesterolemia Type IIA	LDL receptor deficiency	Autosomal recessive	Early OLT may avoid cardiac atherosclerosis. May need heart and liver TX
Gaucher's Disease	Glucocerebrosidase deficiency	Autosomal recessive	Widespread extrahepatic enzyme defect. OLT alone does not present reaccumulation of storage material. ? OLT combined with BMT
Niemann-Pick Disease	Sphingomyelinase deficiency	Autosomal recessive	
Wolman's Disease	Acid lipase deficiency	Autosomal recessive	
Cholesterol Ester Storage Disease	Acid lipase deficiency	Autosomal recessive	
Crigler Najjar Syndrome Type I	Uridine diphosphate glucuronyl transferase	Autosomal recessive	OLT indicated when outgrows efficacy of phototherapy. Avoid fatal kernicterus
Cystic Fibrosis	Abnormality chloride ion transporter gene	Autosomal recessive	Progressive pulmonary disease and infection limit usefulness of OLT alone
Hyperoxaluria Type I	Alanine glyoxalate aminotransferase deficiency	Autosomal recessive	Combined liver-kidney TX usually indicated
Defects of Mitochondrial Function	Medium and long chain acyl CoA dehydrogenase deficiencies Reye's Syndrome	Autosomal recessive	OLT unlikely to reverse neurologic manifestations
Mucopolysaccharidoses	Lysosomal storage diseases	Autosomal recessive (usual)	OLT alone does not prevent or resolve neurologic sequelae. ? role of BMT
Neonatal Iron Storage Disease	Unknown	Variable	OLT needed in infancy usually
Hemophilia A	Factor VIII deficiency	X-linked	OLT indicated if transfusion-related liver disease also present
Hemophilia B	Factor IX deficiency	X-linked	OLT indicated if transfusion-related liver disease also present
Protein C Deficiency	Low undetectable protein C level	Autosomal recessive	Normal protein C levels post OLT
Disorders of Bile Acid Synthesis (eg Byler's Disease)	Unknown	Variable	OLT only in selected cases with associated end stage liver disease

Abbreviations: OLT indicates orthotopic liver transplantation; TX, transplantation; BMT, bone marrow transplantation

fined to the liver, causes profound central nervous system (CNS) damage in the neonatal period. If the infant can be aggressively supported until OLT is performed (ideally within the first few weeks of life), the infant is effectively cured and can grow and develop normally. Diagnosis within hours of birth is essential.

Fulminant Liver Failure

Other metabolic disease causing a fulminant liver failure presentation in the neonatal period are galactosemia and fructosemia. The latter presents usually after the second or third month of life when fruit sugars are first introduced into the diet, the former within the first few days of life with the institution of milk feedings. Another important cause of severe liver injury in the neonatal period is the poorly understood entity of neonatal iron storage disease. The spectrum of presentation is variable ranging from infants born with hydrops, synthetic function defects, established cirrhosis, and liver failure, to an initially milder form that shows rapid progression to liver failure in the first weeks of life. Chelation therapy with antioxidants has been advocated by some, but in general these profoundly ill infants will require aggressive medical management until transplantation can be performed in the first weeks of life. The diagnosis is made by demonstrating an elevated serum ferritin level, increased transferrin saturation and an increased iron content by magnetic resonance imaging of the liver and other extra-hepatic organs.

The future for correcting some metabolic defects in the liver may well lie with gene therapy. This is particularly true for single enzyme defects localized to the liver such as Crigler-Najjar syndrome and ornithine transcarbamylase deficiency. Another approach has been the use of auxiliary liver transplantation when a partial graft is placed leaving behind a portion of the native liver. The partial graft provides enough enzyme activity to correct the defect. This approach has been successful in Crigler-Nijjar syndrome.

Accounting for 5% to 7% of pediatric liver transplants, the etiology of fulminant liver failure remains unknown in more then 50%. Apart from the usual serologic tests for viral etiologies, in children, particular attention should be paid to the possibility of accidental acetaminophen overdose. The administration of higher than recommended doses on a regular four to six hourly basis over several days may induce fulminant liver failure. Suicidal acetaminophen overdose occurs in the older age group. Early recognition of acetaminophen overdose is essential to allow for the successful use of N-acetylcysteine. Other drugs that have been commonly associated with fulminant liver in children include isoniazid, and valproic acid.

Chronic active hepatitis with cirrhosis, while the most common indication for transplantation in adults, is

relatively less common in children. Included in this category is neonatal hepatitis, a rather nonspecific diagnostic category that should most properly be reserved for neonatal hepatitis secondary to infectious agents acquired in utero such as cytomegalovirus. Autoimmune hepatitis, while typically occurring in school-aged girls, may occur even in early childhood. This entity may also present as fulminant liver failure as a consequence of previously unrecognized compensated chronic liver disease. Chronic hepatitis C and B while less common in the childhood years, may still present in teenagers as chronic liver disease if acquired in the perinatal period.

While malignancy of the liver is less common in children as compared to adults, hepatoblastoma occurring within the first five years of life is the most common primary liver malignancy in children. Metastatic spread is less common than with hepatocellular carcinoma, and many of these children can be successfully transplanted if the disease is unresectable. The expected long-term disease-free survival is approximately 50%. Hepatocellular carcinoma, usually presenting in the teenage years, carries a much worse prognosis.

An increasingly important cause of end-stage liver disease in children is cirrhosis induced by long-term parental nutrition. Many of these children become candidates for combined liver small bowel transplantation. Another disease in which multi-organ transplant may be indicated is cystic fibrosis, where in selected cases consideration is made for combined liver and lung transplantation. Primary oxalosis, while causing end-stage renal disease, will not be cured by kidney transplantation alone as the enzymatic defect resides in the liver. Combined liver and kidney, or preemptive liver transplantation before kidney failure occurs is indicated.

PRETRANSPLANT EVALUATION AND MANAGEMENT

Children awaiting OLT receive the standard evaluation described above for adults. However, there are several areas of special concern.

Nutritional Assessment and Management

The nutritional status of the child pretransplant is of particular importance. The metabolic cost of chronic disease and the added demands of growth must be satisfied by sufficient caloric intake. Poor nutrition is associated with a higher morbidity (eg, increased infection, increased intensive care unit stay, increased ventilator dependence) and mortality. Malnutrition pretransplantation may also affect long-term growth. The infant with biliary atresia is not only the most common candidate found on a pediatric waiting list, but also the candidate with the constellation of factors most likely to cause malnutrition (Table 79-3). These are: (1) cholestasis leading to malabsorption of fat in fat soluble vitamins; (2) anorexia secondary to chronic disease and enlarged abdominal girth; (3) increased catabolic state from intercurrent infection; and (4) peripheral insulin resistance. Protein calorie malnutrition is the consequence and must be recognized and treated early. Nasogastric or nasojejunal feedings with low-fat high MCT-containing formulas may be attempted but are frequently not tolerated secondary to increased intra-abdominal pressure. Early intervention with parenteral nutrition when enteral support fails becomes essential. Not only can a constant source of adequate calories and vitamins be supplied, but the necessary restriction of both water and salt can be easily controlled.

Congenital Anomalies

This is most relevant to the cardiovascular system. Patency of the portal vein should be assessed by ultrasound in all children pre-OLT. Children with biliary atresia have an increased incidence of congenital heart disease, situs inversus, and paraduodenal portal vein. Alagille's syndrome (hypoplasia of the intrahepatic bile ducts) is associated with pulmonary stenosis and occasionally severe cyanotic heart disease (ie, Tetralogy of Fallot). In addition, renal dysfunction characterized by renal tubular acidosis and impairment of glomerular filtration rate is seen in some children with Alagille's syndrome.

Immunizations

Proper and timely immunizations are a cornerstone of child health, but the schedule is frequently interrupted or overlooked in the sick child awaiting liver transplantation.

KILLED VACCINES. The child awaiting liver transplantation can receive all killed vaccines (diphtheria, tetanus toxoid, killed polio, influenza B, hepatitis B, influenza virus vaccine) according to the recommended schedule. Whenever possible, attempts to catch up missed vaccines should be made pretransplant. Par-

---

Table 79-3. Factors Causing Malnutrition Pre-Orthotopic Liver Transplant in Children

- Malabsorption 2° to cholestasis
- Anorexia of chronic disease
- ↓oral intake + vomiting 2° abdominal distension
- ↑catabolic rate 2° to intercurrent infection, complications
- Peripheral insulin resistance
- → ↓gluconeogenesis, ↓protein synthesis
- Low insulin-like growth factor-1 levels
- End-organ resistance to GH, IGF-1

---

ticular attention should be paid to appropriate hepatitis B vaccination and the administration of Pneumovax™ to children under two years old. Hepatitis A vaccine, while not currently a routinely recommended immunization in children, should be given to all children with liver disease either pretransplant or posttransplant. Once available, the newer conjugate pneumococcal vaccine may be particularly beneficial to children both before transplant, when many have splenic dysfunction, or after transplant when immunosuppression contributes to difficulties with recurrent sinusitis and otitis media.

LIVE VACCINES. The common live vaccines are oral polio, varicella, and the measles/mumps/rubella (MMR) vaccine and the new rotavirus vaccine. As live polio vaccine may be excreted in the stool for more than three months, children awaiting OLT should be given killed polio vaccine. The rotavirus vaccine is currently recommended at two, four and six months of age. Children awaiting transplantation should be immunized if possible. However, a four week period after vaccination is required before liver transplantation to allow clearance of the rotavirus from the stool. Varicella and the MMR vaccine are recommended at 12 months of age in normal children. However, in the young child awaiting transplantation, consideration should be given to immunizing earlier, at even nine months, and checking the antibody response, with the option of providing an early booster six to eight weeks later. If possible, administration of these vaccines should be avoided within four weeks of transplant. In children with a living-related donor, careful coordination of vaccination with transplantation is possible. Table 79-4 summarizes recommendations for live and killed vaccine administration.

Psychosocial Evaluation

As the child is completely dependent on his guardian for posttransplant care, an in-depth assessment of the caretakers must be made. In some cases, it may be important to suggest or even mandate as a prerequisite to listing that the child's guardianship is changed. Special support measures may be needed for single parents and families stressed by socioeconomic disadvantage.

POSTOPERATIVE COMPLICATIONS

The most important postoperative complication distinguishing children from adult liver transplant recipients is the higher incidence of hepatic artery thrombosis (HAT).

Hepatic Artery Thrombosis (see also Vascular Complications – Postoperative Care)

Hepatic Artery Thrombosis (HAT) remains the most common cause of graft loss in children and also the

Table 79-4. Vaccinations
Pretransplant
Killed Vaccines • DPT • Polio • Influenza B • Hepatitis A and B Live Vaccines • Oral polio (avoid within six months of OLT) • Varicella (do not give within four weeks of OLT) • MMR (do not give within four weeks of OLT)
Posttransplant (all indicated)
Killed Vaccines • Influenza Vaccines (give yearly) • Pneumovax® (give every five to ten years when over two years old) Live Vaccines (contraindicated) • Give VZG for Varicella exposure • Give IgG for MMR exposure • Substitute killed polio for oral

single most important precipitating factor for Gram-negative septicemia and subsequent death from multiorgan failure and sepsis. The technical challenge posed by the anastomosis of the small caliber of both the recipient and donor vessels is formidable and is the most important factor contributing to the HAT incidence of 10% to 20% in children. The lowest reported incidence of 1.7% is from the Japanese living-related liver transplant experience. After their first experiences, this program advocated the routine use of the operating microscope, underscoring the importance of surgical technique.

In the postoperative period, an essential principle is the maintenance of an adequate blood flow to the graft. Aggressive efforts should be made to avoid any hypotension, and whenever possible, blood pressure should be supported by volume rather than by vasoconstrictor agents. Few other postoperative strategies have any proven success in decreasing the incidence of HAT. Full heparinization, low-dose heparin, antiplatelet therapies (eg, macrodex, aspirin, dipyridamole) are frequently used.

The presentation, diagnosis, and management of HAT, as described elsewhere, is the same in children as in adults. However, the increased risk in children mandates increased vigilance whenever children after OLT develop sudden graft dysfunction or new onset fevers. Fevers associated with HAT may be caused by abscesses within the liver, bile leaks, cholangitis secondary to biliary strictures, or positive blood cultures for enteric organisms.

Diagnosis of HAT

A high clinical suspicion of HAT may prompt an emergency laparotomy. Occasionally patency of the HAT can be restored by reconstruction of the vessel. The duplex ultrasound provides a quickly obtained and useful screening examination, but may be difficult to interpret in children with small arteries. It has been reported that up to one-third of children show patency of the hepatic artery by ultrasound but have occlusion on angiography. This is particularly true beyond the first few postoperative weeks when signals from collateral vessels that have already formed may be misread as the hepatic artery signal. Angiography remains the "gold standard" to diagnose HAT. Interestingly, there is a subgroup of children in which HAT is diagnosed, but whose graft function normalizes. Presumably such grafts are able to establish sufficient collateral blood supply to avoid ischemic injury.

REJECTION

Children are considered to be more immunoresponsive than adults. Absolute numbers of T cells and response to mitogens have both been reported to be increased in pediatric recipients. Under cyclosporine (CsA) immunosuppression, one center reported a 32% incidence of steroid-resistant rejection. The exception may be very young infants, younger than three months, in whom a lower incidence of rejection has been reported consistent with the hypothesis that the immune response is still immature at this young age. As in adults, early clinical suspicion of rejection, confirmed by liver biopsy, is the cornerstone of successful management. Because of the higher incidence of hepatic artery thrombosis and posttransplant lymphoproliferative disease (PTLD) in children, both of which may mimic rejection by causing fever and increases in transaminases and bilirubin, liver biopsy is essential in the accurate diagnosis and management of graft dysfunction in pediatric liver recipients.

IMMUNOSUPPRESSION AFTER PEDIATRIC LIVER TRANSPLANTATION

In general, centers do not differentiate their induction immunosuppression protocol between pediatric and adult recipients. However, the pharmacokinetics of drugs in children may be quite different from adults, but are frequently not well studied during drug development. This is particularly true if the drug is metabolized in the liver. Hepatic enzyme activity is up-regulated in children leading to increased drug clearance. It is, therefore, erroneous to assume that drug doses recommended in adults will be the same in children to achieve similar blood levels. Dosing recommendations in pediatric liver recipients are shown in Table 79-5.

CsA provides a useful example of this principle. In order to maintain a CsA blood level of 250 to 350 ng/mL, stable adult patients usually require about 3 to 5 mg/kg per day, whereas children may require 10 to 100 mg/kg per day. Increased CsA doses in children with a Roux-en-Y may also be related to poor absorption secondary to shortened bowel length.

The therapeutic target range for CsA is not different in children and adults, 300 to 350 ng/mL in the first postoperative month, decreasing to 150 to 200 ng/mL by the end of the first year. However, CsA levels in children may be more unstable than adults. Gastroenteritis with vomiting and diarrhea, so common in pediatric patients, can markedly decrease CsA levels. In addition, outpatient antibiotics are more often prescribed in children and may contain erythromycin, which precipitates toxic cyclosporine levels.

Neoral®, the microemulsion form of oral CsA, holds advantages for pediatric patients who as a group may be defined as "CsA malabsorbers." Neoral® is absorbed more readily and predictably with less dependence on bile. The C max is the higher, and the time to T max shorter. Trough levels more accurately reflect total exposure to the drug as measured by area under the curve.

The use of monoclonal (ie, muromonab-CD3) and polyclonal antibodies (ie, Atgam®) either as induction therapy or to treat steroid-resistant rejection are generally similar in children compared to adults. Pediatric patients may more readily form antimurine antibodies to muromonab-CD3 and require careful monitoring of peripheral blood CD3 counts and possibly muromonab-CD3 serum levels as well. Dose escalation may be needed as a consequence. Muromonab-CD3 for rescue therapy has also been associated with an increased risk of lymphoproliferative disease.

Table 79-5. Doses of Immunusuppressive Drugs in Pediatric Liver Transplantation

Drug	IV mg/kg per day	p.o. mg/kg per day	Levels
Cyclosporine	1 to 5	5 to 20	250 to 350 ng/mL
Tacrolimus	0.05 to 0.1	0.1 to 0.3	5 to 15 ng/mL
Azathioprine	1 to 2	1 to 2	—
Prednisone (maintenance)	—	0.3	—
Muromonab-CD3	2.5 mg if < 30 kg 5.0 if > 30 kg	—	CD3 # < 25-50/mm3
Mycophenolate mofetil	?	? 20-25	—

NEW IMMUNOSUPPRESSIVE AGENTS

Mycophenolate mofetil (MMF) and tacrolimus are the two new immunosuppressive drugs currently in clinical use after OLT in children. To date, only tacrolimus has been studied in a prospective randomized trial in children after liver transplantation. Pediatric recipients treated with tacrolimus compared to CsA-based primary immunosuppression had a lower overall incidence of rejection, a lower incidence of steroid-resistant rejection requiring muromonab-CD3, and a lower cumulative steroid dose over the first year post-transplant. Between the two drug regimens, there was no difference in patient or graft survival and no significant difference in the incidence or severity of adverse reactions, particularly the incidences of nephrotoxicity and neurotoxicity.

Tacrolimus has also been successfully used as rescue treatment for both chronic rejection and acute rejection following muromonab-CD3 therapy. The increased immunosuppressive efficacy of tacrolimus may carry the disadvantage of an increased risk of PTLD. Under CsA-based immunosuppression, children after OLT have a reported historical incidence of PTLD of about 4%. Under tacrolimus primary therapy, the incidence of PTLD is about 8% to 10%, and after tacrolimus rescue therapy may rise as high as 15% to 20%.

The mg/kg per day dose of oral tacrolimus in children may be quite different from adults due to differences in clearance of the drug. The starting dose of 0.5 to 0.1 mg/kg per day orally on postoperative day one reflects the relatively poor cytochrome P450 activity of the new graft. The dose should be adjusted to maintain a level of 12 to 15 ng/mL in the first postoperative month, 10 to 12 ng/mL in months two and three, and 5 to 10 ng/mL thereafter. The dose may need to be aggressively lowered to achieve levels of less than 5 ng/mL in the face of acute nephrotoxicity, neurotoxicity, systemic infection, cytomegalovirus (CMV) disease, primary Epstein-Barr virus (EBV) infection, or PTLD.

Intravenous tacrolimus has been associated with increased toxicity and is not recommended or required in the early postoperative period. The exception is those children with combined liver and small bowel transplantation in whom a short period of intravenous tacrolimus is required until the transplanted intestine regains adequate absorptive function. Therapeutic levels can be easily achieved with oral tacrolimus even in children with short bowel syndrome, diarrhea, or ileus. The current capsule formulation of tacrolimus is problematic in children. The recently available 0.5 mg capsule is particularly useful for children requiring small doses. Tacrolimus is not able to be formulated as an oral solution. Stability for an oral suspension of tacrolimus has been shown and many pharmacies formulate tacrolimus suspensions, usually at a concentration of 0.5 mg/mL. Failing this, on a dose by dose basis, parents can open the tacrolimus capsule, suspend the contents in saline and draw up the appropriate volume by syringe to be placed directly either in an NG or per os.

MMF, an antipurine with no nephrotoxicity or neurotoxicity, is most often used in conjunction with CsA or FK and may allow lower doses with less toxicity of these two agents, and perhaps a lower incidence of rejection. The most commonly-observed side effects are gastrointestinal.

STEROID WITHDRAWAL

The potential for a detrimental long-term effect of steroid use on growth is particularly concerning in children. All induction regimens children currently used include steroids, although rapid weaning to 0.3 to 0.5 mg/kg per day after the first postoperative week is common. Successful steroid withdrawal under CsA-based immunosuppression is now more often being reported, even as early as three months after transplantation. In a randomized prospective trial, children more than one year posttransplant and without a history of recurrent or severe rejection had no increased rate of rejection after steroid withdrawal. One of the early reported advantages of tacrolimus was early steroid withdrawal in up to 90% of children. This early experience has been confirmed by others. Steroid withdrawal at least by one year post-OLT should now be considered standard care in children after OLT. The possible exceptions are children with autoimmune liver disease and those with multiple or late rejection episodes. Long-term effects on growth and lipid profiles remain to be determined.

LATE COMPLICATIONS IN CHILDREN AFTER LIVER TRANSPLANTATION
Renal Dysfunction

The long-term effect on renal function of CsA and tacrolimus (both equally nephrotoxic) remains unknown. It is well documented that glomerular filtration rate (GFR) falls by as much as 50% after one month of CsA or tacrolimus exposure and remains depressed at a similar level throughout the next one to two years. Renal dysfunction is responsive to lowering of levels early after transplantation, but attempts to manipulate dosing levels in the long-term appear to have little effect on established renal impairment. Of debate is whether there is a slowly progressive loss of renal function. In one pediatric study, children after OLT continued to show a gradual fall-off in GFR beyond one year. If this is validated, a slowly declining GFR over potentially decades of exposure to CsA or tacrolimus in children transplanted at a young age may eventually result in clinically apparent renal failure. Particularly in children, simply following the serum creatinine is a poor predictor of GFR and may not be sufficient to appreciate the degree of renal impairment. Failure to recognize a low GFR may have serious practical implications during the concomitant use of other drugs. Renal failure may be precipitated by a supervening acute dehydrating illness.

Infection

The most serious infectious complication distinguishing children from adults occurring after the first six months is EBV-associated PTLD. The two most important risk factors, young age and primary EBV infection in the early posttransplant period, are common to many children undergoing OLT. Contributing to the risk are increased levels of immunosuppression as a consequence of rejection therapy, the use of older donors (eg, living-related, reduced-size), and newer more potent immunosuppressive drugs.

Apart from the increased incidence of PTLD in children compared to adults, PTLD has several other distinctive features in this age group. Early recognition of a primary EBV infection with subsequent lowering of immunosuppression may help prevent the development of PTLD. Although primary EBV may be asymptomatic, clinical suspicion should be raised during any febrile illness with associated lymphadenopathy, even if subtle, particularly in patients known to be previously EBV seronegative. Aggressive attempts to make an early diagnosis either by the demonstration of EBV antigens (eg, EBER-1) by PCR in the peripheral blood or on tissue samples are essential to allow early lowering of immunosuppression. Seroconversion is usually a later event and is an unreliable marker for infection as immunosuppression may not mount an adequate antibody response. With timely management, the primary EBV infection may regress. However, later progression to PTLD must always be suspected.

New approaches to the prevention of PTLD include a combination of preemptive therapy with antiviral agents such as ganciclovir, or the use of high titre EBV antibody preparations (eg, Cytogam®), combined with serial monitoring of peripheral blood lymphocytes for EBV virus by quantitative PCR techniques. At the first evidence of a rising EBV PCR immunosuppression should be reduced. Such strategies appear to be reducing the incidence of progression of primary infection to EBV disease or PTLD.

PTLD has protean manifestations in children (Table 79-6). Common sites are the lymph nodes, GI tract, CNS, and upper respiratory tract lymphoid tissue. Children may present with fever of unknown origin, anorexia, lymphadenopathy, abdominal pain, diarrhea or bowel obstruction, GI blood loss, seizures, headaches, upper airway obstruction, and failure to thrive. A high index of clinical suspicion is necessary in order to implement early treatment. The principles of treatment in children are the same as in adults. With early diagnosis, more than half of children with PTLD will show regression.

Other more common infections in childhood that can be problematic in the posttransplant period include varicella, which is treated with intravenous acyclovir to avoid systematic dissemination, a high incidence of recurrent sinusitis, and the more recent association of herpes 6 virus with roseola. Herpes virus 6 and the varicella virus may infect the liver and cause hepatitis.

Hyperlipidemia

Usually confined to studies of adult populations, it has been recently appreciated that children after OLT frequently have elevated serum cholesterol and triglyceride levels. In one study, 50% of children were above the 50th percentile, and 20% were above the 90th percentile. Steroids and CsA have both been implicated and adversely affect liver metabolism. Interestingly, children treated with FK after one year had substantially lower mean serum cholesterol than the CsA-treated control group. Awareness of the problem, monitoring, dietary and exercise advice, and possible steroid withdrawal are important long-term strategies to obviate a more serious problem arising in adulthood.

GROWTH AFTER PEDIATRIC LIVER TRANSPLANTATION

Growth after liver transplantation, even with a normally functioning liver allograft, may be impaired. The single most important factor impairing posttransplant growth is poor nutritional status and growth failure pretransplantation. In the pre-OLT period, chronic liver disease may affect normal growth primarily by inducing malnutrition. Cholestasis itself leads to fat malabsorption and deficiencies of fat-soluble vitamins (ie, A, D, E, and K). Chronic liver disease with superimposed complications

---

Table 79-6. Manifestations of Lymphoproliferative Disease in Children

- Fewer of unknown origin
- Upper airway obstruction
- Tracheitis
- Abdominal mass
- Mediastinal mass
- CNS – seizures, vomiting
- GI – ulcers, diarrhea, bleeding, mass, obstruction
- Diffuse pulmonary spread
- Hepatitis
- Splenomegaly

---

such as sepsis both increases the catabolic rate, as well as induces anorexia causing further negative caloric balance. The enlarged abdominal girth so often seen with accumulated ascites may lead to early satiety and vomiting. In addition, the diseased liver may develop peripheral insulin resistance.

Other factors that adversely influence posttransplant growth are high steroid doses and poor graft function. The pretransplant diagnosis can also affect growth. Alagille's syndrome and some of the cholestatic syndromes of infancy are associated with constitutional short stature. Whereas some catch-up growth may be seen with correction of the liver disease, these children generally remain below the 5th percentile for height. A recent study of overall growth in a large population of children undergoing liver transplantation showed that over five years of follow-up for the population as a whole, the height Z score pretransplant of -1.72 (4th percentile) did not significantly improve at five years posttransplant (Z score -1.4).

In general, children younger than two with the diagnosis of biliary atresia, and those children with the most growth delay at the time of transplant, showed the best posttransplant growth.

Perturbations of growth hormones and insulin-like growth factor (IGF) are not yet well understood after liver transplantation in children. There have been reports of depressed IGF I levels, but little experience has been reported describing the role of growth hormone in the posttransplant period.

DEVELOPMENT AND SCHOOL PERFORMANCE

After successful liver transplantation, children generally return to a full and active life. Gross motor development may be impaired pretransplant, and a catch-up period in physical skills is often seen. However, in the few studies of cognitive function and school performance in children post-OLT, it is clear that many children are functioning below average. In one study, 30% had either repeated a grade or needed special education services. Nonverbal intelligence tests and academic achievement were significantly impaired in comparison to age-matched children with cystic fibrosis. There is also an unexplained higher incidence of enuresis in post-OLT children. The most significant factor that correlates with impaired intellectual function is chronic liver dysfunction in the first year of life. As biliary atresia commonly is associated with pronounced liver impairment before the first birthday, these children are at particular risk and in need of further study to understand their long-term potential for cognitive function.

TEENAGE ISSUES

Noncompliance is the most important problem impacting liver function in the teenaged OLT recipient. Denial, depression, and surreptitious avoidance of medication may go unrecognized by parents and physicians alike unless increased vigilance is maintained. More frequent visits and monitoring of immunosuppressive levels may be needed. In addition, drug and alcohol use, contraceptive practices, pregnancy, and fertility issues should be preemptively discussed with teens and their parents.

RECOMMENDED READING

Whitington PF, Balistreri WF. Liver transplantation in pediatrics: indications, contraindications, and pretransplant management. J Pediatr. 1991;118(2):169–177.

Malatack JJ, Schaid DJ, Urbach AH, et al. Choosing a pediatric recipient for orthotopic liver transplantation. J Pediatr. 1987;111(4):479–489.

Moukarzel AA, Najm I, Vargas JV, McDiarmid SV, Busuttil RW, Ament ME. Effect of nutritional status on outcome of orthotopic liver transplantation in pediatric patients. Transplant Proc. 1990;22(4):1560–1563.

Shepherd RW, Chin SE, Cleghorn GJ, et al. Malnutrition in children with chronic liver disease accepted for liver transplantation: clinical profile and effect on outcome. J Paediatrics Child Health. 1991;27(5):295–299.

Kaufman SS, Murray ND, Wood RP, Shaw BW, Vanderhoof JA. Nutritional support for the infant with extrahepatic biliary atresia. J Pediatr. 1987;110(5):679–686.

Goss JA, Shackleton CR, Swenson K, et al. Orthotopic liver transplantation for congenital biliary atresia. Ann Surg. 1996;214(3):276-287.

McDiarmid SV. Risk factors and outcomes after pediatric liver transplantation. Liver Transpl Surg. 1996;2(5 Suppl 1):44-56.

Goss JA, Yersiz H, Shackelton CR, et al. In situ splitting of the cadaveric liver for transplantation. Transplantation. 1997;64(6):871-877.

Goyet JD, Hausleithner V, Reding R, Lerut J, Janssen M, Otte JB. Impact of innovative techniques on the waiting list and results in pediatric liver transplantation. Transplantation. 1993;56(5):1130–1136.

McDiarmid SV. The liver and metabolic diseases of childhood. Liver Transpl Surg. 1998;4(5 Suppl 1):S34-S50.

Goss JA, Shackleton CR, Maggard M, et al. Liver transplantation for fulminant hepatic failure in the pediatric patient. Arch Surg. 1998;133(8):839-846.

Woodle ES, Millis JM, So SK, et al. Liver transplantation in the first three months of life. Transplantation. 1998;66(5):606-609.

Reding R, de Goyet J de V, Delbeke I, et al. Pediatric liver transplantation with cadaveric or living related donors: comparative results in 90 elective recipients of primary grafts. J Pediatr. 1999;134(3):280-286.

Goss JA, Shackleton CR, McDiarmid SV, et al. Long-term results of pediatric liver transplantation: an analysis of 569 transplants. Ann Surg. 1998;28(3):411-20.

McDiarmid SV, Busuttil RW, Terasaki P, Vargas JV, Ament ME. OKT3 treatment of steroid-resistant rejection in pediatric liver transplant recipients. J Pediatr Gastroenterol Nutr. 1992;14(1):86–91.

McDiarmid SV. The use of tacrolimus in pediatric liver transplantation. J Pediatr Gastroenterol Nutr. 1998;26(1):90-102.

Ho M, Jaffe R, Miller G, et al. The frequency of Epstein-Barr virus infection and associated lymphoproliferative syndrome after transplantation and its manifestations in children. Transplantation. 1988;45(4):719–727.

McDiarmid SV, Jordan S, Kim GS, et al. Prevention and preemptive therapy of posttransplant lymphoproliferative disease in pediatric liver recipients. Transplantation. 1998;66(12):1604-1611.

Newell KA, Alonso EM, Whitington PF, et al. Posttransplant lymphoproliferative disease in pediatric liver transplantation. Interplay between primary Epstein-Barr virus infection and immunosuppression. Transplantation. 1996;62(3):370-375.

Cao S, Cox K, Esquivel CO, et al. Posttransplant lymphoproliferative disorders and gastrointestinal manifestations of Epstein-Barr virus infection in children following liver transplantation. Transplantation. 1998;66(7):851-856.

McDiarmid SV, Ettenger RB, Hawkins RA, et al. The impairment of true glomerular filtration rate in long-term cyclosporine-treated pediatric allograft recipients. Transplantation. 1990;49(1):81–85.

McDiarmid SV, Gornbein JA, Fortunat M, et al. Serum lipid abnormalities in pediatric liver transplant patients. Transplantation. 1992;53(1):109–115.

McDiarmid SV, Gornbein JA, DeSilva PJ, et al. Factors affecting growth after pediatric liver transplantation. Transplantation,.1999;67(3):404-411.

Sudan DL, Shaw BW Jr, Langnas AN. Causes of late mortality in pediatric liver transplant recipients. Ann Surg. 1998;227(2):289-295.

Stewart SM, Hiltebeitel C, Nici J, Waller DA, Uauy R, Andrews W. Neuropsychological outcome of pediatric liver transplantation. Pediatrics. 1991;87(3):367–376.

Tornqvist J, Van Broeck N, Finkeenauer C, et al. Long-term psychosocial adjustment following pediatric liver transplantation. Pediatr Transplant. 1999;3(2):115-125.

80 CLINICAL INTESTINAL TRANSPLANTATION: RECENT ADVANCES AND FUTURE CONSIDERATION

Kareem Abu-Elmagd, MD, PhD, FACS
Jorge Reyes, MD, FACS
John J. Fung, MD, PhD, FACS

Intestinal transplantation can be a lifesaving procedure for patients with irreversible intestinal failure who no longer can be maintained on total parenteral nutrition (TPN). Although satisfactory results with this procedure have been achieved, further improvements in survival and cost-effectiveness could be achieved with earlier patient referral, proper candidate selection, better understanding of the graft neuroenteric functions, and new management strategies to overcome some of the immunologic and biologic barriers that currently challenge intestinal transplant physicians.

The purpose of this chapter is to outline current indications for, describe new technical modifications of, and highlight recent advances in the perioperative management of intestinal transplantation.

GASTROINTESTINAL FAILURE

Failure of the gastrointestinal system is defined as the inability to maintain nutrition or adequate fluid and electrolyte balance without special support, due to impairment of the primary enteric digestive, absorptive, neuroendocrine, and motor functions. Surgical removal or congenital absence of a significant length of the intestine (ie, short gut syndrome) are common causes of gastrointestinal insufficiency. The irreversibility of intestinal failure should be declared only after failure of currently available pharmacologic and surgical therapies that may augment the adaptation process and/or treat the primary disease. Resection of over 80% of the small bowel along with most

Kareem Abu-Elmagd, MD, PhD, FACS, Professor of Surgery; Director, Intestinal Rehabilitation and Transplantation Center, University of Pittsburgh, Thomas E. Starzl Transplantation Institute, Pittsburgh, PA

Jorge Reyes, MD, FACS, Professor of Surgery; Director of Pediatric Transplant Program, University of Pittsburgh, Thomas E. Starzl Transplantation Institute, Pittsburgh, PA

John J. Fung, MD, PhD, FACS, Professor of Surgery; Chief, Division of Transplantation Surgery, University of Pittsburgh, Thomas E. Starzl Transplantation Institute, Pittsburgh, PA

of the colon and the ileocecal valve is usually associated with failure of the adaptive process and development of permanent intestinal failure. Functional failure of the gastrointestinal system results from defects of either the enterocyte function or the neuromuscular enteric activity. Microvillus inclusion disease is an example of enterocyte failure, and hollow visceral myopathy and/or neuropathy are examples of gut motility disorders.

The following diseases may cause intestinal failure and are specific indications for intestinal transplant: (1) short gut syndrome: necrotizing enterocolitis, intestinal atresia, midgut volvulus, gastroschisis, trauma, Crohn's disease, surgical adhesions, gardener's syndrome, desmoid tumor, and mesenteric vascular thrombosis; (2) intestinal dysmotility syndrome: hollow visceral myopathy, neuropathy, and total intestinal aganglionosis; (3) enterocyte failure: microvillus inclusion disease, selective autoimmune enteropathy, radiation enteritis, inflammatory bowel disease, and intestinal polyposis.

Since its introduction in 1968, TPN has been a lifesaving treatment for patients with temporary or permanent intestinal failure. Despite the reported high survival rate, most patients do not escape the potential risks of TPN with a therapy-related mortality rate of 7% to 28%. Among the life-threatening complications is the development of cholestatic liver failure, which is more common (30% to 40%) among the pediatric population. Central venous thrombosis, pulmonary embolism and metabolic and trace element disorders are other common morbid events associated with TPN. Equally important are the limited social and personal activities and the overwhelming incidence of psychiatric disturbances and narcotic dependence. Finally, the increasing cost of TPN per patient per year (>$150,000) is a major financial burden at both personal and national levels.

INDICATIONS FOR TRANSPLANTATION

Patients with chronic intestinal failure are candidates for intestinal transplant either alone, combined with liver or as part of a multivisceral graft depending upon the functional status of their liver and other residual abdominal viscera. The currently recommended indications for each of the above including the inclusion and exclusion criteria, are discussed herein.

Isolated Intestinal Transplant

This procedure should be considered for patients with irreversible intestinal failure who no longer can be safely maintained on TPN. Irreversibility is usually declared after failure of the currently available medical and surgical treatments to enhance the three different phases of intestinal adaptation and gut functions. Isolated intestinal transplant is the only available rescue therapy to TPN patients with impending liver failure, vanishing central venous access, multiple line/systemic infections, and frequent episodes of severe dehydration despite intravenous fluid supplementation. The procedure is also of great therapeutic benefit for patients with premalignant intestinal polyposis, and/or locally aggressive mesenteric desmoid tumor. Contraindications, either relative or absolute, include significant cardiopulmonary insufficiency, incurable malignancy, persistent intra-abdominal/systemic infections, and immune deficiency syndromes.

Combined Liver-Intestinal Transplant

This operation is a life-saving treatment for patients with irreversible failure of both organs. The need for hepatic replacement is usually determined by the severity of hepatocellular dysfunction and histopathologic evidence of irreversible liver damage. Most patients have irreversible intestinal failure first and subsequently develop liver failure from TPN-related cholestasis. The procedure should also be considered for patients with liver failure and concomitant thrombosis of the portomesenteric system. Patients with an inherited hypercoagulable state and short gut syndrome due to isolated mesenteric vascular thrombosis and without liver failure should be considered for isolated intestinal transplant with lifelong anticoagulant therapy.

The inclusion criteria include documented end-stage hepatic disease associated with refractory ascites, spontaneous bacterial peritonitis, refractory variceal bleeding, chronic encephalopathy, hepatorenal syndrome, failure to thrive, and a severe compromise in the quality of life. The relative and absolute contraindications are similar to those previously mentioned for the isolated intestine.

Multivisceral Transplant

With full multivisceral transplantation, the stomach, duodenum, and pancreas are transplanted en bloc with the intestine and liver. The procedure can be modified, according to patient need, to contain all of these organs with exclusion of the liver. This operation is quite different from the originally described cluster procedure since the latter includes only the pancreas and duodenum in continuity with the liver. Full or modified multivisceral transplant is the only available treatment for patients with irreversible failure of their abdominal visceral organs including the small bowel. It is indicated for symptomatic extensive thrombosis of the splanchnic vascular system, massive gastrointestinal polyposis or other premalignant neoplasms, and generalized hollow visceral myopathy/neuropathy.

PRETRANSPLANT EVALUATION

The evaluation process must be designed to establish and assess: (1) etiology and extent of gastrointestinal failure; (2) other intra-abdominal and extra-abdominal organ involvement due to the primary disease or long-term use of TPN; and (3) systemic risk factors. Assessment of the etiology, extent, and severity of the primary disease is essential in every case. Of great importance is full evaluation of gastrointestinal functions and nutritional status of the patient. This should include a thorough clinical history, anthropometric measures, and other biochemical and metabolic indices. However, the best practical method to assess the functional capacity and reserve of the gastrointestinal tract is the outcome of several TPN weaning attempts with pharmacologic manipulation of the enterocytes.

The evaluation process is usually guided by the etiology of intestinal failure and clinical manifestations of extra-intestinal diseases. For patients with primary enterocyte disease, full radiologic, endoscopic, and pathologic examination of the residual gastrointestinal tract is essential. Patients with pseudo-obstruction syndrome should undergo esophagogastric and colorectal motility studies to define the type and extent of their disease. Candidates with thrombotic disorders require tests to identify the underlying hypercoagulable state and abdominal visceral angiography to assess patency of the splanchnic vascular system. The hematologic studies should include measurement of protein C, S, and antithrombin III serum levels, lupus anticoagulant, anticardiolipin antibodies and factor II/V mutations. In these and other high-risk patients, imaging of the upper and lower extremity central veins is essential to determine if there will be adequate venous access at the time of surgery. Desmoid tumors should be assessed with one of the newly developed imaging techniques to define the extent of the lesion and its relationship to the adjacent vital structures.

Assessment of hepatic function is the single most important factor in determining the type of intestinal graft required. Patients with biochemical evidence of hepatic injury should undergo percutaneous liver biopsy to assess the extent of liver damage. The abdominal imaging studies are also needed to assess patency of the hepatic vessels and biliary system, degree of portal hypertension, and to identify any concomitant pathology of the solid abdominal organs. The work-up required to assess cardiopulmonary function and other risk factors is usually dictated by patient age, the complexity of medical and surgical history, and nature of the primary disease.

DONOR SELECTION AND MANAGEMENT

A graft of good quality, appropriate size, and proper anatomy is the key to successful intestinal transplantation. Young, hemodynamically stable, and ABO-identical cadaveric donors are preferred. A handful of living-related/identical twin donors have been successfully used, worldwide, for an isolated intestinal transplant. Donors of similar or smaller size to recipients are preferred to compensate for the contracted abdominal cavity because of previous multiple abdominal operations. Because of the current shortage in cadaveric donors, newborn, reduced-sized, and ABO-compatible composite visceral grafts have been used for pediatric recipients. No attempts are being made by most centers to deplete the donor lymphoid mass, using irradiation or antilymphocyte antibodies, or to match donor and recipient HLA. With isolated intestinal transplants, positive lymphocytotoxic crossmatch donors should be avoided, if possible, and cytomegalovirus (CMV) negative recipients should receive CMV negative donors.

Selective gut decontamination should be attempted in all donors. A combination of tobramycin/gentamicin, polymyxin E, and amphotericin B/mycostatin is given through a nasogastric tube once the donor has been accepted and then every six hours if time permits. In addition, standard intravenous antibiotic prophylaxis with cefotaxime and ampicillin is also administered to all donors.

University of Wisconsin (UW) solution is routinely used by all centers for both in situ flushing and cold storage. Flushing is usually achieved through the aortic cannula with 1.5 to 2.5 liters for adults and 50 to 100 cc/kg for pediatric donors. Luminal flushing of the intestine is not required. Cold ischemia time is a major risk factor for survival and should be kept to a minimum. This can be simply achieved by coordinating the timing of the donor and recipient operations.

SURGICAL TECHNIQUES
Donor Operation
The procedure begins with a long midline incision and bilateral subcostal transverse extension to facilitate exposure, dissection, and detachment of the abdominal viscera from the peritoneal reflections. The abdominal organs should be examined thoroughly to evaluate their quality and size and to search for vascular anomalies. A knowledge of the embryonic origin and segmental vascular supply of the different abdominal organs (Figure 80-1) is the key to successful isolated or en bloc retrieval of these organs.

INTESTINE ALONE. After the initial dissection of the hepatic hilus, procurement of the isolated intestinal graft begins. The greater omentum and abdominal colon are dissected and resected using the stapler technique. The duodenum is then kockerized and mobilized until the pedicle of the superior mesenteric vessels is visualized with separation of the root of the mesentery from its retroperitoneal attachments. Next, the proximal jejunum is transected at the duodenojejunal junction after

detaching the ligament of Treitz and dividing the inferior mesenteric vein. To achieve better exposure of the superior mesenteric pedicle, the very proximal jejunal vessels should be divided close to the jejunal wall.

If the pancreas is to be used for another recipient, dissection of the superior mesenteric vessels should be limited to the level of the uncinate process with preservation of the inferior pancreaticoduodenal vascular arcades as recently described (Figure 80-2). If the pancreas is to be sacrificed, the confluence of the superior mesenteric and splenic veins is exposed by transecting the pylorus and neck of the pancreas (Figure 80-3). This step, as well as complete resection of the pancreaticoduodenal segment, can be performed during the back table dissection. Providing there is early control of the aorta, such dissection with intact circulation can be terminated at any time with prompt institution of in situ cooling with essentially no penalty of warm ischemia. Attention should always be paid to the presence of a replaced right hepatic artery that will affect the technique and decision to retrieve both the intestine and pancreas. After the in situ cooling of the subdiaphragmatic organs by aortic infusion of the UW solution and simultaneous exsanguination, the intestine is removed by dividing the superior mesenteric vessels at the site of previous dissection (Figure 80-2). It is important to avoid over perfusion and if the intestine does not feel cold after limited perfusion, this is no cause for concern providing it is blanched. In any event, further surface cooling after immersion in cold UW is rapid because the intestine is a hollow organ. It is essential to obtain a good segment of an arterial and venous graft by harvesting the donor iliac

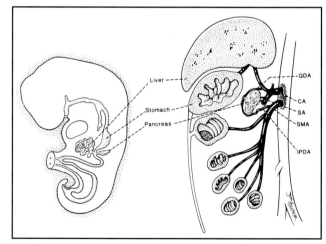

Figure 80-1. The embryonic origin of the liver, pancreas, and alimentary canal. Note the shared axial blood supply and its segmental distribution. CA indicates celiac axis; SMA, superior mesenteric artery; GDA, gastroduodenal artery; SA, splenic artery; IPDA inferior pancreaticoduodenal artery. (From Abu-Elmagd K, Fung J, Bueno J, et al. Logistics and technique for intestinal, pancreatic, and hepatic grafts from the same donor. Ann Surg. 2000;232(5):680-687.

and carotid vessels for vascular reconstruction of the intestine and pancreas as an isolated or en bloc graft (Figure 80-4).

Very little revision of the intestinal graft is needed during the back table procedure. It is preferable to anastomose the vascular conduits for the superior mesenteric vessels to the recipient infrarenal aorta and portal vein or vena cava rather than to the mesenteric vessels on the back table (Figure 80-2). This avoids having to work at close quarters around the bulky visceral allograft.

LIVER PLUS INTESTINE. With combined liver-intestinal retrieval, the initial hilar dissection is eliminated with the exception of assessing the arterial anatomy and flushing the gallbladder without transecting the bile duct. A previously described procurement technique has been recently modified to preserve continuity of the hepatic biliary system with the intestinal graft by harvesting the donor duodenum en bloc with the hepatic-intestinal graft (Figure 80-5). Resection of

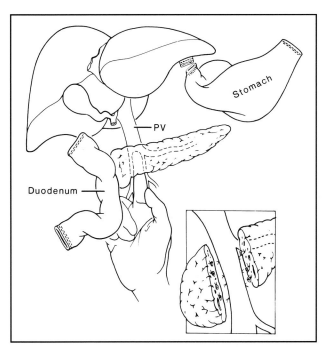

Figure 80-3. Harvesting of the intestinal allograft with transection of the pancreas. PV indicates Portal vein. (From Starzl TE, Todo S, Tzakis A, et al. The many faces of multivisceral transplantation. Surg Gyne Obstet. 1991;172(5):335-344, used by permission).

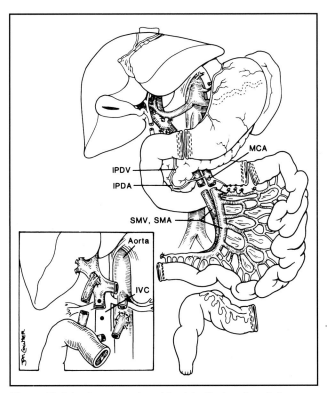

Figure 80-2. In situ separation of the intestinal graft and dissection of the superior mesenteric pedicle. Note preservation of both the inferior pancreaticoduodenal artery (IPDA) and inferior pancreaticoduodenal vein (IPDV) with the pancreatic graft by limiting the dissection of the superior mesenteric vessels below the level of the ligated middle colic artery (MCA). The vascular conduits for the intestinal allograft are anastomosed to the recipient infrarenal aorta and portal vein or inferior vena cava (IVC) rather than to the mesenteric vessels at the back table (insert). (From Abu-Elmagd K, Fung J, Bueno J, et al. Logistics and technique for intestinal, pancreatic, and hepatic grafts from the same donor. Ann Surg. 2000;232(5):680-687.

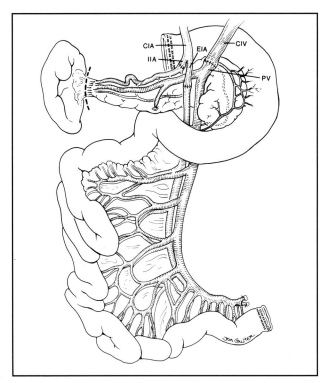

Figure 80-4. Back table vascular reconstruction of the composite intestinal-pancreatic allograft. Note continuity of the pancreas, duodenum and small intestine with intact vascular pedicle. CIA indicates common iliac artery, IIA, internal iliac artery; EIA, external iliac artery; CIV, common iliac vein; portal vein. (From Abu-Elmagd K, Fung J, Bueno J, et al. Logistics and technique for intestinal, pancreatic, and hepatic grafts from the same donor. Ann Surg. 2000;232(5):680-687.

the donor colon and mobilization of the duodenum and root of the mesentery is carried out as described above. No further dissection of the intestine is required and the pylorus is transected using the stapler technique. The next step is to free the spleen and pancreas from their retroperitoneal attachments with medial visceral rotation. Transection of the pancreatic gland to the left of the portal vein can be done at this stage or on the back table after dissecting the splenic vessels from the tail and body of the pancreas. It is essential to preserve the pancreaticoduodenal vascular arcades to maintain viability of the duodenum (Figure 80-5). The left gastric artery is then identified and ligated close to the gastric wall with preservation of the left replaced hepatic artery if present. After in situ perfusion with chilled UW solution is accomplished through the aortic cannula, a Carrel patch is fashioned around the origins of the celiac trunk and superior mesenteric artery and the combined hepatic-intestinal bloc is removed. It is unnecessary to do in situ flushing of the portal system with UW solution through the inferior mesenteric vein.

During the back table dissection, the vena cava margins are prepared as for the isolated liver graft and both the duodenal and pancreatic stumps are oversewn with nonabsorbable sutures. The Carrel patch is revised and sutured to an arterial graft, usually the donor thoracic aorta, as a single vascular conduit to the common origin of the celiac and superior mesenteric trunks. With the rapid en bloc multivisceral harvesting technique, separation of the excess organs during the back table procedure requires proper anatomic orientation and is usually time consuming.

Donor-recipient size mismatch has been a limited factor, in addition to organ shortage, for transplanting children who require composite visceral grafts. To overcome such a barrier, we recently utilized newborn and reduced grafts containing either the right hepatic lobe (Figure 80- 6) or the left lateral hepatic segment in continuity with the intestine (Figure 80-7).

MULTIVISCERAL GRAFT. Retrieval of a multivisceral graft, which usually includes stomach, duodenum, pancreas, intestine, and liver, is an extension of the technique used for multiple abdominal organ procurement. The graft can be modified by excluding the liver (Figure 80-8) or including the kidney (Figure 80-9). The technique used for harvesting a combined liver-intestinal graft is modified for retrieving a full or modi-

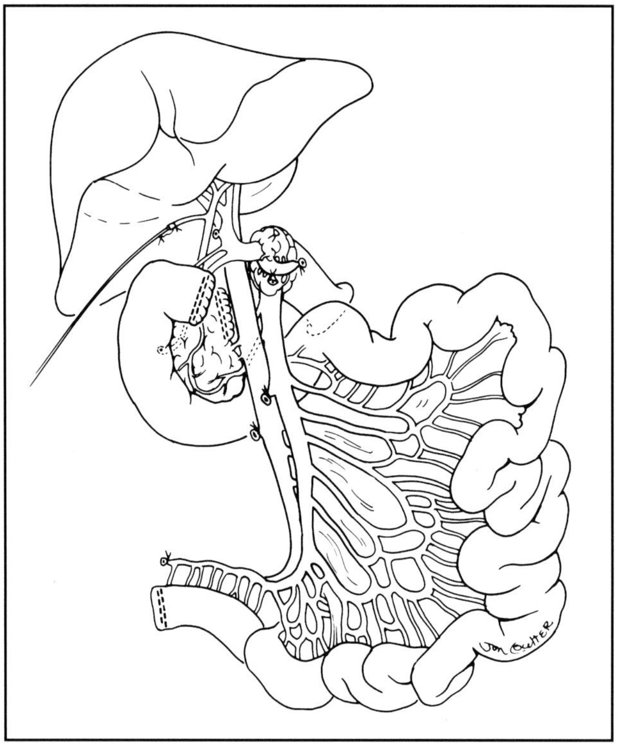

Figure 80-5. Composite liver and intestinal graft with preservation of the duodenum in continuity with the graft jejunum and hepatic biliary system. Note transection of the pancreas to the right of the portal vein with preservation of the pancreatoduodenal arterial and venous arcade. (From Abu-Elmagd K, Reyes J, Todo S, et al. Clinical intestinal transplantation: new perspectives and immunologic considerations. J Am Coll Surg. 1998;186(5):512-527, used by permission).

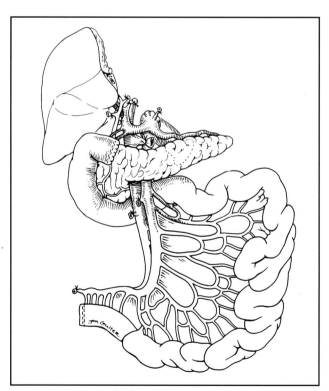

Figure 80-6. Combined liver-intestinal allograft with reduced liver that consists of the right lobe and medial hepatic segment. (From Bueno J, Abu-Elmagd K, Mazariegos G, et al. Composite liver – small bowel allografts with preservation of donor duodenum and hepatic biliary system in children. J Ped Surg. 2000;35(2):291-296, used by permission).

fied multivisceral graft. The gastrohepatic ligament is left intact, but the gallbladder is opened and flushed. The stomach is disconnected from the esophagus by transecting the abdominal esophagus with the stapler technique after division of the greater omentum outside the gastroepiploic arch, resection of the abdominal colon, and ligation, if needed, of the short gastric vessels. The spleen is used as a handle during the in situ dissection and then removed on the back table with ligation of the splenic vessels within the splenic hilus to prevent injury to the tail of the pancreas. The whole abdominal organs are infused with the appropriate volume of UW solution and only through the aortic cannula. The back table procedure is limited to placement of the arterial conduit as with combined liver-intestine, over-sewing the transected gastroesophageal junction, and performing pyloroplasty or pyloromyotomy.

Recipient Operation

The technical steps of implanting the three different types of the intestinal graft start with a generous midline abdominal incision with appropriate unilateral or bilat-

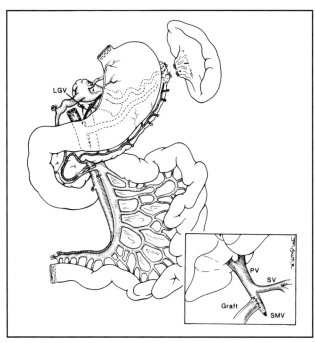

Figure 80-8. Modified multivisceral graft that contains stomach, duodenum, pancreas, and small intestine. Note preservation of the gastroepiploic arcade and left gastric pedicle including the left gastric vein (LGV). Insert, venous drainage of the composite visceral graft to the side of the recipient superior mesenteric vein (SMV) stump by using the donor common iliac vein as extension graft without compromising the recipient portal venous flow during graft implantation.

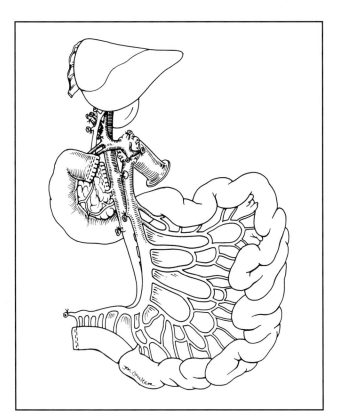

Figure 80-7. Composite liver-intestinal allograft with a reduced liver component that consists of the left lateral hepatic segment. The vascular and biliary structures of the left lateral segment are maintained in continuity with the intestine. (From Bueno J, Abu-Elmagd K, Mazariegos G, et al. Composite liver – small bowel allografts with preservation of donor duodenum and hepatic biliary system in children. J Ped Surg. 2000;35(2):291-296, used by permission).

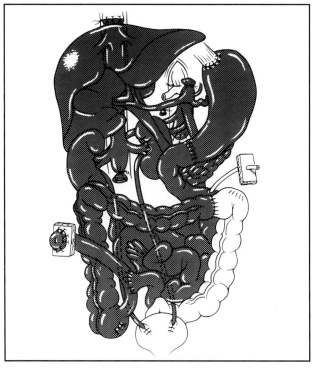

Figure 80-9. Full multivisceral graft with inclusion of the kidney. (From Todo S, Tzakis A, Abu-Elmagd K, et al. Abdominal multivisceral transplantation. Transplantation. 1995;59(2):234-240, used by permission).

eral transverse extensions. The technical challenge in these patients is usually determined by the number of abdominal organs to be replaced, the number of previous abdominal operations, the degree of contracture of the abdominal cavity, the severity of portal hypertension, and the nature of the primary gastrointestinal disease. With combined liver-intestinal transplant, the surgery is more difficult because of the presence of portal hypertension and associated abdominal collaterals. However, the most challenging surgical procedure is the upper abdominal exenteration in patients with thrombosed splanchnic venous system who require multivisceral replacement. In cases with contracted abdominal cavity, small-sized donors and innovative techniques to accommodate the allograft and reconstruct the recipient abdominal wall are needed. Temporary use of synthetic materials and the use of tissue expanders, split thickness grafts, or myocutaneous flaps are valuable options for some patients.

ISOLATED INTESTINAL TRANSPLANT. The most important initial step of the operation is identification and dissection of the recipient infrarenal aorta and a segment of the portomesenteric venous system or infrarenal inferior vena cava for graft revascularization. This usually requires lysis of the abdominal adhesions, kockerization of the duodenum, and careful dissection of the residual intestine. Great attention should be paid to avoid injury of the inferior mesenteric artery and to preserve the residual intestine including the colon, if present. The technique of graft revascularization by anastomosing the conduits to the recipient vessels (Figure 80-2, insert), rather than to the graft mesenteric vessels on the back table, can be used to avoid difficult exposure and possible prolongation of the warm ischemia time. The route of venous drainage of the intestinal graft depends primarily on the technical feasibility of gaining access to the recipient portomesenteric system. Portal venous drainage should always be attempted in patients with caval filters and those with previous splenectomy and inadequate portal venous flow. The systemic caval drainage is used for patients with frozen hepatic hilus, portal vein thrombosis, previous intestinal transplant, and prolonged cold ischemia time.

Reconstruction of gastrointestinal continuity is done using conventional techniques. A vent chimney or simple loop ileostomy is performed to monitor graft rejection and provide easy access for frequent surveillance endoscopy. Surgical closure of these vents is performed 12 to 24 weeks after transplantation guided by the postoperative course and functional recovery of the intestinal graft. One practice is to insert jejunostomy and gastrostomy tubes for postoperative decompression and early enteral feeding.

LIVER-INTESTINAL TRANSPLANT. The phases of hepatic-intestinal transplant are similar to those of isolated liver. The piggyback technique can be used to avoid the venovenous bypass because of the frequent coexistence of upper extremity or central venous stenosis/thrombosis. Equally important is the performance of portocaval shunt during the early phase of the recipient operation to decompress the left portal system and prevent excessive bleeding during dissection and removal of the host organs. The conversion to portoportal shunt after graft reperfusion is not mandatory and should be avoided in cases with a small donor portal vein to eliminate the potential risk of portal vein thrombosis.

The gastrointestinal tract is reconstructed as in isolated intestinal recipients. The newly-adopted technique of combined hepatic-intestinal retrieval with preservation of the duodenum in continuity with the graft jejunum and hepatic biliary system (Figure 80-5) reduces the operative time and avoids the potential complications of biliary reconstruction.

MULTIVISCERAL TRANSPLANT. The operation replaces most of the native gastrointestinal organs en bloc. The graft can be modified according to patient need with exclusion or inclusion of one or more of the abdominal organs including the liver and kidney. Inclusion of the small bowel is essential to consider the graft as multivisceral and differentiates the procedure from the previously described cluster transplantation. The latter includes only liver, pancreas, duodenum, and possibly stomach.

The arterial inflow and venous outflow of the full multivisceral graft are established as in combined liver-intestinal transplant. Total exenteration of the native upper abdominal organs obviously eliminates the need for a portocaval or portoportal shunt. With modified multivisceral transplant, when there is no need for liver replacement or resection of the residual left upper abdominal organs, integrity of the native portomesenteric system can be maintained by draining the graft venous system into the host portal circulation using the piggy-back technique (Figure 80-8).

Continuity of the proximal gastrointestinal tract is established by anastomosing the anterior wall of the donor stomach to the recipient gastric cuff or abdominal esophagus. Reconstruction of the distal gut is established as in isolated intestinal transplant. Because of complete denervation of the donor stomach, a drainage procedure (ie, pyloroplasty or pyloromyotomy) is needed to prevent gastric outlet obstruction. It is optional to temporarily decompress the bile flow with a cannula in the graft common bile duct to minimize the risk of postoperative pancreatitis.

POSTOPERATIVE MANAGEMENT

The difficult task required to manage the three different intestinal transplant recipients stems from the high level of host-graft alloreactivity, the complexity of the graft absorptive and neuroenteric functions, and the high risk of infection because of the heavy bacterial load in the gut. With standard postoperative management being fully described elsewhere in this book, herein the focus will be on the recent advances in the postoperative care of this unique population.

Immunosuppression

The worldwide currently adopted immunosuppression protocol consists primarily of tacrolimus and steroids. Prostaglandin E1 is used intravenously at a dose of 0.6 μg/kg body weight per hour as an adjunct drug therapy during the first postoperative week. Induction therapy with cyclophosphamide or muromonab-CD3 had been previously used by few centers but with unsatisfactory results. Daclizumab, a humanized anti-IL2 receptor antibody, is currently used at the University of Pittsburgh as a prophylactic therapy in an intravenous dose of 1 to 2 mg/kg body weight for a total of five doses. The first dose is usually administered within a few hours before surgery and the remaining four doses were given postoperatively at two, four, six, and eight weeks after transplantation. Azathioprine (100 to 150 mg/day) or mycophenolate mofetil (15 to 30 mg/kg per day) is used from the outset as a third drug in selected patients. A steroid bolus and a five day taper are used to treat rejection episodes along with an increase in the daily tacrolimus dose to achieve higher trough levels. Muromonab-CD3 or thymoglobulin are used to treat steroid-resistant and severe rejection episodes.

In two major intestinal transplant centers, a single (Pittsburgh) or multiple (Miami) doses of unmodified adjunct donor bone marrow cells are currently given perioperatively to the intestinal recipients in order to take advantage of the more tolerogenic profile of bone marrow cells compared to that of the intestinal passenger leukocytes. With informed consent from both donor and recipient families, bone marrow cells are prepared from donor thoraco-lumbar vertebrae and infused at a dose of $3-5 \times 10^8$ cells/kg body weight for 20 minutes during the first 24 hours after revascularization of the intestinal graft.

Host-Graft Alloreactivity

The diagnosis of host vs graft reaction (rejection) is currently achievable with a high index of clinical suspicion and frequent performance of surveillance endoscopic biopsies. The availability of noninvasive, more sensitive, and highly specific tools to detect early intestinal allograft rejection will undoubtedly improve outcome and cost-effectiveness of the procedure. The recent availability of the zoom video endoscopy may help early detection of rejection by a better guidance for random biopsies. However, efforts should be directed toward other biochemical and immunologic serum and tissue markers that can be used to predict or detect the rejection process. Similarly, the early diagnosis of graft-vs-host disease (GVHD) requires a high index of clinical suspicion and availability of a highly advanced immuno-histochemical technology. Prompt adjustment of immunosuppressive therapy with steroid augmentation is usually effective with the early diagnosis of rejection or GVHD. Severe or steroid-resistant rejection episodes are usually treated with a seven to 14 day course of muromonab-CD3 or thymoglobulin.

Graft Functions

The previously adopted measures to assess graft functions, including oral tacrolimus pharmacokinetic studies, D-xylose tolerance test , measurement of serum albumin, fatty acids, vitamin A, D, and E levels, and fecal fat excretion, have been replaced by careful serial clinical, biochemical, and nutritional assessments. Successful complete withdrawal of TPN with establishment of full gastrointestinal nutritional autonomy has been, at the University of Pittsburgh, the most valuable tool in assessing intestinal allograft functions. The neuro-endocrine functions of the residual native and transplanted abdominal viscera have yet to be thoroughly evaluated.

Infections

Protocols for prophylactic and active treatment of viral, bacterial, and fungal infections are adopted from those developed for liver transplantation. In addition, selective gut decontamination is used perioperatively, during severe rejection episodes, and in patients with overt symptoms of bacterial overgrowth. The newly developed technique of quantitative PCR assay of Epstein-Barr virus (EBV) in the peripheral blood is used for early detection and monitoring of EBV viremia, which forewarns of the development of PTLD and initiates pre-emptive antiviral therapy. CMV-specific hyperimmune globulin is used as an adjunct antiviral agent for treatment of CMV and EBV infection in high-risk patients.

The concept of infectious implications of rejection that have been demonstrated with liver transplantation is even more applicable with the intestine because a disrupted mucosal barrier quickly creates a lethal environment for the recipient. The paradoxical therapeutic philosophy of treating infection related to rejection with prompt increase in immunosuppression, in addition to systemic and local antibiotic therapy, is of utmost importance to prevent or stop bacterial translocation among intestinal transplant recipients.

CURRENT CLINICAL EXPERIENCE

Between 1985 and May, 1999, a total of 443 patients received 471 intestinal transplants at 43 transplant centers worldwide. There has been a steady increase in the number of intestinal transplants performed per year as well as the number of transplant centers that perform this operation. The transplanted intestine was an isolated graft in 45%, en bloc with liver in 40%, and part of a multivisceral graft in 15% of the cases. Of the 443 recipients, 55% were male and 62% were children. The causes of intestinal failure and indications for transplant in children were gastroschisis (22%), volvulus (22%), necrotizing enterocolitis (12%), pseudo-obstruction (10%), intestinal atresia (9%), aganglionosis/Hirschsprung's (7%), and others (19%); in adults these were ischemia (19%), Crohn's disease (16%), desmoid tumor (14%), trauma (11%), Gardner's disease/familial polyposis (10%), volvulus (9%), and others (22%). Of the total population, 56% were hospitalized at the time of transplant and 44% were at home.

Survival Outcome

The most recent data of the International Intestinal Transplant Registry showed a 1-year patient survival of 63% with a graft survival rate of 58% for transplants performed after February, 1995. The 3-year patient survival is 51% with a graft survival rate of 45%. The three different types of intestinal allografts experienced a similar actuarial survival rate (P=0.18). The causes of death for the total population were a combination of sepsis (55%), nontransplant organ failure (14%), lymphoma (14%), technical (13%), graft rejection (12%), and others (5%). The main causes of graft loss were rejection (57%) and technical failure (23%).

The database of the Pittsburgh Intestinal Transplant Program, which includes a total of 130 consecutive intestinal transplants that were performed between May, 1990 and May, 1999, showed a 1-year patient survival of 72% with a 5 year survival rate of 48%, (Figure 80-10). Most of the deaths occurred during the first 30 postoperative months. The graft survival rate is 64% at 1-year and 40% at 5-years (Figure 80-10) with achievement of full nutritional autonomy in more than 90% of the current survivors. During the last four years, the intestinal allograft survival has significantly (P=0.04) improved in Pittsburgh with a cumulative rate of 65% (Figure 80-11). Such an achievement reflects recent refinement in operative techniques, immunosuppressive therapy, and management strategies.

The survival benefits of intestinal transplantation have been most evident among children with the best outcome among recipients between two and 17 years old who have a 5-year cumulative survival rate of 68% (Figure 80-12). The best survival rates have been

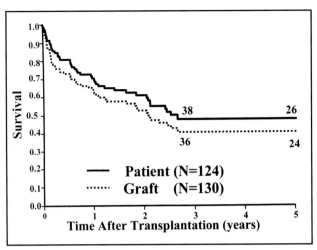

Figure 80-10. The overall Kaplan-Meier patient and graft survival rates in the Pittsburgh series.

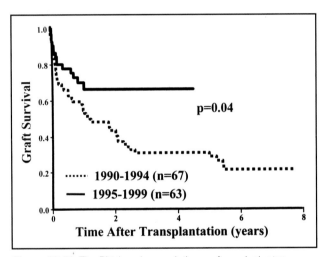

Figure 80-11. The Pittsburgh cumulative graft survival rates before and after the 1994 moratorium.

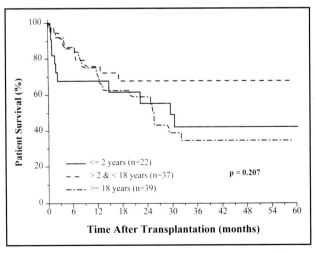

Figure 80-12. Patient survival according to recipient age. (From Abu-Elmagd K, Reyes J, Todo S, et al. Clinical intestinal transplantation: new perspectives and immunologic considerations. J Am Coll Surg. 1998,186(5):512-527, used by permission).

achieved among children with microvillus disease/ gastroschisis and among adults with Crohn's disease/ vascular thrombosis (Figure 80-13). Bone marrow augmentation has yet to significantly improve survival (Figure 80-14). Although both the isolated intestinal and composite visceral grafts have similar survival rates, the cumulative risk of graft loss due to rejection is significantly (P=0.045) higher among the isolated intestine (Figure 80-15). Systemic venous drainage of the isolated intestine does not significantly affect graft survival (Figure 80-16).

Risk Factors

Careful statistical analysis of the largest single center (Pittsburgh) series identified multiple significant risk factors that affect patient and graft survival. The most detrimental variables are frequency of rejection with the need for high levels of maintenance immunosuppression, cold ischemia time, number of previous abdominal opera-

tions, and operative time. Other important risk factors include development of PTLD, CMV disease, and inclusion of a large segment of colon with the graft.

Based upon the 1997 and 1999 reports of the International Intestinal Transplant Registry, the worldwide survival outcome with intestinal transplantation has been influenced by two important factors: era of transplantation, and size of the transplant center. Graft survival has significantly (P=0.005) improved over time and both patient and graft survival outcomes are significantly better at centers that have performed more than a total of ten intestinal transplants with a P value of 0.0005, and 0.0009, respectively. These two variables are surrogate markers for the recent availability of better immunosuppressive drugs and steady improvement in

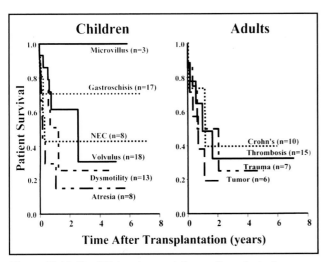

Figure 80-13. The Pittsburgh cumulative graft survival rates according to the native intestinal disease.

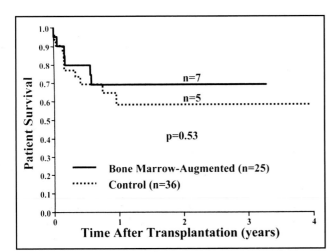

Figure 80-14. The Pittsburgh Kaplan-Meier patient survival rates for the bone marrow-augmented and control groups.

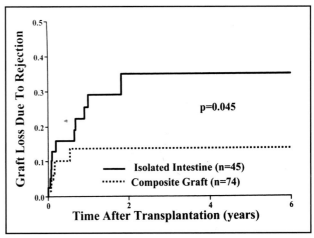

Figure 80-15. Cumulative risk of graft loss from rejection in the intestine-only and composite visceral grafts that contained liver. (From Abu-Elmagd K, Reyes J, Fung JJ, et al. Clinical intestinal transplantation in 1998: Pittsburgh experience. Actoa Gastroenterologica Belgica. 1999;62(2):244-247, used by permission).

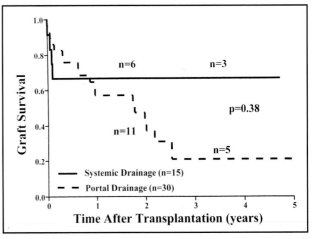

Figure 80-16. Effect of type of venous drainage on intestinal allograft survival. (From Abu-Elmagd K, Reyes J, Fung JJ, et al. Clinical intestinal transplantation in 1998: Pittsburgh experience. Actoa Gastroenterologica Belgica. 1999;62(2):244-247, used by permission).

surgical techniques, perioperative patient management, and physician's experience.

Rejection

Despite the currently adopted powerful immunosuppressive cocktails, intestinal allografts are still more vulnerable to rejection and recipients are still at a relatively higher risk of graft loss with long-term follow-up compared to other solid organ transplants. Acute rejection of the intestinal allograft occurs with a cumulative incidence of 73% to 93%. The diagnosis is usually made by histopathologic studies of random and endoscopically guided multiple mucosal biopsies, mostly of the ileum. The wide range in the incidence of acute rejection reported by different centers could be related to the adoption of different immunosuppressive protocols and variable diagnostic methodology. The histopathologic criteria that has been recently identified and published by Lee et al to diagnose and grade acute intestinal rejection , should be uniformly adopted by all of the intestinal transplant centers.

Based upon the Pittsburgh published data, most of the acute intestinal rejection episodes are mild to moderate, and more than 50% of the episodes occur within the first three months after graft implantation. These episodes are predominantly cellular with significant vascular changes only among a few of the isolated intestinal allografts. The expected effect of the degree of HLA mismatch on the incidence, frequency, and severity of rejection among the intestinal allografts has yet to be seen. Positive T cell lymphocytotoxic crossmatch undoubtedly increases frequency and severity of rejection particularly of the isolated intestine.

The isolated intestinal graft is at a significantly higher risk of acute rejection compared with intestine contained in a composite graft. Although the cumulative risk of rejection of the intestine contained in a composite graft approaches that of the isolated intestine by the end of the first postoperative year (Figure 80-17A), the cumulative rate of graft loss is less than half (Figure 80-15).

With composite hepatic-visceral transplantation, the incidence of liver rejection is less than 50% of that in the intestine (Figure 80-17B), and about only one third of the intestinal grafts that include large intestine shows histologic evidence of acute colonic rejection. Interestingly, the stomach and pancreas have the lowest incidence of rejection with a rate of 12%.

Chronic rejection of the intestinal allografts has been reported at a rate of 7% to 10% with a median onset of diagnosis to time of transplant of 15 months (range: 2 to 75). The diagnosis is suspected in recipients with chronic graft dysfunction concomitant with persistent histopathologic mucosal changes in the form of low grade apoptosis, cryptopenia, and submucosal fibrosis. Segmental arteriolar stenosis can be angiographically demonstrated in some of these grafts (Figure 80-18).

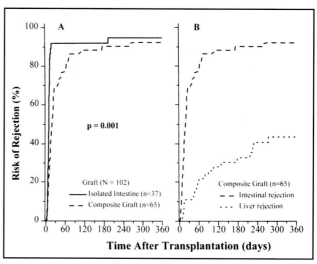

Figure 80-17A. Cumulative risk of intestinal rejection for the isolated intestine and composite grafts that contained liver. (From Abu-Elmagd K, Reyes J, Todo S, et al. Clinical intestinal transplantation: new perspectives and immunologic considerations. J Am Coll Surg. 1998;186(5):512-527, used by permission).

Figure 80-17B. Cumulative risk of both intestinal and hepatic rejection in the composite visceral allografts. (From Abu-Elmagd K, Reyes J, Todo S, et al. Clinical intestinal transplantation: new perspectives and immunologic considerations. J Am Coll Surg. 1998;186(2):512-527, used by permission).

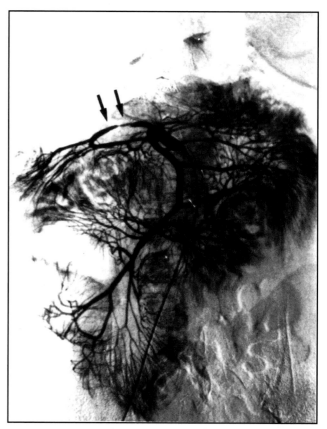

Figure 80-18. Superior mesenteric arteriogram showing segmental narrowing of the jejunal and ileal arterial branches (arrows) in a chronically rejecting intestinal graft.

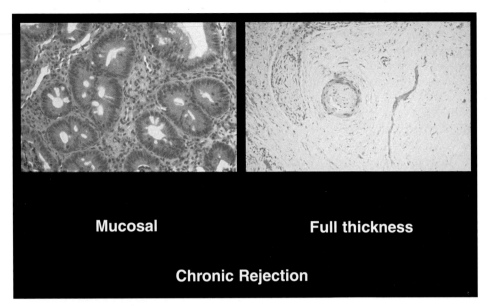

Mucosal

Full thickness

Chronic Rejection

Figure 80-19. The histopathologic picture of a mucosal (left) and a full-thickness (right) intestinal specimen after graft enterectomy. The mucosal biopsy showed persistent apoptosis while examination of arteries in the mesenteric root and bowel serosa revealed obliterative arteriopathy, as is typical of chronic rejection in all vascularized organ allografts (hematoxylin-eosin, X140).

Because a definitive diagnosis requires a transmural specimen that is not deliberately obtained in endoscopic biopsies (Figure 80-19), the incidence of chronic rejection undoubtedly is grossly underestimated. Of great interest is the recently reported higher incidence of chronic rejection among isolated intestinal (23%) compared to liver-intestinal (1.5%) and multivisceral (0%) grafts. Other statistically significant risk factors are frequency/severity of acute rejection and donor age.

Graft-vs-Host Disease

Unexpectedly, the incidence of GVHD has been relatively low despite the large lymphoid mass being contained in the transplanted intestine. In one series, the overall clinical incidence of the disease was 11% with histopathologic confirmation in only half of the cases (5%). It is the practice at the University of Pittsburgh to immediately biopsy any suspected skin or gastrointestinal lesions and to study the biopsy specimen by the conventional histopathologic methods and the currently available immuno histopathologic staining for donor-specific HLA antigen, and, when applicable, the in situ hybridization technique using the Y chromosome-specific probe. Other target organs should be thoroughly evaluated when clinically indicated. With similar incidence among the three different types of intestinal transplantation, the disease is treatable in most cases with steroid therapy and an increase in the level of maintenance immunosuppression. In the University of Pittsburgh study, only one pediatric recipient succumbed to the disease, and one adult patient developed chronic GVHD.

Surgical Infections

Intestinal recipients are usually at high risk for surgical infections. This is essentially related to the frequent existence of preoperative enteric stomata or enterocutaneous fistulae, operative manipulation of the intestinal graft, risk of postoperative enteric leaks and microbial translocation, development of postoperative chylous ascites, failure of complete closure of the recipient abdominal wall, and the need for a central line during the early postoperative period. The most common organisms cultured from intra-abdominal infections are enteric bacterial and/or fungal microorganisms. A high index of clinical suspicion and prompt initiation of antibiotic therapy and radiologic/surgical interventions are essential for successful outcome in these heavily immunosuppressed hosts.

Cytomegaloviral Disease

The overall incidence of de novo or reactivation CMV infection ranges from 23% to 36%. The incidence according to the donor and recipient CMV serologic status is higher for positive-to-negative and positive-to-positive cases. Adults are more susceptible than children and there is no significant difference in the incidence and onset of the disease between the different types of intestinal graft. Avoidance of CMV seropositive grafts in seronegative recipients, and prolonged use of prophylactic antiviral therapy for high/moderate risk patients have recently reduced the risk of CMV disease at Pittsburgh (Figure 80-20).

Lymphoproliferative Disease

The development of PTLD is a significant morbid event among intestinal recipients. According to the most recently published data, the incidence of PTLD ranges from 12% to 20%. The reported higher incidence (20%) in the Pittsburgh series may be related to the longer duration of posttransplant follow-up compared to that of the other intestinal transplant centers. The disease is lethal or mandates enterectomy (isolated intestine) in nearly half of the affected patients. Using multivariate analysis, young age (children), type of intestinal transplant (multivisceral), and recipient splenectomy are the three major significant risk factors for development of PTLD. Bone marrow augmentation does not seem to increase the risk of PTLD. The recent use of PCR technique to serially monitor EBV viremia with prompt initiation of preemptive therapy has reduced the risk of the disease (Figure 80-21). A new management strategy to prevent the need for heavy immunosuppression without the penalty of rejection is necessary to further ameliorate this and other significant morbid events.

Motility Disorders

Delayed emptying of both the native and transplanted stomach has been a common observation during the early postoperative period with spontaneous and complete recovery particularly of the native stomach in all recipients. Graft dysmotility has been documented

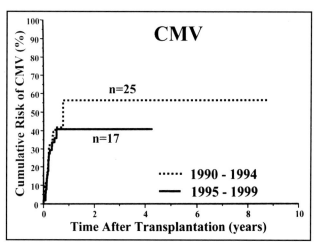

Figure 80-20. Reduction in the cumulative risk of CMV disease during the last four years of the Pittsburgh experience.

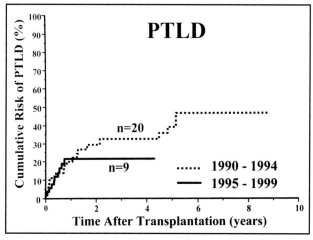

Figure 80-21. Reduction in the cumulative risk of PTLD disease during the last four years of the Pittsburgh experience.

radiographically and by measuring the myoelectric activity among the three different types of intestinal transplant. The predominant pattern is rapid transit with incomplete coordination of the transmitted migrating motor complex activity between the native and transplanted intestine. These abnormalities seem to improve in most patients with longitudinal follow-up.

Microbial Overgrowth

Bacterial and fungal overgrowth is a common finding in the intestinal allografts. Such a change in the ecology of intestinal flora could be related to the surgical manipulations, absence of the ileocecal valve, disruption of the intestinal lymphatics, immunosuppression, gut dysmotility, suppression of gastric acidity, and the need for temporary intravenous nutrition and an enteric-defined formula diet. The loss of an effective mucosal barrier caused by preservation injury, rejection, or PTLD and the impaired host defenses caused by the need for heavy immunosuppression may precipitate the potential deleterious effects of microbial overgrowth. Although it is not always technically feasible to prove, the reported high incidence of systemic infections could be partly related to the development of translocation.

Chylous Ascites and Fat Intolerance

The current lack of surgical ability to reconstruct the lymphatics of the intestinal graft frequently leads to lymphatic leakage and impaired fat absorption particularly during the early postoperative period. The lymphatic leak is commonly noticed after initiation of the enteral feeding with development of chylous ascites, chylothorax, or chylocutaneous fistulae. The latter usually leads to high volume losses that require daily fluid replacement. This is usually self-limited with the judicious use of medium chain triglyceride enteral formula. In a few cases, discontinuation of the enteral feeding and reinstitution of TPN is required until spontaneous reconstitution of the lymphatic collaterals occurs. The limited capacity of the engrafted intestine to absorb fat with impaired tolerance and high fecal fat excretion has been documented in some recipients up to 12 months after transplantation. These two morbid observations could be potentially ameliorated by anastomosing the major donor and recipient lymphatic channel at the time of implantation.

Disease Recurrence

Recurrence of the primary intestinal disease is a potential risk after intestinal transplantation particularly among patients with inflammatory bowel disease and inherited metabolic, vascular, neoplastic, and autoimmune disorders. With follow-up periods ranging from six months to nine years, none of the Pittsburgh recipients showed any clinical or histopathologic evidences of disease recurrence in the visceral graft or elsewhere. However, the Miami group documented recurrence of Crohn's disease in one recipient, and extra-intestinal desmoid tumor in another patient.

Long-Term Rehabilitation and Cost-Effectiveness

The long-term rehabilitation with all three kinds of the intestinal transplant procedure is similar to that achieved with lung transplantation and some other types of thoraco-abdominal organ transplant. Out of a total of 215 worldwide intestinal transplant survivors, 78% maintained fully functioning grafts with complete enteric nutritional autonomy. The remaining recipients either lost the graft (12%), or required intravenous nutritional support (10%). Interestingly enough, 86% of the recipients who survived beyond the sixth postoperative month achieved a modified Karnofsky performance score of 90% to 100%. This therapeutic index is even higher at centers with vast experience.

The cost-effectiveness of a combined intestinal-liver transplant is immeasurable because of the lack of an alternative therapy for hepatic-intestinal failure. With isolated intestinal or modified (without liver) multivisceral transplant, the cost-effectiveness can be examined based upon the availability of chronic TPN as an alternative therapy for patients with irreversible gastrointestinal failure and normal liver functions. Based on Medicare data, the average cost of TPN in 1992 was more than $150,000 per patient per year not including the cost of frequent hospitalization, medical equipment, and nursing care. Based upon a single center (Pittsburgh) experience, the cost of the isolated intestinal transplant has been significantly reduced during the last four years to an average of $132,285. Intestinal transplantation appears to become cost-effective by the second year after surgery.

CONTROVERSIES

The current cumulative experience with clinical intestinal transplantation has either confirmed or brought into question the validity of previously accepted assumptions related to this procedure. Among these are the importance of portal venous drainage of the isolated intestinal graft and the role of simultaneous liver replacement in intestinal engraftment. Other new controversial issues are the therapeutic efficacy of isolated liver transplantation for TPN induced liver failure in patients with short gut syndrome, and the extent of visceral replacement in patients with hollow visceral dysmotility syndromes.

The venous outflow of the isolated intestinal graft can be drained into the recipient portal system or directed into the systemic circulation via the inferior vena cava. Although several experimental studies have proven the superiority of portal drainage, our current clinical results have failed to demonstrate any significant difference in the risk of rejection and survival outcome between the two procedures. Nonetheless, portal drainage should always be considered in the absence of technical difficulties and anatomic abnormalities as described above.

The immunoprotective effect induced by a concomitantly transplanted liver to other organ allografts, procured from the same donor, has been repeatedly demonstrated in numerous animal experiments. Abu-Elmagd et al, however, are the first to clearly demonstrate, in the clinical context of their intestinal transplant series, the consequent protective effect on the intestine of the contemporaneously transplanted liver (Figure 80-15). The mechanism of hepatic tolerance could be better explained by the recently discovered two-way paradigm of transplant immunity with migration of the highly tolerogenic passenger leukocytes from the hepatic allograft into the host organs "microchimerism".

The recent evolution of abdominal visceral transplant has questioned the therapeutic role of isolated liver replacement in children with TPN induced liver failure. This controversial issue is fueled by the previously reported unsatisfactory outcomes with solitary liver transplant, and the recently documented high mortality rate among children waiting for composite visceral grafts. A satisfactory short-term outcome, however, has been recently achieved with isolated liver transplant in a highly select group of children who have shown evidence of increasing enteral feeding tolerance and have sufficient small bowel that complete enteral adaptation can be reasonably expected. Even with such careful selection, some of these isolated liver allografts may not escape the long-term deleterious effects of TPN.

The recently defined syndrome of hollow visceral neuropathy and/or myopathy is not an uncommon indication for intestinal transplant among both the pediatric and adult population. The frequent involvement of the stomach at the time of referral and the well known progressive nature of the disease dictate, in our opinion, the need for full or modified (without liver) multivisceral replacement. Others have advocated a less extensive operation by limiting the visceral replacement to the small intestine with surgical drainage of the native stomach to the proximal jejunum of the transplanted bowel.

FUTURE CONSIDERATIONS

Prediction and/or early detection of allograft rejection are important steps to raise the level of intestinal transplantation to be the standard of care for all patients with chronic intestinal failure. The development of a highly sensitive and specific serum or tissue marker will undoubtedly improve the survival outcomes and the cost-effectiveness of the procedure.

Although donor leukocyte augmentation and enhanced natural chimerism with donor bone marrow infusion has not markedly altered most of the endpoints, establishment of the safety of this adjunct procedure opens the way to further immune-modulation as a novel strategy to overcome the current immunologic barriers with clinical intestinal transplantation. Consequently, it is planned to bring graft cytoreduction with a relatively low-dose of ex vivo irradiation combined with adjunct donor bone marrow infusion to clinical trial.

The temporary and permanent effects of the ischemia-reperfusion injury, the central enteric denervation, and the intestinal lymphatic disruption are important nonimmunologic factors that contribute to the delayed and sometimes incomplete recovery of the graft metabolic and neuroenteric functions. These pathophysiologic and anatomic defects, in addition to the relatively high risk of rejection, have precluded the wide use of clinical intestinal transplantation. Therefore, better understanding of the mechanisms and sequelae of these injuries may increase the practicality of the procedure by opening the way for further refinement in the current implantation techniques and management protocols.

With the achievement of further improvement in survival, intestinal transplantation should be offered to all patients with irreversible intestinal failure including those who can still be maintained on TPN. Early referral for isolated intestinal transplant will undoubtedly reduce the need for combined organ replacement and save a significant number of cadaveric donor livers. This will also improve the perioperative survival and the cost-effectiveness of the procedure

CONCLUSIONS

Intestinal transplantation has become a life-saving procedure for patients with irreversible intestinal failure who cannot be maintained on TPN. With a rehabilitation index similar to other transplant procedures, intestinal transplant should no longer be considered experimental and therefore should be eligible for reimbursement under all third party payers, Medicare, and Medicaid.

Despite the recent improvement in survival and cost-effectiveness, the procedure has yet to become the treatment of choice for all patients with irreversible intestinal failure who can safely be maintained on TPN. The current management difficulties and overall suboptimal results have stemmed largely from the inability to completely control rejection without the long-term need for heavy immunosuppression. Based upon the results of the most recent preclinical trials at the University of Pittsburgh, further improvement in survival and long-term rehabilitation is expected with further immune-modulation strategies that can be added to the current management protocols.

RECOMMENDED READING

Abu-Elmagd K, Reyes J, Todo S, et al. Clinical intestinal transplantation: New perspectives and immunologic considerations. J Am Coll Surg. 1998;186(5):512-527.

Abu-Elmagd KM, Reyes J, Fung JJ, et al. Evolution of clinical intestinal transplantation: improved outcome and cost effectiveness. Transplant Proc. 1999;31 (1-2):582-584.

Abu-Elmagd K, Reyes J, Fung J. Transplantation of the human intestine: the forbidden organ. Curr Opin Organ Transplant. 1998;3:286-292.

Fung JJ, Abu-Elmagd K, Todo S. Intestinal and multivisceral transplantation. In: RH Bell Jr, ed. Digestive Tract Surgery: A Text and Atlas. Philadelphia, Pa: Lippincott Williams & Wilkins; 1996: 1229-1261.

Howard L, Ament M, Fleming CR, Shike M, Steiger E. Current use and clinical outcome of home parenteral and enteral nutrition therapies in the United States. Gastroenterology. 1995;109(2):355-365.

Todo S, Tzakis A, Abu-Elmagd K, Reyes J, Starzl TE. Current status of intestinal transplantation. Adv Surg. 1994;27:295-316.

Abu-Elmagd K, Fung J, Bueno J, et al. Logistics and technique for intestinal, pancreatic, and hepatic grafts from the same donor. Ann Surg. 2000;232(5):680-687.

Casavilla A, Selby R, Abu-Elmagd K, et al. Logistics and technique for combined hepatic-intestinal retrieval. Ann Surg. 1992;216(5):605-609.

Starzl TE, Todo S, Tsakis A, et al. The many faces of multivisceral transplantation. Surg Gynecol Obstet. 1991; 172(5):335-344.

Abu-Elmagd K, Fung JJ, Reyes J, Casavilla A, Van Thiel DH, Iwaki Y, Warty V, Nikolaidis N, Block J, Nakamura K, Goldbach B, Demetris AJ, Tzakis A, Todo S, Starzl TE: Management of intestinal transplantation in humans. Transplant Proc. 1992;24(3):1243-1244.

Abu-Elmagd KM, Tzakis A, Todo S, et al. Monitoring and treatment of intestinal allograft rejection in humans. Transplant Proc. 1993;25(1 Pt 2):1202-1203.

Todo S, Reys J, Furukawa H, et al. Outcome analysis of 71 clinical intestinal transplantations Ann Surg. 1995; 222(3):270-282.

Grant D. Intestinal transplantation: 1997 Report of the international registry. Intestinal Transplant Registry. Transplantation. 1999;67(7):1061-1064.

Lee RG, Nakamura K, Tsamandas AC, et al. Pathology of human intestinal transplantation. Gastroenterology. 1996;110(6):1820-1834.

Reyes J, Todo S, Green M, et al. Graft-versus-host disease after liver and small bowel transplantation in a child. Clin Transplant. 1997;11(5 Pt 1):345-348.

Manez R, Kusne S, Green M, et al. Incidence and risk factors associated with the development of cytomegalovirus disease after intestinal transplantation. Transplantation. 1995; 59(7):1010-1014.

Campbell WL, Abu-Elmagd K, Furukawa H, Todo S. Intestinal and multivisceral transplantation. In: Radiol Clin North Am. 1995;33(3):595-614.

Abu-Elmagd K, Todo S, Tzakis A, et al. Intestinal transplantation and bacterial overgrowth in humans. Transplant Proc. 1994;26(3):1684-1685.

DiMartini A, Rovera GM, Grahm TO, et al. Quality of life after small intestinal transplantation and among home parenteral nutrition patients. J Parent Enteral Nutrit. 1998;22(6):357-362.

Starzl TE, Demetris AJ, Murase N, Ildstad S, Ricordi C, Trucco M. Cell migration, chimerism, and graft acceptance. Lancet. 1992;339(8809):1579-1582.

81   HEPATOCYTE TRANSPLANTATION

Ira J. Fox, MD
Jayanta Roy-Chowdhury, MD, MRCP

Since the development of a method for isolating primary hepatocytes by collagenase perfusion, many investigators have demonstrated the efficacy of hepatocyte transplantation in the treatment of liver failure and inherited metabolic disorders in experimental animals. Treatment of liver diseases with transplantation of isolated hepatocytes, rather than the whole liver, has several theoretical advantages. Unlike the whole liver, isolated hepatocytes could be cryopreserved for instant availability and could be modified genetically or otherwise to enhance specific functions, stimulate proliferation or abrogate allograft rejection. Hepatocyte transplantation should be less stressful than whole liver transplantation because the host organ remains intact. Since the transplanted cells integrate into the host liver, they could provide restorative potential and the consequences of graft loss would be relatively minor. Hepatocyte transplantation would not interfere with subsequent liver transplantation, should that become necessary, and, of particular importance, it would permit liver-directed gene therapy, when it becomes available.

TECHNICAL ASPECTS
Sources of Hepatic Tissue for Transplantation

Genetically-matched primary hepatocytes have been used in experimental transplantation studies because of the ease of evaluating engraftment without concern for immune rejection. In order to avoid the need for immunosuppression in the clinic, autologous hepatocytes have been isolated from resected liver segments and transplanted directly, or used for ex vivo gene transfer, followed by transplantation. In animals, allogeneic hepatocytes have been transplanted in conjunction with immunosuppression to investigate methods for abrogating allograft rejection. The worldwide shortage of donor organs, and particularly good quality tissues for hepatocyte isolation, however, has stimulated exploration of two alternative sources: immortalized hepatocytes and hepatocytes obtained from animal livers. Although cur-

Ira J. Fox, MD, Associate Professor of Surgery, University of Nebraska Medical Center, Omaha, NE

Jayanta Roy-Chowdhury, MD, MRCP, Professor of Medicine and Molecular Genetics, Albert Einstein College of Medicine, Bronx, NY

rent techniques do not permit massive expansion of primary hepatocytes in culture, hepatocytes immortalized by transferring the gene for the simian virus 40 large T antigen can be grown in culture. Laboratory research toward generating hepatocytes, immortalized by this or other methods, that would be safe for transplantation is being explored. Although daunting immunological hurdles and concerns about unmanageable animal-derived infections remain, xenogeneic hepatocytes, usually obtained from porcine sources, are also being investigated for their ability to provide short-term metabolic support in animals and patients with liver failure.

Sites of Hepatocyte Engraftment

The vascular bed of the liver and the splenic pulp are the most effective sites for engraftment and function of transplanted hepatocytes. A number of ectopic sites have also been examined, but appear to be far less hospitable to hepatocyte engraftment. With further development, the peritoneal cavity may provide an alternative site for transplantation of encapsulated or matrix-attached hepatocytes.

The optimal site for hepatocyte engraftment is the liver. Within the liver substance, transplanted hepatocytes receive the benefit of portal nutrients, contact with adjacent hepatocytes and nonparenchymal cells, proximity to paracrine factors, and they can use the native biliary system to excrete bile. Hepatocytes can be seeded into the liver by infusion into the portal vein or by injection into the splenic pulp, from which the cells translocate to the liver through the splenic vein. After introduction into the hepatic sinusoids, the hepatocytes migrate rapidly into the liver parenchyma and integrate into the liver cords, leaving the hepatic architecture intact.

Syngeneic, allogeneic and xenogeneic hepatocytes have been transplanted successfully into the liver and, in rodent recipients, engrafted hepatocytes can survive and function throughout life. Hepatocytes, representing 1% to 4% of the hepatocyte mass, can be transplanted into structurally normal livers with only mild and transient increases in portal pressure, although more serious portal hypertension, portal vein thrombosis and intestinal hemorrhage have been reported in dogs. In contrast to recipients with normal liver architecture, cirrhotic rats develop prolonged portal hypertension and increased right atrial pressure after hepatocyte transplantation. Transplanted hepatocytes do engraft in cirrhotic nodules, but neither the safety nor efficacy of hepatocyte transplantation into the liver of cirrhotic patients has been established.

While the majority of hepatocytes injected into the splenic pulp migrate to the liver, a smaller fraction engraft within the spleen in the spaces of Billroth, giving rise to structures resembling hepatic cords, and replacing up to 40% of the spleen in several months. When a significant hepatocyte mass develops in the spleen, bile canaliculi, sinusoidal structures, and endothelial and stellate cells may also appear, resulting in further morphologic resemblance to the liver. In cirrhotic recipients, the spleen may be considered the most appropriate site for transplantation of hepatocytes.

Because of its large capacity and easy access, the peritoneal cavity is an attractive site for hepatocyte transplantation. Although isolated hepatocytes do not survive after direct injection into the peritoneum, when transplanted after attachment to microcarriers, encasement within hydrogel-based hollow fibers or in combination with nonparenchymal cells, they can survive for months. Encasement in hydrogel-based hollow fibers may also protect the transplanted cells from allograft rejection.

EVALUATION OF THE FUNCTION OF ENGRAFTED HEPATOCYTES
Animal Studies

Disorders caused by single gene mutations offer the best opportunity to evaluate the function of engrafted cells. Rodents with natural mutations have been used extensively for determining the efficacy of hepatocyte transplantation. Gunn rats, which lack hepatic bilirubin glucuronidation, and are models for human Crigler-Najjar syndrome type 1, and the Nagase analbuminemic rat, are among the best-studied models. Intrasplenic, intraperitoneal, or intraportal transplantation of normal donor hepatocytes has been shown to result in excretion of bilirubin glucuronides in the bile and reduced serum bilirubin levels in Gunn rats. Similarly, hepatocyte transplantation increases serum albumin concentrations in Nagase analbuminemic rats. Transplanted hepatocytes completely or partially correct the metabolic abnormalities in animal models of tyrosinemia (fumarylacetoacetate hydrolase deficient mice), familial hypercholesterolemia (LDL receptor deficiency in Watanabe rabbits) and a number of other liver-based metabolic deficiencies.

Hepatocyte transplantation also increases the survival of rodents with acute liver failure experimentally induced by D-galactosamine, dimethylnitrosamine, hepatic ischemia or 90% hepatectomy. Some reports, however, suggest that engraftment is not necessary for improved survival and that hepatocyte-derived substances may be responsible for the beneficial effect. As the regeneration of the host liver has not been significantly inhibited in these studies, such experimental models do not fully represent the clinical situation, where failure of hepatocellular regeneration is a critical prognostic factor. Thus, release of substances, such as glucose, from the injected hepatocytes may be sufficient to provide transient life support until there is adequate hepatic regeneration for survival. Therefore, these studies are not sufficient to permit the prediction that hepatocyte transplantation will improve the survival of patients with acute liver failure.

In rodent models of chronic liver insufficiency, hepatocyte transplantation has been shown to improve physiological function. In rats with hepatic encephalopathy caused by end-to-side portacaval shunt, spontaneous activity and certain reflexes are measurably affected. In this model, injection of hepatocytes into the spleen improves the behavior score and partially corrects the amino acid imbalance. Although the elevation of ammonia levels due to the portacaval shunt is not reversed by hepatocyte transplantation, the procedure protects portacaval-shunted rats from developing hepatic coma induced by an exogenous ammonia load. More recently, intrasplenic hepatocyte transplantation in rats with decompensated liver cirrhosis has been shown to stabilize total bilirubin, and to improve serum albumin and ammonia levels, prothrombin time and encephalopathy scores, as well as prolong survival.

Human Studies

ACUTE LIVER FAILURE. In an initial study performed in India, seven patients with acute liver failure received intraperitoneal injection of approximately 5×10^8 hepatocytes obtained from fetuses of 26 to 34 week gestational age. The overall survival of patients receiving hepatocytes was 43% compared with 33% in matched controls. All patients with grade III hepatic encephalopathy that received hepatocyte transplantation survived, whereas only 50% of matched controls did. Recovery from encephalopathy was observed within 48 hours.

In the United States, hepatocyte transplantation has also been performed for acute liver failure, often as a "bridge" to liver transplantation. In one study, seven potential transplant candidates were infused with 10^7 to 10^9 viable hepatocytes through the splenic artery. Five of these patients survived long enough to receive orthotopic liver transplantation. In another series, five patients, who were not candidates for organ transplantation, were transplanted with as many as 2×10^{10} hepatocytes by infusion into the portal vein via a percutaneous transhepatic or transjugular transhepatic approach. Three additional patients have also been treated by intraportal hepatocyte infusion. In general, engrafted hepatocytes could be found in the spleens of some patients who received intrasplenic transplantation, and in the livers of some patients who received intraportal hepatocyte infusion. Two of the transplant recipients in the entire group recovered without liver transplantation, while others had anecdotal improvement in ammonia, prothrombin time, encephalopathy, cerebral perfusion pressure and cardiovascular stability. Reported complications included: transient hemodynamic instability during intraportal hepatocyte infusion; overwhelming sepsis, which may or may not have been related to hepatocyte transplantation; and translocation of the hepatocytes to the lungs without clinical manifestations of pulmonary embolism. Although the data suggest that the transplanted hepatocytes provided some benefit, convincing evidence of engraftment and function of the transplanted cells has not been obtained. Because some patients with acute liver failure can survive without transplantation, survival rate alone is difficult to use as a definitive indicator of functional engraftment of hepatocytes.

Isolated hepatocytes have also been incorporated into bioartificial liver devices and used to support patients with decompensated acute liver failure. The efficacy of one device, that used cells derived from an immortalized human tumor line, was tested in a single-center prospective study and has been redesigned for further investigation. A second device, that incorporates porcine hepatocytes and charcoal perfusion, has been more extensively studied. While the data indicates that some measures of liver failure may be improved by the use of these devices, more extensive, randomized trials will be needed to determine their true efficacy and role in the management of acute liver failure.

CHRONIC LIVER DISEASE. In a Japanese study, ten patients with chronic hepatitis or cirrhosis were transplanted with hepatocytes isolated from their own left lateral liver segment. Four patients underwent hepatic artery ligation in addition to hepatocyte transplantation to control ascites. Patients received from $1X10^7$ to $6X10^8$ hepatocytes into the spleen, either by direct splenic puncture or via the splenic artery or portal vein. In one patient, hepatocyte engraftment and survival was detected in the spleen by ^{99m}PMT-radioisotope uptake 11 months after transplantation. In this patient the ascites and encephalopathy eventually resolved. The investigators, however, do not believe the patient's improvement can be conclusively attributed to hepatocyte transplantation.

Eight patients with decompensated chronic liver disease have been treated in the United States by transplantation with up to 10^{10} hepatocytes through the splenic artery. One of three patients who was a candidate for organ transplantation was successfully bridged to transplantation. Patients appeared to tolerate the infusions well, and improvement in encephalopathy, as well as synthetic and renal function have been described in a preliminary report. In two patients, scanning for uptake of ^{99m}Tc-labeled glycosylated albumin indicated the presence of engrafted hepatocytes in the spleen.

LIVER-BASED METABOLIC DISEASES. The first attempt to correct a liver-based metabolic disease with hepatocyte transplantation was performed with genetically modified autologous hepatocytes. Familial hypercholesterolemia is caused by an inherited deficiency of

LDL receptors and is associated with severe hypercholesterolemia and premature coronary artery disease. In a single series from the University of Pennsylvania, autologous hepatocytes were recovered from the left lateral hepatic segment of patients with familial hypercholesterolemia and infected ex vivo with a recombinant virus containing the gene encoding a normal LDL receptor. The cells were then transplanted back into the patient's own liver via the portal vein. Improvement in serum cholesterol occurred but was relatively limited.

Patients with ornithine transcarbamylase (OTC) deficiency, alpha-1-antitrypsin deficiency, and Crigler-Najjar syndrome type 1 (bilirubin-uridinediphosphoglucuronate glucuronosyltransferase deficiency) have received unmodified allogeneic hepatocyte transplantation. One child with OTC deficiency had enzyme activity in a posttransplantation liver biopsy specimen, but died following cell transplantation with hyperammonemia. Another child received hepatocyte transplantation at birth, via an umbilical vein catheter and exhibited transient clinical evidence of enzyme activity, maintaining normal ammonia and glutamine levels off phenylbutyrate/phenylacetate while receiving more than 2 grams of protein/kg per day. The cells may have been rejected because of inadequate immunosuppression.

Unequivocal evidence of function of transplanted human hepatocytes has been obtained only in one patient with Crigler-Najjar syndrome type 1, who had significant reduction of serum bilirubin levels after hepatocyte transplantation. The patient, a ten year-old girl, had required ten to 12 hours of phototherapy daily before transplantation to keep her serum unconjugated bilirubin level between 24 and 27 mg/dL. She received an infusion of $7.5X10^9$ hepatocytes into the portal vein through a percutaneously placed catheter. The child remained conscious during the cell infusion and was discharged 20 hours after it was completed. After transplantation, the serum bilirubin level was reduced to 10.6 to 14 mg/dL and remained at that level for more than a year, despite reduction in phototherapy. Hepatic bilirubin-UGT activity increased from barely detectable (0.4% of normal) levels to 5.5% of normal and more than 30% of the pigments excreted in bile are bilirubin glucuronides.

TECHNICAL BARRIERS THAT NEED TO BE OVERCOME

A number of problems impede wider application of hepatocyte transplantation. At this time, organs that are not suitable for transplantation because of excess macrovesicular fat are the usual source of hepatocytes. These livers do not consistently yield cells sufficient in quality or quantity for transplantation. Residual segments from reduced liver transplants and tissues obtained from hepatic resection for trauma provide better cells, but such tissues are not commonly available. The ability to cryopreserve hepatocytes is a principle attraction of hepatocyte transplantation, but the efficacy of cryopreservation is variable, and depends on the initial quality of the hepatocytes and possibly other factors that are not well understood. Finally, isolation of human hepatocytes is expensive and inefficient. Research on cell isolation, cryopreservation and expansion of human hepatocytes in vitro using growth factors or by genetic engineering should address these issues. Studies concerning the feasibility of transplanting hepatocytes from other species may also alleviate the shortage of human organs.

The maximum number of hepatocytes that can be transplanted at one time needs to be better defined. Currently, only 30% or less of the transplanted hepatocytes engraft. A better understanding of factors that allow hepatocyte integration may lead to techniques for transplanting a larger number of hepatocytes. In diseases such as hereditary tyrosinemia or progressive intrahepatic cholestasis type 3 (MDR3 deficiency), the host cells die spontaneously and therefore the transplanted normal cells eventually repopulate the entire liver. In most cases, however, transplanted hepatocytes do not have a survival advantage over the host cells. In experimental animals, a selective growth advantage can be provided to transplanted hepatocytes by inhibiting the regeneration of host hepatocytes by preparative irradiation of the liver, delivery of suicide genes to the liver, or chemicals, such as retrorsine, that block the hepatocyte cell cycle.

It is likely that gene therapy will eventually supplant hepatocyte transplantation for the treatment of liver-based diseases caused by single gene disorders. Therefore, the future of hepatocyte transplantation appears to be in the treatment of liver failure. While hepatocyte transplantation is not expected to ameliorate portal hypertension or prevent liver cancer, improvement in liver function, quality of life and patient survival may be possible. For this purpose, safe methods and optimal sites of transplanting hepatocytes must continue to be explored.

Evaluation of engraftment and function of transplanted hepatocytes in the human liver remains challenging. For liver-based metabolic disease, biopsy measurement of enzyme activity in the liver can be useful; however, to assess whether rejection is taking place, less cumbersome methods of identifying the transplanted hepatocytes will be needed.

SUMMARY

At this time, hepatocyte transplantation offers hope to children with debilitating metabolic diseases until effective gene therapy methods become available. Hepato-cyte transplantation is expected to benefit patients with acute and chronic liver disease although definitive evidence is not yet available. Further research on proliferation of hepatocytes or its progenitors in culture, cryopreservation, abrogation of allograft and xenograft rejection and massive repopulation of the liver may herald a broader use of this tantalizing therapeutic modality.

RECOMMENDED READING

Gupta S, Aragona E, Vemuru RP, Bhargava KK, Burk RD, Roy-Chowdhury J. Permanent engraftment and function of hepatocytes delivered to the liver: implications for gene therapy and liver repopulation. Hepatology. 1991;14(1): 144-149.

Demetriou AA, Whiting JF, Feldman D, et al. Replacement of liver function in rats by transplantation of microcarrier-attached hepatocytes. Science. 1986; 233(4769):1190-1192.

Roger V, Balladur P, Honiger J, et al. Internal bioartificial liver with xenogeneic hepatocytes prevents death from acute liver failure: an experimental study. Ann Surg. 1998;228(1):1-7.

Ribeiro J, Nordlinger B, Ballet F, et al. Intrasplenic hepatocellular transplantation corrects hepatic encephalopathy in portacaval-shunted rats. Hepatology. 1992;15(1): 12-18.

Habibullah CM, Syed IH, Qamar A, Taher-Uz Z. Human fetal hepatocyte transplantation in patients with fulminant hepatic failure. Transplantation. 1994;58(8); 951-952.

Strom SC, Roy-Chowdhury J, Fox IJ. Hepatocyte transplantation for the treatment of human disease. Sem Liver Dis. 1999;19(1):39-48.

Mito M, Kusano M, Kawaura Y. Hepatocyte transplantation in man. Transplant Proc. 1992;24(6):3052-3053.

Fox IJ, Roy-Chowdhury J, Kaufman SS, et al. Treatment of the Crigler-Najjar syndrome type I with hepatocyte transplantation. New Eng J Med . 1998;338(20):1422-1426.

Laconi E, Oren R, Mukhopadhyay D, et al. Long-term, near-total liver replacement by transplantation of isolated hepatocytes in rats treated with retrorsine. Am J Pathol. 1998;153(1):319-329.

Section VIII

LUNG TRANSPLANTATION

82 LUNG TRANSPLANTATION – HISTORICAL PERSPECTIVE

G.A. Patterson, MD

During the past fifteen years, lung transplantation has become a successful treatment option for patients with a variety of end-stage lung diseases. There are active and successful lung transplant programs in many centers throughout the western world. The International Society for Heart and Lung Transplantation maintains an accurate worldwide registry of lung transplant results compiled from more than 1,200 cases performed annually.

The technical feasibility of lung transplantation was established in canine experiments performed by Metras, Hardin and Kittle during the 1950s. These technical principles were used by Hardy when his team performed the first human lung transplant in 1963. Although this patient survived only 18 days, the experience demonstrated the feasibility of human lung transplantation. During the next two decades there were approximately 45 subsequent attempts at human lung transplantation with the longest survivor a patient who survived ten months following the procedure. All of these other attempts proved unsuccessful. The majority of these patients died as a result of complications from donor bronchial ischemia.

In 1982, Reitz and his colleagues reported the first long-term successful pulmonary transplantation: a series of patients undergoing combined heart-lung transplantation. One advantage of this combined procedure was that the viability of the donor tracheobronchial tree was virtually assured as a result of reliable collateral circulation through the pericardium between the coronary and bronchial circulations. However, by this time, Cooper and his colleagues had demonstrated that high-dose corticosteroid therapy had an adverse effect on experimental bronchial anastomotic healing and that a pedicled flap of abdominal omentum could be used to support and revascularize the ischemic donor bronchus within a period of several days. Using these principles, the Toronto group conducted the first single lung transplant procedure associated with long-term success. Subsequently, the Toronto group reported the first successful en bloc double-lung transplant procedure, performed in 1986. While this en bloc double-lung procedure had the obvious attraction of preserving the

Joseph C. Bancroft Professor of Surgery, Division of Cardiothoracic Surgery, Washington University School of Medicine, St. Louis, MO

native heart, it was associated with a significant incidence of ischemic donor airway complications. In 1989, Pasque and his colleagues at Washington University described a bilateral sequential single-lung transplant procedure that avoids the tracheal complications of the en bloc double-lung technique. This bilateral sequential procedure with minor modifications has evolved as the procedure of choice for bilateral lung replacement.

During these early years of successful lung transplantation, most attention was directed to resolution of technical problems and perioperative complications such as reperfusion injury and donor airway complications. Griffith and his colleagues reported a 10-year experience ending in 1992 with 232 lung transplant recipients, noting an improvement in 1-year survival from 53% to 70% in early and later transplants, respectively. These improved results are due to a number of developments that occurred in experienced transplant centers.

Surgical technique improved to enable more expeditious conduct of harvest and implantation, thereby shortening allograft warm ischemic time. Better strategies of graft preservation and avoidance of reperfusion injury have resulted in much more predictable satisfactory early allograft function. In the early experience, immunosuppression was imprecise, as was the diagnosis and treatment of acute lung allograft rejection. This situation was improved dramatically with the widespread acceptance of transbronchial lung biopsy as the standard for diagnosis of acute lung allograft rejection. Opportunistic infection has become less of a problem with the routine use of effective antiviral agents such as acyclovir and ganciclovir. Cytomegalovirus (CMV) infection has been reduced significantly by policies of donor-to-recipient CMV matching and CMV prophylaxis. In addition, progress has been made in expanding the donor pool. Starnes and his colleagues have pioneered the application of living lobar transplant using lower lobes from two recipients as bilateral grafts in a single recipient. It has been demonstrated that early and late allograft function is not adversely affected by using marginal donor lungs or by long distance donor harvest. These significant improvements have led to an overall improvement in early and late survival. In a recent 10-year review comprising 450 lung transplant procedures, an overall 1- and 5-year survival of 83% and 54%, respectively, was noted.

Unfortunately, long-term survival is compromised by the frequent development of chronic lung allograft rejection manifested by bronchiolitis obliterans syndrome. To date, there has been limited progress in understanding the pathogenesis of this condition or developing effective treatment strategies. This progressive, usually fatal, obliterative small airways disease represents the single biggest obstacle to the long-term success of lung transplantation.

RECOMMENDED READING

Metras H. Note preliminare sur la greffe totale du poumon chez le chien. C R Acad Sci.(Paris). 1950;231:1176.

Hardin CA, Kittle CF. Experiences with transplantation of the lung. Science. 1954;119:97.

Hardy JD, Webb WR, Dalton ML, et al. Lung homotransplantation in man. JAMA. 1963;186(12):1065.

Derom F, Barbier F, Ringoir S, et al. Ten-month survival after lung homotransplantation in man. J Thorac Cardiovasc Surg. 1971;61(6):835-846.

Reitz BA, Wallwork JL, Hunt SA, et al. Heart-lung transplantation: successful therapy for patients with pulmonary vascular disease. N Engl J Med. 1982;306(10):557-564.

Lima O, Cooper JD, Peters WJ, et al. Effects of methylprednisolone and azathioprine on bronchial healing following lung autotransplantation. J Thorac Cardiovasc Surg. 1981;82(2):211-215.

Morgan E, Lima OJ, Goldberg M, Ferdman A, Luk SK, Cooper JD. Successful revascularization of totally ischemic bronchial autografts with omental pedicle flaps in dogs. J Thorac Cardiovasc Surg. 1982;84(2):204-210.

Anonymous. Unilateral lung transplantation for pulmonary fibrosis. Toronto Lung Transplantation Group. N Engl J Med. 1986;314(18):1140-1145.

Patterson GA, Cooper JD, Goldman B, et al. Technique of successful clinical double-lung transplantation. Ann Thorac Surg. 1988;45(6):626-633.

Patterson GA, Todd TR, Cooper JD, Pearson FG, Winton TL, Maurer J. Airway complications after double lung transplantation. Toronto Lung Transplant Group. J Thorac Cardiovasc Surg. 1990;99(1):14-20.

Pasque MK, Cooper JD, Kaiser LR, Haydock DA, Triantafillou A, Trulock EP. An improved technique for bilateral lung transplantation: rationale and initial clinical experience. Ann Thorac Surg. 1990;49(5):785-791.

Griffith BP, Hardesty RL, Armitage JM, et al. A decade of lung transplantation. Ann Surg. 1993;218(3):310-320.

Higenbottam T, Stewart S, Penketh A, Wallwork J. Transbronchial lung biopsy for the diagnosis of rejection in heart-lung transplant patients. Transplantation. 1988;46:532-539.

Starnes VA, Barr ML, Cohen RG, et al. Living-donor lobar lung transplantation experience: intermediate results. J Thorac Cardiovasc Surg. 1996;112(5):1284-1290.

Meyers BF, Lynch J, Trulock EP, et al. Lung transplantation: a decade experience. Ann Surg. 1999;239(3):362-370.

Cooper JD, Billingham M, Egan T, et al. A working formulation for the standardization of nomenclature and for clinical staging of chronic dysfunction in lung allografts. International Society for Heart & Lung Transplantation. J Heart Lung Transplant. 1993;12(5):713-716.

83 EVALUATION AND MANAGEMENT OF PROSPECTIVE LUNG AND HEART-LUNG RECIPIENTS

Janet R. Maurer, MD

INTRODUCTION

At the end of 1998, the International Registry of Heart and Lung Transplantation reported a cumulative total of almost 9,000 solitary lung and 2,350 heart-lung transplants. After a rapid annual increase in the number of solitary unilateral and bilateral lung transplant procedures in the early 1990s, the international yearly total of approximately 1,200 to 1,300 operations has remained stable since the mid-1990s. Despite the leveling off of the number of transplants performed, the number of potential recipients has steadily risen, so that now the US waiting list is more than 3,000 patients and the average wait for an acceptable graft is more than one and one-half years.

As the donor source becomes more and more limited relative to the demand, it has become increasingly important to not only select candidates that have an optimum chance of survival, but also to ensure that selection procedures are as fair as possible. In this environment, representatives from a number of lung transplant centers around the world, supported by four pulmonary and transplant societies in addition to the American Society of Transplantation, met in 1997 to produce a uniform set of guidelines for selection of lung transplant candidates. These guidelines were published in four journals in 1998. This chapter summarizes both the general medical selection criteria thought important by this group, as well as diagnosis-specific markers of advanced disease. In addition, this chapter will review some of the considerations that went into arriving at these criteria and the investigations that are useful in deciding both whether a patient might be a good transplant candidate, and also appropriate time of referral.

GENERAL CONSIDERATION IN END-STAGE LUNG DISEASE

Different chronic pulmonary processes have variable rates of progression and often require a follow-up period of months to years to determine the speed at which lung function is being lost, and whether pharmacological or

Head, Section of Lung Transplantation, Department of Pulmonary and Critical Care Medicine; Associate Medical Director, Transplant Center, Cleveland Clinic Foundation, Cleveland, OH

surgical treatments short of transplant are effective. It is important for the treating physician to monitor appropriate parameters (ie, pulmonary function studies and/or measures of exercise capability) over time to establish the course of the disease. In this context, it is important that usual medical therapies to treat the disease progress, and improved pulmonary function or functional capacity be implemented before the patient is deemed a potential transplant candidate. This requirement is at times problematic. Patients often receive high doses of corticosteroids, which is a common medical therapy for many types of progressive lung disease. By the time the clinician has established that treatment is ineffective, the disease may have so progressed that the patient is no longer a good candidate, or complications from the medical therapy may have rendered the patient a high-risk candidate for transplant.

Many patients presenting for lung transplantation are in their 60s and 70s, which is the usual age of onset of pulmonary fibrosis and the most common age at which obstructive lung disease becomes severe enough to warrant transplant. Thus, many of the patients presenting for lung transplant have comorbid illnesses such as obesity, systemic hypertension, diabetes mellitus, peptic ulcer disease and gastroesophageal reflux disease, which require ongoing therapy. While these and other medical conditions generally do not contraindicate transplant, patients should receive, prior to referral, optimal treatment for these as well as investigations to rule out any vital end-organ damage from the diseases that might impact posttransplant survival. Of particular importance are a thorough investigation of renal, cardiac and hepatic function in at-risk patients.

Patients with pulmonary fibrosis and smoking-related emphysema or chronic bronchitis have an increased risk of lung cancers. Careful attention should be paid to screening chest CT scans to avoid overlooking "hidden" or small malignancies.

Patients with cystic fibrosis, though generally younger at the time of presentation, also have a number of potential comorbidities that may require investigation. Diabetes mellitus is common, and while end-organ dysfunction is not, patients who have had very brittle diabetes may present unacceptable management issues. Significant hepatic dysfunction secondary to focal biliary cirrhosis and portal hypertension is found in a small subgroup of potential candidates. Though not generally prohibitive issues, gastrointestinal problems with malabsorption, distal intestinal obstruction syndrome, a history of chronic nausea and vomiting or a family history of colon malignancy require careful screening and proactive management plans.

In all pretransplant patients over 45 years old (and in all posttransplant patients) yearly preventive health maintenance, including mammograms and Pap smears in female patients and colon cancer screening in all patients, should be part of routine care. All immunizations, including up-to-date tetanus, hepatitis B, influenza, and Pneumovax vaccinations, should be administered and/or documented.

GENERAL MEDICAL CONDITIONS OFTEN ASSOCIATED WITH POOR OUTCOMES

As lung transplant centers have gained experience in working with increasing numbers of mid-term and long-term post-lung transplant survivors, a variety of preexisting conditions have been recognized that have a particularly frequent negative impact either on survival or on the quality of life. This has led to recommendations for selection of candidates who have the following common medical problems.

Metabolic Bone Disease

Information about osteopenia and osteoporosis in advanced organ disease of all types has increased remarkably in the last five years. At least half of patients with obstructive lung disease and cystic fibrosis coming to transplant have moderate to severe metabolic bone disease. In addition, in the first six months following transplant a dramatic loss of bone has been documented in both heart and kidney recipients. This is likely due to immunosuppressive medications and almost certainly occurs to the same degree in lung transplant recipients. Vertebral compression fractures are the most common fracture associated with severe osteoporosis and have been reported as a common complication in lung recipients. Not only does the severe pain usually associated with these fractures impact on lung function, it also results in greatly impaired quality of life. Thus, it is currently recommended that all patients presenting for lung transplant consideration have a bone mineral density scan. Patients who have osteopenia or osteoporosis as defined by WHO criteria should be started on antiresorptive treatment, of which bisphosphonates appear the most effective. In addition, patients deficient in hormones should have them replaced and dietary recommendations should include 1,000 mg of calcium and 15 to 20 micrograms of 25-OH vitamin D daily. Pretransplant symptomatic osteoporosis should be considered a relative contraindication, particularly if the patient cannot participate fully in preoperative rehabilitation or the bone disease otherwise impairs ambulation. Bone density should be reassessed on a yearly basis.

Non-Ambulatory Status

Functional status has been shown to be a predictor of survival to lung transplant and the highest studied risk

for poor postoperative survival is the requirement for preoperative invasive ventilation. Reports from various centers document a 1-year survival in such patients of less than 50 percent. Data on survival of patients receiving noninvasive ventilation (eg, nighttime CPAP or BIPAP) is not available, but is not thought to impact upon survival as long as patients remain ambulatory. Currently ventilated patients are considered only rarely to be appropriate candidates and then only if ventilated for very short time periods and in addition must meet all other criteria.

Musculoskeletal Disease

Progressive musculoskeletal disease resulting in poor lung function is not treatable by lung transplant and therefore is an absolute contraindication to transplantation. Kyphoscoliosis and other thoracic deformities are much more problematic and difficult to assess. In cases of kyphoscoliosis, full lung function studies including assessment of diffusing capacity along with routine and high-resolution chest CT scans may be helpful in trying to decide how much of the functional impairment is due to lung disease and how much is due to fixation of the thorax. When skeletal disease is the primary abnormality it is unlikely transplant will be successful and should be considered a relative contraindication.

Nutrition

Nutrition has been noted for some time to be a predictor of surgical outcome. Obesity has been documented as a potential negative outcome predictor in heart and kidney transplant, but no data is available in lung transplant recipients. Controversy exists as to the impact of low body weight in cystic fibrosis patients on outcomes. Overall, transplant physicians generally feel that severe malnutrition (either over or under weight) is a relative contraindication to lung transplantation. Both morbid obesity (IBW >130 percent of ideal) and severe undernutrition (IBW <70 percent of ideal) require preoperative intervention and in many centers are a relative contraindication, though one that can usually be effectively addressed.

Colonization

The thought on several issues in selection has evolved considerably as more experience has been accumulated in working with transplant candidates and recipients. Among these are issues of colonization of the potential candidate's lungs with potentially pathogenic bacteria. Cystic fibrosis patients and other patients with bronchiectasis are universally colonized as are varying proportions of other diagnoses at end-stage (eg, COPD patients). Recent data suggests that colonization with many organisms including even relatively resistant *pseudomonal sp* does not necessarily confer a negative survival risk. The same appears to be true of most fungi and atypical mycobacteria. However, the presence of these organisms preoperatively, especially *aspergillus sp*, often mandates either bilateral lung transplant or perioperative specific prophylaxis. The one organism that has almost universally been associated with a worse outcome and high levels of resistance is *B cepacia* and many programs consider presence of resistant strains of this organism an absolute contraindication. In the international guidelines, *pan resistance* is defined as resistance in vitro to all groups of antibiotics and *multiply resistant* as resistant to all agents in two of the following classes of antibiotics: the beta-lactams, aminoglycosides, and quinolones. Treated *M tuberculosis* infection is not a contraindication to lung transplantation; in general, patients who have positive tuberculin skin tests or have a history of old untreated or incompletely treated tuberculosis should have prophylaxis initiated when selected as candidates. Finally, a history of x-ray or serologic findings consistent with endemic fungal infections, principally histoplasmosis, blastomycosis and coccidiomycoses, do not contraindicate lung transplantation but specific perioperative prophylaxis should be considered in many cases.

Steroids

A second area where the approach to potential candidates has evolved considerably is in the use of perioperative steroids. In the early era of lung transplantation (1980s), oral steroids were felt to be a significant risk for bronchial anastomotic dehiscence; however, several studies have failed to confirm that theoretical threat. The greatest threat from prolonged oral steroid use is the myriad side effects that the medication causes: principally osteoporosis, myopathy, hyperglycemia, and obesity. Current recommendations are that the steroids should be reduced to the lowest dose possible, preferably to under 20 mg/day of predisone (or equivalent).

Psychosocial Issues and Drug Abuse

A third area that has been increasingly recognized as vital to the outcome of the transplant recipient is that of psychosocial health. Outcomes are critically dependent upon a recipient's ability and willingness to adhere to complex medication regimens, to cope with sudden and potentially fatal changes in clinical status and to do this within the framework of trying to maintain as normal a life as possible. Clearly, achieving all this is not simple or easy and requires patients with considerable coping skills and willing support systems. It also requires significant motivation, a desire and ability to be compliant with a structured care program and often considerable financial resources. Thus, relative contraindications include documented psychiatric problems that are not responsive to intervention, documented histories of medical noncompliance and active substance abuse. Candidates for lung transplant should be free of tobacco, alcohol or narcotic abuse for at least six months before being considered. Benzodiazepines can be used in moderation by potential candidates since these drugs are often helpful in managing the anxiety that many end-stage patients with severe dyspnea experience.

CONTRAINDICATIONS TO LUNG TRANSPLANTATION
Nonpulmonary Organ Dysfunction

In general, significant nonpulmonary organ dysfunction is an absolute contraindication to lung transplantation. Of particular importance is kidney function, since both the primary immunosuppressive drugs, cyclosporine and tacrolimus, universally reduce kidney function over time. Thus, creatinine clearances of less than half normal (<50 mg/mL per min) generally contraindicate transplant. Untreatable coronary disease or left ventricular dysfunction is also a general contraindication unless the patient is considered for heart-lung transplant.

Hepatic disease in which there is histologic evidence of fibrosis/cirrhosis is also often considered a contraindication. Other contraindications include the presence of hepatitis B antigen positivity and the presence of hepatitis C *if* it is accompanied by biopsy-proven histologic evidence of liver disease. Thus, the candidate presenting for evaluation who has hepatitis C should undergo liver biopsy to assess the health of the liver.

Malignancy

One of the murkiest areas in transplant candidate assessment is how to deal with the presence of a history of malignancy. The most complete compendium of post-transplant malignancies is kept in a registry in Ohio by Dr. I. Penn who has reported results from his data on a number of occasions. He also has data on outcomes of transplant recipients who had malignancies prior to transplantation and their subsequent outcomes. Unfortunately, reporting to this registry is completely voluntary and the information, while valuable, may not be completely accurate in terms of rates of recurrence of pretransplant disease. In general, Dr. Penn's data suggests that with the exception of basal and squamous cell carcinoma of the skin, patients with malignancy should not be considered for transplant within two years of the active malignancy. Tumors that have a propensity for late occurrence should probably have a longer disease-free period. These include lymphomas, most carcinomas of the breast, prostate or colon or large (>5 cm) symptomatic renal carcinomas. Patients with bronchoalveolar cell carcinoma have been transplanted with disappointing results.

SYSTEMIC DISEASE WITH SINGLE ORGAN FAILURE. Patients with a variety of diseases that are systemic, but that can result in isolated pulmonary failure, have been often referred and considered for lung transplantation. The number of transplants performed on such patients is small and outcome data are limited. Nevertheless systemic illness per se is not considered a contraindication to transplant as long as organs other than the lung have not been significantly damaged by the disease process. On rare occasions, a patient with isolated pulmonary plus one other organ failure (eg, a cystic fibrosis patient with pulmonary and hepatic disease) may be considered for a "multi organ" transplant. The most often-referred patients with systemic disease are those with collagen vascular processes, sarcoidosis, and cystic fibrosis. In these illnesses, care must be taken to assess the vital organs known to be often affected by the disease process and decisions regarding transplant candidacy made on an individual basis.

A second group of patients presenting for transplant are those who have systemic illness such as diabetes mellitus and who happen to have a progressive pulmonary disease not resulting from the systemic illness. In general, the same rules apply to these patients in that a careful search should be made for target organ damage and cases should be individually evaluated according to the general medical criteria described above.

TIMING OF PATIENT REFERRAL: DISEASE-SPECIFIC GUIDELINES

Since lung transplantation is limited by availability of donors and since there are many, many more candidates for lung grafts than there are organs available, it is important to choose candidates for the procedure who truly are very advanced in their illnesses, yet who are likely to survive the transplant experience. Because the wait for a donor organ(s) often exceeds a year and is usually at least several months, potential candidates for transplant are generally chosen when it is felt they have less than two years to live, yet are not so ill that they are not likely to survive the operation. While defining this stage of a patient's disease may sound – and sometimes is – difficult, data regarding prognosis and survival statistics are becoming increasingly available. Table 83-1 outlines specific pulmonary function and, in some cases, hemodynamic or supportive data that has been found helpful in estimating very limited survivals. These are guidelines recommended for referral of potential transplant candidates to transplant centers. Some of the other issues that are relevant to specific diagnoses are discussed below.

Nonbronchiectatic Chronic Obstructive Lung Disease

This category of pulmonary illness includes a number of diagnoses, but by far the largest group is smoking-related emphysema/chronic bronchitis in some combination. In this group of patients, it is important to ensure that maximal medical therapy of the underlying disease is in place, since a number of these patients will have significant reversible airways disease. Pulmonary rehabilitation and supplemental oxygen therapy may also make a significant impact upon the patient's quality of life and may influence a decision to go forward with transplant evaluation. In some patients who have predominant emphysema and who have particularly amenable disease, volume reduction surgery may be an option. While it is true that the long-term outcomes of volume reduction surgery are not yet clear, the less-than-50% survival of lung transplant recipients, along

Table 83-1. Diagnosis-Specific Parameters for Referral

Chronic Obstructive Airways Disease	Cystic Fibrosis/Bronchiectasis
FEV_1 <25% (Pred) and/or $PaCO_2$ >55 mmHg Elevated PAP	FEV_1 <30% (Pred) or FEV_1 >30% predicted and falling FEV_1 or Massive hemoptysis or cachexia or increasing hospitalizations $PaCO_2$ >55 mmHg PaO_2 <55 mmHg
Idiopathic Pulmonary Fibrosis	
Symptomatic, Progressive Reassess q 3 mos Rest or exercise desaturation VC <60% to 70% predicted D_L CO <50% to 60% predicted	Primary Pulmonary Hypertension
	NYHA III or IV despite optimum therapy CI <2L/min per m² RAP >15 mmHg PAP >55 mmHg
Eisenmenger's Syndrome	
Progressive symptoms NYHA III or IV	

with the huge financial burden and potential complications, can make the former a preferred choice, especially for older patients.

In this disease category, whether the diagnosis is emphysema/chronic bronchitis or the other most common obstructive process, bronchiolitis obliterans, survival times are the hardest to predict. Those patients with hypercapnia and progressive deterioration seem to have a poorer prognosis than those who have cor pulmonale. In general, however, patients with severe obstructive lung disease and marked limitation of activity to the point of having difficulty with routine activities of daily living may have rather prolonged survivals. In addition, registry data has shown that patients with this diagnostic category may not experience a survival benefit with transplant. Transplant centers and referring physicians should recognize this fact and clarify to their patients that transplant in this population often results in much improved functional ability and quality of life, but may not confer an increased survival.

Many of the patients undergoing lung transplant for obstructive lung disease receive unilateral grafts and have a significant cigarette smoking history. Computed tomography (see section below) is particularly important in this group of patients, as that modality can apparently pick up many early lung cancers not apparent on chest x-ray.

Cystic Fibrosis and Other Diseases with Bronchiectasis

The primary issue of concern in these populations are the organisms with which the patients are colonized. However, as noted earlier in this chapter, even panresistance is no longer a contraindication in and of itself, except in the case of *Burkholderia sp* in most centers. The most widely quoted survival data comes from a Canadian longitudinal study published by Kerem et al. This data may be somewhat biased since a number of the patients in that population were colonized with a relatively virulent strain of *B cepacia*. Newer US data suggests that in the absence of that organism, survivals with similar FEV_1s might be much better than that suggested by Kerem et al. In the absence of *B cepacia,* factors other than an FEV_1 of under 30% may be more important criteria for initiating transplant referral. Such factors include rate of deterioration, increasing oxygen requirements and frequency of hospital admissions. More data on survivals in non-cepacia colonized will undoubtedly be forthcoming and should help to revise referral recommendations.

A second factor that is occasionally important in the evaluation of cystic fibrosis patients is liver disease with portal hypertension, since most adult cystic fibrosis patients have some degree of focal biliary cirrhosis. Unless the patient is a candidate for liver-lung trans-

plant, symptomatic liver disease is a contraindication to lung transplantation in most centers. Other common issues in this group of patients, like diabetes mellitus, sinus disease, and malnutrition are rarely absolute contraindications to transplant.

Idiopathic Pulmonary Fibrosis

The main concern with this group of patients is late referral. Because of the high rates of death in patients with pulmonary fibrosis, the United Network for Organ Sharing now affords these patients a 'handicap' of 90 days when they are listed for transplant. It is not clear whether primary care physicians wait until too late in the illness to refer patients for transplant, or whether it is simply the rapid progression of disease that makes survival to transplant so difficult. Probably the more common scenario is that patients are relatively asymptomatic until very late in the illness and the degree of disease that is present is not appreciated either by patient or physician. Numerous articles have sought to define good prognostic criteria for patients with pulmonary fibrosis, but such criteria have been elusive. The guidelines suggested in Table 83-1 are aimed to encourage early referral of patients, as early as within a few months of diagnosis if there is not a measurable positive response to treatment or even at the time of diagnosis if certain pulmonary function criteria are met.

Pulmonary fibrosis patients are often near the upper age limit for lung transplant recipients and as such may have a number of comorbidities. Potential comorbidities related to their lung disease include bronchogenic carcinoma, areas of traction bronchiectasis and/or large cystic areas colonized with pathogenic bacteria or fungi. Computed tomography in this disease category, as in the obstructive lung disease group, is very important. Here, high-resolution images in addition to the usual scan are useful.

Other morbidities in pulmonary fibrosis patients are those of the normal aging population and those that are related to attempted therapy for the underlying pulmonary disease. Steroids and cytotoxic therapy are effective in probably no more than about 20% of patients, yet have a very important toxicity profile. Significant complications of these drugs include osteoporosis, obesity, diabetes mellitus and hemorrhagic cystitis. In cases in which these therapies are not ameliorating the pulmonary disease, it is important to withdraw the drugs or minimize doses to reduce the medical complications. Probably of most importance in the therapy of these patients is adequate supplemental oxygen, both at rest and with exercise, and a pulmonary rehabilitation program to maintain mobility as long as possible. Frequent reassessment (ie, every three months) is warranted because of the rapid progression of the disease.

Primary Pulmonary Hypertension

When the National Institutes of Health pulmonary hypertension registry information was gathered in the late 1980s, the reported outcomes were dismal, with a mean survival of all patients of about 2.8 years. The hemodynamic data that predicted poor survival were collected and are reproduced in Table 83-1. However, the outlook for these patients changed significantly in the mid- and late-1990s. Calcium channel blocker trials are often still tried in these patients, but the use of epoprostenol (Flolan®) as a continuous intravenous infusion treatment has become the "gold standard" of care for these patients in institutions where it is available, and appears not only to increase the functional capacity of most patients but also to benefit survival. Patients who have been listed for transplant frequently request that they be inactivated once starting on Flolan®. No data is yet available to tell whether the benefit of this drug is sustained over extended periods, and increasing doses are required on a regular basis in virtually all patients. Patients who do not do well with epoprostenol, or who initially do well and then deteriorate despite appropriate dosing, should be carefully evaluated so that the window of opportunity for transplant is not missed. The use of epoprostenol is fraught with a number of complications including recurrent line infections and distressing side-effects of the drug. On occasion, these may mandate early consideration for transplant rather than disease progression during treatment.

Another alternative therapy that has been suggested, and may be appropriate for palliative care in some patients who are rapidly deteriorating, is atrial septostomy.

Systemic Diseases Associated with Pulmonary Disease

Pulmonary fibrosis along with pulmonary hypertension (to be described later) are the two most common end-stage pulmonary processes found in systemic disease.

PULMONARY FIBROSIS. Underlying illnesses that can have pulmonary fibrosis as a primary end-organ manifestation include scleroderma, systemic lupus erythematosis, combined connective tissue disease, rheumatoid arthritis, and sarcoidosis among others. The manifestations of these diseases can be highly variable and each patient must be considered on an individual basis. In the autoimmune diseases, progressive pulmonary fibrosis tends to behave much like idiopathic pulmonary fibrosis and the guidelines in Table 83-1 are useful.

Sarcoidosis, on the other hand, which is probably the most commonly-referred systemic disease with end-stage pulmonary pathology, has a much more difficult-to-predict course. It is often many years before

a patient with sarcoidosis reaches end-stage. In addition, the pulmonary functions may be both obstructive and restrictive, or primarily obstructive. The end-stage sarcoid patient often has very low diffusing capacity and pulmonary hypertension. Though it usually takes many more years to get to end-stage with a diagnosis of sarcoidosis, as compared to idiopathic pulmonary fibrosis, the terminal phase of the disease is often not recognized until the patient is near death. Again, prognostic criteria are virtually nonexistent. The best approach for patients with sarcoid, as for patients with idiopathic pulmonary fibrosis, is to err on the side of early referral. Referral is appropriate when sarcoid patients begin to require supplemental oxygen or develop symptomatic disease that is no longer responsive to steroid or cytotoxic therapy.

Other primarily interstitial processes, that may or may not have a systemic component and present as end-stage lung disease include lymphangioleiomyomatosis and eosinophilic granuloma. These diseases also do not have well-described predictors for survival and patients are considered individually with decisions for listing made primarily based on an assessment of progressive functional deterioration.

It is of interest that a number of diseases have been reported to recur posttransplant and nearly all of these have been in the category of interstitial disease. Sarcoid is the most commonly recurring, though usually subclinical, disease. Other recurring diseases include lymphangioleiomyomatosis, eosinophilic granuloma, panbronchiolitis, giant cell interstitial pneumonia and desquamative interstitial pneumonitis.

Pulmonary Hypertension in Systemic Illness

Along with pulmonary fibrosis, pulmonary hypertension is a frequent manifestation in systemic disease. Among those diseases are scleroderma, systemic lupus erythematosis, sarcoidosis, and thromboembolic disease, and those that are medication-related. In general, pulmonary hypertension in these diagnoses has the same prognosis as in primary disease. As with primary disease, calcium channel blockers and, more recently, epoprostenol have been employed therapeutically. Little data is available on the usefulness of vasodilator therapy in these situations. If available and appropriate, alternative therapeutic interventions should be used. Thromboendarterectomy may be an option in selected patients with thromboembolic disease, for example. When considering patients with systemic disease for lung transplantation, it is important to remember that candidates should be eligible by all the general medical criteria outlined earlier in this chapter.

Eisenmenger's Syndrome

Pulmonary hypertension resulting from congenital heart disease behaves differently from primary pulmonary hypertension or pulmonary hypertension in systemic disease. Often these patients have as high as or higher pulmonary artery pressures than those of patients with primary disease, but right atrial pressures are lower and cardiac output is higher. Whether these slightly different hemodynamics are the reason or whether it is some other factor(s), these patients do not have the same prognosis as those with primary disease. In general, survival is much better in Eisenmenger patients than in those with primary or secondary disease with the same degree of pulmonary hypertension. Thus, predictors of survival are less reliable and it is unclear what criteria should be used. In addition, the role of vasodilator therapy in these patients is unclear. Because no other good predictors are available, patients are usually listed when they reach New York Heart Association class III or class IV status.

EVALUATION OF CANDIDATES

The evaluation of the transplant candidate includes blood and urine tests, imaging studies, pulmonary function studies, measures of exercise capacity, nutritional, financial and psychosocial assessments (Table 83-2). Many of these, usually with the exception of the psychosocial and financial assessments, can be done by the primary physician and do not need to be repeated at the transplant center.

BLOOD AND URINE TESTS

Testing can be divided into two areas: assessment of organ function and a measurement of serologies that reflect exposure to infectious agents. Abnormal values should precipitate further evaluations. For example, an abnormal liver function study may precipitate an ultrasound or other evaluation or an abnormal creatinine may mandate a creatinine clearance. Some centers

---

Table 83-2. Recommended Investigations in Transplant Candidates

Full pulmonary function studies
6-minute walk test or other study of exercise capacity
Electrocardiogram
Echocardiogram
Computed tomography of chest with high-resolution images
Stress echocardiogram or angiography in high-risk patients
Bone mineral density study
24-hour creatinine clearance
Liver function studies

---

require 24-hour creatinine clearance in all patients because of the universal nephrotoxicity of immunosuppressive agents.

The blood tests required for assessment of target organs are routine renal and hepatic panels. In addition, complete blood counts of electrolytes and minerals are measured. Serologies looking for exposure to cytomegalovirus, herpes simplex, Epstein-Barr virus, hepatitis B and hepatitis C are obtained. If the patient is ultimately found to be a suitable candidate for transplant, tissue typing will also be done.

PULMONARY FUNCTIONS AND EXERCISE CAPACITY

Full pulmonary function studies including reliable lung volumes should be done within the three to six months prior to referral. In addition, some measure of exercise capacity is very useful since it has been associated with survival while awaiting a transplant. The most commonly-used test of exercise capacity is the 6-minute walk test, as it can be done by most patients even with well-advanced disease and can be repeated with subsequent preoperative visits easily. During these tests, oxygen saturation should be measured to ensure that the patient is on adequate amounts of supplemental oxygen.

IMAGING STUDIES: LUNGS, HEART, BONE

Imaging studies of both the heart and lungs are required in most patients presenting for transplant. The most important study of the lungs is computed tomography with some high-resolution slices. This study can help to characterize pleural and parenchymal disease as well as any mediastinal abnormalities. Unsuspected nodules, areas of bronchiectasis, bullae or cystic areas are all readily identified on these scans. For patients who will receive unilateral grafts, often one side will be identified as preferable for transplant. Some centers perform quantitative ventilation/perfusion scans in addition to the CT scans. They find this useful in deciding which lung to transplant in the cases of unilateral transplants or, alternatively, which lung to transplant first in bilateral transplants especially if there is a desire to avoid cardiopulmonary bypass.

Cardiac disease must be excluded in lung transplant recipients. Electrocardiograms and echocardiograms are performed in all potential candidates. Of particular importance in the echocardiographic data is left ventricular size and function, right ventricular size and function, and estimate of right ventricular systolic pressure and any evidence of intracardiac shunting. Stress echocardiograms and/or coronary arteriography are performed in patients over 40 or who have risk factors or symptoms suggestive of coronary artery disease. Recent recommendations from the American College of Cardiology suggest that coronary arteriography in assessing patients for noncardiac solid organ transplant should be limited to this latter high-risk group.

In nearly all lung transplant centers, bone mineral density measurements are now required of patients being evaluated for lung transplantation. These studies are done to document the status of the bones and to guide replacement therapy preoperatively and post-operatively. Since most patients experience a significant bone loss in the first six months posttransplant, it is appropriate to initiate antiresorptive therapy in patients who have osteopenia or more severe bone disease pre-transplant. Appropriate therapy includes hormone replacement therapy in both female and male patients who are deficient and bisphosphonate or other treatment as well. In osteopenic patients, oral therapy in addition to appropriate calcium and vitamin D intake is probably sufficient, whereas, in osteoporotic patients, intravenous therapy may address the problem more quickly and effectively.

NUTRITIONAL ASSESSMENT

Patients who fall outside the recommended variation from ideal body weight should have nutritional counseling. In the case of obese patients, the institution of a proper diet and increased exercise as well as a reduction in steroid dose (when possible) usually results in the person attaining adequate weight loss to be listed for transplant. Very malnourished patients may require supplemental feeding via a nasogastric tube or a PEG placed directly into the stomach. Cystic fibrosis patients in particular appear to benefit from these feeding approaches and often can gain significant amounts of weight with nighttime feedings.

PSYCHOSOCIAL ASSESSMENT

Probably no assessment is more important in the evaluation of the prospective lung transplant candidate than the psychosocial assessment. The major areas addressed in this assessment are those of substance abuse, limiting anxiety and depression, issues of medical compliance, coping skills and support system adequacy. Major psychiatric diagnoses are rarely an issue though borderline personality traits that may impact upon long-term outcome are sometimes identified. The purpose of this assessment is not only to identify areas that might impact long-term outcome, but also areas for which positive interventions (eg, antidepressants) can improve the patient's quality of life and status as a potential recipient. It is also an important part of this assessment to identify active substance abuse issues and to initiate appropriate treatment if necessary.

Patients deemed to have untreatable or unresponsive psychosocial barriers to a successful outcome should not be transplanted.

FINANCIAL ASSESSMENT

The financial impact of transplant extends far beyond the perioperative period. Many insurance companies have a fixed amount than can be spent on transplant or have a cap on the amount that will be spent for drugs. Some patients who are no longer able to work have ongoing insurance for a limited period which, when it lapses, leaves them completely uncovered. Patients need to be counseled that the ongoing cost of drugs can be as much as $1,000 to $2,000 per month and that these costs will continue into the indefinite future. In addition, complications are frequent and many visits to the transplant center are likely. While many posttransplant patients will be well enough to work, finding suitable employment may be difficult. Significant costs related to the transplant will continue for the rest of their lives.

FINAL SELECTION AND EDUCATION

When all data is gathered regarding a potential candidate it should be reviewed by members of the transplant team and a decision made by the team as to the patient's candidacy. The transplant review board/committee is usually comprised of the transplant pulmonologist, transplant surgeon, social worker, transplant coordinator, relevant subspecialty representation (eg, transplant cardiologist, nephrologist). Before transplant, it is essential that the patient is fully educated as to the entire transplant process: what the transplant process will entail, what will be expected of him, what will be required in terms of follow-up and compliance, what the costs will be, what the complications, risks and survivals are, etc.

PRETRANSPLANT PERIOD

Periodic follow-up during the pretransplant period ensures that the patient remains a viable candidate and helps the team and the patient stay "connected." These visits are handled in different ways at different centers. It is useful to periodically repeat exercise capacity tests, assess oxygen requirements and the overall nutritional and psychosocial status of the patient. If patients are on the wait list for more than a year it may be useful to repeat the echocardiogram and the CT scan.

RECOMMENDED READING

Hosenpud JD, Bennett LE, Keck BM, Fiol B, Boucek MM, Novick RJ. The Registry of the International Society for Heart and Lung Transplantation: fifteenth official report – 1998. J Heart Lung Transplant. 1998;17(7):656-661.

Panos RJ, Mortenson RL, Niccoli SA, King TE Jr. Clinical deterioration in patients with idiopathic pulmonary fibrosis: causes and assessment. Am J Med. 1990;88(4): 396-404.

Julian BA, Laskow DA, Dubovsky J, Dubovsky EV, Curtis JJ, Quarles LD. Rapid loss of vertebral mineral density after renal transplantation. N Engl J Med. 1991;325(8): 544-550.

Aris RM, Neuringer IP, Weiner MA, Egan TM, Ontjes D. Severe osteoporosis before and after lung transplantation. Chest. 1996;109(5):1176-1183.

Sharples L, Hathaway T, Dennis C, Caine N, Higenbottam T, Wallwork J. Prognosis of patients with cystic fibrosis awaiting heart and lung transplantation. J Heart Lung Transplant. 1993;12(4):669-674.

Plochl W, Pezawas L, Artemiou O, Grimm M, Klepetko W, Hiesmayr M. Nutritional status, ICU duration and ICU mortality in lung transplant recipients. Intensive Care Med. 1996;22(11):1179-1185.

Grady KL, Costanzo MR, Fisher S, Koch D. Preoperative obesity is associated with decreased survival after heart transplantation. J Heart Lung Transplant. 1996;15(9): 863-871.

Aris RM, Gilligan PH, Neuringer IP, Gott KK, Rea J, Kankaskas JR. The effects of panresistant bacteria in cystic fibrosis patients on lung transplant outcome. Am J Resp Crit Care Med. 1997;155(5):1699-1704.

Penn I. Posttransplant malignancies. Transplant Proc. 1999;31(1-2):1260-1262.

Penn I. Evaluation of transplant candidates with pre-existing malignancies. Ann Transplant. 1997;2(4): 14-17.

Yeatman M, McNeil K, Smith JA, et al. Lung transplantation in patients with systemic diseases: an eleven-year experience at Papworth Hospital. J Heart Lung Transplant. 1996;15(2):144-149.

Moy ML, Ingenito EP, Mentzer SJ, Evans RB, Reilly JJ Jr. Health-related quality of life improves following pulmonary rehabilitation and lung volume reduction surgery. Chest. 1999;115(2):383-389.

Anthonisen NR. Prognosis in chronic obstructive pulmonary disease: results from multi center clinical trials. Am Rev Resp Dis. 1989;140(3pt2):S95-S99.

Hosenpud JD, Bennett LE, Keck BM, Edwards EB, Novick RJ. Effect of diagnosis on survival benefit of lung transplantation for end-stage lung disease. Lancet. 1998;351(9095):24-27.

Kerem E, Reisman J, Corey M, Canny GT, Levison H. Prediction of mortality in patients with cystic fibrosis. N Engl J Med. 1992;326(18):1187-1191.

Doershuk CF, Stern RC. Timing of referral for lung transplantation for cystic fibrosis: overemphasis on FEV may adversely affect overall survival. Chest. 1999;115(3): 782-787.

Turner-Warwick M, Burrows B, Johnson A. Cryptogenic fibrosing alveolitis: response to corticosteroid treatment and its effect on survival. Thorax. 1980;35(8):593-599.

Hanson D, Winterbauer RH, Kirtland SH, Wu R Changes in pulmonary function test results after 1 year of therapy as predictors of survival in patients with idiopathic pulmonary fibrosis. Chest. 1995;108(2):305-310.

Schwartz DA, Helmers RA, Galvin JR, et al. Determinants of survival in idiopathic pulmonary fibrosis. Am J Respir Crit Care Med. 1994;149(2 Pt 1):450-454.

Vestbo J, Viskum K. Respiratory symptoms at presentation and long-term vital prognosis in patients with pulmonary sarcoidosis. Sarcoidosis. 1994;11(2):123-125.

Mana J, Salazar A, Pujol R, Manresa F. Are the pulmonary function tests and the markers of activity helpful to establish the prognosis of sarcoidosis? Respiration. 1996;63(5):298-303.

Padilla ML, Schilero GJ, Teirstein AS. Sarcoidosis and transplantation. Sarcoidosis Vasc Diffuse Lung Dis. 1997;14(1):16-22.

Nine JS, Yousem SA, Paradis IL, Keenan R, Griffith BP. Lymphangioleiomyomatosis: recurrence after lung transplantation. J Heart Lung Transplant. 1994;13(4): 714-719.

Baz MA, Kussin PS, Van Trigt P, Davis RD, Roggli VL, Tapson VF. Recurrence of diffuse panbronchiolitis after lung transplantation. Am J Respir Crit Care Med. 1995:151(3 Pt 1):895-898.

Gabbay E, Dark JH, Ashcroft T, et al. Recurrence of Langerhan's cell granulomatosis following lung transplantation. Thorax. 1998;53(4):326-327.

Frost AE, Keller CA, Brown RW, et al. Giant cell interstitial pneumonitis. Disease recurrence in the transplanted lung. Am Rev Respir Dis. 1993;148(5):1401-1404.

King MB, Jessurun J, Hertz MI. Recurrence of desquamative interstitial pneumonia after lung transplantation. Am J Respir Crit Care Med. 1997;156(6):2003-2005.

D'Alonzo GE, Barst RJ, Ayers SM, et al. Survival in patients with primary pulmonary hypertension. Results from a national prospective registry. Ann Intern Med. 1991;115(5):343-349.

Hopkins WE, Ochoa LL, Richardson GW, Trulock EP. Comparison of the hemodynamics and survival of adults with severe primary pulmonary hypertension or Eisenmenger syndrome. J Heart Lung Transplant. 1996;15(1 Pt 1):100-105.

84 LIVING-DONOR LOBAR LUNG TRANSPLANTATION: DONOR EVALUATION AND SELECTION

Felicia A. Schenkel, RN, BS, CCTC
Mark L. Barr, MD
Vaughn A. Starnes, MD

Over the past three decades, the field of lung transplantation has undergone steady development in the areas of donor and recipient operative techniques, organ preservation, immunosuppressive drug management, and prevention and control of infectious complications. However, the availability of cadaveric donor lungs has failed to match the dramatic increase in the number of potential recipients referred for lung transplantation. For those patients who require bilateral lung transplantation due to the nature of their underlying pulmonary disease, this donor/recipient disparity is even further exaggerated. The increasing number of deaths on the lung transplant waiting list led to the development of living-donor lobar lung transplantation, in which the adult or pediatric recipient receives the right and left lower lobes from a pair of living adult donors. This chapter will focus on the living-donor lobar evaluation and selection process, and postoperative results.

EVALUATION OF POTENTIAL DONORS
Selection

Although immediate family members were initially the only donors considered, lobes from extended family members and unrelated individuals who can demonstrate an emotional attachment to the recipient are currently being used routinely. Potential recipients are encouraged to provide a list of all potential willing donors with information on height, weight, age, relationship, and smoking history. Donors must be between the ages of 18 and 55, have had no thoracic procedures

Felicia A. Schenkel, RN, BS, CCTC, Senior Cardiothoracic Transplant Coordinator, Department of Cardiothoracic Surgery, University of Southern California School of Medicine, Los Angeles, CA

Mark L. Barr, MD, Associate Professor of Cardiothoracic Surgery, Department of Cardiothoracic Surgery, University of Southern California and Children's Hospital Los Angeles, Los Angeles, CA

Vaughn A. Starnes, MD, Hastings Professor and Chairman, Department of Cardiothoracic Surgery, University of Southern California and Children's Hospital Los Angeles, Los Angeles, CA

on the side to be donated, and be in good general health. Donors taller than the recipient are favored over donors of the same or lesser height than the recipient to provide more lung reserve. Several potential donors are selected from that list by the transplant team and are contacted for a preliminary psychosocial evaluation to evaluate their desire to donate. Subsequently, they undergo preliminary screening with blood typing for compatibility, a chest x-ray to assess size, and spirometry to assure normal or supernormal pulmonary function. A more thorough medical work-up is completed after the preliminary screening results are evaluated (Table 84-1). Since many patients are referred from outside the geographic vicinity, the majority of potential donors are evaluated at outlying institutions, thereby limiting pretransplant stay and minimizing time away from work, family and home. In addition, a preliminary screening process allows for evaluation of a limited number of potential donors, thereby reducing costs. Unfortunately, an outside hospital evaluation has the disadvantage of decreasing the interaction between the potential donor and the transplant team. Thus, intense communication is required between the referring institution, insurance carrier and transplant center to facilitate the evaluation process for both the medical staff and family.

After two suitable donors have been identified, one donor is chosen to undergo removal of the right lower lobe and the other for removal of the left lower lobe. If an acceptable donor has a history of thoracic procedures, trauma or infections, the contralateral side is chosen for donation. Otherwise, the larger donor is selected for donation of the right lobe because it is usually smaller than the left lobe. If the two donors are the same height, the donor with the most complete fissure on the left is chosen to donate that side. HLA-matching is not

Table 84-1. Medical Screening for Potential Donors
Spirometry with arterial blood gas (forced vital capacity and forced expiratory volume in one second must be greater than 85% predicted and arterial oxygenation must be greater than 80 mmHg on room air)
Chest x-ray
Routine transplant serologies, including HIV, VDRL, CMV, EBV, and hepatitis serologies
Electrocardiogram and echocardiogram (stress testing for donors over age 40)
Quantitative ventilation/perfusion scan with differential split and segmental analysis
High-resolution chest computerized tomography

required for donor selection. In the series at the University of Southern California, the donor cohort of 174 patients (60% male and 40% female) had a mean age of 39 years (range 18-55), a mean height of 170 cm (range 155-191), and a mean weight of 72 kg (range 50-105).

Psychosocial Evaluation

Concurrent with the medical evaluation, a thorough psychosocial evaluation is performed. Initially, only the mother and father of the recipient were considered for donation. However, many of the older cystic fibrosis patients had parents who were too old for donation. Subsequently, siblings were added to the list of potential donors. This group has created concerns regarding potential coercion of the donor because some felt that they had no choice other than donation to remain integrated in the family. After careful consultation and explanation of the procedure, those patients who still feel pressured to donate are denied on the basis of unspecified reasons. This prevents any untoward feelings between the family, recipient, and potential donor. Currently, extended family and friends who can demonstrate a close relationship or emotional attachment to the recipient are considered suitable donors. Interestingly, friends appear to be the group with the least concern regarding coercion to donate, as they have volunteered to donate out of concern for the recipient rather than out of a feeling of responsibility. Table 84-2 shows the relationship of the donor to the recipient in the USC cohort.

Potential donors are interviewed both separately (to assess for signs of coercion) and with the recipient and family to ascertain family dynamics. All potential donors meet with the team social worker and transplant coordinator. Key issues include the donor's motivation to donate, pain tolerance, feelings regarding donation

Table 84-2. Donor Relationship to Recipient

Related	N	(%)	Nonrelated	N	(%)
Mother	33	-19	Friend	30	-17.1
Brother	27	-15.5	Husband	1	-0.6
Father	25	-14.4			
Sister	14	-8			
Cousin	19	-10.9			
Uncle	13	-7.5			
Aunt	5	-2.9			
Distant family	4	-2.3			
Son	1	-0.6			
Niece	1	-0.6			
Grandmother	1	-0.6			
N = 174					

should the recipient expire, and their ability to be separated from family and career obligations. Spouses and other key family members of the donor are also interviewed to obtain their opinions regarding the potential donation. Donors and their spouses meet patients who have previously donated a lobe to ask questions regarding medical issues, family relationships and financial concerns. This can also familiarize the potential donor with the incision and the medical equipment that they will encounter during their stay. All patients take a tour of the postoperative unit prior to hospitalization to become familiar with their surroundings. Issues that arise in many interviews concern the ability to return to work and the loss of income during this time. Many patients' employers provide short-term disability policies, which lessens donors' concerns. Some donors have fears regarding the long-term effect on their careers, such as pilots and police officers. Prior to donation, the appropriate agencies are consulted regarding their policies concerning lobectomy and return to work. Other concerns include the costs of relocating to the area during the donation and for subsequent aftercare. A social worker is available to help facilitate housing and travel arrangements for both donors and their families during their stay in the area.

POSTOPERATIVE DONOR MANAGEMENT

Following the lobectomy, donors are transported to the recovery room with epidural catheters in place for pain management via a patient-controlled analgesia unit. They are then transferred to the cardiothoracic floor where many patients prefer to share a semi-private room with the other donor so they may share concerns with each other and support from family and friends. This has led to a healthy competition between the donors allowing them to encourage each other to walk and exercise. Two chest tubes are required until any air leak has stopped, chest tube output is acceptable, and the remaining lung tissue fills the hemithorax. Respiratory therapy consists of frequent intermittent positive pressure breathing and the use of an incentive spirometer. Physical therapy is consulted to provide exercises to encourage the patients to mobilize the upper extremity on the surgical side. Patients are also encouraged to ambulate in the halls and outside as tolerated. Oral analgesics are administered upon removal of the chest tubes and are continued for a short time at home.

DONOR OUTCOME
Morbidity

There have been no cases of donor mortality and a relatively low incidence of donor morbidity (Table 84-3). The most common "complication" has consisted of prolonged air leaks resulting in increased chest tube duration. The average hospital length of stay for donors is approximately eight days. Four donors have required surgical re-exploration during the initial hospitalization, none of which resulted in long-term complications. Six patients developed post-pericardiotomy syndrome (two patients required corticosteroids and one required a pericardial window). The most serious complication seen to date has been thrombus in the pulmonary artery that resulted in significant acute respiratory distress. Both patients with this complication were treated with intravenous heparin followed by oral anticoagulation, and have had no long-term sequelae.

Donors are instructed to stay in the local region for one week to have a follow-up clinic visit and chest x-ray. One and two year postoperative pulmonary function testing has demonstrated an average decrease of 17% in forced vital capacity, 15% in forced expiratory volume in one second and 16% in total lung capacity from preoperative values. All donors have returned to their activities of daily living without restrictions.

Quality of Life Issues Following Donation

To evaluate the long-term perceptions regarding physical functioning, personal and emotional health, social interactions, and changes in health status, the donors have been followed using a modified RAND 36-item survey. There were 137 patients involved in this substudy: 99% of the donors had no regrets about donating, 97% felt no pressure regarding donation, and 99% of donors felt the donation had either not changed or had

strengthened their relationships with the recipient, other donors and family members. In addition, 85% of donors surveyed rated their health no different or improved following their donation. This survey included donors for recipients who died after the operation.

SUMMARY

Lobar lung transplantation using living donors provides a reasonable alternative for both adult and pediatric patients for whom a cadaveric organ is not available. Because the procedure presents risks to the donors, both recipient and donor selection must be performed carefully. Close monitoring of the donors in regard to postoperative pulmonary function and exercise capability has demonstrated that this procedure is well-tolerated from a physiologic standpoint. Quality of life studies have revealed that the great majority of donors have been extremely satisfied with their decision to donate. Despite the concerns regarding risks to the living healthy donors, the results of the USC experience have demonstrated the safety of this procedure. Living-donor lobar donation provides organ availability that can be life saving in severely ill patients who will either die or become unsuitable recipients before a cadaveric organ becomes available.

RECOMMENDED READING

Schenkel FA, Barr ML, Starnes VA. Living related lobar transplantation. In: Williams BAH, Sandiford-Guttenbeil DM, eds. Trends in Organ Transplantation. New York, NY: Springer Publishing Co., Inc.; 1996:179-187.

Cohen RG, Barr ML, Schenkel FA, DeMeester TR, Wells WG, Starnes VA. Living-related donor lobectomy for bilateral lobar transplantation in patients with cystic fibrosis. Ann Thorac Surg. 1994;57(6):1423-1428.

Starnes VA, Barr ML, Cohen RG, et al. Living-donor lobar lung transplantation experience: intermediate results. J Thorac Cardiovasc Surg. 1996;112(5):1284-1291.

Barr ML, Schenkel FA, Cohen RG, et al. Recipient and donor outcomes in living related and unrelated lobar transplantation. Transplant Proc. 1998;30(5):2261-2263.

Table 84-3. Donor Complications		
	N	**(%)**
Dressler's Syndrome	6	-3
Re-explorations	4	-2
Sterile empyema (1)		
Bleeding (2)		
Persistent air leak (1)		
Pulmonary artery thrombosis / embolism	2	-1
N = 174		

85 LIVING-DONOR LOBAR LUNG TRANSPLANTATION: SURGICAL TECHNIQUE AND PERIOPERATIVE MANAGEMENT

Craig J. Baker, MD
Mark L. Barr, MD
Vaughn A. Starnes, MD

Live donor lobar transplantation has surgically evolved to avoid morbidity to the healthy volunteer while allowing adequate tissue margins for implantation in the recipient. Lobar vascular and bronchial anatomy, along with sufficient pulmonary volume, has led to the routine use of the right and left lower lobes. Explantation of the upper lobes involves multiple arteries, whereas the middle lobe, while easily removed, frequently performs segmentally upon implantation, often incapable of accepting a full cardiac output in conditions associated with pulmonary hypertension. These circumstances, in addition to the variability of middle lobe venous drainage, suggest that lower lobe donation is associated with the fewest potential complications. The anatomy of these lobes has permitted their removal with minimal complications in the donor and has provided adequate pulmonary reserve in the recipient. The optimal method to determine an appropriate size match between the donor and recipient has yet to be determined. Currently, computed tomographic scans and spirometry are used to estimate lung volumes. Further improvements in this methodology are warranted.

DONOR SURGICAL TECHNIQUE

The donors are placed in separate operating rooms and epidural catheters are inserted for postoperative pain control. After induction of anesthesia, fiberoptic bronchoscopy is performed to exclude infection, inflammation or alterations in bronchial anatomy. The single-lumen endotracheal tube is subsequently replaced with a

Craig J. Baker, MD, Senior Research Fellow, Department of Cardiothoracic Surgery, University of Southern California and Children's Hospital Los Angeles, Los Angeles, CA

Mark L. Barr, MD, Associate Professor of Cardiothoracic Surgery, Department of Cardiothoracic Surgery, University of Southern California and Children's Hospital Los Angeles, Los Angeles, CA

Vaughn A. Starnes, MD, Hastings Professor and Chairman, Department of Cardiothoracic Surgery, University of Southern California and Children's Hospital Los Angeles, Los Angeles, CA

double-lumen tube, and the patient is positioned in the appropriate lateral decubitus position. Prostaglandin E1 is administered intravenously to dilate the pulmonary bed and the dosage is adjusted to maintain a systolic blood pressure of 90 to 100 mmHg. There are important differences in performing a lobectomy for lobar transplantation in comparison with that for cancer or infection. The lobe must be removed with an adequate cuff of bronchus and pulmonary artery and vein to allow for successful implantation into the recipient. In general, all dissection in the donor is performed on the side of the remaining lung to minimize trauma to the lobar graft.

Donor Right Lower Lobectomy

After the donor lung is deflated, the chest is entered through a standard posterolateral thoracotomy incision and the lung is carefully inspected to exclude unsuspected pathology. Excellent exposure is mandatory, allowing dissection of hilar structures without excessive manipulation or clamping of the graft. The inferior pulmonary ligament is incised with electrocautery, and the mediastinal pleura is dissected to the superior pulmonary vein anteriorly and the lower margin of the takeoff of the right upper lobe bronchus posteriorly. Dissection in the fissure characterizes anatomic variants and identifies the pulmonary arteries to the right lower lobe and right middle lobe. The relationship between the superior segmental artery to the right lower lobe and middle lobe artery should be visualized. Commonly, the middle lobe has two arteries, with the smaller artery having a more distal origin than the superior segmental artery to the lower lobe. In this case, the smaller artery may be divided. Ideally, there will be sufficient distance between the take-off of the middle lobe artery and the superior segmental artery of the right lower lobe to allow placement of a vascular clamp distal to the middle lobe artery (Figure 85-1). This enables a sufficient vascular cuff for the pulmonary arterial anastomosis at implantation.

After confirming that the inferior pulmonary vein does not receive venous drainage from the right middle lobe, the pericardium surrounding the inferior pulmonary vein is incised. This dissection allows a vascular clamp to be placed on the left atrium and the inferior pulmonary vein cut with an adequate cuff on the donor lobe (Figure 85-2). When the vascular dissections are complete, the fissures are stapled using a 75 mm nonvascular stapler and raw areas of pulmonary parenchyma are cauterized.

The lung is reinflated and ventilated for five to ten minutes. Ten thousand units of heparin and 500 mg of methylprednisolone are administered intravenously after reinflation and allowed to circulate while the lung is inspected for air leaks. The lung is then deflated. To avoid vascular congestion of the pulmonary allograft, a vascular clamp is placed first on the pulmonary artery and subsequently on the left atrial side of the inferior pul-

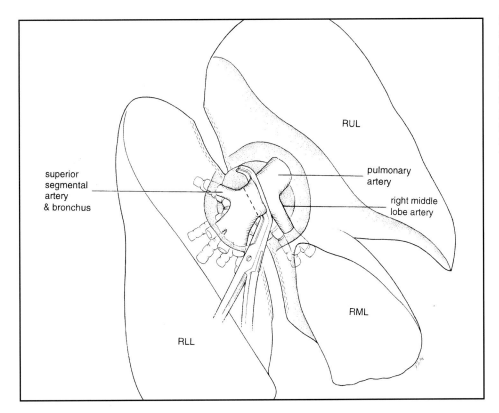

Figure 85-1. Dissection and division of the pulmonary artery for donor right lower lobectomy. Reprinted with permission from Cohen RG, Barr ML, Schenkel FA, DeMeester TR, Wells WG, Starnes VA. Living-related donor lobectomy for bilateral lobar transplantation in patients with cystic fibrosis. Ann Thorac Surg. 1994;57(6):1423-1427.

monary vein, optimizing the length of the venous cuff for pulmonary venous anastomosis. The pulmonary artery is transected at a point that will allow an adequate vascular cuff for anastomosis while leaving enough length to permit repair without compromising the remaining pulmonary arterial branches. The inferior pulmonary vein is transected with a small cuff of left atrium.

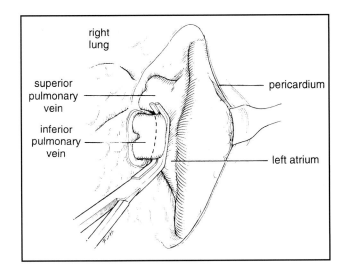

Figure 85-2. Dissection of the right inferior pulmonary vein so that a vascular clamp can be placed on the intrapericardial left atrium. Reprinted with permission from Cohen RG, Barr ML, Schenkel FA, DeMeester TR, Wells WG, Starnes VA. Living-related donor lobectomy for bilateral lobar transplantation in patients with cystic fibrosis. Ann Thorac Surg. 1994;57(6):1423-1427.

The bronchus to the right lower lobe should now be exposed. Minimizing dissection around the bronchus preserves blood supply to both the donor lobe and the remaining lung. The right middle lobe bronchus is identified and a no. 15 blade is used to tangentially transect the bronchus to the lower lobe. The incision begins in the bronchus intermedius above the bronchus to the superior segment of the right lower lobe, and moves obliquely to a point just below the takeoff of the right middle lobe bronchus (Figure 85-3).

Division of the pulmonary vessels and bronchus should be performed expeditiously to limit the warm ischemic time of the allograft. When separated, the donor lobe is wrapped in a cold, moist sponge and taken to a separate, sterile table for preservation. The donor's pulmonary artery is repaired in two layers with a running polypropylene suture and the pulmonary vein/left atrium is closed in a similar fashion. The bronchus is closed with interrupted polypropylene, being careful to avoid narrowing of the bronchus intermedius or infolding of the middle lobe carina. The bronchial suture line is covered with a pleural flap to separate the arterial and bronchial suture lines. Two chest tubes are placed in the pleural space and the chest is closed in the standard fashion.

Donor Left Lower Lobectomy

The chest is opened in a similar fashion to that described for the right side. The inferior pulmonary ligament is incised and dissection in the fissure defines vascular

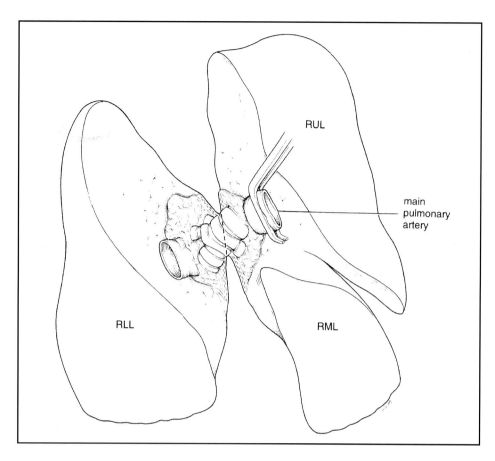

RUL

main
pulmonary
artery

RLL

RML

Figure 85-3. Dissection and division of the bronchus to the right lower lobe. Reprinted with permission from Cohen RG, Barr ML, Schenkel FA, DeMeester TR, Wells WG, Starnes VA. Living-related donor lobectomy for bilateral lobar transplantation in patients with cystic fibrosis. Ann Thorac Surg. 1994;57(6):1423-1427.

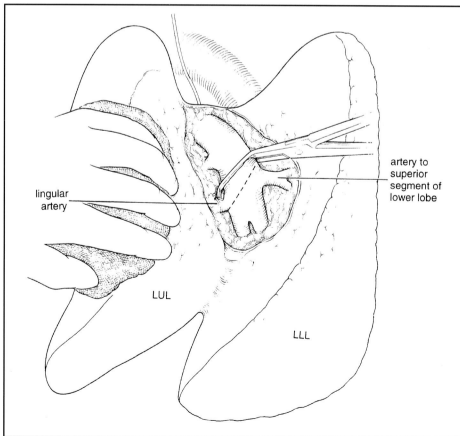

lingular
artery

artery to
superior
segment of
lower lobe

LUL

LLL

Figure 85-4. Dissection and division of the pulmonary artery for donor left lower lobectomy. Reprinted with permission from Cohen RG, Barr ML, Schenkel FA, DeMeester TR, Wells WG, Starnes VA. Living-related donor lobectomy for bilateral lobar transplantation in patients with cystic fibrosis. Ann Thorac Surg. 1994;57(6):1423-1426.

anatomy. The relationship between the superior segmental artery to the lower lobe and the anteriorly positioned lingular artery is evaluated. The lingular artery may be ligated and divided if it is of small size and its origin is too far distal to the artery to the superior segment of the lower lobe. If the significance of this artery is uncertain, the anesthesiologist can inflate the lung and subsequently deflate while this artery is being occluded. If the lingular segment does not become atelectatic, reflecting impaired absorption atelectasis secondary to poor blood flow, reimplantation of the lingular artery is suggested. Dissection of the pulmonary artery to the lower lobe should enable placement of a vascular clamp proximal to the artery supplying the superior segment of the lower lobe (Figure 85-4). The pericardium around the inferior pulmonary vein is opened circumferentially and the fissures are completed with a nonvascular stapler.

When the dissection is complete, the lung is reinflated and ventilated for five to ten minutes as described for the right side. Heparin and methylprednisolone are administered. The lung is subsequently deflated and the pulmonary artery and vein are clamped and transected in the sequence described for the right lung. The exposed bronchus is followed upward until the lingular bronchus is identified. The tangential transection begins at the base of the upper lobe bronchus and ends superiorly to the bronchus to the superior segment of the left lower lobe (Figure 85-5). The donor lobe is

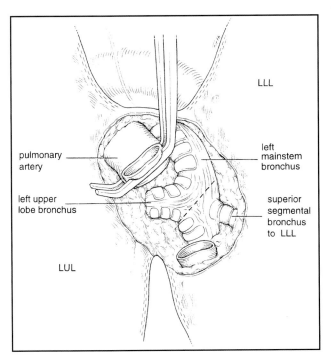

Figure 85-5. Dissection and division of the bronchus to the left lower lobe. Reprinted with permission from Cohen RG, Barr ML, Schenkel FA, DeMeester TR, Wells WG, Starnes VA. Living-related donor lobectomy for bilateral lobar transplantation in patients with cystic fibrosis. Ann Thorac Surg. 1994;57(6):1423-1427.

then taken to a separate table for preservation and storage. The pulmonary vessels and bronchus are repaired in a manner similar to that previously described.

ALLOGRAFT PRESERVATION

Preparation of the donor lobe begins at the start of the donor operation with a continuous prostaglandin infusion and meticulous attention to operative technique during the lobectomy. In contrast to cadaveric lung explantation, preservation of the live donor lobe does not permit in vivo flushing and cooling of the graft with high potassium-containing preservation solutions. Therefore, after the donor lobe is removed, it is taken to a separate, sterile table for preservation. The allograft is immersed in cold crystalloid solution. The pulmonary artery and vein are cannulated in an alternating fashion and flushed with one to two liters of cold, pulmonoplegic solution until the pulmonary venous and arterial effluent is clear and the parenchyma is blanched white. During perfusion, the lobe is gently ventilated with room air. A ventilation bag with different-sized endotracheal tubes should be available. Using an appropriately-sized endotracheal tube will allow an adequate seal to be formed while ventilating the bronchus and will prevent potential damage to the bronchus caused by crushing or squeezing the bronchus in order to obtain an adequate seal. Depending on the length of the bronchus, it may be necessary to intubate the superior segment bronchus separately with a smaller tube to ventilate that portion of the lobe. The superior segment artery may have to be perfused separately as well. Care must be taken to prevent the crystalloid bath or the preservation solution effluent from entering the bronchus. In addition, a manometer is fastened to the ventilation apparatus and the lobe is inflated to a pressure of 20 to 25 mmHg, being careful to avoid overpressurizing the lung. After adequate perfusion and ventilation, a final breath is administered to achieve approximately 75% maximum inflation, the endotracheal tube is quickly removed, and the bronchus is occluded with a noncrushing clamp. The donor lobe is placed in sterile bags with cold storage solution, and transported to the recipient operating room in an ice-filled cooler.

RECIPIENT SURGICAL TECHNIQUE
Recipient Pneumonectomy

While the donor operations are being performed, the recipient operation commences in a third operating room. The operation is performed through a transverse thoracosternotomy (clamshell) incision, which provides exposure for cardiac cannulation and adequate access to the pleural spaces. The clamshell incision is preferred over a standard median sternotomy because many of the recipients, especially those with cystic fibrosis, have extensive pleural adhesions from chronic infections or prior thoracic procedures. Procedures are performed with cardiopulmonary bypass because of the recipient's critical condition as well as the risk of reperfusion pulmonary edema while exposing one lobe to the entire cardiac output while the other lobe is being implanted. Cardiopulmonary bypass allows simultaneous reperfusion of both lobes in a controlled fashion. Hilar dissection and lysis of adhesions are completed prior to heparinization and cardiopulmonary bypass. The pleural cavity of cystic fibrosis patients is irrigated with an aminoglycoside and amphotericin B solution. Dissection of the pulmonary artery and veins is performed as distally as possible to optimize cuff length for the anastomosis (Figure 85-6). When the dissection is complete, cardiopulmonary bypass is initiated and the pulmonary vasculature is divided. The pulmonary veins are divided between stapling devices while the pulmonary artery is doubly ligated and divided. The bronchus is divided with a stapling device at the level of the takeoff of the upper lobe bronchus. After the onset of bypass, the anesthesiologist suctions the lungs and removes the endotracheal tube.

Allograft Implantation

The first allograft is placed on a cooling jacket within the pleural space and the exposed lung is wrapped in iced-saline-soaked sponges. The bronchial anastomosis is performed with running 4-0 polypropylene suture (Figure 85-7). The donor bronchus is usually slightly telescoped into the recipient. Care is taken to limit the amount of peribronchial dissection. The bronchial anastomosis places the donor lobar vein in close approxima-

tion to the superior pulmonary vein of the recipient, and the venous anastomosis is performed in a running fashion with 5-0 polypropylene suture (Figure 85-8). The short length of the donor vein makes anastomosis directly to the left atrium difficult and underscores the importance of leaving an adequate length of recipient pulmonary vein during pneumonectomy. The pulmonary artery anastomosis is performed end-to-end with 5-0 polypropylene suture (Figure 85-9). A similar procedure is performed for the second allograft.

After completing the bilateral implantations, the vascular clamps are removed and ventilation is begun. Continuous nitric oxide starting at 20 ppm and intermittent aerosolized bronchodilator therapy are both administered via the anesthesia circuit. Blood volume is

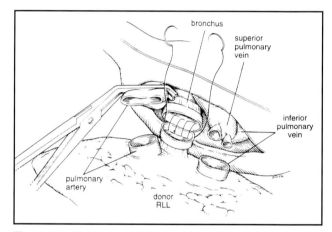

Figure 85-7. Right lower lobe implantation: bronchial anastomosis. Reprinted with permission from Starnes VA, Barr ML, Cohen RG. Lobar transplantation. Indications, technique, and outcome. J Thorac Cardiovasc Surg. 1994;108(3):403-410.

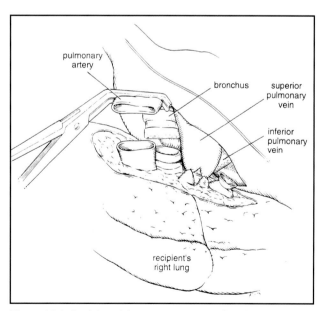

Figure 85-6. Recipient right pneumonectomy. Reprinted with permission from Starnes VA, Barr ML, Cohen RG. Lobar transplantation. Indications, technique, and outcome. J Thorac Cardiovasc Surg. 1994;108(3):403-410.

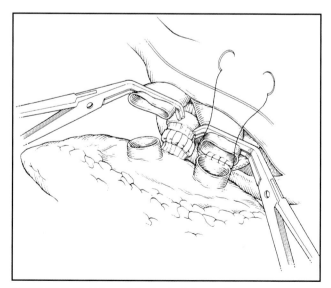

Figure 85-8. Right lower lobe implantation: pulmonary venous anastomosis. Reprinted with permission from Starnes VA, Barr ML, Cohen RG. Lobar transplantation. Indications, technique, and outcome. J Thorac Cardiovasc Surg. 1994;108(3):403-410.

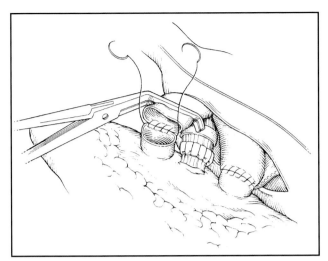

Figure 85-9. Right lower lobe implantation: pulmonary arterial anastomosis. Reprinted with permission from Starnes VA, Barr ML, Cohen RG. Lobar transplantation. Indications, technique, and outcome. J Thorac Cardiovasc Surg. 1994;108(3):403-410.

gradually returned allowing increased cardiac ejection and pulmonary blood flow to occur with subsequent weaning from cardiopulmonary bypass. At the completion of implantation, transesophageal echocardiography (checking for patency of the one pulmonary vein on each side draining into the left atrium) and bronchoscopy are performed to exclude technical complications.

SPECIAL ISSUES IN PERIOPERATIVE RECIPIENT MANAGEMENT

Perioperative management of the lobar recipient may present unique challenges compared with standard cadaveric lung transplantation. The recipient is ventilated through a single lumen endotracheal tube with positive end-expiratory pressures of 5 to 10 cm H_2O, for at least 48 to 72 hours. This prolonged ventilatory support is used in an attempt to decrease atelectasis and optimize expansion of the relatively undersized lobes. Depending on the degree of size mismatch between the donor lobe and the recipient pleural cavity, conventional chest tube suction in the perioperative and acute postoperative phases can result in impaired deflation mechanics. Subsequent air trapping with increasing airway pressures, and a resulting rise in pulmonary vascular resistance with an acute rise in pulmonary arterial pressures can occur. This problem is exaggerated as the dis-

crepancy between the size of the lobe and the thoracic cavity increases. Therefore, suction is applied at low levels (10 cm H_2O) to each tube sequentially, for 1-hour intervals, in a rotational fashion for the first 24 hours postoperatively. Subsequently, each of the four chest tubes is placed on continuous suction that is gradually increased to 20 cm H_2O over the next 48 hours. As the entire cardiac output is flowing through only two lobes, efforts to minimize the risk of reperfusion injury, pulmonary vascular hypertension, and pulmonary edema are undertaken. These include maintenance of the recipient in a relatively hypovolemic state and continuous infusion of nitroglycerin to minimize pulmonary arterial pressures. Additionally, aerosolized nitric oxide, which was started in the operating room, is continued for the first 48 to 72 hours. Finally, the recipient may have prolonged, high-output chest tube drainage which is exacerbated by greater size and topographic mismatches. The question of whether these tubes can be removed despite these higher than normal outputs is unclear as there is an obligatory space-filling of the pleural cavity with fluid. However, because of concerns of lobe compression by the pleural fluid, the chest tubes are left in place for two to three weeks, which is significantly longer than in conventional cadaveric transplantation.

RECOMMENDED READING

Cohen RG, Barr ML, Schenkel FA, DeMeester TR, Wells WG, Starnes VA. Living-related donor lobectomy for bilateral lobar transplantation in patients with cystic fibrosis. Ann Thorac Surg. 1994;57(6):1423-1427.

Starnes VA, Barr ML, Cohen RG. Lobar transplantation. Indications, technique, and outcome. J Thorac Cardiovasc Surg. 1994;108(3):403-410.

Starnes VA, Barr ML, Cohen RG, et al. Living-donor lobar lung transplantation experience: intermediate results. J Thorac Cardiovasc Surg. 1996;112(5):1284-1290.

Starnes VA, Barr ML, Schenkel FA, et al. Experience with living-donor lobar lung transplantation for indications other than cystic fibrosis. J Thorac Cardiovasc Surg. 1997;114(6):917-921.

Barr ML, Schenkel FA, Cohen RG, et al. Recipient and donor outcomes in living related and unrelated lobar transplantation. Transplant Proc. 1998;30(5):2261-2263.

86 CADAVER LUNG DONOR SELECTION CRITERIA

Edward R. Garrity, Jr., MD
Wickii T. Vigneswaran, MD
Sangeeta M. Bhorade, MD

Chief among donor-related obligations is the careful selection and management of the donor to optimize recipient outcome while enhancing maximal utilization of a scarce resource. The availability of suitable donor lungs is the sole current limitation to the number of lung transplants that can be performed. In the coming year, an estimated 300 to 500 potential recipients will die awaiting viable lungs. This section will deal with donor issues and with increasing the usable donor pool.

CADAVER LUNG DONOR SELECTION CRITERIA

The current reliance on cadaver donors introduces time and availability as risk factors for the recipient. One estimate of donor pool size, derived from hospital deaths, suggested a possible 59 donors per million population or more than 15,000 per year. Yet only about 15 donors per million are identified and used annually. Factors involved in nonuse of potential donor organs include denial of consent by next-of-kin and medical examiners, failure to request donation by medical personnel, and the presence or development of medical unsuitability. Donors and organs deteriorate rapidly, especially the lungs.

Brain death of a potential donor should be determined by the physician who is caring for the patient. Brain death criteria were initially developed at Harvard Medical School in 1968 and modified in 1981 by the President's Commission for the Study of Ethical Problems in Medicine.

The transplant team plays no part in the declaration of brain death. After brain death criteria have been fulfilled, early identification of a potential donor is

Edward R. Garrity, Jr., MD, Professor of Medicine; Pulmonary & Critical Care; Medical Director, Lung Transplantation Program, Loyola University Medical Center, Maywood, IL

Wickii T. Vigneswaran, MD, Professor of Surgery; Chief, Thoracic Surgery; Surgical Director, Lung Transplantation Program, Loyola University Medical Center, Maywood, IL

Sangeeta M. Bhorade, MD, Pulmonary & Critical Care Medicine Program, and Lung Transplantation Program, Loyola University Medical Center, Maywood, IL

extremely important. Once a potential donor is identified, the local organ procurement organization should be informed quickly and the request for tissue and organ donation should be coordinated by a trained specialist from this organization.

ISSUES RELATED TO DONOR SUITABILITY

The cause of death impacts on transplantability of the lung (eg, multiple trauma or motor vehicle accidents are less likely to yield usable lungs; drowning virtually excludes lung donation). In the US, a large percentage of lung donors result from head injuries, particularly gunshot wounds to the head and intracerebral hemorrhages.

Potential donor lung disease is considered. A history of smoking would not prevent use of a donor, but historical organ dysfunction, with the exception of the young mild asthmatic donor, would make lung donation less likely. Presently, lungs from donors over age 55 are infrequently used, but there is no inherent reason to discard healthy older lungs in this life-saving situation. Finally, donors are assessed for infection, historical and current, to avoid acute recipient pneumonia or later problems with tuberculosis or other pathogens.

Of immediate concern are the issues of donor intubation, assessment of chest x-rays, arterial blood gases, and size matching. Circumstances of donor intubation can greatly influence organ function, as in witnessed or suspected aspiration of gastric contents or improper tube placement with compromise of airway drainage and subsequent obstruction and atelectasis. "In the field" intubations of unstable donors are more often associated with the above outcomes than elective intubations of the conscious patient. Though the incidence of nosocomial infections increases with prolonged intubation, aspiration pneumonias may take five to nine days to be recognized radiologically, so a "clear" chest x-ray at five days post-intubation may actually be preferable to a clear x-ray one day after an emergent intubation. Second, the ideal donor will have a clear chest x-ray or atelectasis resolvable by bronchoscopy. Even mild pulmonary edema may not eliminate a donor from consideration. Minor shadows may not rule out use, but need to be investigated thoroughly by a donor management team familiar with the appearance of acute aspiration.

The presence of many polymorphonuclear leukocytes (PMNs) on a Gram stain of suctioned sputum or bronchial wash, coupled with the erythematous edematous airways seen with a relatively fresh aspiration, or PMNs and multiple bacteria imply pneumonia, either nosocomial or aspiration, would preclude the use of the donor in many circumstances. Bronchoscopy should be early and rapid, visualizing all the airways, noting color, edema, and the presence of secretions. Trauma to the airways with suction or the introduction of saline should be minimized or avoided altogether, as such intervention alters the epithelial surface adhesiveness for pathogens such as pseudomonas. However, bronchial hygiene must be maintained. While of minimal importance in a stable, nonimmunosuppressed patient, in the denervated, reperfused, and immunosuppressed recipient of the organ such interventions can have theoretically greater impact.

Arterial blood gases are measured on tidal volumes of 5 to 10 mL/kg ideal body weight, PEEP 5 cm, and a rate appropriate to the donor's pH. The range of acceptable values varies among centers but generally a PaO_2 of greater-than-or-equal-to 300 mmHg on $FiO_2=1.0$ (Table 86-1) is considered appropriate.

Next, recipient/donor size match is important to avoid hyperinflation or atelectasis with resultant compromise of function, increased work of breathing, and/or pleural space problems. This is currently accomplished by use of the well-established, published predicted normal values based on age, sex, height and race. Weight is not a significant factor. Historically, size matching had been accomplished by the comparison of chest x-rays and thoracic measurement, and this still may play a role. The current approach is to estimate the total lung capacity (TLC) of both donor and recipient and match within approximately 25% of predicted TLC (Table 86-2).

Other contraindications include systemic sepsis and identification of the human immunodeficiency virus (HIV) infection or high-risk behavior frequently associated with AIDS. Organ and tissue recipients have become HIV-positive after grafting from an infected host. Likewise, when a cause of death is obscure, the transplant community tends to refuse donor organs for fear of grafting disease with the tissue. Clearly, however, if a detailed donor evaluation doesn't reveal either a specific cause of death or significant organ impairment, then the donor may well be used, especially in critical need situations. Hepatitis B antigenemia is assessed in the donor population and is considered a contraindication to transplantation (Table 86-3).

Another concern about the donor lung is the estimated ischemia time. While all centers would prefer to receive well-preserved lungs with under four hours ischemia, this is uncommon. The current average lung ischemic time reported to UNOS is four to six hours. Obviously, some ischemic times are substantially longer and yet successful. The key appears to be the quality of the graft, the adequacy of cold preservation, and protection from long warm ischemia (ie, >90 minutes) during reimplantation and reperfusion. A rule of thumb is: good donor, good graft, good operation and good outcome.

Finally, three very common complications of management often raise concern about donor use. First, particularly with serious head injury, disseminated intravascular coagulopathy (DIC) is common. If serious donor hemorrhage or thrombosis is absent, such organs are acceptable. Next, pneumothoraces often occur as a consequence of injury or treatment. If the injury is clean and can be easily treated, the donor lungs may still be salvageable. Lastly, while programs may turn down donor hearts after cardiopulmonary resuscitation, unless contused, infected, or flooded, the lungs may still be suitable for use. In each of these situations, utmost care in evaluation will lead toward optimal donor use and maximal recipient success.

DONOR MANAGEMENT

The management of potential lung donors requires exemplary critical care management where a thorough understanding of cardiopulmonary physiology and hemodynamics is essential, but where attention to preservation of central nervous system (CNS) function and pressures is no longer required. Brain death often

---

Table 86-1. Guidelines for Donor Suitability

Age <55 years
Tobacco history <20 to 30 pack years
Clear chest radiograph
Oxygenation (PaO_2 >300 mmHg on a $FiO_2=1.0$)
Normal bronchoscopic examination
No history of pulmonary disease

Table 86-2. Estimate of Total Lung Capacity (TLC)

Predicted Total Lung Capacity
Male: 0.0795 x H(cm) + 0.0032 (A) - 7.33 = TLC
Female: 0.0590 x H(cm) - 4.537 = TLC

H indicates height; A, age

Table 86-3. Contraindications to Donor Use in Lung Transplantation

Active sepsis syndrome
HIV disease
Viral hepatitis
Guillain-Barre Syndrome
Malignancy*: prone to recurrence or metastasis
Intravenous drug use

*Except localized brain tumor, excised squamous or basal cell skin cancer, localized carcinoma of the cervix.

leads to instability of the respiratory and cardiac systems with resultant changes in temperature control and systemic vascular resistance. Under usual circumstances, donor temperature can be controlled by external heating or by the use of warmed intravenous fluids, crucial for control of coagulopathy. Attempts should be made to keep the central venous pressure (CVP) between 5 and 10 mmHg to maintain adequate tissue perfusion and to allow weaning of α-adrenergic agents. Still, vasodilation will be evident due to the loss of brain stem vasomotor control.

Brain stem demise also leads to dysfunction of the anterior pituitary gland, decreased production of antidiuretic hormone (ADH), and development of diabetes insipidus (DI) in 50% to 70% of multiple organ donors. As urine output rises to extremes (ie, 1 to 2 L/h), dehydration, hypernatremia, hypokalemia, hypocalcemia, and other electrolyte derangements can occur. Most commonly, DI is treated by the administration of desmopressin (DDAVP) 0.5 to 2.0 mg every eight to twelve hours or by titrated infusion to limit urine flow to 100 to 250 mL/hr. Dopamine, in modest doses, can also help with blood pressure maintenance while avoiding massive fluid infusions. The combination of dopamine and DDAVP is preferable to the "drowned" lung of overly vigorous fluid repletion. While a lung with pulmonary edema can be used for transplantation, differentiating fluid from infection can be difficult. Donors are frequent recipients of antibiotics for colonization of the respiratory tract. The benefits of this practice are not clinically established. Another issue after brain death concerns depletion of thyroxine, cortisol, and insulin. Experimental evidence suggests potential benefit from infusion of these agents, but large scale clinical use is still awaiting solid trial data.

The very influential therapy in support of the potential lung donor is tied to respiratory therapy and mechanical ventilation. Careful, aggressive management can lead to optimization of donor utilization, while suboptimal care may predispose to atelectasis and pneumonia leading to loss of organs. Most acceptable donors will have been ventilated for three days or less, but duration of intubation by itself is not a reason to exclude use of a donor if gas exchange is adequate, chest x-ray is reasonably clear, and secretions are minimal and nonpurulent.

The respiratory care should be aimed at avoidance of atelectasis and lung injury. Because PEEP is avoided in the CNS-injured patient, atelectasis may be a problem in the established donor. Also, support has been delivered conventionally with ventilator tidal volumes of 10 to 15 mL/kg. The cycling of the lung through high tidal volumes and partial atelectasis may be injurious and lead to alveolar injury worsened by further ventilation, oxygen, and fluids. Appropriate management should include the use of PEEP to raise end-expiratory lung volume to just above the lower inflection point of the lung pressure-volume curve (Figure 86-1).

This is determined by the addition of PEEP in increments to maximize the lung compliance at the lowest PEEP possible. The best information suggests a tidal volume of 5 to 10 mL/kg at a rate to keep $PaCO_2$ about 40 mmHg and plateau ventilatory pressures less than 30 cm H_2O above PEEP (Figure 86-2). When the liver is being concomitantly harvested, PEEP of less-than-or-equal-to 10 cm is usually preferred. This information is derived from patients with acute lung injury, but it seems reasonable to extrapolate to the donor when avoidance of lung injury is key. FiO_2 should be supplemented as needed to keep adequate PaO_2 and pulse oximetry, but $FiO_2 > 0.40$ suggests a gas exchange problem and may lead to donor exclusion. While ventilated, position changes and chest physiotherapy are integral to donor support.

Aggressive donor resuscitation with hormonal replacement therapy, invasive cardiopulmonary monitoring, and early assessment and intervention by an intrathoracic transplant team may lead to improved salvage of hearts and lungs, as well as other organs.

ORGAN PROCUREMENT AND PRESERVATION

At present, procurement of lungs for transplant remains lowest among the solid organs retrieved, as a result of the tenuous nature of the respiratory function among potential donors. In addition, despite considerable experimental work over the past 15 years, predictable prolonged (ie, >6 hours) lung graft preservation still eludes clinical lung transplantation. The restricted storage time further denies complete access to the available

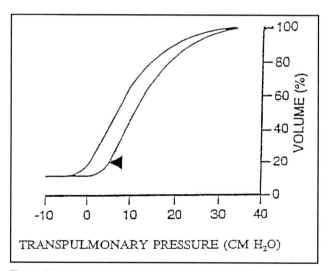

Figure 86-1. Lung pressure-volume curve, from residual volume to total lung capacity. Arrow marks desirable PEEP, so that maximal compliance is achieved over the respiratory cycle, and airways remain open.

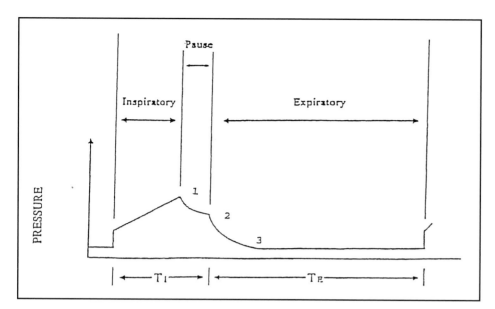

Figure 86-2. Pressure-time waveform of mechanical ventilation. P_1-peak pressure; P_2-plateau pressure; P_3-PEEP; (P_2-P_3-static transpulmonary pressure, ideally under 30 cm H_2O.

donor pool, and causes financial implications for transplantation centers for transportation and personnel. According to the International Society of Heart and Lung Transplantation Registry, in the first three months following lung transplantation, approximately a third of mortality is attributed to nonspecific graft failure, at least partly associated with the preservation/storage process.

Several techniques have been applied for graft preservation during ischemia. Simple cold immersion was the technique used in the early cases reported by the Toronto Lung Transplant Group. This technique provided good results, but topical cooling alone did not address the need for extension of the period of preservation. Autoperfusion of heart-lung blocks was tried, but due to its complexity and increased sharing of intrathoracic donor organs among centers, this technique has been abandoned. Donor core cooling on cardiopulmonary bypass has been used in some selected centers, but this technique is cumbersome with the cooling of the lung inefficient and an unestablished value in prolonging the ischemic time.

From the experience gained in other solid organ preservation, the technique of using a single flush of a cold solution prompted the use of this technique for distant lung procurement by the Stanford group. The technique is simple, requires a minimal amount of specialized equipment and provides efficient cooling of the lungs. Currently, this technique is the most widely practiced method for lung preservation. The number of solutions and additives, along with the rate and volume of administration, may vary from center to center in the search for the ideal. The solutions most commonly used are some modification of Euro-Collins or the University of Wisconsin solutions.

A majority of centers using a single flush perfusion for lung graft preservation use pulmonary vasodilators in the perfusate and/or donor pretreatment. The most popular agents are prostaglandins, either E_2 or I_1. Nitroprusside is also used by some centers, and in addition, acts as a potent nitric oxide donor. These agents are very potent pulmonary vasodilators and facilitate uniform distribution of preservative throughout the lung. The pulmonary vasodilatation also allows for a large volume of flush perfusion at low pressure. The average volume of the crystalloid perfusate used for graft perfusion is about 60 cc/kg and is delivered at normal pulmonary artery pressures. The additional effects of prostaglandins include inhibition of platelet adherence, protection against release of neutrophil-mediated free radicals, reduced endothelial permeability, mediation of immunosuppression by selective B-lymphocyte function, and depressed humoral antibody response. Donor pretreatment with steroids is practiced by some transplant centers for its antiinflammatory and neutrophil stabilizing properties. When used, the steroid is delivered intravenously to the donor.

Pulmonary vascular resistance is lower when the lungs are inflated. During the pulmonary flush perfusion, the lungs are ventilated throughout the period to allow uniform and adequate cooling. Attempts to continue ventilation during storage are cumbersome and provide no additional advantage over an inflated graft. The optimal gas mixture for ventilation and storage has not been established, but experimental work has shown that an $FiO_2=1.0$ is detrimental to the lung. Many centers, therefore, use room air or oxygen concentration of less than 40% in the mixture.

Warm ischemia is well documented to be harmful to the pulmonary graft. Hypothermia significantly reduces

the lung metabolism and is protective during ischemia. Uniform cooling of the donor lung during procurement is one of the major principles of ischemic preservation. It is common practice to perfuse the lungs with solution at 4°C and store for transportation at the same temperature with the graft immersed in ice. Some groups believe a temperature of 10°C is preferable to the 4°C, but if the higher temperature is practiced, addition of a metabolic substrate is important during the ischemic period. The popular substrates are 1% glucose or glutathione and are added to the perfusate to support the metabolism in the graft. Glutathione is an attractive additive, as it is also a powerful free radical scavenger; but use of oxygen free radical scavengers in the perfusate, although attractive, has not been widely adopted. Other agents commonly added for this purpose are allopurinol, mannitol, and desferrioxamine.

Nonspecific graft failure remains responsible for one-third of the deaths within the first three months following transplantation and contributes to morbidity in a significant fraction. It appears that there is room for improvement in the widely practiced techniques of lung graft preservation. Extending the safe ischemic time of the graft will improve access to lungs for transplantation. This still remains a challenge in clinical transplantation.

RECOMMENDED READING

Mackersie RC, Bronsther OL, Shackford SR. Organ Procurement in patients with fatal head injuries. The fate of the potential donor. Ann Surg. 1991;213(2):143-150.

Anonymous. A definition of irreversible coma. Report of the Ad Hoc Committee of the Harvard Medical Schoolto Examine the Definition of Brain Death. JAMA. 1968;205(6):337-340.

Crapo RO, Morris AH, Clayton PD, Nixon CR. Lung volumes in healthy nonsmoking adults. Bull Eur Physiopathol Respir. 1982;18(3):419-425.

Dreyfuss D, Soler P, Saumon G. Mechanical ventilation-induced pulmonary edema. Interaction with previous lung alterations. Am J Respir Crit Care Med. 1995;151(5):1568-1575.

Puskas JD, Cardoso PF, Mayer E, Shi S, Slutsky AS, Patterson GA. Equivalent eighteen-hour lung preservation with low-potassium dextran or Euro-Collins solution after prostaglandin E1 infusion. J Thorac Cardiovasc Surg. 1992;104(1):83-89.

Mayer E, Puskas D, Cardos PF, Shi S, Slutsky AS, Patterson GA. Reliable eighteen-hour lung preservation at 4 and 10 C by pulmonary artery flush after high-dose prostaglandin E1 administration. J Thorac Cardiovasc Surg. 1992;103(6):1136-1142.

Haverich A. Preservation for clinical transplantation. In: Patterson GA, Courad L, eds. Lung Transplantation. Amsterdam, The Netherlands: Elsevier Science BV; 1995:147-155. A review recognized surgical authors of the methods of preservation and results.

Amato MBP, Barbas CSV, Mederios DM, et al. Beneficial effects of the "open lung approach" with low distending pressures in acute respiratory distress syndrome. A prospective randomized study on mechanical ventilation. Am J Respir Crit Care Med. 1995;152(1):1835-1846.

Novitzky D, Cooper DK, Reichart B. Hemodynamic and metabolic responses to hormonal therapy in brain-dead potential organ donors. Transplantation. 1987;43(6):852-854.

Wheeldon DR, Potter CD, Oduro A, Wallwork J, Large SR. Transforming the "unacceptable" donor: outcomes from the adoption of a standardized donor management technique. J Heart Lung Transplant. 1995;14(4):734-742.

Potter CD, Wheeldon DR, Wallwork J. Functional assessment and management of heart donors: a rationale for characterization and a guide to therapy. J Heart Lung Transplant. 1995;14(1 Pt 1):59-65.

Wheeldon DR, Potter CD, Jonas M, Wallwork J, Large SR. Using "unsuitable" hearts for transplantation. Eur J Cardiothorac Surg. 1994;8(1):7-11.

87 CADAVER LUNG DONOR ALLOCATION SCHEME

Sangeeta Bhorade, MD
Edward R. Garrity, Jr., MD

Determination of appropriate organ sharing and donor allocation in lung transplantation is significantly affected by the limited supply of available donors. This discrepancy between the rising number of patients waiting on the lung transplant list and the limited donor supply has led to increasing difficulty in selecting the optimal criteria for lung donor allocation. Clearly, the ideal allocation scheme should enhance the number of successful lung transplants, while minimizing the number of deaths on the waiting list. In order to conduct this process more efficiently, the Organ Procurement and Transplantation Network (OPTN), a national service organization, was developed in 1984 to oversee and optimize donor allocation. OPTN currently determines the national policies and regulations for all the solid organ donor allocation schemes. All active organ procurement organizations (OPOs) and transplant centers are required to be members of OPTN.

Currently, the allocation scheme for lung donors is initiated through the local OPO. After a potential lung donor has been identified, the regional OPO contacts the local lung transplant centers within that specific region. Allocation of organs to the individual centers is determined according to a schedule controlled by the OPO. Each lung transplant center in an OPO has a waiting list for candidates. The center's lists are merged within the OPO based upon UNOS regulations and waiting time. A list of potential recipients is generated when a donor is available, and organs are offered based on accrual of waiting time. Once an individual center has been contacted, the center then determines if they will accept the organ for the recipient highest on their waiting list. If the transplant center deems the donor inappropriate for the designated recipient, the local OPO contacts the next transplant center according to candidate waiting time. If a donor is not accepted by the local transplant centers, the local OPO may contact a nearby OPO within the same region to offer the donor lungs to a transplant center in a different region, and subsequently on a wider basis if organs are not used in the region. A system of concentric circles from the OPO is drawn for sequential offerings outside the region, in increasing radii of 500 miles each.

The primary determinant of lung donor allocation is the accrual of time on the lung transplant waiting list. In comparison to the other solid organ allocation schemes, the severity of illness plays no part in determining a patient's status for lung transplantation. This difference primarily arises from the poor outcome of the most severely ill patients and the significant shortage of available lung donors. Transplant candidates who are on mechanical ventilation or in the intensive care unit (ICU) have suffered increased morbidity and mortality during surgical intervention and the immediate postoperative course. Therefore, in order to use a scarce resource more efficiently, these patients are not given priority over other patients with longer waiting times. Patients with idiopathic pulmonary fibrosis (IPF) are typically referred late in the course of their disease and, as a result, were found to die more frequently on the transplant waiting list. Due to their poor prognosis, these patients are credited with an extra 90 days to their waiting time when they are listed. However, as physicians begin to refer these patients earlier for transplantation, these issues may need to be readdressed.

In addition to accrual of time on the transplant waiting list, compatibility of ABO blood-typing and size-matching are important factors at the time of donor allocation. Ideally, lung donor allocation is based on identical matching of ABO blood type. However, if identical matching is not possible, compatibility of ABO blood type between donor and recipient is acceptable with the recognition of the increased risk of transient hemolytic anemia. Size matching is based upon matching of the donor total lung capacity (TLC) to within approximately 25% of the recipient TLC. A more complete description of appropriate size matching is presented in Chapter 86, Cadaver Lung Donor Selection Criteria.

Allocation of a heart-lung donor is briefly described here and further detailed in Chapter 86. Briefly, when a heart-lung donor becomes available, an initial decision is made whether to use the heart and lungs together for a heart-lung recipient, or separately for two or three recipients. If the decision is made to perform a combined heart-lung transplant, the regional OPO will contact transplant centers within its region in a similar fashion as that described above. Each heart-lung candidate will be listed on both the heart and lung waiting lists separately, according to the criteria specific to the respective organ system. When a heart-lung candidate is eligible to receive the heart from a given donor, the lung will be allocated to the patient from the same donor. If the heart-lung candidate is eligible to receive the lung, the heart will be allo-

Sangeeta Bhorade, MD, Pulmonary & Critical Care Medicine, and Lung Transplantation Program, Loyola University Medical Center, Maywood, IL

Edward R. Garrity, Jr., MD, Professor of Medicine; Pulmonary & Critical Care; Medical Director, Lung Transplantation, Loyola University Medical Center, Maywood, IL

cated to the candidate from the same donor if there are no Status 1A isolated heart candidates eligible to receive the heart. If the organs are not used within a specific region, then the OPO will contact other regional OPOs for the potential use of the heart and/or lungs.

Several issues may limit organ sharing and donor allocation of lungs. First and foremost, while the length of donor lung ischemia time has not been significantly associated with decreased function of the transplanted lung, six hours is commonly felt to be a reasonable ischemic time limit. The injury sustained by the donor lung is presumably secondary to ischemia-reperfusion injury resulting in early graft dysfunction due to cellular injury from oxygen free radicals and other metabolites. This ischemia-reperfusion injury may result in increased vascular permeability, pulmonary edema, impaired gas exchange and overall decreased survival. Currently, acceptable donor ischemia times from the time of harvesting of the donor lungs to reimplantation into the recipient lies between four to ten hours, with six hours felt to be ideal. Due to this time constraint, ischemic time continues to be an impediment for expanding successful donor allocation outside of a given region. As current preservation methods and surgical techniques continue to improve, a more widespread distribution of donor organs, coupled with better donor-recipient matching, may lead to a higher rate of successful lung transplants.

In part due to the limitation of donor ischemic time, human leukocyte antigen (HLA) crossmatching between donor and recipient is not usually available in lung transplant recipients. Fortunately, early retrospective evaluations of lung transplant recipients and donor HLA-mismatch have not shown HLA-mismatch to be an important contributing factor to early lung allograft complications. However, transplant candidates with high levels of HLA alloantibodies as manifested by an elevated panel-reactive antibody titre (PRA) are at increased risk of developing hyperacute rejection if the donor has a reactive antigen to the recipient's HLA alloantibodies. Due to this risk, patients with an elevated PRA should undergo therapy prior to transplantation to reduce the HLA alloreactivity (ie, plasmapheresis, cyclophosphamide and/or intravenous immunoglobulin infusions) or forego transplant.

Several issues have arisen concerning the current organ sharing and donor allocation scheme. One of the major concerns highlights the significant variability in waiting times and waiting list mortality across the different regions and transplant centers. Obviously, the main reason for this discrepancy arises from the local OPOs and the individual transplant centers being the centers of organ distribution. Unfortunately, this system has evolved due to the perceived need to limit donor ischemia time. Thus, although it would be difficult to implement a national list for more optimal donor allocation and distribution, several ideas have been proposed to increase the uniformity of waiting time between centers.

One idea includes the transfer of donor organs from the recipient's home area to the center at which the patient decides to undergo transplantation, including those patients who are undergoing transplantation outside of their home state. Currently, there is no flexibility for the transfer of these donor organs to follow the transplant candidate to the center of his/her choice. Ideally, this method would help to provide some uniformity in waiting time accrual among the candidates. In addition, a candidate would be able to undergo transplantation at the center of his or her preference without compromising waiting time. Another proposal would draw concentric circles around the donor hospital, and transplant centers could choose how far they would be able to travel for donor lungs. This would tend to equalize waiting times, while the recipient would become the focus of allocation, rather than the transplant center.

Ongoing debate of these and other proposals will hopefully equalize waiting times among the various centers. Further discussions regarding the optimal way to allocate and distribute organs will continue as long as there remains a significant shortage of donor organs. After all, there would be no debate on allocation if there were an adequate number of donor organs available.

RECOMMENDED READING

United Network for Organ Sharing, Allocation of Thoracic Organs, Policy 3.7, 11/20/98

United Network for Organ Sharing,, Allocation for Lung Transplantation, Policy 3.7.6, 11/20/98

United Network for Organ Sharing, Allocation for Heart-Lung Transplantation, Policy 3.7.7., 11/20/98

United Network for Organ Sharing, Waiting Time Accrual for Lung Candidates with Idiopathic Pulmonary Fibrosis (IPF), Policy 3.7.9.2., 11/20/98

Kirk AJ, Colquhoun IW, Dark JH. Lung preservation: a review of current practice and future directions. Ann Thorac Surg. 1993;56(4):990-1000.

Hopkinson DN, Bhabra MS, Hooper TL. Pulmonary graft preservation: a world wide survey of current clinical practice. J Heart Lung Transplant. 1998;17(5):525-531.

Hosenpud JD, Bennett LE, Keck BM, Fiol B, Boucek MM, Novick RJ. The Registry of the International Society for Heart and Lung Transplantation: Fifteenth Official Report - 1998. J Heart Lung Transplant. 1998;17(7):656-668.

88 LUNG AND HEART-LUNG TRANSPLANT SURGICAL PROCEDURE

Christine L. Lau, MD
Howard Todd Massey, MD
R. Duane Davis, Jr., MD

Prior to proceeding with an on-site evaluation, the donor's medical history is obtained, with particular emphasis and attention paid to the donor's age, cause of death, timing of death, smoking history, and prior thoracic procedures.

DONOR PROCUREMENT PROCEDURES
Donor Procurement – Lung

Upon arrival of the procurement team to the donor's location, inspection of the donor's most recent chest radiograph is undertaken. Preferably, both lung fields should be free of pulmonary contusions, pneumonia, or atelectasis. Size matching is usually based on donor and recipient heights, but recipient chest radiographs are routinely carried by the harvest team to compare with the donor's chest size. The midclavicular line is used to measure the vertical dimension, and the transverse dimension is measured at the level of the diaphragm domes. Confirmation of satisfactory gas exchange, using the standard gas exchange parameters of PaO_2 >300 mmHg on FIO_2 of 100% and PEEP of 5cm H_2O, is obtained on the donor lungs. If these criteria are not met because one lung is felt to be suboptimal, a blood gas from the contralateral lung's pulmonary vein is obtained. Additionally, lung parameters, including mean airway pressures and compliance, are evaluated. Bronchoscopy is performed to assess the airways. The presence of mucopurulent secretions that are easily cleared are acceptable, but the presence of frank pus, significant airway erythema, or evidence of aspiration contraindicates the use of the lung from which these findings arise (but not necessarily the contralateral lung). Manual examination of the donor lungs at median sternotomy allows

Christine L. Lau, MD, Senior Assistant Resident in General & Thoracic Surgery, Duke University Medical Center, Durham, NC

Howard Todd Massey, MD, Fellow in Cardiothoracic Transplantation, Duke University Medical Center, Durham, NC

R. Duane Davis, Jr., MD, Director, Cardiothoracic Transplantation; Associate Professor of Surgery, Duke University Medical Center, Durham, NC

evaluation of the pulmonary parenchyma for nodules, edema, and evidence of interstitial disease. Pulmonary artery pressures may be measured directly or estimated by palpation.

Sundaresan and colleagues reported the technique of donor lung procurement which allows en bloc removal of the lungs and preservation of the heart, with the potential of performing three separate transplants. Following median sternotomy, the pleural spaces are opened and the lungs are visually inspected. The pericardium is opened and stay sutures are placed allowing exposure of the great vessels. The superior vena cava (SVC) is encircled doubly with silk sutures and the inferior vena cava (IVC) is encircled. The pulmonary artery window is dissected in preparation for placement of the aortic cross clamp. The superior vena cava and the aorta are gently retracted laterally and the posterior pericardium is incised above the right pulmonary artery, allowing access to the trachea. The plane of the trachea is manually partially developed. Following completion of the thoracic dissection and prior to placement of the aortic and pulmonary artery cannulas, the patient is heparinized (250 to 300 units/kg). The ascending aorta is cannulated with a routine cardioplegia cannula for cardiac preservation. At the bifurcation of the main pulmonary artery a Sarns 6.5-mm curved metal cannula is placed and secured with a purse-string prolene suture for pulmonary flush delivery. After placement of the cannulas, a bolus dose of prostaglandin E_1 (PGE_1) (500 μg) is given directly into the pulmonary artery adjacent to the placement of the pulmonary artery catheter using a 25-gauge needle.

Immediately after the PGE_1 is infused, the superior vena cava is ligated, and the inferior vena cava is divided, allowing the right heart to decompress. The aorta is cross clamped, cardioplegia is initiated, and the left atrial appendage is incised, allowing the left side of the heart to decompress (Figure 88-1).

The pulmonary flush is initiated and consists of several liters (50 to 75 cc/kg) of either University of Wisconsin or modified Euro-Collins solution at 4°C. To prevent pulmonary edema, the pulmonary flush bag should be elevated to no more than 30 cm above the pulmonary artery. Retrograde flush through the left atrium has been shown in animal models to be superior to antegrade flush, resulting in improvement in pulmonary edema, airway resistance, and oxygenation during the first several hours after transplantation. Retrograde flush is easily used as an adjunct to antegrade following procurement of the heart by delivery through the pulmonary veins. While the heart and lung preservation fluids are running, the chest cavity is cooled with ice-cold normal saline. Ventilation is continued throughout.

After completion of the pulmonary flush and the cardioplegia, the heart is extracted (Figure 88-2). This is best performed as described by Sundaresan and

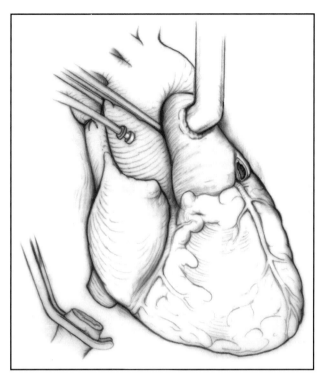

Figure 88-1. Drawing at time of cross clamping showing placement of cannulas and venting of right and left side of the heart (Adapted from Sundaresan S, Trachiotis GD, Aoe M, Patterson GA, Cooper JD. Donor lung procurement: assessment and operative technique. Ann Thorac Surg. 1993;56(6):1412.)

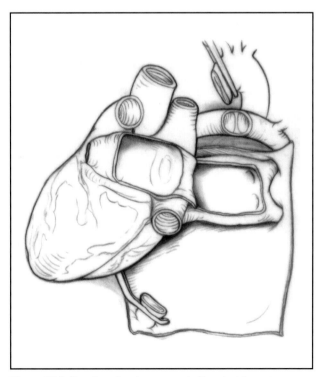

Figure 88-2. Drawing showing removal of heart at thoracic organ harvest (Adapted from Sundaresan S, Trachiotis GD, Aoe M, Patterson GA, Cooper JD. Donor lung procurement: assessment and operative technique. Ann Thorac Surg. 1993;56(6):1412.)

colleagues. The superior vena cava is transected between ties, followed by both division of the aorta proximal to the cross clamp, and the pulmonary artery at the bifurcation of the main pulmonary artery. Division of the left atrium proceeds by carefully dividing the atrium midway between the coronary sinus and the left pulmonary veins. Once the incision has been opened, the remaining cuff of left atrium can be transected while internally visualizing the right pulmonary veins.

Following extraction of the heart, the pulmonary team proceeds with the en bloc lung removal.

En bloc removal of the contents of the thoracic cavity prevents injury to the membranous trachea, pulmonary arteries, and pulmonary veins. The pericardium near the diaphragm is transected and the inferior pulmonary ligaments are divided. Following removal of the gastric tube, the esophagus is bluntly dissected and divided using a gastrointestinal anastomosis stapler (GIA) stapler at the level of the pericardium (Figure 88-3). Mediastinal tissue is divided with the scalpel across the midline and along the spine posterior to the aorta on the left and hemiazygous on the right to a level above the aortic arch. The tissue back along the thoracic spine is sharply dissected. The trachea is com-

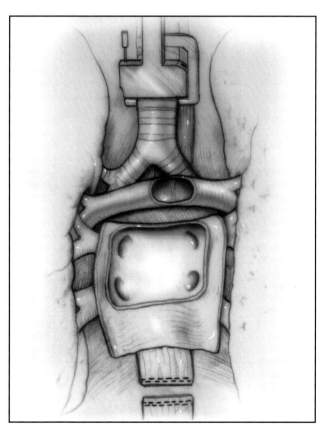

Figure 88-3. Drawing showing thoracic cavity with heart removed, esophagectomy, and division of trachea prior to double-lung bloc extraction.(Adapted from Sundaresan S, Trachiotis GD, Aoe M, Patterson GA, Cooper JD. Donor lung procurement: assessment and operative technique. Ann Thorac Surg. 1993;56(6):1413.)

pletely encircled and umbilical tape is placed around it. While the donor is ventilated with 100% oxygen, and the lungs are inflated to two-thirds maximum, a TA-30 stapler is fired one to two rings above the carina, with attention paid to preventing the endotracheal tube from being incorporated in the staples (Figure 88-3).

Another row of staples is placed slightly more proximally. The trachea is transected between the staple lines using a scalpel blade. It is important to avoid overinflation. Completion of the esophagectomy is performed with a GIA stapler near the level of the transected trachea, and the lungs are removed en bloc. Further dissection is carried out on the back table while the bloc is kept in an ice-cold bath. The donor esophagus and aorta are removed and the pericardium is excised.

An alternative approach to the donor lung harvest can be performed. After the heart has been removed, the posterior pericardium near the diaphragm is divided and the plane between the esophagus and the trachea is bluntly dissected. The posterior mediastinal tissue is sharply transected and the proximal thoracic aorta is divided. Following transection of the trachea as described above, the lungs are removed en bloc.

If the lungs are returning to the same institution, they are tripled-bagged together, with cold preservation solution and transported on ice. Alternatively, if the lungs are to be used at separate institutions they are divided on the back table by division of the posterior pericardium, left atrium between the pulmonary veins, division of the main pulmonary artery at the bifurcation, and division of the left bronchus above the take-off of the upper lobe bronchus. The left bronchus is divided between staples to maintain the inflation of each lung.

Donor Procurement – Heart-Lungs
The donor procurement procedure in heart-lung is similar to the separate procurements for heart and lungs, except the heart and lungs are removed en bloc without prior removal of the heart. Following completion of the pulmonary flush and the cardioplegia, the superior vena cava is transected between ties, followed by division of the aorta proximal to the cross clamp. The trachea is completely encircled, doubly stapled, and transected, again with the lungs inflated to two-thirds maximum. En bloc removal of the contents of the thoracic cavity proceeds as in the lung procurement technique.

RECIPIENT IMPLANTATION PROCEDURES
Single-Lung Implantation Into Recipient
All recipients should have complete hemodynamic monitoring including a Swan-Ganz catheter. Transesophageal echocardiography is routinely performed at many institutions and at a minimum should be available. Double

lumen endotracheal intubation is performed for adults followed by replacement with a single lumen tube at the completion of the procedure. For children and small adults, routine cardiopulmonary bypass may be used.

The choice of side of transplant is based on several factors, but when possible, the side with the poorest function determined by preoperative ventilation-perfusion scanning is transplanted, provided that the thoracic cavity on that side is normal. In patients with pulmonary hypertension with profound hypoxia or hypercarbia, the right side is preferred because cannulation for cardiopulmonary bypass can be easily performed within the chest. The standard incision is the posterolateral thoracotomy.

A pneumonectomy is performed via standard technique. The pulmonary artery, left atrium, and bronchus are mobilized and dissected back toward the mediastinum to prepare for implantation of the donor lung. For right-sided transplants, the left atrial groove requires mobilization to provide an adequate left atrial cuff.

The donor lung is placed within the recipient's chest cavity covered by a cold lap pad. The bronchial anastomosis is usually performed first (Figure 88-4). A continu-

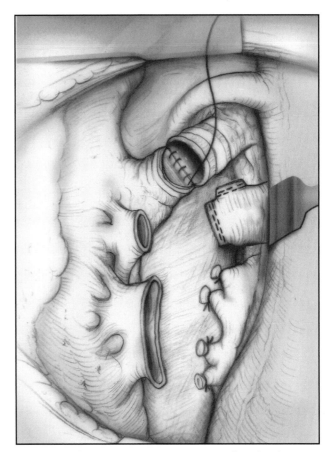

Figure 88-4. Single right lung transplant procedure showing bronchial anastomosis as continuous 4.0 PDS suture (Adapted from Patterson GA, Cooper JD. Lung Transplantation. In: Shields TW, ed. General Thoracic Surgery. Vol.1. Baltimore, Md: Lippincott Williams and Wilkins; 1994:1074.)

ous 4.0 PDS suture is used for the anastomosis, beginning with the posterior membranous trachea and proceeding anteriorly.

Upon completion of the anastomosis, the anterior portion is covered with peribronchial tissue for protection (Figure 88-5).

Following this, the pulmonary artery of the donor and recipient are aligned in proper orientation and trimmed to prevent excessive length and possible kinking of the pulmonary artery postoperatively. The anastomosis is performed end-to-end using 5.0 or 6.0 polypropylene suture as a continuous stitch (Figure 88-6A and 88-6B).

Finally, the left atrial cuff of the donor organ containing superior and inferior pulmonary veins is anastomosed to the recipient's left atrium (Figures 88-7A and 88-7B). Care is taken to incorporate intima without a significant amount of muscle in this anastomosis in order to limit the thrombogenicity of this suture line.

Following completion of the transplant and closure of the incision, and prior to leaving the operating room, bronchoscopy is performed to check for adequacy of the bronchial anastomosis.

Double-Lung Implantation Into Recipient

For sequential double-lung transplantation, bilateral anterior thoracotomies and transverse sternotomy (ie, clamshell incision) are performed to provide excel-

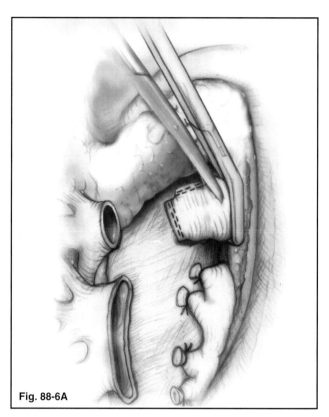

Fig. 88-6A

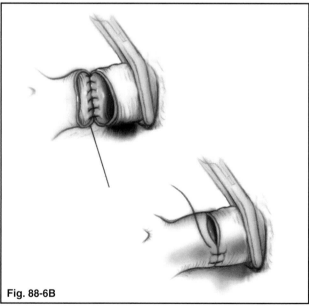

Fig. 88-6B

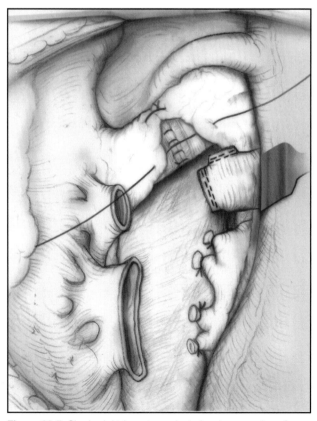

Figure 88-5. Single right lung transplant showing covering of anterior portion of bronchial anastomosis with peribronchial tissue. (Adapted from Patterson GA, Cooper JD. Lung Transplantation. In: Shields TW, ed. General Thoracic Surgery. Vol.1. Baltimore, Md: Lippincott Williams and Wilkins; 1994:1074.)

Figure 88-6. A) Single right lung transplant showing preparation of pulmonary artery for anastomosis. **B)** Continuous end-to-end anastomosis of pulmonary artery using a 5.0 or 6.0 polypropylene suture. (Adapted from Patterson GA, Cooper JD. Lung Transplantation. In: Shields TW, ed. General Thoracic Surgery. Vol.1. Baltimore, Md: Lippincott Williams and Wilkins; 1994:1074.)

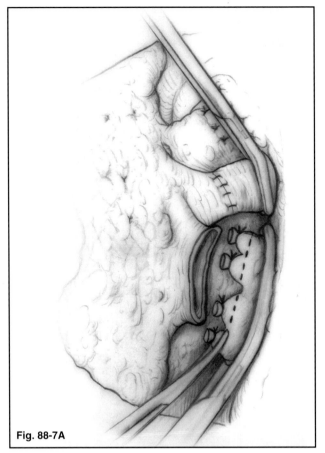

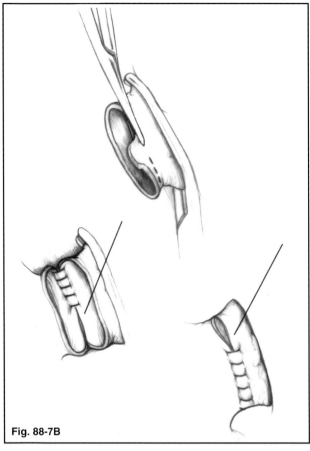

Figure 88-7. A) Single right lung transplant showing preparation of left atrial cuff. **B)** Continuous suture anastomosis of left atrial cuffs. (Adapted from Patterson GA, Cooper JD. Lung Transplantation. In: Shields TW, ed. General Thoracic Surgery. Vol.1. Baltimore, Md: Lippincott Williams and Wilkins; 1994:1075.)

lent exposure to both pleural spaces (Figure 88-8). Alternatively, bilateral anterior thoracotomies without sternal division can be performed with the benefit of avoiding sternal wound problems. The lung with the worst function is gently explanted first. The decision to place the patient on cardiopulmonary bypass is made based on the patient's status (eg, right ventricular failure, hypoxia), or, once the first allograft is in, with the development of pulmonary hypertension or pulmonary edema. The technical procedure is the same as for single lung transplants.

Heart-Lung Implantation Procedure

The recipient is brought to the operating room and anesthetized. Surgical exposure is improved if the recipient is able to tolerate single lung ventilation and a dual lumen endotracheal tube can be used. The type of incision performed is based on the surgeon's preference with either a median sternotomy or an anterotranssternal (ie, clamshell) thoracotomy providing excellent exposure. For patients with prior thoracic surgeries, significant adhesions between lung and chest wall, tracheobronchial collateral or systemic artery-to-pulmonary connections,

the clamshell thoracotomy provides greater visualization and technical ease (Figure 88-8). Mobilization of the IVC, SVC, and ascending aorta is performed. The SVC and aorta are retracted laterally and the posterior pericardium is incised above the right pulmonary artery allowing the trachea to be encircled with umbilical tape. For cardiopulmonary bypass the ascending aorta is cannulated and bicaval cannulation provides venous return. Both pleural spaces are opened and adhesions are divided. The hilar structures are carefully dissected and mobilized, a step that may have to await initiation of cardiopulmonary bypass in patients with pulmonary hypertension.

Following the arrival of the donor organs, cardiopulmonary bypass is initiated by placing a vascular occlusion clamp across the ascending aorta below the aortic cannula. Tapes around the vena cava allow complete occlusion. The recipient is cooled to between 28 to 32°C, and mechanical ventilation is ceased to allow better exposure. The pericardium around the level of the hilum is excised and the pulmonary artery and veins are mobilized in the intrapericardial space. The right atrium is excised adjacent to the atrioventricular groove anteriorly and the excision is extended circumferentially along the atrial septum. The aorta is divided above the aortic valve and retracted superiorly. The remaining pulmonary arteries, left atrium and ventricular structures are dissected free from surrounding mediastinal tissue and the patient's heart is removed (Figure 88-8).

The bronchi on each side are mobilized and ligated proximally using a surgical stapler. Division distal to the staple line allows for removal of the recipient's lungs (Figure 88-9). Importantly, the phrenic nerve must be identified and preserved on both sides.

After removal of the patients lungs, the pericardial opening is extended inferiorly and superiorly, enabling positioning of donor lungs into the appropriate pleural cavities. By retracting the umbilical tape surrounding the trachea, the bronchi and carinal structures are mobilized and the patient's trachea is divided immediately above the carina. A 2.0 silk suture through the anterior aspect of the tracheal wall serves as a traction stitch. Care must be taken to ensure that the large bronchial and systemic arteries are ligated. Obtaining hemostasis before proceeding with anastomosis is critical, as exposure to the posterior mediastinum after heart-lung implantation is difficult and often impossible.

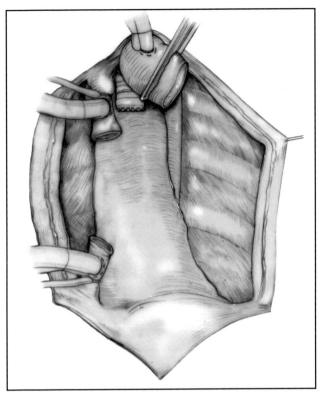

Figure 88-9. Heart-lung transplant procedure with appearance of recipient's chest cavity after removal of heart and lungs. The pericardial-phrenic pedicles are seen in the drawing.

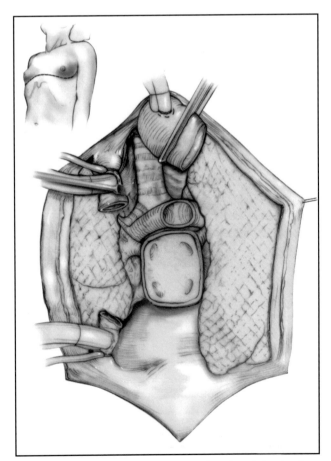

Figure 88-8. Heart-lung transplant procedure, insert showing the typical clamshell incision. Appearance of the recipient's chest after heart removal and prior to lung removal.

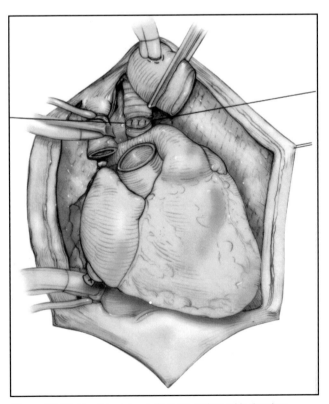

Figure 88-10. Heart-lung transplant procedure with drawing depicting placement of the donor's heart-lung in the recipient and performance of tracheal anastomosis with running 4.0 PDS suture.

The donor heart-lung block is brought into the operative field with a cold lap pad surrounding the organs to maintain topical hypothermia. The donor lungs are passed through the opening in the pericardium into the pleural cavities posterior to the phrenic nerve-pericardial pedicles. The tracheal anastomosis is performed first (Figure 88-10). The donor's trachea is divided one to two rings above the carina. A running 4.0 PDS suture is used.

Over the suture line, peritracheal tissue is approximated to cover the anastomosis (Figure 88-11). Following the tracheal anastomosis, the venous anastomosis is performed either by the bicaval technique or the right cuff technique described by Shumway and Lower. In the bicaval technique the interatrial groove on the recipient heart is developed, the Swan-Ganz catheter removed, and the SVC is transected just above the junction between the cava and right atrium. The inferior aspect of the right atrium is divided above the level where the right inferior pulmonary vein enters the left atrium. Residual areas of right atrial free wall are excised. Control of several vessels transversing the septum and the mediastinum require control with cautery or suture ligation. The IVC anastomosis is performed first, followed by the SVC (Figure 88-11). Both are performed using 5.0 or 6.0 prolene suture in a running fashion. Prior to completion of the SVC anastomosis, the pulmonary artery catheter is advanced through the donor heart. If ischemic time is prolonged, this anastomosis can be performed after the aortic.

In the right atrial cuff technique of Shumway and Lower, the anastomosis is begun along the medial side of the donor's right atrial cuff at the level of the IVC-right atrial juncture, which is anastomosed to the septal portion of the recipient atrium. After this portion is complete, the lateral wall of the donor atrium is anastomosed to the lateral wall of the recipient's right atrial cuff.

The aortic anastomosis is performed using running 4.0 prolene (Figure 88-12). Before tying this anastomosis, the heart-lung block is de-aired. Upon completion, systemic rewarming is initiated. A vent is placed via the right superior pulmonary vein into the left ventricle. When the recipient's temperature reaches 34°C and adequate ventricular function is present, the left ventricular vent is removed. Attention to de-airing the cardiac chambers is imperative and transesophageal echocardiography is extremely useful in assessing amount of residual air. The level of inotropic support required to separate the patient from cardiopulmonary bypass is then assessed.

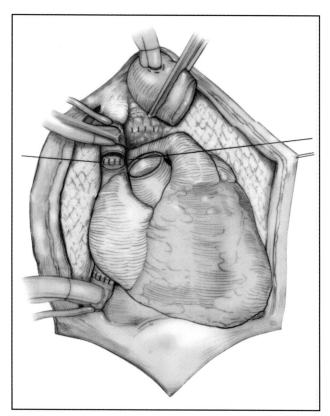

Figure 88-11. Heart-lung transplant procedure with drawing showing tracheal anastomosis covered with peritracheal tissue and completion of IVC anastomosis. The SVC anastomosis is depicted with a running 5.0 prolene.

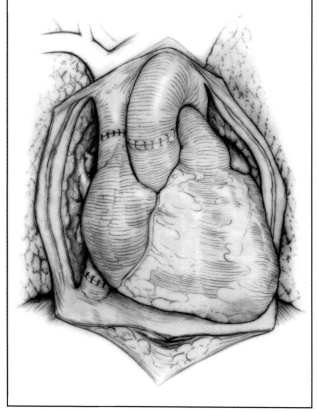

Figure 88-12. Appearance of the recipient chest at the conclusion of the heart-lung transplant. The aortic anastomosis has been completed using a running 4.0 prolene.

LUNG TRANSPLANTATION WITH COEXISTING CORONARY ARTERY DISEASE, VALVULAR HEART DISEASE, OR CONGENITAL HEART DEFECTS

Lung transplantation can be performed in the presence of coexisting correctable cardiac conditions in carefully selected patients. In such patients, surgical treatment should be technically straightforward. When cardiopulmonary bypass is required for the cardiac repair a short bypass and cross clamp time should be expected, excellent cardiac function post repair should be anticipated, and an excellent long-term prognosis with regard to the cardiac condition should be obtainable. Generally, in such patients the surgical results should be predictable. Usually, in these patients, right single lung transplant is preferred. The surgical approach depends on the planned procedure, but for a right single lung transplant, a right anterolateral thoracotomy, a median sternotomy with a T extension, or a right anterolateral thoracotomy with a transsternal extension can be used. When the cardiac repair does not require cardiopulmonary bypass, a minimally invasive technique with a left single lung transplant can be performed. For bilateral lung transplants with repair of cardiac defects, a clamshell incision provides the optimal exposure. After placement of the patient on cardiopulmonary bypass, the necessary bypass grafts are performed. Depending on the status of the patient after the grafts are placed, the decision is made whether to come off cardiopulmonary bypass prior to proceeding with the lung transplant procedure. The lung transplant proceeds as normal.

RECOMMENDED READING

Sundaresan S, Trachiotis GD, Aoe M, Patterson GA, Cooper JD. Donor lung procurement: assessment and operative technique. Ann Thorac Surg. 1993;56(6):1409-1413.

Patterson GA, Cooper JD. Lung Transplantation. In: Pearson FG, Deslauriers J, Ginsberg RJ, Hiebert CA, McKneally MF, Harold C. Urschel J, eds. Thoracic Surgery. Vol. 1. New York, NY: Churchill Livingstone; 1995:931-959.

Lau CL, Palmer SM, D'Amico TA, F Tapson V, Davis RD. Lung Transplantation at Duke University Medical Center. In: Cecka JM, Terasaki PI, eds. Clinical Transplants. Los Angeles, Ca: UCLA Tissue Typing Laboratory; 1998:327-340.

Jhaveri R, Davis RD, Tardiff B, Leone B. Heart and Heart-Lung Transplantation. In: Sharpe MD, Gelb AW, eds. Anesthesia and Transplantation. Boston, Ma: Butterworth and Heinemann; 1999:113-141.

Chen CZ, Gallagher RC, Ardery P, Dyckman W, Low HB. Retrograde versus antegrade flush in canine left lung preservation for six hours. J Heart Lung Transplant. 1996;15(4):395-403.

Meyers BF, Patterson GA. Technical aspects of adult lung transplantation. Semin Thorac Cardiovasc Surg. 1998;10(3):213-200.

89 IMMEDIATE POSTOPERATIVE MANAGEMENT OF THE LUNG TRANSPLANT RECIPIENT

Scott M. Palmer, MD
Victor F. Tapson, MD, FCCP

The care of the lung transplant recipient in the immediate postoperative period presents a number of challenges for surgeons, pulmonologists, anesthesiologists, nurses and other personnel involved. Optimal management of ventilation and hemodynamics is difficult, and careful consideration must be given to the specific underlying lung disease as well as posttransplant allograft function. In this section, the approach to postoperative care in lung transplant recipients is reviewed followed by a discussion of postoperative surgical complications. Pulmonary parenchymal complications, such as reperfusion injury or acute allograft rejection, are discussed elsewhere in the primer and will not be covered in this section.

POSTOPERATIVE MANAGEMENT
Mechanical Ventilation and Respiratory Care

Postoperatively, patients are transported, intubated, to the intensive care unit (ICU) for constant monitoring. Patients typically leave the operating room on an inspired oxygen concentration (FiO2) of 60% to 100% and are in an assist control mode of ventilation (either volume or pressure). An advantage of pressure control ventilation includes the ability to limit peak airway pressures and prevent barotrauma to the bronchial anastomosis. Commonly, attempts are made to limit plateau pressures to no more than 35 mmHg. If the initial postoperative arterial blood gas demonstrates an arterial pO2 of greater than 70 and/or an oxygen saturation greater than 90%, then the FiO2 is gradually weaned, with repeat measurements of arterial oxygenation made after each change. The FiO2 is reduced as tolerated in order to minimize the risk of oxygen toxicity. In most patients without significant reperfusion edema, the FiO2 can be

Scott M. Palmer, MD, Associate in Medicine, Division of Pulmonary and Critical Medicine, Duke University Medical Center, Durham, NC

Victor F. Tapson, MD, FCCP, Associate Professor of Medicine, Division of Pulmonary and Critical Medicine; Medical Director, Duke University Lung Transplant Program, Duke University Medical Center, Durham, NC

weaned successfully to 30% or less within the first 12 to 24 hours after transplantation.

In single lung transplant patients with chronic obstructive pulmonary disease (COPD), zero or minimal positive end expiratory pressure (PEEP) is used, along with an adequate expiratory phase of ventilation to prevent air trapping in the native lung. An expiratory hold maneuver may be useful to detect air trapping in these patients. Only rarely is it necessary to use a dual lumen endotracheal tube to prevent hyperinflation of the native lung with resulting compression of the transplanted lung. These smaller diameter dual lumen tubes are less ideal than single lumen tubes because the smaller diameter of the bifurcated tube makes adequate clearance of secretions more difficult. Furthermore, maintaining the desirable position of the double lumen tubes is more difficult and malposition may occur with subsequent lobar atelectasis. In single lung transplantation for non-obstructive lung disease or bilateral lung transplantation, a small amount of PEEP may be useful to prevent alveolar collapse and improve oxygenation, especially in patients with reperfusion injury.

Nitric oxide may be used in the early postoperative period to decrease pulmonary vascular resistance and improve arterial oxygenation. Although no randomized placebo-controlled trials of nitric oxide have been performed in lung transplant recipients, several anecdotal reports suggest that the early postoperative use of inhaled nitric oxide may be beneficial, especially in patients with reperfusion injury. Once a patient's clinical status improves, attempts are made to wean the nitric oxide. If weaning the nitric oxide proceeds without more than a 10% decrease in arterial oxygenation, or a 10% increase in pulmonary vascular pressures, then weaning should continue.

Once a patient begins to breathe spontaneously, attempts can be made to wean mechanical ventilatory support. The weaning protocol may involve the use of pressure support ventilation. Inspiratory pressure is gradually reduced as tolerated with careful observation of the respiratory rate, tidal volumes, and arterial blood gas. Pulmonary mechanics are usually tested prior to extubation. Patients should have a negative inspiratory force maneuver of greater than -50 and a frequency to tidal volume (f/Vt) ratio of less than 100. Prior to extubation, patients undergo bronchoscopy to assess the anastomosis and ensure adequate clearance of secretions. In approximately half of single or bilateral lung transplant recipients, liberation from mechanical ventilation can be accomplished within 48 hours of transplantation.

Following extubation, the apical chest tubes are removed in the absence of an air-leak, commonly within 48 hours after transplantation. Because of the frequent occurrence of recurrent pleural effusions postoperatively, especially in bilateral lung transplant candidates, the basal chest tubes remain for several days, usually being removed on postoperative day five to seven, depending on the clinical situation. Chest tubes are typically removed when the chest tube drainage decreases to less than 50 cc to 150 cc over 24 hours (this varies between centers).

Vigorous chest physiotherapy, inhaled bronchodilators, and frequent clearance of pulmonary secretions by endotracheal suctioning is required in the postoperative care of these patients. Postural drainage is performed at least three times a day. Early and constant involvement of physical therapy ensures that these patients are out of bed in a chair, ambulating with assistance, and using the treadmill or exercise bicycle as soon as possible, even if they remain intubated.

Phrenic nerve injury with diaphragmatic paralysis should be considered in posttransplant recipients with difficulty weaning, especially in the absence of significant pulmonary parenchymal injury. Phrenic nerve injury is reported to occur in approximately 3% of lung transplant recipients. When suspected, fluoroscopy may be useful to confirm the diagnosis, and treatment is mainly supportive with recovery of function in some patients over several months.

In patients who develop significant reperfusion edema or other early posttransplant complications that prolong the duration of mechanical ventilation, early tracheostomy should be considered to facilitate weaning. There should be a low threshold for performing tracheostomies because they allow easier mobility of the patient, in addition to better oral hygiene and clearance of pulmonary secretions.

Hemodynamic Monitoring and Management

Because of the complexity of the hemodynamic management of lung transplant recipients in the immediate postoperative period, a pulmonary artery catheter should be used to guide patient care. Despite careful operative fluid management, lung transplant recipients frequently arrive in the acute care unit with a significant positive fluid balance. In addition, increased vascular permeability occurs in most patients after transplantation and predisposes the transplanted lung(s) to the development of pulmonary edema. Therefore, a goal of the early postoperative hemodynamic management is to reduce pulmonary capillary filling pressures and minimize pulmonary edema while still maintaining adequate urine output. Combinations of blood, colloid, inotropes and diuretics are employed to maintain the pulmonary capillary wedge pressure at approximately 10 to 12 mmHg. Although controlled data is lacking, dopamine at 2 to 3 µg/kg per minute is often used as a renal vasodilator to increase diuresis. Overly aggressive diuresis, however, can result in renal insufficiency, which may be exacer-

bated by high postoperative cyclosporine levels, and careful monitoring of renal function is essential during the immediate postoperative period. The pulmonary artery catheter is removed when the patient is extubated and sent out of the ICU.

Pain Management

Adequate analgesia is necessary to prevent atelectasis, which develops from poor chest movement and inadequate coughing effort in the setting of postthoracotomy incisional pain. An epidural catheter provides an excellent means of achieving pain control with minimal systemic effects. It appears that the use of an epidural catheter after lung transplantation may be associated with faster extubation and shorter intensive care unit stay compared with the use of intravenous morphine. Patients often require at least some oral narcotics in the first few weeks after transplantation for pain management. Oral narcotics or acetaminophen are preferred over nonsteroidal antiinflammatory agents that could contribute to renal insufficiency in those patients already on cyclosporine and other potentially nephrotoxic drugs.

Infection Prophylaxis

BACTERIAL. Bacterial infection is the leading cause of death in the early posttransplant period and careful selection of prophylactic antibiotic regimens is essential to a successful outcome. At most institutions, lung transplant patients receive a seven to ten day course of broad spectrum antimicrobial prophylaxis, which includes coverage of Gram-positive and Gram-negative organisms. The antibiotic regimen is modified depending on results of the cultures obtained from the donor and recipient prior to transplantation (especially in patients with cystic fibrosis who have preoperative pathogens with known sensitivities). Antibiotics may be continued longer, depending on the recipient's cultures after transplantation. Antibiotic selection at each institution should be determined by the specific isolates and sensitivity patterns observed in their population of patients, with periodic reevaluation of antibiotic selection.

VIRAL INFECTION PROPHYLAXIS. Although cytomegalovirus (CMV) contributed significantly to early posttransplant morbidity and mortality after lung transplantation in the pre-ganciclovir era, current prophylaxis regimens have significantly decreased the frequency and severity of CMV infections. Most institutions use prophylaxis regimens based upon donor and recipient CMV serology. A typical regimen for donor-positive/recipient-positive or donor-negative/recipient-positive patients would include ganciclovir at 5 mg/kg intravenously every 12 hours for one to two weeks followed by 5 mg/kg per day for an additional two to six weeks. Again, these regimens vary from center to center, and are governed by individual center experience, recipient-specific factors such as perioperative immunosuppressant requirements, renal function, and the availability of readily-performed CMV blood screening tests such as CMV-PCR and CMV antigenemia. In donor-positive/recipient-negative patients, CMV hyperimmune globulin (CytoGam®) is usually added at 150 to 200 mg/kg per dose for a total of five to eight doses over eight to 12 weeks. The use of CytoGam® is favored in these high-risk mismatch patients because of evidence for its utility in the prophylaxis of CMV infections in other solid organ transplant recipients. For high-risk patients, ganciclovir is administered for a more prolonged period. A typical regimen would be 5 mg/kg IV every 12 hours for two to four weeks, followed by 5 mg/kg per day IV for a total of six to ten weeks. In donor-negative/recipient-negative patients, ganciclovir administration is not generally employed, but CMV negative and leuko-reduced packed red blood cells are used if transfusion is required. Regimens for CMV prophylaxis are somewhat variable at different medical centers. In the absence of indications for ganciclovir prophylaxis, most centers routinely use acyclovir prophylaxis (200 mg orally or IV bid) to protect the transplant recipient from herpes viral infections. The latter were a frequent cause of morbidity and mortality during the first postoperative months before the routine use of acyclovir or ganciclovir.

FUNGAL PROPHYLAXIS. Although fungal infections are recognized as an important cause of posttransplant morbidity and mortality, prophylaxis regimens vary widely among centers. Some centers rely upon azole antifungal compounds such as fluconazole or itraconazole. However, there are several limitations to the use of these azole drugs. First, there is no currently available broad spectrum azole drug that adequately covers both *Aspergillus* and *Candida* species. Second, increasing resistance among certain *Candida* isolates to fluconazole limits the utility of this drug as a prophylactic agent. Finally, variable absorption, especially with itraconazole, and drug interactions between fluconazole or itraconazole and cyclosporine also complicate the use of these drugs in transplant recipients.

Other centers have employed low-dose systemic amphotericin B as antifungal prophylaxis. However, failures have been reported with this approach as well, which may involve substantial risks of nephrotoxicity given concomitant use of cyclosporine in these patients.

Advantages of aerosolized antifungal prophylaxis include the direct delivery of the antifungal medication to the lungs, allowing for high concentrations in the pulmonary tissues with no significant systemic side effects. Recent reports have suggested aerosolized amphotericin B may provide effective prophylaxis against fungal infec-

tion in lung transplant recipients. Nausea and bronchospasm, however, have been described as common side effects with aerosolized amphotericin B. Preliminary data on the use of aerosolized liposomal amphotericin B (ABLC) in humans is available as part of an ongoing study after lung transplantation. Nebulized ABLC appears to be better-tolerated than aerosolized amphotericin B, and was associated with a dramatic reduction in pulmonary fungal infections. Although further study of aerosolized ABLC is needed in humans, animal data suggests several advantages of liposomal amphotericin B over conventional amphotericin B, including increased pulmonary drug concentrations, longer tissue half-life, and less nephrotoxicity.

***PNEUMOCYSTIS CARINII* PROPHYLAXIS.** At most lung transplant centers, patients receive prophylaxis with trimethoprim/sulfamethoxazole three times per week (or monthly-aerosolized pentamidine if the patient is allergic to sulfa drugs) for the prevention of *Pneumocystis carinii* pneumonia (PCP). To date, there have been no reports of failure of these prophylaxis regimens in transplant recipients in contrast to data from HIV-infected patients.

Gastrointestinal Considerations

Narcotics, calcium channel blockers, immunosuppressive medications and vagal injury after lung transplantation can all contribute to the development of gastrointestinal complications. Several groups have reported early life-threatening gastrointestinal complications after lung transplantation, including bowel obstruction and/or perforation, in addition to the widely reported complication of gastroparesis. The mechanism of gastroparesis is probably related to vagal injury. Gastroparesis can contribute to gastroesophageal reflux (GER), with the associated risks of aspiration, as well as impacting on absorption and therefore blood levels and efficacy of immunosuppressants. Because GER may contribute to postoperative respiratory complications, promotility and acid suppression medications should be employed early in the postoperative period. Aggressive regimens should be instituted postoperatively to initiate and maintain regular bowel movements after transplantation. Multiple laxatives and enemas are often necessary, especially in the early posttransplant period. The issues of gastrointestinal motility are magnified in patients with cystic fibrosis, where aggressive therapy with oral Golitely®, and Hypaque® enemas with Tween® have been required to avoid, or relieve, distal ileal obstruction syndrome – the adult equivalent of meconium ileus.

Postoperative Consultation

Because the postoperative care of the lung transplant recipient involves the coordinated efforts of many different transplant team members, early notification of all involved personnel is crucial. Although the transplant surgeon, pulmonologist and ICU nursing team are all involved in the immediate care of the patient upon arrival from the operating room, transplant infectious disease personnel, the anesthesia pain team, physical therapists, and the nutrition support team should all participate in early posttransplant care. Other team members should be involved as needed in the early postoperative care. For example, early involvement of transplant social workers may facilitate discharge planning. Successful outcomes depend upon the coordinated efforts of the multidisciplinary transplant team and communication among all team members is essential.

EARLY POSTOPERATIVE COMPLICATIONS

Bronchial Anastomotic Complications

Anastomotic complications limited the success of many early attempts at human lung transplantation. Lethal tracheal dehiscence and/or extensive airway necrosis was reported in four of the initial 13 bilateral lung transplant recipients in Toronto, Canada. Anastomotic complications, however, are now infrequent in modern lung transplantation. Bilateral sequential transplantation is preferred to en bloc tracheal anastomosis. Anastomotic healing is improved with bilateral sequential transplantation which employs telescoping anastomoses. Acute bronchial anastomotic complications are now uncommon, although late anastomotic stenosis still occurs in 7% to 14% of patients. Although bronchial dehiscence is now rare, careful attention to the anastomosis is required at all posttransplant bronchoscopies because early posttransplant anastomotic infections have been described. *Aspergillus* and *Candida* have been identified as potential pathogens which can cause life-threatening bronchial anastomotic infection. The presence of extensive anastomotic pseudomembranes, particularly with evidence of necrosis, may indicate that fungal infection is present, and cautious endobronchial biopsies should be considered to rule out an invasive fungal infection. Although the optimal treatment of bronchial anastomotic fungal infection is unknown, a combination of systemic and inhaled antifungal agents should be considered, because aerosolization allows direct drug delivery to the poorly vascularized anastomosis. Success has been reported with such an approach in the treatment of three lung transplant recipients with biopsy-proven invasive *Candida* anastomotic infection.

Pulmonary Vascular Complications

Clinically significant pulmonary vascular complications are rare after lung transplantation, but associated with significant morbidity and mortality when present. Most series suggest the incidence of pulmonary arterial complications is less than 2%, with the incidence of pulmonary venous complications even lower. Vascular anastomotic complications may occur related to technical problems with the donor harvest, but have also been reported in apparently normal anastomoses as well. To evaluate for the presence of vascular anastomotic complications, all patients should undergo a quantitative lung perfusion scan within four hours of transplantation to assess for adequate patency and graft flow. Perfusion of less than 50% to the transplanted lung in a single lung allograft recipient or a significant discrepancy between right and left lung perfusion in a bilateral lung transplant recipient should raise concern for potential pulmonary vascular complications. Alternatively, intraoperative transesophageal echocardiography is used at some centers to assess pulmonary vascular anastomoses, but offers only limited views of the left pulmonary vein, and therefore, is not routinely used. The "gold standard" for the diagnosis of pulmonary arterial complications is pulmonary angiography. The most common findings identified in one series of patients with vascular complications were pulmonary arterial stenosis or thrombosis. In cases of stenosis, several reports suggest that the use of percutaneously delivered endovascular stents can achieve excellent results with significantly less morbidity than reoperation .

As with other surgical patients, lung transplant recipients are at risk of deep venous thrombosis and pulmonary embolism. This has been reported to occur in up to 12% of lung transplant recipients in one series, with pulmonary embolism causing or contributing to several deaths in that series. Patients with severe reperfusion edema and prolonged posttransplant ventilator courses appear to be at the highest risk for venous thromboembolism, and prophylaxis should be strongly considered in those patients. Controlled trials of deep venous thrombosis prophylaxis after lung transplantation, however, have not been performed. The utility of such prophylaxis must be carefully weighed against any risks of postoperative bleeding.

Other Postoperative Complications

Significant ischemia reperfusion injury complicates approximately 10% to 15% of lung transplant operations, and is usually manifest within the first 24 to 48 hours postoperatively. Acute rejection occurs in almost 90% of lung transplant recipients within three months postoperatively. Despite prophylaxis, postoperative infections also occur commonly in the early posttransplant period. Although bacterial infections are most common early after transplantation, fungal infections, CMV, or respiratory viral infections should also be considered. Bronchoscopy with transbronchial biopsy is essential for the diagnosis of early acute complications in the lung transplant recipient with signs or symptoms of allograft dysfunction.

RECOMMENDED READING

Meyer KC, Love RB, and Zimmerman JJ. The therapeutic potential of nitric oxide in lung transplantation. Chest. 1998;113(5):1360-1371.

Maziak DE, Maurer JR, and Kesten S. Diaphragmatic paralysis: a complication of lung transplantation. Ann Thorac Surg. 1996;61(1):170-173.

Triantafillou AN, Heerdt PM, Hogue CW, et al. Epidural vs intravenous morphine for postoperative pain management after lung transplantation. Anesthesiology. 1992;77:A858.

Trulock EP. Lung transplantation 1997. Am J Respir Crit Care Med. 155(3):789-818.

Soghikian MV, Valentine VG, Berry GJ, Patel HR, Robbins RC, Theodore J. Impact of ganciclovir prophylaxis on heart-lung and lung transplant recipients. J Heart Lung Transplant. 1996;15(9):881-887.

Levine MS, Kubak BM, Shipiner RB, et al. The efficacy of antifungal prophylaxis in lung allograft recipients. Chest. 1996 (supplement); 110:227S.

Lubetkin EI, Lipson DA, Palevsky HI, et al. GI complications after lung transplantation. Am J Gastroenterol. 1996;91(11):2382-2390.

Patterson GA, Cooper JD, Kark JH, et al. Airway complications after double lung transplantation in humans. J Thorac Cardiovasc Surg. 1988;95:70-74.

Palmer SM, Perfect JR, Howell DN, et al. Candidal anastomotic infection in lung transplant recipients: successful treatment with a combination of systemic and inhaled antifungal agents. J Heart Lung Transplant. 1998;17(10): 1029-1033.

Clark SC, Levine AJ, Hasan A, Hilton CJ, Forty J, Dark JH. Vascular complications of lung transplantation. Ann Thorac Surg. 1996;61(4):1079-7982.

Hearne SE, O'Laughlin MP, Davis RD, Baker WA, Bashore TM, Harrison JK. Total pulmonary artery occlusion immediately after lung transplantation: successful revascularization with intravascular stents. J Heart Lung Transplant. 1996;15(5):532-535.

Kroshus TJ, Kshettry VR, Hertz MI, Bolman RM 3rd. Deep venous thrombosis and pulmonary embolism after lung transplantation. J Thorac Cardiovasc Surg. 1995;110(2):540-544.

90 PHYSIOLOGY OF THE TRANSPLANTED LUNG

Larry L. Schulman, MD

Successful lung transplantation has enabled pulmonary physiologists to begin to clarify fundamental pathophysiologic problems that were previously unapproachable or available only in animal models. This chapter will deal with issues related to lung denervation, impaired cough and mucociliary clearance, lymphatic interruption, vascular tone, right ventricular function, and pulmonary function in single and bilateral lung allografts. Numerous physiologic questions and studies remain to be addressed in the future.

PULMONARY DENERVATION

Bilateral lung transplantation or combined heart-lung transplantation interrupts the pulmonary branch of the vagus nerve, which is the afferent pathway for stretch receptors in the lung. As a consequence of vagal interruption, the classic Breuer-Hering reflex is abolished. Nevertheless, the resting breathing pattern in lung transplant recipients is no different from normal subjects, provided there are no concurrent restrictive or obstructive ventilatory defects. There are no disturbances in sleep architecture, oxyhemoglobin saturation, or sleep-disordered events compared to normal subjects. Duration of breath-holding time and associated respiratory distress is not substantially modified. Thus, pulmonary vagal afferent information does not appear to contribute significantly to the regulation of resting breathing in humans, either during wakefulness or during sleep.

Interpretation of physiologic studies of the denervated lung requires careful exclusion of associated restrictive or obstructive ventilatory defects. For example, an early study of heart-lung transplant recipients suggested that disruption of vagal pathways blunts the ventilatory response to hypercapnia, whereas the ventilatory response to hypoxia remains intact. These patients, however, had restricted lung volumes (see Pulmonary Function below). A subsequent study of heart-lung recipients with near-normal lung volumes showed normal ventilatory responses to hypercapnia. In fact, the observation that restricted denervated transplant recipients retain the usual "restrictive" response during venti-

Associate Professor of Clinical Medicine; Director, Lung Transplant Service, Columbia University, College of Physicians & Surgeons, New York, NY

latory stimulation (ie, decreased tidal volume and increased frequency), implies that these responses are mediated at least in part by extravagal pathways. Similarly, transplant recipients with airflow obstruction as a consequence of obliterative bronchiolitis retain the typical "obstructive" response to ventilatory stimulation.

A more clinically-relevant consequence of afferent vagal denervation is that the cough response to airway irritants is impaired. During fiberoptic bronchoscopy, mechanical stimulation of the bronchi below the anastomosis between donor and recipient fails to induce coughing. Similarly, the cough response to ultrasonically nebulized distilled water or to extract of red pepper is strikingly diminished compared to normal subjects. Afferent denervation also diminishes the chronic cough associated with gastroesophageal reflux. In contrast, the efferent limb of the cough response appears unaffected, and patients are able to generate sufficient respiratory muscle motor output for coughing after transplantation.

Another potential consequence of vagal disruption is bronchial hyper-reactivity, possibly as a result of denervation hypersensitivity of airway smooth muscle receptors. Some studies have reported bronchial hyper-responsiveness to methacholine in heart-lung and double-lung recipients. Bronchial hyper-responsiveness was unrelated to the level of FEV_1, time after transplantation, presence of airway inflammation, or presence of acute allograft rejection. Other studies have shown hypersensitivity to methacholine or histamine in single-lung recipients to be less marked than in heart-lung or double-lung recipients, presumably reflecting intact innervation of the native lung in single-lung recipients. Other investigators have questioned whether this phenomenon of bronchial hypersensitivity exists at all when they demonstrated normal bronchial responsiveness to methacholine and isocapnic dry air hyperventilation in heart-lung or double-lung recipients. Certainly, bronchial hyper-responsiveness is not a clinical problem after lung or heart-lung transplantation. Diurnal variation in FEV_1 is similar to normal subjects. Even in those studies that demonstrate bronchial hypersensitivity, the presence and degree of hyper-reactivity are highly variable. Furthermore, denervation hypersensitivity, per se, cannot account for the increased cholinergic responsiveness observed in these patients, since pathologic studies demonstrate normally functioning postganglionic nerves and no change in cholinergic responsiveness or cholinergic receptors. Since there is no functional adrenergic innervation of human airway smooth muscle, denervation would not influence β-receptor function. Thus, if posttransplant bronchial hyper-reactivity does exist, future work must focus on other mechanisms, such as the peptidergic neurotransmitters of the nonadrenergic, noncholinergic system.

Finally, it is important to remember that although vagal information is disrupted after lung transplantation, afferent neural information is still transmitted via chest wall or diaphragmatic afferents and by stretch receptors in the airway above the anastomosis (ie, cough reflexes are preserved above the anastomosis). There is also some evidence that the neural pathways may regenerate slowly. Cardiac sympathetic reinnervation occurs after heart transplantation, and pulmonary stretch receptors become reinnervated within two years of vagal interruption in dogs. However, there is no solid evidence yet for vagal reinervation after human lung transplantation.

AIRWAYS
Cough Reflex
As indicated above, the cough response to airway irritants after lung transplantation is markedly impaired. As a consequence, transplant recipients may fail to clear respiratory secretions properly. They may be insensitive to microaspiration, which can occur as a consequence of postoperative gastroparesis. These factors contribute to the high incidence of bacterial infections after lung transplantation.

Mucociliary Clearance
In addition to impaired cough reflexes, there is evidence that mucociliary clearance after lung transplantation is impaired. In one study, the clearance time of a technitium-labeled aerosol was nearly double the clearance rate in normal controls. Of course, loss of cough reflex itself will delay clearance of an aerosol. Moreover, passage across the tracheal or bronchial anastomosis is delayed because of interruption of the ciliary carpet. (Note: even well-healed anastomoses are often covered by a layer of white fibrous tissue replacing normal pink respiratory mucosa. In addition, anastomoses may be "ridged" or narrowed, particularly the "telescoped" anastomosis.) Ciliary function itself (eg, ciliary beat frequency) may be impaired.

Abnormal mucociliary clearance after lung transplantation probably relates to multiple factors including denervation, quantitative alterations in respiratory secretions, airway inflammation related to previous episodes of rejection or infection, and altered immunologic function in the airways related to immunosupprevise therapy and abnormal interactions between circulating host lymphocytes and donor macrophages in the allografted lung. The predisposition to bacterial infection is underscored by the clinical observation that in single-lung transplant recipients, bacterial infections are often limited to the transplanted side.

LYMPHATICS
Formation of Lymph
Fluid normally leaks out of capillaries located in the alveolar wall and moves out of the small septal interstitial spaces to the larger tissue spaces surrounding terminal airways, where it enters lymphatic capillaries. Under normal circumstances, the rate at which filtered proteins and water enter the lymph equals the rate at which they cross the capillary wall. Lymph flow increases approximately 20% for each 1 mmHg change in capillary pressure. Lymph flow changes greatly for similar elevations in capillary pressure under conditions of increased permeability of the capillary walls.

Effect of Lymphatic Interruption
Because lymph removes proteins and fluid from the interstitium, lymphatic vessel interruption would be expected to produce lung edema. In experimental lymphatic ligation, lungs develop slight interstitial edema when capillary pressure is elevated. The maximum increase in tissue water occurs within three days and subsides to normal levels by five days. In experimental lung reimplantation, lung water also reaches its maximal value after three days, and returns to normal levels by six weeks. Some degree of lymphatic function, assessed by injection of blue dye, returns as early as one week after reimplantation, and new lymphatic vessels are visible within 12 days. In experimental lung allotransplantation, lymphatic function, assessed by lymphoscintigraphic visualization of mediastinal nodes, is reestablished in some animals as early as the second postoperative week, and in all animals within two to four weeks.

In human lung transplantation, the incidence of radiographic signs of lung allograft edema in the early postoperative period is highly variable, but in one series was reported to be as high as 97%. The accumulation of lung allograft interstitial edema in the early postoperative period increases the likelihood of atelectasis and infection. In addition to impaired cough and mucous clearance as mentioned before, lymphatic interruption prevents migration of immune effector cells to mediastinal lymph nodes. This interferes with presentation of antigen to antigen-processing cells, thereby impairing the host immune response to microbial pathogens. In one experimental preparation, the major factors increasing the severity of pneumonia after lung transplantation were immunosuppressive medications and lymphatic interruption. Thoracotomy, transplant surgery, and allogenicity itself did not significantly influence the severity of postoperative pneumonia.

Although there is no treatment of pulmonary interstitial edema caused by lymphatic interruption, supportive measures and minimizing pulmonary capillary pressures in the early postoperative period are usually successful in maintaining function of transplanted lungs. The temporary changes in function and increased susceptibility to infection do not preclude successful lung transplantation.

VASOACTIVITY
General Principles

Under normal circumstances, there is low vascular tone in the pulmonary circulation. This is related to basal endogenous elaboration of vasodilators such as prostacyclin. Neurohumoral influences become important when there are perturbations in pulmonary vascular pressures and flow. Denervated lungs after transplantation provide a unique opportunity to examine some of the complex neural, humoral and local regulatory mechanisms in the pulmonary circulation.

Nevertheless, there are major difficulties in studying the behavior of the denervated pulmonary vasculature after lung transplantation, either in humans or in experimental animals. These confounding effects include: lung injury related to tissue ischemia; surgical trauma; immunosuppressive therapy; tissue rejection; effects of anesthetics in experimental models; single point calculations of pulmonary vascular resistance; and "fixed" resistances at the site of the arterial and pulmonary venous anastomoses.

Left Lung Autotransplant Model

The canine left lung autotransplant model of Murray et al has provided a highly versatile model for studying the effects of lung transplantation on pulmonary vasomotor regulation. The preparation involves minimal ischemic time, no immunosuppression, and no tissue rejection. Studies are performed two days to two months after reimplantation. Continuous plots of left lung pulmonary arterial (PA) pressures vs flow allow accurate assessment of vasoreactivity. The data demonstrate increased pulmonary vascular resistance compared to identically instrumented sham-operated control dogs. This vasoconstriction is independent of flow and not related to PA or venous anastomotic sites. In this model, endothelium-dependent pulmonary vasodilation (measured by the response to acetylcholine or bradykinin) is impaired; sympathetic beta-adrenoreceptor function (measured by the response to isoproterenol or propranolol) is unaffected; and sympathetic α-adrenoreceptor function (measured by the response to phenylephrine or prazosin) is enhanced. These data suggest that left lung autotransplantation may induce endothelial dysfunction with reduced endothelium-derived relaxing factor (EDRF), generally accepted as nitric oxide (NO) activity, and denervation-induced supersensitivity of vascular smooth muscle to α-adrenergic activation.

Clinical Pulmonary Vasoreactivity

Pulmonary hypertension is not generally a clinical problem after lung transplantation. Even in patients who underwent transplantation for primary or secondary pulmonary hypertension, there is no evidence that the condition recurs after transplantation. Hypoxic vasoconstriction is intact, and the distribution of pulmonary flow in response to vasoactive stimuli is grossly unimpaired.

Right Ventricular Function

Patients with abnormal left ventricular (LV) function or extensive coronary artery disease are not suitable candidates for lung transplantation. On the other hand, patients with abnormal right ventricular (RV) function or abnormal pulmonary hemodynamics may be suitable candidates for lung transplantation depending on the degree of RV dysfunction or severity of pulmonary hypertension. Predicting the degree of RV functional recovery after lung transplantation remains an important challenge to lung transplant physicians. Early transplant efforts avoided this difficulty by performing combined heart and lung transplantation for patients with severe pulmonary hypertension. This approach was modified when several small studies demonstrated the ability of lung transplantation to restore RV function in patients with pulmonary hypertension. These observations were subsequently confirmed in two larger studies of patients with primary pulmonary hypertension (PPH). Ritchie et al demonstrated significant immediate and short-term (ie, <3 months) improvement in RV function after single-lung transplantation. These effects were sustained up to two years after transplantation. Regression of RV free wall hypertrophy did not occur early after transplantation, but was observed in long-term follow-up, although wall thickness generally did not return to normal levels.

Another study noted variability in the degree of RV functional recovery, especially in patients other than those with PPH. In this study, 14 patients with abnormal preoperative RV function by echocardiography were studied before and after lung transplantation. Mean echocardiographic observations appear in Figure 89-1. These include RV end-diastolic area (EDA), RV end-systolic area (ESA), and RV fractional area change (FAC). Right ventricular fractional area change (RV FAC) is calculated by the formula:

$$RV\ FAC = \left(\frac{EDA - ESA}{EDA}\right) \times 100$$

All three variables improved significantly after transplantation (Figure 90-1). Eight of 14 (57%) patients demonstrated paradoxical septal motion before transplantation, whereas no patients demonstrated paradoxical septal motion after transplantation (P <0.02).

Although the group as a whole showed significant improvement in RV function after lung transplantation, a subgroup of four patients exhibited no change in RV function. Patients who achieved improvement in RV function (n=10) tended to be younger, had shorter duration of disease before transplantation, and had significantly higher PA pressures before transplantation. Eight of ten patients had PPH and two patients with obstructive lung disease had uncharacteristically high pulmonary arterial pressures. In contrast, two of the three patients with emphysema and both patients with IPF who failed to achieve improvement in RV function had only modest elevations of pulmonary arterial pressures.

These observations indicate that patients with the most severe degree of pulmonary hypertension preoperatively experience the greatest degree of reduction of PA pressures postoperatively. Under these circumstances, RV function directly parallels afterload reduction in the pulmonary vascular bed. In fact, in the presence of high pulmonary arterial pressures, echocardiographic parameters do not truly represent RV function, per se, but rather the effects of afterload on RV ejection. More specific indicators of myocardial contractility such as systolic pressure-volume curves might permit distinguishing the effects of afterload from true myocardial impairment. To explain the absence of RV recovery in patients with emphysema and pulmonary fibrosis who

had only modest elevations of PA pressures, we must assume these patients had intrinsic myocardial dysfunction preoperatively. This may relate to the older ages of these patients or to the longer duration of disease process. Alternatively, absence of RV recovery may reflect a different response of the pulmonary vascular bed in parenchymal lung disease vs primary vascular disease.

Some studies have suggested that there may be greater RV afterload reduction after bilateral lung transplants as compared to single-lung transplants, but available data in single-lung transplants indicate that RV function improves in patients with pulmonary hypertension to a similar degree after single-lung or bilateral-lung transplantation.

In summary, there is significant improvement in RV function after lung transplantation in patients with severe RV dysfunction before transplantation. The most important factors determining RV functional recovery are the degree of RV afterload reduction and intrinsic myocardial contractility. RV ejection parameters, however, do not distinguish between these two factors.

SURFACTANT

Alterations in surfactant properties occur during lung preservation and may contribute to impaired gas exchange and graft failure after reperfusion. However, there is increasing data to suggest that disturbances in surfactant properties persist even months to years after successful lung transplantation. In one study, surfactant activity was significantly impaired in transplant recipients who were free of infection or rejection as compared to normal controls. Surfactant-specific proteins (eg, SP-A) may be decreased, and there may be changes in surfactant phospholipid composition. These findings suggest persistent type-II cell dysfunction after lung transplantation. Despite these alterations in surfactant activity, however, graft function is preserved in most instances, and the clinical relevance of disturbed surfactant function after lung transplantation remains to be clarified.

PULMONARY FUNCTION
Spirometry

Pulmonary function measurements in lung transplant recipients are sensitive to intercurrent infection or acute rejection. In addition, a substantial proportion of lung transplant recipients develop obliterative bronchiolitis (OB), generally felt to represent chronic rejection, which results in irreversible airflow obstruction. A retrospective review of sequential spirometry measurements after lung transplantation revealed a high degree of variability during the first postoperative year, due to increasing values for FVC and FEV_1. After the first year, variability in FVC and FEV_1 was generally less than 11% to 12%. A decline in FVC and FEV_1 greater than 11% to 12% strongly sug-

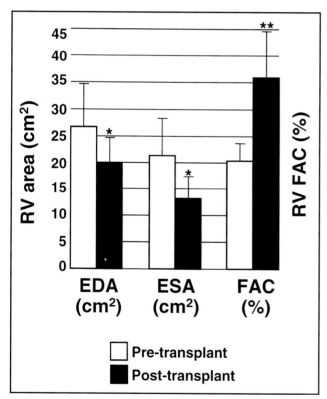

Figure 90-1. Echocardiographic parameters of RV function in 14 patients before and after lung transplantation. Abbreviations: RV indicates right ventricle; FAC, fractional area change; EDA, end diastolic area; ESA, end systolic area; *, *P*-value < 0.01; **, *P* < 0.001. Reprinted with permission from Transplantation. 1996;62:622-625. Lippincott, Williams and Wilkins Publishers, New York, NY.

gests graft dysfunction due to infection or rejection. During the remainder of this section, it will be assumed that the allograft is functioning normally and that there is no intercurrent infection or rejection.

Heart-Lung and Bilateral Lung Transplants

Most heart-lung and bilateral lung transplant recipients achieve normal static and dynamic lung volumes, although FVC and TLC may not completely normalize. This mild "restrictive" defect is partly related to the effects of sternotomy and thoracotomy, since lung volumes tend to improve in the first 12 months after surgery. The persistent restriction observed in some patients after 12 months is not related to increased lung elastic recoil since measured lung compliance in these patients is normal. Although average respiratory muscle strength is normal, a linear correlation between indices of respiratory muscle function (eg, PImax) and TLC suggests that decreased inspiratory force may be responsible for some patients' inability to achieve a normal TLC. In addition, up to 10% of patients may also sustain diaphragmatic dysfunction after lung transplantation.

Static lung volumes after heart-lung or bilateral-lung transplantation are strongly influenced by the preoperative disease for which the transplant was performed. Whereas patients with primary pulmonary hypertension (PPH) have normal or near normal FRC and RV, patients with cystic fibrosis (CF) show a persistent increase in FRC and RV even after transplant. In one study, patients with CF had average values of FRC and RV of 141% and 164%, respectively, at six months after transplant. The increase in FRC was not related to decreased lung elastic recoil since measured lung compliance in these patients was normal. Rather, the increase in FRC appeared to relate to persistent overinflation of the chest wall (ie, a leftward shift of the chest wall pressure-volume curve). Measurement of the anterior diameter of the rib cage at FRC averaged 12.1 cm in patients with CF as compared with only 9.5 cm in patients with PPH (P <0.05). Thus, after transplantation, patients with CF showed persistent hyper-inflation due to rib cage expansion along the anterior diameter.

In patients with emphysema, the available data suggests that FRC and RV do not remain elevated after transplantation. The difference between emphysema and CF may relate to the fact that most of the hyperinflation in emphysema involves downward displacement of the diaphragm. Since emphysema develops in adulthood, the rib cage is not substantially deformed. In contrast, patients with CF develop their disease in childhood when the bony rib cage is still growing and can be remodeled considerably.

Thus, the volume of the thoracic cavity after heart-lung or bilateral-lung transplantation is most affected by the underlying disease of the recipient. If changes in thoracic structure are reversible, then lung volumes after transplantation should reach normal levels regardless of whether the preoperative TLC is elevated as in emphysema, or reduced as in PPH or pulmonary fibrosis. By one year after surgery, lung volumes should return to values predicted by the patient's sex, age and height even if there are large disparities between the donor lung size and the recipient's preoperative TLC. Thus, as recommended by the Cambridge group, it is most appropriate to use the recipient's predicted lung volumes as the normal values after transplantation, and the best method of matching donor and recipient volumes is to use their respective predicted TLC values.

Aside from lung volumes, other parameters of respiratory function after heart-lung or bilateral-lung transplantation are remarkably intact: there is no evidence of airflow obstruction (normal FEV_1/FVC, normal airway resistance); distribution of alveolar ventilation (measured by single breath N2 washout) is normal; muscle pressures are normal; pulmonary arterial pressures are normal; and gas exchange is normal at rest and with exercise.

SINGLE-LUNG TRANSPLANTS

Pulmonary function in single-lung transplant recipients is highly dependent on physiologic interactions with the diseased native lung. For example, in single-lung transplants performed for emphysema, there may be acute mediastinal shift in the early postoperative period (secondary to overdistention of the native emphysematous lung) with impaired gas exchange and even impaired hemodynamics (Figure 90-2A). (Some transplant surgeons prefer to implant an "oversized" lung in patients with emphysema to minimize mediastinal shift.) Later in the postoperative course, the transplant lung still appears radiographically "smaller" than the native, hyperinflated lung (Figure 90-2B). In one study, the volume of the transplant lung was only 33% of TLC, whereas the volume of the native emphysema lung was 75% to 80% of TLC. Overall, the thorax remains hyperinflated and maximal inspiratory muscle pressures are reduced.

Despite these volume discrepancies, however, there is marked clinical improvement. Spirometry and arterial oxygen tension improve considerably (Figure 90-3). Typically, FEV_1 increases by 1.0 to 1.5 liters, whereas FVC increases somewhat less than 1.0 liter. Quantitative ventilation and perfusion studies demonstrate that the transplant lung receives 60% to 80% of the overall ventilation and perfusion. In one study, at six months after single-lung transplantation, FEV_1 increased from 0.49 (16% pred) to 1.8 (60% pred), FVC increased from 1.7 (43% pred) to 2.4 (62% pred), and FEV_1/FVC rose from 0.3 to 0.73. Mean PaO_2 increased from 58 mmHg to 87 mmHg, and no patient required supplemental oxygen

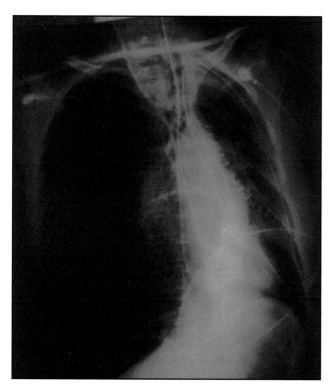

Figure 90-2A. Postoperative mediastinal shift in a 50 year-old woman after left single lung transplantation for severe emphysema. The native right lung has massively overinflated across the midline, displacing both heart and transplanted left lung to the left.

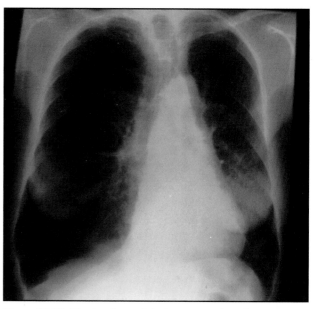

Figure 90-2B. Chest radiograph in the same patient six months after left single transplantation. The native right lung remains hyperinflated compared to the transplanted left lung, but there is no mediastinal shift. Reprinted with permission from Anesthesiology. 1991;74:1144-1148. Lippincott Williams and Wilkins Publishers, New York, NY.

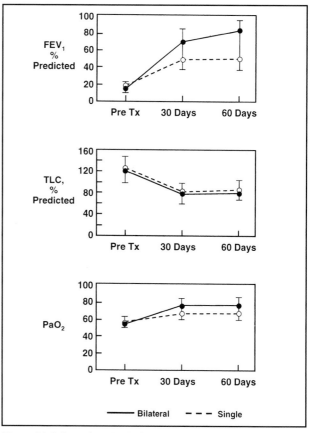

Figure 90-3. Lung function before and after single and bilateral lung transplantation for advanced pulmonary emphysema. Adaptation reprinted with permission from J Thorac Cardiovasc Surg. 1992;103:1119-1126, Mosby Publishers, New York, NY.

at rest or exercise after transplantation. Quantitative ventilation and perfusion to the transplant lung were 85% and 81%, respectively.

There do not appear to be significant differences in physiologic parameters in patients undergoing right vs left single-lung transplantation for emphysema. However, spirometric results for single-lung transplantation do not achieve the normal levels reported for bilateral or heart-lung transplantation. A biphasic pattern of expiratory flow is often observed in the flow-volume curve after single-lung transplantation for emphysema. The initial high flow phase of the flow-volume curve derives from the transplanted lung, and the terminal low flow from the native, emphysematous lung. In the absence of anastomotic stenosis, the flow-limiting segment is located in the native bronchus, immediately proximal to the anastomosis. There is data to suggest that selective assessment of single-lung transplant function by 133Xe radiospirometry may be helpful in distinguishing infection from rejection. During acute rejection, lung transplant perfusion (Qtx) and spirometry selectively decline.

With the advent of lung volume reduction surgery (LVRS), some transplant centers have reported improved allograft function after native lung lobectomy or native lung bullectomy when the native lung is excessively hyperinflated and compromises allograft function. At least one center has reported simultaneous single-lung transplantation for emphysema and native lung volume reduction. These approaches may provide the single-lung transplant recipient with emphysema a degree of respiratory function closer to that achieved after bilateral lung transplantation. There is even data that native lung volume reduction may salvage respiratory function after the onset of chronic allograft rejection, representing another variation in the evolving relationship between lung transplantation for emphysema and LVRS.

In single-lung transplants performed for pulmonary fibrosis, there are fewer adverse physiologic interactions with the diseased native lung, since the latter has reduced compliance and increased vascular resistance. In one study, at one year after transplantation, FVC was 69%, FEV_1 79%, and DLCO 62% of predicted values. Relative perfusion to the transplanted lung was 77%. Arterial oxygen tension was 87 mmHg, and supplemental oxygen was no longer needed by any patient after transplantation.

Single-Lung Vs Bilateral-Lung Transplants

Limited availability of donor lungs dictates wider use of single lung-transplants over bilateral-lung transplantation if possible. Comparison of functional results indicates that patients undergoing bilateral-lung transplantation for emphysema have higher values of FEV_1, PaO_2, and 6-minute walk as compared to single-lung recipients (Figure 89-3). However, patients undergoing bilateral-lung transplantation for emphysema have a higher incidence of postoperative complications and a lower 1-year survival (71% vs 91% in one series).

As previously noted, some transplant centers prefer bilateral-lung over single-lung transplantation for patients with pulmonary hypertension. This is based on clinical experience suggesting overperfusion of the single-lung transplant in the early postoperative period (secondary to high vascular resistance in the native lung). Others have suggested that there may be greater RV afterload reduction after bilateral-lung transplants as compared to single-lung transplants, but available data indicate that RV function improves to a similar degree after single-lung or bilateral-lung transplantation. After single-lung transplantation for pulmonary hypertension, the allograft receives greater than 90% of the pulmonary blood flow because of the high vascular resistance in the native lung. This may have important consequences when the ventilation to the allograft declines as a result of obliterative bronchiolitis, resulting in severe hypoxemia.

Exercise

Despite satisfactory allograft function after lung transplantation, most transplant recipients, including bilateral-lung and heart-lung recipients, are unable to achieve maximal levels of work and O_2 consumption. In one study, bilateral-lung recipients with normal spirometry achieved lower work (62 vs 155 W) and O_2 consumption (0.88 vs 2.26 L/min) than control subjects. Within their limited range of exercise, however, ventilatory responses are normal. These findings are similar to previous findings indicating that lack of vagal innervation is not required for control of ventilation. (Note: the only exception may be regulation of inspiratory time during conditions of exercise with expiratory load.) Poor exercise performance is most clearly related to limb muscle endurance associated with deconditioning, but also possibly to the effects of corticosteroids (myopathy) and cyclosporine (impaired muscle vasodilation). Transplant recipients invariably report leg fatigue and pain as the reason they stop exercising during testing. Abnormal skeletal muscle oxidative capacity after lung transplantation has been superbly demonstrated by 31P-magnetic resonance spectroscopy. Exercise induces a lower pH and greater release of potassium ion than control subjects. Aerobic exercise training increases peak oxygen uptake. In one study, a 6-week aerobic exercise training program improved peak work (66 vs 81 W) and O_2 consumption (1.1 vs 1.3 L/min). Nevertheless, these improved values are still only 55% to 65% compared to control subjects, and all transplant recipients still terminated exercise due to leg pain.

RECOMMENDED READING

Martinez JA, Paradis IL, Dauber JH, et al. Spirometry values in stable lung transplant recipients. Am J Respir Crit Care Med. 1997;155(1):285-290.

Cheriyan AF, Garrity ER Jr, Pifarre R, Fahey PJ, Walsh JM. Reduced transplant lung volumes after single lung transplantation for chronic obstructive pulmonary disease. Am J Respir Crit Care Med. 1995;151(3 Pt 1):851-853.

Schulman LL, Leibowitz DW, Anadarangam T, et al. Variability of right ventricular functional recovery after lung transplantation. Transplantation. 1996;62(5):622-625.

Pellegrino R, Rodarte JR, Frost AE, Reid MB. Breathing by double-lung recipients during exercise: response to expiratory threshold loading. Am J Respir Crit Care Med. 1998;157(1):106-110.

91 INDUCTION IMMUNOSUPPRESSION PROTOCOLS FOR LUNG TRANSPLANTATION

Melissa B. King, MD

INDUCTION THERAPY

Induction therapy refers to the short-term use of augmented or specialized immunosuppression at the time of initial organ transplantation. This practice is prevalent in other solid organ transplant regimens, and has been extrapolated for use in lung transplantation in some centers. However, a lack of randomized studies of induction therapy and reliance on single center data has led to variable and inconclusive results. Consequently, the use of induction therapy and regimens employed by individual transplant centers varies considerably and remains controversial.

The theoretical indications for using induction therapy in an immunosuppressive regimen are also varied. One theory postulates that induction creates a long-lasting immunosuppressive effect by modulating the initial immune response directed against the newly engrafted organ. In this model, a state of relative immunologic unresponsiveness is maintained for a period of time while donor antigens are cleared. For example, passenger leukocytes and macrophages, which have a finite life span, age without interacting with the recipient's lymphocytes, thus decreasing host alloreactivity. Induction therapy is therefore given in addition to triple drug maintenance immunosuppression. This approach suggests that there is an optimal duration of induction therapy that is most effective for long-term graft survival.

Other approaches use induction therapy to protect against drug toxicity during the early posttransplant reperfusion injury phase of early graft dysfunction. This leads to sequential therapy, in which initial immunosuppression consists of a lymphocytolytic agent, corticosteroids and azathioprine, while the addition of cyclosporine or tacrolimus is delayed. This is most relevant in renal transplantation, since nephrotoxicity is a common side effect of standard immunosuppressive regimens. However, since kidney dysfunction is an incremental risk factor for early death after heart transplantation, this rationale may be applicable to lung recipients as well.

Assistant Professor of Medicine, Division of Allergy, Pulmonary and Critical Care, University of Minnesota, Minneapolis, MN

Antibody Induction Regimens

CYTOLYTIC ANTIBODIES. Induction regimens in lung transplantation have classically used lymphocytolytic agents as the cornerstone of therapy. These include the polyclonal antithymocyte and antilymphocyte globulins (ie, ATG, ALG) as well as the muromonab-CD3 monoclonal anti-CD3 antibody. Many of the polyclonal preparations have been produced at and used exclusively by individual transplant centers. Minnesota ALG was one agent that was produced locally, but distributed nationally and used widely, but has been subsequently removed from the market. Currently, the commercially available products are Atgam® (Upjohn), Thymoglobulin® (SangStat) and Orthoclone OKT®3 (Ortho Pharmaceuticals). The activity of these agents relies on their capacity to induce peripheral lymphocytopenia through various mechanisms, and they can all induce long-lasting immunosuppressive activity even after treatment cessation. The dosage and duration of induction therapy varies widely among centers. Table 91-1 outlines the various therapies. Chapters 6 and 7 discuss each agent in detail.

These drugs are generally administered through a central venous catheter to minimize phlebitis and subcutaneous infiltration. Side effects are common, and include chills, flushing and fever. These may be reduced by prophylactic administration of acetaminophen, diphenhydramine and low-dose corticosteroids. Muromonab-CD3 consistently causes a "first dose response" thought to be due to cytokines released from T lymphocytes upon initial exposure to muromonab-CD3. This consists of fever, chills, vomiting and diarrhea; more severe symptoms include hypotension and noncardiogenic pulmonary edema. These effects may be particularly detrimental in patients with preexisting respiratory compromise. Since antilymphocyte preparations are produced in nonhuman species, serum sickness may also develop following exposure to these drugs. Thrombocytopenia and leukopenia can be seen and should prompt a decrease in dosage.

Therapy may be monitored by following the percent and absolute values of lymphocyte subsets in peripheral blood; CD3 is commonly used. Generally, these counts will fall significantly from baseline values after three to five days of therapy. Guidelines for target levels of these cells vary, but range from an absolute number less than $10/mm^3$ to less than $50/mm^3$. Failure to reduce the CD3+ count should lead to consideration of increasing the dosage. Conversely, dramatic reductions in CD3 count may allow lower cumulative dosing, potentially reducing side effects. For muromonab-CD3, failure of the CD3 count to decrease may signify that the patient has developed antibodies to mouse immunoglobulin, which can be measured in serum. Successful reuse of muromonab-CD3 may be limited in patients with high titer (>1:100)

		Dosage (mg/kg per day)	Duration (Days)
Agent	**Type**		
Anti-thymocyte globulin (ATGAM®, Upjohn Co)	Polyclonal horse anti-thymocyte	5 to 20	5 to 21
Rabbit anti-thymocyte globulin (Thymoglobulin®, SangStat Medical Corp)	Polyclonal rabbit anti-thymocyte	1.5	1 to14
Muromonab-CD3 (Orthoclone OKT®3, Ortho Pharmaceutical Corp)	Monoclonal mouse anti-CD3	2.5 to 5	10 to14
Basiliximab (Simulect®, Novartis)	Chimeric monoclonal anti-IL-2 receptor	20 mg dose (Not weight based)	Pre-op, then day 4 or 5
Daclizumab (Zenapax®, Hoffman-LaRoche)	Humanized monoclonal anti-IL-2 receptor	1	Pre-op, then q 7 to 14 days for total of 5 doses

Table 91-1. Agents Used for Induction Therapy

anti-muromonab-CD3 antibodies. The variability of CD3+ depletion has led some centers to abandon immunologic monitoring completely.

INTERLEUKIN-2 RECEPTOR ANTIBODIES. New drugs that appear promising as potential induction agents in lung transplantation are the interleukin-2 (IL-2) receptor antagonists. The IL-2 receptor is present on activated, but not resting, T cells, and the interaction of IL-2 with this receptor is necessary for the clonal expansion and viability of these cells. Targeting this receptor presents an opportunity to selectively deplete the cells thought to be most integral in mediating rejection. Two agents are currently commercially available. Daclizumab is a molecularly engineered human IgG1 which incorporates a murine antigen-binding site directed against the a chain of the IL-2 receptor. Since 90% of the genetic sequence is human, this is often referred to as a "humanized" antibody. Basiliximab is a chimeric monoclonal antibody that contains a murine variable (antigen-binding) and a human constant region. Both agents have been used in renal transplantation, and have been shown to decrease early acute rejection. Importantly, side effects were minimal.

Antibody Free Induction Therapy

When antibody therapy is not included in the postoperative regimen, doses of triple drug immunosuppressives (cyclosporine/tacrolimus, mycophenolate mofetil/ azathioprine and corticosteroids) are generally kept at higher levels for a period of three to six months post-transplant. Other modalities that could potentially be used to augment perioperative immunosuppression include total lymphoid irradiation and photopheresis; however, these therapies are used infrequently and little data is available regarding their efficacy.

INITIATION OF INDUCTION AND EARLY IMMUNOSUPPRESSANT THERAPY

Induction therapy begins preoperatively, with lung transplant recipients receiving a dose of cyclosporine, or tacrolimus and azathioprine, or mycophenolate mofetil, usually upon arrival at the transplant center. Corticosteroids are administered intraoperatively, usually following release of the pulmonary artery clamp.

SELECTION OF INDUCTION PROTOCOL BY PATIENT TYPE
Immunologic High-Risk Patients

Acute rejection occurs in the majority of lung transplant recipients, and is identified as a major risk factor for development of obliterative bronchiolitis. Thus, early intensification of immunosuppression via induction therapy may serve to reduce both acute and chronic rejection episodes. Induction also allows for a window of time to optimize maintenance immunosuppression, especially with regard to cyclosporine and tacrolimus levels. However, there is little data available to evaluate this. Centers report successful and similar outcomes both with and without cytolytic induction therapy. Two studies have shown a decrease in episodes of acute rejection with induction therapy, and one report suggests that bronchiolitis obliterans syndrome is delayed in patients who receive muromonab-CD3 induction.

Despite the paucity of data regarding this, certain patients who have an increased risk of immunologic complications should be seriously considered for induction therapy. These include patients undergoing retransplantation, recipients with underlying immunologic dysfunction (such as connective tissue disorders) and those with high panel-reactive antibody (PRA) levels pretransplant. All patients with elevated PRA levels should undergo donor-recipient crossmatching at the time of transplantation. If the crossmatch is positive, aggressive immunosuppression is indicated, consisting of induction therapy, plasmapheresis and intravenous immunoglobulin. Such patients are at risk for hyperacute rejection, which carries a poor prognosis.

Patients with Preoperative or Perioperative Organ Dysfunction

Side effects of triple drug immunosuppression may cause significant organ dysfunction in the perioperative period which limits patient outcomes. Examples include renal dysfunction from tacrolimus or cyclosporine, hepatic abnormalities from mycophenolate mofetil or azathioprine, and hyperglycemia, poor wound healing and steroid myopathy from corticosteroids. These may be compounded by perioperative stress such as the need for cardiopulmonary bypass. Use of induction therapy can allow reduced or delayed administration of maintenance immunosuppressives postoperatively and potentially reduce these complications.

Patients at Increased Risk of Lymphoproliferative Disorders

Posttransplant lymphoproliferative disorders (PTLD) are recognized as complications of immunosuppression. These disorders are often related to Epstein-Barr virus (EBV) infection, and are thought to result from inadequate T cell control over EBV-related B cell proliferation. The risk of development of this complication is related to the degree of immunosuppression, and may also be increased in EBV-negative recipients. Induction therapy with muromonab-CD3 was shown to increase the incidence of PTLD in heart transplant recipients in a dose-dependent fashion. Consequently, induction therapy may be contraindicated in EBV-negative patients, or patients with other risk factors for lymphoproliferative diseases.

Patients at Increased Risk of Infection

Intensive early immunosuppression can increase the risk of infection, leading to pulmonary dysfunction, sepsis and death. Serious infections with viruses, fungi and bacteria have all been reported following the use of induction therapy. Early concerns regarding severe cytomegalovirus infection have decreased at many centers due to routine use of effective ganciclovir prophylaxis as well as improved diagnostic techniques. Patients who are colonized pretransplant with organisms that are especially difficult to treat (ie, multiply-resistant *Pseudomonas* species or *Aspergillus*) may present a special risk with cytolytic induction therapy.

PERIOPERATIVE CORTICOSTEROID USE

Corticosteroids are valuable agents in immunosuppressive protocols, and most centers consider their use mandatory in lung transplantation. However, during the early experience in lung transplantation, a high incidence of bronchial anastomotic dehiscence was blamed on corticosteroid effects. This led transplant physicians to advocate delayed administration of induction corticosteroids for a period of one to three weeks. As experience in lung transplantation broadened, it became evident that patients could be safely managed using perioperative corticosteroids without increased anastomotic complications. Currently, high-dose Solumedrol® (500 mg to 1 g) given intraoperatively followed by a tapering dosage schedule over weeks to months is common in many transplant centers.

IMMUNOSUPPRESSION IN THE NPO PATIENT

In the postoperative period, many lung transplant recipients are unable to take oral medications due to anesthesia, analgesia, temporary gastroparesis or the presence of an endotracheal tube. Thus, immunosuppressives may need to be given intravenously. All of the commonly used immunosuppressives are available in intravenous form, and Table 91-2 outlines standard dosing regimens. However, shorter operative times and early extubation frequently eliminate the need for parenteral administra-

Table 91-2. Parenteral Dosing of Immunosuppressives

CsA/Neoral or Tacrolimus		AZA or MMF		Steroid
40 μg/kg per hr continuous infusion; usual dose 1,000 to 3,000 μg/hr	1.0 μg/kg per hr continuous infusion; usual dose 50 to 100 μg/hr	1 to 1.25 mg/kg per day IV	1 to 1.5 gm IV bid	Methylprednisolone 0.25 mg/kg IV bid
Titrate dose based on blood concentration monitoring		Monitor WBC count; decrease dose if < 4,000		

tion. In most cases, patients can be given their immuno-suppression through a nasogastric tube by the first post-operative day with adequate adsorption and few side effects.

SUMMARY

Induction therapy is controversial in lung transplantation, and will remain so until multicenter controlled trials are available to evaluate its impact. As our armamentarium of other more effective immunosuppressive agents increases, the need for induction therapy may become less in the future. At the same time, better management and diagnosis of the major complications of induction immunosuppression, as well as availability of safer, better tolerated preparations may improve our ability to administer this therapy safely.

RECOMMENDED READING

Wain JC, Wright CD, Ryan DP, Zorb SL, Mathisen DJ, Ginns LC. Induction immunosuppression for lung transplantation with OKT3. Ann Thorac Surg. 1999;67(1): 187-193.

Ross DJ, Jordan SC, Nathan SD, Kass RM, Koerner SK. Delayed development of obliterative bronchiolitis syndrome with OKT3 after unilateral lung transplantation. A plea for multicenter immunosuppressive trials. Chest. 1996;109(4):870-873.

Kriett JM, Smith CM, Hayden AM, et al. Lung transplantation without the use of antilymphocyte antibody preparations. J Heart Lung Transplant. 1993;12(6 Pt 1): 915-923.

92 DIAGNOSIS AND TREATMENT OF PULMONARY DYSFUNCTION EPISODES

Steven R. Duncan, MD

GENERAL CONSIDERATIONS

The last two decades have seen remarkable advances in the techniques of allogeneic pulmonary transplantation. Lung transplantation remains a complex procedure, however, and episodes of pulmonary dysfunction are extremely frequent among recipients. The unique nature of the transplantation procedure renders patients at considerable risk for the development of surgical complications. Moreover, allograft viability can only be sustained by life-long and nonspecific immunosuppression that often results in opportunistic infections and lymphomas. These regimens are only partly effective, however, and allograft rejection is near ubiquitous among lung transplant recipients.

In addition to complexities imposed by the broad range of potential pathoetiologies, the diagnosis and management of pulmonary dysfunction episodes among lung transplant recipients are further confounded by the often overlapping or nonspecific clinical features of these problems. Furthermore, the ability to rely on empirical therapy or expectant observation may be extremely limited, since many of the pulmonary dysfunction disorders in lung transplant recipients will rapidly progress if mistreated. Accordingly, a very low threshold for early use of definitive diagnostic procedures is most often appropriate in this population.

Nonetheless, a powerful tool in the initial evaluation of pulmonary dysfunction episodes among lung transplant recipients is an appreciation of the posttransplantation intervals, during which particular problems tend to be most prevalent (Figure 92-1). Certain general details, particularly with respect to infectious complications, are similar to those that affect other solid organ transplantation recipients. While reference to these outlines is not intended to supplant diagnostic tests, the ability to assign relative prior probabilities to the many possible complications of transplantation can expedite and focus an appropriate evaluation. This awareness may also enable implementation of rational empirical therapies while awaiting test results, as well as direct subsequent efforts if initial diagnostic tests are unrevealing.

Assistant Professor, Department of Immunology, The Scripps Research Institute; Attending Physician, Chest and Critical Care Medicine, Scripps Green Hospital, La Jolla, CA

EARLY CAUSES OF PULMONARY DYSFUNCTION

The potential range of abnormalities that can result in lung dysfunction is perhaps greatest during the first few days after transplantation. In addition to the usual causes of pulmonary problems associated with major thoracic surgeries (see also Chapter 23), lung transplant recipients are also susceptible to a unique set of complications referable to the airway and vascular anastomoses of the allograft, and the injury responses of a newly-implanted organ. Pulmonary infections are a serious cause of morbidity and mortality in the first few days following transplantation but, unlike later periods, opportunistic pathogens are unusual.

Reperfusion Injury

This poorly understood syndrome, also referred to as reimplantation or preservation injury, is the most frequent early complication of lung transplantation. While mild abnormalities may be occult and are undoubtedly even more common, clinically significant reperfusion injury (RI) occurs in as many as 20% to 40% of lung transplant patients, depending on local techniques and patient populations. Overall mortality figures are highly variable, a likely function of severity biases, but deaths among more advanced cases may approach 50%. Typical episodes are often evident by radiographic and physiologic abnormalities within minutes-to-hours after transplantation, although the full extent of the injury may not be apparent for a few days. Clinical manifestations of early RI largely mimic those of hydrostatic pulmonary edema, with interstitial or patchy infiltrates that often rapidly coalesce and become homogenous (Figure 92-2), decreased compliance, and impaired gas exchange.

Biopsies of severely injured lungs demonstrate nonspecific diffuse alveolar damage, similar to cases of adult respiratory distress syndrome (ARDS). Like ARDS, the cellular pathophysiology of RI can also be simplistically viewed as a manifestation of capillary or small vessel "leakiness". Although intuition and circumstantial evidence suggest that RI is due to ischemic injury associated with organ harvest and preservation, there is only poor correlation between graft ischemic times and severity of the syndrome. Other possible contributing factors have also been proposed, including mechanical trauma of the allograft prior to or during/after procurement (by positive pressure ventilation and rough handling, respectively), disruption of bronchial and lymphatic circulations, or lung denervation. A clear correlation exists between arterial flow/perfusion pressure in the newly-transplanted lung and development of RI, with highest incidences and severity of the syndrome after single lung transplantations into patients with pretransplant pulmonary hypertension.

The diagnosis of RI can usually be established by clinical presentation. Depending on the exact details of an individual case, the differential diagnosis may include hyperacute rejection, vascular anastomotic abnormalities (especially pulmonary venous obstruction), or hydrostatic pulmonary edema. As discussed later, hyperacute rejection is exceedingly rare, and largely preventable by appropriate blood type and antibody screening. Establishing a prior probability of vascular anastomotic prob-

lems can be facilitated by discussions with surgeons regarding intraoperative problems or anatomic anomalies, and these comparatively unusual complications can be further excluded by appropriate diagnostics (below). Hydrostatic edema can be excluded by measurements of pulmonary artery wedge pressures, echocardiography, and refractoriness to diuresis. Lung biopsy is seldom necessary in typical cases of RI, and may be relatively contraindicated when gas exchange is

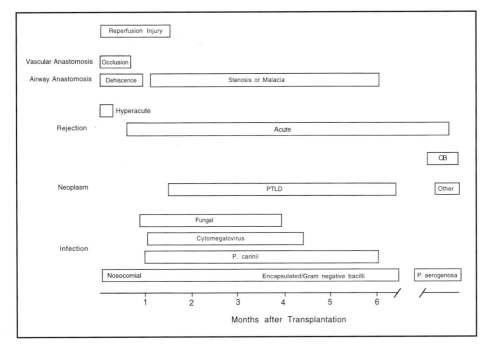

Figure 92-1. Peak prevalences of common pulmonary problems following lung transplantation. Of note, effective prophylaxis may significantly delay onset of infections (and OB).

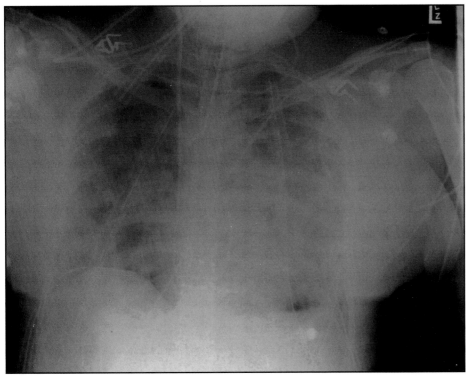

Figure 92-2. Reperfusion injury following double-lung transplantation. Note the diffuse pulmonary edema-like infiltrates. The differential diagnosis based on this radiograph would include hydrostatic pulmonary edema and vascular anastomosis problems (Courtesy of V Valentine).

tenuous. Biopsy by transbronchial biopsy (TBB) or open procedure may be useful later, however, especially among those with a relapsing or worsening course after initial improvement, in order to exclude superimposed acute rejection or pulmonary infection. Evaluation of the latter, however, can usually be more easily accomplished by bronchoalveolar lavage (BAL) or double-lumen protected brush catheter.

In general the mainstay of RI management is supportive. Most cases with mild or moderate manifestations resolve within days-to-a few weeks. The observation of a link between pulmonary artery hypertension and RI has lead to the use of measures to decrease these arterial pressures, including administration of nitric oxide admixed in inspired gases, with often considerable improvements of gas exchange. Extracorporeal membrane oxygenation has been employed in particularly severe cases. Clinical resolution of severe, refractory episodes may require protracted periods of ventilatory support, during which patients are at risk for infections, barotrauma, and other ICU complications. Slow but eventual improvement of pulmonary function, often to normal or near-normal values, can be expected among those who survive.

Airway Anastomosis Problems

The most serious early airway problem stemming from the transplantation procedure is dehiscence of the bronchial anastomosis. Overall incidence of this complication among experienced programs is probably in the range of 1% to 3%, which represents a substantial improvement compared to the early days of lung transplantation. Ischemia is the putative mechanism of most cases of dehiscence, as well as other later-occurring airway anastomosis problems (ie, stenosis and malacia). At best, the blood supply to the proximal donor bronchus is tenuous, being limited to retrograde, low oxygen-tension flow from collaterals of the pulmonary artery. Other contributing factors that may further impair circulation at the anastomosis have been postulated to include edema due to RI or acute allograft rejection, and low cardiac output. The preoperative use of steroids was long considered likely to promote dehiscence and other anastomosis complications by impairment of wound healing, but more recent data suggests minimal deleterious effects of these agents. Surgical airway problems are probably least frequent among en bloc heart-lung recipients, due to increased blood supply at the tracheal anastomosis from collaterals of the coronary arteries.

Minor dehiscences are generally treated by expectant observation. Surgical repair of major disruptions is difficult, although re-anastomosis or emergency re-transplantation has successfully treated occasional cases. Airway obstruction due to necrotic debris with or without edema is readily diagnosed and treated broncho-

scopically. Deaths are usually attributable to mediastinitis or massive hemorrhage from bronchovascular fistulas.

Vascular Anastomosis Problems

Serious vascular complications are now unusual after lung transplantation, and by most accounts develop in less than 2% of anastomoses. However, these infrequent events remain associated with considerable morbidity and a high mortality. The clinical history in many reported cases suggests that risk factors for these complications include difficult surgical exposure of the operative field (usually due to small thoracic size or musculoskeletal deformities), as well as the presence of adhesions from prior invasive procedures. Pulmonary venous obstructions (stenosis or thrombosis) typically present with refractory pulmonary edema, gas exchange abnormalities, and elevated pulmonary artery pressures. The unexplained postoperative occurrence or persistence of pulmonary hypertension or edema should prompt consideration of these complications. Pulmonary artery stenosis may have a similar clinical presentation, or with more occult manifestations of prolonged hypoxemia and ventilator dependence. Anecdotal reports include rare cases of preexistent pulmonary emboli in donor lungs that were not evident prior to organ harvest, including thrombi or cerebral tissue (the latter resulting from head injury). Clinical features of vascular complications are usually evident immediately (or within one to two days) after surgery, although diagnosis is often delayed because the nonspecific manifestations are readily confused with more common disorders, especially RI.

The diagnostic evaluation for suspected pulmonary artery stenoses may include isotope perfusion scans, although abnormal findings are not necessarily diagnostic. Transesophageal echocardiography probably has a relatively high sensitivity and specificity for pulmonary venous obstruction, whereas analogous transthoracic studies have seldom been useful. The definitive test for vascular anastomotic anomalies remains pulmonary angiography.

There are no clear-cut guidelines for management of these complications. Expectant observation in arterial anastomotic obstructions seems to be associated with a high mortality. Data from Schulman et al indicates that degrees of pulmonary venous anastomotic narrowing are more common and can be successfully monitored. Angioplasty and stent insertion has been successfully employed and, if feasible, may be better tolerated than reoperation in pulmonary arterial anastomotic obstructions.

Allograft Rejection

HYPERACUTE REJECTION. These rejection responses are mediated by preexistent recipient antibodies against donor alloantigens, including MHC and ABO blood types. These antibodies bind to corresponding allo-antigens present on endothelial surfaces of the graft, resulting in immediate tissue injury by activation of complement cascades and neutrophils. Extensive platelet and fibrin thrombi form in small arterioles and capillaries, and the allograft becomes edematous and cyanotic. The incidence of hyperacute rejection among lung allograft recipients is exceeding low, due to widespread blood type matching and pretransplant screening of recipient sera against allogeneic cell panels.

ACUTE REJECTION. Although acute rejection (AR) tends to occur early in the posttransplant course, this entity is defined by histologic rather than temporal criteria (see Chapter 93). Nearly every lung transplant recipient will be afflicted by one or more episodes of AR.

The peak prevalence of AR steadily increases approximately one week after transplantation and continues for nearly a year. However, cases have been seen as early as three days following transplantation when induction immunosuppression was omitted or abbreviated, and sporadic episodes may occur several years later. Early and severe AR tends to mimic the nonspecific pulmonary edema presentation of RI (or pulmonary vascular abnormalities). Associated symptoms may include low-grade fever, cough, and dyspnea, usually with some degree of hypoxemia. Asymptomatic cases are frequent, however, particularly in later periods following transplantation. In contrast to early cases, chest radiographs in milder episodes occurring later than one or two months after transplantation are typically unimpressive. The differential diagnosis of AR episodes, depending on the time of onset, should usually include respiratory tract infections.

Clinical assessments are often unable to reliably gauge the presence or severity of AR, nor distinguish this entity from pulmonary infections. Accordingly, the diagnosis of AR is dependent on demonstration of typical histologic abnormalities. TBB is almost invariably the method of choice. The sensitivity of this procedure has been reported to be as great as 94%, but the diagnostic yield of TBB appears to be highly variable among institutions or operators. Current recommendations by the Lung Rejection Study Group include sampling by at least five biopsies that each contain bronchioles and greater than 100 air sacs. Concomitant BAL is useful for exclusion of infections. Given the difficulties inherent in noninvasive clinical diagnoses of AR, many centers employ regularly scheduled TBB in their lung transplant recipients. However, the frequency and utility of these procedures in entirely asymptomatic patients remains disputed.

Many aspects of AR treatment are also controversial. Virtually all transplant centers treat symptomatic patients, and most similarly manage higher grade (ie, > moderate) episodes (Table 92-1). AR usually remits with any number of immunosuppressive treatments, including short courses of high-dose steroids. Other agents that have seen successfully used include anti-T cell antibody preparations, additions or increases of azathioprine, methotrexate, or mycophenolate, replacements of primary immunosuppressant (eg, tacrolimus instead of cyclosporine), aerosolized cyclosporine, extracorporeal photochemotherapy, or total lymphoid irradiation. There is no clear consensus regarding routine treatment of asymptomatic or milder cases (especially later in the posttransplant period), or optimal management of the comparatively unusual patient with refractory AR. The extent of AR correlates strongly with the likelihood for subsequent development of chronic rejection, although it is by no means certain that aggressive early treatment actually lessens this risk. To further confound decisions, the potential for infections and lymphomagenesis is clearly associated with the intensity of immunosuppression.

Somewhat similarly, the optimal management of lymphocytic bronchiolitis ("airway inflammation") has been controversial for years. More recent evidence, however, suggests this entity is also a precursor to chronic rejection, and is probably a subset or analogous manifestation of AR. Accordingly, lymphocytic bronchitis is now most frequently treated interchangeably with classic AR.

Table 92-1. Acute Rejection Grades

Grade	Histology
A0 (normal)	No apparent abnormality
A1 (minimal)	Infrequent perivascular infiltrates
A2 (mild)	Frequent perivascular infiltrates
A3 (moderate)	Dense perivascular infiltrates with extension into alveolar septa
A4 (severe)	Diffuse infiltrates in all lung compartments with pneumocyte damage ± necrosis of parenchyma or vessels
Adapted from Trulock EP, Yousem SA, et al.	

Bronchiolitis obliterans with organizing pneumonia (BOOP) is also occasionally seen in TBB or other lung biopsies. Unlike the aforementioned entities, however, there is as yet no clear picture regarding the pathogenesis or significance of BOOP in this population. Most often, BOOP is seen in early periods after transplantation, may be present as an isolated finding or in association with either AR or infections, and most often appears to be a nonspecific response to diverse injuries.

Pulmonary Infections Occurring During the First Month after Transplantation

BACTERIAL PNEUMONIAS. Pulmonary infections immediately after lung transplantation are, for the most part, similar in etiology and presentation to those seen after other major thoracic or upper abdominal procedures. Bacteria are overwhelmingly the most common early cause of pulmonary infections among lung allograft recipients during the first month after transplantation. Organisms typical for nosocomial infections are predominant (eg, *Enterobacteriaceae, P aeruginosa,* and less often *S aureus*). Truly opportunistic infections (intracellular bacteria, cytomegalovirus [CMV], and *Pneumocystis carinii*) are infrequent during this period.

In addition to the usual factors contributing to development of pneumonias following major surgery (eg, atelectasis, retained airway secretions, diaphragmatic dysfunction), lung transplant recipients are at increased risk for pulmonary infections due to globally depressed mucociliary transport (presumably due to ischemia), as well as mechanical disruptions at the airway anastomosis. Denervation of airways distal to the anastomosis results in loss of cough reflexes, and further hinder secretion clearance. Lung transplant recipients are also unique in that the allograft may be in direct communication with a source of pathogens in the native, residual lung (among single lung recipients) or the upper airways (eg, among cystic fibrosis or dysfunctional cilia patients). In some cases, the source of pulmonary infections can be attributed to organisms colonizing the allograft at the time of harvest. Early (or pretransplant) glucocorticosteroids may hinder defenses against extracellular bacteria and fungi by impairments of phagocytosis and antibody production, and doses of these drugs have been correlated with risks for pneumonias. Other predisposing factors of recipients include older age, antecedent or residual pulmonary problems, and prolonged intubation.

In the absence of ongoing major pulmonary problems (eg, RI), the presentation of bacterial pneumonias tends to be acute, rapidly progressive, and with typical clinical features (ie, a febrile illness with obvious gas exchange or ventilatory impairments, and segmental or focal radiographic infiltrates.) Treatment of bacterial pneumonias in these patients follows conventional approaches, with selection of antibiotics predicated on appropriate cultures whenever possible, or empirical therapy based on the most probable etiologies. The mortality of lung transplant recipients with early bacterial pneumonias, given early and appropriate therapies, does not seem to exceed that of otherwise analogous groups in most published series and anecdotal reports. Mortality is often much greater, however, when infections are due to multiresistant organisms, as typically seen in patients undergoing transplantation for long-term suppurative lung diseases (eg, cystic fibrosis).

Although the incidence of bacterial pneumonias in early series was quite high (often approximating or exceeding 50% of allograft recipients), improvements of postoperative care and prophylaxis with antibiotics have resulted in significant reductions in rates of these infections. Aggressive postoperative secretion clearance (including adequate pain control to improve cough efficacy) and reexpansion maneuvers, in conjunction with early extubation when feasible (Chapter 89) should be standard-of-care for these patients. While there are many differences in prophylactic regimens among transplant centers, initial coverage is often directed against organisms cultured from the remaining lung of single-lung recipients, or proximal airways in those with cystic fibrosis. In the absence of underlying (or residual) suppurative airway colonization, another approach is to use prophylactic agents that have activity against microbes cultured from donor tracheas (obtained during organ procurement). Alternatively, and in cases where cultures are negative or unimpressive, various combinations of empirical antibiotics with broad activity have been successfully employed (eg, clindamycin with ceftriaxone). Obviously, selection of agents should be influenced by knowledge of locally predominant organisms and sensitivities, as well as experiences of the institution. In general, prophylaxis is administered for seven days, although some centers routinely use 10-day or even longer courses, especially in recipients at particularly high risk. Pretransplant irrigation and surgical drainage of sinuses among selected recipients with cystic fibrosis has also been anecdotally reported to decrease early pneumonias in these patients, although the effectiveness with respect to overall/long-term infection rates has not been established.

OTHER CAUSES OF EARLY PNEUMONIAS. Occasional cases of pneumonias due to *Aspergillus* or geographically endemic fungi have been reported during the first month after transplantation. Sporadic cases of *Legionella spp.*, have also occurred during this early period but are avoidable with surveillance of hospital water supplies. A herpes simplex virus (HSV) is fairly commonly isolated during the first few weeks after transplantation, although the majority of these isolations are due to clinically insignificant viral shedding.

Nonetheless, occasional cases of necrotizing tracheitis or other mucocutaneous infections have been attributed to HSV. The virus is susceptible to acyclovir, and prophylaxis with ganciclovir (usually given for prevention of CMV infection) is also highly effective. With routine perioperative use of acyclovir or ganciclovir, HSV infection is now rarely seen immediately postoperatively.

PULMONARY COMPLICATIONS ONE TO SIX MONTHS AFTER TRANSPLANTATION
Pulmonary Infections

Pneumonias during this intermediate period following lung transplantation are marked by an increased proportion of opportunistic infections. Lung transplant recipients are among the most severely immunocompromised patients encountered in clinical practice, and they are at risk for nearly the entire range of respiratory tract pathogens. In early series, prior to more effective preventative and diagnostic techniques, opportunistic organisms accounted for more than 50% of deaths due to infections, and were the most important cause of mortality following the immediate postoperative period.

Evaluations of pulmonary dysfunction episodes that are due to opportunistic infections are often complicated by blunted host defenses that render presentations nonspecific or overtly atypical. Progression of these infections may initially be insidious, although fulminant manifestations later in the course can also be expected. Radiographic features are often highly unusual. For example, a solitary pulmonary nodule can yield CMV, *P. carinii*, or *Aspergillus*, or any combination of these (and other) pathogens. The natural history of these infections with respect to initial manifestations and time of onset following transplantation may be highly altered by previous prophylactic therapy. Because presentations are often nonspecific or otherwise complex, and sensitivities of noninvasive tests are less than optimal, evaluations of lung transplant recipients with possible opportunistic infections are reliant on early BAL (if radiographically diffuse), or fine needle aspiration (FNA) of focal and/or peripheral lesions.

CYTOMEGALOVIRUS. Cytomegalovirus (CMV) is the single most frequent, serious, and complex pathogen of lung transplant recipients. Humans are the only known reservoir for this double-stranded DNA herpes virus, and thousands of genetic and antigenic variants exist worldwide. The virus is transmitted via exchange of any bodily secretion or excretion, and infections can be acquired throughout life. Approximately 50% of adult transplant candidates have serologic evidence of prior infection. Among the immunologically competent, CMV infections range in severity from asymptomatic viral replication to a mild mononucleosis syndrome. Infection leads to life-long persistence of the virus in leukocytes, although the course usually remains dormant as long as immunologic defenses are intact.

Intense immunosuppression resulting in impaired cellular-mediated responses enable reactivation of the virus, however, despite the persistence of anti-CMV antibodies. Reactivation may be triggered by proinflammatory cytokines (eg, TNF- α), which may account for the frequent temporal association of CMV with episodes of allograft rejection or infections. Evidence of CMV infections occur in greater than 75% of lung transplant patients at risk by virtue of prior infection (eg, reactivation) or receipt of a CMV-positive allograft or blood transfusion. Other predisposing factors for CMV infections include age of recipients, extent of donor-recipient MHC mismatching and, most importantly the intensity of immunosuppression. In the absence of effective CMV prophylaxis, the onset of these infections is greatest between one and four months after transplantation.

CMV manifestations among lung transplant recipients may range from asymptomatic viral shedding to fulminant organ dysfunction. Primary infections among serologically negative recipients tend to have a much worse prognosis than most cases of viral reactivation (or superinfections with an antigenically distinct strain). The pulmonary allograft is the predominant site of overt infection, with a presentation of hypoxemia, nonspecific dyspnea, malaise, and radiographic infiltrates that progress in severity over a few hours or days. The typical radiograph shows diffuse interstitial infiltrates, although CMV infections can present with protean radiographic abnormalities.

The natural history of early CMV pulmonary infections in these patients has not been completely delineated. In the absence of typical histologic or cytopathic findings, recovery of virus by immunofluorescence assays or conventional cultures of BAL specimens does not necessarily establish the diagnosis of ongoing pneumonitis (nor obviously exclude the possibility of other concomitant processes). Whereas asymptomatic CMV shedding in BAL of allogeneic bone marrow recipients portends eventual pneumonitis, analogous isolation of virus from the pulmonary allografts of lung transplant recipients does not necessarily predict the development of cytopathic disease. Even asymptomatic viral shedding, however, is a marker for subsequent development of deleterious and often delayed CMV sequelae. In particular, the prevalence and severity of chronic allograft rejection is increased in transplant recipients by prior or concomitant CMV infections. This correlation between OB and CMV is most striking in patients with prior symptomatic viral pneumonitis (demonstrated by organ dysfunction and histologic cytopathic changes). A variety of effects that increase allograft immunogenicity have

been attributed to CMV (Table 92-2). CMV infections are also associated with significantly increased risks for superinfections with *Aspergillus, P. carinii,* and other microbial pathogens.

There are many controversies regarding the management of CMV infections in lung transplantation recipients. Intravenous ganciclovir for two or more weeks is generally the treatment of choice for pneumonias or other serious CMV infections. Resistant strains can be treated with foscarnet, or multidrug combinations, and several other antiviral agents are currently undergoing study. The addition of intravenous immunoglobulin (IVIG) has demonstrably increased the effectiveness of ganciclovir treatment for serious CMV infections in bone marrow transplant (BMT) recipients, presumably by immunomodulation, rather than direct anti-CMV effects. Although lung transplant recipients share certain similarities to BMT patients with respect to lethality of CMV pneumonitis (perhaps since immune effector cells are uniquely allogeneic to lungs among both populations), combined ganciclovir and IVIG therapy has not been systematically studied among pulmonary allograft populations. Anecdotal evidence, however, suggests the combination treatment may have increased efficacy. The optimal management of immunosuppression in the presence of CMV infections is another difficult issue. On the one hand, reductions of immunosuppression should allow recovery of some antiviral cytotoxic T cell function, but this consideration needs to be balanced by the possibility that allograft rejection will be heightened by the infection. The approach to asymptomatic viral shedding is also controversial. Many centers treat these episodes with expectant waiting. In at least some cases, recipients are empirically treated if the viral shedding occurs during or immediately after courses of augmented immunosuppression for rejection. Treatment of viral shedding would seemingly be indicated in many other cases, since the adverse

immunopathic effects of CMV can occur in the absence of extensive or cytopathic disease. However, antiviral therapy is expensive, not without potential toxicity, and may select for drug resistant virus.

Given the considerable potential for delayed immunopathogenic sequelae, primary prevention of the infection has considerable potential value. Several agents have been used for CMV prophylaxis, although comparative trials are few. IVIG has some efficacy, particularly use of high titer anti-CMV preparations. Ganciclovir has demonstrated efficacy for prevention of CMV infections in lung and other transplant populations, and is clearly superior to acyclovir in this indication. There are often considerable variations in prophylaxis protocols among transplant centers. In general, the most favorable results are seen when intravenous ganciclovir is administered daily or three times per week during much or all of the period at greatest risk for viral infection. Prophylaxis is also routinely used in later periods, during or after augmentation of immunosuppression for allograft rejection. CMV infections are unusual during the duration of prophylaxis, but ganciclovir works to prevent replication, rather than elimination of the virus. Accordingly, no long-term protection is conferred, and the cumulative incidence of infections (and secondary sequelae) begins to increase following cessation of prophylaxis. In an effort to prolong the period of protection, some centers have employed even more prolonged courses of oral ganciclovir or other agents following an initial intravenous course. In addition to anti-CMV activity, there are indications that ganciclovir prophylaxis diminishes the incidence of other opportunistic infections, notably including Epstein-Barr virus (EBV) and HSV. Some centers have anecdotally reported a lower incidence of EBV-associated posttransplant lymphoproliferative disease since the introduction of ganciclovir prophylaxis.

Table 92-2. Immunomodulating Sequelae of CMV Infections

Effect	Consequence
Upregulation of allograft MHC molecules	Increased immunogenicity of allografts
Increased expression of cell adhesion molecules	Facilitates function of CD8$^+$ cytotoxicity
Increased elaboration of proinflammatory cytokines	Promotion of multiple immune effector mechanisms

Peptides encoded by CMV genome have Homologies to:
    MHC Class II DR-β
    MHC Class I-α
	Viral mimicry increase immunogenicity of allografts

Super antigenic effects	Promiscuous nonspecific activation of vast numbers of T cells, many of which may then crossreact with alloantigens

PNEUMOCYSTIS CARINII. Although a former scourge of lung and other allograft recipients, the implementation of prophylaxis with trimethoprim-sulfamethoxazole, or other effective agents, has resulted in the near elimination of disease due to *P. carinii*. Another benefit of prophylaxis has also been a reduction in the number of pneumonias due to *Nocardia* and other susceptible bacteria. The relatively rare cases of *P. carinii* today occur primarily among patients with poor medication compliance or intolerance. Like CMV, this opportunist can cause serious disease years after transplantation, if prophylaxis is discontinued. The yield of BAL for *P. carinii* in lung transplant recipients is often less than the near-perfect sensitivities reported in AIDS patients. The comparatively decreased sensitivity of BAL in transplant recipients is probably due to lesser absolute numbers of organisms and a tendency for *P. carinii* to be localized to the interstitium during early infections. Accordingly, the diagnostic sensitivity of bronchoscopy for *P. carinii* in transplant recipients can be considerably improved by concomitant TBB.

FUNGI. Fungal pneumonias continue to have a high mortality in lung transplant recipients. The most frequent of these pathogens is *Aspergillus spp.*, with other comparatively sporadic reports of infections due to endemic fungi. In general, fungal infections tend to have insidious presentations and frequently metastasize to other organs. Radiographs of transplant recipients with fungal pneumonias characteristically reveal peripheral focal or multifocal infiltrates, with upper lobe predominance. Lesions tend to cavitate, reflecting the predilection of these organisms for angiocentric invasion, thrombosis, and necrosis. Chest radiographs of fungal pulmonary infections are frequently atypical, however, and multiple other opportunists may also be concomitantly isolated from the same lesion. In addition to geographically determined susceptibilities, the intensity of immunosuppression is a major risk for fungal infections.

Unlike most other opportunistic pathogens, the predominant interstitial and perivascular locations of *Aspergillus* and other fungi often renders recovery by BAL and TBB somewhat problematic, with false-negative rates of 25% to 50% and 85% to 90%, respectively. FNA has a much higher reported diagnostic sensitivity. To further confound assessments, *Aspergillus* colonizing airways in the absence of overt infection is frequently isolated by BAL. Some small series and anecdotal reports suggest, however, that as many as 50% of transplant recipients with asymptomatic fungal colonization will subsequently develop invasive disease. Accordingly, many centers routinely administer prophylaxis with itraconazole or aerosolized amphotericin to recipients with *Aspergillus* colonization. These cases should be distinguished from colonizations with yeasts

(Candida), which are much less frequently associated with serious pulmonary infections.

EPSTEIN-BARR VIRUS AND POSTTRANSPLANT LYMPHOPROLIFERATIVE DISEASE. Epstein-Barr virus (EBV) is a herpes virus, related to CMV, that also has a ubiquitous distribution and high prevalence among adults. Like CMV, reactivation or primary infections with EBV occur in the majority of susceptible recipients during the first few weeks after transplantation. The target of EBV is limited, however, to human B lymphocytes via binding to their complement receptors. Acute infections with this virus are often asymptomatic, although severe mononucleosis syndromes may occur. The most serious consequence of EBV in recipients is the development of posttransplant lymphoproliferative disorder (PTLD).

In early series, PTLD occurred in from 2% to 10% of adult transplant recipients, and rates were even greater in pediatric patients. The median time of onset is between two and four months after transplantation, although cases have been reported as early as six weeks, or as late as several years. The usual presentation is an insidiously growing mass or nodule(s) (Figure 92-3), but aggressive tumors are not infrequent. Mediastinal or pulmonary involvement is frequent among lung transplant recipients, whereas occasionally some PTLD is predominantly subdiaphragmatic. TBB or FNA can readily diagnose accessible tumors.

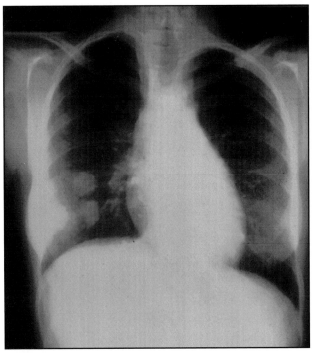

Figure 92-3. Posttransplant lymphoproliferative disease. Slowly growing lymphoma nodules in left lung allograft. Similar lesions have been reported in a variety of fungal and other opportunistic infections. The diagnosis here was established by fine needle aspiration. (Courtesy of V Valentine).

Even though many of the tumors undergo at least partial remissions with decreases of immunosuppression, the eventual mortality among afflicted patients may be in excess of 80%, particularly among those with monoclonal or oligoclonal PTLD. Treatment by conventional lymphoma management stratagems has only been successful in a small proportion of cases. As previously mentioned, CMV prophylaxis with ganciclovir seems to have decreased the incidence of PTLD. While the mechanism is unproven, ganciclovir prophylaxis could be beneficial by either decreasing the number of predisposing CMV infections or, more likely, via a direct suppression of EBV replication.

OTHER VIRUSES. A number of other viral diseases of lung transplant recipients have been infrequently reported during the intermediate posttransplant period. Varicella-zoster virus (VZV) pneumonitis can occur during dissemination of the pathogen, although the most frequent manifestation of this virus is primarily cutaneous lesions and dermatomal pain syndromes with reactivation. Sporadic pneumonias due to parainfluenza and adenoviruses have been observed, and the latter virus is notable for potential transmission via the allograft. Respiratory syncytial virus (RSV) can afflict both adult and pediatric recipients, and these infections are notable as an unusual cause of acute airflow obstruction. Detection of RSV infections is particularly worthwhile since specific antiviral therapies are available.

PULMONARY DYSFUNCTION EPISODES SIX MONTHS OR MORE AFTER TRANSPLANTATION
Pulmonary Infections
While incidences of pneumonia tend to diminish a few months after transplantation, the relative risk of pulmonary infections in lung transplant recipients remains several-fold greater than among normal populations. Accordingly, continued attention and rapid evaluation of symptoms or radiographic changes are indicated. Bacteria are the most frequent cause of pneumonias several months or more after transplantation, and are an especially serious cause of morbidity and mortality in recipients with OB. Bacterial infections among long-term survivors of lung transplantation tend to present with symptoms and signs that are qualitatively similar to those of immunocompetent patients. Sporadic cases due to opportunistic pathogens continue to occur, particularly with the cessation of *P. carinii* or CMV prophylaxis.

Transplant recipients also appear to have some increased risks for mycobacterial infections. These infections can occur anytime, including several months or years after transplantation. Mycobacterial disease often presents with unusual clinical and radiographic features in immunocompromised hosts, and there are increased relative frequencies of atypical organisms. Screening and prophylaxis of patients with prior infections before their transplantation has been shown to lessen risks of tuberculosis. Diagnoses are established using conventional methodologies, and infections usually respond to standard, albeit prolonged, antimicrobial regimens.

Airway Anastomosis Complications
Progressive strictures or bronchomalacia at the airway anastomosis may result in airflow limitation, dyspnea, cough, and/or wheezing several months or years after transplantation. The overall prevalence of airway anastomosis problems in lung transplant recipients may be as great as 20% to 30%, although the seriousness of the problems is highly variable. In general, institution rates of airway complications decrease with continued experience. Ischemic-related mucosal injuries are commonly seen during bronchoscopies in the early postoperative period, and may portend subsequent anastomotic complications. These early assessments tend to be insensitive, however, since the extent of the injury is frequently underestimated.

The *sine qua non* of these complications is direct observation of significant (ie, >50%) luminal obstruction. Assessments of spontaneously breathing patients by fiberoptic bronchoscopy facilitate determinations of dynamic collapse during exhalation. Lesser degrees of luminal obstruction may also warrant treatment, if accompanied by disabling or progressive symptoms, or significant physiologic impairments. Spirometric indices of expiratory airflow obstruction in these patients are similar to those seen with intrinsic pulmonary disease, including OB. Chest radiographs most frequently are also nonspecific, although airtrapping or atelectasis may be present. Chest CT may be a useful adjunct to bronchoscopic evaluations, particularly to determine the length of severe obstructions.

While the morbidity of airway anastomosis problems may be considerable, these lesions are infrequently lethal. Significant bronchomalacia is optimally managed by stent placement, with prolonged or permanent treatment necessary in most cases. Stents are also ultimately necessary for severe strictures, although lesser obstructions have been successfully treated with dilatations. Granulation tissue or other localized fibrotic reactions are often treated by laser excision.

Recurrence of Pulmonary Disease
Evaluations of pulmonary dysfunction episodes should also include considerations that the pretransplant lung disease has recurred in the allograft. Relapses of diverse idiopathic lung disorders with a presumably immunologic pathogenesis have been most often described, including sarcoidosis, desquamative interstitial pneumonitis, Langerhans' cell granulomatosis, talc granulo-

matosis, hard metal pneumoconiosis, and diffuse pan-bronchiolitis. Sporadic cases of recurrent lymphangioleiomyomatosis and pulmonary alveolar proteinosis have also been reported. A small series of lung transplantations for treatment of bronchoalveolar cell carcinoma showed recurrent malignancies among most recipients within two years. In general, recurrences of sarcoidosis have been limited to incidental findings of granulomas on biopsy that were not associated with significant allograft dysfunction. Many of the other disease relapses have been associated with significant graft dysfunction. The diagnosis in most cases has been established by lung biopsies, and treatments are similar to those employed in untransplanted patients.

Neoplasms

The possibility of primary or metastatic neoplasm should also be considered in the differential diagnoses of slowly growing pulmonary infiltrates among lung transplant recipients. As discussed previously, the most common pulmonary malignancies following lung transplantation are EBV-associated lymphomas, and infrequent cases may occur after several years. Recipients of other organ allografts have a somewhat increased incidence of certain carcinomas and Kaposi's sarcoma (the latter associated with Herpesvirus-8), although the numbers of long-term lung transplantation survivors is too limited to assign a definitive relative risk to this population.

Chronic Allograft Rejection, Obliterative Bronchiolitis and Bronchiolitis Obliterans Syndrome

While acute rejection episodes may continue to afflict recipients for months after transplantation, chronic rejection manifested by obliterative bronchiolitis (OB) becomes a far more serious and difficult problem. OB ultimately develops in approximately one-half of long-term lung transplantation survivors, and is the single greatest cause of morbidity and mortality in this population. Biopsy documented cases have occurred as early as six weeks after transplantation, but peak incidences are usually between 12 to 24 months. To a considerable degree, the time of OB onset is conditional on previous treatments, with development of disease somewhat delayed by aggressive early immunosuppression and/or effective (prolonged) CMV and other infection prophylaxis.

Many details of OB pathogenesis remain uncertain. Various cell types, growth/reparative factors, and pro-inflammatory cytokines have been implicated in the airway injuries that typify OB (Chapter 93). The severity and/or frequency of antecedent acute rejection is a major risk factor for OB, as is the extent of MHC or other alloantigen mismatches (including male-specific antigens) between donors and recipients. As noted earlier, prior CMV infections also predispose to OB, presumably

via one or more global immune-activation sequelae. A variety of early nonimmunogenic pulmonary injuries (eg, reperfusion injury) may also increase risks of OB, possibly due to increased release of alloantigens or nonspecific recruitment/activation of immune effector cells.

Although exact details of responsible mechanisms have not been completely delineated, both circumstantial clinical associations (eg, the correlation between AR and OB) and experimental studies strongly implicate T cell allograft recognition and effector responses in the development of OB. T cell depletion in animals with pulmonary allografts prevents OB occurrences, as does induction of central (ie, T cell) tolerance to alloantigens. More recently, alloreactive T cells have been shown in human lung transplant recipients to undergo marked clonal proliferations concomitant with or prior to development of OB. Presumptive evidence based on the number and variety of clonal T cell expansions suggests that indirect alloantigen recognition may play an important role in pathogenesis of OB. It is further tempting to speculate that the typical paucity of infiltrating T cells in biopsies of OB, as well as the usually meager clinical response of OB to anti-T cell therapies, implies that the damage effected by these cells occurred much earlier in the development of the syndrome, and the actual ongoing airway injuries are largely due to secondary effector mechanisms.

The clinical manifestations of OB range from indolent to rapidly progressive. In many cases, the first evidence of OB is an otherwise asymptomatic decrement of expiratory flow, as determined by spirometry. Slightly more advanced or aggressive episodes present with dyspnea, cough, or infection. Patients with OB have greatly increased prevalence of bacterial lower airway infections, especially with *P aeruginosa*. The clinical course of some mimics severe bronchiectasis, ie, recurrent episodes of productive bronchitis that can be ameliorated somewhat by bronchodilators, regular courses of rotating antibiotics, and chest physiotherapy. Overall, the mortality among those with severe or progressive OB is increased several-fold relative to the unafflicted cohort, with deaths attributable to both infections and graft failure.

The diagnosis of OB is highly reliant on spirometry, and virtually all transplant centers incorporate regular spirometry in their routine surveillance of lung transplant recipients. The development of expiratory flow obstruction should prompt further evaluations in order to exclude other and usually more treatable disorders. Chest radiographs typically show a paucity of acute abnormalities, although hyperinflation may be evident. High-resolution chest CT scans show air trapping, bronchiectasis, and mosaic phenomenon, but generally add little to the diagnostic evaluation. The value of CT scans may be increased, however, in cases in which recurrences of the original lung diseases may be a consideration (see above). Occasionally, progressive hyperinflation of the contralateral native lung among single-lung recipients with underlying COPD can present with some similarities, but this particular problem can easily be excluded by chest radiographs. Bronchoscopy plays a role in exclusion of airway anastomosis problems, and BAL is often employed to rule out occult underlying infections.

The role of TBB in the evaluation of OB is controversial. The lesions of OB are often heterogeneously distributed, and easily missed by too few or too minute biopsies. Overall, the reported diagnostic sensitivity of TBB for OB in many published series is as low at 15% to 60%. Nonetheless, TBB and biopsy interpretations are operator-dependent procedures, and the diagnostic yield may be considerably greater in the hands of adept bronchoscopists and experienced lung pathologists. Moreover, repeat TBB in individual cases may increase the sensitivity by ~50%. Other indirect modalities for either prediction or diagnosis of OB, including quantitations of BAL cell counts or differentials, measures of BAL or serum cytokines, or assays of donor T cell alloreactivity, while valuable for experimental studies, uniformly lack the degree of sensitivity and specificity necessary for clinical use.

Given the general difficulty in diagnosis of OB by TBB or other measures, a clinically-validated standard for spirometric abnormalities has been developed and is widely used (Table 92-3). In the absence of other potentially confounding problems (above), a greater-than-or-equal-to 20% decrement of FEV_1 from previous optimal values is generally considered presumptive evidence of chronic rejection and, lacking biopsy confirmation, is specified as bronchiolitis obliterans syndrome (BOS). Other physiologic measures, including decrements of midexpiratory flow (eg, FEF_{25-75}) or increments of airway resistance, may have greater sensitivity, but are also liable to confounding by residual native lungs, may be less reproducible, and have not yet been widely validated.

In practical terms, the difficulty with management of OB is not in establishing a diagnosis, but stems from the inadequacies of current treatments. A large number of immunosuppressive strategies have been suggested,

as previously described for AR. While successes have been reported for all of these treatments, the corresponding reports typically suffer from small numbers of patients with anecdotal or retrospective methodologies. Assessments of therapeutic efficacies in these uncontrolled series are further confounded by the highly variable rate of OB progression. In general, it appears that augmented global immunosuppression may stabilize pulmonary function in a minority of recipients, and occasionally reverse expiratory airflow in a smaller proportion. The course of OB in the majority of recipients seems to be largely unaffected by these treatments, however, and even most "successes" are usually of finite duration. Overall, the limited efficacy of augmented immunosuppressive treatments also needs to be balanced against their predilections to increase risks for infections and lymphomagenesis, although these risks may, in turn, be lessened somewhat by appropriate antimicrobial prophylaxis. The only definitive remedy for OB at this time appears to be re-transplantation. However, re-transplantation is clearly a less-than-optimal approach for universal application, in light of the paucity of donor organs, as well as countless and considerable emotional and financial considerations. Given the many current vagaries, definitive recommendations regarding the treatment of OB cannot be given with overwhelming confidence, but are usually based on a combination of local experiences and biases.

RECOMMENDED READING

Boehler A, Kesten S, Weder W, Speich R. Bronchiolitis obliterans after lung transplantation: a review. Chest. 1998;114(5):1411-1426.

Noble S, Faulds D. Ganciclovir. An update of its use in the prevention of cytomegalovirus infections and disease in transplant recipients. Drugs. 1998;56(1):115-146.

Shennib H, Massard G. Airway complications in lung transplantation. Ann Thorac Surg. 1994;57(2):506-511.

Shepard J-AO. Radiology of lung transplantation. Sem Resp Crit Care Med. 1998;19:533-542.

Trulock EP. Lung transplantation. Am J Respir Crit Care Med. 1997;155(3):789-818.

Yousem SA, Berry GJ, Cagle PT, et al. Revision of the 1990 working formulation for the classification of pulmonary allograft rejection: Lung Rejection Study Group. J Heart Lung Transplant. 1996;15(1 Pt 1):1-15.

Table 92-3. Spirometric Staging of Bronchiolitis Obliterans Syndrome

BOS Stage	Decrement of FEV_1
0 (no significant abnormality)	<20%
1 (mild)	20% to 35%
2 (moderate)	35% to 50%
3 (severe)	> 50%
Adapted from Yousem SA, et al.	

93 PATHOLOGY OF PULMONARY ALLOGRAFT DYSFUNCTION

Aliya N. Husain, MD
Anderson S. Gaweco, MD, PhD

Pulmonary dysfunction after lung transplantation can be evaluated using a number of cytological and histopathological techniques, none of which is ideal in every situation. Depending on the clinical scenario, examination of bronchoalveolar lavage (BAL) fluid, endobronchial biopsy (EBB), transbronchial biopsy (TBB), fine needle aspiration biopsy (FNAB), and/or open lung biopsy (OLB) may be performed. The diagnostic yield, sensitivity and specificity of each of these techniques varies depending upon the clinical setting.

BAL is most useful in providing material for microbiological cultures. After extensive studies of BAL fluid with regard to cellular composition, subtyping of lymphocytes, and molecules derived from activated inflammatory cells, it has been generally concluded that BAL fluid cannot be used to diagnose pulmonary allograft rejection. It has, however, helped in understanding the pathogenesis of both acute and chronic rejection. EBB is invaluable in assessing the bronchial anastomotic site and any other airway lesion that can be seen bronchoscopically. TBB is the most commonly used procedure to obtain lung tissue for histologic evaluation of the allograft. Three to five pieces of alveolated lung parenchyma, each containing bronchioles and more than 100 air sacs, are necessary to confidently diagnose and grade acute and chronic rejection. It may be necessary for the bronchoscopist to obtain more than five biopsies to provide this minimum number of adequate alveolated pieces. Preservation methods vary. Immediately upon collecting the specimens, many centers recommend placement in formalin and gentle agitation to inflate the biopsy fragments. Other centers choose to place the samples in sterile saline first to permit re-expansion of the tissue if needed due to forceps crush artifact, followed by subsequent immersion in formalin. Frozen sections are not performed on TBB specimens. Tissue processing is routinely done overnight, but can be completed in a rush cycle requiring as little as six hours if clinically necessary. FNAB yields the most useful information during the initial evaluation of a mass in either the transplanted or native lung. When correlated with histology, the sensitivity and specificity of FNAB are close to 100%. OLB is useful in those patients with clinical deterioration or with a radiographic mass in whom the results of TBB or FNAB are inconclusive. Finally, it may be that only an examination of the transplanted lung either after re-transplantation or at autopsy will find a specific cause for lung failure. Although such findings will not help in the allograft that has failed, these will certainly provide information relative to the disease processes that accounted for the graft failure and may assist in its prevention should re-transplantation be possible. Moreover, the examination of such specimens will add to the body of information available to the clinician in the future.

VASCULAR COMPLICATIONS

Early and late complications of the pulmonary arterial and venous anastomoses, although uncommon, are an important surgical problem as any delay in their recognition and treatment leads to a high morbidity and mortality rate. Even a minor obstruction at the site of anastomosis, whether due to suture placement or some other anatomic constraint, can lead to thrombus formation with partial or total occlusion of the vascular lumen. On pathologic examination, inflammatory cells and endothelial disruption are seen in the early posttransplant period while stenosis and fibrosis with scattered foreign body giant cells are present in the intermediate to late posttransplant period. A superimposed recent or organizing thrombus is often identifiable irrespective of time after transplant. The lung parenchyma shows both interstitial and intraalveolar edema with areas of recent hemorrhage.

BRONCHIAL ANASTOMOTIC COMPLICATIONS

The frequency of both early ischemic and late stenotic complications of the bronchial anastomosis have markedly decreased as lung transplant programs have gained experience and improved their surgical techniques and postoperative management. The anastomosis heals by formation of granulation tissue, the surface of which re-epithelializes within a few days. Occasionally, exuberant polypoid granulation tissue may form and project into the airway lumen and may need to be removed. Occluded bronchial artery remnants can be easily identified on histologic sections. Micro-revascularization typically occurs over the first few weeks.

Superimposed infection may interrupt the healing process. In a third of EBB specimens obtained from the bronchial anastomosis, specific microorganisms can be identified using either routine or special staining and

Aliya N. Husain, MD, Associate Professor of Pathology; Director, Surgical Pathology, Loyola University Medical Center, Loyola University Chicago, Maywood, IL

Anderson S. Gaweco, MD, PhD, Assistant Professor of Medicine and Pathology, Loyola University Medical Center, Loyola University Chicago, Maywood, IL

appropriate culture techniques. The most common organisms found are fungi, including *Candida sp* and *Aspergillus sp* (Figure 93-1), followed by cytomegalovirus (CMV) and various bacteria. Severe infection may result in dehiscence of the anastomosis, which is only rarely due to ischemia alone. Worse, the infection may extend into the adjacent mediastinum and produce a bronchopulmonary artery fistula. Varying amounts of inflammation and necrosis involving the mucosa, submucosa and cartilage are seen in biopsy specimens from these anastomotic sites.

Bronchial anastomotic stenosis occurring as a result of poor healing secondary to ischemic injury demonstrates nonspecific acute and chronic inflammation. Narrowing of the lumen occurs with formation of granulation tissue and fibrosis of the submucosa. Associated squamous metaplasia and focal erosion of the bronchial epithelium also occurs. Depending on the severity of the underlying ischemic injury, the bronchial cartilage may demonstrate perichondral fibrosis with loss of normal contour of the cartilage plates, sub-perichondral calcification, eosinophilia, ossification and fibrovascular ingrowth.

INTRINSIC PULMONARY DISEASES
Preservation-Reperfusion Injury
Preservation-reperfusion injury clinically manifests as pulmonary edema and occurs in 10% to 20% of patients in the early posttransplant period. Its pathogenesis is multifactorial, including ischemia, surgical trauma, reperfusion injury, denervation and an interruption of the lymphatic drainage of the transplanted lung. The pulmonary endothelium appears to be particularly susceptible to this type of injury, which is mediated by a variety of mechanisms including neutrophil adhesion and transendothelial migration with release of pro-inflammatory mediators and reactive oxygen species. Increased endothelial permeability, rather than hydrostatic pressure, has been shown to be the primary cause of reperfusion-associated interstitial edema. Accumu-

lation of large quantities of interstitial edema results in fluid flow into alveolar spaces. It has been shown that the alveolar epithelium is more resistant to injury than the endothelium in the setting of lung ischemia and reperfusion. In the majority of patients, alveolar epithelial fluid clearance is intact and the endothelial injury appears to be self-limited, thus the alveolar fluid is rapidly removed and the patient recovers.

Fortunately, there are not many opportunities to histologically examine reperfusion injury in human lungs. In the early years of the Loyola University Lung Transplant Program, TBB were performed routinely in the first five to 12 postoperative days to differentiate a reimplantation response from acute rejection. Most of these biopsies showed mild to moderate interstitial and alveolar edema with small numbers of neutrophils in the alveolar septa and alveoli (Figure 93-2).

The absence of a mononuclear cell infiltrate, both in the perivascular area and in the airway, easily distinguishes reperfusion injury from acute rejection. Ultrastructural changes seen as a result of the reperfusion injury consist of endothelial damage manifested by weak intercellular connections, numerous intercellular gaps and widespread endothelial cell detachment.

Rejection
Despite improvements in short-term to medium-term graft survival rates, the long-term results of lung allograft survival remain poor compared to other solid organ transplants with no substantial change in graft attrition rate. Following lung transplantation, chronic allograft rejection remains an important complication in the posttransplant period. It is the primary cause of late graft failure and is the principal indication for re-transplantation. More importantly, antirejection therapy is not without side effects and may result in a high incidence of infections and toxicity in the short-term, as well as development of lymphoproliferative disorders in the long-term. An unequivocal diagnosis of allograft rejection is there-

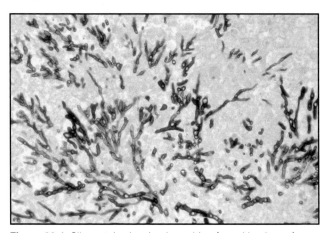

Figure 93-1. Silver stain showing branching fungal hyphae of *Aspergillus* species.

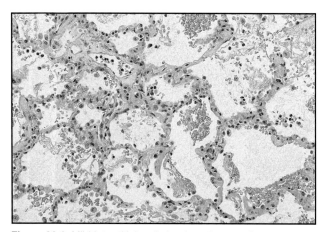

Figure 93-2. Mild interstitial and alveolar edema and acute inflammation characteristic of reimplantation response.

fore critical for timely medical intervention and possible prevention of rejection-related complications. A working formulation for the grading of pulmonary allograft rejection was initially developed in 1990 and revised in 1996. It is a morphology-based system for the interpretation of TBB performed for allograft monitoring of both pediatric and adult patients.

HYPERACUTE REJECTION. Hyperacute or humoral (antibody-mediated) rejection is clinically and pathologically well-characterized in kidney, heart, and liver allografts but has only recently been recognized to occur in lung allografts (partly due to the historically infrequent occurrence of prospective crossmatching). Humoral sensitization is rare in the lung transplant population. Only a single case has been reported wherein a lung transplant recipient developed graft failure consistent with hyperacute rejection. A prospective pathologic study of 55 lung transplant recipients has failed to demonstrate any occurrence of hyperacute rejection. Since its histological features are unclear, hyperacute rejection has not been included in the current working formulation for the classification of lung allograft rejection.

ACUTE REJECTION. Acute rejection of transplant allografts is primarily a lymphocyte-mediated process. The characteristic histological feature of acute rejection

Table 93-1. Working Formulation for Classification and Grading of Pulmonary Allograft Rejection

A. Acute rejection

Grade 0 - None
Grade 1 - Minimal
Grade 2 - Mild
Grade 3 - Moderate
Grade 4 - Severe

B. Airway inflammation – lymphocytic bronchitis/bronchiolitis

Grade 0 - None
Grade 1 - Minimal
Grade 2 - Mild
Grade 3 - Moderate
Grade 4 - Severe

C. Chronic airway rejection – bronchiolitis obliterans

C1. Active
C2. Inactive

D. Chronic vascular rejection – accelerated graft vascular sclerosis

in lung allografts as well as those in other solid organ allografts is the progressive infiltration of the graft by host mononuclear cells. The immune-destructive effector cell responses involve a cascade of both nonspecific and antigen-specific mechanisms. The complex interplay of the host immunological attack against the foreign graft include an afferent and efferent phase. The interaction of circulating host lymphocytes with foreign graft alloantigens on vascular endothelium triggers effector cell activation. This consequently leads to the recruitment of graft-infiltrating cells, the provision of inflammatory mediators such as cytokines, monokines, chemokines and the up-regulation of adhesion molecules, each of which contributes to allograft injury and destruction.

In the first posttransplant year, the most common complications are acute rejection and infection. Both are characterized by fever, dyspnea and decreased lung function. Acute cellular rejection occurs most often in the first six months after transplantation but can occur anytime in the posttransplant period. The severity, timing and frequency of acute rejection episodes have been implicated in the development of chronic rejection. The "gold standard" for the diagnosis of acute rejection is the histologic examination of routinely stained specimens consisting of at least five fragments of lung allograft tissue obtained by transbronchial biopsy. TBB may be performed as indicated by clinical criteria or by surveillance protocol. Acute rejection is characterized by a predominantly lymphocytic infiltrate with scattered eosinophils, neutrophils and plasma cells. The infiltrate may be perivascular with or without extension into the lung parenchyma or peribronchial tissue. Perivascular and peribronchial lesions may not always be seen together or necessarily be of the same grade in a given biopsy specimen. Endothelialitis/vasculitis is often seen but does not influence the grading of acute rejection. Although clinical findings are important in patient management, these are not used for making the definitive histologic diagnosis or in grading the rejection.

The original 1990 Working Formulation for the Classification of Pulmonary Allograft Rejection has been revised by the Lung Rejection Study Group and was published in 1996 (Table 93-1). Airway inflammation, which was initially thought to be a nonspecific histological finding, most likely carries the same implication for graft function as acute perivascular rejection, once infection is excluded.

The grading of acute rejection is based primarily on the finding of a progressively increasing perivascular and airway lymphocytic inflammation. The grading score ranges from Grade A0/B0 (none) (Figures 93-3 and 93-4) through Grade A4/B4 (severe). In minimal acute rejection (Grade A1/B1), there are scattered infrequent perivascular and airway mononuclear infiltrates that are not obvious at low magnification. Blood vessels, particularly venules, are cuffed by small round, plasmacytoid and transformed lymphocytes forming a ring of two to three cells in thickness in the perivascular adventitia (Figure 93-5) and submucosa of bronchi and bronchioles (Figure 93-6). Mild acute rejection (Grade A2/B2) consists of greater than three layer cuffing of activated lympho-

cytes, eosinophils, and neutrophils around small blood vessels (Figure 93-7) or a band-like infiltrate in the airway submucosa (Figure 93-8). Moderate acute rejection (Grade A3/B3) is characterized by an extension of the inflammation into alveolar septa with or without vasculitis (Figure 93-9) or a band-like infiltrate in the submucosa extending into the airway epithelium with focal epithelial necrosis (Figure 93-10). In severe acute rejection (Grade

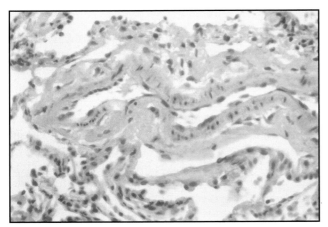

Figure 93-3. Alveolated lung parenchyma with no acute rejection (A0).

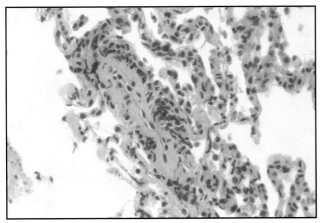

Figure 93-4. Airway and lung parenchyma with no rejection (A0, B0).

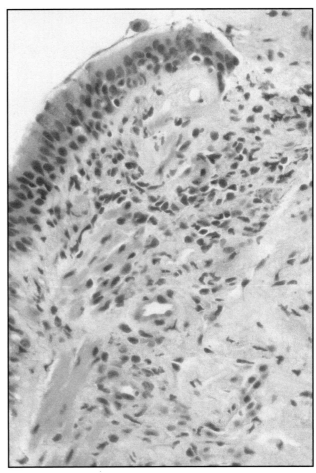

Figure 93-6. Minimal lymphocytic bronchitis/bronchiolitis (B1).

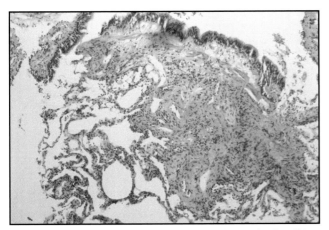

Figure 93-5. Minimal perivascular acute rejection with blood vessel cuffed by two cell layers of mononuclear cells (A1).

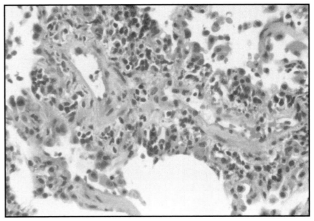

Figure 93-7. Mild perivascular acute rejection with blood vessel cuffed by more than three layers of activated lymphocytes (A2).

A4/B4), diffuse perivascular, interstitial and air space infiltrates associated with pneumocyte damage, macrophages, hyaline membranes, hemorrhage and neutrophils or epithelial ulceration with fibrinopurulent exudates are seen. With current potent immunosuppressive regimens, grades 3 and 4 acute cellular rejection are rarely seen.

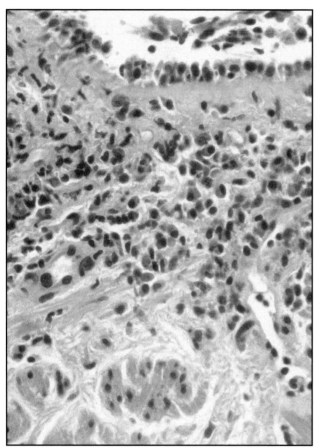

Figure 93-8. Mild airway inflammation with band-like infiltrate of mononuclear cells in the submucosa (B2).

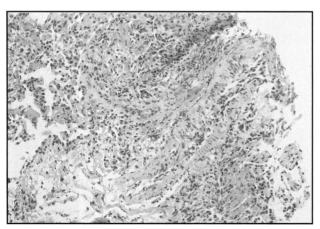

Figure 93-9. Moderate perivascular acute rejection with vasculitis and extension of inflammation into adjacent alveolar septa. Eosinophils and neutrophils are admixed with the mononuclear cells (A3).

CHRONIC REJECTION. Chronic rejection remains a major cause of late graft failure. The underlying pathogenetic mechanisms of chronic allograft rejection, although extensively studied, are still ill-defined. Current concepts of chronic rejection obtained from experimental data implicate a multifactorial pathogenesis that involves primarily alloantigen-dependent mechanisms and a contributory role of alloantigen-independent factors. The process of chronic rejection in general is believed to occur in stages. The initial wave of an antibody-mediated humoral response is paralleled by a cellular-mediated reaction characterized by intense graft mononuclear cell infiltration. Considerable data have implicated a central role of the monocyte/macrophage compartment as the critical effector cells during chronic rejection in contrast to the lymphocyte-mediated acute rejection process. Lastly, the production of inflammatory mediators and growth factors by the profuse graft infiltrates contribute to the observed tissue remodeling and fibroproliferative response of the damaged graft.

Chronic rejection of the transplanted lung allograft presents clinically as bronchiolitis obliterans (BO) syndrome, which is characterized by progressive airflow obstruction and deterioration of graft function. Chronic

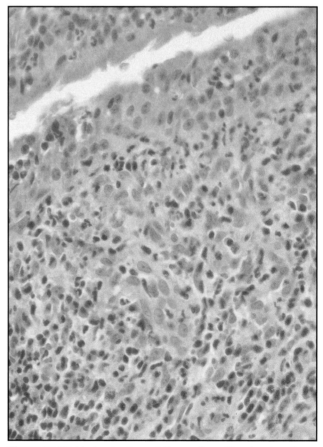

Figure 93-10. Moderate airway inflammation with extension of inflammatory cells into the epithelium. Eosinophils and neutrophils are admixed with the mononuclear cells (B3).

lung allograft dysfunction is characterized primarily by BO. The characteristic damage of epithelial-lined bronchial structures is similarly seen in epithelial-lined conduits of other allografts (ie, bile ducts, renal tubules and pancreatic ducts). The high antigenicity of these epithelial cells through the up-regulated expression of MHC, adhesion and costimulatory molecules, together with the abundance of antigen-presenting cells and circulating lymphocytes, provide an increased propensity to damage of these structures. The initial stages of injury and inflammation of airways progress to a fibroproliferative stage leading to irreversible graft damage. Substantial data implicate an immune-mediated attack directed against bronchiolar structures in the pathogenesis of BO. The most important risk factor for BO is acute allograft rejection.

Although the term "chronic" implies a late temporal process, BO can be seen as early as three to six weeks after transplantation, but primarily occurs one or more years posttransplant. The clinical parameters of BO are well-characterized and histopathological confirmation is not required for either definitive diagnosis or treatment. A biopsy, either transbronchial or wedge, is performed only to exclude other differential diagnoses (ie, infection and PTLD). The sensitivity of a transbronchial biopsy is low; hence, a wedge biopsy is preferable to establish the unequivocal diagnosis of BO. Histologically, BO is a submucosal fibrosing process that predominantly involves bronchioles in a patchy distribution and causes partial or total obliteration of the bronchiolar lumen. The grading of BO takes into account only the presence and absence of mononuclear cells within the fibrous tissue, designated either as active (Figure 93-11) or inactive (Figure 93-12), respectively.

Chronic vascular rejection of the lung is histologically similar to the transplant vasculopathy seen in other solid organ allografts, however, it does not appear to have the same relevance to allograft function. In the lung, chronic rejection is manifested primarily as BO.

Infection

Bacterial infections are seen commonly in both pulmonary allografts and native lungs. Identification of the specific microorganism depends upon culture of either sputum or BAL fluid. Histologically, there is a patchy or confluent neutrophilic inflammation of airways, interstitium and alveolar spaces. In TBB, the presence of numerous neutrophils is highly suggestive of an infection. In the presence of infection, rejection cannot be accurately evaluated, however the pathologist may suggest that coexisting rejection is also present when there are typical perivascular and airway mononuclear inflammatory cell infiltrates.

CMV infection is the most common viral infection of the transplanted lung. A definitive diagnosis of CMV pneumonitis is based on the identification of CMV inclusions, which are easily seen on routine H&E sections of the biopsy and readily identified on cytology. The infected cell is enlarged with a single intranuclear inclusion and multiple small intracytoplasmic inclusions. Multinucleated cells may also be seen with each enlarged nucleus containing an intranuclear inclusion (Figure 93-13).

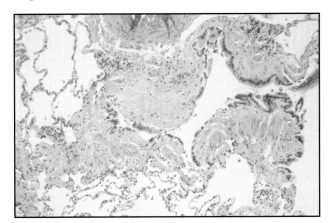

Figure 93-12. Nodule of fibrous tissue is seen bulging into the lumen of a bronchiole. There is no inflammation within the fibrous tissue (bronchiolitis obliterans, inactive Cb).

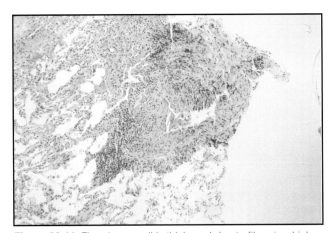

Figure 93-11. The airway wall is thickened due to fibrosis which partially occludes the lumen. Lymphocytes are present within the fibrous tissue (bronchiolitis obliterans, active, Ca).

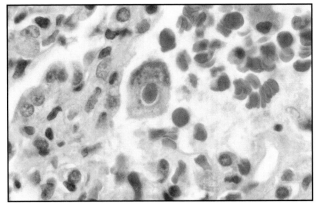

Figure 93-13. Diagnostic cytopathic changes of CMV are present: enlarged cell with single large intranuclear inclusion and multiple small intracytoplasmic inclusions. There is a lack of inflammation in the adjacent lung tissue.

In the very early stage of CMV infection, immuno-histochemical staining against immediate-early antigen may demonstrate positivity in cells lacking cytopathic changes (Figure 93-14).

Adenoviral pneumonia is relatively common in the pediatric transplant population and is a major cause of mortality in this age group. Characteristic smudgy nuclear inclusions, necrotizing bronchitis, bronchiolitis and interstitial pneumonitis are observed in the allograft. Immunohistochemical staining for adenovirus protein, in situ hybridization for viral genome and viral cultures are useful in establishing a diagnosis of adenoviral infection.

The bronchial anastomotic site is predisposed to develop fungal infections, mainly caused by *Candida sp* and *Aspergillus sp,* which can progress to ulcerative tracheobronchitis and fungal pneumonia. The identification of fungal hyphae in the biopsy is facilitated by silver stains such as Gomori methenamine silver. *Pneumocystis carinii* pneumonia (PCP) has been largely eliminated as a clinical problem with the prophylactic use of antibi-otics. When PCP occurs, it is characterized by the presence of an intra-alveolar frothy exudate (Figure 93-15) which on silver staining is seen to contain diagnostic trophozoites and cysts (Figure 93-16).

Bronchiolitis Obliterans Organizing Pneumonia

Bronchiolitis obliterans organizing pneumonia (BOOP), originally described as an idiopathic disease, has been reported in association with a variety of pulmonary diseases, as well as after lung transplantation. In the latter case, it results from acute epithelial injury secondary to acute allograft rejection or an ongoing infection and is not a component of nor does it predispose to chronic rejection (BO). In a study of 115 transplant patients at Loyola, BOOP was seen in 32 at some time in their post-transplant course. Histologically, BOOP is characterized by the presence of nodules of granulation tissue or Masson bodies, which are located within the lumina of small airways and extend into alveolar ducts and alveoli (Figure 93-17).

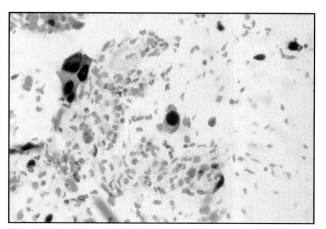

Figure 93-14. Immunohistochemical stain for CMV stains the nucleus brown. In addition to the staining of large cells, note the positive staining of nuclei without cytopathic effect, indicating early infection.

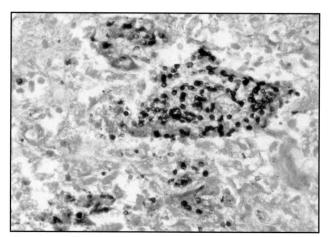

Figure 93-16. Gomori methenamine silver (GMS) stains the *Pneumocystis carinii* black.

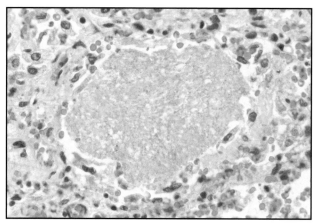

Figure 93-15. Characteristic intra alveolar frothy exudate of PCP is seen on H&E staining.

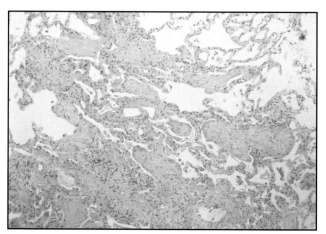

Figure 93-17. Bronchiolitis obliterans organizing pneumonia (BOOP), in contrast to BO, shows intra alveolar nodules of bluish myxoid fibrous tissue.

Other Forms of Lung Injury

Diffuse alveolar damage (DAD), acute interstitial pneumonitis and interstitial fibrosis may all be seen as nonspecific responses to lung injury in the posttransplant patient. The etiology of these responses is diverse and is not specifically related to either acute or chronic rejection.

Recurrent Disease

Up to 80% of patients transplanted for sarcoidosis develop granulomas seen in TBB, but they have not been shown to cause clinical disease. Other recurrent diseases include lymphangioleiomyomatosis, bronchioloalveolar carcinoma and alveolar proteinosis. Histologically, each of these demonstrates typical findings as would be present in a nontransplant setting.

Neoplasia

POSTTRANSPLANT LYMPHOPROLIFERATIVE
DISORDERS . In the lung transplant population, PTLD occurs in 3% to 5% of patients and is a monoclonal or polyclonal B cell expansion caused by the Epstein-Barr virus (EBV). The histological features of PTLD are similar to those seen in any other transplant patient. The unique characteristic of PTLD in lung transplant patients is the almost invariable involvement of the allograft. Several classifications of PTLD have been formulated that are used in different transplant institutions according to preference. PTLD is categorized into plasmacytic hyperplasia, polymorphic PTLD, and malignant lymphoma/multiple myeloma based on morphologic and molecular genetic criteria which include the presence or absence of monoclonality of B cells. Various genetic abnormalities of c-myc, N-ras and p53 have been described. Plasmacytic hyperplasia is predominantly seen in the pediatric group. Only malignant lymphoma has been seen at Loyola since adults comprise the majority of the lung transplant population. Of 250 patients, seven have developed PTLD, all of which were malignant lymphoma and occurred in the allograft with or without systemic involvement.

Early diagnosis of PTLD using monoclonal antibodies IgM, CD19+ B cells and EBV-DNA PCR may prove useful. However, the histopathologic diagnosis of PTLD remains the gold standard. Monomorphic lesions should be classified according to a recognized classification of non-Hodgkin lymphoma. Confluent sheets of atypical B cells infiltrate around the airways and blood vessels with extension into the lung parenchyma (Figures 93-18, 93-19 and 93-20).

The tumor cells are large, blastic cells, with prominent nucleoli, basophilic cytoplasm and a high mitotic rate. Polymorphic lesions should be evaluated for clonality by immunophenotyping and, if necessary, analysis of antigen-receptor and EBV genome. In cases with limited biopsy material, Immunohistochemistry for EBV proteins can be used in paraffin-embedded tissue (Figure 93-21).

In polymorphic lesions, the entire range of B lymphocytes is seen, including small lymphocytes, plasma cells, small lymphoplasmacytoid forms, plasmacytoid immunoblasts and small cleaved and noncleaved lym-

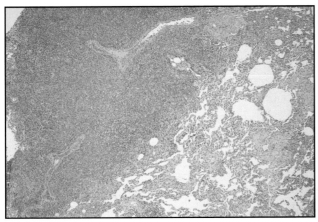

Figure 93-18. At low power, a diffuse infiltrate of hyperchromatic cells (ie, PTLD) can be seen in the lung.

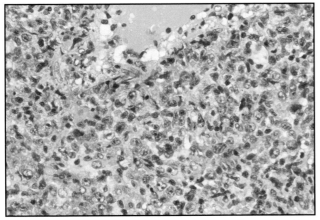

Figure 93-19. At high power, the infiltrate seen in Figure 93-18 is composed of large atypical lymphocytes with mitoses and single cell necrosis. At the top of the picture, the malignant cells are invading a blood vessel.

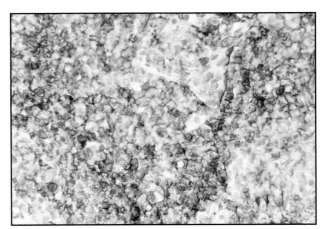

Figure 93-20. Immunohistochemistry shows the cells seen in Figures 93-18 and 93-19 to be B lymphocytes.

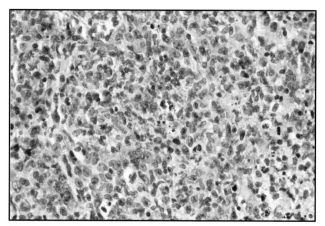

Figure 93-21. Characteristic staining for EBV protein is seen in this case of PTLD by immunohistochemistry.

phoid cells. In plasmacytic hyperplasia, there is a diffuse infiltrate of plasmacytoid lymphocytes associated with plasma cells and sparse immunoblasts.

OTHER NEOPLASMS. Many lung transplant patients have several risk factors for the development of lung carcinoma. Thus, primary squamous cell carcinomas and adenocarcinomas will be found in the native lung.

RECOMMENDED READING

Ware LB, Golden JA, Finkbeiner WE, Matthay MA. Alveolar epithelial fluid transport capacity in reperfusion lung injury after lung transplantation. Am J Respir Crit Care Med. 1999;159(3):980-988.

Saint Martin GA, Reddy VB, Garrity ER, et al. Humoral (antibody-mediated) rejection in lung transplantation. J Heart Lung Transplant. 1996;15(12):1217-1222.

Yousem SA, Berry GJ, Cagle PT, et al. Revision of the 1990 working formulation for the classification of pulmonary allograft rejection: Lung Rejection Study Group. J Heart Lung Transplant. 1996;15(1 Pt 1):1-15.

Tullius SG, Tilney NL. Both alloantigen-dependent and -independent factors influence chronic allograft rejection. Transplantation. 1995;59(3):313-318.

Husain AN, Siddiqui MT, Holmes EW, et al. Analysis of risk factors for the development of bronchiolitis obliterans syndrome. Am J Respir Crit Care Med. 1999;159(3):829-833.

Schlesinger C, Meyer CA, Veeraraghavan S, Koss MN. Constrictive (obliterative) bronchiolitis: diagnosis, etiology, and a critical review of the literature. Ann Diagn Pathol. 1998;2(5):321-334.

Siddiqui MT, Garrity ER, Husain AN. Bronchiolitis obliterans organizing pneumonia-like reactions: a nonspecific response or an atypical form of rejection or infection in lung allograft recipients? Hum Pathol. 1996;27(7): 714-719.

Gabbay E, Dark JH, Ashcroft T, Corris PA. Cryptogenic organizing pneumonia is an important cause of graft dysfunction and should be included in the classification of pulmonary allograft rejection. J Heart Lung Transplant. 1998;17:230-231.

Chadburn A, Chen JM, Hsu DT, et al. The morphologic and molecular genetic categories of posttransplantation lymphoproliferative disorders are clinically relevant. Cancer. 1998;82:1978-1987.

94 LONG-TERM MANAGEMENT ISSUES IN LUNG TRANSPLANTATION

Adaani E. Frost, MD

Long-term management in lung transplantation is focused on early recognition and management of complications in the graft (both immune and nonimmune) and diagnosis and management of the non-pulmonary complications of the transplant.

ASSESSMENT OF GRAFT FUNCTION

The objectives of lung transplantation are both improved pulmonary function and improved survival, and since survival is predicated on the continued optimum functioning of the graft, the emphasis in the long-term management of lung transplantation is on early recognition and prevention of graft dysfunction. To accomplish early recognition of graft dysfunction, four methods are used: scheduled visits at the transplant center; patient self-monitoring; ready access to the transplant coordinator; and phone monitoring. Monitoring includes clinical, laboratory, pulmonary function, and radiological parameters. Current understanding of rejection limits the capacity for its early recognition and treatment. Rejection in its acute and chronic form and its treatment is the most important cause of mortality in the lung transplant recipient. There is as yet no rapid reliable noninvasive diagnostic test that is both specific and sensitive for rejection.

Clinical

Patients are instructed to self-monitor clinical parameters including daily weight, temperature and symptoms. Following discharge from a hospital they are advised that they should experience a slow but steady increase in their functional capacity. Deterioration in their exercise tolerance, temperatures (defined variably by different centers as greater than 99°F to 100°F), sudden increases in weight, visible edema, or new or worsening symptoms of a cough, shortness of breath, or chest discomfort are to be reported immediately to the transplant coordinators. The same symptoms and parameters are routinely explored by the transplant physicians' scheduled visits. The physical assessment of the patient during evaluation should include all the usual features of a physical examination with emphasis on the chest exam, cardiac exam, and presence of a peripheral edema.

Associate Professor, Pulmonary Critical Care, Department of Medicine, Baylor College of Medicine, Houston, TX

Pulmonary Function

Patients are provided at most centers with a method for home monitoring of simple spirometric parameters – FEV_1, and FVC (eg, Micro Spirometer, Micro Medical Ltd). The best of three consecutive reproducible efforts is recorded by the patient in a diary with the clinical parameters mentioned above. At some institutions, weekly downloading of stored data by modem to a central data bank at the transplant center is performed. A 10% decrease from baseline in FEV_1 precipitates notification and evaluation of the patient by the transplant center. This evaluation will usually include a bronchoscopy, and transbronchial lung biopsy (see Chapter 92).

Scheduled visits usually include spirometry or full pulmonary function testing done at the transplant center. While a reduction in midflow (FEF_{25-75}) is the earliest indicator of bronchiolitis obliterans, the variability of this measurement increases reliance on FEV_1. Spirometry has been demonstrated to improve steadily in single-lung recipients transplanted for interstitial lung disease. The rate of improvement for patients with single-lung transplants for emphysema is more variable and the final values achieved (FEV_1 50% ± 8%) are on the average less than that achieved for SLT for pulmonary fibrosis (FEV_1 79 ± 15%).

Spirometry can be used therefore as a "red flag" for individuals who are not improving at the expected rate or to the expected level. This is often indicative of unrecognized rejection, infection or of airway complications, such as anastomotic obstruction(s).

In single-lung transplant recipients for emphysema, declining FEV_1 with relative preservation of FVC and increasing total lung capacity (TLC) can be indicative of disease progression with associated hyperinflation in the native lung with no demonstrable abnormality in the transplanted organ. In these instances, ancillary investigation with CT scan and biopsy will discriminate between pathology in the transplanted lung vs progressive emphysema in the native lung.

Spirometry is used as an indicator of effective therapy, posttreatment for infection or rejection. Declining spirometry in the absence of any other identifiable pathology defines bronchiolitis obliterans syndrome (addressed later in this chapter).

A reduction in FVC with relative preservation of FEV_1 suggests muscle weakness as a factor contributing to graft dysfunction.

Declining oxygen saturation (particularly with effort) is an insensitive, but highly specific, indicator of pathology. Oxygen saturations are routinely tested at rest on scheduled and clinically indicated visits. Desaturation during the 6-minute walk test (done at most centers on an every six-to-12 month basis) again is an insensitive but specific marker of the function of the transplanted organ.

Exercise Testing

The limitation to exercise capacity following lung transplantation is reviewed in Chapter 89 on the Physiology of the Transplanted Lung. Exercise testing is part of routine reassessments at the transplant center. A modified Bruce protocol and a 6-minute walk test are usually undertaken at six, 12, 18, 24, and 36 months, and yearly thereafter. These tests are obviously too cumbersome for use as a routine screen for patient function. They have, however, provided information about the etiology of exercise limitation experienced by single, double and heart-lung transplant recipients. Information points to some respiratory limitation in recipients of single-lung transplants with evidence of exercise-induced shift of perfusion back to the native lung with altered V/Q matching. Recent data suggests that, in addition, altered muscle physiology contributes to this exercise limitation. While conditioning has been demonstrated to improve exercise capacity to some extent, exercise function remains reduced relative to normal individuals. Prior chronic disease, and chronic immunosuppression combined with associated diseases (ie, hypertension, hypercholesterolemia, diabetes) and aging make exercise testing an insensitive and nonspecific indicator of graft dysfunction. Steady improvement in exercise capacity, however, is usually indicative of improving or stable graft function.

Ventilation and Perfusion Lung Scan

In addition to the usual indications for V/Q (Ventilation/Perfusion) lung scanning, differential V/Q scans in single-lung transplant recipients can identify alterations in the relative perfusion in the native vs the transplanted lung. Perfusion should increase steadily in the transplanted lung from about 50:50 in the first few months postoperatively to as much as 80% to 90% perfusion to the graft in single-lung recipients for interstitial disease. In the case of single-lung transplants for severe pulmonary hypertension 90% to 95% of the perfusion will go to the transplanted lung immediately upon completion of the vascular anastomoses. Single-lung transplants for emphysema tend to shift the perfusion more gradually and not often as dramatically to the transplant and often never receive more than 50%. Shift of perfusion back to the native lung in an established graft suggests vascular pathology, often acute rejection.

Radiology

Standard PA and lateral chest x-rays are part of routine screening and clinically indicated visits. After the first three months, postoperative chest x-rays are insensitive indicators of rejection. Prior to that time hazy infiltrates, or pleural effusions can be seen with rejection. Remote from transplant, x-rays can demonstrate all the usual features in the presence of community-acquired infections. Opportunistic infections (eg, cryptococcus, *pneumocystis carinii* pneumonia [PCP], cytomegalovirus) can present with either normal x-rays, or with nodules or infiltrates. Posttransplant lymphoproliferative disorder (PTLD) presenting in the first posttransplant year can manifest nodules, or hazy infiltrates. Later manifestations can include lymphadenopathy with normal parenchyma or nonspecific infiltrates.

CT scans of the chest (usually performed without intravenous contrast to avoid adverse renal impact) can further define pulmonary, mediastinal, and pleural processes. The radiological appearance of many infections can be very atypical in lung transplant recipients relative to the nonimmunosuppressed patient population. This is particularly true of mycobacterial infections, which can present with a variety of unusual x-ray, and CT features including isolated solitary node enlargement, small loculated pleural effusions or lower lobe (basal) consolidation. CT scans are not usually part of the routine monitoring visits, though protocols vary between institutions.

Laboratory Evaluations

There is no readily accomplished laboratory evaluation that is sensitive or specific for graft dysfunction. Elevations of LDH have been seen with graft infections, rejection, and PTLD. Some centers follow circulating levels of soluble receptors of interleukin-2 (IL-2). This is usually elevated in the presence of activated lymphocytes as is seen with rejection. However, this is not a widely used or clinically validated test. IL-2 levels are elevated in CMV and in non-pulmonary infection or insult. The use of IL-2 receptor antagonists (ie, basiliximab, daclizumab) results in very low levels of circulating IL-2 even in the presence of significant rejection. Routine lab monitoring includes evaluations of the white blood cell count (WBC). While the efficacy of azathioprine is not proportional to the reduction in WBC it produces, dosage alterations are required for reductions in WBC less than 4,000. Lymphocytosis or lymphopenia can be indicative of CMV infection. A relative peripheral lymphocytosis or basophilia can also be seen in the presence of early acute rejection. Late rejection has been reported to be associated with a relative increase in peripheral blood neutrophils. Bronchiolitis obliterans has been associated with an increase in bronchoalveolar lavage (BAL) neutrophils, but as yet no such association with peripheral blood neutrophils has been demonstrated.

Cardiac Evaluations

Echocardiographic evaluation is usually reserved for those individuals transplanted for pulmonary hypertension (such as Eisenmenger's patients, and primary pulmonary hypertensives), recipients of heart-lung transplants or in individuals noted pretransplant to have

unexplained reductions in left ventricular function. While patients with a left ventricular ejection fraction of less than 40% are usually denied isolated lung transplantation, marginal echos are occasionally seen prior to transplantation in the presence of normal endomyocardial biopsies and coronary angiography. In such cases, and in individuals who undergo combined lung transplant and coronary revascularization procedures, the echocardiogram is usually followed as part of the routine posttransplant monitoring visits. As reviewed in Chapter 90, individuals with right ventricular overload, and hypertrophy prior to transplant experience a slow improvement in the RVH, and near normalization of pressures in the immediate posttransplant period. Individuals with marginal left ventricular function usually demonstrate normalization of their left ventricular ejection fraction early in the posttransplant period – either immediately postoperatively or shortly thereafter. The mechanisms of this LV dysfunction remains to be elucidated.

Scheduled and Clinically Indicated Bronchoscopy

Bronchoscopic evaluation of the allograft is done frequently during the first year postoperatively. The schedule varies between institutions, but generally every three months a screening bronchoscopy with biopsy is undertaken. After the first year, this schedule is replaced with a semiannual routine, and subsequently by an annual evaluation. Usually three to five alveolated pieces of lung tissue are taken for optimum diagnostic yield. While some centers advocate multiple biopsies from multiple sites (including both lungs in the event of a double-lung or heart-lung transplant) this is not universally accepted, and the yield with repeated biopsies does not increase greatly. In addition, there is data to suggest that biopsies from the lower lobes have the highest yield for diagnosing rejection more readily, and indicating the highest degree of rejection.

Bronchoscopy is clinically indicated for many of the previously mentioned features potentially associated with dysfunction of the allograft. These include low-grade temperature, declining spirometry, decreasing exercise tolerance, cough, shortness of breath, declining resting or exercise oxygen saturation, or failure of the patient to improve at the expected rate. The utility of the BAL cell count in differentiating rejection vs infection has been much discussed. Clinically and statistically significant indices differentiating rejection vs infection have not yet been identified. BAL cytology is useful in broader sampling of the alveoli for infectious diagnoses (eg, CMV, PCP). In the very stable patient remote from transplant (five to ten years out) the utility of screening bronchoscopy becomes hard to validate.

IMPACT OF RECURRENT DISEASE

The recurrence of pulmonary disease following a lung transplant may take several forms: recurrence of disease in the transplant that is histologically identical to the original disease process; progression of disease in the native lung such that it compromises the transplant lung with resultant organ dysfunction and patient deterioration; the development of chronic allograft dysfunction that may leave the patient impaired in a manner comparable to or almost identical to his/her original disease process. This is reviewed later in this chapter, under the Chronic Allograft Dysfunction and Its Management heading.

Recurrence of Histologically Identical Disease

Disease recurrence in the transplanted lung has been reported in a number of conditions including sarcoidosis, lymphangioleiomyomatosis, Langerhans' cell histiocytosis, pulmonary fibrosis/interstitial pneumonia, giant cell interstitial pneumonia, talc granulomatosis, diffuse panbronchiolitis, and alveolar proteinosis. While many of these conditions are rare, and rarely indications for transplant, sarcoid and pulmonary fibrosis are relatively common indications for transplantation. Interestingly, the recurrence of sarcoid in the transplanted organ, which has been identified relatively early (within the first three months) following transplant has not been associated with any major long-term sequelae, although there is some suggestion that it may be associated with an increased incidence of acute rejection. In at least one instance where declining function and worsening x-ray picture was attributed histologically to recurrent sarcoid, signs and symptoms improved with augmented oral steroids. Though histological evidence of sarcoid granulomas persisted, the patient remained clinically asymptomatic with normal chest x-rays and PFTs for the duration of reported follow-up (about two years). The impact of this disease in the posttransplant period, and in pretransplant consideration remains uncertain.

Idiopathic pulmonary fibrosis (IPF) was the condition for which the first successful single-lung transplants were undertaken. It still accounts for approximately 15% to 20% of all single lung transplant procedures. In spite of the frequency of this indication for transplantation, the recurrence of pulmonary fibrosis posttransplant has been infrequently reported. One of the initial cases described was actually giant cell interstitial fibrosis (GIF). Only one case of recurrent IPF has been described. This may reflect in part the nonspecific nature of the fibrotic changes that can occur in both the primary disease, and as a consequence of injury (allogeneic, and nonallogeneic) to the transplanted lung.

GIF as indicated above, an occupational disease related to exposure to tungsten and cobalt, has been shown to recur posttransplant. In those reported cases the disease recurrence has resulted in death. The mechanism is unknown, as the patients were long removed from their environmental exposure, but may reflect the solubilization of these metals, or conversely, an immune-mediated response to the total body load of unexcreted, unaltered dusts.

Lymphangioleiomyomatosis is a multisystem disease of premenopausal women associated with a mixed obstructive and restrictive pulmonary disorder, the development of recurrent pneumothoraces, and chylous pleural effusions, as well as renal angiolipomas. This is a rare indication for lung transplantation, but has been well-recognized to recur in the transplanted organ. The smooth muscle proliferation in the bronchioles, arteries, and veins, as well as the lymphatic spaces have been identified as being of donor origin, suggesting some circulating, systemic stimulus to smooth muscle cell proliferation rather than an end-organ/receptor abnormality. A registry of patients undergoing transplantation has been recently developed to assess the natural history of this disease in the posttransplant period.

Langerhans' cell granulomatosis is a diffuse, smoking-aggravated lung disease characterized pathologically by bronchiolocentric inflammation, with resulting cyst formation that is often detectable by high-resolution CT scan. The pulmonary function and disease manifestations are similar to those of bronchiolitis obliterans and as such can mimic it in the posttransplant period. Only a few cases have been reported to date of recurrence of this disease in the transplanted lung, however, relatively few transplants have been done for this indication. The diagnosis is made by identifying the classical Langerhans' cell on biopsy specimens (accomplished by use of immunophenotypic markers). Appropriate therapy is anecdotal, though a response to cyclophosphamide has been reported. The role of transplantation in this patient population is uncertain.

Diffuse panbronchiolitis is an extremely rare inflammatory airway disease that has until recently been described only in those of Japanese origin, and then in association with HLA Bw54. There are now, however, a handful of cases in the US of non-Asian extraction with DPB, and lacking this genetic marker. There is only one case report of a lung transplant recipient with this diagnosis, and this individual developed recurrent disease, which, as has been reported in the native disease, did respond to therapy with erythromycin, resulting in no adverse long-term sequelae.

Progression of Disease in the Native Lung

This problem has its main impact in the case of patients transplanted for emphysema, where a highly compliant native lung can become progressively more distended with respiratory effort, and with the natural progression of the underlying disease process. Such progressive distension produces further disruption of alveolar septa, hyperinflation of the lung, with actual encroachment of the native lung into the opposite thoracic cavity. The progressive compromise of the transplanted lung leads to gradual atelectasis with further decreases in its compliance. This leads to a snowball effect of progressive compromise of the transplanted lung with hyperinflation of the native lung. To address this problem, several approaches have been undertaken by various transplant centers. These include preferentially undertaking double-lung transplants for those patients where this is thought to pose a particular risk (ie, patients with alpha$_1$ antitrypsin deficiency). Alternatively, this possibility should be considered in the differential diagnosis of any patient who, without histological evidence of rejection, develops progressive loss of volume in the transplanted organ with hyperinflation in the native lung. The pulmonary function tests in these circumstances will show progressive obstruction related to the increasing contribution of the native lung. Occasionally, perfusion to the transplanted lung is inordinately well-preserved: a clue to the absence of vascular compromise as in acute rejection. Once pathology in the transplanted lung has been ruled out with appropriate biopsies, conventional volume reduction, more often lobectomy, or occasionally even pneumonectomy or re-transplant of the native lung has been successfully undertaken.

Williams-Campbell syndrome is a rare disorder characterized by bronchial cartilage deficiency resulting in distal airway collapse, bronchiectasis, and recurrent infections. While it has not been reported to recur in the transplanted lung, the presence of bronchial cartilage collapse in the airways proximal to the bronchial anastomoses following a lung transplant has been reported. The bronchomalacia was apparently refractory to aggressive management with CPAP and stent placements, and the transplant recipient died of recurrent infections.

CHRONIC ALLOGRAFT DYSFUNCTION AND ITS MANAGEMENT

Bronchiolitis obliterans (BO) is extensively described in the pathological portion of this section. It is characterized by progressive airway obstruction with gas trapping. Diffusion capacity, in contrast to emphysema, is usually relatively well-maintained in the absence of associated acute rejection or the consequences of airway obstruction-recurrent pneumonias. This condition physiologically mimics the features of emphysema, the diagnosis for which 40% to 50% of all lung transplant procedures are undertaken. The diagnostic criteria for BO syndrome

is described in Chapters 92 and 93 in this section. Treatment protocols for BO are many, and generally unsuccessful. Since its development is most frequently associated with recurrent episodes of acute rejection (AR), the prevention of BO is predicated on prevention of AR. There is some data to suggest that the frequency of AR may be diminished with immunosuppression protocols that include tacrolimus and mycophenolate mofetil. However, this has not been validated by large multicenter studies. Rapamycin (sirolimus) has been shown, in the only animal model to date of BO, to ameliorate the pathological process, and possibly even reverse the early stages of BO. This data, while encouraging, remains to be validated in studies that are currently ongoing. Antilymphocyte therapy, as described in the section on induction immunosuppression, has also been used in an attempt to arrest the progression of BO, with largely anecdotal, and sporadic results. Similar data or lack thereof is available on photopheresis and the use of total lymphoid irradiation. Most of these therapies result in profound immunocompromise of the patient. The obvious risks vs the potential benefits should be individualized in each patient. BO can progress rapidly and inexorably, or it can have a staccato course with long periods of relative stability and functional compensation. Such a variable course further complicates the evaluation of any of these treatments.

NONPULMONARY ISSUES
Cardiac Disease and Systemic Hypertension
Patients posttransplant commonly have systemic hypertension (66% develop it de novo posttransplant and a significant number of patients have controlled hypertension prior to transplant), and frequently experience hypercholesterolemia, and diabetes – risk factors for coronary artery disease. In addition, the heart is commonly denervated following a lung transplant (either single or double). Therefore, atypical chest discomfort, unexplained shortness of breath or limitations in exercise tolerance should include a cardiac evaluation in patients with these risk factors. Such evaluations should include EKG, echocardiogram, and noninvasive evaluations (such as dobutamine thallium or dobutamine echocardiography). While coronary angiograms may ultimately be necessary, the avoidance of dye in these patients who always have some degree (usually underestimated) of renal compromise is advisable.

Management of systemic hypertension follows the same guidelines as seen with other organ transplants. Calcium channel blockers are the first line of defense recognizing that the dihydropyridine group (eg, amlodipine, felodipine) have little impact on the metabolism of calcineurin inhibitors. The use of diltiazem and similar calcium channel blockers increases cyclosporine and tacrolimus levels. Their use, therefore, requires monitoring and dose adjustments of these drugs. Alternatives or additional therapy include the use of clonidine patches, ACE inhibitors and angiotensin II receptor antagonists. Beta blockers can be used, although they are not first line drugs. As the main potential adverse impact of antihypertensive therapy is on renal blood flow in calcineurin-treated patients, the management of hypertension in lung transplant patients is not vastly different from that of other solid organ transplants. Increased airway reactivity has been reported in the early posttransplant period, but this is so far only a theoretical consideration in the choice of antihypertensive agents (such as ACE inhibitors and beta blockers).

Renal Dysfunction
Direct effects of calcineurin inhibitors on renal blood flow, and indirect effects mediated by increased sympathetic tone, increased circulating catecholamines and the associated development of hypertension result in a significant number of lung transplant recipients developing renal impairment over time. This can lead ultimately to the need for renal transplantation or dialysis. Hemolytic uremic syndrome has, to date, been reported in only one recipient of lung transplantation, probably reflecting the infrequent occurrence of this calcineurin inhibitor-associated complication in all solid organ transplants (0.5% to 3.4%). The mechanisms and management of these renal complications are addressed in detail in Chapter 21.

Gastrointestinal Dysfunction
Gastrointestinal (GI) complications of lung and heart-lung transplantation are being recognized with increasing frequency and can pose a significant risk to the outcome of the transplant. Some of the conditions necessitating lung transplantation are themselves associated with GI dysfunction, notably cystic fibrosis, and scleroderma/CREST. The presence of a systemic disease is no longer considered to be a contraindication to transplantation in the absence of demonstrable major end-organ damage. However, the disorders of motility and absorption associated with these diseases and with diabetes (a common complication of prolonged steroid use, inactivity, obesity and cystic fibrosis) can impact both pretransplant nutritional status and posttransplant absorption of medications. In addition, delayed gastric emptying and/or disorders of esophageal motility can predispose to reflux and aspiration. This can pose a major threat to the integrity of the transplanted organ in the presence of immunosuppression, coupled with denervation and altered mucociliary clearance. Some of these problems can be anticipated prior to transplant, and many centers undertake gastric and esophageal

motility studies as a prerequisite prior to transplantation. The presence of free reflux, or an immotile esophagus (as seen in CREST) is considered at some institutions a contraindication to transplantation. The very frequent disruption of the vagus nerve posttransplant results in delayed gastric emptying, which further increases the risk of aspiration.

In a series of 133 heart or heart-lung transplant recipients, 21% experienced a gastrointestinal complication. These complications included visceral perforation, retroperitoneal abscess, cholecystitis, gastric atony, perianal abscess, gastrointestinal bleeding, esophagitis, pancreatitis, pancreatic abscess, hepatitis, and diarrhea. Almost half of the complications resulted in surgical intervention and the surgical mortality rate was 8%.

Gastrointestinal complications are often atypical in presentation. It is not unheard of for a patient who has suffered a free intestinal perforation complicated by fecal soiling of the peritoneal cavity to look relatively well, with a remarkably benign abdominal examination.

Bowel obstructions can be seen frequently, particularly (but not exclusively), in the cystic fibrosis patient population. The use of narcotics, bed rest and calcium channel blockers for control of hypertension are common predisposing factors for the development of such obstructions. Recognized early they can be treated with aggressive purgatives using Golitely®, magnesium citrate, and if necessary Hypaque® enema coupled with Tween®. Surgical decompression may be required.

Gastric atony with the development of bezoars in the stomach has been reported, again predominantly but not exclusively, in the cystic fibrosis population. The presence of an unrecognized gastric concretion containing calcineurin inhibitors can lead to wild swings in the levels of these drugs that would otherwise be inexplicable. There is no large body of literature on the management of these bezoars, but conventional management with papain and lavage has not appeared successful in the literature. Recognition and consideration of early pyloroplasty should be entertained.

Many institutions consider documented significant prior pancreatitis (as seen in cystic fibrosis) a relative contraindication to transplantation. Pancreatitis posttransplant can be a manifestation of pretransplant disease, or can occur as a complication of cholelithiasis, hypercholesterolemia (as is seen frequently with conventional calcineurin inhibitor-based immunotherapy, and most recently with the use of sirolimus and its analogues), refeeding, and azathioprine. It can also be associated with cardiopulmonary bypass, hypoperfusion, and splanchnic vasoconstriction (related to vasopressors).

Cholecystitis may present with nothing more than mild elevation of alkaline phosphatase, and persistent anorexia and/or nausea. Pretransplant ultrasound visualization of the gall bladder is routine, but does not necessarily predict the development of symptomatic gall bladder disease in the postoperative period. Acute cholecystitis can complicate the immediate postoperative period, retarding perioperative convalescence. The enterohepatic recirculation of cyclosporine has been suggested to contribute to the development of cholelithiasis following transplantation.

Diarrhea and weight loss can be a manifestation of infection, certain drug (eg, mycophenolate mofetil) side effects or PTLD. Refractory diarrhea with stools negative for fecal leukocytes, particularly if associated with elevations of peripheral blood LDH should raise suspicion of the latter possibility. Cultures negative for the usual pathogens (eg, *C difficile*) should precipitate a GI consult and colonoscopy. This will readily identify CMV colitis and PTLD. The former, while a frequent manifestation of CMV infection in renal patients, is seen relatively infrequently in the lung transplant population. The consequences of severe CMV, and *C difficile* (such as toxic megacolon) are rare occurrences in the lung transplant patient. The differential diagnosis of toxic megacolon in the lung transplant population should include vascular compromise.

Anemia, Thrombocytopenia and Leukopenia

Anemia in the perioperative period is not uncommon, due to operative blood loss complicating the pretransplant treatment and disease process (eg, cachexia, anorexia, hypoxemia-associated increased GI blood loss). Remote from transplant, it can be a manifestation of chronic iron deficiency, or due to marrow suppression by immunosuppressive drugs (eg, azathioprine, methotrexate, antilymphocyte products) or therapies (eg, total lymphoid irradiation for refractory rejection). Pancytopenia is infrequently reported with sirolimus and mycophenolate. The routine use of ganciclovir for treatment or prevention of CMV can also result in significant depression of marrow function with resulting pancytopenia. Anemia of any cause in posttransplant patients is associated with inappropriately low production of erythropoietin, which does not appear to be related to renal dysfunction, and may reflect an isolated effect of calcineurin inhibitors on juxtaglomerular cells responsible for its production. Use of erythropoietin to treat anemia under these circumstances may avoid undesirable transfusions.

Osteoporosis and Osteonecrosis

Many recipients of lung transplantation have significant osteoporosis as a consequence of prolonged inanition, lack of exercise, steroids, and in some cases chronic disturbance of calcium and vitamin D metabolism (as is the case in patients with cystic fibrosis). Severe osteoporosis has been reported pretransplant in the lumbar spines with a frequency of 30%, and in the femoral heads 49%, in patients awaiting transplantation. It is particularly severe in cystic fibrosis patients in whom vitamin D levels are significantly reduced. While painful osteoporosis is considered a relative contraindication to transplantation, careful pretransplant screening and management with calcium, calcitriol, and diphosphonates does not always prevent the development of osteoporosis, and osteonecrosis. The latter commonly involves the femoral heads, knees, and ankles. Painful fractures of the pelvis have also been reported, and are a significant cause of morbidity. Atraumatic fractures occurred in 37% of patients being evaluated following transplant. Most occurred in women, and in the presence of pretransplant glucocorticoid therapy. Management is directed toward prevention. Most centers use a regimen of calcium replacement (1 to 1.5 gm po qd), coupled with calcitriol (0.25 mcg po qd-bid). Estrogen replacement is indicated in postmenopausal females coupled with careful gynecological follow-up and routine mammography. Biphosphonates can be used, but it is sometimes difficult to time the oral biphosphonates such that they do not interfere with the absorption of the many other medications the patients are required to take. Calcitonin (nasal spray) has also been used to relieve the bone pain associated with osteonecrosis, sacral, pelvic and vertebral fractures. In the presence of established osteonecrosis of a weight-bearing area, management includes resting the area (non-weight-bearing), usually followed by surgical replacement of the joint. The success of decompression in this population has been limited.

EVALUATION FOR AND ROLE OF RE-TRANSPLANTATION.

The role of re-transplantation following a failed lung transplant is a difficult medical and ethical decision, and practices vary between centers. Despite improving survival with lung transplantation and remote from transplant as a consequence of BO, graft loss and dysfunction in the immediate perioperative period is a significant cause of morbidity and mortality. There is extensive experience in pulmonary re-transplantation in both pediatric and adult recipients. The Pulmonary Retransplant Registry has developed a database since 1991 for analysis of outcomes of re-transplantation. Analysis of data from this registry concluded that overall Kaplan-Meier survival was 47%, 40% and 33% at one, two, and three years, respectively. However within this larger group of re-transplant recipients, the subgroup of patients who were ambulatory and ventilatory independent had a 64% 1-year survival compared to 33% for those patients who were nonambulatory, and ventilated. While 64% is still well below the usual accepted standard for 1-year survival following lung transplantation, it

is better than the 1-year survival for African-American patients transplanted for sarcoidosis (50% 1-year survival; unpublished UNOS data), and approximately the same as 1-year survival for patients with primary pulmonary hypertension or idiopathic pulmonary fibrosis. While the limited donor pool and optimum use of health care dollars raises serious questions about the validity and ethics of giving one patient two transplants, the success of the procedure in carefully selected patients is hard to dispute. Initial data suggested a higher incidence of BO in recipients of re-transplantation. Eighty-one percent (81%), 70%, 62% and 56% of survivors were BO free at one, two, three and four years after re-transplantation, respectively. The incidence of BO stage 3 at two years was greater in those with an interval of less than two years from primary to re-transplant, and less in those patients independent of the ventilator prior to re-transplantation. Considering that, for the most part, re-transplantation is reserved for those who have already sustained BO, the fact that not all patients develop BO rapidly is encouraging, and might suggest a role for avoidance of shared antigens between 1st and 2nd donor organs.

ROLE OF PRIMARY CARE PHYSICIANS IN LONG-TERM MANAGEMENT

This is a very difficult role to determine. Lung transplant recipients are complicated patients, on multiple medications, many of which have major interactions with each other, and are used to treat common ailments for which one would consult a primary care physician. Examples of these are many, and are included in the section on pharmacology of immunosuppressive drugs. The role of the primary physician should be worked out carefully between that physician and the transplant pulmonologist and surgeon, prior to return of the patient to his/her original environment. As this can be remote from the transplant center, it is reasonable to have a first line of defense for the patient other than the transplant center. This should usually be a combination of the primary care physician and the original referring pulmonologist. It is critical that a summary of relevant events about the transplant, current functional status, and a list of all medications be provided for both of these physicians upon return of the patient to the home environment. Many centers provide a detailed list of all the potential drug interactions that can confound immunosuppressive drugs, and aggravate their adverse effects on bone marrow, liver, and most importantly kidney. The primary physicians should be encouraged, and the patient should be advised to encourage them, to call the transplant center for any concerns related to the patient's condition or about introduction of new pharmacotherapies. A cordial and collegial relationship between the transplant physicians and the local care providers is essential to the success of the transplant, and the survival of the patient. The level of involvement in long-term follow-up (eg, PFT's, echocardiograms, laboratory analyses, exercise testing) is best determined by a joint decision between the transplant center and the local physicians, and should respect the needs of the transplant patient, recognizing, however, that for both survival statistics and experimental protocols to evaluate new and different immunosuppressive protocols, follow-up at the transplant center will be necessary. More remote from transplant, this may become a less critical and controversial management issue.

RECOMMENDED READING

Tikkanen J, Lemstrom K, Halme M, Pakkala S, Taskinne, Koskinen P. Detailed analysis of cell profiles in peripheral blood, bronchoalveolar lavage fluid, and transbronchial biopsy specimens during acute rejection and CMV infection in lung and heart-lung allograft recipients. Transplant Proc. 1999;31(1-2):163-164.

Johnson BA, Duncan SR, Ohori NP, et al. Recurrence of sarcoidosis in pulmonary allograft recipients. Am Rev Respir Dis. 1993;148(5):1373-1377.

Nine JS, Yousem SA, Paradis IL, Keenan R, Griffith BP. Lymphangioleiomyomatosis: recurrence after lung transplantation. J Heart Lung Transplant. 1994;13(4): 714-719.

Anderson MB, Kriett JM, Kapelanski DP, Perricone A, Smith CM, Jamieson SW. Volume reduction surgery in the native lung after single lung transplantation for emphysema. J Heart Lung Transplant. 1997;16(7): 752-757.

Augustine SM, Yeo CJ, Buchman TG, Achuff SC, Baumgartner WA. Gastrointestinal complications in heart and in heart-lung transplant patients. J Heart Lung Transplant. 1991;10(4):547-555.

Berkowitz N, Schulman LL, McGregor C, Markowitz D. Gastroparesis after lung transplantation. Potential role in postoperative respiratory complications. Chest. 1995;108(6):1602-1607.

Morrison RJ, Short HD, Noon GP, Frost AE. Hypertension after lung transplantation. J Heart Lung Transplant. 1993;12(6 Pt 1):928-931.

Novick RJ, Stitt LW, Al-Kattan K, et al Pulmonary retransplantation: predictors of graft function and survival in 230 patients. Pulmonary Retransplant Registry. Ann Thorac Surg. 1998; 65(1):227-234.

95 MAINTENANCE IMMUNOSUPPRESSION PROTOCOLS FOR LUNG TRANSPLANTATION

Marshall I. Hertz, MD

ROUTINE MAINTENANCE IMMUNE SUPPRESSION

Most lung transplant patients are maintained on triple-drug immune suppression (ie, a calcineurin inhibitor, either cyclosporine [CsA] or tacrolimus) plus a purine synthesis inhibitor (ie, either azathioprine [AZA] or mycophenolate mofetil [MMF]) plus a corticosteroid (ie, either prednisone or prednisolone). The exact doses and target levels of these medications vary somewhat from institution to institution; the regimen followed at the University of Minnesota is summarized in Table 95-1.

Calcineurin Inhibitors

The calcineurin inhibitors, tacrolimus and cyclosporine, work by similar mechanisms to inhibit transcription of genes that are critical for T cell activation. It is, therefore, not unexpected that their efficacy and spectrum of toxicities are similar. In a controlled trial comparing tacrolimus to CsA after lung transplantation, Griffith et al reported a lower rate of acute rejection episodes in tacrolimus-treated recipients, although survival rates were similar. Current UNOS/International Society of Heart and Lung Transplantation registry data indicate that 20% to 30% of lung transplant recipients are treated with tacrolimus. Tacrolimus has also been used successfully as a "rescue" therapy for patients with persistent or recurrent acute rejection episodes after lung transplantation. Similar studies of CsA rescue of tacrolimus-treated patients have not been carried out.

The spectra of toxicities of tacrolimus and CsA are similar, but their occurrence in individual patients is variable; therefore, individualized therapies are required. In some cases, special clinical circumstances favor treatment with tacrolimus or CsA. For example, cystic fibrosis patients are often treated with tacrolimus due to impaired intestinal absorption of CsA. Some centers treat women preferentially with tacrolimus to avoid the hirsutism often associated with CsA. Finally, tacrolimus, which can induce hyperglycemia, is often avoided in diabetic lung transplant recipients.

Professor of Medicine, Pulmonary/Critical Care Medicine Division, University of Minnesota, Minneapolis, MN

Because of the variable absorption of tacrolimus and CsA, measurement of blood levels is essential to monitor therapy. Predose trough levels are employed for patients taking oral tacrolimus or CsA to minimize the effect of erratic absorption and variable timing of administration. Because several assays are available, note must be taken of the method used for blood level measurement when comparing results from different transplant centers.

As discussed in Section II, Chapter 12, the intestinal absorption of the calcineurin inhibitors is affected by many other medications. Commonly used drugs that increase absorption of calcineurin inhibitors include: the macrolide antibiotics erythromycin, azithromycin, clarithromycin; doxycycline; the azole antifungal agents ketoconazole, fluconazole and itraconazole; the calcium channel blockers diltiazem, verapamil, nicardipine; and some H2 blockers. Commonly used medications that decrease calcineurin inhibitor absorption include the antiseizure medications phenytoin, phenobarbital and carbamazepine; the antituberculous medications INH and rifampin; and octreotide. Many additional medications potentiate the nephrotoxicity of calcineurin inhibitors including acyclovir, ganciclovir, aminoglycosides, ciprofloxacin, amphotericin B, ACE inhibitors, colchicine, erythromycin, H2-blockers and NSAIDs. Caution must be used, and blood levels followed carefully, when using any of these medications. The absorption-enhancing properties of the calcium channel-blocking agents and azole antifungal agents has been used to advantage by some centers that treat patients with one of them to enhance absorption, thereby decreasing the dosage requirement and related expense of calcineurin inhibitors.

Purine Synthesis Inhibitors

Historically, the purine synthesis inhibitor azathioprine has been used in lung transplant patients. However, MMF has recently had increasing use as a result of promising studies in renal and heart transplantation and preliminary studies in lung transplantation. Current UNOS/International Society of Heart and Lung Transplantation registry data indicate that approximately 20% of lung transplant recipients are treated with mycophenolate mofetil. MMF has been reported to stabilize patients with recurrent acute rejection and those with bronchiolitis obliterans syndrome. Recently, Ross et al reported a small randomized comparison of azathioprine and MMF; the MMF-treated recipients demonstrated less acute rejection and better pulmonary function tests after one year. Based on the available information, MMF is currently used by some centers as primary immune suppression, by other centers during the first posttransplant year only, and by some centers as "rescue therapy" for patients with recurrent or refractory acute rejection.

Table 95-1. Routine Lung Transplant Immunosuppression at the University of Minnesota

Time	Neoral or Tacrolimus		Azathioprine or MMF		Steroid
Preoperative (one oral dose)	5 mg	0.05 mg/kg	2.5 mg/kg	BW <50 kg = 750 mg BW >50 kg = 1,000 mg	None
Intraoperative	None	None	None	None	Methylprednisolone 500 mg/kg IV at release of pulmonary artery clamp
Immediately postoperative, if, po/ng admin. feasible	4 mg/kg bid	0.05 mg/kg bid	2.5 mg/kg per day	BW <50kg = 1,000 mg bid BW >50kg = 1,500 mg bid	Methylprednisolone 125 mg IV q8h x 3 doses, then prednisone 0.25 mg/kg bid
Immediately postoperative, if po/ng admin. not feasible	40 μg/kg per hour continuous infusion; usual dose 1,000-3,000 μg/hr	1 microgram/kg per hour continuous infusion; usual dose 50 to 100 μg/hr	1 to 1.25 mg/kg day IV	1 to 1.5 gm IV bid	Methylprednisolone 0.25 mg/kg IV bid
Monitoring/ dose adjustments	Monitor pre-dose blood levels (max. 3X weekly). First 9 to 12 months: Aim for blood level 200 ng/mL (HPLC, whole blood method) Maintenance: Reduce target level by 25%	Monitor pre-dose blood levels (max. 3X weekly). First 9 to 12 months: Aim for blood level 10 to 15 ng/mL (Abbott TDx method) Maintenance: reduce target level by 25%	Monitor WBC Adjust dose downward, if necessary to maintain WBC>4000	Monitor WBC Adjust dose downward, if necessary, to maintain WBC>4000 and for GI side effects	Taper prednisone over six months to 0.1 mg/kg po qd

Abbreviations: CsA indicates cyclosporine; MMF, mycophenolate mofetil; BW, body weight.

The primary toxicity of AZA and MMF is bone marrow suppression, particularly leukopenia, and, to a lesser extent, thrombocytopenia and anemia. MMF causes much more gastrointestinal toxicity than AZA; this may be ameliorated somewhat by three times daily dosing compared with twice daily dosing. When changing patients from AZA to MMF and vice-versa, a "washout" period is not necessary.

Corticosteroids

Corticosteroids are routinely used as maintenance immune suppression by most lung transplant centers. Dosage and tapering schedules vary widely from center to center, but a typical regimen would include methylprednisolone 125 mg IV every eight hours immediately after transplantation, followed by oral prednisone 0.5 mg/kg per day, and tapering to 0.1 mg/kg per day by three to six months after transplantation. A few centers initiate immune suppression using perioperative steroids only, and then add prednisone in patients demonstrating acute rejection; published data are lacking comparing this approach with maintenance corticosteroid treatment in all patients. As with other corticosteroid-treated patients, lung transplant recipients undergoing surgery or other major physiologic stress are treated with increased "stress" doses of corticosteroids for a short period of time.

ADDITIONAL MAINTENANCE THERAPIES FOR PATIENTS WITH RECURRENT OR CHRONIC REJECTION
Methotrexate

The addition of maintenance methotrexate can be beneficial for patients with recurrent acute rejection or with bronchiolitis obliterans syndrome. Oral treatment is usually prescribed in three divided doses taken 12 hours apart once weekly; the total weekly dose varies from 5 mg to 22.5 mg depending on side effects and efficacy. The most common side effects of methotrexate are leukopenia and stomatitis. Folic acid, 5 mg/day, on non-methotrexate days, has been reported to reduce methotrexate-induced toxicity. Most patients require reduction or elimination of purine synthesis inhibitors while taking methotrexate. Increased rates of opportunistic infections have been reported in methotrexate-treated patients.

Photopheresis

Photopheresis, which involves ex vivo treatment of white blood cells with 8-methoxypsoralen, followed by reinfusion into the patient, has been reported to reduce acute rejection in heart transplant recipients and to help stabilize lung transplant recipients with bronchiolitis obliterans syndrome. Photopheresis typically is continued for six to 12 months and, therefore, can be considered a form of maintenance immune suppression. Side effects and toxicities are minimal and photopheresis has not been associated with an increased propensity for infection.

CONDITIONS REQUIRING REDUCED IMMUNE SUPPRESSION

Reduction of immune suppression must always be undertaken with caution. In patients with medication-induced leukopenia, temporary dose reduction or elimination of AZA or MMF may be necessary. At some centers, long-term transplant survivors have had corticosteroids weaned or have been maintained on lower serum concentration of calcineurin inhibitors; however, these approaches have not been rigorously tested. In patients with neoplasia, particularly transplant-induced EBV lymphoproliferative disorders and lymphoma, reduction of immune suppression may be helpful. Finally, in patients with severe or recurrent infections, careful reduction of immune suppressive medication may be indicated; this must be considered on a case-by-case basis.

RECOMMENDED READING

Cahill BC, O'Rourke MK, Strasburg KA, et al. Methotrexate for lung transplant recipients with steroid-resistant acute rejection. J Heart Lung Transplant. 1996;15(11):1130-1137.

Dusmet M, Maurer J, Winton T, Kesten S. Methotrexate can halt the progression of bronchiolitis obliterans syndrome in lung transplant recipients. J Heart Lung Transplant. 1996;15(9):948-954.

Griffith BP, Bando K, Hardesty RL, et al. A prospective randomized trial of FK506 versus cyclosporine after human pulmonary transplantation. Transplantation. 1994;57(6):848-851.

Horning NR, Lynch JP, Sundaresan SR, Patterson GA, Trulock EP. Tacrolimus therapy for persistent or recurrent acute rejection after lung transplantation. J Heart Lung Transplant. 1998;17(8):761-767.

Mentzer RM, Jr., Jahania MS, Lasley RD. Tacrolimus as a rescue immunosuppressant after heart and lung transplantation. The U.S. Multicenter FK506 Study Group. Transplantation. 1998;65(1):109-113.

Ross DJ, Waters PF, Levine M, Kramer M, Ruzevich S, Kass RM. Mycophenolate mofetil versus azathioprine immunosuppressive regimens after lung transplantation: preliminary experience. J Heart Lung Transplant. 1998;17(8):768-774.

Ross DJ, Lewis MI, Kramer M, Vo A, Kass RM. FK 506 'rescue' immunosuppression for obliterative bronchiolitis after lung transplantation. Chest. 1997;112(5):1175-1179.

Whyte RI, Rossi SJ, Mulligan MS, et al. Mycophenolate mofetil for obliterative bronchiolitis syndrome after lung transplantation. Ann Thorac Surg. 1997;64(4):945-948.

96 LUNG TRANSPLANTATION: OUTCOMES

Elbert P. Trulock, MD

Information about the outcomes of lung transplantation is available from both national and international registries. In the US, the scientific registry is maintained by the United Network for Organ Sharing (UNOS); results are available in the annual report and through the UNOS World Wide Web site (http://www.unos.org/). The International Society for Heart and Lung Transplantation (ISHLT) publishes an annual summary of its international registry, and information is accessible via the internet from the ISHLT homepage (http://www.ishlt.org/).

The indications for lung and heart-lung transplantation (HLT) are shown in Table 96-1. Although primary pulmonary hypertension was a common indication for HLT in the 1980s, complex congenital heart disease with Eisenmenger's syndrome is the most frequent pretransplantation diagnosis in heart-lung recipients now. Chronic obstructive pulmonary disease (COPD) remains the leading indication for isolated lung transplantation, with COPD and α_1-antitrypsin deficiency emphysema together accounting for almost one-half of all lung transplants. In recent years, cystic fibrosis has emerged as the second most common underlying disease in lung transplant recipients.

After increasing steadily for many years, activity in lung transplantation appears to have reached a plateau both nationally (Figure 96-1) and internationally, probably because the number of transplants has approached the current supply of useable donor lungs. The number of registrations on the US national waiting list for lung transplantation has continued to increase, but, in spite of this rising demand, the median waiting time for lung transplantation was relatively stable at 535 to 566 days for patients who entered the waiting list from 1994 to 1996.

The outcome of lung transplantation can be gauged by several endpoints. The major outcome measures are actuarial survival, physiologic function, quality of life, and cost-effectiveness. National and international registries have recorded actuarial survival, and, as more recipients have been accrued, some risk factor analyses have been possible. Excellent physiologic function has been reported after both heart-lung and single or bilateral lung transplantation for a variety of diseases, and these results are summarized separately in Chapter 89,

"Physiology of the Transplanted Lung." Quality of life has been less extensively studied, but some limited results are available. The cost-effectiveness of lung transplantation is difficult to measure and recommended references are provided for the reader at the end of this chapter.

ACTUARIAL SURVIVAL AND DETERMINANTS OF OUTCOME

Actuarial survival after lung and heart-lung transplantation is shown from the ISHLT registry in Figure 96-2.

Table 96-1. Indications for Heart-Lung and Lung Transplantation by Type of Procedure

Disease	Percentage of Procedures		
	HLT (n=2428)	SLT (n=4777)	BLT (n=3278)
COPD	4	44.1	18.2
α_1-antitrypsin deficiency emphysema	2.3	11.1	10.5
Cystic fibrosis	15.5	2	33.6
Idiopathic pulmonary fibrosis	2.7	20.9	7.5
Primary pulmonary hypertension	25.9	5.2	10.2
Eisenmenger's syndrome	27.6		
Re-transplantation	2.8	3	2.2
Other	19.2	13.7	17.7

Data from the Registry of the International Society for Heart and Lung Transplantation, Fifteenth Official Report, 1998. HLT indicates heart-lung transplantation; SLT, single-lung transplantation; BLT, bilateral lung transplantation.

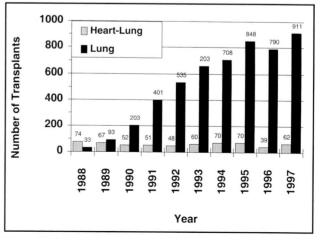

Figure 96-1. Annual activity in heart-lung and lung transplantation in the US. Data from the UNOS registry (August 1998).

Professor of Medicine, Division of Pulmonary and Critical Care Medicine, Washington University School of Medicine, St. Louis, MO

Center-specific outcomes for US programs are available through the UNOS website. Heart-lung transplantation has had a higher early mortality rate than isolated lung transplantation, mostly related to postoperative complications. However, the early advantage of lung transplantation gradually dissipates, and actuarial survival for heart-lung and lung recipients is nearly identical five years after transplantation.

Survival rates after single and bilateral lung transplantation have been comparable during the first three years and have diverged thereafter (Figure 96-3), but the difference in actuarial survival between single and bilateral transplantation has not reached statistical significance. Bilateral lung transplantation theoretically provides more reserve lung function than single lung transplantation, and this buffer is potentially advantageous against late complications, especially chronic allograft rejection. Indeed, the annual proportion of lung transplant operations that are bilateral has increased from approximately 30% in the early 1990s to almost 50% now.

Actuarial survival after lung transplantation is tabulated by pretransplantation diagnosis in Table 96-2. Stratification in the 1-month survival rates is related primarily to operative and postoperative complications. The transplant surgery is usually simplest in patients with COPD and α_1-antitrypsin deficiency emphysema, and mortality in the first month is relatively low. In contrast, the operation always requires cardiopulmonary bypass for recipients with primary pulmonary hypertension or congenital heart disease with Eisenmenger's syndrome. Perioperative mortality is higher, and the 1-month survival rates lower, in these transplant recipients. Beyond the perioperative period, transplantation itself is the great equalizer. There is a steady, slow attrition caused mainly by the complications of transplantation that affect all recipients similarly, regardless of their pretransplantation diagnosis.

A spectrum of donor and recipient variables has been examined as risk factors for death after lung transplantation. In the analysis of the ISHLT registry, independent predictors of death during the first year after transplantation included ventilator dependence at the time of transplantation, re-transplantation, an underlying disease other than COPD (especially congenital heart disease with Eisenmenger's syndrome), and older age (especially >60 years). Donor age was also a risk factor in the first year; mortality was higher in recipients of organs from donors over age 50. Fewer risk factors were influential in the outcome at five years. However, age over 60, a primary diagnosis of idiopathic pulmonary fibrosis, and re-transplantation were associated with increased mortality.

The other major determinants of outcome are posttransplantation complications. The causes of death after lung transplantation are presented in Table 96-3. In the first three months after surgery, infections (other than cytomegalovirus [CMV]) and primary graft failure, which is usually related to ischemia-reperfusion injury, have been the principal causes of death. Although acute rejection has been prevalent, it has rarely been fatal. Later, chronic rejection (bronchiolitis obliterans syndrome) or infection has caused most deaths. The morbidity and mortality associated with rejection and infection are often interdependent. When rejection occurs, immunosuppression is usually intensified, and the risk of an infectious complication increases concomitantly.

Time-dependent risk factors for death after transplantation have been examined in one institutional series. The risk of death was highest in the first 100 days, but a second period of increased risk occurred around 800 days after transplantation. Multivariate analysis determined that significant risk factors for early death

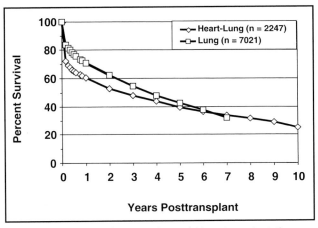

Figure 96-2. Survival after heart-lung and lung transplantation. Data from the Registry of the International Society for Heart and Lung Transplantation, Fifteenth Official Report - 1998.

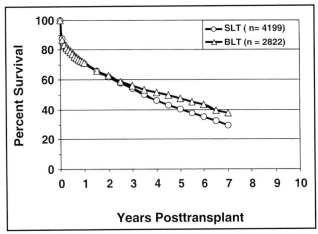

Figure 96-3. Actuarial survival after single (SLT) and bilateral (BLT) lung transplantation. Data from the Registry of the International Society for Heart and Lung Transplantation, Fifteenth Official Report - 1998.

Table 96-2. Actuarial Survival, by Diagnosis, after Lung Transplantation

Diagnosis	Survival (%)			Survival (%)		
	N_{94-95}	1 Mo.	1 Yr.	N	3 Yr.	5 Yr.
COPD	572	95	82	1193	62	41
α_1-antitrypsin deficiency emphysema	130	94	75	407	59	46
Cystic fibrosis	210	91	80	454	58	53
Idiopathic pulmonary fibrosis	179	88	74	425	52	33
Primary pulmonary hypertension	107	82	73	309	56	45
Other	171	84	69	454	54	46
Overall	1412	91	77	3283	58	43

Data from 1997 Annual Report, US Scientific Registry. N indicates number of transplants from October, 1987-December, 1995; N_{94-95}, number of transplants from 1994-1995.

(<100 days) were CMV serologic mismatch (ie, donor-positive, recipient-negative), no prophylaxis against CMV infection, and an infection other than CMV. The risk factors associated with later death included CMV serologic mismatch; no prophylaxis against CMV infection; an episode of CMV disease; the use of cyclosporine-based immunosuppression (vs tacrolimus); the presence of diffuse alveolar damage or adult respiratory distress syndrome (usually an early acute lung injury that extended into this period); a preformed recipient anti-HLA antibody that was positive against more than 10% of the standard lymphocyte test panel (panel-reactive antibody); and an HLA-DR mismatch.

Chronic allograft rejection, which is manifested clinically as progressive airflow limitation and histologically as bronchiolitis obliterans, has emerged as the major impediment to better medium-term survival after lung transplantation. Its prevalence in two large single-institution series was 34% and 41%, with case fatality rates of 25% and 29%, respectively. In contrast, overall mortality in recipients without chronic rejection was only 7% in one of these series.

Several studies have examined potential risk factors for the development of chronic rejection, and antecedent acute rejection has been identified as the most important precursor. Unfortunately, the prevalence of acute rejection has been relatively high with most immunosuppressive protocols; hence, the die for late morbidity and mortality may actually be cast rather early. Other factors, such as previous bouts of CMV pneumonitis or organizing pneumonia, have also been associated with an increased risk of chronic rejection in some reports, but the correlation between chronic rejection and variables other than acute rejection has been inconsistent.

QUALITY OF LIFE

While traditional measures like survival and lung function have often been emphasized, quality of life is an equally important measure of outcome. Even if the survival advantage of lung transplantation is marginal, the improvement in quality-adjusted survival has suggested that many patients "will trade quantity for quality of life." Almost 90% of recipients have expressed satisfaction with their decision to have a transplant and would encourage a friend with a similar problem to seek transplantation.

Table 96-3. Indications for Heart-Lung and Lung Transplantation by Type of Procedure

Cause of Death	Percentage of Deaths* Time after Transplantation		
	≤30 Days	31 Days- 1 Yr	>1 Year
Nonspecific graft failure	23.4		
Acute rejection	4.1		
Bronchiolitis (chronic rejection)		5.3	33.6
CMV infection		4.3	
Infection, other than CMV	16	34.1	15.5
Malignancy			2.2
Hemorrhage	3.7		
Other thoracic complication	4.6	4	5.2
Multiorgan failure		4.4	2.5
Other	48.2	47.9	41

Data from the Registry of the International Society for Heart and Lung Transplantation, Fifteenth Official Report-1998.
*Percentage of deaths with known causes only.

Although studies have been limited by relatively small numbers of patients and by cross-sectional rather than longitudinal design, several have documented a significant improvement in both overall and health-related quality of life after heart-lung and lung transplantation. With multidimensional profiles, the improvement has extended across most quality of life domains, including perceptions of physical function, social function, role activity, and general and mental health, except pain. Not surprisingly, this enhancement in quality of life may not be noticeable during the first few months of recuperation. Thereafter, however, it is consistent, and it does not deteriorate unless a complication, such as chronic rejection, arises. In the ISHLT registry, for example, 82% and 89% of lung transplant recipients were portrayed as having no limitations to activity at one and three years after transplantation, respectively.

COST AND COST-EFFECTIVENESS

Only pilot studies of the cost and cost-effectiveness of heart-lung and lung transplantation have been done. In a survey from the University of Washington Medical Center, the mean charge for lung transplantation was $164,989; the elements were organ acquisition (15.9%), physician fees (18.2%), and hospital and pharmacy charges (65.9%). The average charges for posttransplantation care were $16,628 per month during the first six months, $5,440 per month during the second six months, and $4,525 per month after the first year; medication charges alone frequently exceeded $1,000 per month. On the basis of current survival rates, the lifetime cost for the care of a lung transplant recipient was projected to be $424,853, and the incremental cost per quality-adjusted life year gained through lung transplantation was calculated to be $176,817. Prolonging posttransplantation survival and reducing the cost of postrecovery care were suggested as the two factors that would most improve the cost-effectiveness of the sprocedure.

Wage effects are not included in the cost-effectiveness analysis in most studies, and, if recipients returned to work, this would be an obvious asset. Employment patterns did not change after transplantation in one institutional study that specifically addressed this issue, but there are obstacles other than health to employment after transplantation. Disappointingly, only 38% of the recipients in this study said they felt able to work. Likewise, while 82% and 89% of recipients in the ISHLT registry were characterized as having "no activity limitations," only 33% and 39% were described as working, either part-time or full-time, at their 1-year and 3-year follow-ups, respectively.

RE-TRANSPLANTATION

Re-transplantation has been performed infrequently. In the US registry, re-transplantation comprised 2% to 6% of lung transplants annually from 1990 through 1996, and, in the ISHLT registry, re-transplantation has been the indication for approximately 2% of all heart-lung and lung transplantations. The most common reasons for re-transplantation have been early graft failure, intractable airway complications and chronic rejection.

Overall, the results of re-transplantation have been poor in comparison with primary transplantation. In the latest summary of the voluntary re-transplantation registry, actuarial survival in the cohort of 230 re-transplant recipients was 47% at one year, 40% at two years, and 33% at three years. The three leading causes of death and their respective contribution to mortality after re-transplantation were opportunistic infection, 42%; acute graft failure, 29%; and chronic rejection, 21%. However, bronchiolitis obliterans syndrome (BOS) developed after re-transplantation in a pattern similar to its evolution after primary transplantation; the prevalence of BOS (stages 1 to 3) was 19% at one year, 38% at three years, and 50% at five years after re-transplantation.

In a univariate analysis, factors associated with survival after re-transplantation included a longer interval between transplants (especially >2 years), ventilator independence and ambulatory status before re-transplantation. The importance of recipients being ambulatory and ventilator-independent before re-transplantation was corroborated by the multivariate model, and, in addition, survival was significantly better for re-transplantations after 1991. In the subset of recipients who were both ambulatory and ventilator-independent before re-transplantation, survival rates during the first three years after re-transplantation approached those of primary transplantation. Hence, recipient selection for re-transplantation is a key determinant of outcome.

Because of high prevalence of chronic graft failure among primary transplant recipients, the shortage of donor organs and the generally inferior results of re-transplantation in comparison with first transplants, re-transplantation has raised many ethical issues. Nevertheless, the re-transplant registry has validated a reasonable prospect for success for appropriately-selected recipients.

LIVING DONOR TRANSPLANTATION

During the last few years, lobar transplantation from a living donor has become an option for selected recipients when a cadaveric organ is not expected to become available in time to save the patient's life. The ethical issues surrounding transplantation from living donors have been debated. Nevertheless, recipient outcomes have been satisfactory, and donor morbidity has been minimal.

In the largest single center experience, 41 recipients had undergone lobar transplantation from living donors between January 1993 and May 1997. Most of the patients were children or young adults with cystic fibrosis. The majority of donors were parents or siblings of the recipient, but other relatives and 14 nonrelatives were donors, too. Actuarial survival during the first two years was comparable to the results for cadaveric lung recipients in the ISHLT registry. Acute rejection occurred at a rate of 0.8 episodes per recipient, and more episodes of histologic acute rejection were detected in recipients with four to six HLA mismatches than in those with zero to three mismatches. Chronic rejection had been diagnosed in seven recipients for a prevalence of 16%, but the average follow-up in the recipients who were still alive was less than two years. No mortality or serious morbidity was reported among the donors.

SUMMARY

The results of heart-lung and lung transplantation have been good, but better outcomes are the goal. Ischemia-reperfusion injury, which causes most early graft dysfunction or failure, and rejection remain the main obstacles to better short-term and intermediate-term results.

RECOMMENDED READING

1997 Annual Report of the US Scientific Registry for Transplant Recipients and the Organ Procurement and Transplantation Network – Transplant Data: 1988-1996. UNOS; Richmond, VA; and the Division of Transplantation, Office of Special Programs, Health Resources and Services Administration, US Department of Health and Human Services; Rockville, MD.

Hosenpud JD, Bennett LE, Keck BM, Fiol B, Boucek MM, Novick RJ. The Registry of the International Society for Heart and Lung Transplantation: fifteenth official report – 1998. J Heart Lung Transplant. 1998;17(7):656-668.

Bando K, Paradis IL, Komatsu K, et al. Analysis of time-dependent risks for infection, rejection and death after pulmonary transplantation. J Thorac Cardiovasc Surg. 1995;109(1):49-59.

Sundaresan RS, Trulock EP, Mohanakumar T, Cooper JD, Patterson GA. Prevalence and outcome of bronchiolitis obliterans syndrome after lung transplantation. Washington University Lung Transplant Group. Ann Thorac Surg. 1995;60(5):1341-1347.

Sharples LD, Tamm M, McNeil K, Higenbottam TW, Stewart S, Wallwork J. Development of bronchiolitis obliterans syndrome in recipients of heart-lung transplantation – early risk factors. Transplantation. 1996;61(4):560-566.

Duncan SR, Paradis IL, Yousem SA, et al. Sequelae of cytomegalovirus pulmonary infections in lung allograft recipients. Am Rev Respir Dis. 1992;146(6):1419-1425.

Ramsey SD, Patrick DL, Albert RK, Larson EB, Wood DE, Raghu G. The cost-effectiveness of lung transplantation: a pilot study. University of Washington Medical Center Lung Transplant Study Group. Chest. 1995;108(6):1594-1601.

Gross CR, Savik K, Bolman RM 3rd, Hertz MI. Long-term health status and quality of life outcomes of lung transplant recipients. Chest. 1995;108(6):1587-1593.

Ramsey SD, Patrick DL, Lewis S, Albert RK, Raghu G. Improvement in quality of life after lung transplantation: a preliminary study. The University of Washington Medical Center Lung Transplant Study Group. J Heart Lung Transplant. 1995;14(5):870-877.

Novick RJ, Stitt LW, Al-Kattan K, et al. Pulmonary retransplantation: predictors of graft function and survival in 230 patients. Pulmonary Retransplant Registery. Ann Thorac Surg. 1998;65(1):227-234.

Starnes VA, Barr ML, Cohen RG, et al. Living-donor lobar lung transplantation experience: intermediate results. J Thorac Cardiovasc Surg. 1996;112(5):1284-1290.

97 PEDIATRIC LUNG TRANSPLANTATION: SPECIAL CONSIDERATIONS AND REMAINING HURDLES

George B. Mallory, Jr., MD

For technical, practical and ethical reasons, solid organ transplantation has historically been performed in adult patients before its use in infants and children. The era of modern lung transplantation was ushered in by Dr. Joel Cooper at the University of Toronto in 1983. Since the late 1980s, pediatric lung transplantation has been practiced in selected centers in the USA and Europe. Published reports from a number of pediatric lung transplant centers indicate success in adapting surgical techniques, immunosuppression and posttransplant care to infants and children. Death from acute and chronic pulmonary and pulmonary-vascular disease remain the most common categories of mortality in the younger segment of the population. Thus, there is and will continue to be a clear clinical indication for this therapeutic procedure.

The most recent United States data available from the United Network for Organ Sharing (UNOS) show that lung transplantation remains relatively limited within the pediatric age group. As of August 31, 2000, registrations for lung transplantation showed that only 2.5% of lung transplant candidates were 17 years and older compared with 6.1% of liver and 5.8% of heart transplant candidates. Interestingly, 64.4% of heart-lung transplant candidates fell within the pediatric age group, with the majority being adolescents. It should be noted that the volume of heart-lung transplants performed within the US has continued to fall dramatically as organ blocks have become less available and isolated lung and heart transplantation are being successfully applied to clinical problems that heretofore led to heart-lung transplantation. When actual numbers of transplants performed within the US is examined, pediatric patients are somewhat more heavily represented with 11.3% of heart transplants, 7.3% of lung transplants, and 12.4% of liver transplant patients in the calendar year 1998. Over time, the number of pediatric lung transplants has gradually increased. In 1993, 36 pediatric patients underwent lung transplantation and in 1998 there were 62 patients. The International Society for Heart and Lung Transplantation (ISHLT) reported 80 total pediatric lung transplants performed in 1998 worldwide, or 18 pediatric patients outside the US. In a few leading centers where transplantation for end-stage lung disease is performed, heart-lung transplantation remains the preferred operation. However, this phenomenon is becoming less common. In 1998, there were a total of 20 heart-lung transplant operations performed in pediatric patients worldwide, compared with the 265 pediatric heart transplants and 552 pediatric liver transplants.

From a practical point of view, there are very few active and experienced pediatric lung transplant centers in the US and perhaps even fewer outside the US. From 1995 through 1998, there were only three US centers that performed three or more lung transplant procedures in pediatric patients each of those four years: Los Angeles Children's Hospital with 30, Children's Hospital of Philadelphia also with 30, and St. Louis Children's Hospital with 109 pediatric patients. In short, pediatric lung transplantation has been established as an accepted therapy but in total numbers of transplants, patients on the waiting list, and number of experienced and active centers, it lags behind adult lung transplantation and other pediatric solid organ transplantation.

Disease entities predisposing to death from respiratory failure and pulmonary vascular disease that have proven to be suitable for lung transplantation are shown in Table 97-1. This international cumulative data from the ISHLT demonstrates that "miscellaneous" is the largest category for the ten years and younger group whereas cystic fibrosis is the indication in almost 60% of the older group. Since the most common form of pulmonary hypertension is not primary pulmonary hypertension, but instead pulmonary hypertension associated with a variety of repaired or unrepaired congenital heart

Associate Professor of Clinical Pediatrics, Washington University School of Medicine, St. Louis Children's Hospital, St. Louis, MO; Consultant Physician, Cardiopulmonary Transplantation Programme, Great Ormond Street Hospital for Children NHS Trust, London, United Kingdom

Table 97-1. Diagnosis of Pediatric Lung Transplant Recipients Transplanted between 1987 and 1998*

Diagnostic Category	0 to 10 Years	11 to 17 Years
Congenital problems	4.4%	2.4%
Primary pulmonary hypertension	12.7%	10.5%
Cystic fibrosis	20.4%	64.2%
Pulmonary fibrosis	6.6%	5.4%
Miscellaneous causes	44.8%	11.5%
Re-transplant	11%	6.1%

*Data obtained from the International Society of Heart and Lung Transplantation website in September, 2000.

defects, these children would fall into the miscellaneous group. As well, infantile pulmonary alveolar proteinosis has become the most common indication for infantile lung transplantation in St. Louis and would fall into the miscellaneous group. Other miscellaneous but uncommon disease entities leading to lung transplantation in the younger age group include infantile or early childhood interstitial lung disease, post-viral bronchiolitis obliterans, bronchopulmonary dysplasia, respiratory insufficiency after bone marrow transplantation, pulmonary hemosiderosis, and intrapulmonary vascular shunts. Meaningful statistical information about the underlying diagnoses leading to lung transplantation from the data compiled both by UNOS and ISHLT will be limited as long as adult disease categorization remains the norm. Nonetheless, it is clear that cystic fibrosis is the dominant underlying diagnosis leading to lung transplantation in older children and adolescents.

The general criteria for lung and heart-lung transplantation are similar in infants and children to be used in adults: those who are at risk of dying from single organ failure (in this case the lung) within a finite period of time and who are clinically stable enough so that organ procurement is possible. In infants for whom organ procurement within days or weeks is currently possible in some regions of the US, and in whom recuperation is often gratifyingly rapid, a candidate on mechanical ventilation and technologic support including nitric oxide inhalation and extracorporeal membrane oxygenation (ECMO) may sometimes be appropriate for listing and transplantation. Older children are usually considered candidates if death within months to two years seems likely. For children with rare diseases or atypical courses of more common diseases, prognostication will depend on careful serial measurements of cardiopulmonary function to ascertain the natural history of the underlying disease process.

Medical and surgical contraindications for lung transplantation in children are listed in Table 97-2. In the current era, most contraindications are relative, and those that are absolute are rare in the population at risk. Nonmedical contraindications include financial and psychosocial factors. Although most insurers cover lung transplantation at the present time, many policies do not provide for travel and living expenses. Community fundraising may be necessary for many families to afford the heavy uncovered costs. Psychosocial factors are critically important to assess both by the transplant center team and the family in light of the uncertainties, complexities and rigors of life after lung transplantation. It would seem obvious that serious mental health disorders or disability that would obviate cooperation with the administration of medication and/or follow-up testing are contraindications to transplantation. Family dysfunction manifest as repeated nonadherence to medical regimens in the past

is also considered a relative or absolute contraindication depending on the center and the seriousness of the nonadherence. A thorough evaluation of the child and family by a child psychologist, pediatric social worker, and the team of transplant caregivers is required before accepting or rejecting any individual candidate. Transplant centers depend on the integrity and truthfulness of referring physicians and caregivers in receiving all relevant information about patients and families that bear on past and future health behaviors. In some borderline situations, probationary listing of a child with a clear contract of expectations may be appropriate.

Like their adult counterparts in the USA, pediatric candidates for lung transplantation are listed by ABO blood group, height and the date of initial listing. Waiting period is highly variable from region to region and center to center depending on a variety of factors. Size considerations are clearly more important for pediatric recipients and donors because of the wide variability in size of the thorax and lungs during the span of childhood. Lobar transplantation and down-sizing of donor lungs with a

Table 97-2. Medical and Surgical Contraindications to Pediatric Lung Transplantaiton

Absolute
Severe scoliosis or thoracic cage deformity
Pneumonectomy (unless volume-occupying device in place)
Severe tracheomegaly and/or tracheomalacia, unamenable to therapy
Hepatic, renal, left ventricular failure*
Active malignancy
HIV infection
Active viral infection
Active mycobacterial infection
Bacteremia or septicemia
Irreversible and significant respiratory muscle dysfunction

Relative
Symptomatic osteoporosis or osteopenia
Panresistant micro-organisms within the respiratory tract
Burkholderia cepacia lower respiratory infection
Daily systemic corticosteroids
Severe malnutrition
*potentially amenable to multi-organ transplantation

surgical stapling device are options for the transplant surgeon in the event that over-sized lungs are offered.

The pediatric anesthesiologist must approach each patient individually. More pediatric patients are likely to be in intensive care units at the time that organs become available than adult candidates. The transition from the ICU to the operating room must be managed with careful attention to the time required, the need for line placement, and the condition and therapy of the child candidate. A high percentage of pediatric patients with end-stage pulmonary vascular disease have had previous thoracic surgical procedures, which predisposes to longer surgery and more bleeding at the time of transplantation. Some pediatric transplant surgeons elect cardiopulmonary bypass (CPB) for all lung transplant procedures. The disadvantages of CPB are the associated coagulopathy that accompanies heparinization and the capillary leak syndrome that affects all organs to a variable degree after CPB. The advantages of CPB include improved access to dissection of the lung and hilum, the ability to clamp and cleanse (with aminoglycoside in cystic fibrosis patients) the proximal bronchial airway, and a minimization of ischemic time. Clearly, operative and anesthetic approaches will be specific to each institution.

Immediate postoperative issues are graft function, bleeding and stabilization of a critically ill patient. An initial chest radiograph, early bedside radionuclide lung perfusion scan, and serial measures of blood pressure, central venous pressures, arterial blood gases, and urine output are critical in assessing the integrity of graft function. Fluid administration including the administration of blood products (always irradiated) and inotropic agents are administered accordingly. In St. Louis, within the first 24 hours, flexible bronchoscopy is used to inspect the anastomosis and the vascular supply of the bronchial mucosa beyond the anastomoses and to perform bronchoalveolar lavage (BAL) for the diagnosis of infection. Experience at St. Louis Children's Hospital has taught us that infants often spend a considerably longer time in ventilatory failure than older children. In addition, they have a greater likelihood of having been sicker and on ventilatory support with heavy sedation and neuromuscular blockade prior to transplant. The weaning and rehabilitation process must be based on objective data and should not be reckless in expectation or elaboration. Infants may have more easily fatigued respiratory muscles and the hypercompliance of the thorax contributes to an inefficiency of ventilatory effort that would naturally lead to a more prolonged rehabilitation. Infant airway cartilage is more compliant than the cartilage in older patients as well, which can lead to an exaggerated collapsibility (malacia) of the intrathoracic airways, particularly around the anastomoses, leading to increased work of breathing and a limited respiratory

reserve. With a healthy graft, weaning from mechanical ventilatory support can always succeed, but may occasionally take weeks instead of days in older children and hours in adolescents or adults.

Immunosuppression is often begun with a dose of cyclosporine or tacrolimus and intravenous corticosteroids just prior to surgery. A regimen of immunosuppression and appropriate antibiotics are begun immediately after transplantation. At St. Louis Children's Hospital, cyclosporine remains the calcineurin inhibitor of choice with an initial intravenous loading dose of 0.5 mg/kg over two hours followed by an infusion at 0.1 mg/kg per hour (maximum dose = 4 mg/hr) titrated to a steady state or trough level of 300 to 400 ng/mL on whole blood samples. However, it may be more efficacious to give the same total daily dose in two 4-hour infusions separated by twelve hours to obtain the same kind of pharmacokinetic profile as would occur with the oral administration of Neoral. A change to oral dosing is begun after oral function and gastric emptying have been established. Some centers have embraced tacrolimus as the calcineurin inhibitor of choice for initial immunosuppression. Initial tacrolimus dosing may be by intravenous drip or oral or nasogastric tube bolus dosing. Tacrolimus trough levels are titrated to 10 to 15 ng/mL on whole blood samples. Azathioprine has been traditionally used as part of a three drug strategy with dosing at 2.0 to 3.0 mg/kg per day initially given intravenously. Several centers have changed to mycophenolate mofetil (MMF) as the second agent in a triumvirate of immunosuppressants. Although pediatric dosing has not been universally established, adult dosing would suggest a pediatric dose of 15 mg/kg twice daily. Corticosteroid dosing also varies by center. In some programs, a dose of intravenous methylprednisolone is given pretransplant and continued in moderate dosing the first three days posttransplant. There is broad consensus that the appropriate early dose, beyond the first 72 hours, of methylprednisolone or oral prednisone/prednisolone is 0.5 mg/kg per day. Tapering of corticosteroid dosing usually begins at the earliest in the second to third month posttransplant.

Antibiotic treatment before and after transplantation is not, in the strict sense, prophylaxis. Most donor lungs, if cultured, grow one or more potential pathogens. Cystic fibrosis patients have intrathoracic airways, including the proximal trachea and bronchi, infected by typical organisms. Therefore, it is universal practice to choose an antibiotic regimen before, during and after lung transplantation geared to the likely pathogens. At St. Louis Children's Hospital in the year 2000, the initial antibiotic choice in non-cystic fibrosis patients is limited to a first generation cephalosporin. In cystic fibrosis patients, at least two intravenous antipseudomonal antibiotics should be chosen based on the most recent respiratory microbiological specimen. Other agents are chosen if *Pseudomonas aeruginosa* is either not present or not the exclusive pathogen. Two agents are chosen, as is the usual practice in cystic fibrosis care, to seek synergy between antibiotics and to lessen the chance of emergence of antibiotic resistance of Gram-negative organisms. In CF patients with a history of *Aspergillus* infection, allergic bronchopulmonary aspergillosis, or recent sputum cultures positive for *Aspergillus fumigatus,* antifungal therapy with relatively low dose Amphotericin (0.25 mg/kg per day) is begun by the intravenous route. Depending on clinical course and the results of respiratory culture at the time of transplant and the first bronchoalveolar lavage culture at 24 hours posttransplant, the intravenous amphotericin may be changed within three to ten days to the nebulized route, usually 10 mg in 5 to 10 cc sterile water three times daily, for an additional one to two weeks. Lung transplant recipients who have circulating antibody for cytomegalovirus (CMV) before transplantation or who receive an organ from a donor with positive CMV serology are treated with IV ganciclovir for the first six weeks posttransplant. Trimethoprim-sulfamethoxazole is commenced in the first week after transplantation as prophylaxis for *pneumocystis carinii* pneumonia (PCP). Some programs continue PCP prophylaxis long-term; others discontinue after three months. Oral nystatin is commonly prescribed to reduce the likelihood of clinically significant oral candidiasis. Oral acyclovir is used in some programs routinely as prophylactic treatment for herpes simplex infection.

Careful and frequent posttransplant assessment of graft and patient function is the key to maximizing long-term survival. There are practical issues such as cost, expertise and degree of involvement by hometown primary care physicians and regional specialists, distance from the transplant center, and preference either by the patient and family or the insurer that will serve to inform the actual protocol for reassessments. The major medical issues in children as well as adults after lung transplantation are those related to infection and graft rejection. Issues of particular importance in infants and young children are somatic growth, social and neurologic development, obvious or occult aspiration of gastric contents, and susceptibility to community viral infections. Life-threatening episodes of aspiration have occurred in the first weeks after lung transplantation in several infants in St. Louis. Older children may demonstrate bronchoscopic or biopsy evidence of aspiration during or after acute respiratory illnesses. As with most medical complications, caregivers must have a high degree of suspicion and a low threshold for medical or surgical interventions with possible gastroesophageal reflux-related pulmonary complications. The use of daily corticosteroids at significant doses inhibits skeletal growth

and anabolism in general. Although the transplant physician's highest priority in the early months after transplantation is to enhance and protect graft function, growth becomes a legitimate concern beyond the first few months after transplantation. In St. Louis, prednisone dosage is rarely reduced below 0.25 mg/kg per day in the first months after transplantation. However, some children, including many infants, will resume growth even at this dosage. Depending on the number and severity of episodes of graft rejection, corticosteroid dosing should be tapered during the second six month period after transplant. It is standard practice, barring continuing graft rejection, for prednisone to be weaned to 0.15-0.20 mg/kg per day by one year and to 0.1 mg/kg per day at two years posttransplant. It is uncommon in St. Louis to revert to every other day steroid dosing and a patient has never been weaned entirely off corticosteroids.

The methods used for graft surveillance are similar in children and adults. It is common sense and straightforward to use serial historical information, physical exam including auscultation and periodic chest radiograph in these patients. In St. Louis, it has become routine to procure a pulse oximeter for daily monitoring of oxygen saturation in all pediatric recipients of lung transplantation. The baseline range is established in the hospital or in the clinic and the family is given a "threshold of concern" which should prompt a phone call to a physician or the transplant nurse. Standard spirometry can be performed in most children aged six years and older. Home spirometers are procured for daily use at home after discharge. Once again, a "threshold of concern" should be established. We have found it important for children and adolescents to have a periodic critique of technique and refresher course in the hospital pulmonary function laboratory. Infant lung function testing is now available in many medical centers but requires sedation. Therefore, infants are only periodically reassessed at defined intervals and potentially with illnesses. Flexible bronchoscopy with bronchoalveolar lavage (BAL) and transbronchial biopsy (TBB) has been the standard method for diagnosing graft rejection in children as well as adults. In St. Louis, regularly scheduled bronchoscopy has remained a hallmark of the surveillance program for all pediatric patients. The procedures are scheduled at 24 hours after transplant (without TBB), one to two weeks, six weeks, three, six, nine, 12, 18, 24, 30, 36, 48 …months after transplant and at any time of significant respiratory illness. Techniques have been developed that are suitable for infants and young children in whom standard pediatric equipment does not permit TBB. The recent availability of small caliber forceps for use in the pediatric 3.7 mm bronchoscope has made the obtaining of biopsies in infants more possible. Experience has shown that diligence and special skill is required to get adequate tissue specimens.

The pharmacologic regimen of most patients after transplantation is complex. The fact that the calcineurin inhibitors have a narrow therapeutic index, frequently results in reduction in renal function, and adverse drug interactions. For these reasons, complications of pharmacologic therapy need to be anticipated. Important complications of cyclosporine are hirsutism, gingival hypertrophy, lowering of the seizure threshold, systemic hypertension, hypercholesterolemia, and reduction in glomerular filtration rate. The accumulated clinical experience at St. Louis Children's Hospital is that approximately 20% of lung and heart-lung transplant recipients will develop seizures, most in the first several weeks after transplant. The seizures are generally short-lived. Some patients do not require anticonvulsants and in those who do, the anticonvulsant can often be discontinued within a few weeks. Phenytoin has been one drug of choice. Tacrolimus does not result in hirsutism and gingival hypertrophy, which may be of serious significance to adolescent girls. However, tacrolimus does cause hypertension and reduction in renal function, at least comparable to cyclosporine, and may cause more headache and certainly is more diabetogenic than cyclosporine. Azathioprine is occasionally associated with neutropenia. Dosage is not changed unless the absolute neutrophil count is less than 1,500 cells/mL. With regard to prednisone, there is concern about retardation of skeletal growth, but with previously chronically ill children involved, osteoporosis with or without vertebral compression fractures is an additional more recent concern.

Infection is a major risk factor for lung transplant recipients because of the anatomic exposure of the lung. Pediatric patients are at greater risk than adults because of their immunologic immaturity and their exposure to siblings and peers. Viral infections are particularly common within the younger portion of any community. Among the respiratory viruses of concern are respiratory syncytial virus, adenovirus and parainfluenza virus. Serious life-threatening infections may be seen with each of these viruses, particularly in infants or in young children recently transplanted. Current therapies including aerosolized ribavirin and systemic cidofovir for adenovirus must be given early in the course of infection to be effective. The herpes family viruses are of additional concern after transplant because of their immortalized status after primary infection. Pediatric patients are at greater risk of primary infection after transplantation, which brings greater disease risk than reactivation. Herpes simplex occasionally causes pneumonia, whereas cytomegalovirus (CMV) usually does in the lung transplant recipient. Varicella is a particularly pernicious pulmonary infection in the immunosuppressed patient although preventable via hyperimmune globulin after exposure or vaccine. No controlled studies of varicella vaccine in immunosuppressed patients has been performed, but vaccination is almost certainly much safer than natural infection. Acyclovir could be used in the event of the earliest sign of illness in a vaccine recipient. Primary EBV infection is probably a risk factor for post-transplant lymphoproliferative disease, a neoplastic complication with high morbidity and substantial mortality after solid organ transplantation. The key to the clinical approach of herpes family viruses is a high index of suspicion, frequent scheduled surveillance by culture and serologic testing, and prompt treatment.

The lung appears to be less "immunologically privileged" than other solid organs. Consequently, the incidence and severity of graft rejection is greater within the lung than heart, liver or kidney transplantation. There are cogent reasons to explain the predilection of the lung to immune attack after transplantation. First, the lung has the largest endothelial surface of any organ. Since major histocompatibility complex antigen expression on the endothelial surface is the primary signal for host immune recognition, the lung might then be the most "exposed" transplantable organ. Second, the lung is equipped with an elaborate array of antigen-presenting cells, giving a superior skill in antigen presentation to host effector cells. Donor dendritic cells and macrophages are largely replaced by recipient cells within a few weeks after transplantation, providing a battlefield for short-term and long-term immunologic warfare. Acute graft rejection is commonly diagnosed in most children in the first months after lung or heart-lung transplantation, but usually can be treated. However, the number and severity of episodes of acute graft rejection appear to be the most accurate predictor of chronic rejection or bronchiolitis obliterans (BO). BO remains the single most imposing barrier to long-term survival in pediatric lung transplant patients. There are no published studies comparing pediatric and adult lung transplant recipients with respect to graft rejection to know if there is a greater propensity to rejection in children who are perhaps at the peak of immunologic activity of life.

In summary, infants, children and adolescents die from progressive pulmonary and pulmonary vascular disease at a detectable rate. Many of these patients would have no significant contraindication to transplantation. Lung transplantation as a surgical and medical therapy has been shown to be a viable option with acceptable and slowly improving survival rates in children as in adults. Perhaps because of the daunting nature of the work and the requisite resources, only a few pediatric centers for lung and heart-lung transplantation have been developed over the past decade. Technical hurdles can be surmounted with experience. The remaining challenges remain the accurate and timely diagnosis of infection and graft rejection and application of therapies. The enhanced rate of infection and the unique needs of growth and development add to the difficulty of providing comprehensive care for these patients. As with other organ transplant programs in pediatric and adult populations, a more effective and less toxic immunosuppressive or immunomodulatory therapeutic strategy needs to be developed to reduce graft reduction and improve graft tolerance.

RECOMMENDED READING

Noyes BE, Kurland G, Orenstein DM. Lung and heart-lung transplantation in children. Pediatr Pulmonol. 1997;23(1):39-48.

Gaynor JW, Bridges ND, Clark BJ, Spray TL. Update on lung transplantation in children. Curr Opin Pediatr. 1998;10(3):256-261.

These reviews are the most recently published overviews in the North American medical literature.

Sweet SC, Spray TL, Huddleston CB, et al. Pediatric lung transplantation at St. Louis Children's Hospital 1990-1995. Am J Resp Crit Care Med. 1997;155(3):1027-1035.

This series review is the most recent from the large St. Louis Children's Hospital program demonstrating the various diagnostic approaches to pediatric lung and heart-lung transplantation.

Mendeloff EN, Huddleston CB, Mallory GB, et al. Pediatric and adult lung transplantation for cystic fibrosis. J Thorac Cardiovasc Surg. 1998;115(2):404-413.

This retrospective review demonstrates that pediatric CF lung transplant recipients survive at least as well, if not better than adult counterparts, from a single university medical center.

Cohen AH, Sweet SC, Mendeloff EN, et al. High incidence of posttransplant lymphoproliferative disease in pediatric patients with cystic fibrosis. Am J Respir Crit Care Med. 2000;161(4 Pt 1):1252-1255.

Boyle GJ, Michaels MG, Webber SA, et al. Post-transplantation lymphoproliferative disorders in pediatric thoracic organ recipients. J Pediatr. 1998;131(2): 309-313.

PTLD is a particularly devastating complication of solid lung transplantation. These series suggest that the incidence may be particularly high in CF pediatric lung transplant recipients.

Wong M, Mallory GB Jr, Goldstein J, Goyal M, Yamada KA. Neurologic complications of pediatric lung transplantation. Neurology. 1999;53(7):1542-1549.

This series from St. Louis shows a high incidence of neurologic complications, especially seizures in pediatric lung transplant recipients.

Bridges ND, Spray TL, Collins MH, Bowles NE, Towbin JA. Adenovirus infection in the lung results in graft failure after lung transplantation. J Thorac Cardiovasc Surg. 1998;116(4):617-623.

Evidence presented here from one of the active US pediatric lung transplant programs that adenovirus is a particularly virulent viral pathogen in this clinical setting.

INDEX